New Advances on Zika Virus Research

New Advances on Zika Virus Research

Special Issue Editors

Luis Martinez-Sobrido
Fernando Almazán

MDPI • Basel • Beijing • Wuhan • Barcelona • Belgrade

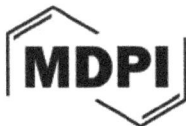

MDPI

Special Issue Editors

Luis Martinez-Sobrido
University of Rochester Medical Center
USA

Fernando Almazán
National Centre for Biotechnology (CNB-CSIC)
Spain

Editorial Office
MDPI
St. Alban-Anlage 66
4052 Basel, Switzerland

This is a reprint of articles from the Special Issue published online in the open access journal *Viruses* (ISSN 1999-4915) from 2018 to 2019 (available at: https://www.mdpi.com/journal/viruses/special_issues/Zika)

For citation purposes, cite each article independently as indicated on the article page online and as indicated below:

LastName, A.A.; LastName, B.B.; LastName, C.C. Article Title. *Journal Name* **Year**, *Article Number*, Page Range.

ISBN 978-3-03897-764-3 (Pbk)
ISBN 978-3-03897-765-0 (PDF)

Cover image courtesy of Luis Martinez-Sobrido and Fernando Almazán.

Contents

About the Special Issue Editors ix

Luis Martinez-Sobrido and Fernando Almazán
New Advances on Zika Virus Research
Reprinted from: *Viruses* 2019, *11*, 258, doi:10.3390/v11030258 1

Ginés Ávila-Pérez, Aitor Nogales, Verónica Martín, Fernando Almazán and
Luis Martínez-Sobrido
Reverse Genetic Approaches for the Generation of Recombinant Zika Virus
Reprinted from: *Viruses* 2018, *10*, 597, doi:10.3390/v10110597 5

Maximilian Münster, Anna Płaszczyca, Mirko Cortese, Christopher John Neufeldt,
Sarah Goellner, Gang Long and Ralf Bartenschlager
A Reverse Genetics System for Zika Virus Based on a Simple Molecular Cloning Strategy
Reprinted from: *Viruses* 2018, *10*, 368, doi:10.3390/v10070368 27

Lizhou Zhang, Wei Ji, Shuang Lyu, Luhua Qiao and Guangxiang Luo
Tet-Inducible Production of Infectious Zika Virus from the Full-Length cDNA Clones of African-
and Asian-Lineage Strains
Reprinted from: *Viruses* 2018, *10*, 700, doi:10.3390/v10120700 44

Trisha R. Barnard, Maaran M. Rajah and Selena M. Sagan
Contemporary Zika Virus Isolates Induce More dsRNA and Produce More Negative-Strand
Intermediate in Human Astrocytoma Cells
Reprinted from: *Viruses* 2018, *10*, 728, doi:10.3390/v10120728 60

Luwanika Mlera and Marshall E. Bloom
Differential Zika Virus Infection of Testicular Cell Lines
Reprinted from: *Viruses* 2019, *11*, 42, doi:10.3390/v11010042 77

Danielle B. L. Oliveira, Giuliana S. Durigon, Érica A. Mendes, Jason T. Ladner,
Robert Andreata-Santos, Danielle B. Araujo, Viviane F. Botosso, Nicholas D. Paola,
Daniel F. L. Neto, Marielton P. Cunha, Carla T. Braconi, Rúbens P. S. Alves,
Monica R. Jesus, Lennon R. Pereira, Stella R. Melo, Flávio S. Mesquita,
Vanessa B. Silveira, Luciano M. Thomazelli, Silvana R. Favoretto, Franciane B. Almonfrey,
Regina C. R. M. Abdulkader, Joel M. Gabrili, Denise V. Tambourgi, Sérgio F. Oliveira,
Karla Prieto, Michael R. Wiley, Luís C. S. Ferreira, Marcos V. Silva, Gustavo F. Palacios,
Paolo M. A. Zanotto and Edison L. Durigon
Persistence and Intra-Host Genetic Evolution of Zika Virus Infection in Symptomatic Adults:
A Special View in the Male Reproductive System
Reprinted from: *Viruses* 2018, *10*, 615, doi:10.3390/v10110615 88

Ina Lee, Sandra Bos, Ge Li, Shusheng Wang, Gilles Gadea, Philippe Desprès and
Richard Y. Zhao
Probing Molecular Insights into Zika Virus–Host Interactions
Reprinted from: *Viruses* 2018, *10*, 233, doi:10.3390/v10050233 104

Stephanie Thurmond, Boxiao Wang, Jikui Song and Rong Hai
Suppression of Type I Interferon Signaling by *Flavivirus* NS5
Reprinted from: *Viruses* 2018, *10*, 712, doi:10.3390/v10120712 130

Sang-Im Yun, Byung-Hak Song, Jordan C. Frank, Justin G. Julander, Aaron L. Olsen, Irina A. Polejaeva, Christopher J. Davies, Kenneth L. White and Young-Min Lee
Functional Genomics and Immunologic Tools: The Impact of Viral and Host Genetic Variations on the Outcome of Zika Virus Infection
Reprinted from: *Viruses* **2018**, *10*, 422, doi:10.3390/v10080422 . . . . **146**

Chaker El Kalamouni, Etienne Frumence, Sandra Bos, Jonathan Turpin, Brice Nativel, Wissal Harrabi, David A. Wilkinson, Olivier Meilhac, Gilles Gadea, Philippe Desprès, Pascale Krejbich-Trotot and Wildriss Viranaïcken
Subversion of the Heme Oxygenase-1 Antiviral Activity by Zika Virus
Reprinted from: *Viruses* **2019**, *11*, 2, doi:10.3390/v11010002 . . . . **174**

Maria del Pilar Martinez Viedma and Brett E. Pickett
Characterizing the Different Effects of Zika Virus Infection in Placenta and Microglia Cells
Reprinted from: *Viruses* **2018**, *10*, 649, doi:10.3390/v10110649 . . . . **187**

Liming Zhao, Barry W. Alto, Dongyoung Shin and Fahong Yu
The Effect of Permethrin Resistance on *Aedes aegypti* Transcriptome Following Ingestion of Zika Virus Infected Blood
Reprinted from: *Viruses* **2018**, *10*, 470, doi:10.3390/v10090470 . . . . **203**

Francine Azouz, Komal Arora, Keeton Krause, Vivek R. Nerurkar and Mukesh Kumar
Integrated MicroRNA and mRNA Profiling in Zika Virus-Infected Neurons
Reprinted from: *Viruses* **2019**, *11*, 162, doi:10.3390/v11020162 . . . . **221**

Liesel Stassen, Charles W. Armitage, David J. van der Heide, Kenneth W. Beagley and Francesca D. Frentiu
New Advances on Zika Virus Research
Reprinted from: *Viruses* **2018**, *10*, 198, doi:10.3390/v10040198 . . . . **243**

Sneha Singh and Ashok Kumar
Ocular Manifestations of Emerging Flaviviruses and the Blood-Retinal Barrier
Reprinted from: *Viruses* **2018**, *10*, 530, doi:10.3390/v10100530 . . . . **258**

Yin Xiang Setoh, Nias Y. Peng, Eri Nakayama, Alberto A. Amarilla, Natalie A. Prow, Andreas Suhrbier and Alexander A. Khromykh
Fetal Brain Infection Is Not a Unique Characteristic of Brazilian Zika Viruses
Reprinted from: *Viruses* **2018**, *10*, 541, doi:10.3390/v10100541 . . . . **278**

Jonathan O. Rayner, Raj Kalkeri, Scott Goebel, Zhaohui Cai, Brian Green, Shuling Lin, Beth Snyder, Kimberly Hagelin, Kevin B. Walters and Fusataka Koide
Comparative Pathogenesis of Asian and African-Lineage Zika Virus in Indian Rhesus Macaque's and Development of a Non-Human Primate Model Suitable for the Evaluation of New Drugs and Vaccines
Reprinted from: *Viruses* **2018**, *10*, 229, doi:10.3390/v10050229 . . . . **288**

Forrest T. Goodfellow, Katherine A. Willard, Xian Wu, Shelley Scoville, Steven L. Stice and Melinda A. Brindley
Strain-Dependent Consequences of Zika Virus Infection and Differential Impact on Neural Development
Reprinted from: *Viruses* **2018**, *10*, 550, doi:10.3390/v10100550 . . . . **304**

Silvia Márquez-Jurado, Aitor Nogales, Ginés Ávila-Pérez, Francisco J. Iborra, Luis Martínez-Sobrido and Fernando Almazán
An Alanine-to-Valine Substitution in the Residue 175 of Zika Virus NS2A Protein Affects Viral RNA Synthesis and Attenuates the Virus In Vivo
Reprinted from: *Viruses* **2018**, *10*, 547, doi:10.3390/v10100547 319

Ge Li, Sandra Bos, Konstantin A. Tsetsarkin, Alexander G. Pletnev, Philippe Desprès, Gilles Gadea and Richard Y. Zhao
The Roles of prM-E Proteins in Historical and Epidemic Zika Virus-Mediated Infection and Neurocytotoxicity
Reprinted from: *Viruses* **2019**, *11*, 157, doi:10.3390/v11020157 340

Diego Simón, Alvaro Fajardo, Pilar Moreno, Gonzalo Moratorio and Juan Cristina
An Evolutionary Insight into Zika Virus Strains Isolated in the Latin American Region
Reprinted from: *Viruses* **2018**, *10*, 698, doi:10.3390/v10120698 361

Himanshu Garg, Tugba Mehmetoglu-Gurbuz and Anjali Joshi
Recent Advances in Zika Virus Vaccines
Reprinted from: *Viruses* **2018**, *10*, 631, doi:10.3390/v10110631 372

Marco P. Alves, Nathalie J. Vielle, Volker Thiel and Stephanie Pfaender
Research Models and Tools for the Identification of Antivirals and Therapeutics against Zika Virus Infection
Reprinted from: *Viruses* **2018**, *10*, 593, doi:10.3390/v10110593 385

Juan-Carlos Saiz, Nereida Jiménez de Oya, Ana-Belén Blázquez, Estela Escribano-Romero and Miguel A. Martín-Acebes
Host-Directed Antivirals: A Realistic Alternative to Fight Zika Virus
Reprinted from: *Viruses* **2018**, *10*, 453, doi:10.3390/v10090453 415

Fabian Elgner, Catarina Sabino, Michael Basic, Daniela Ploen, Arnold Grünweller and Eberhard Hildt
Inhibition of Zika Virus Replication by Silvestrol
Reprinted from: *Viruses* **2018**, *10*, 149, doi:10.3390/v10040149 433

Katherine A. Willard, Christina L. Elling, Steven L. Stice and Melinda A. Brindley
The Oxysterol 7-Ketocholesterol Reduces Zika Virus Titers in Vero Cells and Human Neurons
Reprinted from: *Viruses* **2019**, *11*, 20, doi:10.3390/v11010002 447

Oliver Donoso Mantke, Elaine McCulloch, Paul S. Wallace, Constanze Yue, Sally A. Baylis and Matthias Niedrig
External Quality Assessment (EQA) for Molecular Diagnostics of Zika Virus: Experiences from an International EQA Programme, 2016–2018
Reprinted from: *Viruses* **2018**, *10*, 491, doi:10.3390/v10090491 464

Sanchita Bhadra, Miguel A. Saldaña, Hannah Grace Han, Grant L. Hughes and Andrew D. Ellington
Simultaneous Detection of Different Zika Virus Lineages via Molecular Computation in a Point-of-Care Assay
Reprinted from: *Viruses* **2018**, *10*, 714, doi:10.3390/v10120714 471

Fernando De Ory, María Paz Sánchez-Seco, Ana Vázquez, María Dolores Montero, Elena Sulleiro, Miguel J. Martínez, Lurdes Matas, Francisco J. Merino and Working Group for the Study of Zika Virus Infections
Comparative Evaluation of Indirect Immunofluorescence and NS-1-Based ELISA to Determine Zika Virus-Specific IgM
Reprinted from: *Viruses* **2018**, *10*, 379, doi:10.3390/v10070379 . . . . **493**

Liding Zhang, Xuewei Du, Congjie Chen, Zhixin Chen, Li Zhang, Qinqin Han, Xueshan Xia, Yuzhu Song and Jinyang Zhang
Development and Characterization of Double-Antibody Sandwich ELISA for Detection of Zika Virus Infection
Reprinted from: *Viruses* **2018**, *10*, 634, doi:10.3390/v10110634 . . . . **502**

Carmel T. Taylor, Ian M. Mackay, Jamie L. McMahon, Sarah L. Wheatley, Peter R. Moore, Mitchell J. Finger, Glen R. Hewitson and Frederick A. Moore
Detection of Specific ZIKV IgM in Travelers Using a Multiplexed Flavivirus Microsphere Immunoassay
Reprinted from: *Viruses* **2018**, *10*, 253, doi:10.3390/v10050253 . . . . **514**

Fátima Amaro, María P. Sánchez-Seco, Ana Vázquez, Maria J. Alves, Líbia Zé-Zé, Maria T. Luz, Teodora Minguito, Jesús De La Fuente and Fernando De Ory
The Application and Interpretation of IgG Avidity and IgA ELISA Tests to Characterize Zika Virus Infections
Reprinted from: *Viruses* **2019**, *11*, 179, doi:10.3390/v11020179 . . . . **529**

About the Special Issue Editors

Luis Martinez-Sobrido, Ph.D., is currently an Associate Professor in the Department of Microbiology and Immunology at University of Rochester. His Ph.D. research focused on the study of viral replication and transcription of respiratory syncytial virus under the guidance of Dr. Jose Antonio Melero at the Instituto de Salud Carlos III in Madrid, Spain. He also conducted post-doctoral research on the molecular biology of influenza viruses under the supervision of Dr. Adolfo Garcia-Sastre at the Icahn School of Medicine at Mount Sinai in New York, USA. His research interest has been focused on the molecular biology, immunology, and pathogenesis of negative-stranded (influenza viruses, respiratory syncytial virus, human metapneumovirus, arenavirus, thogotovirus, Ebola virus, Crimean Congo hemorrhagic fever virus) and positive-stranded (dengue virus, SARS coronavirus, mouse hepatitis virus) RNA and DNA (human cytomegalovirus and vaccinia) viruses. His current research interest focuses on the molecular biology of RNA viruses—mainly influenza, arenaviruses and Zika virus.

Fernando Almazán, Ph.D., is currently a Research Leader in the Department of Molecular and Cell Biology at the National Centre for Biotechnology (CNB-CSIC) in Madrid, Spain. He obtained his Ph.D. degree in Biology at the Centre for Molecular Biology "Severo Ochoa" (Madrid, Spain) in 1991 under the supervision of Dr. Eladio Viñuela. In 1998, he moved to Oxford University, where he completed an EMBO postdoctoral fellowship in the laboratory of Dr. Geoffrey L. Smith. Upon completing his postdoctoral studies, he joined the laboratory of Dr. Luis Enjuanes at the National Centre for Biotechnology (Madrid, Spain) as a "Ramon y Cajal" researcher. Finally, in 2008 he was appointed as Permanent Scientist of the Spanish National Research Council (CSIC) in the National Centre for Biotechnology (Madrid, Spain). During his scientific career, his research interest has focused on the molecular biology, immunology, virus–host interaction, and pathogenesis of complex DNA viruses (ASFV and vaccinia virus) and positive-stranded RNA viruses, including coronaviruses (TGEV, SARS-CoV, MERS-CoV, HCoV-OC43, and FIPV) and flaviviruses (Dengue and Zika viruses). Currently, his research interest is focused on the study of the molecular bases of Zika virus pathogenesis.

![viruses logo] *viruses*

MDPI

Editorial

New Advances on Zika Virus Research

Luis Martinez-Sobrido [1,*] and **Fernando Almazán [2]**

1   Department of Microbiology and Immunology, School of Medicine and Dentistry, University of Rochester, Rochester, New York, NY 14642, USA
2   Department of Molecular and Cell Biology, Centro Nacional de Biotecnología (CNB-CSIC), Campus Universidad Autónoma de Madrid, 3 Darwin street, 28049 Madrid, Spain; falmazan@cnb.csic.es
*   Correspondence: Luis_Martinez@URMC.Rochester.edu

Received: 11 March 2019; Accepted: 11 March 2019; Published: 14 March 2019

Zika virus (ZIKV) is an emerging mosquito-borne member of the *Flaviviridae* family that has historically been known to cause sporadic outbreaks, associated with a mild febrile illness, in Africa and Southeast Asia. However, the recent outbreaks of ZIKV in the Americas and its association with severe neurological disorders, including fetal microcephaly, Guillain-Barré syndrome, and ocular abnormalities, have caused a great social and sanitary alarm. The significance of ZIKV in human health, together with a lack of approved therapeutic (antivirals) or prophylactic (vaccines) interventions, has triggered a global effort to develop effective countermeasures against this pathogen, which has the potential to affect millions of people worldwide.

Since the re-emergence of the virus in 2015 in Brazil, massive advances have been made in practically all areas of the biology of ZIKV. In this Special Issue, we have assembled a collection of 32 research papers and reviews that cover recent advances on ZIKV research in molecular biology, replication and transmission, virus-host interactions, pathogenesis, epidemiology, vaccine development, antivirals, and diagnosis.

The first part of this Special Issue focuses on the development of ZIKV reverse genetic approaches, which constitute a powerful tool to answer important questions on the biology of ZIKV and for vaccine development. This theme is covered by a complete review of all ZIKV reverse genetic systems developed in the last years (Ávila-Pérez et al. [1]) and two research papers describing the generation of a ZIKV infectious clone by the mutational silencing of cryptical bacterial promoters present in the viral genome (Münster et al. [2]) and a Tet-inducible ZIKV infectious clone (Zhang et al. [3]).

The second topic of the Special Issue addresses recent advances in viral replication and transmission and is covered by three research articles (Barnard et al. [4]; Mlera and Bloom [5]; and Oliveira et al. [6]).

The third topic, virus-host interactions, includes two comprehensive reviews, one describing the molecular insights into ZIKV-host interactions (Lee et al. [7]) and other discussing the type I interferon (IFN) antagonist mechanisms used by flaviviruses, with a focus on the non-structural (NS)5 protein (Thurmond et al. [8]). In addition, this topic includes five research manuscripts that describe the impact of viral and host genetic variations on ZIKV infection (Yun et al. [9]), the effect of ZIKV infection on Heme Oxygenase expression (Kalamouni et al. [10]), the different effects of ZIKV infection in placenta and microglia cells (Martinez-Viedma and Pickett [11]), the effect of permethrin resistance on the vector transcriptome after ZIKV infection (Zhao et al. [12]), and the microRNA and mRNA profiling in infected neurons (Azouz et al. [13]).

The fourth subject area address new advances in ZIKV pathogenesis. This theme is covered by two reviews that describe ZIKV pathogenesis in the male reproductive tract (Stassen et al. [14]) and the ocular abnormalities induced by flavivirus infection (Singh et al. [15]), and five research articles that define fetal brain infection with ZIKV isolates not associated with microcephaly (Setoh et al. [16]), the pathogenesis of Asian and African ZIKV isolates in Indian Rhesus macaques (Rayner et al. [17]), the consequences of ZIKV infection in human pluripotent stem cell-derived neural progenitor cells and neurons (Goodfellow et al. [18]), the effect of a single mutation in the NS2A protein in virus pathogenesis (Márquez-Jurado et al. [19]), and the roles of the premembrane (prM) and envelop (E) proteins in ZIKV-mediated infection and neurocytotoxicity (Li et al. [20]).

The fifth section in the Special Issue covers the new advances in epidemiology and virus evolution, including a manuscript describing the evolutionary insight of ZIKV strains isolated in Latin America (Simón et al. [21]).

The next section focuses on ZIKV vaccines and antivirals, and contains three review documents (Garg et al. [22]; Alves et al. [23]; Saiz et al. [24]) and two research articles that describe the antiviral effect of silvestrol (Elgner et al. [25]) and oxysterol 7-ketocholesterol (Willard et al. [26]) in ZIKV replication.

The last section in this Special Issue covers new advances in the molecular diagnostic of ZIKV, and includes a comprehensive review (Mantke et al. [27]) and five research articles that describe the development and characterization of several ZIKV diagnostic methods (Bhadra et al. [28]; de Ory et al. [29]; Zhang et al. [30]; Taylor et al. [31]; Amaro et al. [32]).

We would like to thank all contributing authors for their participation, effort and hard work in putting together this Special Issue. We would also like to thank the Editorial Office at *Viruses* for all the help, support, and advice with this Special Issue. We hope this Special Issue offers a comprehensive view of the recent advances in ZIKV research and stimulates research for future studies aimed at understanding ZIKV evolution, virus-host-interaction, pathogenesis, and the development of effective countermeasures to combat ZIKV infection.

Conflicts of Interest: The authors declare no conflict of interest.

References

1. Ávila-Pérez, G.; Nogales, A.; Martín, V.; Almazán, F.; Martínez-Sobrido, L. Reverse Genetic Approaches for the Generation of Recombinant Zika Virus. *Viruses* **2018**, *10*, 597. [CrossRef]
2. Münster, M.; Płaszczyca, A.; Cortese, M.; Neufeldt, C.J.; Goellner, S.; Long, G.; Bartenschlager, R. A Reverse Genetics System for Zika Virus Based on a Simple Molecular Cloning Strategy. *Viruses* **2018**, *10*, 368. [CrossRef]
3. Zhang, L.; Ji, W.; Lyu, S.; Qiao, L.; Luo, G. Tet-Inducible Production of Infectious Zika Virus from the Full-Length cDNA Clones of African- and Asian-Lineage Strains. *Viruses* **2018**, *10*, 700. [CrossRef] [PubMed]
4. Barnard, T.R.; Rajah, M.M.; Sagan, S.M. Contemporary Zika Virus Isolates Induce More dsRNA and Produce More Negative-Strand Intermediate in Human Astrocytoma Cells. *Viruses* **2018**, *10*, 728. [CrossRef] [PubMed]
5. Mlera, L.; Bloom, M.E. Differential Zika Virus Infection of Testicular Cell Lines. *Viruses* **2019**, *11*, 42. [CrossRef] [PubMed]
6. Oliveira, D.B.L.; Durigon, G.S.; Mendes, É.A.; Ladner, J.T.; Andreata-Santos, R.; Araujo, D.B.; Botosso, V.F.; Paola, N.D.; Neto, D.F.L.; Cunha, M.P.; et al. Persistence and Intra-Host Genetic Evolution of Zika Virus Infection in Symptomatic Adults: A Special View in the Male Reproductive System. *Viruses* **2018**, *10*, 615. [CrossRef] [PubMed]
7. Lee, I.; Bos, S.; Li, G.; Wang, S.; Gadea, G.; Desprès, P.; Zhao, R.Y. Probing Molecular Insights into Zika Virus–Host Interactions. *Viruses* **2018**, *10*, 233. [CrossRef]
8. Thurmond, S.; Wang, B.; Song, J.; Hai, R. Suppression of Type I Interferon Signaling by *Flavivirus* NS5. *Viruses* **2018**, *10*, 712. [CrossRef] [PubMed]
9. Yun, S.-I.; Song, B.-H.; Frank, J.C.; Julander, J.G.; Olsen, A.L.; Polejaeva, I.A.; Davies, C.J.; White, K.L.; Lee, Y.-M. Functional Genomics and Immunologic Tools: The Impact of Viral and Host Genetic Variations on the Outcome of Zika Virus Infection. *Viruses* **2018**, *10*, 422. [CrossRef]
10. El Kalamouni, C.; Frumence, E.; Bos, S.; Turpin, J.; Nativel, B.; Harrabi, W.; Wilkinson, D.A.; Meilhac, O.; Gadea, G.; Desprès, P.; et al. Subversion of the Heme Oxygenase-1 Antiviral Activity by Zika Virus. *Viruses* **2019**, *11*, 2. [CrossRef]

11. Martinez Viedma, M.P.; Pickett, B.E. Characterizing the Different Effects of Zika Virus Infection in Placenta and Microglia Cells. *Viruses* **2018**, *10*, 649. [CrossRef]

12. Zhao, L.; Alto, B.W.; Shin, D.; Yu, F. The Effect of Permethrin Resistance on *Aedes aegypti* Transcriptome Following Ingestion of Zika Virus Infected Blood. *Viruses* **2018**, *10*, 470. [CrossRef]

13. Azouz, F.; Arora, K.; Krause, K.; Nerurkar, V.R.; Kumar, M. Integrated MicroRNA and mRNA Profiling in Zika Virus-Infected Neurons. *Viruses* **2019**, *11*, 162. [CrossRef]

14. Stassen, L.; Armitage, C.W.; Van der Heide, D.J.; Beagley, K.W.; Frentiu, F.D. Zika Virus in the Male Reproductive Tract. *Viruses* **2018**, *10*, 198. [CrossRef]

15. Singh, S.; Kumar, A. Ocular Manifestations of Emerging Flaviviruses and the Blood-Retinal Barrier. *Viruses* **2018**, *10*, 530. [CrossRef]

16. Setoh, Y.X.; Peng, N.Y.; Nakayama, E.; Amarilla, A.A.; Prow, N.A.; Suhrbier, A.; Khromykh, A.A. Fetal Brain Infection Is Not a Unique Characteristic of Brazilian Zika Viruses. *Viruses* **2018**, *10*, 541. [CrossRef]

17. Rayner, J.O.; Kalkeri, R.; Goebel, S.; Cai, Z.; Green, B.; Lin, S.; Snyder, B.; Hagelin, K.; Walters, K.B.; Koide, F. Comparative Pathogenesis of Asian and African-Lineage Zika Virus in Indian Rhesus Macaque's and Development of a Non-Human Primate Model Suitable for the Evaluation of New Drugs and Vaccines. *Viruses* **2018**, *10*, 229. [CrossRef]

18. Goodfellow, F.T.; Willard, K.A.; Wu, X.; Scoville, S.; Stice, S.L.; Brindley, M.A. Strain-Dependent Consequences of Zika Virus Infection and Differential Impact on Neural Development. *Viruses* **2018**, *10*, 550. [CrossRef]

19. Márquez-Jurado, S.; Nogales, A.; Ávila-Pérez, G.; Iborra, F.J.; Martínez-Sobrido, L.; Almazán, F. An Alanine-to-Valine Substitution in the Residue 175 of Zika Virus NS2A Protein Affects Viral RNA Synthesis and Attenuates the Virus In Vivo. *Viruses* **2018**, *10*, 547. [CrossRef]

20. Li, G.; Bos, S.; Tsetsarkin, K.A.; Pletnev, A.G.; Desprès, P.; Gadea, G.; Zhao, R.Y. The Roles of prM-E Proteins in Historical and Epidemic Zika Virus-mediated Infection and Neurocytotoxicity. *Viruses* **2019**, *11*, 157. [CrossRef]

21. Simón, D.; Fajardo, A.; Moreno, P.; Moratorio, G.; Cristina, J. An Evolutionary Insight into Zika Virus Strains Isolated in the Latin American Region. *Viruses* **2018**, *10*, 698. [CrossRef] [PubMed]

22. Garg, H.; Mehmetoglu-Gurbuz, T.; Joshi, A. Recent Advances in Zika Virus Vaccines. *Viruses* **2018**, *10*, 631. [CrossRef] [PubMed]

23. Alves, M.P.; Vielle, N.J.; Thiel, V.; Pfaender, S. Research Models and Tools for the Identification of Antivirals and Therapeutics against Zika Virus Infection. *Viruses* **2018**, *10*, 593. [CrossRef] [PubMed]

24. Saiz, J.-C.; Oya, N.J.; Blázquez, A.-B.; Escribano-Romero, E.; Martín-Acebes, M.A. Host-Directed Antivirals: A Realistic Alternative to Fight Zika Virus. *Viruses* **2018**, *10*, 453. [CrossRef] [PubMed]

25. Elgner, F.; Sabino, C.; Basic, M.; Ploen, D.; Grünweller, A.; Hildt, E. Inhibition of Zika Virus Replication by Silvestrol. *Viruses* **2018**, *10*, 149. [CrossRef]

26. Willard, K.A.; Elling, C.L.; Stice, S.L.; Brindley, M.A. The Oxysterol 7-Ketocholesterol Reduces Zika Virus Titers in Vero Cells and Human Neurons. *Viruses* **2019**, *11*, 20. [CrossRef] [PubMed]

27. Donoso Mantke, O.; McCulloch, E.; Wallace, P.S.; Yue, C.; Baylis, S.A.; Niedrig, M. External Quality Assessment (EQA) for Molecular Diagnostics of Zika Virus: Experiences from an International EQA Programme, 2016–2018. *Viruses* **2018**, *10*, 491. [CrossRef]

28. Bhadra, S.; Saldaña, M.A.; Han, H.G.; Hughes, G.L.; Ellington, A.D. Simultaneous Detection of Different Zika Virus Lineages via Molecular Computation in a Point-of-Care Assay. *Viruses* **2018**, *10*, 714. [CrossRef]

29. De Ory, F.; Sánchez-Seco, M.P.; Vázquez, A.; Montero, M.D.; Sulleiro, E.; Martínez, M.J.; Matas, L.; Merino, F.J.; Working Group for the Study of Zika Virus Infections. Comparative Evaluation of Indirect Immunofluorescence and NS-1-Based ELISA to Determine Zika Virus-Specific IgM. *Viruses* **2018**, *10*, 379. [CrossRef]

30. Zhang, L.; Du, X.; Chen, C.; Chen, Z.; Zhang, L.; Han, Q.; Xia, X.; Song, Y.; Zhang, J. Development and Characterization of Double-Antibody Sandwich ELISA for Detection of Zika Virus Infection. *Viruses* **2018**, *10*, 634. [CrossRef]

31. Taylor, C.T.; Mackay, I.M.; McMahon, J.L.; Wheatley, S.L.; Moore, P.R.; Finger, M.J.; Hewitson, G.R.; Moore, F.A. Detection of Specific ZIKV IgM in Travelers Using a Multiplexed Flavivirus Microsphere Immunoassay. *Viruses* **2018**, *10*, 253. [CrossRef]
32. Amaro, F.; Sánchez-Seco, M.P.; Vázquez, A.; Alves, M.J.; Zé-Zé, L.; Luz, M.T.; Minguito, T.; De La Fuente, J.; De Ory, F. The Application and Interpretation of IgG Avidity and IgA ELISA Tests to Characterize Zika Virus Infections. *Viruses* **2019**, *11*, 179. [CrossRef]

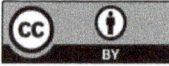

viruses

MDPI

Review

Reverse Genetic Approaches for the Generation of Recombinant Zika Virus

Ginés Ávila-Pérez [1], Aitor Nogales [1], Verónica Martín [2], Fernando Almazán [2,*] and Luis Martínez-Sobrido [1,*]

1   Department of Microbiology and Immunology, University of Rochester Medical Center,
    601 Elmwood Avenue, Rochester, NY 14642, USA; Gines_Perez@urmc.rochester.edu (G.A.-P.);
    aitor_nogales@urmc.rochester.edu (A.N.)
2   Department of Molecular and Cell Biology, Centro Nacional de Biotecnología (CNB-CSIC), Campus
    Universidad Autónoma de Madrid, 3 Darwin street, 28049 Madrid, Spain; veronica.martin@inia.es
*   Correspondence: falmazan@cnb.csic.es (F.A.); luis_martinez@urmc.rochester.edu (L.M.-S.)

Received: 10 October 2018; Accepted: 28 October 2018; Published: 31 October 2018

Abstract: Zika virus (ZIKV) is an emergent mosquito-borne member of the *Flaviviridae* family that was responsible for a recent epidemic in the Americas. ZIKV has been associated with severe clinical complications, including neurological disorder such as Guillain-Barré syndrome in adults and severe fetal abnormalities and microcephaly in newborn infants. Given the significance of these clinical manifestations, the development of tools and reagents to study the pathogenesis of ZIKV and to develop new therapeutic options are urgently needed. In this respect, the implementation of reverse genetic techniques has allowed the direct manipulation of the viral genome to generate recombinant (r)ZIKVs, which have provided investigators with powerful systems to answer important questions about the biology of ZIKV, including virus-host interactions, the mechanism of transmission and pathogenesis or the function of viral proteins. In this review, we will summarize the different reverse genetic strategies that have been implemented, to date, for the generation of rZIKVs and the applications of these platforms for the development of replicon systems or reporter-expressing viruses.

Keywords: flavivirus; Zika virus (ZIKV); reverse genetics; infectious clone; full-length molecular clone; bacterial artificial chromosome; replicon; infectious RNA

1. Introduction

1.1. Importance of Zika Virus in Human Health

Zika virus (ZIKV) is a recently emerged mosquito-borne virus, which in 2016 was declared as an international public health emergency by the World Health Organization (WHO, http://www.who.int/csr/en/) [1]. ZIKV is a member of the Flavivirus genus that belongs to the *Flaviviridae* family and is closely related to other mosquitoes-transmitted flaviviruses of public health relevance such as Dengue virus (DENV), Yellow fever virus (YFV), Japanese encephalitis virus (JEV) and West Nile virus (WNV) [2,3]. ZIKV was first isolated in 1947 of a sentinel rhesus monkey in the Zika forest of Uganda [4] and has been associated with sporadic human cases detected across Africa and Asia, resembling a mild version of DENV or Chikungunya virus (CHIKV) [5]. These similarities with DENV and CHIKV has interfered with ZIKV diagnosis and most probably underestimated the number of cases for ZIKV infections [6]. Symptomatic disease generally is present with a mild febrile illness characterized by fever, rash, muscle pain, headache and conjunctivitis, although as up to 80% of the ZIKV cases are asymptomatic [7–9]. However, the outbreak in the island of Yap in 2007 [10], French Polynesia in 2013–2014 [11,12] and the massive epidemic that emerge in Brazil in 2015 [13,14] have caused major concerns due to the association of ZIKV infection with severe congenital abnormalities, including microcephaly in infants and an increased risk of Guillain-Barré syndrome in adults [15–18]. ZIKV is mainly transmitted to people through the bite of an infected *Aedes* spp. mosquito (*Ae. Aegypti* and *Ae. Albopictus*) [19], which carries a high risk for pregnant woman due to the ability to cross the placenta and infected fetal nervous tissues [20]. In addition to maternal-fetal transmission, ZIKV can also be transmitted from mother to child during pregnancy or spread through sexual contact, breastfeeding, blood transfusion and non-human primate bites [21–23].

1.2. ZIKV Biology

ZIKV is an enveloped virus containing three structural proteins (Figure 1): the capsid (C) protein, the membrane (M) protein and the envelope (E) glycoprotein (Figure 1A). Inside the virion, the viral (v)RNA genome is complexed with multiple copies of the C protein, surrounded by the E and M proteins, which are anchored in a lipid membrane (Figure 1A). The surface of the mature virion has a icosahedral shell consisting of 90 E:M heterodimers (Figure 1A) [24]. The viral genome is made of a positive single-stranded RNA molecule of approximately 10.8 kb with a single open reading frame, flanked at the 5'- and 3'-ends by the viral untranslated regions (UTRs) (Figure 1B). ZIKV vRNA is translated by cap-dependent initiation producing a single polyprotein of approximately 3423 amino acids, which is co- and post-transcriptionally processed by both viral and cellular proteases into the three structural proteins (C, pre-Membrane (prM) and E) and seven non-structural (NS) proteins (NS1, NS2A, NS2B, NS3, NS4A, NS4B, NS5) (Figure 1B). The structural proteins are essential components of the virion and are involved in viral entry, fusion and assembly. The NS proteins are mainly involved in vRNA synthesis, assembly and regulation of the host cell responses [25]. Phylogenetic analysis of ZIKV have revealed two major genetic lineages (African and Asian), which have undergone substantial changes during the past 50 years. Sequence homology analysis indicated that the strains that have been responsible for the recent human outbreaks throughout the Pacific and the Americas are phylogenetically related to the most recent Asian lineage [26,27].

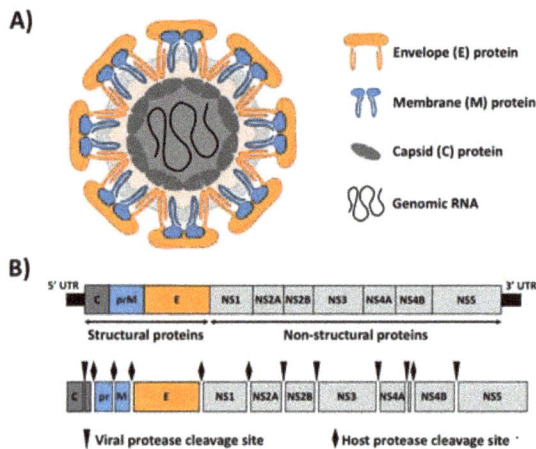

Figure 1. Zika virus (ZIKV) virion structure and genome organization. (**A**) Schematic representation of ZIKV virion structure: ZIKV virion surface is decorated with the E and M proteins, anchored in a lipid bilayer with an icosahedral-like symmetry. Under the viral lipid bilayer is the nucleocapsid composed of the vRNA genome associated with the C protein. (**B**) Genome organization and polyprotein processing: ZIKV genome (approximately 10.8 kb) is translated as a single polyprotein that is cleaved co- and post-translationally by viral (arrows) and host (diamonds) proteases to yield the three structural proteins C, M and E; and seven NS proteins NS1, NS2A, NS2B, NS3, NS4A, NS4B and NS5. The 5′ and 3′ untranslated regions (UTR) are indicated as black lines at the end of the viral genome.

Like other flaviviruses, ZIKV entry occurs via attachment of the virions to the cell surface, a mechanism mediated by the viral E glycoprotein, followed by internalization by receptor-mediated endocytosis [28]. After virus internalization, the acid environment inside the endosome induces major conformational changes in the E glycoprotein that promote fusion of the viral and endosome membranes and the subsequent release of the viral genome into the cytoplasm of the infected cell. Once the genomic vRNA is released, it is translated to the viral polyprotein. As other positive-stranded RNA viruses, flaviviruses replication occurs on virus-induced host cell membranes, mainly characterized by invaginations of the endoplasmic reticulum (ER) membrane termed vesicle packets, which serve as scaffold for anchoring the viral replication complexes [29–31]. The immature viral particles are assembled within the ER, where the genomic vRNA is associated with the C protein and is packaged into ER-derived membranes containing the prM and E proteins. Virion maturation occurs in the *trans*-Golgi network during its transit through the cellular secretory pathway. Cellular furin protease mediate the cleavage of the prM, resulting in the release of the pr peptide and formation of mature virions containing the M protein that will be released from infected cells [32–34].

Because the very recent emergence of ZIKV, there are not currently approved vaccines or antivirals available to combat infection by this important human pathogen. Therefore, the generation of prophylactic (vaccines) and therapeutic (antivirals) options for the treatment of ZIKV are urgently required. The development of ZIKV reverse genetic systems provide investigators with a powerful tool for the development of vaccines and antivirals to counteract disease caused by this important human pathogen.

2. ZIKV Reverse Genetics

In 1981, Racaniello et al. reported, for the first time, the production of infectious virus by transfecting mammalian cells with a DNA plasmid containing the entire viral genome of poliovirus [35]. Since then, numerous reverse genetic technologies have been employed to recover recombinant viruses for the majority of viral families, including positive-sense RNA viruses such as coronavirus [36], picornavirus [37,38], flavivirus [39]; or negative-sense RNA viruses such as influenza [40] and arenavirus [41,42], among many others. Reverse genetic techniques have allowed investigators to generate recombinant viruses containing specific mutations to evaluate their contribution in viral replication and transcription, pathogenicity, virus-host interactions, inhibition of host cellular responses and host range or transmissibility [37]. Importantly, reverse genetic approaches have also been used for the developing of vaccines based on attenuated forms of the virus [37,40] and the generation of recombinant viruses harboring reporter genes to easily track viral infection, which have been resourceful to identify antivirals, host factors or for the in vitro and in vivo study of viral infections [43,44]. Viral reverse genetic approaches allow to recover infectious recombinant viruses upon transfection of a single (non-segmented viruses) or multiple (segmented viruses) DNAs into susceptible cells [40].

Similar to other viruses, the recent emergence of ZIKV as an important human pathogen, has promoted the rapid development of numerous reverse genetic approaches to increase our knowledge of the molecular biology and pathogenesis of ZIKV. To date, three major reverse genetic strategies have been described to generate rZIKVs: (i) infectious RNA transcripts from a full-length complementary (c)DNA copy; (ii) DNA plasmids that are directly transfected to produce infectious ZIKV; and (iii) Infectious Subgenomic Amplicons (ISA) (Figure 2 and Table 1). The first strategy involves the in vitro transcription of an infectious RNA genome from a full-length cDNA copy containing the ZIKV genome under the control of a prokaryotic RNA polymerase promoter (e.g., T7 or SP6) (Figure 2A). In this case, the last nucleotide of the viral genome is followed by the hepatitis delta virus ribozyme (HDVr) sequence to produce synthetic RNAs bearing an accurate 3′ end (Figure 2A). Once transcribed, the vRNA is transfected into susceptible cells to recover infectious rZIKV. The second approach consist in the construction of a full-length infectious cDNA clone containing the viral genome flanked by a eukaryotic polymerase II-driven promoter at the 5′ end, mainly the cytomegalovirus (CMV) promoter and the HDVr sequence followed by a polymerase II terminator and polyadenylation signal (pA) at the 3' end of the viral genome (Figure 2B). The full-length cDNA is usually assembled in a low-copy plasmid for its stable propagation in bacteria. In this system, the full-length infectious cDNA clone is directly transfected into susceptible cells where the vRNA is primarily transcribed in the nucleus by the cellular RNA polymerase II with further amplification steps in the cytoplasm driven by the viral polymerase. The last approach is based on the generation of overlapping double-stranded (ds)DNA fragments, covering the entire genome of ZIKV. In this case, the 5' end fragment contains a polymerase II driven promoter (e.g., CMV) and the 3' end fragment a HDVr sequence followed by a polymerase II terminator and polyadenylation signal (Figure 2C). This ISA approach involves the co-transfection of all the cDNA fragments into susceptible cells followed by the self-assembly of a full-length cDNA copy inside of the transfected cells by homologous recombination.

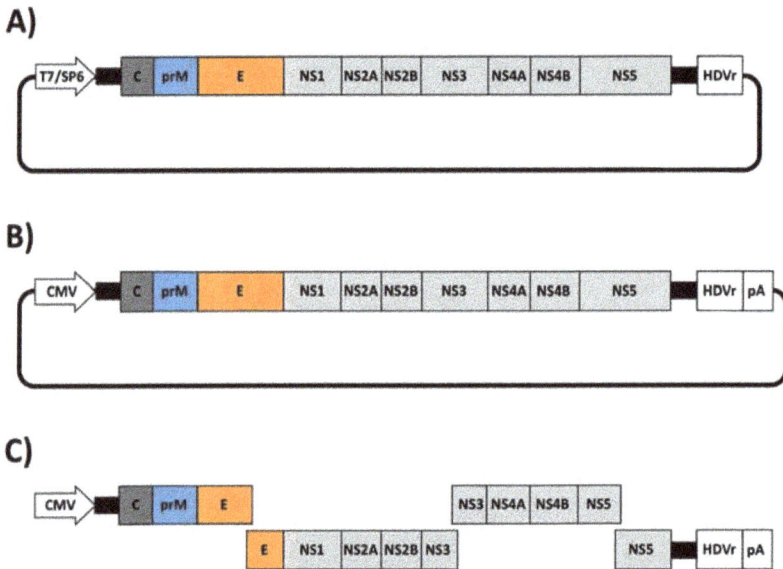

Figure 2. Schematic representation of ZIKV reverse genetic approaches. (**A**) Infectious RNA transcripts from full-length cDNA clones: A full-length genomic cDNA clone containing the ZIKV genome flanked by a prokaryotic promoter (e.g., T7 or SP6) and the hepatitis delta virus ribozyme (HDVr) is usually assembled in a low-copy plasmid. In this approach, in vitro transcription is required to produce viral RNA that is transfected into susceptible cells to initiate viral replication and transcription in the cytoplasm of transfected cells. (**B**) Full-length infectious genomic cDNA clones: A full-length infectious genomic cDNA clone containing the viral genome flanked by a polymerase II-driven promoter from cytomegalovirus (CMV) and the HDVr followed by a polymerase II terminator and polyadenylation signal (pA) is assembled in a low-copy plasmid. In this case, the full-length cDNA clone is transcribed in the nucleus of transfected cells by the cellular RNA polymerase II. Primary transcripts are translocated to the cytoplasm where further amplifications steps are conducted by the viral polymerase. (**C**) Infectious Subgenomic Amplicons (ISA): The ISA approach can be used for the production of infectious viruses from genomic DNA material, including pre-existing infectious cDNA clones, viral RNA or *de novo* synthesized DNA genomic sequences. The entire viral genome is amplified by overlapping PCR reactions with each PCR product containing 30–40 base pairs overlapping regions [45]. The first and last PCR products are flanked by the CMV promoter and the HDVr followed by a polymerase II terminator and pA signal, respectively. Co-transfected cDNAs result in self-assembly in the cytoplasm of susceptible cells and virus production.

Table 1. ZIKV reverse genetics techniques.

Approaches	Advantages	Disadvantages	Ref.
Infectious RNA transcripts from full-length ZIKV cDNAs	○ vRNAs are directly electroporated into cells ○ RNA electroporation is generally more efficient than transfection	○ Need an in vitro RNA transcription step ○ Genome instability of flavivirus cDNA clones in bacteria ○ Error rate of RNA in vitro transcription can produce undesired mutation	[42,46–55]
Full-length infectious ZIKV cDNA clones	○ Plasmid containing the viral genome is directly transfected into the cells ○ In vitro transcription is not required	○ Genome instability of flavivirus cDNA clones in bacteria	[48,56–59]
Infectious subgenomic amplicons (ISA)	○ Rapid and easy construction ○ cDNA assembly occurs into the cells	○ Nonhomogeneous populations by error in the recombination events	[45,60,61]

The construction of full-length cDNA clones for ZIKV has been hampered due to the toxicity of the viral genome, similar to other flavivirus, which is known to be toxic and unstable during its propagation in bacteria using standard plasmids [62–65]. This is attributed to the leaky expression of toxic viral proteins from cryptic prokaryotic promoters within the E and the NS1 coding sequences [66]. Therefore, several approaches have been developed to overcome the genome instability of flavivirus cDNA clones, including ZIKV. Those methods are summarized in Table 2 and described in detail in the following sections.

Table 2. Strategies to avoid toxicity of full-length constructs.

Approaches	Advantages	Disadvantages	Ref.
Low-copy number plasmid	Cryptic promoters are maintained at low level of expression	Low plasmid yield Flavivirus genome are often unstable	[46–49]
Bacterial artificial chromosome (BAC)	Minimization of toxicity by a strictly controlled replication leading to only one plasmid per cell. Stable maintenance of large DNA fragments	Low plasmid yield Manipulation of big DNA constructs	[48,56]
Inactivation of cryptic *E. coli* promoters (CEP)	CPEs are inactivated	Introduction of punctual mutation can disrupt the viral RNA structure and viral fitness	[50,51]
Intron insertion	Expression of toxic regions is interrupted in bacteria	Introduction of external sequences in the viral genome	[42,57,58]
In vitro ligation	Non-required propagation of full-length cDNA in bacteria	Viral genome is maintained in multiple fragments in bacteria Low ligation efficiency Low virus recovery efficiency	[52,53]
Gibson assembly or Circular polymerase extension cloning (CPEC)	Non-required propagation of full-length cDNA in bacteria Rapid assembly in one step	Viral genome is maintained in multiple fragments in bacteria Low virus recovery efficiency Error rate of the reaction can produce undesired mutations	[54,55,59]

2.1. Infectious RNA Transcripts from Full-Length ZIKV cDNAs

In the last two years, several approaches based on the use of infectious RNA transcripts from full-length ZIKV cDNAs have been developed to overcome the toxicity problems associated with several sequences of ZIKV genome when amplified in bacteria. Those methods involve the use of low-copy number plasmids [46–51], the incorporation of an intron in the genome to disrupt toxic regions [42], in vitro ligation of cDNA fragments [52,53] and Gibson assembly [54,55], amount others.

2.1.1. Construction of Full-Length ZIKV cDNA Clones Using Low-Copy Number Plasmids

A widely employed approach to overcome the toxicity of ZIKV and facilitate the stability of full-length cDNA clones consist in the use of low-copy number plasmids in which the cryptic prokaryotic promoters are maintained at a low level of expression, along with the use of prokaryotic transcription terminators to prevent the spurious transcription of foreign DNA sequences in bacterial host cells [63] (Table 2). Following this strategy, Shan-June et al. in 2016 [46] engineered the first ZIKV reverse genetic approach for the ZIKV FSS13025 strain that was isolated in 2010 from a 3-year-old patient from Cambodia [67]. In this approach, five RT-PCR fragments spanning the complete viral genome were individually cloned and assembled into a low-copy number plasmid using unique restriction sites present in the viral genome. Authors chose the low-copy number plasmid pACYC177 (15 copies of plasmid per cell) because it was previously used with other flavivirus cDNA clones [68,69]. Importantly, during the cloning procedure, the fragment spanning the viral prM-E-NS1 genes was reported to be toxic using a high-copy number plasmid. The T7 promoter and the HDVr sequence were engineered at the 5' and 3' ends of the ZIKV cDNA for in vitro transcription and the generation of the authentic 5' and 3' ends of the viral RNA, respectively. Using this approach, a rZIKV was successfully recovery after transfection of the infectious in vitro transcribed RNA in mammalian Vero cells. However, in vitro analysis showed that the rZIKV replicated at lower efficiency than the natural ZIKV isolate in both mammalian (Vero) and mosquito (C6/36) cells. Moreover, whereas the rZIKV produced plaques with homogenous morphology in Vero cells, the parental viral strain formed plaques with heterogeneous sizes. This phenotype correlated with what was observed in vivo using interferon receptor deficient (IFNAR−/−) A129 mice, where rZIKV was less virulent that the parental ZIKV.

In 2017, Mutso et al. [48] constructed a reverse genetic system based on the ZIKV Brazilian BeH81915 strain using a single low-copy plasmid. In this case, the bacterial artificial chromosome (BAC) plasmid pCC1-BAC was used to assemble the ZIKV genome under the control of a bacterial SP6 promoter. Notably, the rescued rZIKV showed similar in vitro grow kinetics in mammalian Vero cells, human brain endothelial cells (hCMEC/D3) or human choriocarcinoma placental epithelial (BeWo) cells than the natural ZIKV strain PRVABC59 isolated in Puerto Rico in 2015 [70].

Similarly, Nannamaliai et al. in 2017 [49] described the construction of a full-length cDNA clone of the historical 1947 Uganda ZIKV strain MR766 using a low-copy number plasmid. To that end, four RT-PCR fragments spanning the complete ZIKV MR766 genome were assembled in the plasmid pBR322 (around 20 copies per cell). However, the fragment containing the NS1 coding region was systematically instable during its propagation in bacteria, introducing deletion of 1 or 2 nucleotides. To bypass this problem, they cloned the toxic fragment in the linear vector pJAZZ-OC [71], which was used to assemble the full-length cDNA clone. pJAZZ-OC plasmid is derived from the linear dsDNA genome of coliphage N15 and can be maintained with 2–4 copies/cells [71] in the bacteria host. This plasmid has prokaryotic transcription terminators flanking the cloning site to eliminate the transcription into and out of the insert, which increases the stability of the insert in the bacterial host. Viral RNA transcripts were produced in vitro using the T7 RNA polymerase and infectious virus was obtained from RNA-transfected Vero cells. Importantly, the rZIKV MR766 showed similar grow kinetics in vitro in mammalian Vero or mosquito C6/36 cells than the parental MR766 ZIKV strain. Moreover, rZIKV MR766 recapitulated the pathogenic properties in vivo of the parental MR766 virus (IFNAR−/− A129 mice).

2.1.2. Stabilization of Full-Length ZIKV cDNA by Mutational Inactivation of Cryptic *E. coli* Promoters (CEPs)

An alternative approach to reduce the toxicity related with the expression of CEPs consist in the inactivation of these sequences by the introduction of punctual silent mutations in the viral genome (Table 2). This approach was previously described to stabilize the full-length cDNA clones of JEV and DENV-2 [66]. Following this strategy, Münters et al. in 2018 [50] described the construction of full-length cDNA clones of the African 1947 Uganda MR766 and the Asian French Polynesia 2013 (H/PF/2013) strains of ZIKV. In this case, four fragments spanning the entire ZIKV genomes were assemble into the low-copy pFK plasmid [72] under the control of the phage T7 promoter using unique restriction sites. However, they consistently observed that the full-length cDNA clones were unstable during their propagation in bacteria. This problem was avoided with the introduction of punctual silent mutations to disrupt the CEPs present in the viral genome. Mutational inactivation of these cryptic promoters, which were predicted in silico to reside in the structural regions of MR766 and H/PF/2013 genomes, was sufficient to stabilize the full-length cDNA clones of both ZIKV strains. Furthermore, ZIKV cDNA clones were stable after five serial passages in *E. coli*. Both viruses were successfully rescue after transfection of Vero cells with RNA produced in vitro using the T7 RNA polymerase.

Recently, Zhao et al. in 2018 [51] also described the stabilization of a full-length cDNA clone from a ZIKV Brazilian isolated (SPH2015) by introducing silent mutations into the ZIKV genome to eliminate the activity of CEPs. However, one potential problem in this approach is that the introduction of multiple silent mutations can disrupt the viral RNA structure and affect viral replication and transcription, affecting the successful rescue or the phenotype of the recovered virus in cultured cells or in vivo (Table 2).

2.1.3. Stabilization of Full-Length ZIKV cDNA Clones Using Intron Insertions

The introduction of short eukaryotic introns in the viral genome to disrupt toxic regions has been previously described to stabilize flavivirus cDNA clones [73]. Following this strategy, a full length cDNA clone of ZIKV GZ01, a virus strain isolated from a patient in China [74], was successful assembled by Liu Z-Y et al. [42] in 2017 to successfully rescue a rZIKV. Authors introduced a modified version of the group II self-splicing *P.li.LSUI2* intron [75,76] between the E and NS1 ZIKV coding regions to disrupt the toxic regions located in that region of the viral genome. The intronic sequences generally contain multiple stop codons, which interrupt the translation of the gene in bacteria (Table 2). The *P.li.LSUI2* intron, from the brown alga *Pylaiella littoralis* [77], was shown to have the ability to carry out efficient self-splicing under in vitro conditions [75]. Thus, authors used this *P.li.LSUI2* intron to produce vRNA transcripts with an intact ZIKV sequence. To construct the full-length cDNA clone, four RT-PCR fragments covering the entire full-length ZIKV genome were assembled under the control of the SP6 promoter in the low-copy plasmid pACNR1180 [78]. The intron sequence was chemically synthesized and cloned into the first fragment using overlapping PCR. Importantly, the intron-encoded protein sequence, required for self-splicing, was removed to prevent the splicing of the ZIKV cDNA in bacteria cells. In addition, the exon binding sequences of the inserted intron were modified to recognize the flanking ZIKV sequences in order to ensure the correct splicing. Using this approach, a rZIKV GZ01 was successfully recovered after the transfection of the in vitro-spliced RNA in BHK-21 cells (baby hamster kidney cell line). The recovered rZIKV GZ01 and the parental virus had similar grown kinetics and plaque morphology in vitro in both mammalian BHK-21 and mosquito C6/36 cells. Moreover, both viruses caused similar levels of neurovirulence in neonatal BALB/c mice, demonstrating that this approach can be a feasible option for rescue rZIKV [42].

2.1.4. Construction of Full-Length ZIKV cDNA Clones Using In Vitro Ligation

A common strategy to overcome the instability associated with the construction of full-length cDNA clones of some flaviviruses has been the transfection of infectious vRNA transcripts from a full-length cDNA template, which is produced by in vitro ligation [79]. This method involved the partition of the viral genome in multiples fragments flanked by natural or engineered specific restriction sites that allows the systematic and precise assembly of a full-length cDNA by in vitro ligation. Following this method, Widman et al. [52] described in 2017 the successfully rescue of representative strains of ZIKV from the African (MR766) and Asian (H/PF/2013) lineages. In addition, they were able to rescue two rZIKV from two strains (SPH2015 and BEH819015) isolated in Brazil [52]. Authors generated a quadripartite system to disrupt the toxic ZIKV genomic regions by cloning the genome in four stable plasmids. Furthermore, natural nonpalindromic restriction endonuclease sites located near of toxic regions [52,80] were used to allow the directional ligation of the digested subgenomic fragments to generate a full-length cDNA clone. The resulting assembled product was then transcribed into RNA in vitro using the T7 polymerase. This method avoids the use of a bacterial host for the propagation of the full-length cDNA and therefore overcome the problems associated with cDNA instability (Table 2). Importantly, rZIKVs generated using this approach replicate in cultured cells similarly than their parental viral isolates. Moreover, rZIKVs were virulent in type I and type III interferon deficient AG129 mice, although slightly attenuated compared to their natural viral isolates [52].

Recently, the same reverse genetic approach was used by Gorman et al. in 2018 to rescue the African ZIKV strain Dakar 41525 [53]. Likewise, Deng et al. in 2017 also described the successful rescue of rZIKV SZ-WIV01, a ZIKV strain belonging to the Asian lineage [81]. In this case, authors combined the use of a quadripartite system with BglI overhang restrictions sites for in vitro ligation and assembly of the full-length cDNA clone.

2.1.5. Construction of Full-Length ZIKV cDNA Clones Using Gibson Assembly

Gibson assembly is a molecular cloning method which allows the assembly of multiple overlapping DNA molecules in one reaction using a 5′ exonuclease, a DNA polymerase and a DNA ligase [82]. Like the in vitro ligation method described above, the entire viral genome is generated and maintained in multiples overlapping fragments to disrupt the toxic regions present in the viral genome (Table 2) [82]. Following this approach, in 2017, Weger-Lucarelli et al. developed a reverse genetic system for the ZIKV PRVABC59 strain [54]. In this manuscript, the viral genome of PRVABC59 was cloned in two separated pieces into the pACYC177 vector to disrupt the unstable NS1 region. To that end, the authors generated one vector with the T7 polymerase promoter sequence followed by the first third of the ZIKV genome. A second pACYC177 vector with the rest of the viral genome followed by the HDVr sequence was also generated. Both pACYC177 plasmids were engineered containing overlapping regions with unique restriction sites to allow reassemble of the viral genome. The full-length cDNA of ZIKV PRVABC59 was then generated by digestion and ligation using the Gibson assembly method. The resulting assembled product was then transcribed into RNA using the phage T7 polymerase and the product was transfected in Vero cells for the successful rescue of rZIKV PRVABC59. Like in the in vitro ligation approach described above, this method avoids the need to use a bacterial host for the propagation of the cDNA after the final assembly (Table 2). Importantly, the rZIKV PRVABC59 was able to replicate at similar levels to the natural virus isolate in both mammalian (Vero cells, BHK-21 cells, Huh7 human hepatoma cell line, JAR human placental cell line, amount others) or mosquito (C6/36 or Aag2) cells. Moreover, the levels of transmission in mosquitos and pathogenesis in type I and type III interferon deficient AG129 mice were also comparable between the genetically engineered and the natural ZIKVs isolates.

2.2. Full-Length Infectious ZIKV cDNA Clones

The use of reverse genetic approaches containing eukaryotic polymerase II-dependent promoters significantly simplifies the recovery of recombinant viruses as compared to the previously described procedures using phage T7 or SP6 RNA polymerase-based promoters, since direct plasmid transfection in susceptible cultured cells allows the rescue of recombinant viruses (Table 1). This approach involves the expression of the viral RNA in the nucleus of transfected cells from a polymerase II-dependent promoter with subsequent amplification steps in the cytoplasm by the viral polymerase. However, as described above, the main concern with this approach is the construction of full-length infectious ZIKV cDNA clones and the problems associated with stability of the viral genome during its propagation in bacteria. Several approaches have been developed to overcome the problems associated with genome instability of full-length infectious ZIKV cDNAs, including the use of intron sequences [57,58], assembly by circular polymerase extension cloning [59] or the use of BACs [48,56] (Table 2).

2.2.1. Stabilization of Infectious Full-Length ZIKV cDNA Clones Using Introns

The first reverse genetic approach for the construction of a full-length infectious ZIKV cDNA clone was reported by Tsetsarkin et al. in 2016 [57]. Authors described the generation of an infectious cDNA clone for ZIKV Paraiba_01/2015, a virus isolated from serum of a febrile female subject in the Paraiba state in Brazil during the 2015 epidemic. To that end, four overlapping cDNA fragments spanning the entire ZIKV genome were individually cloned and assembled into the low-copy number plasmid pACNR1811 using conventional molecular cloning techniques. To restrict plasmid toxicity during the propagation of the cDNA in bacteria, they inserted two intron sequences in the NS1 and NS5 regions of the viral genome. Authors observed that the insertion of a single intron into the NS1 was sufficient for stable propagation of the infectious ZIKV cDNA clone but insertion of a second intron copy into the NS5 region was necessary to increase the plasmid yield in *E. coli*. The RNA polymerase II dependent CMV promoter and the HCVr sequences were engineered to flank the complete viral cDNA genome to ensure the successful rescue of the virus after plasmid transfection in Vero cells. Excision of the introns was carried out by the cellular machinery in the nucleus of transfected cells and, therefore, the resulting RNA was identical to the virus sequence and could initiate the replication/transcription steps in the cytoplasm (Table 2). The cDNA-derived rZIKV replicated efficiently in multiple cell lines, including those of placental and neuronal origin. Likewise, Schwarz et al. in 2016 also reported the construction of a plasmid carrying the complete genome of the prototype MR766 ZIKV African strain under the control of a CMV promoter [58]. In this case, the full-length cDNA clone was toxic during propagation in bacteria but incorporation of an intron in the NS1 region was sufficient to stabilize the cDNA clone.

2.2.2. Assembly of Full-Length Infectious ZIKV cDNA Clones Using Circular Polymerase Extension Cloning (CPEC)

As an alternative to bypass the inherent problem associated with the toxicity of ZIKV cDNA genomes during the propagation in bacteria, Setoh et al. in 2017 used a CPEC reaction approach [83] to construct a full-length infectious cDNA clone of the Brazilian ZIKV strain Rio Grande do Natal (RGN) [59]. The approach is based on the assembling of multiple cDNA fragments in the right order using a polymerase extension mechanism (Table 2). Briefly, eight overlapping cDNA fragments covering the entire viral genome flanked by the CMV promoter (5′ end) and HDVr and pA signal (3′ end), were mixed and subjected to a CPEC reaction using the Q5 high fidelity DNA polymerase. During the denaturalization step associated with the PCR reaction, the overlapping ends of contiguous cDNA anneal to each other and the PCR reaction generates a circular end product. The CPEC products were then used to directly transfect Vero cells without any additional manipulations, allowing the rescue of the rZIKV. The rZIKV-RGN was able to replicate in Vero, human A459 and mosquito C6/36 cells. Due to the absence of an RGN natural isolated, the author compared the replication of the rZIKV-RGN with the Asian strain ZIKV MR766, showing that rZIKV-RGN replicated less efficiently than ZIKV MR766. Moreover, ZIKV-RGN was detected in serum of infected IFNAR−/− A129 mice after 4-5 days, however the infection was asymptomatic with 100% of survival. In contrast, ZIKV-RGN infection of pregnant IFNAR−/− A129 dams showed severe fetal disorder.

2.2.3. Construction of Full-Length Infectious ZIKV cDNA Clones Using BACs

Another strategy used to engineer infectious full-length cDNA clones of positive-strand RNA viruses is the use of BACs [62,84–88]. Following this strategy, we have recently developed an infectious cDNA clone of ZIKV RGN strain [56]. To that end, the full-length cDNA copy of the ZIKV RGN genome was assembled in the BAC plasmid pBeloBac11 [89], a synthetic low-copy number plasmid based on the *E. coli* F-Factor [90]. This plasmid allows the stable maintenance of large DNA fragments and minimizes the toxicity associated with the propagation of full-length viral genomes in bacteria (Table 2). The full-length copy of the viral genome was cloned using four overlapping synthesized individual cDNA fragments and assembled into the pBeloBac11 using conventional cloning methods and unique restriction sites present in the viral genome. In this case, the viral genome was flanked at the 5′ end by the CMV promoter and at the 3′ end by the HDVr followed by the bovine growth hormone (BGH) termination and polyadenylation sequence to produce synthetic RNAs bearing authentic 3′-ends of the viral genome. The ZIKV-RGN clone was highly stable during passage in *E. coli* and infectious virus was recovered after direct transfection of susceptible Vero cells. Grown kinetics and plaque morphology showed than the recover rZIKV-RGN replicated efficiently in Vero and human A549 cells, with a homogeneous plaque morphology. Importantly, IFNAR−/− A129 mice succumbed to infection with the rZIKV-RGN in a dose-dependent manner. As the manipulation of BAC cDNA clones is relatively easy, we also used our system to construct a full-length infectious rZIKV clone containing an amino acid change (A175V) in the viral NS2A protein. Notably, this single and conserved amino acid change impaired viral RNA synthesis and viral production in cultured cells and attenuated the virus in vivo.

Likewise, Mutso et al. [48] in 2017 used a similar strategy to construct an infectious full-length cDNA clone based on the Brazilian ZIKV strain BeH81915. To that end, four DNA fragments spanning the entire viral genome were assembled into the BAC plasmid pCC1-BAC. In this case, the second intron of the human beta globin gen was introduced in the capsid region to increase the stability of the cDNA clone.

2.3. Infectious Subgenomic Amplicons (ISA) for the Generation of rZIKVs

ISA reverse genetics were development a few years ago by Aubry et al. [91]. In this approach, simple transfection of overlapping dsDNA fragments, covering the entire genome of an RNA virus flanked at the 5′ end by a CMV promoter and at the 3′ end by the HDVr sequence and pA signals, were sufficient to rescue multiple flaviviruses, including DENV, JEV or WNV [91,92]. This approach is based on spontaneous recombination between the overlapping cDNA fragments that allows the assembly and synthesis of a full-length cDNA copy of the complete viral genome in transfected cells. This approach could facilitate the rescue of recombinant RNA viruses from cDNA without requiring propagation in bacteria or in vitro RNA transcription. Following this strategy, Gadea et al. described in 2016 the rescue of rZIKV MR766 African [45] and BeH819015 Asian [61] strains. In addition, Atieh et al. in 2016 used the ISA technology for the generation of two reverse genetic systems based on the genome of ZIKV H/PF/2013 and Dakar 1984, representative members of Asian and African ZIKV lineages, respectively [60]. However, a potential concern with this method could be associated to a low efficiency of recombination of the cDNA fragments into transfected cells. Therefore, the amount of virus produced after the transfection using the ISA approach could be low, negatively impacting the successful rescue of recombinant viruses harboring, for instance, mutations that affect one or several steps in the replication cycle of the virus.

3. Rescue of rZIKVs Using Reverse Genetics Approaches

The generation of rZIKVs using reverse genetic approaches is currently well established and although is used by multiple laboratories worldwide, it is possible to find multiple variations between these approaches among different research groups. Moreover, the origin of the ZIKV strain used and the reverse genetic approach selected might require introducing modifications and/or optimization procedures for the successful rescue of rZIKVs.

To generate rZIKVs (Figure 3), susceptible cells (commonly mammalian Vero cells) are transiently transfected with the genetic material encoding the viral genome, as infectious RNA transcribed in vitro from a full-length cDNA clone (Figure 2A), full-length infectious cDNA clones (Figure 2B) or using infectious subgenomic amplicons (Figure 2C). Like the viral RNAs, the infectious RNA transcripts are directly expressed into the cytoplasm producing the viral proteins required for viral replication and transcription. However, both full-length infectious clones and subgenomic amplicons require a primary transcription in the nucleus by the cellular RNA polymerase II and the successive translocation of the vRNA into the cytoplasm. In general, after transfection of either cDNA clones or infectious RNAs, a clear cytopathic effect is observed at 3-4 days post-transfection with viral titers ranging between 1×10^4 and 1×10^7 plaque forming units (PFU) per mL in the tissue culture supernatants of transfected cells. However, both time and titers will depend on the viral strain and the reverse genetic approach used to generate the rZIKVs. Moreover, after transfection, one or multiple steps of viral amplification in mammalian (e.g., Vero) or mosquito (e.g., C6/36) cells could be required to obtain a working stock with higher viral titers (Figure 3). The successful rescue of rZIKVs using reverse genetic approaches can be evaluated by performing classical plaque (PFU/mL) or immunofluorescence (immunofluorescent forming units, FFU/mL) assays.

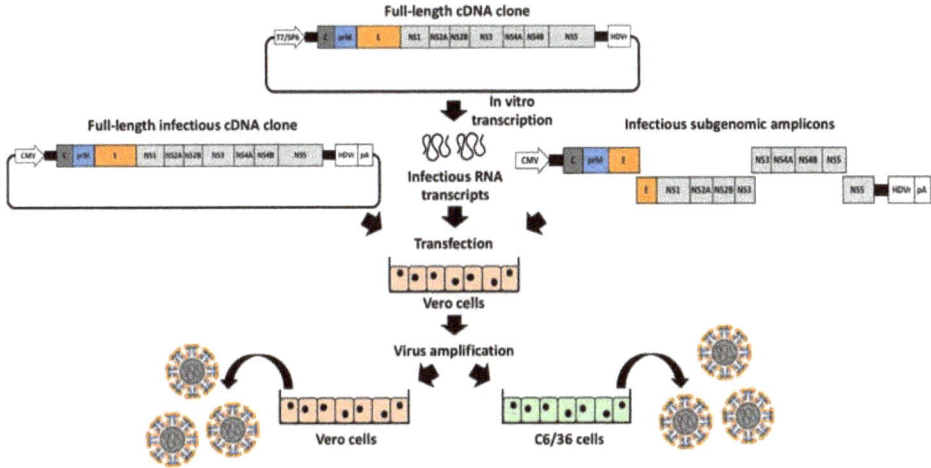

Figure 3. Schematic representation for the generation of rZIKV: Mammalian Vero cells are transiently transfected with infectious RNA transcribed in vitro from a full-length cDNA clone (top), full-length infectious cDNA clones (**left**) or infectious subgenomic amplicons (**right**) (see also Figure 2). After 3–4 days post-transfection, when cytopathic effect is observed, rZIKVs present in tissue-culture supernatants can be recover for titration or viral amplification in mammalian (Vero, **left**) or insect (C6/36, **right**) cells.

4. Applications of ZIKV Reverse Genetic Approaches

4.1. ZIKV Replicons

Subgenomic replicons systems are powerful tools to study viral replication in the absence of virus entry or virion assembly, since they contain all the elements needed to produce effective viral replication in susceptible host cells but lack one or multiple viral structural genes [36,72,93–95]. Due to the lack of viral structural genes, these replicon systems are non-infectious, allowing the study of viral replication without biosafety concerns associated with the work of infectious viruses [85,96]. Thus, replicons represent a safe tool to study, among others, viral replication, transcription or the subcellular localization of the viral replication complexes. Moreover, replicons systems have been used for the identification of compounds with antiviral activity or host factors involved in viral replication using high-throughput screening settings [97–100].

The first ZIKV replicon was described by Xie et al. in 2016 [101] (Figure 4A). The replicon was constructed using the infectious cDNA clone of ZIKV FSS13025 strain by replacing the viral structural genes with the Renilla luciferase (Rluc) reporter gene, followed by the foot-and-mouse disease virus (FMDV) 2A protease sequence to allow the cleavage of Rluc from the viral polyprotein. Importantly, the Rluc-2A cassette was flanked by the first 38 amino acids of the viral C protein (C_{38}) that contain the flavivirus-conserved cyclization sequence required for viral RNA replication [102,103] and the last 30 amino acids of E protein (E_{30}) fused in-frame with the downstream NS1 protein (Figure 4A). The E_{30} region was maintained to ensure proper translocation of the NS1 protein into the lumen of the ER [103]. To evaluate viral replication, in vitro RNA transcripts synthesized by the T7 RNA polymerase were electroporated into Huh-7 cells and Rluc signal was evaluated. As a proof of concept and to demonstrate the susceptibility of this replicon approach to identify compounds with anti-ZIKV activity, the authors showed that Rluc signal was suppressed using the broad antiviral NITD-008 in a dose-dependent manner [104]. Moreover and to obtain a Huh-7 stable cell line expressing the viral replicon, they engineered a second ZIKV replicon containing Rluc and the Neomycin (Neo) resistance gene (Figure 4B). The Neo gene driven by an encephalomyocarditis virus internal ribosomal entry site (IRES) was introduced downstream of the first 28 nucleotides of 3′ UTR. Importantly, authors demonstrated that the generated Neo resistant stable cell line maintains the ZIKV replicon for several passages and expressed high levels of Rluc.

An alternative strategy was performed by Li et al. in 2017 [105] (Figure 4C). Authors generated a bicistronic ZIKV replicon of SZ-WIV001 strain [81], in which the selection gene puromycin *N*-acetyl-transferase (PAC) and the reporter Rluc were separated by a FMDV 2A protease sequence (Figure 4C). In this case, the PAC-2A-Rluc construct was followed by a second 2A protease sequence and the cassette was introduced, in frame, between the C_{38} and the E_{30} sequences (C_{38}-PAC-2A-Rluc-2A-E_{30}) (Figure 4C). Murine BHK-21 stable cell lines constitutively expressing the viral replicon were produced after transfection of the ZIKV RNA replicon produced in vitro (T7) and selection with puromycin. In addition, the replicon was stably maintained in BHK-21 cells during multiple passages. Importantly, authors were able to adapt this technology to evaluate ZIKV inhibitors using a high throughput screening assay.

Recently, in 2018, Münters et al. described the construction of a set of Rluc ZIKV replicons using the full-length cDNA clones of ZIKV Asian H/PF/2013 or African MR766 strains, which contained silent mutation to disrupt the CEPs [50]. The viral structural proteins were replaced by the Rluc-2A cassette flanked by the first 34 amino acids of ZIKV C protein (C_{34}) and the last 24 amino acids of the E protein (E_{24}). Authors found that Rluc signal correlated with the amount of viral NS proteins. Moreover, the replicon induced morphological changes resembling ZIKV infection, highlighting the potential of this approach to study some steps of ZIKV infection.

Lastly, a ZIKV replicon expressing the Gaussian luciferase (Gluc) reporter gene was designed by Mutso et al. in 2017 using the full-length cDNA clone of the Brazilian ZIKV strain BeH819015 (Figure 4D) [48]. In this case, the Gluc reporter gene was inserted followed by the FMVD 2A protease sequence between the C protein and the last 30 amino acids of the E protein (E_{30}) fused in-frame with the NS1 protein. The activity of the replicon was demonstrated in mammalian (BHK-21 and Vero) and mosquito (C6/36) cells.

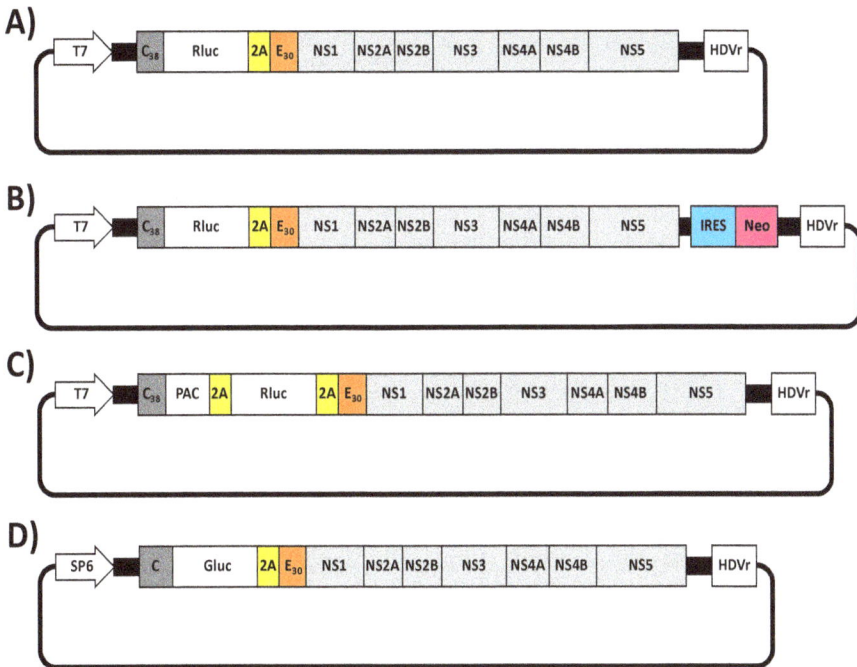

Figure 4. ZIKV replicons. (A,B) Schematic diagram of Rluc-expressing ZIKV replicons: ZIKV replicons expressing Rluc constructed by Xie et al. [101] are shown. In these replicons, ZIKV structural proteins were replaced by the Rluc reporter gene followed by the FMDV 2A protease sequence (2A, yellow). This cassette was flanking by the N-terminal 38 amino acids of C protein (C_{38}, dark gray) and the last 30 amino acids of E protein (E_{30}, orange) fused in-frame with the viral downstream NS proteins (A). A stable reporter ZIKV Rluc-expressing replicon was constructed inserting the encephalomyocarditis virus internal ribosomal site (IRES, blue) followed by a neomycin resistance gene (Neo, pink) into the first 28 nucleotides of 3′ UTR (B). (C) Schematic representation of a PAC- and Rluc-expressing ZIKV replicon: The ZIKV replicon expressing a PAC and a Rluc genes separated by the FMDV 2A protease sequence is shown [105]. Both foreign viral genes, PAC and Rluc, followed by the FMDV 2A protease sequence were introduced between of the first N-terminal 38 amino acids of C protein (C_{38}, dark gray) and the last 30 amino acids of E protein (E_{30}, orange) in-frame with the viral NS1 protein. (D) Schematic diagram of a Gluc-expressing ZIKV replicon: The ZIKV replicon expressing the Gluc reporter gene constructed by Mutso et al. is indicated [48]. The Gluc reporter gene followed by the FMDV 2A protease sequence was introduced downstream of the C protein (dark gray) and the last N-terminal 30 amino acids of E protein (E_{30}, orange) fused in-frame with the NS1 ZIKV protein. T7 and SP6: prokaryotic T7 or SP6 promoters. HDVr: Hepatitis delta virus ribozyme sequence.

4.2. Replicating Competent, Reporter Gene-Expressing rZIKVs

The development of reverse genetic approaches has provided investigators with the possibility of generating replication-competent viruses expressing fluorescent or luminescent reporter genes [106]. The stable incorporation of foreign reporter genes in viruses have allowed the effective tracking of viral infection in vitro and in vivo without the need of laborious secondary approaches to identify the presence of the virus [43,44,106]. Moreover, recombinant reporter-expressing viruses have the advantage that they can be used in high throughput screenings assays for multiple applications, including the identification of compounds with antiviral activity [107,108], host factor involved in viral infection [109,110] and the presence of neutralizing antibodies [111–114], among others. To date, several rZIKVs expressing reporter genes have been described [45,46,48,50]. In all cases, independently of the reverse genetic approach used to generate the reporter gene expressing rZIKV, a similar strategy was used, consisting in the introduction of the reporter genes followed by the FMDV 2A protease sequence upstream of the viral open reading frame. In addition, a copy of the C protein or part of the its N-terminal region that contains the flavivirus-conserved cyclization sequence [102,103] was introduced upstream of the reporter gene to allow successful viral replication (Figure 5).

Shan et al. in 2016 engineered a full-length cDNA ZIKV FSS13025 infectious clone expressing Rluc (rZIKV-Rluc) (Figure 5A) [46]. In this system, Rluc was introduced downstream of the first 25 amino acid of the C protein (C_{25}) followed by the FMDV 2A protease sequence and in frame with the ZIKV downstream proteins (Figure 5A). Importantly, silent mutations were introduced into the original C protein in the flavivirus-cyclization sequence (amino acids 14–17) to reduce the potential recombination between the parental and the duplicated C protein regions (Figure 5A). The rZIKV-Rluc was successful rescued after transient transfection in Vero cells of the full-length in vitro transcribed (T7) ZIKV RNA. However, the rZIKV-Rluc had a reduced plaque size phenotype compared with the parental rZIKV, indicating that insertion of Rluc was deleterious for the virus.

Münters et al. in 2018, described the construction of two Rluc-expressing rZIKVs using the full-length cDNA clones of ZIKV MR766 and H/PF/2013 [50]. In this case, the Rluc-2A cassette was introduced downstream of the first 34 amino acids of the C protein (C_{34}) and in frame with the ZIKV downstream proteins (Figure 5B). In this case, the duplicated region of the C protein was not altered. Expression of Rluc was confirmed for both rescued viruses. However, as in the previous case, rZIKV-Rluc (MR766 or H/PF/2013) replicated at lower extend as compare to non Rluc-expressing rZIKV MR766 or H/PF/2013, further suggesting that insertion of Rluc affected viral fitness. Notably, the reporter gene was unstable and lost after 3 passages. In this case, the rapid loss of the Rluc could be due to recombination events between the partial duplication of the capsid regions. To have a system suitable for microscopy, Münters et al. replaced the Rluc reporter gene by the coding sequence of turbo far-red fluorescent protein FP635, a mutant version of the red fluorescent protein from the sea anemone *Entacmaea quadricolor* [115]. In this case, a SV40 nuclear localization sequence was introduced in frame with the FP635 protein for nuclear export of the fluorescent protein and to avoid interference with viral replication events in the cytoplasm of infected cells. Although, authors did not evaluate the replication properties of these viruses, they demonstrated that FP635-expressing rZIKVs were suitable for live cell imaging.

Using the ISA method, Gadea et al. described in 2016 the generation of a rZIKV MR766 expressing the green fluorescent protein (GFP) reporter gene (rZIKV-GFP) [45] (Figure 5C). GFP was introduced downstream of the first 33 amino acids of C protein (C_{33}) followed by the FMDV 2A protease sequence in-frame with the viral ORF (Figure 5C) [45]. The rZIKV-GFP was successfully rescued after electroporation of several fragments covering the complete genome under the control of the CMV promoter. However, rZIKV-GFP titers were ~1.5 log lower compared with the rZIKV without GFP. Likewise, the plaque phenotype of the rZIKV-GFP was smaller than rZIKV without GFP, indicating that insertion of GFP resulted in viral attenuation. Moreover, rZIKV-GFP was unstable and the virus lost GFP expression after a limited number of passages on Vero cells.

More recently, Mutso et al. described the construction of several reporter-expressing rZIKVs using a BAC system and a SP6 promoter (Figure 5D) [48]. They inserted the sequences of the foreign reporter genes fused to the FMDV 2A protease sequence between two copies of C protein, altering the codon usage of the downstream copy to reduce potential recombination events (Figure 5D). Using this strategy, they generated rZIKVs expressing Firefly luciferase (FlLuc), red shift luciferase from *Luciola italica* (RSLuc) [116], NanoLuc, mCherry or GFP (Figure 5D). Moreover, they inserted a ubiquitin sequence between the FMDV 2A protease sequence and the viral polyprotein in order to help the proteolytic cleavage. However, inclusion of the ubiquitin sequence after the 2A protease sequence was irrelevant for viral rescue and stability. Although the replication of these reporter-expressing rZIKVs were not directly compared with either a rZIKV or a natural isolated, as previously described for the other reporter-expressing rZIKVs, limited stability of the rZIKVs expressing reporter genes was observed, except for NanoLuc which remained stable during four serial passages in cultured cells. These and previous results highlight the important concerns related to the instability of reporter-expressing rZIKVs. Further investigation, including new approaches for the expression of reporter genes in the viral genome are necessary to generate stable rZIKV expressing reporter genes for their use as valid viral surrogates to study ZIKV infection in cultured cells or in validated animal models of infection.

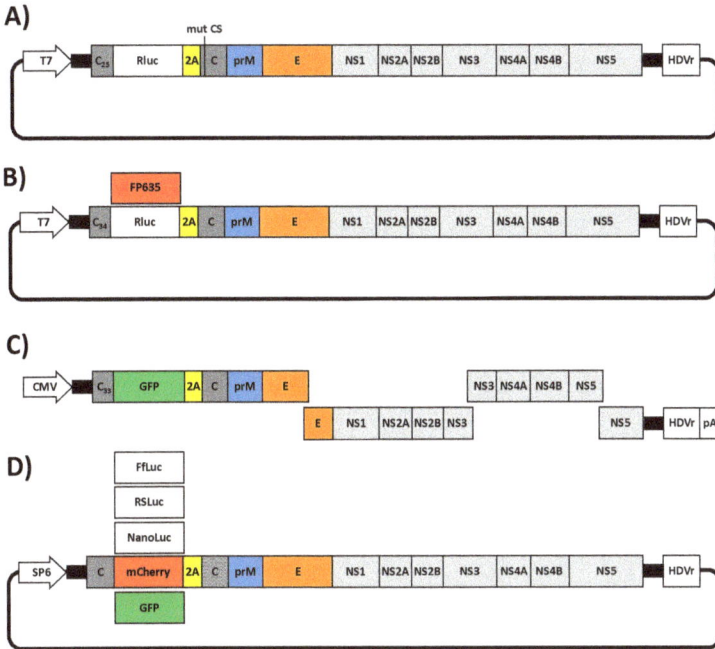

Figure 5. Reporter gene-expressing rZIKVs. (**A**) Schematic diagram of a Rluc-expressing ZIKV cDNA clone: A full-length cDNA clone expressing the Rluc reporter gene (white box) was constructed by Shan et al. [46]. Rluc was introduced downstream of the first 25 amino acids of the C protein (C_{25}, dark gray) followed by the FMDV 2A protease sequence (yellow box) fused in-frame with the viral ORF. Silent mutations changing the flavivirus-cyclization sequence were introduced in the full-length C protein (mut CS). (**B**) Schematic representation of a full-length ZIKV cDNA expressing Rluc or FP635: Full-length cDNA clones expressing Rluc (white box) or FP635 (red box) were generated by Münters et al. [50]. Reporter genes were introduced downstream the first 34 amino acid of the C protein (C_{34}, dark gray) followed by the FMDV 2A protease sequence in-frame with the viral downstream proteins. (**C**) Schematic diagram of a GFP-expressing ZIKV generated by ISA: A ZIKV cDNA clone expressing GFP was constructed by Gadea et al. [45] using the ISA approach. The GFP was introduced downstream of the first 33 amino acid of the C protein (C_{33}, dark gray) followed by the FMDV 2A protease sequence in-frame with the viral ORF. (**D**) Representation of full-length ZIKV cDNAs expressing luciferase and fluorescent proteins: Full-length ZIKV cDNA clones expressing NanoLuc, FfLuc, RSLuc (white boxes), GFP (green box) or mCherry (red box) were constructed by Mutso et al. [48]. Reporter genes were individually introduced downstream of the complete C protein followed by the FMDV 2A protease sequence fused in-frame with the downstream viral ORF. The codon sequence of the downstream copy of the viral C protein was altered to reduce potential recombination (dotted gray). T7 and SP6: prokaryotic T7 or SP6 promoters. CMV: cytomegalovirus promoter. HDVr: Hepatitis delta virus ribozyme sequence. pA: simian virus 40 late polyadenylation signal.

5. Conclusions

The development of ZIKV reverse genetic systems has provided researchers with powerful methods to study multiple aspects of the biology and pathogenesis of ZIKV in vitro and in vivo. For instance, the ability to manipulate the genome of ZIKV to generate recombinant viruses with specific mutations have allowed investigators to gain a detailed understanding of the ZIKV-host interactions and associated disease [49,56,57]. Moreover, reverse genetic approaches have been essential to develop novel and more effective strategies to prevent and control ZIKV infections [117–119]. Likewise, generation of ZIKV replicons or replicating-competent rZIKV expressing reporter genes represent and excellent approach for the identification of compounds with anti-viral activity for the treatment of ZIKV infection [45,46,101,105]. In this review, we have discussed the three major strategies that have been reporter for the generation of rZIKVs: i) generation of infectious RNA transcripts from a full-length cDNA copy; ii) full-length infectious genomic cDNA clones; and, iii) Infectious Subgenomic Amplicons (ISA) (Figure 2 and Table 1). Like other flavivirus, ZIKV cDNA sequences in bacterial has been hindered by the presence of cryptic bacterial promoter in the viral genome. To overcome the problems associated with the instability of ZIKV cDNA clones, several approaches based on the use of low-copy number plasmids, BACs, intron-insertion, in vitro ligation of cDNA fragments and in vitro assembly by Gibson method or by CPEC have been used. Although all those approaches have their advantages and disadvantages (Table 2), they have been not compared side by side. Therefore, it cannot be possible to determine which systems are better for the genetic stability and successful generation of rZIKV. Moreover, successful rescue of rZIKVs could strongly dependent of several biological factors such as the viral strain selected and technical factors such as transfection methods. Finally, the generation of rZIKVs expressing reporter genes, together with the development of ZIKV replicons, constitute important tools for the identification of antiviral drugs against this important human pathogen that are compatible with the use of high throughput screenings settings. However, to date, there are some concerns regarding the stability of currently available reporter-expressing rZIKVs, which will require and guarantee further investigation.

Funding: ZIKV research in LMS and FAT laboratories is partially funded by the Spanish Ministry of Economy and Competitiveness (MINECO) (grant number BFU2016-79127-R) and the National Institute of Allergy and Infectious Diseases (NIAID), National Institutes of Health (NIH) (grant number R21 AI130500).

Acknowledgments: We want to thank all the work conducted by ZIKV researchers that has contributed to the establishment and implementation of reverse genetics approaches for the generation of rZIKVs. We want to apologize if we inadvertently omitted any manuscript(s) describing the generation of recombinant ZIKV using reverse genetic techniques.

Conflicts of Interest: The authors declare no conflict of interest.

References

1. Gulland, A. Who warns of risk of zika virus in europe. *BMJ* **2016**, *353*, i2887. [CrossRef] [PubMed]
2. Valderrama, A.; Díaz, Y.; López-Vergès, S. Interaction of flavivirus with their mosquito vectors and their impact on the human health in the americas. *Biochem. Biophys. Res. Commun.* **2017**, *492*, 541–547. [CrossRef] [PubMed]
3. Huang, Y.-J.S.; Higgs, S.; Horne, K.M.; Vanlandingham, D.L. Flavivirus-mosquito interactions. *Viruses* **2014**, *6*, 4703–4730. [CrossRef] [PubMed]
4. Dick, G.W.; Kitchen, S.F.; Haddow, A.J. Zika virus. I. Isolations and serological specificity. *Trans. R. Soc. Trop. Med. Hyg.* **1952**, *46*, 509–520. [CrossRef]
5. Moulin, E.; Selby, K.; Cherpillod, P.; Kaiser, L.; Boillat-Blanco, N. Simultaneous outbreaks of dengue, chikungunya and zika virus infections: Diagnosis challenge in a returning traveller with nonspecific febrile illness. *New Microbe. New Infect.* **2016**, *11*, 6–7. [CrossRef] [PubMed]
6. Samarasekera, U.; Triunfol, M. Concern over zika virus grips the world. *Lancet* **2016**, *387*, 521–524. [CrossRef]
7. Ioos, S.; Mallet, H.P.; Leparc Goffart, I.; Gauthier, V.; Cardoso, T.; Herida, M. Current zika virus epidemiology and recent epidemics. *Med. Mal. Infect.* **2014**, *44*, 302–307. [CrossRef] [PubMed]

8. Chang, C.; Ortiz, K.; Ansari, A.; Gershwin, M.E. The zika outbreak of the 21st century. *J. Autoimmun.* **2016**, *68*, 1–13. [CrossRef] [PubMed]

9. Eppes, C.; Rac, M.; Dunn, J.; Versalovic, J.; Murray, K.O.; Suter, M.A.; Sanz Cortes, M.; Espinoza, J.; Seferovic, M.D.; Lee, W.; et al. Testing for zika virus infection in pregnancy: Key concepts to deal with an emerging epidemic. *Am. J. Obstet. Gynecol.* **2017**, *216*, 209–225. [CrossRef] [PubMed]

10. Duffy, M.R.; Chen, T.H.; Hancock, W.T.; Powers, A.M.; Kool, J.L.; Lanciotti, R.S.; Pretrick, M.; Marfel, M.; Holzbauer, S.; Dubray, C.; et al. Zika virus outbreak on Yap Island, federated states of Micronesia. *N. Engl. J. Med.* **2009**, *360*, 2536–2543. [CrossRef] [PubMed]

11. Oehler, E.; Watrin, L.; Larre, P.; Leparc-Goffart, I.; Lastere, S.; Valour, F.; Baudouin, L.; Mallet, H.; Musso, D.; Ghawche, F. Zika virus infection complicated by guillain-barre syndrome—Case report, French Polynesia, December 2013. *Euro Surveill.* **2014**, *19*, 20720. [CrossRef] [PubMed]

12. Besnard, M.; Lastere, S.; Teissier, A.; Cao-Lormeau, V.; Musso, D. Evidence of perinatal transmission of zika virus, french polynesia, december 2013 and february 2014. *Euro Surveill* **2014**, *19*, 20751. [CrossRef] [PubMed]

13. Oliveira Melo, A.S.; Malinger, G.; Ximenes, R.; Szejnfeld, P.O.; Alves Sampaio, S.; Bispo de Filippis, A.M. Zika virus intrauterine infection causes fetal brain abnormality and microcephaly: Tip of the iceberg? *Ultrasound Obstet. Gynecol.* **2016**, *47*, 6–7. [CrossRef] [PubMed]

14. Campos, G.S.; Bandeira, A.C.; Sardi, S.I. Zika virus outbreak, Bahia, Brazil. *Emerg. Infect. Dis.* **2015**, *21*, 1885–1886. [CrossRef] [PubMed]

15. Mlakar, J.; Korva, M.; Tul, N.; Popovic, M.; Poljsak-Prijatelj, M.; Mraz, J.; Kolenc, M.; Resman Rus, K.; Vesnaver Vipotnik, T.; Fabjan Vodusek, V.; et al. Zika virus associated with microcephaly. *N. Engl. J. Med.* **2016**, *374*, 951–958. [CrossRef] [PubMed]

16. Costello, A.; Dua, T.; Duran, P.; Gulmezoglu, M.; Oladapo, O.T.; Perea, W.; Pires, J.; Ramon-Pardo, P.; Rollins, N.; Saxena, S. Defining the syndrome associated with congenital zika virus infection. *Bull. World Health Organ.* **2016**, *94*, 406–406A. [CrossRef] [PubMed]

17. Krauer, F.; Riesen, M.; Reveiz, L.; Oladapo, O.T.; Martinez-Vega, R.; Porgo, T.V.; Haefliger, A.; Broutet, N.J.; Low, N. Zika virus infection as a cause of congenital brain abnormalities and guillain-barre syndrome: Systematic review. *PLoS Med.* **2017**, *14*, e1002203. [CrossRef] [PubMed]

18. Miner, J.J.; Cao, B.; Govero, J.; Smith, A.M.; Fernandez, E.; Cabrera, O.H.; Garber, C.; Noll, M.; Klein, R.S.; Noguchi, K.K.; et al. Zika virus infection during pregnancy in mice causes placental damage and fetal demise. *Cell* **2016**, *165*, 1081–1091. [CrossRef] [PubMed]

19. Tham, H.W.; Balasubramaniam, V.; Ooi, M.K.; Chew, M.F. Viral determinants and vector competence of zika virus transmission. *Front. Microbiol.* **2018**, *9*, 1040. [CrossRef] [PubMed]

20. Calvet, G.; Aguiar, R.S.; Melo, A.S.O.; Sampaio, S.A.; de Filippis, I.; Fabri, A.; Araujo, E.S.M.; de Sequeira, P.C.; de Mendonca, M.C.L.; de Oliveira, L.; et al. Detection and sequencing of zika virus from amniotic fluid of fetuses with microcephaly in Brazil: A case study. *Lancet Infect. Dis.* **2016**, *16*, 653–660. [CrossRef]

21. Baud, D.; Gubler, D.J.; Schaub, B.; Lanteri, M.C.; Musso, D. An update on zika virus infection. *Lancet* **2017**, *390*, 2099–2109. [CrossRef]

22. Colt, S.; Garcia-Casal, M.N.; Pena-Rosas, J.P.; Finkelstein, J.L.; Rayco-Solon, P.; Weise Prinzo, Z.C.; Mehta, S. Transmission of zika virus through breast milk and other breastfeeding-related bodily-fluids: A systematic review. *PLoS Negl. Trop. Dis.* **2017**, *11*, e0005528. [CrossRef] [PubMed]

23. Rodriguez-Morales, A.J.; Bandeira, A.C.; Franco-Paredes, C. The expanding spectrum of modes of transmission of zika virus: A global concern. *Ann. Clin. Microbiol. Antimicrob.* **2016**, *15*, 13. [CrossRef] [PubMed]

24. Sirohi, D.; Chen, Z.; Sun, L.; Klose, T.; Pierson, T.C.; Rossmann, M.G.; Kuhn, R.J. The 3.8 Å resolution cryo-EM structure of zika virus. *Science* **2016**, *352*, 467–470. [CrossRef] [PubMed]

25. Lindebach, B.D.; Thiel, H.J.; Rice, C.M. *Fields Virology*, 5th ed.; Knipe, D.M., Howley, P.M., Eds.; Wolters Kluwer Health/Lippincott Williams & Wilkins: Philadelphia, PA, USA, 2007; pp. 1101–1151.

26. Faye, O.; Freire, C.C.; Iamarino, A.; Faye, O.; de Oliveira, J.V.; Diallo, M.; Zanotto, P.M.; Sall, A.A. Molecular evolution of zika virus during its emergence in the 20th century. *PLoS Negl. Trop. Dis.* **2014**, *8*, e2636. [CrossRef] [PubMed]

27. Haddow, A.D.; Schuh, A.J.; Yasuda, C.Y.; Kasper, M.R.; Heang, V.; Huy, R.; Guzman, H.; Tesh, R.B.; Weaver, S.C. Genetic characterization of zika virus strains: Geographic expansion of the asian lineage. *PLoS Negl. Trop. Dis.* **2012**, *6*, e1477. [CrossRef] [PubMed]

28. Rey, F.A.; Stiasny, K.; Heinz, F.X. Flavivirus structural heterogeneity: Implications for cell entry. *Curr. Opin. Virol.* **2017**, *24*, 132–139. [CrossRef] [PubMed]

29. Cortese, M.; Goellner, S.; Acosta, E.G.; Neufeldt, C.J.; Oleksiuk, O.; Lampe, M.; Haselmann, U.; Funaya, C.; Schieber, N.; Ronchi, P.; et al. Ultrastructural characterization of zika virus replication factories. *Cell Rep.* **2017**, *18*, 2113–2123. [CrossRef] [PubMed]

30. Romero-Brey, I.; Bartenschlager, R. Membranous replication factories induced by plus-strand RNA viruses. *Viruses* **2014**, *6*, 2826–2857. [CrossRef] [PubMed]

31. Nogales, A.; Marquez-Jurado, S.; Galan, C.; Enjuanes, L.; Almazan, F. Transmissible gastroenteritis coronavirus RNA-dependent RNA polymerase and nonstructural proteins 2, 3, and 8 are incorporated into viral particles. *J. Virol.* **2012**, *86*, 1261–1266. [CrossRef] [PubMed]

32. Yu, I.-M.; Zhang, W.; Holdaway, H.A.; Li, L.; Kostyuchenko, V.A.; Chipman, P.R.; Kuhn, R.J.; Rossmann, M.G.; Chen, J. Structure of the immature dengue virus at low pH primes proteolytic maturation. *Science* **2008**, *319*, 1834–1837. [CrossRef] [PubMed]

33. Li, L.; Lok, S.-M.; Yu, I.-M.; Zhang, Y.; Kuhn, R.J.; Chen, J.; Rossmann, M.G. The flavivirus precursor membrane-envelope protein complex: Structure and maturation. *Science* **2008**, *319*, 1830–1834. [CrossRef] [PubMed]

34. Prasad, V.M.; Miller, A.S.; Klose, T.; Sirohi, D.; Buda, G.; Jiang, W.; Kuhn, R.J.; Rossmann, M.G. Structure of the immature zika virus at 9 Å resolution. *Nat. Struct. Mol. Biol.* **2017**, *24*, 184. [CrossRef] [PubMed]

35. Stobart, C.C.; Moore, M.L. RNA virus reverse genetics and vaccine design. *Viruses* **2014**, *6*, 2531–2550. [CrossRef] [PubMed]

36. Nogales, A.; Martinez-Sobrido, L. Reverse genetics approaches for the development of influenza vaccines. *Int. J. Mol. Sci.* **2016**, *18*, 20. [CrossRef] [PubMed]

37. Martinez-Sobrido, L.; de la Torre, J.C. Reporter-expressing, replicating-competent recombinant arenaviruses. *Viruses* **2016**, *8*, 197. [CrossRef] [PubMed]

38. Breen, M.; Nogales, A.; Baker, S.F.; Martinez-Sobrido, L. Replication-competent influenza A viruses expressing reporter genes. *Viruses* **2016**, *8*, 179. [CrossRef] [PubMed]

39. Racaniello, V.; Baltimore, D. Cloned poliovirus complementary DNA is infectious in mammalian cells. *Science* **1981**, *214*, 916–919. [CrossRef] [PubMed]

40. Almazan, F.; Sola, I.; Zuniga, S.; Marquez-Jurado, S.; Morales, L.; Becares, M.; Enjuanes, L. Coronavirus reverse genetic systems: Infectious clones and replicons. *Virus Res.* **2014**, *189*, 262–270. [CrossRef] [PubMed]

41. Rieder, E.; Bunch, T.; Brown, F.; Mason, P.W. Genetically engineered foot-and-mouth disease viruses with poly(C) tracts of two nucleotides are virulent in mice. *J. Virol.* **1993**, *67*, 5139–5145. [PubMed]

42. Aubry, F.; Nougairède, A.; Gould, E.A.; de Lamballerie, X. Flavivirus reverse genetic systems, construction techniques and applications: A historical perspective. *Antiviral Res.* **2015**, *114*, 67–85. [CrossRef] [PubMed]

43. Martínez-Sobrido, L.; Paessler, S.; de la Torre, J.C. Lassa virus reverse genetics. In *Reverse Genetics of RNA Viruses: Methods and Protocols*; Perez, D.R., Ed.; Springer New York: New York, NY, USA, 2017; pp. 185–204.

44. Martínez-Sobrido, L.; Cheng, B.Y.H.; de la Torre, J.C. Reverse genetics approaches to control arenavirus. *Methods Mol. Biol.* **2016**, *1403*, 313–351. [PubMed]

45. Usme-Ciro, J.A.; Lopera, J.A.; Enjuanes, L.; Almazan, F.; Gallego-Gomez, J.C. Development of a novel DNA-launched dengue virus type 2 infectious clone assembled in a bacterial artificial chromosome. *Virus Res.* **2014**, *180*, 12–22. [CrossRef] [PubMed]

46. Blaney, J.E.; Hanson, C.T.; Firestone, C.-Y.; Hanley, K.A.; Murphy, B.R.; Whitehead, S.S. Genetically modified, live attenuated dengue virus type 3 vaccine candidates. *Am. J. Trop. Med. Hyg.* **2004**, *71*, 811–821. [CrossRef] [PubMed]

47. Bredenbeek, P.J.; Kooi, E.A.; Lindenbach, B.; Huijkman, N.; Rice, C.M.; Spaan, W.J.M. A stable full-length yellow fever virus cDNA clone and the role of conserved RNA elements in flavivirus replication. *J. Gen. Virol.* **2003**, *84*, 1261–1268. [CrossRef] [PubMed]

48. Liu, Z.Y.; Yu, J.Y.; Huang, X.Y.; Fan, H.; Li, X.F.; Deng, Y.Q.; Ji, X.; Cheng, M.L.; Ye, Q.; Zhao, H.; et al. Characterization of cis-acting RNA elements of zika virus by using a self-splicing ribozyme-dependent infectious clone. *J. Virol.* **2017**, *91*. [CrossRef] [PubMed]

49. Shan, C.; Xie, X.; Muruato, A.E.; Rossi, S.L.; Roundy, C.M.; Azar, S.R.; Yang, Y.; Tesh, R.B.; Bourne, N.; Barrett, A.D.; et al. An infectious cDNA clone of zika virus to study viral virulence, mosquito transmission, and antiviral inhibitors. *Cell Host Microbe* **2016**, *19*, 891–900. [CrossRef] [PubMed]

50. Shan, C.; Xie, X.; Shi, P.-Y. Reverse genetics of zika virus. In *Reverse Genetics of RNA Viruses: Methods and Protocols*; Perez, D.R., Ed.; Springer New York: New York, NY, USA, 2017; pp. 47–58.

51. Mutso, M.; Saul, S.; Rausalu, K.; Susova, O.; Zusinaite, E.; Mahalingam, S.; Merits, A. Reverse genetic system, genetically stable reporter viruses and packaged subgenomic replicon based on a brazilian zika virus isolate. *J. Gen. Virol.* **2017**, *98*, 2712–2724. [CrossRef] [PubMed]

52. Annamalai, A.S.; Pattnaik, A.; Sahoo, B.R.; Muthukrishnan, E.; Natarajan, S.K.; Steffen, D.; Vu, H.L.X.; Delhon, G.; Osorio, F.A.; Petro, T.M.; et al. Zika virus encoding non-glycosylated envelope protein is attenuated and defective in neuroinvasion. *J. Virol.* **2017**, *91*. [CrossRef] [PubMed]

53. Munster, M.; Plaszczyca, A.; Cortese, M.; Neufeldt, C.J.; Goellner, S.; Long, G.; Bartenschlager, R. A reverse genetics system for zika virus based on a simple molecular cloning strategy. *Viruses* **2018**, *10*, 368. [CrossRef] [PubMed]

54. Zhao, F.; Xu, Y.; Lavillette, D.; Zhong, J.; Zou, G.; Long, G. Negligible contribution of M2634V substitution to ZIKV pathogenesis in AG6 mice revealed by a bacterial promoter activity reduced infectious clone. *Sci. Rep.* **2018**, *8*, 10491. [CrossRef] [PubMed]

55. Widman, D.G.; Young, E.; Yount, B.L.; Plante, K.S.; Gallichotte, E.N.; Carbaugh, D.L.; Peck, K.M.; Plante, J.; Swanstrom, J.; Heise, M.T.; et al. A reverse genetics platform that spans the zika virus family tree. *mBio* **2017**, *8*. [CrossRef] [PubMed]

56. Gorman, M.J.; Caine, E.A.; Zaitsev, K.; Begley, M.C.; Weger-Lucarelli, J.; Uccellini, M.B.; Tripathi, S.; Morrison, J.; Yount, B.L.; Dinnon, K.H., 3rd; et al. An immunocompetent mouse model of zika virus infection. *Cell Host Microbe* **2018**, *23*, 672–685. [CrossRef] [PubMed]

57. Weger-Lucarelli, J.; Duggal, N.K.; Bullard-Feibelman, K.; Veselinovic, M.; Romo, H.; Nguyen, C.; Ruckert, C.; Brault, A.C.; Bowen, R.A.; Stenglein, M.; et al. Development and characterization of recombinant virus generated from a new world zika virus infectious clone. *J. Virol.* **2017**, *91*, e01765-16. [CrossRef] [PubMed]

58. Weger-Lucarelli, J.; Duggal, N.K.; Brault, A.C.; Geiss, B.J.; Ebel, G.D. Rescue and characterization of recombinant virus from a new world Zika virus infectious clone. *J. Vis. Exp.* **2017**, *124*, e55857. [CrossRef] [PubMed]

59. Márquez-Jurado, S.; Nogales, A.; Ávila-Pérez, G.; Iborra, F.; Martínez-Sobrido, L.; Almazán, F. An alanine-to-valine substitution in the residue 175 of zika virus NS2A protein affects viral RNA synthesis and attenuates the virus in vivo. *Viruses* **2018**, *10*, 547. [CrossRef] [PubMed]

60. Tsetsarkin, K.A.; Kenney, H.; Chen, R.; Liu, G.; Manukyan, H.; Whitehead, S.S.; Laassri, M.; Chumakov, K.; Pletnev, A.G. A full-length infectious cDNA clone of Zika virus from the 2015 epidemic in Brazil as a genetic platform for studies of virus-host interactions and vaccine development. *mBio* **2016**, *7*. [CrossRef] [PubMed]

61. Schwarz, M.C.; Sourisseau, M.; Espino, M.M.; Gray, E.S.; Chambers, M.T.; Tortorella, D.; Evans, M.J. Rescue of the 1947 Zika virus prototype strain with a cytomegalovirus promoter-driven cDNA clone. *mSphere* **2016**, *1*. [CrossRef] [PubMed]

62. Setoh, Y.X.; Prow, N.A.; Peng, N.; Hugo, L.E.; Devine, G.; Hazlewood, J.E.; Suhrbier, A.; Khromykh, A.A. De novo generation and characterization of new zika virus isolate using sequence data from a microcephaly case. *mSphere* **2017**, *2*. [CrossRef] [PubMed]

63. Gadea, G.; Bos, S.; Krejbich-Trotot, P.; Clain, E.; Viranaicken, W.; El-Kalamouni, C.; Mavingui, P.; Despres, P. A robust method for the rapid generation of recombinant Zika virus expressing the GFP reporter gene. *Virology* **2016**, *497*, 157–162. [CrossRef] [PubMed]

64. Atieh, T.; Baronti, C.; de Lamballerie, X.; Nougairede, A. Simple reverse genetics systems for Asian and African Zika viruses. *Sci. Rep.* **2016**, *6*, 39384. [CrossRef] [PubMed]

65. Bos, S.; Viranaicken, W.; Turpin, J.; El-Kalamouni, C.; Roche, M.; Krejbich-Trotot, P.; Despres, P.; Gadea, G. The structural proteins of epidemic and historical strains of zika virus differ in their ability to initiate viral infection in human host cells. *Virology* **2018**, *516*, 265–273. [CrossRef] [PubMed]

66. Pu, S.-Y.; Wu, R.-H.; Yang, C.-C.; Jao, T.-M.; Tsai, M.-H.; Wang, J.-C.; Lin, H.-M.; Chao, Y.-S.; Yueh, A. Successful propagation of flavivirus infectious cDNA s by a novel method to reduce the cryptic bacterial promoter activity of virus genomes. *J. Virol.* **2011**, *85*, 2927–2941. [CrossRef] [PubMed]

67. Heang, V.; Yasuda, C.Y.; Sovann, L.; Haddow, A.D.; da Rosa, A.P.T.; Tesh, R.B.; Kasper, M.R. Zika virus infection, Cambodia, 2010. *Emerg. Infect. Dis.* **2012**, *18*, 349–351. [CrossRef] [PubMed]

68. Li, X.D.; Li, X.F.; Ye, H.Q.; Deng, C.L.; Ye, Q.; Shan, C.; Shang, B.D.; Xu, L.L.; Li, S.H.; Cao, S.B.; et al. Recovery of a chemically synthesized Japanese encephalitis virus reveals two critical adaptive mutations in NS2B and NS4A. *J. Gen. Virol.* **2014**, *95*, 806–815. [CrossRef] [PubMed]

69. Zou, G.; Xu, H.Y.; Qing, M.; Wang, Q.Y.; Shi, P.Y. Development and characterization of a stable luciferase dengue virus for high-throughput screening. *Antiviral Res.* **2011**, *91*, 11–19. [CrossRef] [PubMed]

70. Lanciotti, R.S.; Lambert, A.J.; Holodniy, M.; Saavedra, S.; Signor Ldel, C. Phylogeny of zika virus in western hemisphere, 2015. *Emerg. Infect. Dis.* **2016**, *22*, 933–935. [CrossRef] [PubMed]

71. Godiska, R.; Mead, D.; Dhodda, V.; Wu, C.; Hochstein, R.; Karsi, A.; Usdin, K.; Entezam, A.; Ravin, N. Linear plasmid vector for cloning of repetitive or unstable sequences in *Escherichia coli*. *Nucleic Acids Res* **2010**, *38*, e88. [CrossRef] [PubMed]

72. Lohmann, V.; Körner, F.; Koch, J.-O.; Herian, U.; Theilmann, L.; Bartenschlager, R. Replication of subgenomic hepatitis C virus RNAs in a hepatoma cell line. *Science* **1999**, *285*, 110–113. [CrossRef] [PubMed]

73. Yamshchikov, V.; Mishin, V.; Cominelli, F. A new strategy in design of (+)RNA virus infectious clones enabling their stable propagation in *E. coli*. *Virology* **2001**, *281*, 272–280. [CrossRef] [PubMed]

74. Zhang, F.C.; Li, X.F.; Deng, Y.Q.; Tong, Y.G.; Qin, C.F. Excretion of infectious Zika virus in urine. *Lancet Infect. Dis.* **2016**, *16*, 641–642. [CrossRef]

75. Costa, M.; Fontaine, J.-M.; Goër, S.L.-D.; Michel, F. A group II self-splicing intron from the brown alga *Pylaiella littoralis* is active at unusually low magnesium concentrations and forms populations of molecules with a uniform conformation. *J. Mol. Biol.* **1997**, *274*, 353–364. [CrossRef] [PubMed]

76. Zerbato, M.; Holic, N.; Moniot-Frin, S.; Ingrao, D.; Galy, A.; Perea, J. The brown algae PI.LSU/2 group II intron-encoded protein has functional reverse transcriptase and maturase activities. *PLoS ONE* **2013**, *8*, e58263. [CrossRef] [PubMed]

77. Fontaine, J.M.; Rousvoal, S.; Leblanc, C.; Kloareg, B.; Loiseaux-de Goer, S. The mitochondrial LSU rDNA of the brown alga *Pylaiella littoralis* reveals α-proteobacterial features and is split by four group IIB introns with an atypical phylogeny. *J. Mol. Biol.* **1995**, *251*, 378–389. [CrossRef] [PubMed]

78. Ruggli, N.; Tratschin, J.D.; Mittelholzer, C.; Hofmann, M.A. Nucleotide sequence of classical swine fever virus strain Alfort/187 and transcription of infectious RNA from stably cloned full-length cDNA. *J. Virol.* **1996**, *70*, 3478–3487. [PubMed]

79. Rice, C.M.; Grakoui, A.; Galler, R.; Chambers, T.J. Transcription of infectious yellow fever RNA from full-length cDNA templates produced by in vitro ligation. *New Biol.* **1989**, *1*, 285–296. [PubMed]

80. Messer, W.B.; Yount, B.; Hacker, K.E.; Donaldson, E.F.; Huynh, J.P.; de Silva, A.M.; Baric, R.S. Development and characterization of a reverse genetic system for studying dengue virus serotype 3 strain variation and neutralization. *PLoS Negl. Trop. Dis.* **2012**, *6*, e1486. [CrossRef] [PubMed]

81. Deng, C.L.; Zhang, Q.Y.; Chen, D.D.; Liu, S.Q.; Qin, C.F.; Zhang, B.; Ye, H.Q. Recovery of the zika virus through an in vitro ligation approach. *J. Gen. Virol.* **2017**, *98*, 1739–1743. [CrossRef] [PubMed]

82. Gibson, D.G.; Young, L.; Chuang, R.Y.; Venter, J.C.; Hutchison, C.A.; Smith, H.O. Enzymatic assembly of DNA molecules up to several hundred kilobases. *Nat. Methods* **2009**, *6*, 343–345. [CrossRef] [PubMed]

83. Quan, J.; Tian, J. Circular polymerase extension cloning of complex gene libraries and pathways. *PLoS ONE* **2009**, *4*, e6441. [CrossRef] [PubMed]

84. Almazan, F.; Gonzalez, J.M.; Penzes, Z.; Izeta, A.; Calvo, E.; Plana-Duran, J.; Enjuanes, L. Engineering the largest RNA virus genome as an infectious bacterial artificial chromosome. *Proc. Natl. Acad. Sci. USA* **2000**, *97*, 5516–5521. [CrossRef] [PubMed]

85. Almazan, F.; Dediego, M.L.; Galan, C.; Escors, D.; Alvarez, E.; Ortego, J.; Sola, I.; Zuniga, S.; Alonso, S.; Moreno, J.L.; et al. Construction of a severe acute respiratory syndrome coronavirus infectious cDNA clone and a replicon to study coronavirus RNA synthesis. *J. Virol.* **2006**, *80*, 10900–10906. [CrossRef] [PubMed]

86. Yun, S.-I.; Kim, S.-Y.; Rice, C.M.; Lee, Y.-M. Development and application of a reverse genetics system for Japanese encephalitis virus. *J. Virol.* **2003**, *77*, 6450–6465. [CrossRef] [PubMed]

87. Suzuki, R.; de Borba, L.; Duarte dos Santos, C.N.; Mason, P.W. Construction of an infectious cDNA clone for a Brazilian prototype strain of dengue virus type 1: Characterization of a temperature-sensitive mutation in NS1. *Virology* **2007**, *362*, 374–383. [CrossRef] [PubMed]

88. Pierro, D.J.; Salazar, M.I.; Beaty, B.J.; Olson, K.E. Infectious clone construction of dengue virus type 2, strain Jamaican 1409, and characterization of a conditional E6 mutation. *J. Gen. Virol.* **2006**, *87*, 2263–2268. [CrossRef] [PubMed]

89. Wang, K.; Boysen, C.; Shizuya, H.; Simon, M.I.; Hood, L. Complete nucleotide sequence of two generations of a bacterial artificial chromosome cloning vector. *BioTechniques* **1997**, *23*, 992–994. [CrossRef] [PubMed]

90. Shizuya, H.; Birren, B.; Kim, U.J.; Mancino, V.; Slepak, T.; Tachiiri, Y.; Simon, M. Cloning and stable maintenance of 300-kilobase-pair fragments of human DNA in *Escherichia coli* using an F-factor-based vector. *Proc. Natl. Acad. Sci. USA* **1992**, *89*, 8794–8797. [CrossRef] [PubMed]

91. Aubry, F.; Nougairede, A.; de Fabritus, L.; Querat, G.; Gould, E.A.; de Lamballerie, X. Single-stranded positive-sense RNA viruses generated in days using infectious subgenomic amplicons. *J. Gen. Virol.* **2014**, *95*, 2462–2467. [CrossRef] [PubMed]

92. De Wispelaere, M.; Frenkiel, M.-P.; Després, P. A Japanese encephalitis virus genotype 5 molecular clone is highly neuropathogenic in a mouse model: Impact of the structural protein region on virulence. *J. Virol.* **2015**, *89*, 5862–5875. [CrossRef] [PubMed]

93. Bartenschlager, R. Hepatitis C virus replicons: Potential role for drug development. *Nat. Rev. Drug Discov.* **2002**, *1*, 911. [CrossRef] [PubMed]

94. Khromykh, A.A.; Westaway, E.G. Subgenomic replicons of the flavivirus Kunjin: Construction and applications. *J. Virol.* **1997**, *71*, 1497–1505. [PubMed]

95. Xiong, C.; Levis, R.; Shen, P.; Schlesinger, S.; Rice, C.; Huang, H. Sindbis virus: An efficient, broad host range vector for gene expression in animal cells. *Science* **1989**, *243*, 1188–1191. [CrossRef] [PubMed]

96. Li, W.; Ma, L.; Guo, L.-P.; Wang, X.-L.; Zhang, J.-W.; Bu, Z.-G.; Hua, R.-H. West nile virus infectious replicon particles generated using a packaging-restricted cell line is a safe reporter system. *Sci. Rep.* **2017**, *7*, 3286. [CrossRef] [PubMed]

97. Kato, F.; Hishiki, T. Dengue virus reporter replicon is a valuable tool for antiviral drug discovery and analysis of virus replication mechanisms. *Viruses* **2016**, *8*, 122. [CrossRef] [PubMed]

98. Puig-Basagoiti, F.; Deas, T.S.; Ren, P.; Tilgner, M.; Ferguson, D.M.; Shi, P.-Y. High-throughput assays using a luciferase-expressing replicon, virus-like particles, and full-length virus for west nile virus drug discovery. *Antimicrob. Agents Chemother.* **2005**, *49*, 4980–4988. [CrossRef] [PubMed]

99. Ge, F.; Luo, Y.; Liew, P.X.; Hung, E. Derivation of a novel SARS–coronavirus replicon cell line and its application for anti-SARS drug screening. *Virology* **2007**, *360*, 150–158. [CrossRef] [PubMed]

100. Hao, W.; Herlihy, K.J.; Zhang, N.J.; Fuhrman, S.A.; Doan, C.; Patick, A.K.; Duggal, R. Development of a novel dicistronic reporter-selectable hepatitis C virus replicon suitable for high-throughput inhibitor screening. *Antimicrob. Agents Chemother.* **2007**, *51*, 95–102. [CrossRef] [PubMed]

101. Xie, X.; Zou, J.; Shan, C.; Yang, Y.; Kum, D.B.; Dallmeier, K.; Neyts, J.; Shi, P.Y. Zika virus replicons for drug discovery. *EBioMedicine* **2016**, *12*, 156–160. [CrossRef] [PubMed]

102. Hahn, C.S.; Hahn, Y.S.; Rice, C.M.; Lee, E.; Dalgarno, L.; Strauss, E.G.; Strauss, J.H. Conserved elements in the 3′ untranslated region of flavivirus RNAs and potential cyclization sequences. *J. Mol. Biol.* **1987**, *198*, 33–41. [CrossRef]

103. Khromykh, A.A.; Meka, H.; Guyatt, K.J.; Westaway, E.G. Essential role of cyclization sequences in flavivirus RNA replication. *J. Virol.* **2001**, *75*, 6719–6728. [CrossRef] [PubMed]

104. Deng, Y.Q.; Zhang, N.N.; Li, C.F.; Tian, M.; Hao, J.N.; Xie, X.P.; Shi, P.Y.; Qin, C.F. Adenosine analog NITD008 is a potent inhibitor of Zika virus. *Open Forum Infect. Dis.* **2016**, *3*, ofw175. [CrossRef] [PubMed]

105. Li, J.Q.; Deng, C.L.; Gu, D.; Li, X.; Shi, L.; He, J.; Zhang, Q.Y.; Zhang, B.; Ye, H.Q. Development of a replicon cell line-based high throughput antiviral assay for screening inhibitors of zika virus. *Antiviral Res.* **2018**, *150*, 148–154. [CrossRef] [PubMed]

106. Li, Y.; Li, L.-F.; Yu, S.; Wang, X.; Zhang, L.; Yu, J.; Xie, L.; Li, W.; Ali, R.; Qiu, H.-J. Applications of replicating-competent reporter-expressing viruses in diagnostic and molecular virology. *Viruses* **2016**, *8*, 127. [CrossRef] [PubMed]

107. Hu, Z.; Lan, K.-H.; He, S.; Swaroop, M.; Hu, X.; Southall, N.; Zheng, W.; Liang, T.J. Novel cell-based hepatitis C virus infection assay for quantitative high-throughput screening of anti-hepatitis C virus compounds. *Antimicrob. Agents Chemother.* **2014**, *58*, 995–1004. [CrossRef] [PubMed]

108. Towner, J.S.; Paragas, J.; Dover, J.E.; Gupta, M.; Goldsmith, C.S.; Huggins, J.W.; Nichol, S.T. Generation of eGFP expressing recombinant Zaire ebolavirus for analysis of early pathogenesis events and high-throughput antiviral drug screening. *Virology* **2005**, *332*, 20–27. [CrossRef] [PubMed]

109. DiPiazza, A.; Nogales, A.; Poulton, N.; Wilson, P.C.; Martínez-Sobrido, L.; Sant, A.J. Pandemic 2009 H1N1 influenza venus reporter virus reveals broad diversity of mhc class II-positive antigen-bearing cells following infection in vivo. *Sci. Rep.* **2017**, *7*, 10857. [CrossRef] [PubMed]

110. Breen, M.; Nogales, A.; Baker, S.F.; Perez, D.R.; Martínez-Sobrido, L. Replication-competent influenza A and B viruses expressing a fluorescent dynamic timer protein for in vitro and in vivo studies. *PLoS ONE* **2016**, *11*, e0147723. [CrossRef] [PubMed]

111. Fuentes, S.; Crim, R.L.; Beeler, J.; Teng, M.N.; Golding, H.; Khurana, S. Development of a simple, rapid, sensitive, high-throughput luciferase reporter based microneutralization test for measurement of virus neutralizing antibodies following respiratory syncytial virus vaccination and infection. *Vaccine* **2013**, *31*, 3987–3994. [CrossRef] [PubMed]

112. Song, K.-Y.; Zhao, H.; Jiang, Z.-Y.; Li, X.-F.; Deng, Y.-Q.; Jiang, T.; Zhu, S.-Y.; Shi, P.-Y.; Zhang, B.; Zhang, F.-C.; et al. A novel reporter system for neutralizing and enhancing antibody assay against dengue virus. *BMC Microbiol.* **2014**, *14*, 44. [CrossRef] [PubMed]

113. Deng, C.-L.; Liu, S.-Q.; Zhou, D.-G.; Xu, L.-L.; Li, X.-D.; Zhang, P.-T.; Li, P.-H.; Ye, H.-Q.; Wei, H.-P.; Yuan, Z.-M.; et al. Development of neutralization assay using an eGFP chikungunya virus. *Viruses* **2016**, *8*, 181. [CrossRef] [PubMed]

114. Nogales, A.; Rodríguez-Sánchez, I.; Monte, K.; Lenschow, D.J.; Perez, D.R.; Martínez-Sobrido, L. Replication-competent fluorescent-expressing influenza B virus. *Virus Res.* **2016**, *213*, 69–81. [CrossRef] [PubMed]

115. Shcherbo, D.; Merzlyak, E.M.; Chepurnykh, T.V.; Fradkov, A.F.; Ermakova, G.V.; Solovieva, E.A.; Lukyanov, K.A.; Bogdanova, E.A.; Zaraisky, A.G.; Lukyanov, S.; et al. Bright far-red fluorescent protein for whole-body imaging. *Nat. Methods* **2007**, *4*, 741–746. [CrossRef] [PubMed]

116. Maguire, C.A.; van der Mijn, J.C.; Degeling, M.H.; Morse, D.; Tannous, B.A. Codon-optimized *Luciola italica* Luciferase variants for mammalian gene expression in culture and in vivo. *Mol. Imaging* **2012**, *11*, 13–21. [CrossRef] [PubMed]

117. Shan, C.; Muruato, A.E.; Nunes, B.T.D.; Luo, H.; Xie, X.; Medeiros, D.B.A.; Wakamiya, M.; Tesh, R.B.; Barrett, A.D.; Wang, T.; et al. A live-attenuated zika virus vaccine candidate induces sterilizing immunity in mouse models. *Nat. Med.* **2017**, *23*, 763. [CrossRef] [PubMed]

118. Xie, X.; Yang, Y.; Muruato, A.E.; Zou, J.; Shan, C.; Nunes, B.T.D.; Medeiros, D.B.A.; Vasconcelos, P.F.C.; Weaver, S.C.; Rossi, S.L.; et al. Understanding Zika virus stability and developing a chimeric vaccine through functional analysis. *mBio* **2017**, *8*. [CrossRef] [PubMed]

119. Yang, Y.; Shan, C.; Zou, J.; Muruato, A.E.; Bruno, D.N.; de Almeida Medeiros Daniele, B.; Vasconcelos, P.F.C.; Rossi, S.L.; Weaver, S.C.; Xie, X.; et al. A cDNA clone-launched platform for high-yield production of inactivated zika vaccine. *EBioMedicine* **2017**, *17*, 145–156. [CrossRef] [PubMed]

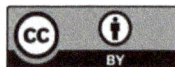

![viruses logo] *viruses*

MDPI

Article

A Reverse Genetics System for Zika Virus Based on a Simple Molecular Cloning Strategy

Maximilian Münster [1,†], **Anna Płaszczyca** [1,†], **Mirko Cortese** [1], **Christopher John Neufeldt** [1], **Sarah Goellner** [1], **Gang Long** [2] and **Ralf Bartenschlager** [1,3,*]

[1] Department of Infectious Diseases, Molecular Virology, Heidelberg University, Centre for Integrative Infectious Disease Research, Im Neuenheimer Feld 344, 69120 Heidelberg, Germany; max.muenster1991@googlemail.com (M.M.); anna.plaszczyca@med.uni-heidelberg.de (A.P.); mirko.cortese@med.uni-heidelberg.de (M.C.); Christopher.Neufeldt@med.uni-heidelberg.de (C.J.N.); sarah.goellner@med.uni-heidelberg.de (S.G.)

[2] Key Laboratory of Molecular Virology and Immunology, Institute Pasteur of Shanghai, Chinese Academy of Sciences, Shanghai 200031, China; glong@ips.ac.cn

[3] German Center for Infection Research, Heidelberg Partner Site, Im Neuenheimer Feld 344, 69120 Heidelberg, Germany

*   Correspondence: ralf.bartenschlager@med.uni-heidelberg.de; Tel.: +49-(0)-6221-56-4225

†   These authors contributed equally to this work.

Received: 1 May 2018; Accepted: 9 July 2018; Published: 12 July 2018

Abstract: The Zika virus (ZIKV) has recently attracted major research interest as infection was unexpectedly associated with neurological manifestations in developing foetuses and with Guillain-Barré syndrome in infected adults. Understanding the underlying molecular mechanisms requires reverse genetic systems, which allow manipulation of infectious cDNA clones at will. In the case of flaviviruses, to which ZIKV belongs, several reports have indicated that the construction of full-length cDNA clones is difficult due to toxicity during plasmid amplification in *Escherichia coli*. Toxicity of flaviviral cDNAs has been linked to the activity of cryptic prokaryotic promoters within the region encoding the structural proteins leading to spurious transcription and expression of toxic viral proteins. Here, we employ an approach based on in silico prediction and mutational silencing of putative promoters to generate full-length cDNA clones of the historical MR766 strain and the contemporary French Polynesian strain H/PF/2013 of ZIKV. While for both strains construction of full-length cDNA clones has failed in the past, we show that our approach generates cDNA clones that are stable on single bacterial plasmids and give rise to infectious viruses with properties similar to those generated by other more complex assembly strategies. Further, we generate luciferase and fluorescent reporter viruses as well as sub-genomic replicons that are fully functional and suitable for various research and drug screening applications. Taken together, this study confirms that in silico prediction and silencing of cryptic prokaryotic promoters is an efficient strategy to generate full-length cDNA clones of flaviviruses and reports novel tools that will facilitate research on ZIKV biology and development of antiviral strategies.

Keywords: ZIKV; reporter virus; cryptic promoter silencing; full-length molecular clone; subgenomic replicon; plasmid toxicity

1. Introduction

The Zika virus (ZIKV), a member of the *Flavivirus* genus within the *Flaviviridae* family, was identified almost 70 years ago in Uganda [1] but until recently was not associated with severe symptoms. However, outbreaks outside of Africa and Asia, in the Yap Islands (2007) [2], French Polynesia (2013) [3] and the Americas (2015) [4], raised major interest as infection was associated with an increased incidence of microcephaly and other neurological manifestations in developing foetuses as well as Guillain-Barré syndrome in infected adults [5,6]. Two lineages of ZIKV have been identified, African and Asian, with the currently circulating strains belonging to the Asian lineage [7]. Although 48 countries have confirmed ZIKV infections associated with *Aedes* mosquito-borne transmission of the virus, neither a prophylactic vaccine nor antiviral therapies are available to date [8]. As a consequence, there is an urgent need for tools, which facilitate studying the molecular determinants that underlie ZIKV pathogenesis and allow testing of potential antiviral therapies. In this respect, stable and traceable reverse genetic systems to generate isogenic mutants, are of great advantage [9,10]. However, construction of ZIKV molecular clones has been hampered by the instability of the viral cDNA genome during propagation via bacterial plasmids. The instability of flaviviral cDNA clones in *Escherichia coli* (*E. coli*) has been linked to the expression of toxic viral proteins from cryptic *E. coli* promoters (CEPs) encoded in the flavivirus genome [11,12]. Strategies to disrupt toxic protein expression and to overcome these toxicity problems include insertion of introns into the viral open-reading frame [13,14] or propagation of ZIKV genome fragments on multiple plasmids and subsequent assembly of the fragments [15–19]. Those strategies, however, have some disadvantages compared to a single plasmid system that allows in vitro transcription of full-length infectious viral RNAs. For instance, the intron insertion method requires nuclear transcription to generate the viral genome with the risk of undesired splicing rendering the RNA non-functional. In the case of multi-plasmid systems, laborious and potentially error prone in vitro assembly steps complicate the protocol. Although Shan and co-workers were able to amplify a full-length ZIKV cDNA clone from Cambodia (FSS13025 strain, isolated in 2010) on a single plasmid in *E. coli*, ours and others' data indicate that this is neither possible for the prototypic African strain MR766 nor for the French Polynesian strain H/PF/2013 (Asian lineage) or isolates from the Americas [13,15–17].

Here we present a different approach that overcomes these problems and is based on the observation that full-length Japanese encephalitis virus (JEV) and Dengue virus 2 (DENV2) infectious cDNAs could be stabilized by CEP silencing [11]. We show that mutational inactivation of multiple CEPs predicted in silico to reside in the structural regions of the MR766 and H/PF/2013 genomes is sufficient to stabilize the full-length cDNA genomes of both ZIKV strains enabling the construction of a single-plasmid based reverse genetic system. Authentic virus genomes and engineered reporter viruses generated with this approach are fully functional in cell culture and suitable for multiple research and development purposes.

2. Materials and Methods

2.1. Cell Lines and Antibodies

VeroE6 and Huh7 cells were cultured at 37 °C and 5% CO_2 in Dulbecco's modified Eagle's medium (DMEM) (Life Technologies, Darmstadt, Germany), supplemented with 10% foetal calf serum (FBS; Sigma-Aldrich, Taufkirchen, Germany), 2 mM L-glutamine, nonessential amino acids (all from Gibco, Life Technologies, Darmstadt, Germany), 100 U/mL penicillin and 100 µg/mL streptomycin (DMEMcplt). Primary antibodies used in this study were: rabbit anti-ZIKV NS3 and anti-NS4B (both from GeneTex, Irvine, CA, USA), mouse pan-flavivirus-anti-E (4G2, ATCC®, Manassas, VA, USA), mouse J2 anti-dsRNA antibody (Scicons, Szirák, Hungary), mouse anti-glyceraldehyde-3-phosphate dehydrogenase (GAPDH, Santa Cruz Biotechnology, Heidelberg, Germany). Secondary horseradish peroxidase-conjugated antibodies were purchased from Sigma-Aldrich. AlexaFluor-conjugated secondary antibodies were obtained from Life Technologies.

2.2. Source of Virus Sequences

For the construction of the ZIKV genome we used the reference genomes KJ776791 (H/PF/2013, accession date August 2016) and DQ859059 (MR766, accession date August 2016). In addition, we amplified the MR766 and the H/PF/2013 strains (obtained from the European Virus Archive;

Marseille, France) by passaging once in C6/36 mosquito cells and once in VeroE6 cells. Viral RNA was isolated from cell lysates using the NucleoSpin RNA II kit (Machery-Nagel, Düren, Germany) and reverse transcribed using SuperScript III RT (Thermo Fisher Scientific Waltham, MA, USA). cDNA was amplified by PCR and amplicons were sequenced by Sanger sequencing (GATC Biotech, Constance, Germany) using primers spanning the complete ZIKV genome. Sequences of the 5′ and 3′UTRs were obtained by the rapid amplification of cDNA ends (RACE) using the 5′/3′ RACE second generation kit (Roche, Basel, Switzerland) with a polyA-tail added to the cDNA prior to the 3′ RACE reaction by using the poly(A) polymerase (New England Biolabs, Ipswich, MA, USA).

2.3. In Silico Prediction of CEPs and Sequence Modifications

Cryptic *E. coli* promoters were predicted with the publicly available Neural Network promoter program from the Berkeley Drosophila Genome Project [20,21] similar to an earlier report [11]. The ZIKV sequences were analysed for CEPs from nucleotide position 1–2683 for H/PF/2013 and 1–2664 for MR766. Putative promoters with a score >0.85 were eliminated by silent nucleotide exchanges introduced into the −10 regions (Pribnow/Schaller box) and/or the −35 regions (Figure S1). CEPs in the 5′UTR were not modified to avoid changes in RNA secondary structures (Acosta et al., 2014 [22]). In addition, in order to facilitate assembly and reverse genetic studies, several restriction sites were inserted or removed by silent nucleotide exchanges (Tables S1 and S2). The T7 promoter sequence (5′-TAATACGACTCACTATAG-3′) was inserted upstream of the 5′UTR to allow for in vitro transcription of viral RNA. The final sequences were re-analysed with the Neural Network promoter program to confirm that the scores were below 0.85. The sequences were ordered as synthetic DNA fragments (four fragments/strain) from the GeneArt Gene Synthesis service (Invitrogen, Darmstadt, Germany).

2.4. Generation of synZIKV Constructs

The pFK vector used for the assembly of the synthetic ZIKV (synZIKV) sequences has been described previously (Lohmann et al., 1999 [23]). A synthetic DNA linker encoding the restriction sites required for assembly of the synZIKV cDNA clones (Figure 1A) was inserted into the vector via HindIII and SpeI. For assembly of the full-length wild-type synZIKV plasmids (pFK-synZIKV) the synthetic DNA fragments were inserted into the modified pFK vector using the indicated restriction enzymes (Figure 1A) and in four steps in the order of fragment 4 to fragment 1. Plasmids were amplified in dcm⁺/dam⁺ DH5α cells. To generate full-length *Renilla* luciferase (RLuc) reporter constructs (pFK-synZIKV-R2A), we used a construct design similar to the one reported by us for the synthetic DENV-2 16681 reporter genome [10]. In brief, we constructed a synthetic DNA fragment encoding the T7 promoter followed by the 5′UTR of ZIKV, the first 102 nts of Capsid required for genome circularization, the *RLuc* gene flanked by NotI and NruI restriction sites and the auto-proteolytic FMDV 2A peptide directly fused to the first nucleotide of the ZIKV coding region. This fragment was inserted into the pFK-synZIKV plasmid via MluI/KpnI restriction sites. Sub-genomic synZIKV RLuc reporter replicons (pFK-synZIKV-sgR2A) were constructed in an analogous way but with the difference that the reporter cassette was inserted between the last 24 codons of E that we retained to ensure proper membrane insertion of NS1 (cloning via MluI and AgeI restriction sites). To generate turbo far-red fluorescent protein FP635 expressing viruses (pFK-synZIKV-FP635 constructs), the reporter gene was amplified by PCR using the FP635-encoding DENV2 16681 construct reported earlier [24] and inserted into the pFK-synZIKV-R2A plasmids via the NotI and NruI restriction sites flanking the *RLuc* gene. Note that a coding sequence for the SV40 NLS (PKKKRKV) was fused in frame to the 3′end of the turbo far-red fluorescent protein FP635-encoding sequence by using PCR (primer sequences available on request). All nucleotide sequences of the final constructs were validated by using Sanger sequencing (GATC Biotech).

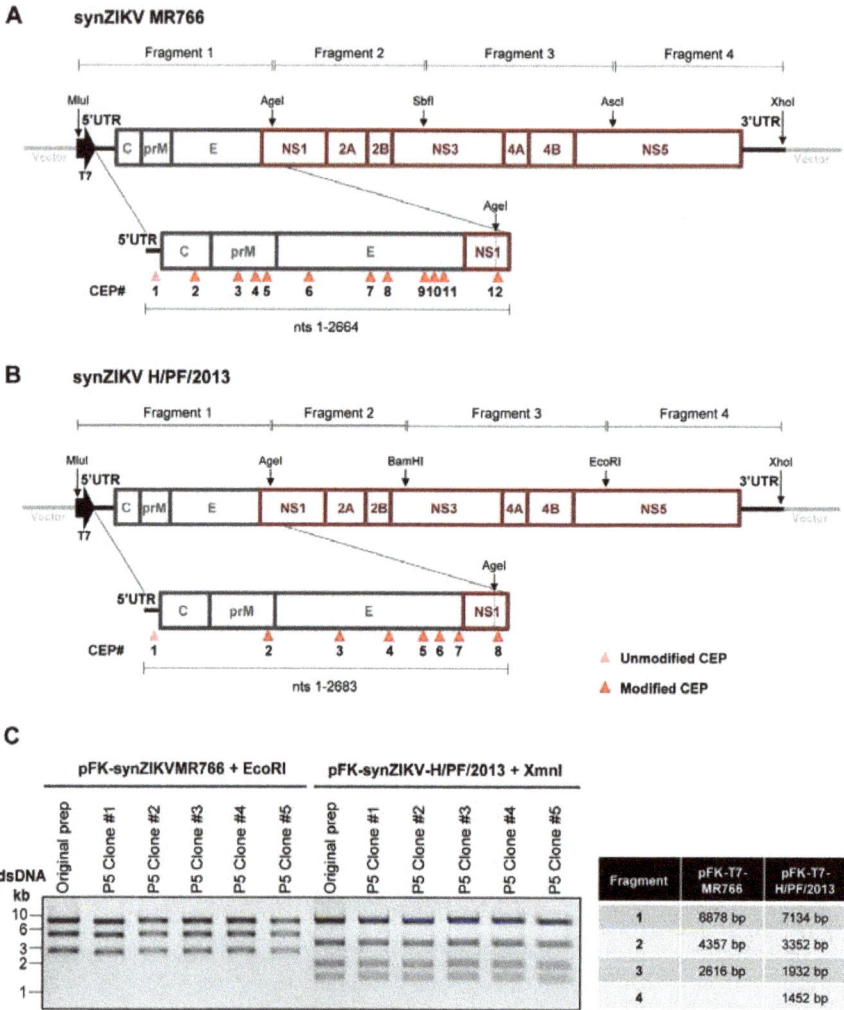

Figure 1. Construction and stability of synthetic full length Zika virus (synZIKV) cDNA clones. (**A**) Schematic representation of the synZIKV MR766 construct and the four fragments used to assemble the genome. The 5′ and 3′UTRs are indicated with bold black lines, the promoter for the T7 RNA polymerase with a black arrow. Restriction sites used for the assembly of the fragments are indicated. An enlargement of fragment #1 is shown below with putative CEPs (score > 0.85) indicated by red arrow heads. CEP 1 was not mutated (indicated with the pink arrow head). (**B**) Same as in panel (**A**) but for synZIKV-H/PF/2013. (**C**) Restriction patterns of pFK-synZIKV constructs obtained after digest with EcoRI (MR766) or XmnI (H/PF/2013) and agarose gel electrophoresis. Plasmids were analysed directly after assembly (original prep) and after five passages (P5) in *E. coli* (five DNA clones of P5 are shown).

2.5. In Vitro Transcription and RNA Transfection

The protocol for in vitro transcription has been described earlier [23]. Briefly, synZIKV sequences were linearized with XhoI (located at the end of the 3′UTR of the viral genome) and the DNA purified with the Nucleo-Spin Extract II kit (Macherey-Nagel, Düren, Germany). The in vitro transcription reaction was carried out with 10 μg of linearized plasmid DNA in a total volume of 100 μL containing 20 μL 5× RRL buffer (400 mM HEPES (pH 7.5), 60 mM MgCl$_2$, 10 mM spermidine and 200 mM DTT), NTP-Mix (3.125 mM ATP, CTP and UTP and 1.56 mM GTP), 1 U/μL RNasin (Promega, Madison, WI, USA), 2 U/μL T7 RNA polymerase (New England Biolabs) and 1 mM anti-reverse cap analogue (ARCA; 3′-O-Me- m7G(5′)ppp(5′)G; New England Biolabs). After incubation at 37 °C for 2.5 h, 1 U/μL T7 RNA polymerase was added followed by additional 2.5 h incubation at 37 °C. DNA was digested with DNaseI for one hour and RNA was purified by acidic phenol-chloroform extraction and isopropanol precipitation. The integrity and size of the RNAs was validated by agarose gel electrophoresis. For electroporation, subconfluent and trypsinized cells were collected in DMEMcplt, washed once with PBS and resuspended in cytomix buffer (120 mM KCl, 0.15 mM CaCl$_2$, 10 mM potassium phosphate buffer, 25 mM HEPES (pH 7.6), 2 mM EGTA, 5 mM MgCl$_2$, freshly supplemented with 2 mM ATP and 5 mM glutathione) at a concentration of 1×10^7 cells/mL for Huh7 and 1.5×10^7 cells/mL for VeroE6 cells. Four hundred μL of the cell suspension was mixed with 10 μg of in vitro transcribed RNA, transferred into an electroporation cuvette (Bio-Rad, Hercules, CA, USA; 0.4-cm gap width) and pulsed once with a Gene Pulser II system (Bio-Rad) at 975 μF and 270 V. Finally, the cells were transferred into pre-warmed DMEMcplt in case of synZIKV-sgR2A replicons or DMEMcplt supplemented with 15 mM HEPES (pH 7.5) in case of the full-length synZIKV. For replication assays, Huh7 cells transfected with synZIKV-sgR2A RNAs were seeded into 12-well plates at a density of 2×10^5 cells/well. VeroE6 cells transfected with full-length synZIKV RNAs were seeded into 24-well plates at a density of 2×10^5 cells/well.

2.6. Virus Stocks and Passaging

Stocks of parental ZIKV strains were produced exactly as described [25]. For production of wild-type synZIKV stocks, two electroporation reactions of the same construct were pooled in 20 mL DMEMcplt and seeded into a single 15 cm-diameter dish. After 48 h, the medium was changed to DMEMcplt containing 15 mM HEPES (pH 7.5). Supernatants were harvested at least twice (between 72–96 h for synZIKV-MR766 and 96–120 h for synZIKV-H/PF/2013). Virus-containing cell culture supernatants were filtered through a 0.45 μm syringe filter and plaque-forming units (PFU) were determined. For final stock production, 7×10^6 VeroE6 cells were seeded into 15 cm-diameter dishes and infected at a multiplicity of infection (MOI) of 0.1 on the next day. Infected cells were cultured in DMEMcplt containing 15 mM HEPES (pH 7.5) and supernatants were collected from day 3–7 post-infection as described above. Aliquots of the virus stocks were stored at −80 °C. For cell culture adaptation of the synZIKVs, multiple rounds of infection were performed in Huh7 cells. Virus stocks (passage 0; P0) were prepared as described above and used to infect Huh7 cells at MOI = 0.1. Virus containing supernatants were harvested at 72 h post infection (P1) and passaged two more times in 72 h hour intervals (P2–P3).

2.7. Virus Titration by Plaque Assay

For titration of wild-type viruses, VeroE6 cells were seeded into 24-well plates at a density of 2.5×10^5 cells/well one day prior to infection. The cells were infected with serial 10-fold dilutions of virus containing supernatants for one hour at 37 °C. All plaque assays were performed in duplicates. After infection, the inoculum was removed and replaced with serum-free MEM (Gibco, Life Technologies) containing 1.5% carboxy-methylcellulose (Sigma-Aldrich). After four days, cells were fixed by the addition of 5% formaldehyde for at least 2 h at room temperature. Fixed cells were washed with water and stained with 1% crystal violet in 10% ethanol for at least 15 min. After rinsing the cells with water, the number of plaques was counted and virus titres were calculated as plaque forming units/mL (PFU/mL).

2.8. RLuc Assays

RLuc activity was determined as previously described [26]. At the indicated time points cells were lysed by addition of 100 μL (full-length synZIKV-R2A) or 125 μL (synZIKV-sgR2A replicons) luciferase lysis buffer (25 mM Glycine-Glycine (pH 7.8), 15 mM $MgSO_4$; 4 mM EGTA, 10% (*v/v*) glycerol, 0.1% (*v/v*) Triton X-100, freshly added 1 mM DTT) to each well. The lysates were stored at −80 °C until use for luciferase assays. Luciferase activity was determined with a Lumat LB9507 luminometer (Berthold Technologies, Bad Wildbad, Germany). For each sample, 20 μL of cell lysate were mixed with 100 μL freshly prepared luciferase assay buffer (25 mM Glycine-Glycine (pH 7.8), 15 mM K_4PO_4 buffer (pH 7.8), 15 mM $MgSO_4$, 4 mM EGTA, 1.42 μM coelenterazine).

2.9. Antiviral Assays and Stability of synZIKV-R2A Viruses

For characterization of RLuc-encoding synZIKV-R2A clones, VeroE6 cells transfected with the respective in vitro transcripts were seeded into 24-well plates at densities of 2×10^5 cells/well. Supernatants were collected 72 h post-electroporation (Passage 0; P0) and stored at −80 °C until use for antiviral assays or further passaging. For antiviral assays VeroE6 cells were seeded into 24-well plates at a density of 1×10^5 cells/well and on the next day infected with a 1:10 dilution of P0 of the respective virus at 37 °C. One hour later the inoculum was removed and replaced with DMEMcplt containing the indicated concentrations of 2′-C-methylcytidine (2′CMC; Sigma-Aldrich). RLuc activities were determined 72 h post-infection. For assessment of the stability, synZIKV-R2A P0 reporter viruses were subjected to multiple rounds of infection of VeroE6 cells (72 h infection/passage). To determine reporter virus stability, Huh7 cells were seeded into 24-well plates at a density of 7.5×10^4 cells/well and infected on the next day with supernatants from each passage as described above. After 72 h supernatants were collected and subjected to plaque assay analysis. Cells were lysed in luciferase lysis buffer and RLuc activities were determined as described above. To check for the integrity of the reporter genomes, RNA was isolated from P0–P3 virus-containing supernatants using NucleoSpin RNA II kit (Machery Nagel, Düren, Germany), reverse transcribed with SuperScript III RT using random hexamer primer (Thermo Fisher Scientific) and amplified by PCR using the forward primer 5′CGACAGTTCGAGTTTGAAGC3′ hybridizing to the 5′UTR of both strains and the reverse primers 5′AGGCTAGAATCGCCAAGACC3′ and 5′GTTGATGAGGCCCAGTGATG3′ complementary to the capsid coding region of H/PF/2013 and MR766, respectively. Amplicons were analysed by agarose gel electrophoresis using Midori Green (Biozym, Hessisch Oldendorf, Germany) staining of DNA.

2.10. Immunofluorescence Microscopy and Western Blotting

For immunofluorescence microscopy 2.5–3.5 $\times 10^4$ cells/well were seeded in DMEMcplt into 24-well plates containing glass coverslips. At the indicated time points the cells were washed twice with PBS and fixed for 20 min by addition of 500 μL PBS containing 4% paraformaldehyde. After three washes with PBS, the cells were permeabilized with 0.2% Triton-X100 in PBS for 5 min. Permeabilized cells were blocked for one hour in PBS containing 0.01% Tween20 (PBS-T-0.01%) and 5% bovine serum albumin (BSA). The cells were incubated with the respective primary antibodies at appropriate concentrations for 2 h at room temperature. After three washes, the cells were incubated with the respective AlexaFluor (488, 568)-conjugated anti-mouse or anti-rabbit secondary antibodies (Life Technologies), respectively, diluted in PBS-T-0.01% containing 5% BSA. After three washes the nuclear DNA was stained with DAPI (Sigma-Aldrich) for 10 min. Finally, the coverslips were mounted on slides with FluoromountG (SouthernBiotech, Birmingham, AL, USA). The images were acquired with a Nikon Eclipse Ti microscope (Nikon, Tokyo, Japan) or a Leica SP8 (Leica, Wetzlar, Germany) confocal microscope. Western blotting was performed exactly as described earlier [27].

3. Results

3.1. In Silico Prediction of CEPs and Assembly of Synthetic Full Length ZIKV cDNAs

We focused on the development of infectious clones for two different ZIKV strains: MR766, which is a historical strain isolated from a rhesus monkey in 1947 [28] and H/PF/2013, a clinical isolate obtained in 2013 from a patient returning from French Polynesia [29]. Nucleotide sequences of the clones were based on the reference sequence DQ859059 for MR766 and KJ776791 for H/PF/2013. In addition, we determined the nucleotide sequences of these two virus strains that we propagated once in C6/36 mosquito cells and once in VeroE6 cells. We found that the H/PF/2013 isolate cultured in our cells was almost identical to the reference sequence with the exception of one nucleotide exchange resulting in an E1399Q amino acid substitution residing in NS2B, while the MR766 isolate differed by four nucleotide changes, two of them leading to E2197G and T3078A amino acid substitutions, residing in the NS4A and the NS5 coding region, respectively.

To assemble the complete genomes of these two strains, we introduced the mutations found in the viruses propagated in our laboratory and inserted in addition several silent nucleotide substitutions removing or creating restriction sites for convenient DNA cloning (Tables S1 and S2). These two sequences were dissected into 4 fragments that were generated by DNA synthesis (Figure 1A,B). The synthetic DNA fragments were assembled and inserted into a pFK-based vector via unique restriction sites [23]. A T7 promoter was inserted upstream of the ZIKV-5'UTR to allow for in vitro transcription of viral RNA. However, while fragments #2–#4 could be combined and amplified in *E. coli* with ease, insertion of fragment #1 repeatedly failed as we were not able to propagate a full-length ligation product. We reasoned that toxicity associated with fragment #1 might be the reason for our failure. In fact, for ZIKV it has been hypothesized that translation products generated from transcripts initiated at CEPs present in the structural region and NS1 might cause toxicity in bacteria [13]. Therefore, we decided to inactivate these bacterial promoters, a strategy successfully applied to the molecular cloning of DENV2 and JEV [11] and analysed our ZIKV sequences by using the promoter prediction tool from the Berkeley Drosophila Genome Project [20,21]. For MR766, 12 putative CEPs with a score >0.85 were detected within the first 2664 nucleotides (Figure 1A,B; Figure S1). By contrast, only eight putative CEPs were predicted within the first 2683 nucleotides of the H/PF/2013 genome (Figure 1B; Figures S1 and S2). To inactive these CEPs, nucleotide substitutions were inserted affecting the -10 region (Pribnow/ Schaller box) and/or the −35 region of all but one putative promoter. We did not alter the CEPs in the 5' untranslated region (5'UTR) of our ZIKV strains because they contain complex RNA structures essential for RNA replication [22]. In total, 18 point mutations were introduced for MR766 and 12 for H/PF/2013 (Figures S1 and S2). For both strains, the modified sequence of fragment #1 was generated synthetically and inserted into the corresponding preassembled ZIKV constructs containing fragments #2–#4 without notable problems (Figure 1A,B). To confirm the stability of these synthetic full length ZIKV (synZIKV) cDNAs, the plasmids were passaged five times in *E. coli* and 5 clones of passage 5 were analysed by analytical restriction digest in comparison to the parental clone (Figure 1C). No obvious changes of the restriction patterns were found. Importantly, nucleotide sequences of the ZIKV genomes isolated after five bacterial passages were identical to the original genome and matched exactly the one generated in silico. Together, this result demonstrates that the synZIKV cDNA clones contained in the single bacterial plasmid vector are stable and that CEP silencing is a very simple and versatile approach to overcome stability problems of difficult-to-clone sequences.

3.2. Functionality of Full-Length synZIKV Wild-Type Genomes

With the aim to determine functionality of the cloned full length synZIKV genomes VeroE6 cells were transfected with in vitro transcripts of synZIKV-MR766 and synZIKV-H/PF/2013. Peak virus titres of about 10^6 plaque-forming units (PFU/mL) were detected in cell culture supernatants; maximum titres were reached faster by the MR766 strain than the HP/F/2013 strain arguing for different replication kinetics (Figure 2A). A comparison of the replication kinetics of the two synZIKV strains with the parental strains in Huh7 cells revealed virtually identical viral fitness in the case of the MR766 strain (Figure 2B). By contrast, wild-type synZIKV-H/PF/2013 replication was attenuated in this cell line relative to the parental H/PF/2013 strain but titres still reached ~10^6 PFU/mL (Figure 2C). Similar results were obtained after infection with lower MOI [30]. Irrespective of that, plaque morphology was well comparable between the two synZIKVs and their parental strains (Figure 2D). The synMR766 strain formed smaller and more defined plaques, whereas synZIKV-H/PF/2013 formed large more diffuse and heterogeneous plaques but in both cases just like the corresponding WT strains (Figure 2D).

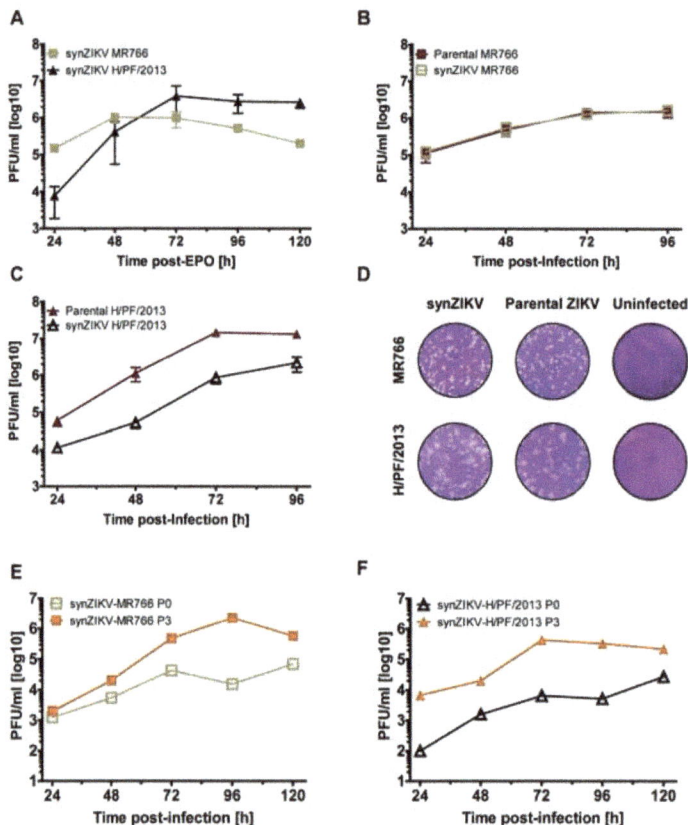

Figure 2. Replication kinetics of viruses obtained with the full-length synZIKV clones. (**A**) Replication kinetics of the two synZIKV clones as determined by plaque assay. VeroE6 cells were transfected with in vitro transcribed synZIKV RNAs and virus contained in culture supernatant at different time points after transfection was measured. Mean ± SEM of two independent experiments is shown. (**B,C**) Comparison of replication kinetics of synZIKV and parental viruses. Huh7 cells were infected with either ZIKV using a multiplicity of infection (MOI) of 1. Supernatants from infected cells were harvested at indicated times post-infection and titres were determined by plaque assay. Mean ± SEM of three independent experiments is shown. (**D**) Comparison of plaque morphology of synZIKV and the parental viruses. (**E,F**) Replication kinetics of passaged synZIKVs. Virus stocks were prepared as described in Materials and methods (P0). Huh7 cells were infected with MOI = 0.1 of P0 virus, cell culture supernatants were collected 72 h post-infection (P1) and passaged two more times by infection of Huh7 cells (P2–P3) in 72 h intervals. Huh7 cells were then infected using a MOI of 0.01 of P0 and P3 virus, respectively and virus titres were measured at indicated time points by plaque assay.

To determine whether passaging in cell culture could increase the fitness of our synZIKVs, we performed three serial passages in Huh7 cells and compared the replication kinetics of P0 and P3 viruses (Figure 2E,F). For both strains titres obtained with passaged viruses were higher than the ones of the corresponding P0 stock arguing for rapid adaptation of synZIKVs to cell culture conditions. Whether distinct adaptive mutations or the viral quasispecies in P3 virus cultures were responsible for increased fitness remains to be determined.

3.3. Replication and Stability of synZIKV Luciferase Reporter Virus Genomes

Reverse genetic systems are powerful tools to study virus biology and pathogenesis but for some applications such as high-content screens reporter systems are superior because of the ease to measure virus replication in high-throughput formats [10]. We therefore manipulated both synZIKV genomes by insertion of a *Renilla luciferase* (*RLuc*) reporter gene (Figure 3A). In these genomes, the 5′ UTR is followed by the first 102 nts of the C-coding region containing an element that is required for genome circularization (CAE; capsid-circularization sequence). Downstream of the CAE we inserted the *RLuc* gene via engineered NotI and NruI restriction sites followed by the ribosome-skipping 2A sequence of the foot-mouth-disease virus (FMDV) to allow the release of the RLuc protein from the viral polyprotein. The functionality of these two synZIKV-R2A genomes was evaluated by electroporation of in vitro transcripts into VeroE6 cells. Virus replication was confirmed in transfected cells by E-specific immunofluorescence (Figure 3B) and quantified by measuring RLuc reporter activity in lysates of cells harvested at different time points after transfection (Figure 3C). As a reference, we constructed for both synZIKV-R2A clones a mutant, in which the catalytic site of the RNA-dependent-RNA-polymerase was inactivated by site-directed mutagenesis (mutants "GAA"). In addition, values were normalized to the 4 h-value reflecting transfection efficiency. For both synZIKV-R2A clones, robust replication was detected with faster kinetics in the case of the MR766 strain (Figure 3C) but comparable values detected at later time points after transfection (>96 h). However, as reported earlier [31], synZIKV-R2A viruses did not form plaques when harvested at early times post-transfection arguing that the insertion of the reporter gene caused attenuation [32].

Therefore, we determined the stability of the reporter virus genomes by multiple passaging of synZIKV-R2A particles collected 72 h post-transfection in VeroE6 cells. Virus contained in supernatants of each passage was used to infect Huh7 cells to determine RLuc reporter activity and plaque formation (Figure 3D,E). While RLuc activities were steadily decreasing with each passage and lost after passage 3 (Figure 3D), virus titres (PFU/mL) were increasing (Figure 3E) indicating a loss of the reporter gene and selection for synZIKV viruses with high replication fitness and plaque forming capability.

To support this assumption, synZIKV-R2A viruses released into culture supernatants were harvested after each passage, RNA was isolated and the region encompassing the RLuc coding sequence was amplified by RT-PCR (Figure 3F). In virus released from transfected cells (P0 supernatant), the amplicon had the expected size for the luciferase reporter gene (~1350 bp) although trace amounts of a smaller amplicon were also detected. However, already in P1 supernatant we could only amplify a fragment with a size expected for a WT clone (~250 bp). Sequence analysis of this PCR product confirmed a perfect match to the WT clone sequence, consistent with a rapid loss of the reporter gene. Nevertheless, by using virus contained in the supernatant of synZIKV-R2A transfected cells (i.e., P0 virus), virus replication was robustly detected and could be used for various assays, including antiviral drug testing. For instance, in line with a previous report [33], we found that the nucleoside 2′CMC strongly reduced the replication of both reporter viruses, thus demonstrating the versatility of our synZIKV system (Figure 3F).

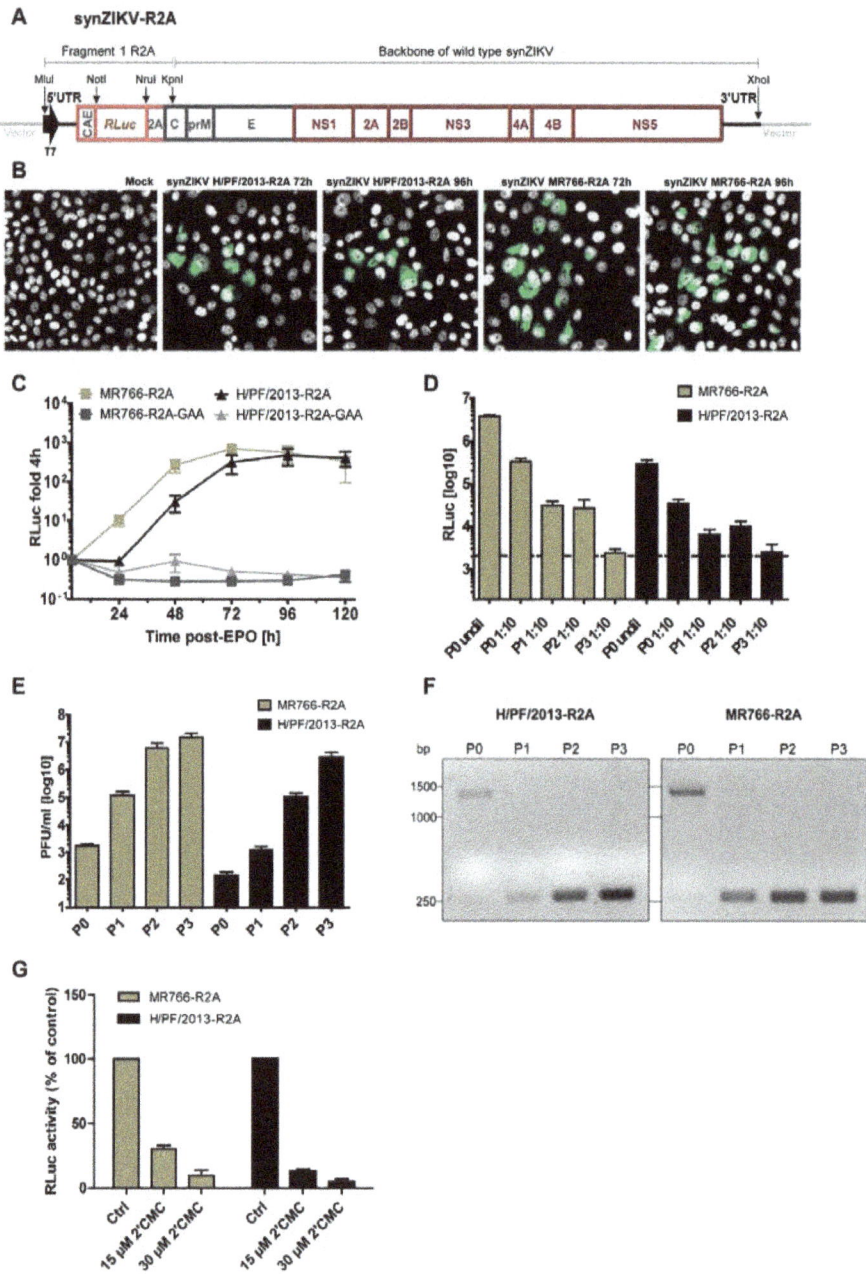

Figure 3. Construction and characterization of synZIKV-R2A reporter virus genomes. (**A**) Schematic representation of the synZIKV-R2A reporter virus genomes. For both strains the R2A reporter cassette (light red) was inserted into the wild-type pFK-synZIKV plasmids via MLuI/KpnI restriction sites. The NotI/NruI sites flanking the *RLuc* gene allow for the exchange of the reporter gene. (**B**) Immunofluorescence analysis of VeroE6 cells transfected with synZIKV-R2A in vitro transcripts. Cells were grown on coverslips, fixed 72 h and 96 h after transfection and stained with E-specific antibody (green). Nuclear DNA was counterstained with DAPI (grey). Scale bar = 15 µm. (**C**) Replication kinetics

of the synZIKV-R2A reporter viruses in VeroE6 cells. After electroporation (EPO) cells were harvested at given time points and RLuc activity was determined. Values were normalized to the 4 h-value reflecting transfection efficiency. Mean ± SEM of three independent experiments is shown. Replication deficient mutants containing two mutations affecting the active site of the RNA-dependent-RNA polymerase in NS5 (GAA) served as negative controls. (**D**) VeroE6 cells were transfected with synZIKV-R2A RNAs, cell culture supernatants were collected 72 h post- transfection (P0) and passaged three times by infection of VeroE6 cells (P1-P3) in 72 h intervals. Culture supernatants obtained from each passage were used to inoculate Huh7 cells. In the case of supernatant obtained directly from transfected VeroE6 cells (P0), Huh7 cells were inoculated with undiluted (undil) or 1:10 diluted supernatant. After 72 h cells were harvested and RLuc activity in cell lysates was determined. Mean ± SEM from two independent experiments is shown. (**E**) Virus titres as determined by plaque assay for each synZIKV-R2A passage; values are mean ± SEM of two independent experiments. (**F**) Stability of the reporter gene. SynZIKV-R2A viruses released into culture supernatants were harvested after each passage as described in panel D, RNA was isolated and the region encompassing the RLuc coding sequence was amplified by using random hexamer primers for reverse transcription and specific primers for subsequent PCR. The ~1350 bp long DNA fragment in the P0 virus sample corresponds to the reporter gene, while the ~250 bp long fragment corresponds to the WT sequence. (**G**) Antiviral assay using synZIKV-R2A viruses. VeroE6 cells were inoculated with a 1:10 dilution of a P0 stock and one hour later the medium was replaced with DMEM containing the indicated amount of 2'CMC. RLuc activity was measured in cell lysates 72 h post-infection. Mean ± SEM from two independent experiments is shown.

3.4. SynZIKV Reporter Viruses Suitable for Live Cell Imaging

In order to have at hand an easy to handle ZIKV system suitable for microscopy-based studies such as live-cell imaging, we replaced the *RLuc* reporter gene by a gene encoding the turbo far-red fluorescent protein FP635 (Figure 4A) [24]. Since ZIKV replicates in the cytoplasm we added a nuclear localization sequence (NLS) to the FP635 marker protein to avoid interference with imaging of cytoplasmic events. We used the well-studied NLS of the Simian Virus 40 (SV40) large T antigen that was fused to the C-terminus of FP635. Ninety-six hours after transfection with synZIKV-FP635 in vitro transcripts, cells were analysed by immune fluorescence to detect the E protein whereas FP635 was detected by its fluorescence (Figure 4B). Virtually all of the E-positive cells also expressed detectable amounts of FP635 (Figure 4B,C) suggesting that the synZIKV-FP635 reporter genomes are functional and allow the detection of infected cells just by means of the fluorescent marker protein. We noted that FP635 primarily accumulated within defined sub-nuclear regions, in line with a previous study reporting the accumulation of a GFP-SV40-NLS fusion protein in the nucleoli [34].

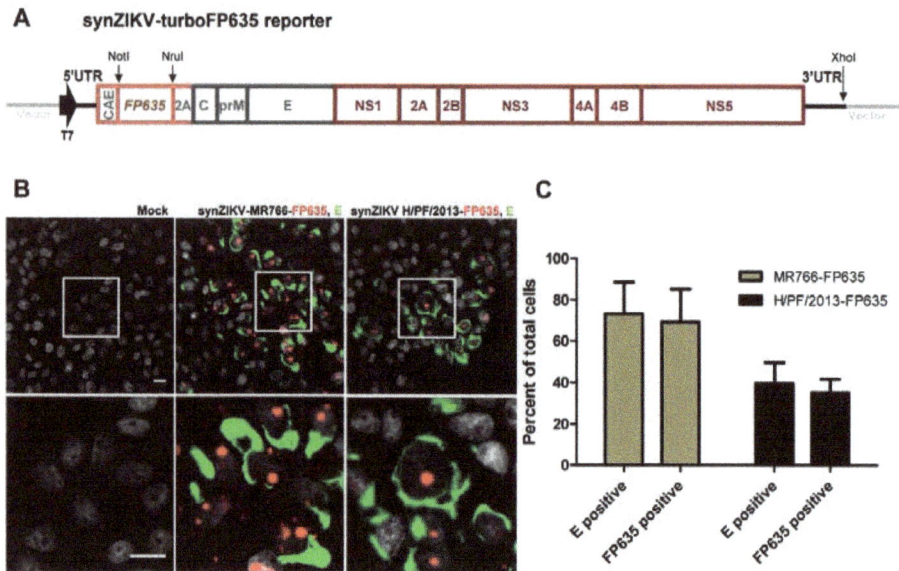

Figure 4. Construction and characterization of synZIKV-FP635 reporter viruses suitable for live cell imaging. (**A**) Schematic representation of the synZIKV-FP635 reporter genomes. The *FP635* gene fused at the 3′ end to the coding sequence of the SV40 NLS (not indicated) was inserted into the synZIKV constructs via NotI/NruI restriction sites. (**B**) Detection of E-antigen by immunofluorescence analysis of VeroE6 cells 96 h post-transfection with synZIKV-FP635 RNAs. The FP635 signal (red) was detected by its fluorescence. Note the accumulation of FP635 in distinct nuclear sites, most likely corresponding to nucleoli. Nuclear DNA was counterstained with DAPI (grey). Scale bar = 15 μm. (**C**) Quantification of E- and FP635-positive VeroE6 cells 96 h post-transfection with synZIKV-FP635 RNAs. Results show the mean from two independent experiments ± SEM. At least 150 cells per condition were counted.

3.5. Sub-Genomic synZIKV Replicons

In addition to full-length reporter viruses, sub-genomic replicons are powerful tools as they allow studying virus replication without biosafety concerns. Therefore, by using our full-length synZIKV molecular clones, we established sub-genomic RLuc reporter replicons. The overall construct design was analogous to the one of the synZIKV-R2A reporter genomes but the replicons lacked the region encoding the ZIKV structural proteins (Figure 5A). Replication of these sgR2A-synZIKV replicons was assessed in Huh7 cells (Figure 5B). RLuc activities detectable in the cell lysates at different time points after transfection correlated well with the amounts of ZIKV NS3 and NS4B proteins detectable by Western blot revealing that also in this case replication kinetics of the MR766 strain was faster than the H/PF/2013 strain (Figure 5C). NS3 as well as double-stranded RNA (dsRNA), a replication intermediate [22], were detectable by immunofluorescence (Figure 5C). As described for ZIKV-infected Huh7 cells, sgR2A-synZIKV-transfected cells had a kidney shaped nucleus [25]. This observation suggests that the non-structural proteins of ZIKV are sufficient to induce changes of nucleus morphology. In summary, these results show that sgR2A-synZIKV replicons are functional and induce morphological changes resembling a ZIKV infection.

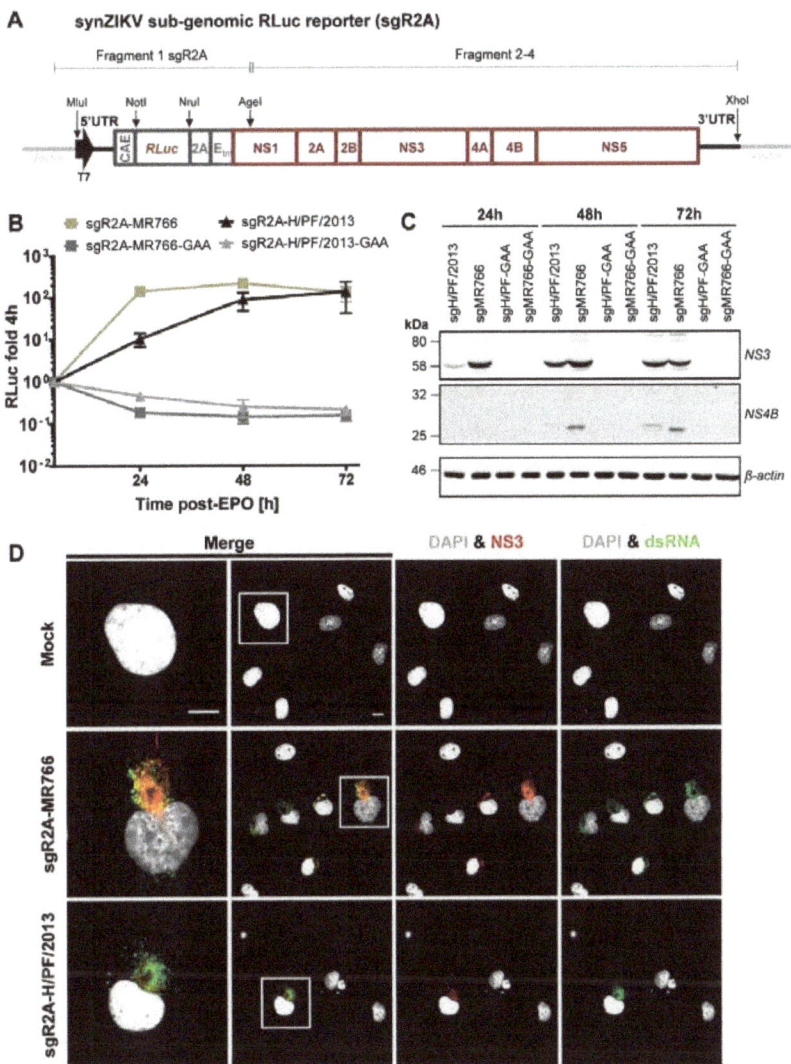

Figure 5. Properties of synZIKV sub-genomic reporter replicons. (**A**) Schematic representation of the synZIKV-sgR2A subgenomic reporter replicons. The reporter cassette (grey) was inserted into the synZIKV genomes via the MluI and AgeI restriction sites and replaces the region encoding the structural proteins. (**B**) RLuc activity in Huh7 cells transfected with wild-type or replication-deficient (mutant GAA) synZIKV-sgR2A replicon RNAs measured at given times post-transfection. Shown RLuc values were normalized to the 4 h value to correct for transfection efficiency. Mean ± SEM of three independent experiments is presented. (**C**) Western blot showing the abundance of ZIKV NS3 and NS4B proteins in Huh7 cells transfected with synZIKV-sgR2A replicon RNAs. Cells were lysed at indicated times post-transfection and ZIKV-specific antibodies were used to detect viral proteins. β actin served as loading control. Numbers on the left refer to the positions of marker proteins that are given in kilodalton (kDa). (**D**) Immunofluorescence analysis of Huh7 cells 48 h post-transfection of synZIKV-sgR2A RNAs. Cells were stained with a dsRNA- (green) and a NS3-specific antibody (red). Nuclear DNA was stained with DAPI (grey). Scale bars = 15 μm. Boxed areas indicate regions that are shown in the left panels as enlargements.

4. Discussion

Here we describe a straightforward and very simple approach to establish a ZIKV reverse genetics system. The key feature is to remove CEPs, responsible for genome instability [9], by using in silico prediction with an open-access online tool and subsequent elimination in the virus sequence by silent nucleotide substitutions. This strategy was successfully applied to two different ZIKV strains—MR766 and H/PF/2013—for which construction of full-length cDNA clones has failed in the past [13,15,17,18] (A.P. and R.B., unpublished). Our approach allows the amplification of functional ZIKV infectious clones on a single, low-copy plasmid, which is superior to time consuming and error prone multi-vector systems reported earlier [15–19]. Moreover, in vitro transcripts generated from our synZIKV clones are infectious, thus mimicking an infection better than DNA-launched systems requiring nuclear transcription of the viral RNA genome. Finally, the possibility to stably propagate the ZIKV genome in a pBR-derived vector circumvents several disadvantages inherent to the use of bacterial artificial chromosome (BAC) systems, such as low DNA yield and complicated procedures to introduce mutations into the genome [35–37].

We did not observe a difference in replication dynamics between the wild-type synZIKV-MR766 molecular clone and the parental MR766 virus, suggesting that the molecular clone fully recapitulates the properties of the parental strain. Also, the plaque morphologies produced by both synZIKV-MR766 and synZIKV-H/PF/2013 closely resembled those of reference viruses. However, we observed that the synZIKV-H/PF/2013 molecular clone was attenuated (Figure 2E). The reasons underlying the reduced fitness are currently unknown. Although the sequence of the synZIKV-H/PF/2013 clone was modified to silence the CEPs and introduce unique restriction sites, these changes are unlikely to contribute to decreased viral fitness as all of the inserted mutations were silent and the regions known to contain regulatory RNA elements were omitted. We note however, that the attenuation observed by us is in line with the study of Widman and co-workers who constructed an H/PF/2013 molecular clone by using an in vitro ligation strategy and observed a similar degree of attenuation [15]. The fitness difference between the synZIKV-H/PF/2013 clone and the reference strain might be due to the genetic homogeneity of the molecular clone whereas the genome population of the H/PF/2013 isolate most likely is more heterogeneous, thus allowing for faster adaption to the cell culture conditions. Additionally, studies on poliovirus and influenza viruses showed that individual variants within viral quasispecies can cooperate to increase the fitness of the total virus population [38,39]. For MR766 this might not apply because this virus has been well adapted to cell culture conditions through intensive passaging since its isolation in 1947 [7]. This adaptation probably is already reflected in the cDNA sequence that served as reference for our clone (DQ859059). Nevertheless, fitness of both synZIKVs could be increased by cell culture passaging, arguing for rapid adaptation of both synZIKV strains and selection for variants with fitness even higher than the parental strains. Although we do not know whether distinct mutations in these synZIKV genomes or the -most likely- higher genetic heterogeneity in P3 stocks account for increased fitness, the use of extensively cell culture passaged virus is less desirable as it might have altered in vivo properties that are not necessarily detectable in vitro. Therefore, it is preferable to work with strains of low passage and defined sequence, which is the case with molecular clones as described here. Moreover, we note that the MR766 strain belongs to the early ZIKV isolates whereas H/PF/2013 is a more recent clinical strain that is closely related to strains isolated during the ZIKV epidemic in Brazil. For instance, the HP/F/2013 strain that we constructed has ~99.5% nucleotide sequence identity with the PE243 strain isolated from a Brazilian patient in 2015 (accession number KX197192) and only one amino acid change. Thus, our synZIKV clones should be useful for comparative studies between historical and contemporary ZIKV strains.

Owing to the reduction of replication fitness by the insertion of the *RLuc* reporter gene this ZIKV reporter virus was rather unstable and reporter-less variants with higher replication fitness were rapidly enriched during cell passage and already after one passage WT was the predominant species. This rapid deletion might be due to recombination occurring in *E. coli* during plasmid amplification and being facilitated by the partial duplication of the capsid coding region (i.e., the first

103 nts containing important *cis*-acting sequences of ZIKV), up- and downstream of the reporter gene. Alternatively, recombination might occur during virus propagation in cell culture. In any case, owing to higher fitness the WT virus rapidly out-competes the reporter virus and becomes the predominant species. Although this problem can be overcome by using ZIKV RLuc reporter viruses contained in culture supernatant of transfected (producer) cells, in which WT virus was not detected (Figure 3D,F), long-term propagation is not possible, which is a limitation when large stocks of reporter viruses are required. Therefore, further attempts are required to stabilize the inserted reporter gene, for example, by altering the sequences flanking the reporter gene, or inserting it into another region of the ZIKV genome. An alternative strategy might be the use of *trans*-complemented particles as we have developed for hepatitis C virus and DENV [40,41]. In this case the subgenomic replicon is transfected into a packaging cell line stably expressing the structural proteins. Virus-like particles are released from these cells that retain infectivity but contain the subgenomic RNA, thus requiring only low biosafety level. Importantly, since the size of the subgenomic replicon is much smaller than the complete genome it allows the insertion of rather long heterologous sequences without exceeding the size of the full-length genome.

In summary, this study reports a comprehensive toolbox for ZIKV research and an easy ZIKV cloning strategy that is based on CEP silencing, initially described for DENV2 and JEV [11]. As continuing globalization supports spreading of flaviviruses and their arthropod hosts, it is possible that outbreaks of other poorly characterized flaviviruses might occur in the future. Therefore, the strategy described here for ZIKV should allow the rapid construction and stable propagation of functional molecular clones of potentially emerging flaviviruses and other difficult-to-clone viruses.

Supplementary Materials: The following are available online at http://www.mdpi.com/1999-4915/10/7/368/s1. Figure S1: Results of in silico prediction of cryptic prokaryotic promoters in the MR766 sequence. Figure S2: Results of in silico prediction of cryptic prokaryotic promoters in the H/PF/2013 sequence. Table S1: Modified restriction sites in the MR766 syn-sequence. Table S2: Modified restriction sites in the H/PF/2013 syn-sequence.

Author Contributions: Conceived and designed the study: A.P. and R.B.; performed the experiments: M.M., A.P., C.J.N., S.G., M.C.; analysed and interpreted the data: M.M., A.P., M.C.; provided important advice: G.L.; wrote the manuscript: M.M., A.P. and R.B.

Funding: This research was funded by the Bundesministerium für Bildung und Forschung (project TTU 01.911) and the Deutsche Forschungsgemeinschaft (Ba1505/8-1). A.P. was funded via the European Union's Horizon 2020 research and innovation programme under the Marie Skłodowska-Curie grant agreement No 642434 (to R.B.). C.J.N was funded by a European Molecular Biology Organization (EMBO) Long-Term Fellowship (ALTF 466-2016). The funding institutions had no role in the design of the study; in the collection, analyses, or interpretation of data; in the writing of the manuscript and in the decision to publish the results.

Acknowledgments: We are grateful to Marie Bartenschlager and Ulrike Herian for excellent technical support. We also thank the European Virus Archive (EVAg) for the provision of the MR766 and the HP/F/2013 strains.

Conflicts of Interest: The authors declare no conflict of interest.

References

1. Dick, G.W.; Kitchen, S.F.; Haddow, A.J. Zika virus (I). Isolations and serological specificity. *Trans. R. Soc. Trop. Med. Hyg.* **1952**, *46*, 509–520. [CrossRef]
2. Duffy, M.R.; Chen, T.H.; Hancock, W.; Powers, A.M.; Kool, J.L.; Lanciotti, R.S.; Pretrick, M.; Marfel, M.; Holzbauer, S.; Dubray, C.; et al. Zika virus outbreak on Yap Island, Federated States of Micronesia. *N. Engl. J. Med.* **2009**, *360*, 2536–2543. [CrossRef] [PubMed]
3. Cao-Lormeau, V.M.; Roche, C.; Teissier, A.; Robin, E.; Berry, A.L.; Mallet, H.P.; Sall, A.L.; Musso, D. Zika virus, French Polynesia, South Pacific, 2013. *Emerg. Infect. Dis.* **2014**, *20*, 1085–1086. [CrossRef] [PubMed]
4. Brasil, P.; Calvet, G.A.; Siqueira, A.M.; Wakimoto, M.; de Sequeira, P.C.; Nobre, A.; de Mendonça, M.C.L.; Lupi, O.; de Souza, R.V.; Romero, C.; et al. Zika Virus Outbreak in Rio de Janeiro, Brazil: Clinical Characterization, Epidemiological and Virological Aspects. *PLoS Negl. Trop. Dis.* **2016**, *10*, e0004636. [CrossRef] [PubMed]

5. Do Rosario, M.S.; de Jesus, P.A.; Vasilakis, N.; Farias, D.S.; Novaes, M.A.; Rodrigues, S.G.; Martins, L.C.; da Costa Vasconcelos, P.F.; Ko, A.I.; Alcântara, L.C., Jr.; et al. Guillain-Barre Syndrome After Zika Virus Infection in Brazil. *Am. J. Trop. Med. Hyg.* **2016**, *95*, 1157–1160. [CrossRef] [PubMed]
6. Mlakar, J.; Korva, M.; Tul, N.; Popovic, M.; Poljsak-Prijatelj, M.; Mraz, J.; Kolenc, M.; Rus, K.R.; Vipotnik, T.V.; Vodušek, V.F.; et al. Zika Virus Associated with Microcephaly. *N. Engl. J. Med.* **2016**, *374*, 951–958. [CrossRef] [PubMed]
7. Haddow, A.D.; Schuh, A.J.; Yasuda, C.Y.; Kasper, M.R.; Heang, V.; Huy, R.; Guzman, H.; Tesh, R.B.; Weaver, S.C. Genetic characterization of Zika virus strains: Geographic expansion of the Asian lineage. *PLoS Negl. Trop. Dis.* **2012**, *6*, e1477. [CrossRef] [PubMed]
8. Diamond, M.S.; Coyne, C.B. Vaccines in 2017: Closing in on a Zika virus vaccine. *Nat. Rev. Immunol.* **2018**, *18*, 89–90. [CrossRef] [PubMed]
9. Aubry, F.; Nougairede, A.; Gould, E.A.; de Lamballerie, X. Flavivirus reverse genetic systems, construction techniques and applications: A historical perspective. *Antivir. Res.* **2015**, *114*, 67–85. [CrossRef] [PubMed]
10. Fischl, W.; Bartenschlager, R. High-Throughput Screening Using Dengue Virus Reporter Genomes. In *Antiviral Methods and Protocols*; Humana Press: Totowa, NJ, USA, 2013; Volume 1030, pp. 205–219.
11. Pu, S.Y.; Wu, R.H.; Yang, C.C.; Jao, T.M.; Tsai, M.H.; Wang, J.C.; Lin, H.M.; Chao, Y.S. Successful propagation of flavivirus infectious cDNAs by a novel method to reduce the cryptic bacterial promoter activity of virus genomes. *J. Virol.* **2011**, *85*, 2927–2941. [CrossRef] [PubMed]
12. Ruggli, N.; Rice, C.M. Functional cDNA Clones of the Flaviviridae: Strategies and Applications. In *Advances in Virus Research*; Academic Press: Cambridge, MA, USA, 1999; Volume 53, pp. 183–207.
13. Schwarz, M.C.; Sourisseau, M.; Espino, M.M.; Gray, E.S.; Chambers, M.T.; Tortorella, D.; Evans, M.J. Rescue of the 1947 Zika Virus Prototype Strain with a Cytomegalovirus Promoter-Driven cDNA Clone. *mSphere* **2016**, *1*, e00246-16. [CrossRef] [PubMed]
14. Tsetsarkin, K.A.; Kenney, H.; Chen, R.; Liu, G.; Manukyan, H.; Whitehead, S.S.; Laassric, M.; Chumakovc, K.; Pletneva, A.G. A Full-Length Infectious cDNA Clone of Zika Virus from the 2015 Epidemic in Brazil as a Genetic Platform for Studies of Virus-Host Interactions and Vaccine Development. *mBio* **2016**, *7*, e01114-16. [CrossRef] [PubMed]
15. Widman, D.G.; Young, E.; Yount, B.L.; Plante, K.S.; Gallichotte, E.N.; Carbaugh, D.L.; Peck, K.M.; Plante, J.; Swanstrom, J.; Heise, M.T.; et al. A Reverse Genetics Platform That Spans the Zika Virus Family Tree. *MBio* **2017**, *8*, e02014-16. [CrossRef] [PubMed]
16. Weger-Lucarelli, J.; Duggal, N.K.; Bullard-Feibelman, K.; Veselinovic, M.; Romo, H.; Nguyen, C.; Rückert, C.; Brault, A.C.; Bowen, R.A.; Stenglein, M.; et al. Development and Characterization of Recombinant Virus Generated from a New World Zika Virus Infectious Clone. *J. Virol.* **2017**, *91*, JVI-01765. [CrossRef] [PubMed]
17. Gadea, G.; Bos, S.; Krejbich-Trotot, P.; Clain, E.; Viranaicken, W.; El-Kalamouni, C.; Mavingui, P.; Desprès, P. A robust method for the rapid generation of recombinant Zika virus expressing the *GFP* reporter gene. *Virology* **2016**, *497*, 157–162. [CrossRef] [PubMed]
18. Atieh, T.; Baronti, C.; de Lamballerie, X.; Nougairede, A. Simple reverse genetics systems for Asian and African Zika viruses. *Sci. Rep.* **2016**, *6*, 39384. [CrossRef] [PubMed]
19. Setoh, Y.X.; Prow, N.A.; Peng, N.; Hugo, L.E.; Devine, G.; Hazlewood, J.E.; Suhrbier, A.; Khromykh, A.A. De Novo Generation and Characterization of New Zika Virus Isolate Using Sequence Data from a Microcephaly Case. *mSphere* **2017**, *2*, e00190-17. [CrossRef] [PubMed]
20. Berkeley Drosophila Genome Project, Neural Network Promoter Prediction. Available online: http://www.fruitfly.org/seq_tools/promoter.html (accessed on 15 May 2017).
21. Reese, M.G. Application of a time-delay neural network to promoter annotation in the Drosophila melanogaster genome. *Comput. Chem.* **2001**, *26*, 51–56. [CrossRef]
22. Acosta, E.G.; Kumar, A.; Bartenschlager, R. Revisiting Dengue Virus-Host Cell Interaction: New Insights into Molecular and Cellular Virology. In *Advances in Virus Research*; Academic Press: Cambridge, MA, USA, 2014; Volume 88, pp. 1–109.
23. Lohmann, V.; Korner, F.; Koch, J.; Herian, U.; Theilmann, L.; Bartenschlager, R. Replication of subgenomic hepatitis C virus RNAs in a hepatoma cell line. *Science* **1999**, *285*, 110–113. [CrossRef] [PubMed]

24. Schmid, B.; Rinas, M.; Ruggieri, A.; Acosta, E.G.; Bartenschlager, M.; Reuter, A.; Fischl, W.; Harder, N.; Bergeest, J.-P.; Flossdorf, M.; et al. Live Cell Analysis and Mathematical Modeling Identify Determinants of Attenuation of Dengue Virus 2'-O-Methylation Mutant. *PLoS Pathog.* **2015**, *11*, e1005345. [CrossRef] [PubMed]

25. Cortese, M.; Goellner, S.; Acosta, E.G.; Neufeldt, C.J.; Oleksiuk, O.; Lampe, M.; Haselmann, U.; Funaya, C.; Schieber, N.; Ronchi, P.; et al. Ultrastructural Characterization of Zika Virus Replication Factories. *Cell. Rep.* **2017**, *18*, 2113–2123. [CrossRef] [PubMed]

26. Kumar, A.; Buhler, S.; Selisko, B.; Davidson, A.; Mulder, K.; Canard, B.; Miller, S.; Bartenschlager, R. Nuclear localization of dengue virus nonstructural protein 5 does not strictly correlate with efficient viral RNA replication and inhibition of type I interferon signaling. *J. Virol.* **2013**, *87*, 4545–4557. [CrossRef] [PubMed]

27. Chatel-Chaix, L.; Fischl, W.; Scaturro, P.; Cortese, M.; Kallis, S.; Bartenschlager, M.; Fischer, B.; Bartenschlager, R. A Combined Genetic-Proteomic Approach Identifies Residues within Dengue Virus NS4B Critical for Interaction with NS3 and Viral Replication. *J. Virol.* **2015**, *89*, 7170–7186. [CrossRef] [PubMed]

28. Kuno, G.; Chang, G.J. Full-length sequencing and genomic characterization of Bagaza, Kedougou, and Zika viruses. *Arch. Virol.* **2007**, *152*, 687–696. [CrossRef] [PubMed]

29. Baronti, C.; Piorkowski, G.; Charrel, R.N.; Boubis, L.; Leparc-Goffart, I.; de Lamballerie, X. Complete coding sequence of zika virus from a French polynesia outbreak in 2013. *Genome Announc.* **2014**, *2*, e00500-14. [CrossRef] [PubMed]

30. Płaszczyca, A.; Bartenschlager, R. Heidelberg University, Heidelberg, Germany. Replication kinetics of synZIKVs in Huh7 cells. Unpublished work. 2018.

31. Shan, C.; Xie, X.; Muruato, A.E.; Rossi, S.L.; Roundy, C.M.; Azar, S.R.; Yang, Y.; Tesh, R.B.; Bourne, N.; Barrett, A.D.; et al. An Infectious cDNA Clone of Zika Virus to Study Viral Virulence, Mosquito Transmission, and Antiviral Inhibitors. *Cell Host Microbe* **2016**, *19*, 891–900. [CrossRef] [PubMed]

32. Münster, M.; Bartenschlager, R. Heidelberg University, Heidelberg, Germany. Titration of synZIKV-R2A viruses. Unpublished work. 2017.

33. Zmurko, J.; Marques, R.E.; Schols, D.; Verbeken, E.; Kaptein, S.J.; Neyts, J. The Viral Polymerase Inhibitor 7-Deaza-2'-C-Methyladenosine Is a Potent Inhibitor of In Vitro Zika Virus Replication and Delays Disease Progression in a Robust Mouse Infection Model. *PLoS Negl. Trop. Dis.* **2016**, *10*, e0004695. [CrossRef] [PubMed]

34. Kitamura, A.; Nakayama, Y.; Kinjo, M. Efficient and dynamic nuclear localization of green fluorescent protein via RNA binding. *Biochem. Biophys. Res. Commun.* **2015**, *463*, 401–406. [CrossRef] [PubMed]

35. Mutso, M.; Saul, S.; Rausalu, K.; Susova, O.; Zusinaite, E.; Mahalingam, S.; Merits, A. Reverse genetic system, genetically stable reporter viruses and packaged subgenomic replicon based on a Brazilian Zika virus isolate. *J. Gen. Virol.* **2017**, *98*, 2712–2724. [CrossRef] [PubMed]

36. Tischer, B.K.; Kaufer, B.B. Viral bacterial artificial chromosomes: Generation, mutagenesis, and removal of mini-F sequences. *BioMed Res. Int.* **2012**, *2012*, 472537. [CrossRef] [PubMed]

37. Yang, Y.; Shan, C.; Zou, J.; Muruato, A.E.; Bruno, D.N.; de Almeida Medeiros, D.B.; Vasconcelos, P.F.C.; Rossi, S.L.; Weaver, S.C.; Xie, X.; et al. A cDNA Clone-Launched Platform for High-Yield Production of Inactivated Zika Vaccine. *EBioMedicine* **2017**, *17*, 145–156. [CrossRef] [PubMed]

38. Vignuzzi, M.; Stone, J.K.; Arnold, J.J.; Cameron, C.E.; Andino, R. Quasispecies diversity determines pathogenesis through cooperative interactions in a viral population. *Nature* **2006**, *439*, 344–348. [CrossRef] [PubMed]

39. Xue, K.S.; Hooper, K.A.; Ollodart, A.R.; Dingens, A.S.; Bloom, J.D. Cooperation between distinct viral variants promotes growth of H3N2 influenza in cell culture. *eLife* **2016**, *5*, e13974. [CrossRef] [PubMed]

40. Scaturro, P.; Trist, I.M.; Paul, D.; Kumar, A.; Acosta, E.G.; Byrd, C.M.; Jordan, R.; Brancale, A.; Bartenschlager, R. Characterization of the mode of action of a potent dengue virus capsid inhibitor. *J. Virol.* **2014**, *88*, 11540–11555. [CrossRef] [PubMed]

41. Steinmann, E.; Brohm, C.; Kallis, S.; Bartenschlager, R.; Pietschmann, T. Efficient trans-encapsidation of hepatitis C virus RNAs into infectious virus-like particles. *J. Virol.* **2008**, *82*, 7034–7046. [CrossRef] [PubMed]

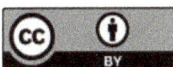

viruses

MDPI

Article

Tet-Inducible Production of Infectious Zika Virus from the Full-Length cDNA Clones of African- and Asian-Lineage Strains

Lizhou Zhang [1], Wei Ji [2], Shuang Lyu [1], Luhua Qiao [1] and Guangxiang Luo [1,2,*

[1] Department of Microbiology, University of Alabama at Birmingham School of Medicine, Birmingham, AL 35294, USA; lizhou8728@gmail.com (L.Z.); shuanglv@uab.edu (S.L.); luhuaq@gmail.com (L.Q.)
[2] Department of Microbiology, Peking University Health Science Center School of Basic Medical Sciences, Beijing 100191, China; jiwei_yunlong@126.com
* Correspondence: gluo@uab.edu; Tel.: +1-(205)-975-2936

Received: 14 September 2018; Accepted: 5 December 2018; Published: 9 December 2018

Abstract: Zika virus (ZIKV) is a mosquito-borne flavivirus that has emerged as an important human viral pathogen, causing congenital malformation including microcephaly among infants born to mothers infected with the virus during pregnancy. Phylogenetic analysis suggested that ZIKV can be classified into African and Asian lineages. In this study, we have developed a stable plasmid-based reverse genetic system for robust production of both ZIKV prototype African-lineage MR766 and clinical Asian-lineage FSS13025 strains using a tetracycline (Tet)-controlled gene expression vector. Transcription of the full-length ZIKV RNA is under the control of the Tet-responsive P_{tight} promoter at the 5′ end and an antigenomic ribozyme of hepatitis delta virus at the 3′ end. The transcription of infectious ZIKV RNA genome was efficiently induced by doxycycline. This novel ZIKV reverse genetics system will be valuable for the study of molecular viral pathogenesis of ZIKV and the development of new vaccines against ZIKV infection.

Keywords: Zika virus; reverse genetics; infectious cDNA; Tet-inducible; MR766; FSS13025

1. Introduction

Zika virus (ZIKV), an arthropod-borne virus, belongs to the *Flavivirus* genus of the Flaviviridae family, which includes several other important human pathogens such as yellow fever virus (YFV), dengue virus (DENV), and West Nile virus (WNV). ZIKV was first discovered in the Zika forest area of Uganda in 1947 [1]. In recent years, it has emerged as an important human viral pathogen, causing several major epidemics in Yap Island and Micronesia, French Polynesia, and South America [2]. Although ZIKV infection is often asymptomatic or mild in clinical manifestation, it can cause congenital malformations, including microcephaly, intrauterine growth retardation, and neurodevelopmental delays, in infants born to mothers infected with the virus during pregnancy [3]. Its infection is also associated with the neurologic disorder Guillain–Barre syndrome in adults [4]. In contrast to other mosquito-borne flaviviruses, ZIKV can cause persistent infection in humans and primates [5,6] and can be transmitted sexually [7–9]. Currently, there are no antiviral drugs or vaccines for the control of ZIKV infection.

ZIKV is an enveloped RNA virus with a positive-sense and single-stranded RNA genome of about 10,800 nucleotides. The viral genomic RNA contains a single open reading frame encoding a large viral polyprotein of 3423 amino acids. Upon translation, the viral polyprotein is cleaved by host and viral proteases into structural proteins (capsid [C], premembrane [prM], and envelope [E]) and nonstructural (NS) proteins (NS1, NS2A, NS2B, NS3, NS4A, NS4B, and NS5) [10,11]. Phylogenetic analysis classified

ZIKV into two major lineages: African lineage and Asian lineage, which exhibit different growth capacity and virulence in vitro and in vivo [12–15]. However, the underlying molecular aspects for distinct viral growth and pathogenesis between African and Asian lineages remain unknown.

The recent development of ZIKV reverse genetics systems has made it possible to determine the role and underlying molecular mechanism of viral proteins in viral replication and pathogenesis as well as for attenuated virus vaccine development [16–21]. Over the course of ZIKV cDNA construction, its genetic instability and toxicity in bacteria were found to be major obstacles to obtaining the full-length infectious cDNA, particularly for the prototype MR766 virus. It was speculated that the presence of cryptic bacterial promoters permits expression of viral peptides/proteins that are toxic to bacteria [22–24]. Several strategies have been explored to overcome the problems associated with viral toxicity and genetic instability in bacteria. The first full-length cDNA of ZIKV (Asian-lineage FSS13025 strain) was successfully constructed by using a very-low-copy plasmid as the vector in conjunction with a T7 promoter for in vitro transcription of ZIKV RNA by a T7 RNA polymerase [18]. Similarly, another group used an SP6 promoter to drive in vitro transcription of the full-length ZIKV RNA. In the latter case, a self-splicing intron was inserted into the C-terminal coding region of the E protein. The SP6 RNA transcripts were subjected to in vitro splicing in order to produce the infectious ZIKV RNA [25]. Alternatively, ZIKV cDNA fragments were amplified separately and cloned into different plasmids, followed by Gibson assembly or DNA ligation in vitro to produce the full-length ZIKV cDNA [20,21,26]. The resulting full-length cDNA was subsequently used as the template for in vitro T7 transcription to produce infectious ZIKV RNAs. Apart from in vitro transcription of infectious ZIKV RNA, infectious ZIKV RNA could be directly produced in the cell by cloning its cDNA into a mammalian expression vector. Transcription of infectious ZIKV RNA is driven by a polymerase II promoter at the $5'$ end of ZIKV cDNA. In the case of infectious ZIKV cDNA, a synthetic intron sequence had to be inserted into the *NS1* or *NS5* gene in order to avoid viral toxicity to bacteria [16,19]. The silence of the cryptic bacterial promoters was also reported to get around toxicity [23]. In present study, we have constructed infectious ZIKV cDNA independent of in vitro RNA transcription or intron insertion using a tetracycline (Tet)-controlled transcription vector. The full-length ZIKV cDNAs were cloned into the pTRE-Tight vector under the control of the Tet-responsive P_{tight} promoter and the antigenomic ribozyme of hepatitis delta virus (HDV). Both African- and Asian-lineage ZIKV were robustly produced upon DNA transfection and treatment with doxycycline. This novel ZIKV reverse genetics system will facilitate genetic determination of the underlying molecular mechanism of ZIKV replication and pathogenesis as well as genetic manipulation of infectious ZIKV for vaccine development.

2. Materials and Methods

2.1. Cell Culture and Virus

Vero and C6/36 (CRL-1660) cell lines were obtained from America type culture collection (ATCC, Manassas, VA, USA) and cultured in Dulbecco's modified Eagle's medium (DMEM) supplemented with 10% fetal bovine serum (FBS) (Atlanta Biologicals, Atlanta, GA, USA), 0.1 mM nonessential amino acids, penicillin-streptomycin (Sigma-Aldrich, St. Louis, MO, USA and HyClone, Logan, UT, USA) at 37 °C in a 5% CO_2 incubator. ZIKV African-lineage MR766 strain was obtained from ATCC and propagated in C6/36 and Vero cells.

2.2. DNA Construction

pTRE-Tight vector containing the Tet-responsive element and a minimal cytomegalovirus (CMV) promoter (P_{tight}) was described previously [27]. pTet-On vector expressing a reverse Tet-responsive transcriptional activator (rtTA) was from Takara Bio. The full-length infectious cDNA of ZIKV/MR766 was amplified by reverse transcription polymerase chain reaction (RT-PCR) similar to the methods used previously by others [16,18]. The virion RNA (vRNA) was isolated from the supernatant of the

ZIKV/MR766-infected Vero cells using QIAamp Viral RNA Kits (Qiagen, Inc., Valencia, CA, USA). The full-length viral cDNA was initially amplified as five subgenomic cDNA fragments by RT-PCR using specific primers containing unique restriction enzyme sites and cloned into the pEASY-Blunt vector (Transgen Biotech, Beijing, China), resulting in five subgenomic cDNA clones, which were confirmed by DNA sequence analysis. These five cDNA fragments were sequentially inserted into a modified pTRE-Tight vector that allows inducible transcription of infectious ZIKV RNA in the cell. Initially, the pTRE-Tight vector was modified by replacing the high-copy-number ColE1 origin of replication with the low-copy-number p15A origin of replication from the vector pACYC177 [18]. For construction of infectious ZIKV/MR766 cDNA, a DNA fragment containing a unique *Sbf* I restriction enzyme site, partial 3′ end sequence (nucleotides 10,779–10,807 with a unique *Eag* I site) of the MR766 genome, and the antigenomic ribozyme of HDV were amplified by PCR and introduced into the low-copy pTRE-Tight vector between the restriction enzyme sites *Sac* I and *Xba* I. Lastly, the nucleotides 1 to 1711 of the MR766 cDNA were fused with the minimal CMV promoter sequence by PCR using synthetic primers containing unique *Sac* I and *Sbf* I sites and inserted into the above modified pTRE-Tight vector, resulting in the pTight-ZIKV/MR766 entry vector. For subsequent cloning of other cDNA fragments excised from subgenomic cDNA clones, partial Fragment 1 between *EcoR* I and *Age* I sites and Fragment 2 between *Age* I and *Sbf* I sites were simultaneously inserted into the pTight-ZIKV/MR766 Entry Vector digested with restriction enzymes *EcoR* I and *Sbf* I. The rest of the three cDNA fragments (3, 4, and 5) were then cloned into the *Sbf* I/*Eag* I-digested pTight-ZIKV/MR766 Entry vector containing Fragments 1 and 2, resulting in a full-length MR766 cDNA clone. Similarly, the Asian-lineage ZIKV strain FSS13025 cDNA was cloned into the pTRE-Tight vector, resulting in pTight-ZIKV/FSS13025. The full-length FSS13025 cDNA (GenBank number KU955593.1) was synthesized and cloned into the vector pCCI-Brick by GenScript, resulting in a plasmid designated pCCI-Brick-ZIKV_FSS13025. The FSS13025 cDNA between restriction enzyme sites *Nhe* I and *Eag* I was excised from the synthetic pCCI-Brick-ZIKV_FSS13025 vector and inserted into the pTight-ZIKV/FSS13025 entry vector cut by the same *Nhe* I and *Eag* I enzymes. The pTight-ZIKV/FSS13025 entry vector was modified from the pTight-ZIKV/MR766 Entry vector by replacing the DNA fragment between restriction enzyme sites *Sac* I and *Eag* I with a synthetic DNA fragment containing part of the minimal CMV promoter and 5′ end nucleotides 1–57 of the FSS13025 genome. DNA ligation was carried out by incubation of the above-described DNA vectors and inserts with T4 DNA ligase (NEB, M0202) at 16 °C overnight. The ligated DNA was concentrated by ethanol precipitation and resuspended in distilled water prior to DNA transformation. One Shot TOP10 Electrocomp *Escherichia coli* (*E. coli*) was from Invitrogen (cat. no. C404052, Carlsbad, CA, USA) and used for DNA transformation by electroporation, which was carried out in a 2 mm cuvette in the following conditions: 2500 V, 25 µF, 200 Ω. The DNA-transformed *E. coli* was spread onto lysogeny broth (LB) plate containing 100 µg/mL of Ampicillin with about 20-h incubation at 30 °C. The clones were cultured in LB medium by shaking (170 rpm) at 30 °C overnight. Plasmid DNA was extracted using QIAGEN kits and confirmed by DNA sequence analysis.

2.3. DNA Mutagenesis

To engineer a genetic marker for rescued MR766 virus, the restriction enzyme *Nhe* I site at the nucleotide 3862 of the MR766 cDNA was mutated by an overlapping PCR method using synthetic oligonucleotide primers containing nucleotide mutations that did not change amino acid sequence (silent mutation). The PCR products were digested by *Sal* I and *Sbf* I and inserted into the infectious cDNA clone pTight-ZIKV/MR766 which was similarly cut by *Sal* I and *Sbf* I. Likewise, the *Nsi* I site at the nucleotide 7178 of the FSS13025 cDNA was destroyed by introducing silent mutations into the DNA fragment between *Kas* I and *Afl* II sites of the infectious FSS13025 cDNA vector pTight-ZIKV/FSS13025.

2.4. DNA Transfection and Virus Production

Vero cells were seeded in a 12-well plate at a density of 2.5×10^5 per well and cultured in DMEM containing 10% FBS overnight. After washing with $1\times$ Phosphate-buffered saline (PBS) twice, Vero cells were transfected with 1 μg of pTight-ZIKV/MR766 or pTight-ZIKV/FSS13025 DNA with 1 μg of either pTRE-Tight or pTet-On vector DNA in Opti-MEM containing 4 μL lipofectamine 2000 (Invitrogen, cat. no. 11668019, Carlsbad, CA, USA). At 4 h post-transfection (p.t.), Opti-MEM was replaced with 1 mL of DMEM containing 3% FBS and 1 μg/mL of doxycycline (Sigma, D9891). The supernatants from DNA-transfected Vero cells were collected at 3 (MR766) or 6 (FSS13025) days after DNA transfection for determining the titers of infectious ZIKV.

2.5. Immunofluorescence Assay (IFA)

The expression of ZIKV proteins in the DNA-transfected or virus-infected Vero cells was determined by immunofluorescence assay (IFA) using a monoclonal antibody specific to the envelope protein (EMD Millipore, clone D1-4G2-4-15, Billerica, MA, USA). The DNA-transfected or virus-infected Vero cells were fixed with methanol at $-20\,^{\circ}\text{C}$ for 15 min and then blocked with a PBS buffer containing 1% FBS, 1% BSA, and 0.05% Tween-20 at room temperature (RT) for 1 h. Cells were then incubated with the E monoclonal antibody at RT for 2 h, followed by incubation with a goat anti-mouse secondary antibody conjugated with Alexa Fluor 488 (Life Technologies, cat. no. A21202, Carlsbad, CA, USA) at RT for 1 h. The cell nucleus was stained with Hoechst 33342 at RT for 10 min. Fluorescent images were captured using Nikon Eclipse Ti microscope.

2.6. Virus Titration and Plaque Assay

A plaque assay was used to determine the titer of infectious ZIKV recovered from Vero cells transfected with infectious ZIKV cDNA clones as described above. Infectious ZIKV in the cell culture supernatant was titrated by a 10-fold serial dilution. Vero cells in 12-well cell culture plates were infected with 10-fold serially diluted ZIKV in triplicate. The virus-infected cells were incubated at $37\,^{\circ}\text{C}$ for two hours with gentle swirling several times. The virus-infected cells were then grown in DMEM containing 5% FBS and 1% of methyl cellulose at $37\,^{\circ}\text{C}$. At 4 to 6 days post-infection, the virus-infected cells were fixed with 4% formaldehyde solution at RT for 1 h. Viable cells were stained with 1% crystal violet solution at RT for 15 min. The numbers of plaques were manually counted and converted to infectious virus titers per milliliter.

2.7. Determination of the Stability of Infectious Zika Virus (ZIKV) cDNA Clone

To determine the stability of infectious ZIKV cDNA clones pTight-ZIKV/MR766 and pTight-ZIKV/FSS13025 in *E. coli*, the plasmid DNA was amplified in TOP10 Electrocomp *E. coli* by several rounds of DNA transformation and amplification. Purified plasmid DNA after each round of amplification was initially validated by restriction enzyme digestion to determine the sizes of plasmid DNA. Purified plasmid DNA after each round of transformation and amplification was also used for DNA transfection into Vero cells to determine its ability to produce infectious ZIKV.

2.8. Statistical Analysis

Graphical representation and statistical analyses were performed by Prism6 software (GraphPad Software, La Jolla, CA, USA). Mean values and standard deviation (SD) were calculated from at least three independent experiments. Comparisons between samples were done using the Students *t*-test. $p < 0.05$ was considered statistically significant.

3. Results

3.1. Construction of the Full-Length Infectious ZIKV cDNA

Genetic instability of Flavivirus cDNA in bacteria is a common problem encountered during the course of developing reverse genetics for certain members of the Flaviviridae family. The full-length cDNA clones of different ZIKV strains have been constructed recently by others using a T7/SP6 transcription vector or a mammalian expression vector that requires the insertion of intron sequence into the NS1 or NS5 gene in order to obtain the infectious cDNA clones [16,18–21]. In the present study, we sought to develop a more convenient and robust reverse genetics system for inducible production and genetic manipulation of infectious ZIKV of various lineages independent of in vitro T7/SP6 polymerase transcription or insertion of intron sequence using a strategy similar to our previous work on the hepatitis C virus (HCV) [28]. The construction of infectious cDNAs of MR766 and FSS13025 strains is described in materials and methods. The full-length cDNA of MR766 was sequentially spliced from 5 subgenomic cDNAs (Figure 1A) and cloned into pTight-ZIKV/MR766 entry vector (Figure 1B), whereas the full-length cDNA of FSS13025 strain was chemically synthesized by GenScript (Figure 1C) and cloned into pTight-ZIKV/FSS13025 entry vector (Figure 1D). The transcription of the full-length ZIKV RNA genome is under the control of the Tet-responsive P_{tight} promoter, and the HDV antigenomic ribozyme is placed immediately downstream of the $3'$ end of ZIKV RNA genome (Figure 1B). Since P_{tight} promoter contains $7\times$ repeat tetracycline responsive operator, the ZIKV RNA transcription would be driven by the binding of reverse Tet-responsive transcriptional activator (rtTA) to the operator in the presence of tetracycline or its derivatives doxycycline. Upon co-transfection of pTight-ZIKV with pTet-On which express rtTA and the addition of doxycycline, the full-length ZIKV RNA genome is transcribed and further processed by the HDV ribozyme-mediated cleavage at the $3'$ end, resulting in an infectious RNA with precise $5'$ and $3'$ ends in the cell. This vector design was successfully used for the construction of the full-length cDNAs of both African-lineage MR766 and Asian-lineage FSS13025 strains of ZIKV, which exhibited genetic instability in bacteria as reported by others [16,18].

3.2. Tet-Inducible Production of Infectious ZIKV from Its cDNA

To demonstrate the functionality of the full-length ZIKV cDNA constructs described above, we have carried out DNA transfection experiments and determined the production of infectious ZIKV. We also sought to determine the Tet-inducible production of infectious ZIKV by co-transfection of Vero cells with both pTight-ZIKV/MR766 and pTet-On with and without the addition of doxycycline, a tetracycline analogue. Initially, the pTight-ZIKV/MR766 DNA was transfected into Vero cells with or without co-transfection with the pTet-On vector. The DNA-transfected Vero cells were then cultured in DMEM medium with or without doxycycline (1 μg/mL). At 3 days post-transfection (p.t.), the cytopathic effect (CPE) could be observed in the DNA-transfected Vero cells when doxycycline was added. The cell culture supernatants were harvested for the determination of infectious ZIKV, whereas the DNA-transfected cells were fixed and stained with a monoclonal antibody specific to the ZIKV E protein (Figure 2A). The expression of viral E protein was detected in cells transfected with the pTight-ZIKV/MR766 DNA regardless of co-transfection with the pTet-On vector or presence of doxycycline, suggesting leaky transcription from the P_{Tight} promoter (Figure 2A). However, the number of E-positive cells and the level of E protein expression were the highest in the cells co-transfected with the pTet-On vector and cultured in the presence of doxycycline (top-right corner, Figure 2A), demonstrating Tet-inducible expression of ZIKV RNA from its cDNA vector. Likewise, infectious ZIKV in the cell culture supernatant was detected by IFA (bottom images of Figure 2A). At 3 days post-infection (p.i.), CPE was observed in Vero cells infected with the cell culture supernatants from the pTight-ZIKV/MR766 DNA-transfected cells (middle panels of Figure 2A). Again, infectious ZIKV in the supernatant of the cells co-transfected with pTight-ZIKV/MR766 and pTet-On in the presence of doxycycline resulted in the highest level of CPE. Similarly, the E protein was detected by IFA staining in the ZIKV-infected cells (bottom panel of Figure 2A). It should be noted that fewer

E-positive cells observed in the cells infected with the supernatants from Vero cells co-transfected with both pTight-ZIKV/MR766 and pTet-On were due to cell death caused by more infectious virus (detached from the plate). Taken together, these findings demonstrate that the full-length cDNA of the African-lineage MR766 strain is able to produce infectious virus in a Tet-inducible manner.

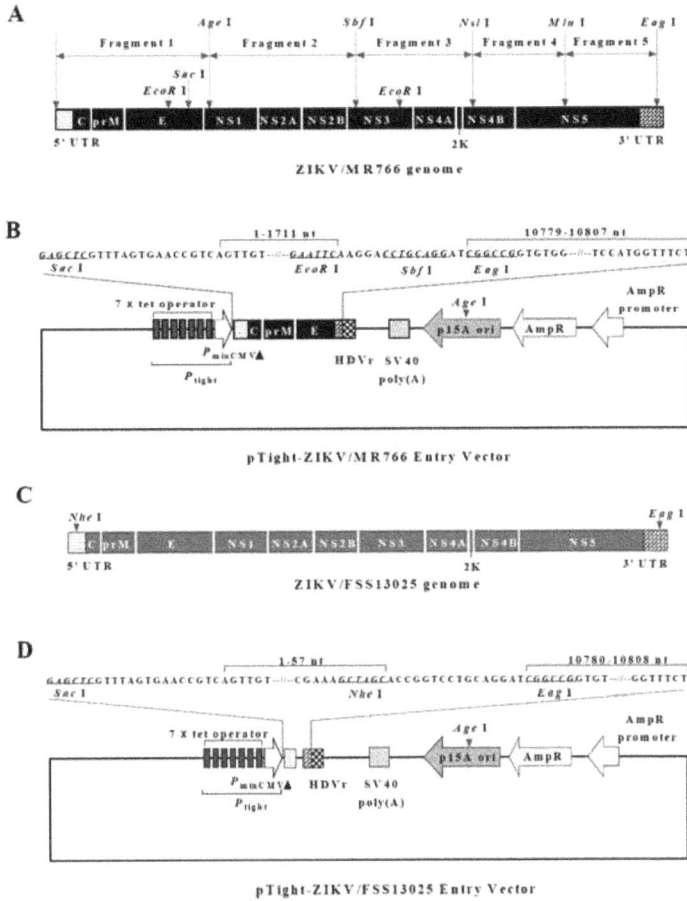

Figure 1. Schematic diagrams of the infectious Zika virus (ZIKV) cDNA amplification and cloning. (**A**) Illustration of subgenomic cDNA amplification and cloning of the African-lineage ZIKV/MR766 strain. Five subgenomic cDNA fragments (1 to 5) of the full-length MR766 genome were initially amplified from its vRNA by reverse transcription polymerase chain reaction (RT-PCR) using specific primers containing unique restriction enzyme sites highlighted in bold on the top. (**B**) Diagram of the pTight-ZIKV/MR766 entry vector. The entry vector was modified from pTRE-Tight by replacing the high-copy-number ColE1 origin of replication with the low-copy-number p15A origin and then inserting the partial MR766 genomic sequence with *EcoR* I, *Sbf* I and *Eag* I sites and hepatitis delta virus (HDV) antigenomic ribozyme sequence at the multiple clone sites region. The rest of the subgenomic cDNA fragments were sequentially inserted into the pTight-ZIKV/MR766 entry vector through the unique enzyme sites, resulting in an infectious MR766 cDNA clone designated pTight-ZIKV/MR766. (**C**) Diagram of the FSS13025 ZIKV genome organization. Two unique restriction enzyme sites *Nhe* I and *Eag* I at the 5′ and 3′ ends are highlighted in bold on the top. (**D**) Schematic map of the pTight-ZIKV/FSS13025 entry vector. A DNA fragment containing the 3′ end 21 nucleotides of the minimal CMV promoter, the 5′ end 57 nucleotides and the 3′ end 29 nucleotides of the FSS13025 cDNA

with a 16-nucleotides spacer, and the HDV antigenomic ribozyme were inserted into the low-copy-number pTRE-Tight vector, resulting in the pTight-ZIKV/FSS13025 entry vector. The FSS13025 cDNA between *Nhe* I and *Eag* I sites was released from the full-length FSS13025 cDNA vector pCCI-Brick-ZIKV_FSS13025 (synthesized by GenScript) and cloned into the pTight-ZIKV/FSS13025 entry vector, resulting in an infectious FSS13025 cDNA clone designated pTight-ZIKV/FSS13025.

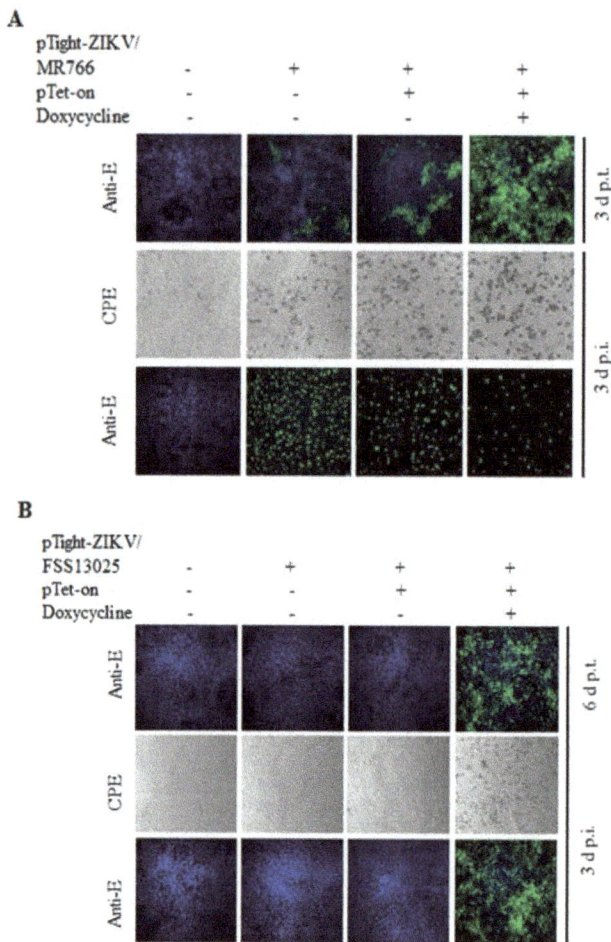

Figure 2. Production of cDNA-derived infectious ZIKV. (**A**) Production of infectious ZIKV/MR766 virus upon DNA transfection with or without Tet-induction. Vero cells (2.5×10^5/well) in 12-well cell culture plates were transfected with 1 µg of pTight-ZIKV/MR766 DNA and 1 µg of empty vector or pTet-On vector using lipofectamine 2000. At 3 days p.t., the viral E protein in the DNA-transfected cells was detected by immunofluorescence assay (IFA) using an E-specific monoclonal antibody (D1-4G2-4-15). At the same time, the supernatants were used to infect fresh Vero cells. At 3 days p.i., the cytopathic effect (CPE) was recorded and the E protein in the ZIKV/MR766-infected cells was determined by IFA. (**B**) Determination of cDNA-derived ZIKV/FSS13025 replication and production by CPE and IFA. Experiments were carried out in the same way as in (**A**) except that the pTight-ZIKV/FSS13025 DNA was used. At 6 days p.t., the E protein was detected by IFA in the pTight-ZIKV/FSS13025 DNA-transfected Vero cells. The ZIKV/FSS13025 in the supernatant was used to infect Vero cells. At 3 days p.i., CPE was photographed and the E protein was measured by IFA as described in (**A**). Images in (**A**,**B**) were 200× magnification.

Similar to MR766 cDNA clone, the Asian-lineage FSS13025 cDNA also resulted in the expression of E protein and production of infectious virus upon DNA transfection into Vero cells although at a much later time (6 days post-transfection), as determined by IFA (Figure 2B). In contrast to MR766 cDNA, transfection with FSS13025 cDNA per se failed to express the E protein or produce infectious virus. The expression of E protein and the production of infectious virus were only detected in Vero cells co-transfected with pTight-ZIKV/FSS13025 and pTet-On DNAs in the presence of doxycycline (Figure 2B). CPE and E protein could only be seen in Vero cells infected with the cell culture supernatant derived from cells co-transfected with pTight-ZIKV/FSS13025 and pTet-On in the presence of doxycycline (Figure 2B). These results suggest that the transcription and expression of infectious FSS13025 RNA from its cDNA clone in the cell are highly dependent on the expression of rtTA and the presence of doxycycline.

To further determine the Tet-inducible expression and production of infectious ZIKV from its cDNA, Vero cells were co-transfected with the pTight-ZIKV/MR766 or pTight-ZIKV/FSS13025 and pTet-On with addition of varying concentrations (0, 0.5, and 1 µg/mL) of doxycycline. The expression of the E protein in the DNA-transfected or virus-infected cells was determined by IFA using an E-specific monoclonal antibody. CPE formation in the virus-infected cells was documented by photography under an optical microscope. Indeed, the E protein expression in the pTight-ZIKV/MR766 DNA-transfected cells was significantly enhanced by increasing concentrations of doxycycline (top images, Figure 3A). CPE in the supernatant-infected cells was also increased in proportion to doxycycline concentrations. More importantly, the titers of infectious ZIKV/MR766 virus were significantly higher when doxycycline was added to the cell culture medium (Figure 3C). More significantly, the E protein expression and infectious virus production from the ZIKV/FSS13025 cDNA were strictly dependent on the presence of doxycycline in a dose-dependent manner (Figure 3B,C). Collectively, these findings demonstrate the Tet-inducible production of infectious ZIKV from its cDNA under the control of a Tet-responsive promoter, especially for ZIKV with less replication efficiency like the Asian-lineage FSS13025 strain.

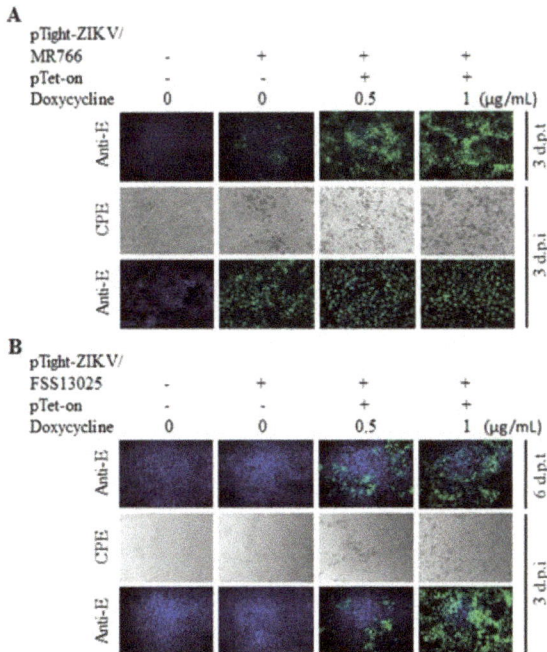

Figure 3. *Cont.*

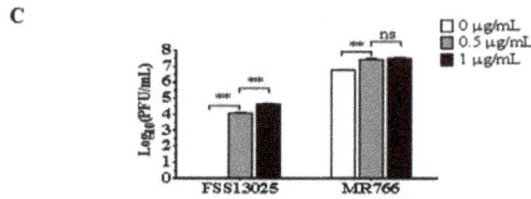

Figure 3. Doxycycline dose-dependent production of cDNA-derived ZIKV. Vero cells in 12-well plates were co-transfected with 1 µg of pTight-ZIKV/MR766 or pTight-ZIKV/FSS13025 DNA and 1 µg of an empty vector or pTet-On. The DNA-transfected Vero cells were cultured with different concentrations (0, 0.5, and 1 µg/mL) of doxycycline. The viral E protein in the DNA-transfected cells was determined by IFA at 3 d p.t. (for MR766) or 6 d p.t. (for FSS13025). The supernatants harvested at 3 d p.t. (MR766) or 6 d p.t. (FSS13025) were used to infect naïve Vero cells. CPE formation was recorded and the E protein was detected by IFA in the virus-infected cells at 3 d p.i. Infectious virus titers were quantified by a limiting dilution and plaque assay in the same way as Figure 3. (**A**) Determination of the E protein in Vero cells co-transfected with pTight-ZIKV/MR766 DNA and vector or pTet-On or infected with cDNA-derived ZIKV/MR766 virus by IFA. CPE formation was also documented in the cDNA-derived ZIKV/MR766 virus. (**B**) IFA detection of the E protein in Vero cells co-transfected with pTight-ZIKV/FSS13025 and pTet-On DNAs or infected with cDNA-derived ZIKV/FSS13025 virus. CPE formed by the cDNA-derived ZIKV/FSS13025 virus is shown in the middle. The images of (**A,B**) were taken under 200× magnification. (**C**) Doxycycline dose-dependent production of cDNA-derived ZIKV between the pTight-ZIKV/MR766 and pTight-ZIKV/FSS13025 DNAs. The supernatants from the DNA-transfected Vero cells as described in (**A,B**) were 10-fold serially diluted and were used for plaque assay. Infectious ZIKV titers were converted from plaque numbers and calculated as plaque-forming units per milliliter (PFU/mL). Values represent the means ± standard deviations (SD) from three independent experiments. Statistical significance was analyzed by Student's *t*-test: ** $p < 0.01$. ns indicates no significant difference.

3.3. Comparison of Virus Growth between the cDNA-Derived MR766 and FSS13025 Viruses

Transfection of pTight-ZIKV/MR766 cDNA into Vero cells resulted in higher titers of infectious virus than that of pTight-ZIKV/FSS13025 cDNA (Figure 3C), suggesting that MR766 grows more efficiently than the FSS133025 virus. To compare their growth capacity in Vero cells, we have determined the plaque-forming ability and growth curves of the cDNA-derived MR766 and FSS13025 ZIKVs. As shown in Figure 4A, MR766 virus formed bigger plaques than FSS13025 virus (Figure 4A). Likewise, MR766 virus grew to 6-, 9-, and 35-times higher titers than FSS13025 virus after 1, 2, and 3 days p.i. (Figure 4B). These results are consistent with the previous findings that African-lineage ZIKVs are more virulent and have higher growth capacity than Asian-lineage ZIKVs [15,29–31]. These observations may partially explain the higher titers of infectious MR766 virus and leaking transcription of MR766 RNA upon DNA transfection compared to FSS13025 virus (Figures 2 and 4).

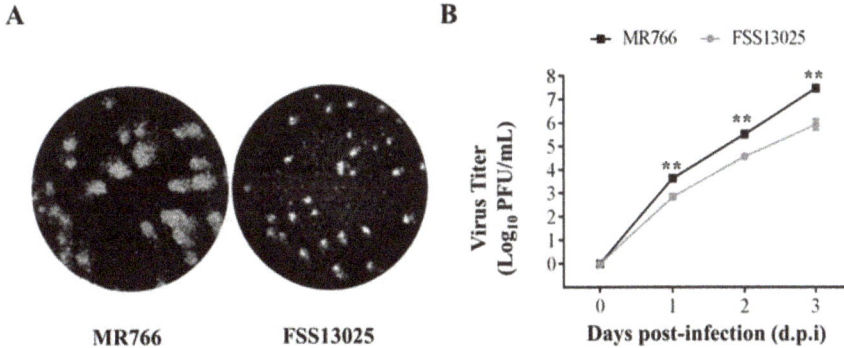

Figure 4. Comparison of cDNA-derived MR766 and FSS13025 virus growth. Vero cells (2.5×10^5/well) in 12-well plates were co-transfected with 1 μg pTight-ZIKV/MR766 or pTight-ZIKV/FSS13025 DNA and 1 μg pTet-On vector, followed by the addition of 1 μg/mL Doxycycline to cell culture media. Infectious virus titers in the supernatants collected at day 3 (MR766) or day 6 (FSS13025) were quantified by a plaque assay. (**A**) Plaque formation by cDNA-derived ZIKV/MR766 and ZIKV/FSS13025 viruses. Vero cells in 12-well cell culture plate were infected with 30 PFU of either MR766 or FSS13025. Plaques were stained and visualized after 4 days (for MR766) or 6 days (for FSS13025) p.i. (**B**) Growth curves of cDNA-derived MR766 and FSS13025 viruses. To compare the growth ability between MR766 and FSS13025, 4×10^5 Vero cells seeded in 6-well plates were infected with MR766 or FSS13025 virus at 0.01 MOI at 37 °C for 1 h. Upon washing with phosphate-buffered saline (PBS) three times, infected Vero cells were incubated with 2 mL DMEM containing 10% FBS. At day 1, 2, and 3 post-infection, virus in the supernatant was collected and stored at −80 °C. Virus yields at different time points were determined by a plaque assay. Data points represent the mean titer of triplicates. Statistical significance was analyzed by Student's *t*-test: ** $p < 0.01$.

3.4. Validation of Infectious ZIKV by the Identification of Genetic Markers

To discriminate cDNA-derived recombinant virus from potentially contaminated ZIKV, one of the two *Nhe* I sites present in the MR766 cDNA was mutated by introducing silent nucleotide mutations as genetic markers for the cDNA-derived ZIKV (Figure 5A). Similarly, one of the two *Nsi* I sites found in the FSS13025 cDNA was mutated (Figure 5B). Upon DNA transfection, resulting infectious MR766 (Figure 5C) and FSS13025 virus (Figure 5D) were confirmed by RT-PCR (Figure 5E) and digestion with restriction enzymes *Nhe* I for MR766 virus (Figure 5F) and *Nsi* I for FSS13025 virus (Figure 5G). The RT-PCR DNAs amplified from wild type but not recombinant viruses were digested with *Nhe* I (MR766) or *Nsi* I (FSS13025). The presence of genetic markers introduced into viral cDNA confirms the authenticity of the cDNA-derived ZIKV.

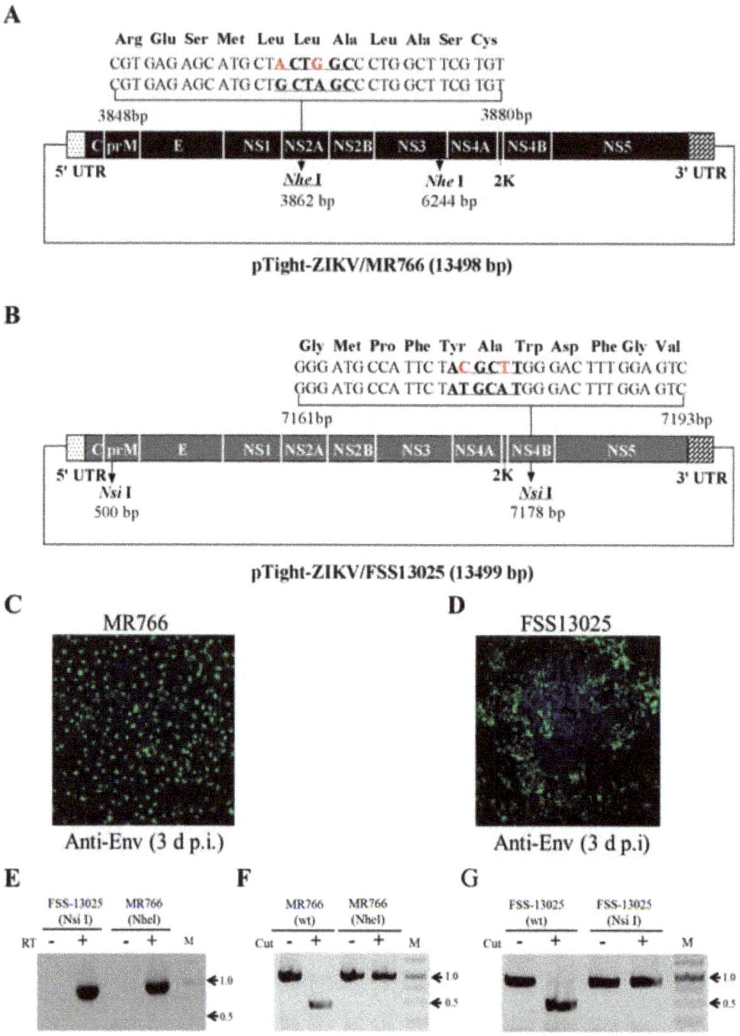

Figure 5. Confirmation of cDNA-derived ZIKV by detection of genetic markers. (**A**) Diagram of the pTight-ZIKV/MR766 DNA containing two nucleotide mutations as genetic markers. The *Nhe* I site at the nucleotide 3862 of the MR766 cDNA was mutated by changing two nucleotides (red) that do not alter amino acids (shown on the top). (**B**) Diagram of the pTight-ZIKV/FSS13025 DNA containing two nucleotide mutations at the [7178]*Nsi* I site of the FSS13025 cDNA as genetic markers. (**C**,**D**) Validation of cDNA-derived infectious ZIKV by IFA. The genetic markers-harboring pTight-ZIKV/MR766 and pTight-ZIKV/FSS13025 DNAs were co-transfected into Vero cells as described in Figure 3. The supernatants of the DNA-transfected cells were used for infection of Vero cells. At 3 d p.i., the expression of the E protein of MR766 (**C**) or FSS13025 (**D**) was detected by IFA. The images of (**C**,**D**) were taken under 200× magnification. The vRNAs were extracted from the supernatants using a Qiagen viral RNA isolation kit and used for reverse transcription (RT, indicated by +). The RT products were amplified by PCR using vRNA without RT as controls (**E**). The RT-PCR products from MR766 vRNA were digested with the restriction enzyme *Nhe* I (**F**), whereas the RT-PCR products of FSS13025 were cut with *Nsi* I (**G**). Wild type MR766 and FSS13025 RT-PCR products were used as controls.

3.5. Stability of Infectious ZIKV cDNA in E. coli

Previous studies by others suggested that infectious ZIKV cDNA is genetically unstable during amplification in bacteria. To determine the genetic stability of our infectious MR766 and FSS13025 cDNA clones based on the Tet-On system, the pTight-ZIKV/MR766 and pTight-ZIKV/FSS13025 plasmids were sequentially transformed to and amplified in *E. coli* up to 5 rounds, similar to the study described previously by others [18]. Plasmid DNA extracted at each round of transformation and amplification was digested with restriction enzyme *EcoR* I (for MR766 cDNA) or *Nhe* I and *Eag* I (for FSS13025 cDNA). The patterns of restriction enzyme digestion remained the same between different rounds of transformation and amplification in *E. coli* (Figure 6A,D), suggesting that there was no large DNA deletion or insertion during plasmid DNA amplification in *E. coli*. More importantly, transfection of Vero cells with plasmid DNA purified from the first round (R1) and fifth round (R5) of transformation resulted in similar levels of the E protein expression and comparable plaque size and numbers (Figure 6B,E) as well as the same titers of infectious ZIKV (Figure 6C,F). These results demonstrate the genetic stability of the infectious ZIKV cDNA cloned into the Tet-inducible vector modified in the lab.

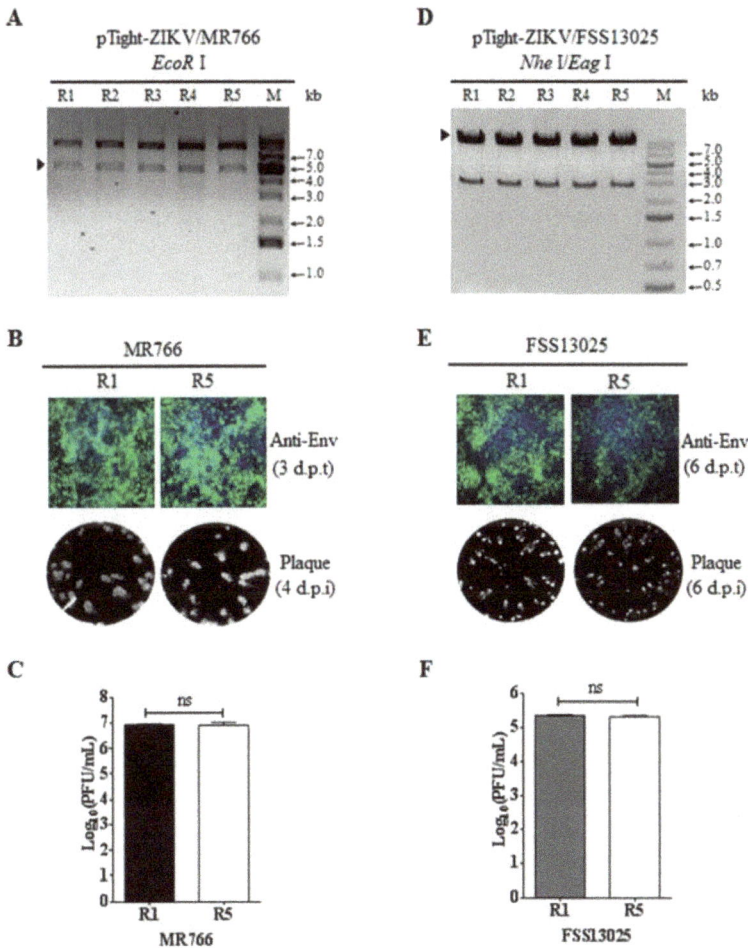

Figure 6. Determination of genetic stability of infectious ZIKV cDNA clones in *E. coli*. (**A**) Analysis of the pTight-ZIKV/MR766 DNA stability by *EcoR* I digestion. The pTight-ZIKV/MR766 plasmid was

sequentially transformed to and amplified in *E. coli* for five consecutive rounds (R1 to R5). The Plasmid DNA purified from each round was digested with *EcoR* I and analyzed by electrophoresis on 1% of agarose gel. The DNA fragment released from ZIKV/MR766 cDNA upon *EcoR* I digestion is indicated by a solid arrow on the left. GeneRuler 1 kb plus DNA ladder (Fisher Scientific, Waltham, MA, USA) is used as DNA size marker (M) shown on the right. (**B**) Confirmation of the pTight-ZIKV/MR766 DNA stability by functional analysis in Vero cells. 1 μg of pTight-ZIKV/MR766 DNAs purified from the first (R1) and fifth (R5) rounds of amplification were co-transfected with 1 μg of pTet-On into Vero cells with the addition of 1 μg/mL of doxycycline to cell culture medium. At 3 d p.t., the viral E protein expression was detected by IFA (up panel, 200× magnification), whereas infectious virus in the supernatant was measured by a plaque assay (lower panel). (**C**) Comparison of infectious virus titers resulting from the pTight-ZIKV/MR766 DNA between R1 and R5. (**D**) Analysis of genetic stability of the pTight-ZIKV/FSS13025 DNA by digestion with restriction enzymes *Nhe* I and *Eag* I. The FSS13025 cDNA released from the pTight-ZIKV/FSS13025 DNA upon digestion with *Nhe* I and *Eag* I (Figure 1C) is indicated by a solid arrow on the left. (**E**) Validation of cDNA-derived ZIKV/FSS13025 upon transfection with R1 and R5 pTight-ZIKV/FSS13025 DNA. Experiments were the same as B except R1 and R5 pTight-ZIKV/FSS13025 DNAs were used. (**F**) Comparison of infectious ZIKV/FSS13025 tiers resulting from R1 and R5 DNA transfection. Values represent the means ± standard deviations (SD) from three independent experiments. Statistical significance was analyzed by Student's *t*-test. ns indicates no significant difference.

4. Discussion

In the present study, we have developed a robust reverse genetics system for production and genetic manipulation of infectious ZIKV using the Tet-inducible (Tet-On) gene expression strategy [32]. The Tet-inducible ZIKV reverse genetics system is superior in many respects to previous ones based on the in vitro T7/SP6 transcription [18,25], in vitro DNA ligation or recombination from multiple DNA fragments [20,21,26], and the insertion of the intron sequence into the *NS1* or *NS5* gene of ZIKV cDNA [16,19]. The Tet-responsive P_{tight} promoter used in our ZIKV cDNA constructs is able to drive the transcription of infectious ZIKV RNA in the cell upon DNA transfection. In the case of T7/SP6 promoter-based vectors, in vitro transcription of infectious ZIKV RNA by T7/SP6 RNA polymerases requires the use of a 7-methyl guanosine nucleotide (m7G(5′)ppp(5′)G) or cap structure derivative [18,25]. The low efficiency of incorporation of the cap structure into T7/SP6 transcripts could affect the quantity of infectious RNA transcripts. Also, RNA transfection is less efficient than DNA transfection. Similarly, in vitro DNA ligation or recombination from multiple subgenomic cDNAs for construction of infectious ZIKV cDNA are laborious, time-consuming, and very inefficient [20,21,26]. Comparing to in vitro RNA transcription methods, our DNA-based vectors for the production of infectious ZIKV in the cell are robust, convenient, and cost-effective. More importantly, the Tet-inducible production of infectious ZIKV from the DNA-based vector transfected into the cell is highly efficient and can be induced by the addition of doxycycline. Although mammalian gene expression vectors were successfully used for production of infectious ZIKV, they require the insertion of the intron sequence into the NS1 or NS5 gene in order to be genetically stable in *E. coli* [16,19]. Subsequent production of infectious ZIKV depends on the splicing of RNA transcripts to remove the intron sequence inserted into the *NS1* or *NS5* gene. It is not clear whether the intron sequence inserted into the ZIKV cDNA will affect the efficiency of virus production in the cell. It was recently found that dengue virus NS5 protein is predominantly localized in the nucleus and is able to suppress RNA splicing by binding to core components of the spliceosome [33]. Although the ZIKV NS5 protein is also exclusively localized in the nucleus [34], its role in RNA splicing has not been determined. This appeared not to be a problem for production of more infectious ZIKV like MR766 strain from its cDNA in the cell given the facts that leaky RNA transcription from the pTight-ZIKV/MR766 DNA was sufficient to produce infectious virus (Figures 2A and 3A). This could be partially due to higher growth capacity of ZIKV/MR766 in the cell (Figure 4). A higher efficiency of RNA transcription is likely required for the production of those ZIKV strains with lower replication efficiency like the FSS13025 strain. Unlike MR766, FSS13025 virus production from its cDNA requires co-transfection with the pTet-On vector and the addition of doxycycline (Figures 2B and 4). In this aspect, the newly developed reverse genetics system through this study will be particularly useful for pathogenesis study and genetic manipulation of clinical isolates of ZIKV. Inducible production of the recombinant virus of clinical ZIKV isolates will be suitable for the study of viral pathogenesis in transgenic animals, which can be controlled by treatment with doxycycline. For instance, transgenic mice carrying the full-length cDNA of ZIKV under the control of pTight promoter can be used for studying congenital ZIKV infection by administrating animals with doxycycline. For genetic studies, robust production of infectious ZIKV as shown by our system may facilitate the study of virus–host interaction and the development of attenuated viruses. This may explain why the intron-based DNA vector for transposon mutagenesis of the ZIKV/MR766 resulted in fewer transposon insertion mutants [35]. Future investigations are warranted to determine if the Tet-inducible ZIKV reverse genetics system will be more efficient than the intron-based system for genome-wide analysis of viral sequence and proteins in viral replication and pathogenesis. Taken together, our findings suggest that the newly developed Tet-inducible ZIKV cDNA vector is highly efficient and robust for the production of infectious ZIKV, especially for attenuated viruses or virus strains with lower replication efficiency. This new DNA-based ZIKV reverse genetics system will facilitate genetic analysis and genetic manipulation of various ZIKV strains regardless of their replication efficiency.

Over the years, the development of reverse genetics systems for flaviviruses has been proven difficult due to their genetic instability in and/or toxicity to *E. coli* during cDNA cloning [36]. The underlying molecular mechanism of viral genetic instability and/or toxicity in *E. coli.* remains elusive. In general, it is believed that cryptic bacterial promoters present in viral cDNA or promoters used to drive the transcription of viral RNA are active in *E. coli*, resulting in the expression of toxic peptides or proteins [22,24,36]. To circumvent the difficulties in ZIKV cDNA cloning, several strategies have been used, including but not limited to the use of low-copy plasmids as vectors for in vitro RNA transcription; the separate cloning of the full-length cDNA as subgenomic DNA fragments in conjunction with in vitro DNA ligation or assembly; the insertion of a spacer sequence such as the intron to disrupt the open-reading frame [36]; and the silencing of cryptic prokaryotic promoters [23]. The immediate early CMV promoter was previously shown to be able to initiate gene expression in *E. coli* [37]. This may explain the viral toxicity observed during the MR766 cDNA cloning to a vector under the control of a CMV promoter, resulting in large deletions in the *NS1* to *NS3* coding regions [16]. To avoid this potential problem, we decided to choose the Tet-responsive P_{tight} promoter, which contains the minimal CMV promoter sequence of 59 nucleotides and can inducibly initiate the transcription of infectious ZIKV RNA. Additionally, we have replaced the high copy-number origin of replication present in the pTRE-Tight vector with the low-copy-number origin sequence of the vector pACYC177, which was successfully used for cloning of the first ZIKV cDNA [18]. It is most likely that the combination of the P_{tight} promoter and the low-copy-number origin of replication eliminated viral toxicity and, therefore, confer genetic stability of the pTight-ZIKV/MR766 and pTight-ZIKV/FSS13025 DNA vectors in *E. coli* (Figure 6). The modified pTight-ZIKV entry vectors (Figure 1) can be used for the construction of infectious cDNAs of all other ZIKV strains.

Author Contributions: L.Z. and G.L. designed experiments. L.Z., W.J., S.L., L.Q. carried out all experiments. L.Z. and G.L. analyzed the data, prepared the figures, and wrote the manuscript.

Funding: This work was partially supported by Development Fund from the University of Alabama at Birmingham and the Development Program (973) of China (2012CB518900).

Conflicts of Interest: The authors declare no conflict of interest.

References

1. Dick, G.W.; Kitchen, S.F.; Haddow, A.J. *Zika virus* I. Isolations and serological specificity. *Trans. R. Soc. Trop. Med. Hyg.* **1952**, *46*, 509–520. [CrossRef]
2. Abushouk, A.I.; Negida, A.; Ahmed, H. An updated review of *Zika virus*. *J. Clin. Virol.* **2016**, *84*, 53–58. [CrossRef] [PubMed]
3. Krauer, F.; Riesen, M.; Reveiz, L.; Oladapo, O.T.; Martinez-Vega, R.; Porgo, T.V.; Haefliger, A.; Broutet, N.J.; Low, N.; Group WHOZCW. *Zika virus* Infection as a Cause of Congenital Brain Abnormalities and Guillain-Barre Syndrome: Systematic Review. *PLoS Med.* **2017**, *14*, e1002203. [CrossRef] [PubMed]
4. Brasil, P.; Sequeira, P.C.; Freitas, A.D.; Zogbi, H.E.; Calvet, G.A.; de Souza, R.V.; Siqueira, A.M.; de Mendonca, M.C.; Nogueira, R.M.; de Filippis, A.M.; et al. Guillain-Barre syndrome associated with *Zika virus* infection. *Lancet* **2016**, *387*, 1482. [CrossRef]
5. Aid, M.; Abbink, P.; Larocca, R.A.; Boyd, M.; Nityanandam, R.; Nanayakkara, O.; Martinot, A.J.; Moseley, E.T.; Blass, E.; Borducchi, E.N.; et al. Zika Virus Persistence in the Central Nervous System and Lymph Nodes of Rhesus Monkeys. *Cell* **2017**, *169*, 610–620. [CrossRef] [PubMed]
6. Paz-Bailey, G.; Rosenberg, E.S.; Doyle, K.; Munoz-Jordan, J.; Santiago, G.A.; Klein, L.; Perez-Padilla, J.; Medina, F.A.; Waterman, S.H.; Gubern, C.G.; et al. Persistence of Zika Virus in Body Fluids—Preliminary Report. *N. Engl. J. Med.* **2018**, *379*, 1234–1243. [CrossRef] [PubMed]
7. Musso, D. *Zika virus* Transmission from French Polynesia to Brazil. *Emerg. Infect. Dis.* **2015**, *21*, 1887. [CrossRef] [PubMed]
8. Tang, W.W.; Young, M.P.; Mamidi, A.; Regla-Nava, J.A.; Kim, K.; Shresta, S. A Mouse Model of Zika Virus Sexual Transmission and Vaginal Viral Replication. *Cell Rep.* **2016**, *17*, 3091–3098. [CrossRef] [PubMed]
9. Uraki, R.; Jurado, K.A.; Hwang, J.; Szigeti-Buck, K.; Horvath, T.L.; Iwasaki, A.; Fikrig, E. Fetal Growth Restriction Caused by Sexual Transmission of Zika Virus in Mice. *J. Infect. Dis.* **2017**, *215*, 1720–1724. [CrossRef] [PubMed]
10. Miner, J.J.; Diamond, M.S. *Zika virus* Pathogenesis and Tissue Tropism. *Cell Host Microbe* **2017**, *21*, 134–142. [CrossRef] [PubMed]
11. Weaver, S.C.; Costa, F.; Garcia-Blanco, M.A.; Ko, A.I.; Ribeiro, G.S.; Saade, G.; Shi, P.Y.; Vasilakis, N. *Zika virus*: History, emergence, biology, and prospects for control. *Antivir. Res.* **2016**, *130*, 69–80. [CrossRef] [PubMed]
12. Bowen, J.R.; Quicke, K.M.; Maddur, M.S.; O'Neal, J.T.; McDonald, C.E.; Fedorova, N.B.; Puri, V.; Shabman, R.S.; Pulendran, B.; Suthar, M.S. Zika Virus Antagonizes Type I Interferon Responses during Infection of Human Dendritic Cells. *PLoS Pathog.* **2017**, *13*, e1006164. [CrossRef]
13. Duggal, N.K.; Ritter, J.M.; McDonald, E.M.; Romo, H.; Guirakhoo, F.; Davis, B.S.; Chang, G.J.; Brault, A.C. Differential Neurovirulence of African and Asian Genotype *Zika virus* Isolates in Outbred Immunocompetent Mice. *Am. J. Trop. Med. Hyg.* **2017**, *97*, 1410–1417. [CrossRef] [PubMed]
14. Govero, J.; Esakky, P.; Scheaffer, S.M.; Fernandez, E.; Drury, A.; Platt, D.J.; Gorman, M.J.; Richner, J.M.; Caine, E.A.; Salazar, V.; et al. *Zika virus* infection damages the testes in mice. *Nature* **2016**, *540*, 438–442. [CrossRef] [PubMed]
15. Simonin, Y.; van Riel, D.; Van de Perre, P.; Rockx, B.; Salinas, S. Differential virulence between Asian and African lineages of Zika virus. *PLoS Negl. Trop. Dis.* **2017**, *11*, e0005821. [CrossRef] [PubMed]
16. Schwarz, M.C.; Sourisseau, M.; Espino, M.M.; Gray, E.S.; Chambers, M.T.; Tortorella, D.; Evans, M.J. Rescue of the 1947 Zika Virus Prototype Strain with a Cytomegalovirus Promoter-Driven cDNA Clone. *mSphere* **2016**, *1*. [CrossRef]
17. Shan, C.; Muruato, A.E.; Nunes, B.T.D.; Luo, H.; Xie, X.; Medeiros, D.B.A.; Wakamiya, M.; Tesh, R.B.; Barrett, A.D.; Wang, T.; et al. A live-attenuated Zika virus vaccine candidate induces sterilizing immunity in mouse models. *Nat. Med.* **2017**, *23*, 763–767. [CrossRef]
18. Shan, C.; Xie, X.; Muruato, A.E.; Rossi, S.L.; Roundy, C.M.; Azar, S.R.; Yang, Y.; Tesh, R.B.; Bourne, N.; Barrett, A.D.; et al. An Infectious cDNA Clone of Zika Virus to Study Viral Virulence, Mosquito Transmission, and Antiviral Inhibitors. *Cell Host Microbe* **2016**, *19*, 891–900. [CrossRef]
19. Tsetsarkin, K.A.; Kenney, H.; Chen, R.; Liu, G.; Manukyan, H.; Whitehead, S.S.; Laassri, M.; Chumakov, K.; Pletnev, A.G. A Full-Length Infectious cDNA Clone of Zika Virus from the 2015 Epidemic in Brazil as a Genetic Platform for Studies of Virus-Host Interactions and Vaccine Development. *mBio* **2016**, *7*. [CrossRef]

20. Weger-Lucarelli, J.; Duggal, N.K.; Bullard-Feibelman, K.; Veselinovic, M.; Romo, H.; Nguyen, C.; Ruckert, C.; Brault, A.C.; Bowen, R.A.; Stenglein, M.; et al. Development and Characterization of Recombinant Virus Generated from a New World Zika Virus Infectious Clone. *J. Virol.* **2017**, *91*. [CrossRef]

21. Widman, D.G.; Young, E.; Yount, B.L.; Plante, K.S.; Gallichotte, E.N.; Carbaugh, D.L.; Peck, K.M.; Plante, J.; Swanstrom, J.; Heise, M.T.; et al. A Reverse Genetics Platform That Spans the Zika Virus Family Tree. *mBio* **2017**, *8*. [CrossRef] [PubMed]

22. Li, D.; Aaskov, J.; Lott, W.B. Identification of a cryptic prokaryotic promoter within the cDNA encoding the 5′ end of dengue virus RNA genome. *PLoS ONE* **2011**, *6*, e18197. [CrossRef] [PubMed]

23. Munster, M.; Plaszczyca, A.; Cortese, M.; Neufeldt, C.J.; Goellner, S.; Long, G.; Bartenschlager, R. A Reverse Genetics System for Zika Virus Based on a Simple Molecular Cloning Strategy. *Viruses* **2018**, *10*, 368. [CrossRef] [PubMed]

24. Ruggli, N.; Rice, C.M. Functional cDNA clones of the Flaviviridae: Strategies and applications. *Adv. Virus Res.* **1999**, *53*, 183–207. [PubMed]

25. Liu, Z.Y.; Yu, J.Y.; Huang, X.Y.; Fan, H.; Li, X.F.; Deng, Y.Q.; Ji, X.; Cheng, M.L.; Ye, Q.; Zhao, H.; et al. Characterization of cis-Acting RNA Elements of Zika Virus by Using a Self-Splicing Ribozyme-Dependent Infectious Clone. *J. Virol.* **2017**, *91*. [CrossRef] [PubMed]

26. Deng, C.L.; Zhang, Q.Y.; Chen, D.D.; Liu, S.Q.; Qin, C.F.; Zhang, B.; Ye, H.Q. Recovery of the Zika virus through an in vitro ligation approach. *J. Gen. Virol.* **2017**, *98*, 1739–1743. [CrossRef]

27. Gossen, M.; Freundlieb, S.; Bender, G.; Muller, G.; Hillen, W.; Bujard, H. Transcriptional activation by tetracyclines in mammalian cells. *Science* **1995**, *268*, 1766–1769. [CrossRef]

28. Cai, Z.; Zhang, C.; Chang, K.S.; Jiang, J.; Ahn, B.C.; Wakita, T.; Liang, T.J.; Luo, G. Robust production of infectious hepatitis C virus (HCV) from stably HCV cDNA-transfected human hepatoma cells. *J. Virol.* **2005**, *79*, 13963–13973. [CrossRef]

29. Anfasa, F.; Siegers, J.Y.; van der Kroeg, M.; Mumtaz, N.; Stalin Raj, V.; de Vrij, F.M.S.; Widagdo, W.; Gabriel, G.; Salinas, S.; Simonin, Y.; et al. Phenotypic Differences between Asian and African Lineage Zika Viruses in Human Neural Progenitor Cells. *mSphere* **2017**, *2*. [CrossRef]

30. Sheridan, M.A.; Balaraman, V.; Schust, D.J.; Ezashi, T.; Roberts, R.M.; Franz, A.W.E. African and Asian strains of Zika virus differ in their ability to infect and lyse primitive human placental trophoblast. *PLoS ONE* **2018**, *13*, e0200086. [CrossRef]

31. Simonin, Y.; Loustalot, F.; Desmetz, C.; Foulongne, V.; Constant, O.; Fournier-Wirth, C.; Leon, F.; Moles, J.P.; Goubaud, A.; Lemaitre, J.M.; et al. Zika Virus Strains Potentially Display Different Infectious Profiles in Human Neural Cells. *EBioMedicine* **2016**, *12*, 161–169. [CrossRef] [PubMed]

32. Das, A.T.; Tenenbaum, L.; Berkhout, B. Tet-On Systems For Doxycycline-inducible Gene Expression. *Curr. Gene Ther.* **2016**, *16*, 156–167. [CrossRef] [PubMed]

33. De Maio, F.A.; Risso, G.; Iglesias, N.G.; Shah, P.; Pozzi, B.; Gebhard, L.G.; Mammi, P.; Mancini, E.; Yanovsky, M.J.; Andino, R.; et al. The Dengue Virus NS5 Protein Intrudes in the Cellular Spliceosome and Modulates Splicing. *PLoS Pathog.* **2016**, *12*, e1005841. [CrossRef] [PubMed]

34. Hou, W.; Cruz-Cosme, R.; Armstrong, N.; Obwolo, L.A.; Wen, F.; Hu, W.; Luo, M.H.; Tang, Q. Molecular cloning and characterization of the genes encoding the proteins of Zika virus. *Gene* **2017**, *628*, 117–128. [CrossRef] [PubMed]

35. Fulton, B.O.; Sachs, D.; Schwarz, M.C.; Palese, P.; Evans, M.J. Transposon mutagenesis of the Zika virus genome highlights regions essential for RNA replication and restricted for immune evasion. *J. Virol.* **2017**. [CrossRef] [PubMed]

36. Aubry, F.; Nougairede, A.; Gould, E.A.; de Lamballerie, X. Flavivirus reverse genetic systems, construction techniques and applications: A historical perspective. *Antivir. Res.* **2015**, *114*, 67–85. [CrossRef]

37. Lewin, A.; Mayer, M.; Chusainow, J.; Jacob, D.; Appel, B. Viral promoters can initiate expression of toxin genes introduced into *Escherichia coli*. *BMC Biotechnol.* **2005**, *5*, 19. [CrossRef]

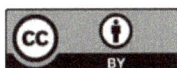

viruses

MDPI

Article

Contemporary Zika Virus Isolates Induce More dsRNA and Produce More Negative-Strand Intermediate in Human Astrocytoma Cells

Trisha R. Barnard [1], Maaran M. Rajah [1] and Selena M. Sagan [1,2,]*

[1] Department of Microbiology and Immunology, McGill University, Montreal, QC H3A 2B4, Canada; trisha.barnard@mail.mcgill.ca (T.R.B.); michael.rajah@mail.mcgill.ca (M.M.R.)
[2] Department of Biochemistry, McGill University, Montreal, QC H3A 2B4, Canada
* Correspondence: selena.sagan@mcgill.ca; Tel.: +1-514-398-8110

Received: 22 October 2018; Accepted: 18 December 2018; Published: 19 December 2018

Abstract: The recent emergence and rapid geographic expansion of Zika virus (ZIKV) poses a significant challenge for public health. Although historically causing only mild febrile illness, recent ZIKV outbreaks have been associated with more severe neurological complications, such as Guillain-Barré syndrome and fetal microcephaly. Here we demonstrate that two contemporary (2015) ZIKV isolates from Puerto Rico and Brazil may have increased replicative fitness in human astrocytoma cells. Over a single infectious cycle, the Brazilian isolate replicates to higher titers and induces more severe cytopathic effects in human astrocytoma cells than the historical African reference strain or an early Asian lineage isolate. In addition, both contemporary isolates induce significantly more double-stranded RNA in infected astrocytoma cells, despite similar numbers of infected cells across isolates. Moreover, when we quantified positive- and negative-strand viral RNA, we found that the Asian lineage isolates displayed substantially more negative-strand replicative intermediates than the African lineage isolate in human astrocytoma cells. However, over multiple rounds of infection, the contemporary ZIKV isolates appear to be impaired in cell spread, infecting a lower proportion of cells at a low MOI despite replicating to similar or higher titers. Taken together, our data suggests that contemporary ZIKV isolates may have evolved mechanisms that allow them to replicate with increased efficiency in certain cell types, thereby highlighting the importance of cell-intrinsic factors in studies of viral replicative fitness.

Keywords: Zika virus; flavivirus; astrocytomas; dsRNA; viral fitness

1. Introduction

The recent emergence and rapid geographic expansion of the mosquito-borne Zika Virus (ZIKV) poses a significant burden on the global health infrastructure [1]. The virus was initially isolated in 1947 from sentinel rhesus macaques in the Zika forest region of Uganda [2]. ZIKV circulated throughout Africa as well as in Southeast Asia over the latter half of the twentieth century, where it caused sporadic infections resulting in mild febrile illness [3,4]. The first major transmission of ZIKV outside of its endemic zone occurred in 2007, where 73% of the population of Yap Island, Federated States of Micronesia contracted the virus within a four-month period [4,5]. However, the clinical manifestations of ZIKV infection during the Yap Island epidemic were relatively similar to historical descriptions; resulting in mild, self-limiting, febrile illness characterized by rash, arthralgia, conjunctivitis, and headaches [3,5]. Interestingly, the continued geographic expansion of the ZIKV epidemic coincided with reports of novel neurological pathogenesis, starting with the 2013 French Polynesian epidemic, which saw a drastic increase in reports of Guillain-Barré syndrome [6].

Following the French Polynesian outbreak, the trans-Pacific transmission of ZIKV resulted in several epidemics throughout the Americas, the most salient being the Brazilian epidemic (2014–2016), which coincided with a 20-fold increase in incidence of congenital malformations, including fetal microcephaly from 2014 to 2015 [7]. Notably, ZIKV outbreaks in South America were also associated with neurological complications, and several investigations now suggest a connection between ZIKV infection and the development of Guillain-Barré syndrome, as well as congenital birth defects, including fetal microcephaly [4,8–12]. In addition to epidemiological factors, such as the increased mobility of infected individuals and the immunological naivety of recently-afflicted human populations, novel genomic polymorphisms acquired by contemporary outbreak strains likely contributed to ZIKV pathogenicity and dissemination in recent outbreaks [13]. Studies conducted in human neurospheres, cerebral organoids, and primary astrocytes, as well as in murine models of infection, have demonstrated differences in neurotropism, pathogenicity, and the antiviral responses between Asian and African lineage isolates [14–17]. Furthermore, a recent investigation uncovered a single nucleotide substitution in the prM region of the viral polyprotein that increases ZIKV infectivity in human and mouse neural progenitor cells and leads to significant fetal microcephaly in mice, resulting in greater mortality of neonatal mice [18]. Additionally, another polymorphism found in the NS1 region of contemporary ZIKV isolates results in increased NS1 antigenemia in mice, enhanced infectivity in *Aedes* mosquitoes, and reduced induction of antiviral signaling in human cells [19,20]. Thus, characterizing the difference in viral replicative fitness between the contemporary epidemic strains to the pre-epidemic strains could help to provide an evolutionary context for the emergence and rapid dissemination of ZIKV in the recent outbreaks.

Herein, we sought to compare viral replicative fitness by investigating viral growth kinetics, cytopathicity, and viral RNA accumulation of contemporary epidemic (2015–2016) and pre-epidemic ZIKV isolates in two cell culture models of ZIKV infection. First, we chose to use the A549 human lung epithelial carcinoma cells in order to contextualize our results within the literature, since A549 cells are widely used in ZIKV research [21–23]. Although A549 cells were reported to be a resilient model of ZIKV infection [21], the lung is not a target of ZIKV infection in vivo [24]. In contrast, several studies have shown that astrocytes are a primary target of ZIKV infection in vivo [16,25,26], and a recent study demonstrated that the U-251 MG human astrocytoma cell line is more permissive to ZIKV infection than A549 cells [27]. Therefore, we chose to use the U-251 MG cell line because an astrocyte-derived cell type may be a more relevant model for ZIKV-induced neuropathology and be better able to distinguish differences between ZIKV isolates. We found that contemporary ZIKV isolates (from Puerto Rico and Brazil) appear to have an increase in viral replicative fitness in astrocytoma cells over a single infectious cycle, with significantly more double-stranded RNA (dsRNA)-positive cells when compared to pre-epidemic isolates, despite similar numbers of infected cells. Moreover, when we investigated viral RNA accumulation, we found that the Asian lineage isolates had a substantially greater proportion of negative-strand intermediates than the African lineage isolate in both A549 and astrocytoma cells. However, over multiple rounds of infection, the contemporary ZIKV isolates appear to be impaired in cell spread, infecting a lower proportion of cells, despite the production of similar or higher titers. Our results suggest that the contemporary ZIKV isolates may have evolved mechanisms that allow them to replicate with increased efficiency in certain cell types and highlight the importance of cell-intrinsic factors in studies of viral replicative fitness.

2. Materials and Methods

2.1. Phylogenetic Analysis

Translated amino acid sequences of 50 ZIKV polyproteins (Table S1) were aligned using ClustalW [28]. Trees were constructed by neighbor joining of pairwise amino acid distances with the program MEGA7 (according to the distance scale provided) [29]. Bootstrap resampling was used to determine robustness of branches; values of $\geq$50% (from 1000 replicates) were used.

2.2. Cells and Viruses

African green monkey kidney (Vero) cells, human embryonic kidney (293T) cells, human lung carcinoma (A549) cells, and human astrocytoma (U-251 MG) cells were kindly provided by Martin J. Richer (McGill University, Montreal, QC, Canada), Connie Krawczyk (McGill University, Montreal, QC, Canada), Russell Jones (McGill University, Montreal, QC, Canada), and Anne Gatignol (Lady Davis Research Institute, Montreal, QC, Canada), respectively. All cells were maintained in Dulbecco's modified Eagle's medium (DMEM) supplemented with 10% fetal bovine serum (FBS), 1% nonessential amino acids, 1% L-glutamine, and 1% penicillin/streptomycin at 37 °C/5% CO_2.

An infectious cDNA of ZIKV strain MR-766 (ZIKV^{AF}; Genbank accession: HQ234498.1) was kindly provided by Matthew Evans (Mount Sinai, NY, USA) [30]. ZIKV^{AF} viral stocks were generated by transfection of 293T cells with the infectious cDNA using Lipofectamine 2000 (Life Technologies, Thermo Fisher Scientific, Waltham, MA, USA) followed by a single passage in Vero cells. ZIKV isolate PLCal_ZV (ZIKV^{CDN}; Genbank accession: KF99378) was generously provided by David Safronetz (National Microbiology Laboratories, Winnipeg, MB, Canada) [31]. Isolates PRVABC59 (ZIKV^{PR}; Genbank accession: KU501215) and HS-2015-BA-01 (ZIKV^{BR}; Genbank accession: KX520666) were provided by Tom Hobman (University of Alberta, Edmonton, AB, Canada) and Mauro Teixeira (Universidade Federal de Minas Gerais, Belo Horizonte, Brazil), respectively. The passage history of each ZIKV isolate is described in Table S2.

2.3. ZIKV Infections

A549 and U-251 MG cells were seeded at a density of 4×10^4 cells per well in 12-well plates the day before infection. Virus was diluted to the indicated MOI in Eagle's minimum essential medium (EMEM; Wisent Inc., St-Bruno, QC, Canada) and was allowed to bind to cells for 1 h at 37 °C/5% CO_2, after which the inoculum was removed, cells were washed with PBS, and media was replaced with fresh media containing 15 mM HEPES (Wisent Inc.) and 2% FBS. At the specified time points, the supernatant was collected and clarified by centrifugation at 4 °C for 10 min at $3000 \times g$, and stored at -80 °C prior to titration.

Viral titers were determined by plaque forming unit (PFU) assay on Vero cells. Briefly, 500 µL of 10-fold serial dilutions were incubated for 2 h on Vero cell monolayers in 12-well plates. The virus inoculum was removed, and the cells were overlaid with DMEM containing 1.2% Carboxymethyl cellulose (Sigma-Aldrich, Oakville, ON, Canada), 2% FBS, and 1% penicillin/streptomycin. Four days post-infection, cells were fixed with 5% formaldehyde and stained with 0.1% crystal violet (Sigma-Aldrich) to visualize plaques.

2.4. Cell Viability

Cell viability was monitored using a modified 3-(4,5-dimethylthiazol-2-yl)-2,5- diphenyltetrazolium bromide (MTT) assay similar to what has been previously described [32]. Briefly, cells were plated at density of 2000 cells per well in flat-bottom 96-well plates and allowed to adhere overnight. Ten wells per strain were infected with 100 µL of ZIKV diluted to the indicated MOI. At the specified time points, 10 µL of 5 mg/mL MTT salt (Sigma-Aldrich) in EMEM solution was added to each well and incubated for 4 h at 37 °C, after which 100 µL of 10% SDS in 0.01 M HCl was added per well and the plates were incubated overnight at 37 °C. Absorbance at 550 nm with a reference wavelength of 650 nm was read on a Spark 10M plate reader (Tecan, Männedorf, Switzerland). The average absorbance of 10 wells was used and viability experiments were carried out in triplicate. The data was expressed in % Cytopathicity, which was defined as: % Cytopathicity = 100% − ((Uninfected Absorbance − Infected Absorbance)/(Uninfected Absorbance) × 100%).

2.5. Flow Cytometry

A549 and U-251 MG cells were seeded at a density of 1×10^6 cells per 15-cm^2 plate the day before infection. Cells were infected with ZIKV at indicated MOI as described above and harvested at the indicated time points. Prior to fixation, cells were stained with Fixable Viability Dye eFluor 780 (Thermo Fisher Scientific, Waltham, MA, USA) according to the manufacturer's instructions. Cells were fixed using Cytofix/Cytoperm (BD Bioscience, Mississauga, ON, Canada) for 20 min and then stained with anti-J2 dsRNA (Scicons, Szirák, Hungary) diluted 1:1000, anti-4G2 (Millipore, Etobicoke, ON, Canada) diluted 1:200, or anti-cleaved Caspase-3 (Cell Signaling, Danvers, MA, USA) diluted 1:800 in PermWash (BD Bioscience) for 1 h followed by secondary staining with goat anti-mouse Alexafluor 488 or goat anti-rabbit Alexafluor A546 (Thermo Fisher Scientific, Waltham, MA, USA) diluted 1:300 for dsRNA or 1:500 for 4G2 and Caspase-3 in PermWash. Data were acquired on an LSRFortessa Analyzer (BD Bioscience) with BD FACSDiva software. Data analysis was performed using FlowJo software version 10.5 (BD Bioscience, Mississauga, ON, Canada). Debris and doublets were excluded from the analysis using forward-scatter width discrimination, and the percentage of dsRNA-, 4G2-, or Caspase-3-positive cells was determined by comparison to mock-infected cells.

2.6. Immunofluorescence Microscopy

A549 and U-251 MG cells were seeded at a density of 2×10^4 cells per well in eight-well chamber slides the day before infection. Cells were infected with ZIKV at indicated MOI as described above and harvested at the indicated time points. Cells were fixed in 4% formaldehyde in $1\times$ PBS, washed three times in PBS, and blocked with 0.3% Triton X-100 and 5% FBS in PBS for 1 h at room temperature. Samples were incubated with anti-J2 dsRNA (Scicons) diluted 1:1000 in PBS containing 1% BSA and 0.3% Triton X-100 at room temperature for 1 h followed by washing three times in PBS. Samples were then incubated with goat anti-mouse Alexafluor 488 (Thermo Fisher Scientific) diluted 1:300 in PBS containing 1% BSA and 0.3% Triton X-100 followed by three PBS washes before mounting with VectaShield containing DAPI (Cedarlane, Burlington, ON, Canada). Z-stack images were acquired using a Zeiss AxioObserver inverted microscope with a $63\times$ oil objective. The number of dsRNA foci per cell was quantified using Imaris version 9.1.2 (Bitplane Inc., South Windsor, CT, USA). Foci of size $0.3 \times 0.3 \times 4$ µm above quality 17.0 were automatically detected using the spot detection function and manually verified for at least 100 cells per condition.

2.7. Quantitative Reverse-Transcription PCR

Total RNA was extracted from cells using Trizol reagent (Thermo Fisher Scientific) following the manufacturer's protocol. Quantification of positive- and negative-strand intracellular viral RNA was determined by quantitative reverse-transcription PCR (qRT-PCR) on a Bio-Rad CFX96 Touch Real-Time System using the iTaQ Universal Probe One-Step Kit (Bio-Rad, Mississauga, ON, Canada) with 0.5 µL of PrimePCR GAPDH primers and probe (HEX, Bio-Rad) per reaction. The primers used to detect ZIKV RNA were as follows: forward, 5′-CCG CTG CCC AAC ACA AG-3′; reverse, 5′-CCA CTA ACG TTC TTT TGC AGA CAT-3′; probe, 5′-/56-FAM/AGC CTA CCT/ZEN/TGA CAA GCA ATC AGA CAC TCA A/3IABkFQ/-3′ [33]. A strand-specific reverse transcription (RT) reaction was carried out by addition of either the forward or the reverse primer during RT at 50 °C for 10 min, after which the other ZIKV primer and ZIKV probe was added to the reaction. The cycling conditions were: 95 °C for 3 min, then 45 cycles of 95 °C for 5 s and 60 °C for 60 s. The amount of viral RNA was normalized to GAPDH using the ΔCt method, and compared to a standard curve of $\log_{10}$ (PFU equivalents) which was extracted from cell culture supernatants [8], using the NucleoSpin RNA virus kit (Macherey-Nagel, Bethlehem, PA, USA) following the manufacturer's instructions. The relative amount of positive- and negative-strand viral RNA was calculated using the $2^{(-\Delta\Delta CT)}$ method using GAPDH as the internal control after normalization to the relative PCR efficiencies of the different ZIKV isolates.

2.8. Statistical Analysis

All statistical analyses were performed using Prism 6 software (GraphPad, San Diego, CA, USA). At each time point, viral titers from growth curves, % cytopathicity, % infected cells, or viral RNA were compared using a one-way analysis of variance (ANOVA) with Tukey's multiple-comparison test.

3. Results

3.1. Phylogenetic and Amino Acid Variance across ZIKV Isolates Selected for Comparative Analyses

Phylogenetic analyses demonstrate that ZIKV can be divided into two main lineages: African and Asian (Figure S1) [34,35]. The African lineage has caused sporadic infections over the last century, typically resulting in mild, febrile illness [1]. All of the strains identified in the 2014–2016 epidemic are of the Asian lineage and are more closely related to the H/PF/2013 French Polynesia strains than the FSM/2007 Micronesia (Yap Island) strain, suggesting that these sub-lineages may have evolved independently from a common ancestor, anchored by the P6-740 strain (Malaysia, 1966) (Figure S1) [34]. Notably, ZIKV outbreaks in French Polynesia and South America were the first to be associated with neurological symptoms, including Guillain-Barré syndrome and fetal microcephaly [4,9,36]. As such, we sought to perform a comparative analysis of historical and contemporary ZIKV isolates to study the impact of genetic polymorphisms on viral replicative fitness and cytopathicity in cell culture. We chose a panel of ZIKV isolates including: Uganda 1947 (MR766, ZIKV^{AF}); an early Asian lineage strain, isolated from a Canadian traveller whom returned from Thailand viremic in 2013 (PLCal_ZV, ZIKV^{CDN}); and two isolates from the 2015 outbreaks in Puerto Rico (PRVABC59, ZIKV^{PR}) and Brazil (HS-2015-BA-01, ZIKV^{BR}). Notably, ZIKV^{AF} was mouse passaged and all of the other viral isolates were passaged through Vero cells or a combination of Vero and C6/36 mosquito cells (Table S2). A detailed amino acid sequence comparison of these strains is available in File S1. Comparison of the overall amino acid composition across strains demonstrates that the maximum amino acid differences are between the ZIKV^{AF} and ZIKV^{PR} isolates (Table S3). Polymorphisms are located throughout the viral polyprotein; however, several regions (prM, E, NS2A, NS4B, and NS5 proteins) have a higher accumulation of amino acid polymorphisms, particularly between the African and Asian lineages (File S1).

3.2. Zika Virus Isolates Display Unique Plaque Morphology and Different Growth Kinetics in Cell Culture

While preparing viral stocks we noticed differences in plaque morphology on Vero cells between the four ZIKV isolates (Figure 1). Plaques from the historical ZIKV^{AF} were smaller than plaques from the Asian lineage isolates and were more uniform in size (Figure 1A). Of the Asian lineage isolates, both ZIKV^{CDN} and ZIKV^{PR} produced plaques with indefinite borders, whereas the plaques from the ZIKV^{BR} had clearly defined edges (Figure 1A). In order to better characterize each viral isolate, we investigated strain-specific differences in growth kinetics, cytopathicity, infectivity, and viral RNA accumulation.

We first sought to determine the viral growth kinetics for each of the four ZIKV isolates (Figure 1B–E). Viral titers were assessed using both one-step and multi-step growth curves after infection at an MOI of 10 and 0.01, respectively (Figure 1B–E). At MOI of 10, ZIKV^{BR} grew to significantly higher titers at 8 h post-infection in both cell types, suggesting that ZIKV^{BR} has an advantage in terms of growth kinetics (Figure 1B,C). In A549 cells, the increased titer of ZIKV^{BR} was much less pronounced by 24 h post-infection, at which time the titers of the other isolates have nearly caught up to within 1-log of ZIKV^{BR} (Figure 1B). In contrast, in U-251 MG cells, ZIKV^{BR} continues to replicate to significantly higher titers than all other isolates at all time points post-infection, even when titers have begun to plateau by 24 h post-infection (Figure 1C). Interestingly, the ZIKV^{BR} titers are already increasing by 8 h post-infection, whereas titers for the other isolates do not increase until after 8 h post-infection based on titers at 0 h [37]. Overall, this suggests that ZIKV^{BR} replicates to higher titers in U-251 MG cells, with faster replication kinetics over a single infectious cycle.

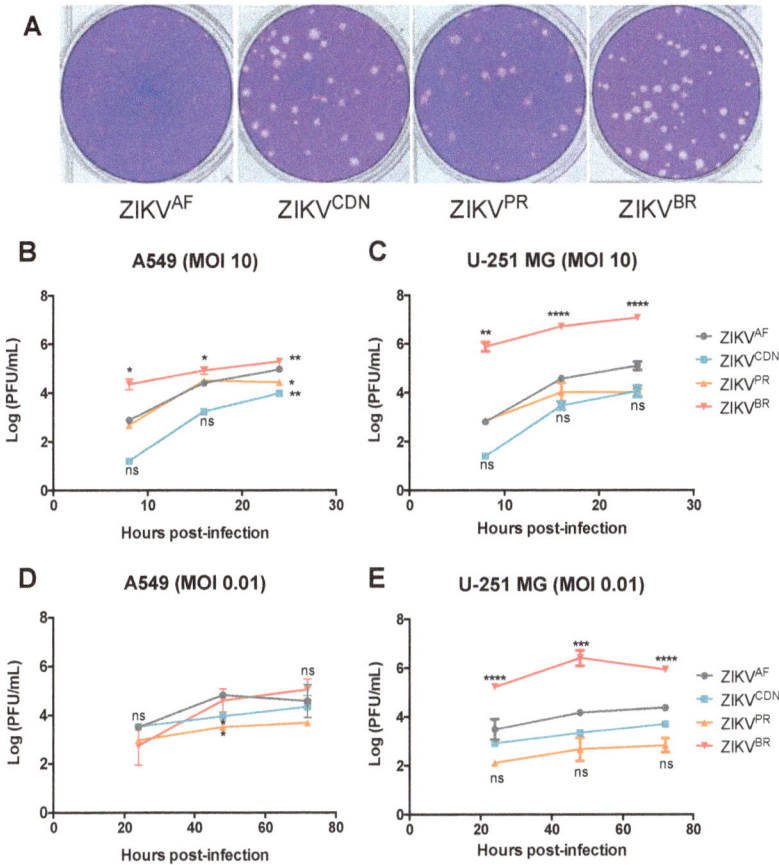

Figure 1. ZIKV isolates demonstrate unique plaque morphology and different growth kinetics in A549 and U-251 MG cell lines. (**A**) Representative images of Vero cell plaque assays of the indicated ZIKV isolates. (**B–E**) Cell culture supernatants were collected at the indicated time points and viral titer was determined by plaque assay. (**B**) A549 and (**C**) U-251 MG cells were infected with ZIKV at MOI = 10. (**D**) A549, and (**E**) U-251 MG cells were infected with ZIKV at MOI = 0.01. Values represent mean $\pm$ SD of at least three independent experiments. Asterisks indicate significant differences in viral titer relative to ZIKV^{AF}: * $p < 0.05$, ** $p < 0.01$, *** $p < 0.001$, **** $p < 0.0001$.

To further investigate the differences in viral replication kinetics between isolates, we also performed a multi-step growth curve at MOI of 0.01 (Figure 1D,E). In A549 cells, although at 48 h post-infection ZIKV^{CDN} and ZIKV^{PR} have lower titers than ZIKV^{AF}, there are no significant strain-dependent differences in viral titers at any other time point post-infection (Figure 1D). In contrast, in the U-251 MG cells, ZIKV^{BR} grew to significantly higher titers at all time points post-infection when compared to all other viral isolates (Figure 1E). There were no significant differences in viral titers between the remaining isolates in U-251 MG cells, although ZIKV^{AF} tended to have slightly higher titers than ZIKV^{CDN} and ZIKV^{PR} (Figure 1E). Overall, the data demonstrates that over multiple rounds of infection, ZIKV^{BR} appears to have a significant replicative advantage in U-251 MG cells, growing to higher titers than all other ZIKV isolates.

3.3. Cytopathic Effects Induced by ZIKV Isolates in Cell Culture Depends on MOI

We next wanted to determine whether there was a connection between viral particle production and the ability to induce cytopathic effects (CPE) in cell culture. Using an MTT assay to investigate strain-specific differences in cytopathicity, we observed that when cells were infected at MOI of 10, CPE induced by the four ZIKV isolates was consistent with the viral load (Figure 2). More specifically, in the A549 cells, all isolates induced similar CPEs with approximately 25% cytopathicity, which represents a 25% reduction in cell viability at 24 h post-infection (Figure 2A), with similar viral titers at this time point (Figure 1B). In contrast, in the U-251 MG cells, ZIKV^{BR} was significantly more cytopathic at the high MOI, inducing approximately 37% cytopathicity compared with an average of 18% cytopathicity at 24 h post-infection induced by the other ZIKV isolates (Figure 2B). Again, this finding is in good agreement with the relative viral titers at this time point (Figure 1C). To determine whether CPEs were apoptosis-driven or due to other forms of cell death, we quantified cleaved caspase-3 positive cells by flow cytometry at MOI of 10 in both cell types (Figure S2). In A549 cells, apoptosis appears to account for a small proportion of cell death with 3.5%, 1.9%, and 7.2% cleaved caspase-3-positive cells during ZIKV^{AF}, ZIKV^{CDN}, and ZIKV^{PR} infection, respectively; however, during ZIKV^{BR} infection approximately 47% of cells stained positive for cleaved caspase-3 (Figure S2A). In U251-MG cells, a similar pattern was observed with fewer cells staining positive for cleaved caspase-3 (between 0.6–1.43% for ZIKV^{AF}, ZIKV^{CDN} and ZIKV^{PR}), whereas approximately 17.1% of cells were cleaved caspase-3-positive during ZIKV^{BR} infection (Figure S2B). This suggests that, at least for ZIKV^{AF}, ZIKV^{CDN,} and ZIKV^{PR}, apoptosis is not the main driver of CPEs during ZIKV infection, and thus, other forms of cell death are likely to contribute to this phenotype. However, apoptosis appears to have a greater contribution to CPEs observed during infection with ZIKV^{BR}. Taken together, this suggests that over a single infectious cycle, ZIKV^{BR} induces more CPEs in U-251 MG cells than the other ZIKV isolates, likely due to an increase in apoptosis. In addition, at least at an MOI of 10, CPEs appear to be directly correlated with the viral titer for all four ZIKV isolates.

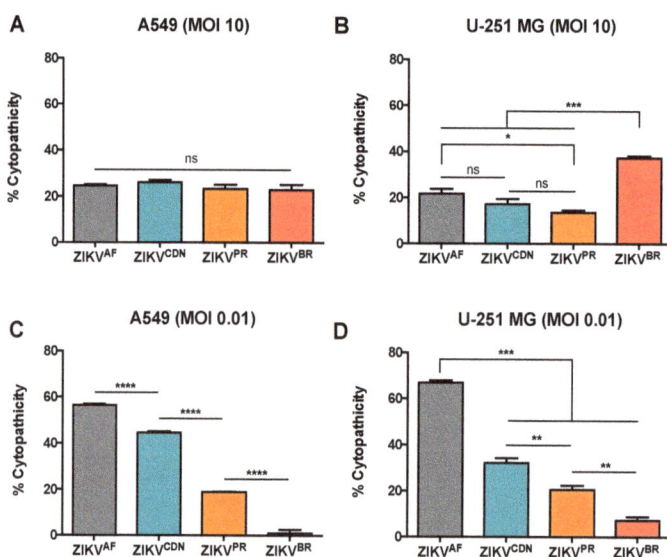

Figure 2. ZIKV isolates elicit different cytopathic effects in A549 and U-251 MG cell lines. (**A**) A549 and (**B**) U-251 MG cells were infected with ZIKV at MOI = 10 and cell viability was determined by MTT assay at 24 h post-infection. (**C**) A549 and (**D**) U-251 MG cells were infected with ZIKV at MOI = 0.01 and cell viability was determined by MTT assay 72 h post-infection. % Cytopathicity = 100% − ((Uninfected Absorbance − Infected Absorbance)/(Uninfected Absorbance) × 100%). Values represent the mean ± SEM of three independent experiments. Asterisks indicate significant differences in % cytopathicity: * $p < 0.05$, ** $p < 0.01$, *** $p < 0.001$, **** $p < 0.0001$.

Next, we determined the relative CPEs induced by the four ZIKV isolates over multiple rounds of infection at a low MOI. In contrast to the high MOI condition, where strain-specific differences in CPE were dependent on cell type, at low MOI, the strain-specific trend in CPE was consistent across cell lines (Figure 2C,D). At 72 h post-infection with MOI 0.01, ZIKV^{BR} induced the least CPEs in both A549 and U-251 MG cells with approximately 2% and 7% cytopathicity, respectively (Figure 2C,D), despite generating similar or higher titers at this time point (Figure 1D,E). ZIKV^{PR} and ZIKV^{CDN} induced intermediate CPE in both cell types (approximately 40% and 20% cytopathicity, respectively). However, ZIKV^{AF} induced the greatest CPE of all isolates at 72 h post-infection at MOI 0.01, with approximately 60% cytopathicity in both A549 and U-251 MG cells (Figure 2C,D). Taken together, these results suggest that although ZIKV^{BR} appears to have a replicative advantage that is more pronounced in astrocytoma cells, this advantage is likely due to increased viral replication in the initial infection rather than to increases over subsequent rounds of infection. As this could imply differences in cell spread across the ZIKV isolates, we next wanted to assess the percentage of infected cells across isolates.

3.4. Flow Cytometry Analysis Reveals Strain-Specific Differences in Viral Infectivity and Cell Spread

Due to the discrepancies in CPEs elicited at different MOIs, we set out to determine the percent of ZIKV-infected cells at high and low MOI using flow cytometry (Figure 3 and Figure S3). We initially determined the % infected cells by staining for the envelope glycoprotein using a pan-flavivirus (4G2) antibody (Figure 3A,B). At MOI 10, ZIKV^{CDN} infected a lower proportion of A549 cells (36%) when compared to ZIKV^{AF} (82%) and ZIKV^{PR} (61%) at 24 h post-infection (Figure 3A). A similar trend was observed in the U251-MG cells, where ZIKV^{AF}, ZIKV^{CDN}, and ZIKV^{PR} infected 88%, 60%, and 72% of cells, respectively (Figure 3B). However, we were unable to detect ZIKV^{BR} using the envelope antibody in either cell line. Given that viral epitopes may have changed over the course of the viral evolutionary history, we stained for dsRNA as a marker for active viral replication, to ensure similar sensitivity of detection across all isolates. At MOI 10, we detected significantly more dsRNA in a higher proportion of A549 cells during ZIKV^{PR} infection (40%), whereas only approximately 7% of A549 cells were dsRNA-positive in the other three isolates (ZIKV^{AF}, ZIKV^{CDN}, and ZIKV^{BR}) at 24 h post-infection (Figure 3C). In the U251-MG cells, the rate of infection was similar to that in A549 cells for ZIKV^{AF} and ZIKV^{CDN}, with approximately 10% and 6% dsRNA-positive cells, respectively (Figure 4D). However, for both the contemporary isolates (ZIKV^{PR} and ZIKV^{BR}), a significantly higher percentage of cells were dsRNA-positive in U-251 MG cells, with approximately 36% and 51% dsRNA-positive cells, respectively (Figure 3D). These results suggest that ZIKV^{PR} may induce more viral RNA replication (as indicated by dsRNA staining) than ZIKV^{AF} and ZIKV^{CDN}, since all three isolates display a similar % of infected cells when staining for the viral envelope, but vastly different amounts of dsRNA-positive cells. This may also be true for ZIKV^{BR}, which had a similar percentage of dsRNA-positive cells; however, we were not able to assess the % infected cells for this isolate using the envelope antibody. Taken together, these results suggest that over a single infectious cycle, ZIKV^{PR} infection results in a greater proportion of dsRNA-positive cells in both cell types, while ZIKV^{BR} selectively induces more dsRNA-positive cells in U-251 MG cells.

At the low MOI (0.01), the trend in % of dsRNA-positive cells closely mirrored the trend in cytopathicity (Figure 2 and Figure S3). At 72 h post-infection at MOI 0.01, ZIKV^{AF} has the highest % of dsRNA-positive cells in both the A549 and U-251-MG cells, with 30% and 15% dsRNA-positive cells, respectively (Figure S3A,B). All of the other ZIKV isolates had a lower % dsRNA-positive cells in both cell types (Figure S3A,B), consistent with the intermediate or low CPEs observed at this MOI (Figure 2C,D). However, dsRNA staining is likely an underestimation the % infected cells if the viral isolates do not induce high levels of dsRNA. Nonetheless, these results suggest that although ZIKV^{BR}, and possibly also ZIKV^{PR}, appear to have a replicative fitness advantage over a single infectious cycle that is more pronounced in astrocytoma cells, they appear to be impaired in cell spread when subjected to multiple rounds of infection at low MOI.

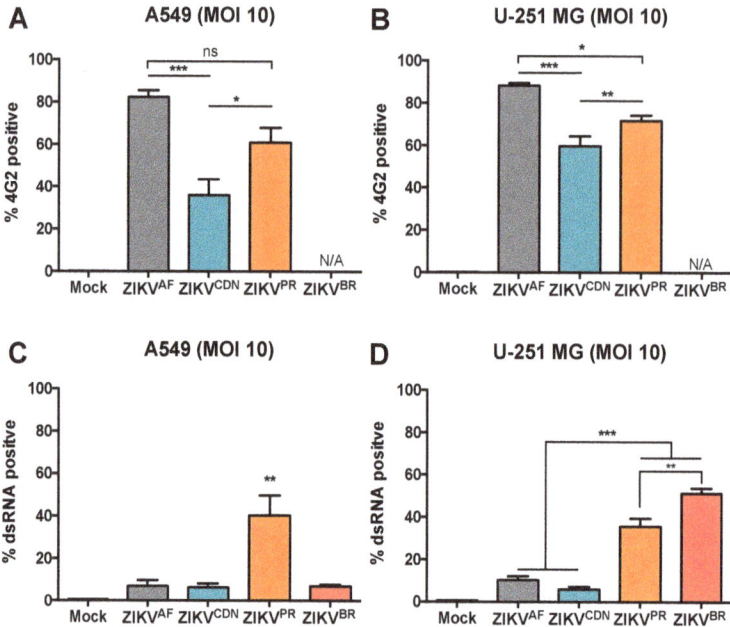

Figure 3. Contemporary ZIKV isolates induce more dsRNA than pre-epidemic isolates, despite similar numbers of infected cells. (**A**) A549 and (**B**) U-251 MG cells were infected with ZIKV at MOI = 10 and at 24 h post-infection cells were stained with the pan-flavivirus (4G2) antibody and the percentage of infected cells was determined by flow cytometry. (**C**) A549 and (**D**) U-251 MG cells were infected with ZIKV at MOI = 10 and 24 h post-infection the percentage of dsRNA-positive cells was determined by flow cytometry. The percentage of positive cells was determined by comparison to mock-infected cells. Values represent mean ± SEM of at least three independent experiments. Asterisks indicate significant differences in % infected cells: * $p < 0.05$, ** $p < 0.01$, *** $p < 0.001$.

3.5. The Number of dsRNA Foci and Ratio of Negative- to Positive-Strand RNA Differ across African and Asian Lineage Isolates

We next wanted to determine whether the increase in the % of dsRNA-positive cells observed during ZIKV[PR] and ZIKV[BR] infection was due to an increased number of replication complexes induced per cell. Thus, we quantified the number of dsRNA foci by immunofluorescence microscopy and image analyses at MOI of 10 in A549 and U-251 MG cells (Figure 4A,B). In A549 cells, ZIKV[AF] yielded the greatest number of dsRNA foci per infected cell, with on average >250 dsRNA foci/cell, while the Asian lineage isolates had, on average, approximately 124–166 dsRNA foci/cell (Figure 4C). In contrast, in the U-251 MG cells, the Brazilian isolate had the greatest number of dsRNA-positive foci, with >225 dsRNA-positive foci/cell, while all other isolates had <100 dsRNA foci/cell on average (Figure 4D). To further confirm these findings, we calculated the mean fluorescence intensity (MFI) of dsRNA-positive cells by flow cytometry (Figure 4E,F). The MFI revealed similar fluorescent intensities across ZIKV isolates in A549 cells, with the exception of ZIKV[PR], which were significantly more intense in this cell type (Figure 4E). Moreover, in U-251 MG cells, the contemporary isolates displayed a higher MFI for dsRNA-positive cells, suggesting that there were greater amounts of dsRNA per cell (Figure 4F). Taken together, this suggests that although the ZIKV[AF] isolate induced more dsRNA foci in A549 cells, they were on average of low fluorescence intensity. In contrast, in U-251 MG cells, ZIKV[BR] produced substantially more dsRNA-positive foci, and together with ZIKV[PR], the foci were brighter than those of the ZIKV[AF] and ZIKV[CDN] isolates. However, we cannot rule out the existence of a larger proportion of small dsRNA foci in these cells as our image analysis relied on a minimum foci size ($0.3 \times 0.3 \times 4$ µm) for quantification.

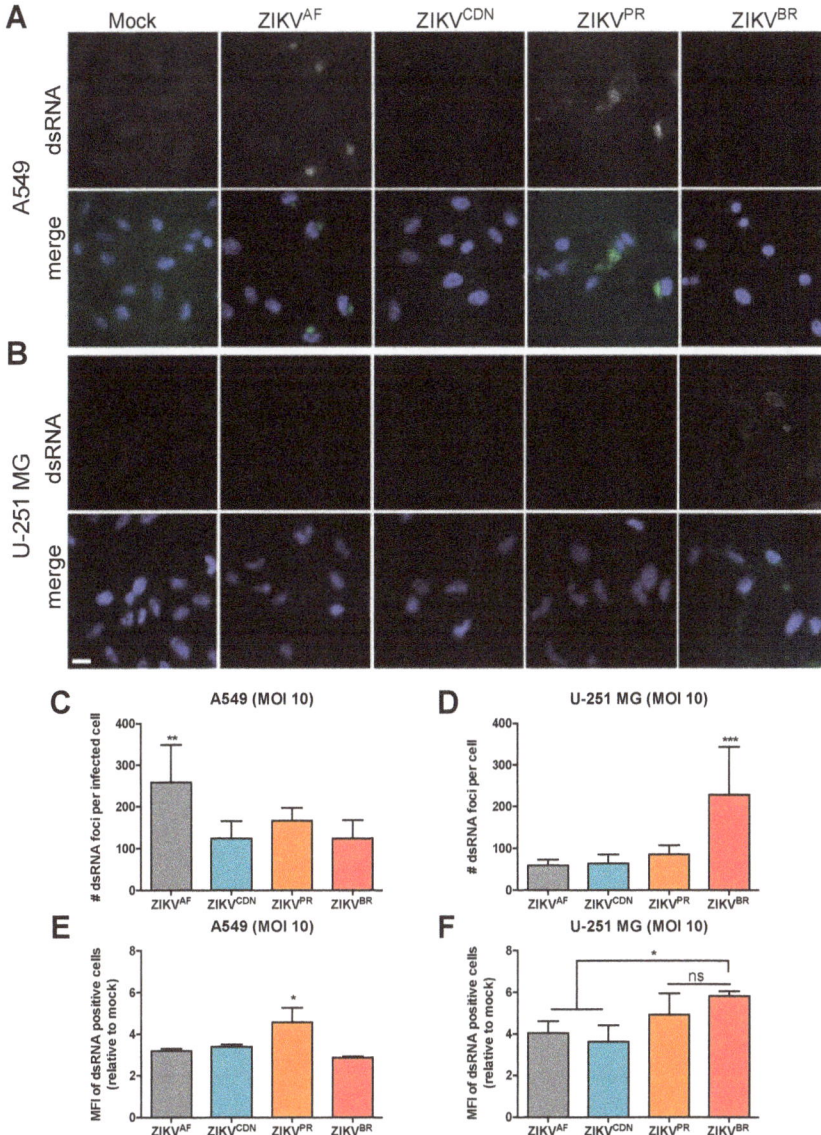

Figure 4. Isolate-specific differences are observed in number and fluorescence intensity of dsRNA foci in infected cell. (**A**) A549 and (**B**) U-251 MG cells were infected with ZIKV at MOI = 10 and 24 h post-infection dsRNA expression was analyzed by immunofluorescence microscopy. Scale bar, 20 µm. The number of dsRNA foci per cell in (**C**) A549 and (**D**) U-251 MG cells was quantified using Imaris software (>100 cells/condition). (**E**) A549 and (**F**) U-251 MG cells were infected with ZIKV at MOI = 10 and 24 h post-infection the mean fluorescence intensity (MFI) of dsRNA-positive cells was determined by flow cytometry. Values represent mean ± SEM of at least three independent experiments. Asterisks indicate significant differences: * $p < 0.05$, ** $p < 0.01$, *** $p < 0.001$.

Finally, to further investigate whether the number and brightness of dsRNA foci was related to an increase in viral replication, we also quantified negative- and positive-strand viral RNA (vRNA) by qRT-PCR analyses (Figure 5). Given that three of the ZIKV isolates used in this study are patient isolates and therefore we are not able to determine absolute vRNA copy numbers using a standard curve of in vitro-transcribed RNA, we quantified positive-strand vRNA relative to a standard curve of vRNA from ZIKV stocks of known titer (log PFU equivalents) as has been done previously [8]. While ZIKV^{CDN} produced less positive-strand vRNA than ZIKV^{AF} in A549 cells, possibly due to the lower proportion of ZIKV^{CDN}-infected cells (Figure 3A), there were no other statistically significant differences in intracellular positive-strand vRNA across ZIKV isolates in either cell type. This indicates that all of the ZIKV isolates produce similar levels of intracellular positive-strand vRNA after infection at high MOI.

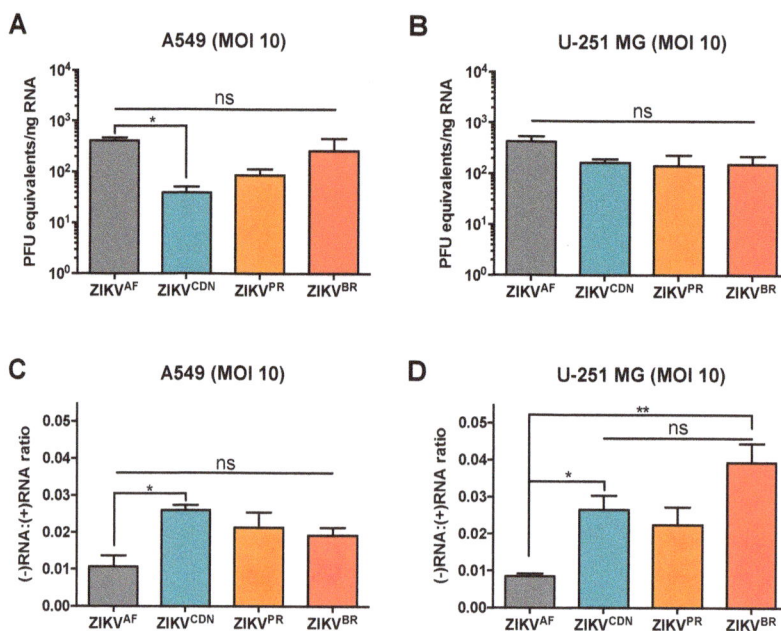

Figure 5. Asian lineage ZIKV isolates induce a higher ratio of negative:positive strand RNA. (**A**) A549 and (**B**) U-251 MG cells were infected with ZIKV at MOI = 10 and 24 h post-infection intracellular positive strand viral RNA was quantified by qRT-PCR. Data are normalized to GAPDH and expressed relative to a standard curve of PFU equivalents per ng input RNA. (**C**) A549 cells and (**D**) U-251 MG cells were infected with ZIKV at MOI = 10 and 24 h post-infection the relative amounts of positive and negative strand ZIKV genomes was quantified by qRT-PCR. Data are expressed as a ratio of negative:positive strand RNA. Values represent mean ± SEM of two or three independent experiments. Asterisks indicate significant differences: * $p < 0.05$, ** $p < 0.01$.

Next, we wanted to determine the relative amount of the replicative intermediate, negative-strand vRNA (Figure 5C,D). Interestingly, on average ZIKV^{AF} produced approximately one copy of negative-strand intermediate vRNA for every 100 positive-strand vRNAs in both A549 and U-251 MG cells. In contrast, the Asian lineage isolates produced 1.9 to 2.6 negative strands for every 100 positive-strand vRNAs in A549 cells, and 2.2 to 3.9 negative-strands for every 100 positive strands in U-251 MG cells. This indicates that approximately 1.8 to 4.5-fold more negative-strand intermediate RNA is produced during infection with Asian lineage isolates when compared with ZIKV^{AF}. Taken together, this data suggests that the Asian lineage isolates are able to produce more negative-strand intermediate vRNA than the African lineage isolate, and that the contemporary isolates, particularly ZIKV^{BR}, induce more dsRNA in U-251 MG cells.

4. Discussion

The recent expansion of the previously obscure ZIKV beyond its historical endemic range in equatorial Africa and Southeast Asia has piqued scientific and public health interest in emerging viral diseases. Phylogenetic analyses and investigations into recently acquired genetic polymorphisms suggest that recent evolutionary changes may have contributed to the rapid emergence and novel neurological pathogenesis observed in contemporary ZIKV outbreaks in the Americas [1,18]. In this study, we selected four ZIKV isolates from different points in its phylogenetic history (Figure S1) and compared viral replicative fitness in human lung carcinoma (A549) and human astrocytoma (U-251 MG) cell lines. We compared two ZIKV isolates from the 2015–2016 outbreaks in Puerto Rico and Brazil (ZIKV^{PR} and ZIKV^{BR}) to an earlier Asian lineage isolate (ZIKV^{CDN}) and the historical Uganda 1947 reference isolate (ZIKV^{AF}). We found that Asian lineage isolates produce more negative-strand intermediate vRNA, and that the contemporary ZIKV isolates, and in particular ZIKV^{BR}, produce more dsRNA and significantly higher viral titers over a single infectious cycle (which was more pronounced in U-251 MG cells), although these contemporary isolates may be impaired in cell spread over multiple infectious cycles.

Several groups have shown strain-dependent differences in ZIKV infection in cell culture and mouse models of infection, albeit with conflicting results [38]. Our data suggests that strain-dependent differences in viral replicative fitness are highly dependent on both cell type and the MOI used, which may explain some of these discrepancies in the literature. For example, several groups have demonstrated enhanced infectivity and replication by contemporary American ZIKV isolates, similar to what we observed herein at high MOI [39,40]. In contrast, other groups have shown that African lineage ZIKV isolates display higher infectivity and increased cytopathicity in cell culture than Asian lineage isolates when low MOIs ($\leq$1) were used, where few cells are predicted to be infected, similar to what we observed herein [41–44]. Although it is postulated that the highly-passaged African lineage isolate (MR766) may not accurately represent the phenotype of circulating African lineage ZIKV isolates, it should be noted that a recent study suggests that MR766 behaves similarly to other low-passage African lineage isolates in cell culture, and that all African lineage ZIKV isolates tested were more cytopathic than Asian lineage isolates at low MOIs [42]. The observed trend in relative CPEs is consistent with our flow cytometry data and the viral titers observed herein, suggesting that there is not an inherent difference in cytopathicity of the four ZIKV isolates, but rather CPE elicited is a consequence of active viral replication. Notably, we found that apoptosis does not appear to be the main driver of cell death during infection, with the exception of ZIKV^{BR}, which induced substantially more cleaved caspase-3 positive cells in both cell types. Moreover, we found that ZIKV infection induced more apoptosis in A549 cells than the U-251 MG cells, which is consistent with a recent study that suggests that human fetal astrocytes are resistant to ZIKV-induced apoptosis [16]. However, we cannot rule out the possibility that apoptosis may be more prevalent at later time points post-infection, as a recent study suggests a higher proportion of activated caspase-3 positive cells at later time points in both A549 cells and human fetal astrocytes with proportions similar to what we report here at earlier time points [16].

In addition, our data suggests that contemporary ZIKV isolates may be impaired in cell spread when compared with the African and early Asian ZIKV isolates, resulting in lower CPE in cell culture when infected at a low MOI. Several factors may contribute to this reduced infectivity and our results do not exclude the possibility that reduced viral binding may account for the differences in cell spread. Correspondingly, a recent study suggests that the structural proteins of a Brazilian ZIKV isolate are impaired in their ability to initiate an infection [41]. Moreover, it is also possible that the increased viral replication induced by the contemporary isolates in the initial round of infection induces a more robust antiviral response in bystander cells, which then restricts viral spread. Further research into strain-dependent differences in induction of innate immune responses may thus help to elucidate mechanisms by which the antiviral response is able to restrict ZIKV infection and whether the contemporary isolates are altered in their abilities to counter host antiviral defenses.

Interestingly, we noticed that both the contemporary isolates induced significantly higher amounts of dsRNA in the U-251 MG astrocytoma cells, while ZIKV^{BR} specifically was able to replicate to significantly higher titers in these cells. Moreover, the contemporary isolates had a higher MFI of dsRNA-positive cells, with ZIKV^{BR} in particular having a greater number of dsRNA foci per cell in the astrocytomas. Further quantification of positive- and negative-strand vRNA during infection revealed that the Asian lineage isolates generate more negative-strand replicative intermediate RNA than the African lineage isolate. Overall, this data supports the hypothesis that Asian lineage isolates may have a higher replicative fitness in astrocytoma cells. This is supported by the greater ratio of negative-strand replicative intermediate vRNA, and greater amounts of dsRNA foci per cell, as well as the significant increase in titer observed in ZIKV^{BR} in this cell type (which correlates well with the increase in negative-strand vRNA and dsRNA foci). On the other hand, it could be argued that ZIKV^{AF} may have the replicative advantage since it produces similar levels of positive-strand vRNA from fewer negative-strand intermediates; however, this does not appear to translate into higher viral infectious titers for this isolate. In addition to the higher infectious titers observed in ZIKV^{BR} infection, it is also possible that, consistent with the greater amount of dsRNA-positive cells during ZIKV^{PR} infection, this isolate may also mirror the increase in titer observed at later time points post-infection. However, our data suggests that ZIKV^{PR} titers have plateaued by 24 h post-infection at MOI 10 in both cell types (Figure 1B,C). As such, ZIKV^{BR} may have an additional advantage over ZIKV^{PR} in a post-replication step of the viral life cycle. In addition to the kinetic advantage ZIKV^{BR} has over a single infectious cycle, this isolate also appears to have a viral replicative fitness advantage over the other ZIKV isolates at low MOI when fewer cells are infected. The similar or higher viral titers produced by ZIKV^{BR} at the low MOI implies more infectious particles are released per cell during infection with this isolate. However, the higher titers of ZIKV^{BR} observed in the multistep growth curve, even when the % infected cells are low, may be due to compounded differences in replication kinetics over several rounds of viral replication.

An increase in viral replicative fitness of contemporary ZIKV isolates in astrocyte-derived cell types may translate into more severe neurological pathogenesis over the course of an infection. A current perspective on the neurotropic potential of ZIKV suggests that infected macrophages could potentially carry the virus into the developing brain through a "Trojan-horse" mechanism [45]. Once the virus is in the brain, other investigations conducted in mice and primary human tissue samples suggest that ZIKV preferentially infects astrocytes [16,25,26]. In concordance with these studies, all of the ZIKV isolates examined herein were able to efficiently infect and replicate in human astrocytoma cells. This affinity for astrocytes is likely due to their high expression of AXL, a putative receptor for ZIKV, which interacts with Gas6 to promote ZIKV infection [46,47]. Thus, examining the differential affinity displayed by different isolates in binding to the AXL/Gas6 viral entry receptor(s) may help to further elucidate the mechanism by which the contemporary strains elicit increased infection kinetics.

Taken together, our data suggests that the contemporary American ZIKV isolates may have evolved mechanisms to increase viral replication and/or infectious particle production in astrocyte-derived cell types. Furthermore, our comparative analysis in human lung carcinoma (A549) and astrocytoma (U-251 MG) cells further highlights the importance of cell-intrinsic factors in studies of ZIKV replicative fitness. Although similar levels of positive-strand intracellular vRNA were observed across isolates, the Asian lineage isolates had substantially more negative-strand replicative intermediate vRNA when compared with the African lineage isolate, suggesting that the Asian lineage isolates may have a greater replicative fitness. The strain-specific differences in ZIKV replication were more pronounced in astrocytoma cells than in the lung carcinoma cells, and thus, the U-251 MG astrocytoma cells may serve as a more appropriate cell culture model for investigating isolate-dependent differences in ZIKV replicative fitness. However, it is important to note that with the exception of ZIKV^{AF}, which was derived from an infectious cDNA, all other isolates were low passage patient isolates and, hence, we cannot rule out the possibility that they may harbor additional mutations resulting from adaptation to and/or propagation in cell culture. Thus, further investigations of these strain-specific polymorphisms that contribute to the observed differences in viral replicative fitness will be conducted by introduction of polymorphisms into infectious cDNAs that are now available for some of the isolates used herein [30,48]. Moreover, thorough investigation of cell-type-specific responses to infection may help elucidate the propensity for ZIKV to invade placental and neural tissues. Future studies must therefore consider the relationship between cell-intrinsic and strain-specific factors when examining ZIKV-host interactions.

Supplementary Materials: The following are available online at http://www.mdpi.com/1999-4915/10/12/728/s1, **Table S1.** List of ZIKV Genbank accession numbers of sequences used in phylogenetic analysis, **Table S2.** Source host, isolation, and passage history of ZIKV strains used in this study, **Table S3.** Percent amino acid identity matrix of the ZIKV isolates used in this study, **Figure S1.** Phylogenetic analysis of ZIKV isolates, **Figure S2.** ZIKV isolates differentially induce apoptosis, **Figure S3.** ZIKV isolates differ in infectivity at low MOI, **File S1.** Amino acid sequence alignment of the ZIKV isolates used in this study.

Author Contributions: T.R.B., M.M.R., and S.M.S. conceived of the study and designed the experiments. T.R.B. and M.M.R. performed the experiments. T.R.B., M.M.R., and S.M.S. analyzed the data and wrote the paper. The final manuscript was edited and approved by all authors. S.M.S. supervised the study and secured funding.

Funding: This work was supported by the Radcliffe Bequeath, operating funds from the Fonds de Recherche du Québec Nature et Technologies (#189120), and start-up funds provided by McGill University (S.M.S.). In addition, this research was undertaken, in part, thanks to funding from the Canada Research Chairs program.

Acknowledgments: We thank David Safronetz (Public Health Agency of Canada), Tom Hobman (University of Alberta, Canada), Mauro Teixeira (Universidade Federal de Minas Gerais, Brazil), and Matthew J. Evans (Icahn School of Medicine at Mount Sinai, New York, NY, USA) for providing ZIKV strains. We also thank Anne Gatignol (Lady Davis Research Institute, Montreal, QC, Canada) for providing U-251 MG cells. T.R.B. would like to thank the Frederick Banting and Charles Best Canada Graduate Scholarships—Doctoral Award (CGS-D) for graduate support. M.M.R. would like to thank the McGill University Faculty of Medicine, Max E. Binz Fellowship for graduate support. The authors acknowledge the McGill Flow Cytometry and Cell Sorting Facility for assistance with the flow cytometry experiments; the facility's infrastructure is supported by the Canada Foundation for Innovation (CFI), as well as the McGill University Life Sciences Complex Advanced BioImaging Facility for assistance with the microscopy experiments.

Conflicts of Interest: The authors declare no conflict of interest. The funders had no role in the design of the study; in the collection, analyses, or interpretation of data; in the writing of the manuscript, or in the decision to publish the results.

References

1. Rajah, M.M.; Pardy, R.D.; Condotta, S.A.; Richer, M.J.; Sagan, S.M. Zika Virus: Emergence, Phylogenetics, Challenges and Opportunities. *ACS Infect. Dis.* **2016**. [CrossRef]
2. Dick, G.W.; Kitchen, S.F.; Haddow, A.J. Zika virus (I). Isolations and serological specificity. *Trans. R. Soc. Trop. Med. Hyg.* **1952**, *46*, 509–520. [CrossRef]
3. Hayes, E.B. Zika virus outside Africa. *Emerg. Infect. Dis.* **2009**, *15*, 1347–1350. [CrossRef] [PubMed]
4. Chang, C.; Ortiz, K.; Ansari, A.; Gershwin, M.E. The Zika outbreak of the 21st century. *J. Autoimmun.* **2016**, *68*, 1–13. [CrossRef]
5. Duffy, M.R.; Chen, T.H.; Hancock, W.T.; Powers, A.M.; Kool, J.L.; Lanciotti, R.S.; Pretrick, M.; Marfel, M.; Holzbauer, S.; Dubray, C.; et al. Zika virus outbreak on Yap Island, Federated States of Micronesia. *N. Engl. J. Med.* **2009**, *360*, 2536–2543. [CrossRef] [PubMed]
6. Cao-Lormeau, V.M.; Blake, A.; Mons, S.; Lastere, S.; Roche, C.; Vanhomwegen, J.; Dub, T.; Baudouin, L.; Teissier, A.; Larre, P.; et al. Guillain-Barre Syndrome outbreak associated with Zika virus infection in French Polynesia: A case-control study. *Lancet* **2016**, *387*, 1531–1539. [CrossRef]
7. Fauci, A.S.; Morens, D.M. Zika Virus in the Americas—Yet Another Arbovirus Threat. *N. Engl. J. Med.* **2016**, *374*, 601–604. [CrossRef]
8. Lazear, H.M.; Govero, J.; Smith, A.M.; Platt, D.J.; Fernandez, E.; Miner, J.J.; Diamond, M.S. A Mouse Model of Zika Virus Pathogenesis. *Cell Host Microbe* **2016**. [CrossRef]

9.   Wakerley, B.R.; Yuki, N. Guillain-Barre syndrome. *Expert Rev. Neurother.* **2015**, *15*, 847–849. [CrossRef]

10.   Mlakar, J.; Korva, M.; Tul, N.; Popovic, M.; Poljsak-Prijatelj, M.; Mraz, J.; Kolenc, M.; Resman Rus, K.; Vesnaver Vipotnik, T.; Fabjan Vodusek, V.; et al. Zika Virus Associated with Microcephaly. *N. Engl. J. Med.* **2016**, *374*, 951–958. [CrossRef]

11.   Wise, J. Study links Zika virus to Guillain-Barre syndrome. *BMJ* **2016**, *352*, i1242. [CrossRef] [PubMed]

12.   Adams Waldorf, K.M.; Stencel-Baerenwald, J.E.; Kapur, R.P.; Studholme, C.; Boldenow, E.; Vornhagen, J.; Baldessari, A.; Dighe, M.K.; Thiel, J.; Merillat, S.; et al. Fetal brain lesions after subcutaneous inoculation of Zika virus in a pregnant nonhuman primate. *Nat. Med.* **2016**. [CrossRef] [PubMed]

13.   Weaver, S.C. Emergence of Epidemic Zika Virus Transmission and Congenital Zika Syndrome: Are Recently Evolved Traits to Blame? *mBio* **2017**, *8*. [CrossRef] [PubMed]

14.   Cugola, F.R.; Fernandes, I.R.; Russo, F.B.; Freitas, B.C.; Dias, J.L.; Guimaraes, K.P.; Benazzato, C.; Almeida, N.; Pignatari, G.C.; Romero, S.; et al. The Brazilian Zika virus strain causes birth defects in experimental models. *Nature* **2016**, *534*, 267–271. [CrossRef]

15.   Hamel, R.; Ferraris, P.; Wichit, S.; Diop, F.; Talignani, L.; Pompon, J.; Garcia, D.; Liegeois, F.; Sall, A.A.; Yssel, H.; et al. African and Asian Zika virus strains differentially induce early antiviral responses in primary human astrocytes. *Infect. Genet. Evol.* **2017**, *49*, 134–137. [CrossRef] [PubMed]

16.   Limonta, D.; Jovel, J.; Kumar, A.; Airo, A.M.; Hou, S.; Saito, L.; Branton, W.; Ka-Shu Wong, G.; Mason, A.; Power, C.; et al. Human Fetal Astrocytes Infected with Zika Virus Exhibit Delayed Apoptosis and Resistance to Interferon: Implications for Persistence. *Viruses* **2018**, *10*, 646. [CrossRef]

17.   Tripathi, S.; Balasubramaniam, V.R.; Brown, J.A.; Mena, I.; Grant, A.; Bardina, S.V.; Maringer, K.; Schwarz, M.C.; Maestre, A.M.; Sourisseau, M.; et al. A novel Zika virus mouse model reveals strain specific differences in virus pathogenesis and host inflammatory immune responses. *PLoS Pathog.* **2017**, *13*, e1006258. [CrossRef]

18.   Yuan, L.; Huang, X.Y.; Liu, Z.Y.; Zhang, F.; Zhu, X.L.; Yu, J.Y.; Ji, X.; Xu, Y.P.; Li, G.; Li, C.; et al. A single mutation in the prM protein of Zika virus contributes to fetal microcephaly. *Science* **2017**. [CrossRef]

19.   Xia, H.; Luo, H.; Shan, C.; Muruato, A.E.; Nunes, B.T.D.; Medeiros, D.B.A.; Zou, J.; Xie, X.; Giraldo, M.I.; Vasconcelos, P.F.C.; et al. An evolutionary NS1 mutation enhances Zika virus evasion of host interferon induction. *Nat. Commun.* **2018**, *9*, 414. [CrossRef]

20.   Liu, Y.; Liu, J.; Du, S.; Shan, C.; Nie, K.; Zhang, R.; Li, X.F.; Zhang, R.; Wang, T.; Qin, C.F.; et al. Evolutionary enhancement of Zika virus infectivity in Aedes aegypti mosquitoes. *Nature* **2017**, *545*, 482–486. [CrossRef]

21.   Frumence, E.; Roche, M.; Krejbich-Trotot, P.; El-Kalamouni, C.; Nativel, B.; Rondeau, P.; Misse, D.; Gadea, G.; Viranaicken, W.; Despres, P. The South Pacific epidemic strain of Zika virus replicates efficiently in human epithelial A549 cells leading to IFN-beta production and apoptosis induction. *Virology* **2016**, *493*, 217–226. [CrossRef]

22.   Airo, A.M.; Urbanowski, M.D.; Lopez-Orozco, J.; You, J.H.; Skene-Arnold, T.D.; Holmes, C.; Yamshchikov, V.; Malik-Soni, N.; Frappier, L.; Hobman, T.C. Expression of flavivirus capsids enhance the cellular environment for viral replication by activating Akt-signalling pathways. *Virology* **2018**, *516*, 147–157. [CrossRef]

23.   Kumar, A.; Hou, S.; Airo, A.M.; Limonta, D.; Mancinelli, V.; Branton, W.; Power, C.; Hobman, T.C. Zika virus inhibits type-I interferon production and downstream signaling. *EMBO Rep.* **2016**, *17*, 1766–1775. [CrossRef] [PubMed]

24.   Hirsch, A.J.; Smith, J.L.; Haese, N.N.; Broeckel, R.M.; Parkins, C.J.; Kreklywich, C.; DeFilippis, V.R.; Denton, M.; Smith, P.P.; Messer, W.B.; et al. Zika Virus infection of rhesus macaques leads to viral persistence in multiple tissues. *PLoS Pathog.* **2017**, *13*, e1006219. [CrossRef] [PubMed]

25.   Retallack, H.; Di Lullo, E.; Arias, C.; Knopp, K.A.; Laurie, M.T.; Sandoval-Espinosa, C.; Mancia Leon, W.R.; Krencik, R.; Ullian, E.M.; Spatazza, J.; et al. Zika virus cell tropism in the developing human brain and inhibition by azithromycin. *Proc. Natl. Acad. Sci. USA* **2016**, *113*, 14408–14413. [CrossRef] [PubMed]

26.   Van den Pol, A.N.; Mao, G.; Yang, Y.; Ornaghi, S.; Davis, J.N. Zika Virus Targeting in the Developing Brain. *J. Neurosci.* **2017**, *37*, 2161–2175. [CrossRef]

27.   Hou, W.; Armstrong, N.; Obwolo, L.A.; Thomas, M.; Pang, X.; Jones, K.S.; Tang, Q. Determination of the Cell Permissiveness Spectrum, Mode of RNA Replication, and RNA-Protein Interaction of Zika Virus. *BMC Infect. Dis.* **2017**, *17*, 239. [CrossRef] [PubMed]

28. Larkin, M.A.; Blackshields, G.; Brown, N.P.; Chenna, R.; McGettigan, P.A.; McWilliam, H.; Valentin, F.; Wallace, I.M.; Wilm, A.; Lopez, R.; et al. Clustal W and Clustal X version 2.0. *Bioinformatics* **2007**, *23*, 2947–2948. [CrossRef] [PubMed]

29. Kumar, S.; Stecher, G.; Tamura, K. MEGA7: Molecular Evolutionary Genetics Analysis Version 7.0 for Bigger Datasets. *Mol Biol Evol* **2016**, *33*, 1870–1874. [CrossRef]

30. Schwarz, M.C.; Sourisseau, M.; Espinosa, M.M.; Gray, E.S.; Chambers, M.T. Rescue of the 1947 Zika Virus Prototype Strain with a Cytomegalovirus Promoter-Driven cDNA Clone. *mSphere* **2016**, *1*, e00246-16. [CrossRef] [PubMed]

31. Fonseca, K.; Meatherall, B.; Zarra, D.; Drebot, M.; MacDonald, J.; Pabbaraju, K.; Wong, S.; Webster, P.; Lindsay, R.; Tellier, R. First case of Zika virus infection in a returning Canadian traveler. *Am. J. Trop. Med. Hyg.* **2014**, *91*, 1035–1038. [CrossRef] [PubMed]

32. Heldt, C.L.; Hernandez, R.; Mudiganti, U.; Gurgel, P.V.; Brown, D.T.; Carbonell, R.G. A colorimetric assay for viral agents that produce cytopathic effects. *J. Virol. Methods* **2006**, *135*, 56–65. [CrossRef] [PubMed]

33. Lanciotti, R.S.; Kosoy, O.L.; Laven, J.J.; Velez, J.O.; Lambert, A.J.; Johnson, A.J.; Stanfield, S.M.; Duffy, M.R. Genetic and serologic properties of Zika virus associated with an epidemic, Yap State, Micronesia, 2007. *Emerg. Infect. Dis.* **2008**, *14*, 1232–1239. [CrossRef] [PubMed]

34. Wang, L.; Valderramos, S.G.; Wu, A.; Ouyang, S.; Li, C.; Brasil, P.; Bonaldo, M.; Coates, T.; Nielsen-Saines, K.; Jiang, T.; et al. From Mosquitos to Humans: Genetic Evolution of Zika Virus. *Cell Host Microbe* **2016**. [CrossRef]

35. Beaver, J.T.; Lelutiu, N.; Habib, R.; Skountzou, I. Evolution of Two Major Zika Virus Lineages: Implications for Pathology, Immune Response, and Vaccine Development. *Front. Immunol.* **2018**, *9*, 1640. [CrossRef] [PubMed]

36. Lazear, H.M.; Diamond, M.S. Zika Virus: New Clinical Syndromes and Its Emergence in the Western Hemisphere. *J. Virol.* **2016**, *90*, 4864–4875. [CrossRef]

37. Barnard, T.R.; Sagan, S.M. (McGill University, Montreal, QC, Canada). Personal Communication, 2018.

38. Simonin, Y.; van Riel, D.; Van de Perre, P.; Rockx, B.; Salinas, S. Differential virulence between Asian and African lineages of Zika virus. *PLoS Negl. Trop. Dis.* **2017**, *11*, e0005821. [CrossRef]

39. Alpuche-Lazcano, S.P.; McCullogh, C.R.; Del Corpo, O.; Rance, E.; Scarborough, R.J.; Mouland, A.J.; Sagan, S.M.; Teixeira, M.M.; Gatignol, A. Higher Cytopathic Effects of a Zika Virus Brazilian Isolate from Bahia Compared to a Canadian-Imported Thai Strain. *Viruses* **2018**, *10*, 53. [CrossRef]

40. Kuivanen, S.; Korhonen, E.M.; Helisten, A.A.; Huhtamo, E.; Smura, T.; Vapalahti, O. Differences in the growth properties of Zika virus foetal brain isolate and related epidemic strains in vitro. *J. Gen. Virol.* **2017**, *98*, 1744–1748. [CrossRef]

41. Bos, S.; Viranaicken, W.; Turpin, J.; El-Kalamouni, C.; Roche, M.; Krejbich-Trotot, P.; Despres, P.; Gadea, G. The structural proteins of epidemic and historical strains of Zika virus differ in their ability to initiate viral infection in human host cells. *Virology* **2018**, *516*, 265–273. [CrossRef]

42. Sheridan, M.A.; Balaraman, V.; Schust, D.J.; Ezashi, T.; Roberts, R.M.; Franz, A.W.E. African and Asian strains of Zika virus differ in their ability to infect and lyse primitive human placental trophoblast. *PLoS ONE* **2018**, *13*, e0200086. [CrossRef] [PubMed]

43. Smith, D.R.; Sprague, T.R.; Hollidge, B.S.; Valdez, S.M.; Padilla, S.L.; Bellanca, S.A.; Golden, J.W.; Coyne, S.R.; Kulesh, D.A.; Miller, L.J.; et al. African and Asian Zika Virus Isolates Display Phenotypic Differences Both In Vitro and In Vivo. *Am. J. Trop. Med. Hyg.* **2018**, *98*, 432–444. [CrossRef] [PubMed]

44. Simonin, Y.; Loustalot, F.; Desmetz, C.; Foulongne, V.; Constant, O.; Fournier-Wirth, C.; Leon, F.; Moles, J.P.; Goubaud, A.; Lemaitre, J.M.; et al. Zika Virus Strains Potentially Display Different Infectious Profiles in Human Neural Cells. *EBioMedicine* **2016**, *12*, 161–169. [CrossRef] [PubMed]

45. Quicke, K.M.; Bowen, J.R.; Johnson, E.L.; McDonald, C.E.; Ma, H.; O'Neal, J.T.; Rajakumar, A.; Wrammert, J.; Rimawi, B.H.; Pulendran, B.; et al. Zika Virus Infects Human Placental Macrophages. *Cell Host Microbe* **2016**, *20*, 83–90. [CrossRef]

46. Nowakowski, T.J.; Pollen, A.A.; Di Lullo, E.; Sandoval-Espinosa, C.; Bershteyn, M.; Kriegstein, A.R. Expression Analysis Highlights AXL as a Candidate Zika Virus Entry Receptor in Neural Stem Cells. *Cell Stem Cell* **2016**, *18*, 591–596. [CrossRef] [PubMed]

47. Meertens, L.; Labeau, A.; Dejarnac, O.; Cipriani, S.; Sinigaglia, L.; Bonnet-Madin, L.; Le Charpentier, T.; Hafirassou, M.L.; Zamborlini, A.; Cao-Lormeau, V.M.; et al. Axl Mediates ZIKA Virus Entry in Human Glial Cells and Modulates Innate Immune Responses. *Cell Rep.* **2017**, *18*, 324–333. [CrossRef]

48. Yun, S.I.; Song, B.H.; Frank, J.C.; Julander, J.G.; Olsen, A.L.; Polejaeva, I.A.; Davies, C.J.; White, K.L.; Lee, Y.M. Functional Genomics and Immunologic Tools: The Impact of Viral and Host Genetic Variations on the Outcome of Zika Virus Infection. *Viruses* **2018**, *10*, 422. [CrossRef] [PubMed]

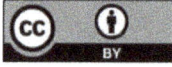

viruses

MDPI

Communication

Differential Zika Virus Infection of Testicular Cell Lines

Luwanika Mlera [†] and Marshall E. Bloom *

Biology of Vector-Borne Viruses Section, Laboratory of Virology, Rocky Mountain Laboratories, NIAID/NIH, Hamilton, MT 59840, USA; Luwanika.Mlera@gmail.com

* Correspondence: mbloom@niaid.nih.gov; Tel.: +1-406-375-9707

† Present address: BIO5 Institute, University of Arizona, Tucson, AZ 85721, USA.

Received: 7 December 2018; Accepted: 5 January 2019; Published: 9 January 2019

Abstract: Background: Zika virus is a mosquito-borne flavivirus responsible for recent outbreaks of epidemic proportions in Latin America. Sexual transmission of the virus has been reported in 13 countries and may be an important route of infection. Sexual transmission of ZIKV has mostly been male-to-female, and persistence of viral RNA in semen for up to 370 days has been recorded. The susceptibility to ZIKV of different testicular cell types merits investigation. Methods: We infected primary Sertoli cells, a primary testicular fibroblast Hs1.Tes, and 2 seminoma cell lines SEM-1 and TCam-2 cells with ZIKV Paraiba and the prototype ZIKV MR766 to evaluate their susceptibility and to look for viral persistence. A human neuroblastoma cell line SK-N-SH served as a control cell type. Results: Both virus strains were able to replicate in all cell lines tested, but ZIKV MR766 attained higher titers. Initiation of viral persistence by ZIKV Paraiba was observed in Sertoli, Hs1.Tes, SEM-1 and TCam-2 cells, but was of limited duration due to delayed cell death. ZIKV MR766 persisted only in Hs1.Tes and Sertoli cells, and persistence was also limited. In contrast, SK-N-SH cells were killed by both ZIKV MR766 and ZIKV Paraiba and persistence could not be established in these cells. Conclusions: ZIKV prototype strain MR766 and the clinically relevant Paraiba strain replicated in several testicular cell types. Persistence of ZIKV MR766 was only observed in Hs1.Tes and Sertoli cells, but the persistence did not last more than 3 or 4 passages, respectively. ZIKV Paraiba persisted in TCam-2, Hs1.Tes, Sertoli and SEM-1 cells for up to 5 passages, depending on cell type. TCam-2 cells appeared to clear persistent infection by ZIKV Paraiba.

Keywords: flavivirus; Zika virus; viral persistence; testicular cells; testes

1. Introduction

Zika virus (ZIKV) is a mosquito-borne flavivirus originally described in captive *Macaca mulatta* monkeys in Uganda [1]. ZIKV recently caused an outbreak of epidemic proportions in Latin American countries and was associated with devastating microcephaly in neonates that contracted the infection in utero [2]. Other complications of ZIKV are varied and include Guillian Barre syndrome [3–6].

Although ZIKV is primarily transmitted by *Aedes* mosquito bites, sexual transmission is now well-documented. The first description of sexual transmission is probably that of 2 American scientists who were bitten by *Aedes* mosquitoes while working in Senegal in 2008 [7]. The male transmitted ZIKV to his wife and she presented clinical signs of disease consistent with ZIKV infection [7]. Additional recent reports described infection in partners following travel to outbreak regions [8,9]. An interesting example is that of an asymptomatic French couple who were only diagnosed when they sought assisted reproductive health services after returning from the French island of Martinique [8]. Most of the sexual transmission cases reported have been male-to-female, but a suspected female-to-male case has been reported [10]. To date, 13 countries have documented sexual transmission of ZIKV [11]. In the US in 2016, 47/5168 ZIKV cases were attributed to sexual transmission [12], whereas 8/451 cases could have been sexually transmitted in 2017 [13]. Thus, sexual transmission may be an important route of acquiring infection although it would be difficult to assess such transmission in the face of a large vector-borne outbreak [14].

The testes are male organs that contain germ cells which differentiate into mature spermatozoa. Sertoli cells are interspaced between germinal epithelial cells and provide support for the germ cells. Leydig cells are irregularly shaped interstitial cells that produce the hormone testosterone. Sexual transmission of ZIKV by males and the presence of virus in semen suggests that cells in the male genitourinary tract are infected [15]. Animal studies have also shown that the testes are infected with various consequences, including testicular atrophy with implications in male fertility [16,17]. Virus was reported to be mainly in the interstitial Leydig cells and Sertoli cells, but this varied from study to study [16,18,19]. Govero and colleagues showed that Sertoli cells detached from the basement membrane and that there was a decline in the germ cell population in ZIKV infected mice [17]. Thus, the different cells in the testes may play different roles in harboring virus for transmission or pathogenesis, which leads to the destruction of organ integrity.

In this paper, we infected several human testicular cells lines to evaluate the extent to which the cells permitted ZIKV replication in vitro; primary Sertoli cells, a primary testicular fibroblast Hs1.Tes and the 2 seminoma cell lines SEM-1 and TCam-2. The infection in the testicular cell lines was compared to infection in a human neuroblastoma cell line SK-N-SH. We were also interested in determining if ZIKV would persist in any of these cell lines. Our results showed that ZIKV differentially infected the testicular cell lines tested and could persist in some cells in a strain-dependent manner. Delayed apoptotic cell death was observed during viral persistence, thus limiting duration of persistence to 5 passages at most.

2. Materials and Methods

2.1. Viruses and Cells

The Ugandan ZIKV strain MR766 were generously provided by Dr. Stephen Whitehead (Laboratory of Infectious Disease, NIAID/NIH). The Brazilian ZIKV Paraiba was isolated by Dr. Pedro F.C Vasconcelos, Instituto Evandro Chagas, Brazil and it was a kind gift from Dr. Stephen Whitehead (Laboratory of Infectious Disease, NIAID/NIH). Virus stocks were prepared by infecting Vero (ATCC) cells and harvesting the supernatants 3 days post infection. Virus in the supernatants was semi-purified by ultracentrifugation over a 20% sucrose solution, followed by quantification using a plaque assay on Vero cells.

The neuroblastoma SK-N-SH cell line [20] was purchased from ATCC and maintained in antibiotic-free Eagle's minimum essential medium (EMEM; Gibco, Hampton, NH, USA) containing 10% fetal bovine serum (FBS). Fibroblast Hs1.Tes cells (ATCC) and the TCam-2 seminoma cell line (a kind gift from Dr. Constantine Stratakis, NICHD/NIH) were maintained in Dulbecco's modified Eagle's medium (DMEM) supplemented with 10% FBS and $1\times$ antibiotic-antimycotic (Gibco). Doubling time for the TCam-2 seminoma cell line in culture is approximately 50 h. Sertoli cells (Lonza, Basel, Switzerland) were grown in DMEM/F12 medium with 10% FBS and penicillin/streptomycin (Gibco) and the cells grow to confluence in 7–10 days when seeded at 450–500 cells/cm^2. SEM-1 seminoma cells were a kind gift from Dr. Alan Epstein (USC Keck School of Medicine, Los Angeles, CA, USA), and they were maintained in RPMI 1640 (Gibco/ThermoFischer) supplemented with 10% FBS and penicillin/streptomycin. SEM-1 cell doubling time is 50 h.

2.2. ZIKV Infection

Two million cells were seeded in 75 cm^2 flasks a day before the infection and allowed to grow at 37 °C and 5% CO$_2$. ZIKV infections with either MR766 or Paraiba strains were performed at a multiplicity of infection of 0.1 with adsorption at 37 °C and rocking for 1 h. All infections were performed in triplicate (biologically independent replicates). The inoculum was removed, and cells were washed 3 times with phosphate buffered saline (PBS; Gibco). Twenty mL of the appropriate cell culture medium was added prior to incubation at 37 °C and 5% CO_2. Supernatant aliquots were removed daily for 7 days and stored at −80 °C until virus titration. The infected cells were also microscopically observed daily for the development of cytopathic effect (CPE). At 7 dpi, intact cell monolayers were washed twice in PBS, trypsinized and passaged at 1:10 in new flasks with fresh culture media.

2.3. ZIKV Titration by Immunofocus Assay

Supernatants from infected cultures were harvested at different time points post infection. Serial 10-fold dilutions were carried out and 250 μL of each dilution was plated onto confluent Vero cells (ATCC) in 12-well plates. Each dilution was plated in duplicate. ZIKV was adsorbed for 1 h at 37 °C with rocking, followed by washing twice with PBS. The infected monolayer was overlaid with DMEM containing 0.8% methylcellulose, 2% FBA and antibiotics. Plates were incubated at 37 °C for 3 days after which the overlay was removed, and the cells were washed with PBS twice. The cells were fixed with 100% methanol for 15 min, washed twice with PBS and probed with an anti-ZIKV E antibody (BioFront Technologies, Tallahassee, FL, USA) at a 1:1000 dilution. Cells in the primary antibody were incubated at 37 °C for 1 h. Following primary antibody incubation, cells were washed twice with PBS and an anti-mouse secondary antibody (Dako, Santa Clara, CA, USA) was added at a 1:1000 dilution and incubated with the cells at 37 °C for 1 h. Next, the cells were washed twice with PBS followed by development of immunofoci with a diaminobenzidine/peroxide substrate (Sigma-Aldrich, St. Louis, MO, USA) and enumeration.

2.4. Monolayer Staining with Giemsa Stain

To visualize the cytopathic effect of ZIKV on infected cell monolayers, cells were washed twice in PBS and fixed with 4% paraformaldehyde (PFA) for 10 min at room temperature. The PFA was aspirated followed by washing twice with PBS. Cells were stained with a 1:5 Giemsa stain for 30 min. The stain was removed, and cells were washed twice with PBS and imaged using an AxioVert.A1 microscope equipped with Zeiss Axiocam 503 monochromatic camera.

2.5. Immunofluorescence Microscopy

ZIKV-infected Sertoli cells at P1 were plated into a 4-well chamber slide at 1×10^4 cells/well and allowed to attach overnight at 37 °C in 5% CO_2. The medium was aspirated, and cells were washed twice with PBS. The cells were fixed with 4% paraformaldehyde/5% sucrose in PBS for 10 min. The fixed cells were permeabilized with 0.1% Triton X/4% PFA in PBS for 10 min with shaking. Aldehydes were quenched using 50 mM glycine for 10 min. Blocking was done with 2% bovine serum albumin for 1 h. Cells were probed with a mouse anti-ZIKV E monoclonal antibody (BioFront Technologies) at 1:1000 dilution, and a rabbit anti-cleaved caspase 3 (BD Biosciences, San Jose, CA, USA) at 1:1000 dilution. The primary antibodies were detected with anti-mouse (conjugated with Alexa Flour 647) and Alexa Flour 488-conjugated anti-rabbit antibodies (Invitrogen, Carlsbad, CA, USA). Images were captured using a Laser Scanning Microscope (LSM) 710 (Zeiss, Oberkochen, Germany) at 40× magnification.

3. Results

3.1. ZIKV Infection of the Fibroblast Hs1.Tes Cell Line

The Hs1.Tes cell line is a fibroblast which represents testicular connective tissue. Both ZIKV MR766 and Paraiba strains were able to infect this cell line in culture, and ZIKV MR766 replicated to higher titers than ZIKV Paraiba (Figure 1). The ZIKV MR766 titer peaked to 1.8×10^7 ffu/mL at 4 dpi, whereas ZIKV Paraiba titers peaked to 1.0×10^6 at 5 dpi (Figure 1). Infection of Hs1.Tes cells with either ZIKV Paraiba or ZIKV MR766 did not result in any obvious cytopathic effect (CPE) by 7 dpi (Figures 2 and 3).

To determine if ZIKV could persist in Hs1.Tes fibroblast cell line, we passaged the ZIKV infected cells after 7 dpi. Infectious ZIKV Paraiba and ZIKV MR766 was recovered from the Hs1.Tes supernatants at each passage for 3 passages, suggesting that ZIKV could persist in these cells (Figure 4). However, we observed a decline in the cell population upon passage each, suggesting delayed and slowly progressive cell death and a 4th passage was not possible (Figure 5a,b). Thus, the duration of ZIKV persistence in Hs1.Tes cells was limited by continued cell death.

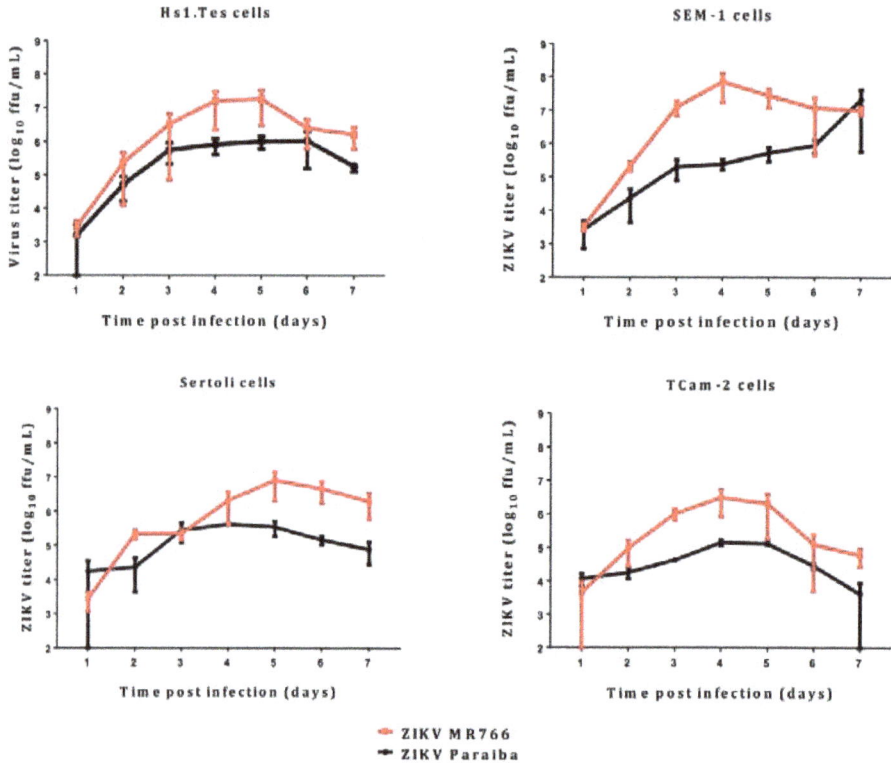

Figure 1. Replication kinetics of ZIKV MR766 and Paraiba over the course of 7 days. Error bars represent standard deviation (SD) from the mean for 3 independent replicates.

3.2. ZIKV Infection of Sertoli Cells

Sertoli cells are testicular cells, which support the germ cells. In culture, we observed that these cells were also permissive to infection by both ZIKV Paraiba and MR766 strains, which replicated to maximal titers at 4 and 5 dpi, respectively (Figure 1). The ZIKV Paraiba titers did not proceed beyond 10^6 ffu/mL for 7 dpi, but MR766 titers neared 10^7 ffu/mL at 5 dpi. Similar to Hs1.Tes cells, infection of Sertoli cells with ZIKV Paraiba did not cause an observable cytopathic effect (CPE) by 7 dpi (Figure 2), but ZIKV MR766 caused minimal CPE which was observed at 7 dpi (Figure 3).

After 7 dpi, we passaged Sertoli cells infected with either ZIKV Paraiba or ZIKV MR766 and observed that ZIKV Paraiba persistently infected Sertoli cells for up to 5 passages before the delayed cell death, like that observed in Hs1.Tes cells, rendered the cells unfit for a 6th passage. Detection of cleaved caspase 3 by immunofluorescence (Figure 5c) suggested that cell death was via apoptosis. We also observed that not all ZIKV-infected cells stained positive for cleaved caspase 3 (Figure 5c).

The progressive cell death was accompanied by a decline in the ZIKV Paraiba titers from 1.0×10^6 ffu/mL at passage 1, to 1.5×10^4 ffu/mL at passage 5 (Figure 4). ZIKV MR766 infection persisted in Sertoli cells for only 4 passages and the viral titers were constant at $\sim 10^5$ ffu/mL from passage 1 to passage 3, but the titer declined to 1.6×10^4 at the 4th passage (Figure 4).

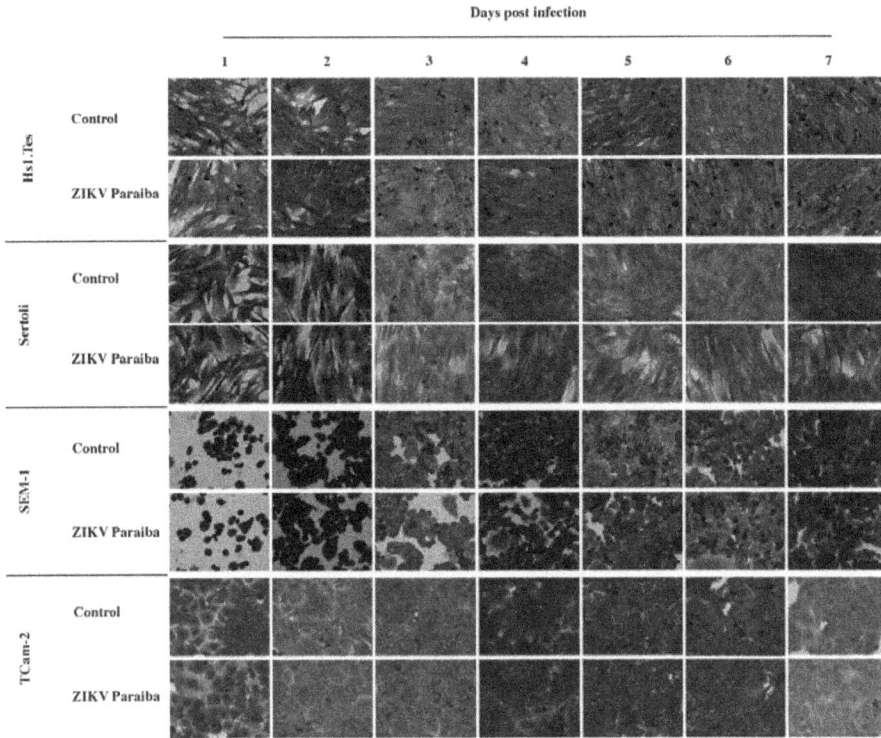

Figure 2. Microscopic evaluation of testicular cell lines infected with ZIKV Paraiba. No obvious cytopathic effect was observed in all testicular cell lines infected with ZIKV Paraiba. Images were captured at a magnification of 400×.

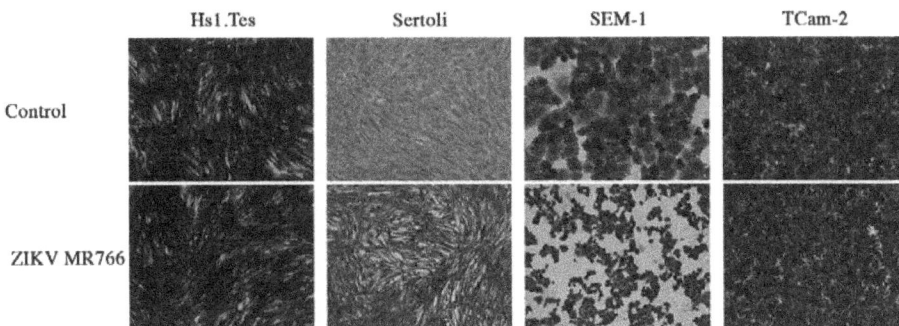

Figure 3. Cytopathic effect of ZIKV MR766 on testicular cell lines at 7 dpi. We noted that ZIKV MR766-infected Sertoli and SEM-1 cells appeared smaller than uninfected controls. TCam-2 and Hs1.Tes cells did show any CPE at 7 dpi. Images were obtained at a magnification of 400×.

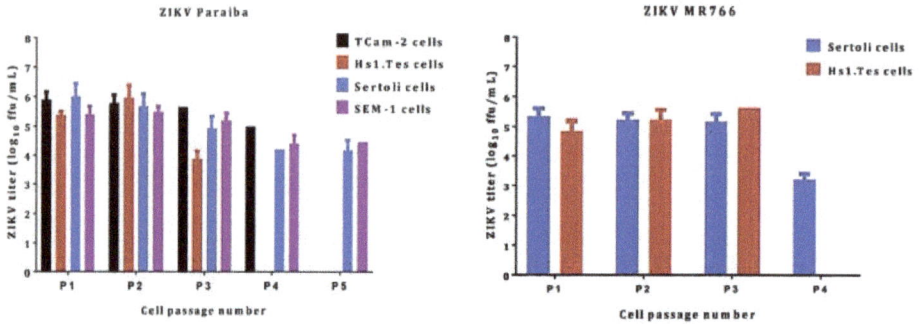

Figure 4. ZIKV titers in persistently infected testicular cell lines. The clinical isolate ZIKV Paraiba was able to persist in all cell lines tested for up to 5 passages (P1 through to P5), depending on cell line. ZIKV MR766 was only able to persist in Sertoli and Hs1.Tes cells. Virus titration was performed using supernatants collected at the end of each 7-day period and each data point represents an average of 3 biological replicates. Error bars represent standard deviation from the mean. Each passage was done after 7 days by washing the monolayer twice with PBS, trypsinizing the cells and seeding into new flasks with fresh culture medium at 1:10.

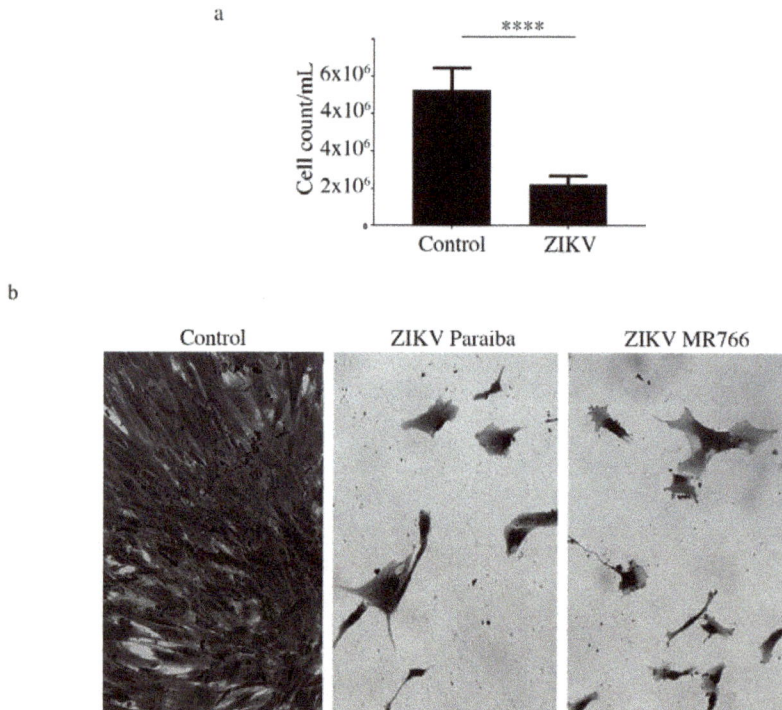

Figure 5. *Cont.*

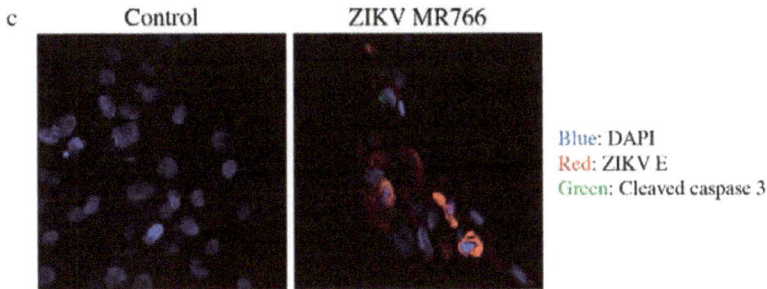

Figure 5. Analysis of continued cell death in ZIKV-infected testicular cells. (**a**) Cell count graph showing that there were 2-times more cells in the uninfected Hs1.Tes control, compared to ZIKV Paraiba-infected Hs1.Tes cells at P1. For both control and ZIKV-infected cells, the count was done after 7 days of cell passage. ****, $p < 0.0001$ (unpaired t-test). (**b**) Microscopic images showing loss of the Hs1.Tes monolayer in ZIKV-infected cells at P3. The morphology of infected cells at this time point appeared grossly aberrant and pleomorphic when compared to that of uninfected control cells. Cells were imaged at a magnification of 400×. (**c**) Confocal microscopy images showing cleaved caspase 3 in some ZIKV-infected Sertoli cells at P1. Not all ZIKV E protein-expressing cells stained positive for cleaved caspase 3, supporting the notion that cell death in persistently infected cells was progressive. Cells were imaged at a magnification of 400×.

3.3. ZIKV Infection of Seminoma Cell Lines

TCam-2 cells are a germ cell seminoma cell line, and SEM-1 cells are a testicular cell line which is an intermediate between a non-seminoma and a true seminoma [21,22]. Compared to all cell lines tested, SEM-1 seminoma cells supported the highest titers of both ZIKV MR766 and ZIKV Paraiba replication (Figure 1). The ZIKV MR766 titer peaked to 7.1×10^7 at 4 dpi, whereas the peak ZIKV Paraiba titer was attained at 7 dpi (Figure 1). Interestingly, the ZIKV replication graph in SEM-1 cells suggested that ZIKV Paraiba was still replicating upwards of the peak attained at 7 dpi. No obvious CPE was observed in ZIKV Paraiba-infected SEM-1 cells (Figure 2), but ZIKV MR766 caused notable cell death by 7 dpi and the infected cells appeared smaller in comparison to uninfected controls (Figure 3). Upon a single passage, ZIKV MR766 infection induced a lytic crisis in SEM-1 seminoma cells. The culture of ZIKV MR766 infected cells did not recover, and thus, a persistent ZIKV MR76 6 infection of SEM-1 cells could not be established. However, a persistent ZIKV Paraiba infection was maintained in SEM-1 cells up to 5 passages (Figure 4).

In TCam-2 seminoma cells, ZIKV titers peaked at 4 dpi, with the MR766 strain at 3×10^6 ffu/mL and the Paraiba strain at 1.4×10^5 ffu/mL (Figure 1). By 7 dpi, ZIKV MR766 and ZIKV Paraiba titers declined to 6×10^4 ffu/mL and 4×10^3 ffu/mL, respectively. Interestingly, both ZIKV strains did not cause any CPE in TCam-2 cells by 7 dpi (Figures 2 and 3). Although ZIKV Paraiba persisted in TCam-2 cells for 4 passages, ZIKV MR766 killed the cells upon passage into P1, suggesting a strain-dependent delayed cell death mechanism.

3.4. ZIKV Infection in a Human Neuroblastoma SK-N-SH Cell Line

Our laboratory has previously reported infection of the human neuroblastoma SK-N-SH cell line [23]. We used the SK-N-SH cells to compare ZIKV infection in testicular cells lines, and to determine if ZIKV would also persist in these cells. ZIKV MR766 replicated to higher titers than ZIKV Paraiba (Fig 6a) as expected [23]. Infection of SK-N-SH cells with either ZIKV MR766 or ZIKV Paraiba resulted in extensive CPE by day 4 or 5, respectively (Figure 6b). Following the lytic crises, the few remaining cells (Figure 6b) died a few days after media replenishment. Thus, no persistent ZIKV infection of SK-N-SH cells could be established.

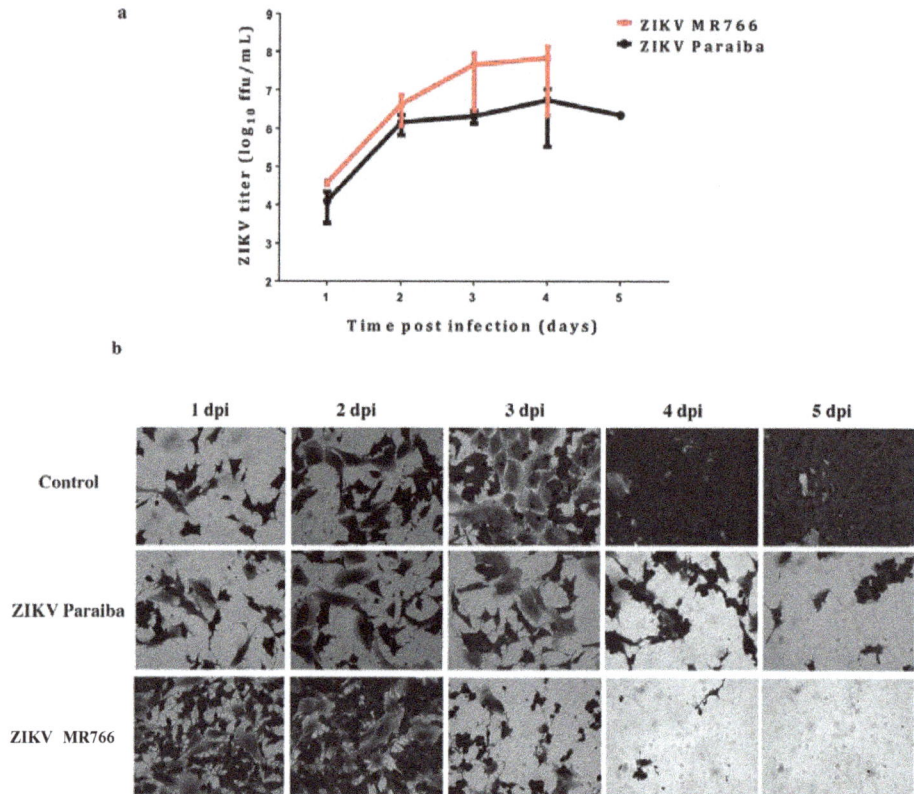

Figure 6. ZIKV infection in a human neuroblastoma SK-N-SH cell line. (**a**) Replication kinetics of ZIKV MR766 and Paraiba strains in SK-N-SH cells. Error bars represent SD from the mean for 3 independent experiments. (**b**) Cell death in SK-N-SH cell monolayers infected with ZIKV Paraiba or ZIKV MR766. ZIKV MR766 was more aggressive at killing SK-N-SH cells. Images of the SK-N-SH monolayer were acquired at a magnification of 400×.

4. Discussion

ZIKV has recently been shown to cause devastating effects in neonates following in utero infection [2,24]. In adults, sexual transmission has been well documented and was associated with testicular atrophy and male sterility [16,17,25,26]. A few reports have subsequently reported infection of testicular cells lines, particularly Sertoli cells [27–29]. In order to further evaluate these reports, we infected 4 testicular cell lines representing connective tissue (Hs1.Tes cells) and germ cells (SEM-1 and TCam-2 cells) as well as Sertoli cells with the prototype ZIKV MR766 and a clinical isolate ZIKV Paraiba to determine the extent to which the viruses would persist in these cells.

All the cells we tested were permissive to both ZIKV MR766 and ZIKV Paraiba, but the former replicated to higher titers than the clinical isolate (Figure 1). These results suggested that any of the testicular cells may be responsible for disseminating virus in the infected organ. However, Leydig cells were reportedly less susceptible to ZIKV infection [27], and their role in virus dissemination may be limited. The higher replication levels of ZIKV MR766 could be related to the fact that this strain has been passaged extensively in mouse brains [1,30]. In addition, ZIKV MR766 and ZIKV Paraiba are 89% identical at nucleotide sequence level and 97% (3313/3423) identical at amino acid level (BLAST; https://blast.ncbi.nlm.nih.gov/Blast.cgi). Thus, the ZIKV MR766 strain may have adapted to mammalian cell culture better than the ZIKV Paraiba strain which was passaged only <5 times. However, replication kinetics of ZIKV Paraiba and ZIKV MR766 in Vero E6 cells is similar from 24 to 60 hpi, but ZIKV MR766 replicates to higher titers from 72 to 96 hpi [31]. Therefore, the MR766 replication advantage may be time and cell-type dependent.

Our primary aim was to establish ZIKV persistence in the testicular cell culture systems. All the cells were able to support persistent infection for a few passages, but ZIKV MR766 was more aggressive at killing cells during persistence. ZIKV MR766 persistence in Sertoli cells has been reported for up to 6 weeks [27], but we only observed persistence of this strain for only 4 weeks. This could be a result of the higher ZIKV MR766 titers, which may trigger the host-cell responses leading to cell death. Persistence of ZIKV Paraiba was also limited to a few passages (5 at most in Sertoli and SEM-1 cells; Figure 4). In humans and animals, ZIKV persistence has been reported for time periods longer than the ones we observed in vitro and persistence was mostly of viral RNA in the absence of infectious virus [15,26,32]. In addition, the testes as an organ is immune privileged to protect the organ from highly inflammatory immune reactions [26]. The cells in our study were infected in the absence of the other cells they would normally be associated with in an organ/tissue context, making them more susceptible to rampant virus replication, which kills the cells faster. This notion is supported by a previous report showing that Sertoli cells infected with ZIKV were less adept at mounting an innate immune response in comparison to A549 cells [27].

It is noteworthy that the cell death we observed was slow and progressive until there were not enough cells for continued culture. In vivo, testicular atrophy and associated male infertility has been reported in mice [16,25]. The mechanism of slow cell death we observed in vitro in Hs1.Tes and Sertoli cells persistently infected with ZIKV may be comparable to the mechanism by which testicular atrophy occurs in vivo. Using Sertoli cells, we showed that cell death was via apoptosis because we could detect cleaved caspase 3 by immunofluorescence. Interestingly, not all ZIKV E protein-positive cells were positive for cleaved caspase 3, suggesting that the death signal(s) were not transmitted or activated uniformly in all virus-infected cells. Kumar et al. also showed that the level of apoptosis in Sertoli cells was lower (4–10%) than in A549 cells (58–72%) when infected with ZIKV at 72 hpi [27]. In another study, it was demonstrated that early ZIKV infection was associated with the suppression of cellular growth and proliferation, but antiviral responses were predominate in later stages of infection [28]. However, the specific mechanism which prevents overt apoptosis in testicular cells is yet to be elucidated and this will be an interesting avenue for further investigation using single cell sequencing approaches.

We were puzzled that TCam-2 seminoma cells infected with ZIKV MR766 prevailed up to 7 dpi without CPE, but the cells died upon passage. This intriguing result contrasted with that observed in SEM-1 cells, an intermediate seminoma cells line, which underwent extensive cell death by 7 dpi. These observations supported the hypothesis that ZIKV MR766 was more of an aggressive strain and the phenotype was also dependent on cell type.

We also attempted to comparatively establish a persistent infection of the neuroblastoma cell line (SK-N-SH) cells, but both ZIKV MR766 and ZIKV Paraiba killed the cells leaving no surviving cells. Thus, these observations further indicated that the outcome of ZIKV infection and persistence is cell type dependent.

In summary, we infected several testicular cell lines with ZIKV MR766 and ZIKV Paraiba with the aim of establishing persistent viral infection. The testicular cell lines we used represented germ cells (SEM-1 and TCam-2) and the connective tissue in the form of the fibroblast Hs1.Tes cell line. We also infected germ cell-supporting Sertoli cells, which have been shown to be permissive to ZIKV replication [28,29]. All the cells we tested allowed ZIKV replication and the prototype MR766 strain replicated to higher titers, compared to ZIKV Paraiba. ZIKV Paraiba persisted in Hs1.Tes, TCam-2, SEM-1 and Sertoli cells for up to 5 passages. ZIKV MR766 killed both TCam-2 and SEM-1 seminoma cells but persisted for 3 passages in Hs1.Tes cells and 4 passages in Sertoli cells. Compared to testicular cell lines, the neuroblastoma SK-N-SH cells were killed by both ZIKV strains, thus preventing viral persistence. Our results are consistent with reports that ZIKV persists in testicular cells and suggest that testicular atrophy may be a result of a slow and progressive cell death.

Author Contributions: Conceptualization, L.M. and M.E.B.; Experiments, L.M.; Writing—Original Draft Preparation, L.M.; Writing—Review & Editing, L.M. and M.E.B.

Funding: This study was supported by the Division of Intramural Research program of the National Institute of Allergy and Infectious Diseases at the National Institutes of Health.

Acknowledgments: We thank members of the Biology of Vector-Borne Viruses section for useful discussions.

Conflicts of Interest: The authors declare no conflict of interest.

References

1. Dick, G.W.A.; Kitchen, S.F.; Haddow, A.J. Zika Virus (I). Isolations and serological specificity. *Trans. R. Soc. Trop. Med. Hyg.* **1952**, *46*, 509–520. [CrossRef]
2. Mlakar, J.; Korva, M.; Tul, N.; Popović, M.; Poljšak-Prijatelj, M.; Mraz, J.; Kolenc, M.; Resman Rus, K.; Vesnaver Vipotnik, T.; Fabjan Vodušek, V.; et al. Zika Virus Associated with Microcephaly. *N. Engl. J. Med.* **2016**, *374*, 951–958. [CrossRef] [PubMed]
3. Nascimento, O.J.M.; da Silva, I.R.F. Guillain–Barré syndrome and Zika virus outbreaks. *Curr. Opin. Neurol.* **2017**, *30*, 500–507. [CrossRef] [PubMed]
4. Roze, B.; Najioullah, F.; Ferge, J.L.; Apetse, K.; Brouste, Y.; Cesaire, R.; Fagour, C.; Fagour, L.; Hochedez, P.; Jeannin, S.; et al. Zika virus detection in urine from patients with Guillain-Barre syndrome on Martinique, January 2016. *Euro Surveill.* **2016**, *21*, 30154. [CrossRef] [PubMed]
5. Rozé, B.; Najioullah, F.; Fergé, J.-L.; Dorléans, F.; Apetse, K.; Barnay, J.-L.; Daudens-Vaysse, E.; Brouste, Y.; Césaire, R.; Fagour, L.; et al. Guillain-Barré Syndrome Associated With Zika Virus Infection in Martinique in 2016: A Prospective Study. *Clin. Infect. Dis.* **2017**, *65*, 1462–1468. [CrossRef] [PubMed]
6. Read, J.S.; Torres-Velasquez, B.; Lorenzi, O.; Rivera Sanchez, A.; Torres-Torres, S.; Rivera, L.V.; Capre-Franceschi, S.M.; Garcia-Gubern, C.; Munoz-Jordan, J.; Santiago, G.A.; et al. Symptomatic zika virus infection in infants, children, and adolescents living in puerto rico. *JAMA Pediatr.* **2018**, *172*, 686–693. [CrossRef]
7. Foy, B.D.; Kobylinski, K.C.; Foy, J.L.C.; Blitvich, B.J.; Travassos da Rosa, A.; Haddow, A.D.; Lanciotti, R.S.; Tesh, R.B. Probable Non–Vector-borne Transmission of Zika Virus, Colorado, USA. *Emerg. Infect. Dis.* **2011**, *17*, 880–882. [CrossRef]
8. Fréour, T.; Mirallié, S.; Hubert, B.; Splingart, C.; Barrière, P.; Maquart, M.; Leparc-Goffart, I. Sexual transmission of Zika virus in an entirely asymptomatic couple returning from a Zika epidemic area, France, April 2016. *Euro Surveill.* **2016**, *21*, 30254. [CrossRef]
9. Nicastri, E.; Castilletti, C.; Liuzzi, G.; Iannetta, M.; Capobianchi, M.R.; Ippolito, G. Persistent detection of Zika virus RNA in semen for six months after symptom onset in a traveller returning from Haiti to Italy, February 2016. *Euro Surveill.* **2016**, *21*. [CrossRef]
10. Davidson, A.; Slavinski, S.; Komoto, K.; Rakeman, J.; Weiss, D. Suspected Female-to-Male Sexual Transmission of Zika Virus—New York City, 2016. *MMWR Morb. Mortal. Wkly. Rep.* **2016**, *65*, 716–717. [CrossRef]
11. Zika Situation Report. Available online: http://www.who.int/emergencies/zika-virus/situation-report/10-march-2017/en/ (accessed on 8 January 2019).
12. 2016 Case Counts in the US. Available online: https://www.cdc.gov/zika/reporting/2016-case-counts.html (accessed on 8 January 2019).
13. 2017 Case Counts in the US. Available online: https://www.cdc.gov/zika/reporting/2017-case-counts.html (accessed on 8 January 2019).
14. Hastings, A.K.; Fikrig, E. Zika Virus and Sexual Transmission: A New Route of Transmission for Mosquito-borne Flaviviruses. *Yale J. Biol. Med.* **2017**, *90*, 325–330. [PubMed]
15. Mead, P.S.; Duggal, N.K.; Hook, S.A.; Delorey, M.; Fischer, M.; Olzenak McGuire, D.; Becksted, H.; Max, R.J.; Anishchenko, M.; Schwartz, A.M.; et al. Zika Virus Shedding in Semen of Symptomatic Infected Men. *N. Engl. J. Med.* **2018**, *378*, 1377–1385. [CrossRef] [PubMed]

16. Uraki, R.; Hwang, J.; Jurado, K.A.; Householder, S.; Yockey, L.J.; Hastings, A.K.; Homer, R.J.; Iwasaki, A.; Fikrig, E. Zika virus causes testicular atrophy. *Sci. Adv.* **2017**, *3*, e1602899. [CrossRef] [PubMed]

17. Govero, J.; Esakky, P.; Scheaffer, S.M.; Fernandez, E.; Drury, A.; Platt, D.J.; Gorman, M.J.; Richner, J.M.; Caine, E.A.; Salazar, V.; et al. Zika virus infection damages the testes in mice. *Nature* **2016**, *540*, 438–442. [CrossRef] [PubMed]

18. Sheng, Z.-Y.; Gao, N.; Wang, Z.-Y.; Cui, X.-Y.; Zhou, D.-S.; Fan, D.-Y.; Chen, H.; Wang, P.-G.; An, J. Sertoli Cells Are Susceptible to ZIKV Infection in Mouse Testis. *Front. Cell. Infect. Microbiol.* **2017**, *7*, 272. [CrossRef] [PubMed]

19. Müller, J.A.; Harms, M.; Krüger, F.; Groß, R.; Joas, S.; Hayn, M.; Dietz, A.N.; Lippold, S.; von Einem, J.; Schubert, A.; et al. Semen inhibits Zika virus infection of cells and tissues from the anogenital region. *Nature Commun.* **2018**, *9*, 2207. [CrossRef] [PubMed]

20. Biedler, J.L.; Helson, L.; Spengler, B.A. Morphology and Growth, Tumorigenicity, and Cytogenetics of Human Neuroblastoma Cells in Continuous Culture. *Cancer Res.* **1973**, *33*, 2643–2652.

21. Mizuno, Y.; Gotoh, A.; Kamidono, S.; Kitazawa, S. Establishment and characterization of a new human testicukar germ cell tumor cell line (TCam-2). *Jpn. J. Urol.* **1993**, *84*, 1211–1218. [CrossRef]

22. Russell, S.M.; Lechner, M.G.; Mokashi, A.; Megiel, C.; Jang, J.K.; Taylor, C.R.; Looijenga, L.H.J.; French, C.A.; Epstein, A.L. Establishment and Characterization of a new Human Extragonadal Germ Cell Line, SEM-1, and its Comparison With TCam-2 and JKT-1. *Urology* **2013**, *81*, 464.e1–464.e9. [CrossRef]

23. Offerdahl, D.K.; Dorward, D.W.; Hansen, B.T.; Bloom, M.E. Cytoarchitecture of Zika virus infection in human neuroblastoma and Aedes albopictus cell lines. *Virology* **2017**, *501*, 54–62. [CrossRef]

24. Tang, H.; Hammack, C.; Ogden, S.C.; Wen, Z.; Qian, X.; Li, Y.; Yao, B.; Shin, J.; Zhang, F.; Lee, E.M.; et al. Zika Virus Infects Human Cortical Neural Precursors and Attenuates Their Growth. *Cell Stem Cell* **2016**, *18*, 587–590. [CrossRef] [PubMed]

25. Ma, W.; Li, S.; Ma, S.; Jia, L.; Zhang, F.; Zhang, Y.; Zhang, J.; Wong, G.; Zhang, S.; Lu, X.; et al. Zika Virus Causes Testis Damage and Leads to Male Infertility in Mice. *Cell* **2016**, *167*, 1511–1524.e10. [CrossRef] [PubMed]

26. Stassen, L.; Armitage, C.; van der Heide, D.; Beagley, K.; Frentiu, F. Zika Virus in the Male Reproductive Tract. *Viruses* **2018**, *10*, 198. [CrossRef]

27. Kumar, A.; Jovel, J.; Lopez-Orozco, J.; Limonta, D.; Airo, A.M.; Hou, S.; Stryapunina, I.; Fibke, C.; Moore, R.B.; Hobman, T.C. Human Sertoli cells support high levels of Zika virus replication and persistence. *Sci. Rep.* **2018**, *8*, 5477. [CrossRef] [PubMed]

28. Strange, D.P.; Green, R.; Siemann, D.N.; Gale, M.; Verma, S. Immunoprofiles of human Sertoli cells infected with Zika virus reveals unique insights into host-pathogen crosstalk. *Sci. Rep.* **2018**, *8*, 8702. [CrossRef]

29. Siemann, D.N.; Strange, D.P.; Maharaj, P.N.; Shi, P.-Y.; Verma, S. Zika Virus Infects Human Sertoli Cells and Modulates the Integrity of the In Vitro Blood-Testis Barrier Model. *J. Virol.* **2017**, *91*, e00623-17. [CrossRef] [PubMed]

30. Haddow, A.D.; Schuh, A.J.; Yasuda, C.Y.; Kasper, M.R.; Heang, V.; Huy, R.; Guzman, H.; Tesh, R.B.; Weaver, S.C. Genetic Characterization of Zika Virus Strains: Geographic Expansion of the Asian Lineage. *PLoS Negl. Trop. Dis.* **2012**, *6*, e1477. [CrossRef]

31. Marzi, A.; Emanuel, J.; Callison, J.; McNally, K.L.; Arndt, N.; Chadinha, S.; Martellaro, C.; Rosenke, R.; Scott, D.P.; Safronetz, D.; Whitehead, S.S.; et al. Lethal Zika Virus Disease Models in Young and Older Interferon α/β Receptor Knock Out Mice. *Front. Cell. Infect. Microbiol.* **2018**, *8*, 117. [CrossRef]

32. Duggal, N.K.; Ritter, J.M.; Pestorius, S.E.; Zaki, S.R.; Davis, B.S.; Chang, G.-J.J.; Bowen, R.A.; Brault, A.C. Frequent Zika Virus Sexual Transmission and Prolonged Viral RNA Shedding in an Immunodeficient Mouse Model. *Cell Rep.* **2017**, *18*, 1751–1760. [CrossRef]

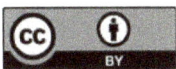

![viruses logo] *viruses*

MDPI

Article

Persistence and Intra-Host Genetic Evolution of Zika Virus Infection in Symptomatic Adults: A Special View in the Male Reproductive System

Danielle B. L. Oliveira [1,†] , Giuliana S. Durigon [2,†], Érica A. Mendes [1,†] , Jason T. Ladner [3,4,†] , Robert Andreata-Santos [1,†] , Danielle B. Araujo [1], Viviane F. Botosso [5], Nicholas D. Paola [1], Daniel F. L. Neto [1], Marielton P. Cunha [1] , Carla T. Braconi [1] , Rúbens P. S. Alves [1], Monica R. Jesus [1], Lennon R. Pereira [1], Stella R. Melo [1], Flávio S. Mesquita [1] , Vanessa B. Silveira [1], Luciano M. Thomazelli [1] , Silvana R. Favoretto [6], Franciane B. Almonfrey [2], Regina C. R. M. Abdulkader [2], Joel M. Gabrili [5,7], Denise V. Tambourgi [5] , Sérgio F. Oliveira [8], Karla Prieto [3,9], Michael R. Wiley [3,9], Luís C. S. Ferreira [1] , Marcos V. Silva [10], Gustavo F. Palacios [3,‡], Paolo M. A. Zanotto [1,‡] and Edison L. Durigon [1,*,‡]

[1]   Department of Microbiology, Institute of Biomedical Sciences, University of São Paulo, São Paulo, SP 05508-000, Brazil; danibruna@gmail.com (D.B.L.O.); ericaarmendes@gmail.com (É.A.M.); robert_andreata@hotmail.com (R.A.-S.); daniellebastos@yahoo.com.br (D.B.A.); nicholasdipaola@gmail.com (N.D.P.); danielviro@gmail.com (D.F.L.N.); marieltondospassos@gmail.com (M.P.C.); cabraconi@gmail.com (C.T.B.); rubens.bmc@gmail.com (R.P.S.A.); modrigues4@gmail.com (M.R.J.); lennon_rp@hotmail.com (L.R.P.); stellmelo@gmail.com (S.R.M.); flavio.mesquita@usp.br (F.S.M.); vanessa.silveirabio@gmail.com (V.B.S.); lucmt@usp.br (L.M.T.); lcsf@usp.br (L.C.S.F.); pzanotto@usp.br (P.M.A.Z.)

[2]   Medical School Clinic Hospital, University of São Paulo, São Paulo, SP 05403-000, Brazil; giuliana.durigon@gmail.com (G.S.D.); fran_almonfrey@hotmail.com (F.B.A.); kader@usp.br (R.C.R.M.A.)

[3]   Center for Genome Sciences, US Army Medical Research Institute of Infectious Diseases, Frederick, MD 21702, USA; jtladner@gmail.com (J.T.L.); karla.prieto.ctr@mail.mil (K.P.); michael.r.wiley19.ctr@mail.mil (M.R.W.); gustavo.f.palacios.ctr@mail.mil (G.F.P.)

[4]   The Pathogen and Microbiome Institute, Northern Arizona University, Flagstaff, AZ 86011-4073, USA

[5]   Virology Laboratory, Butantan Institute, São Paulo, SP 05503-900, Brazil; viviane.botosso@butantan.gov.br (V.F.B.); joel.megalegabrili@gmail.com (J.M.G.); denise.tambourgi@butantan.gov.br (D.V.T.)

[6]   Pasteur Institute, State Health Department, São Paulo, SP 1103-000, Brazil; srfavoretto@usp.br

[7]   Immunochemistry Laboratory, Butantan Institute, São Paulo, SP 05503-900, Brazil

[8]   Department of Cellular and Developmental Biology, Institute of Biomedical Sciences, University of São Paulo, São Paulo, SP 05508-000, Brazil; sfolivei@gmail.com

[9]   Department of Environmental, Agricultural and Occupational Health, University of Nebraska Medical Center, Omaha, NE 68198-4388, USA

[10] Institute of Infectology Emílio Ribas e Pontifícia Universidade Católica (PUC-SP), São Paulo, SP 01246-900, Brazil; mvsilva@pucsp.br

*   Correspondence: eldurigo@usp.br

†   These authors contributed equally for the paper.

‡   These authors contributed equally for the paper.

Received: 22 August 2018; Accepted: 20 October 2018; Published: 7 November 2018

Abstract: We followed the presence of Zika virus (ZIKV) in four healthy adults (two men and two women), for periods ranging from 78 to 298 days post symptom onset. The patients were evaluated regarding the presence of the virus in different body fluids (blood, saliva, urine and semen), development of immune responses (including antibodies, cytokines and chemokines), and virus genetic variation within samples collected from semen and urine during the infection course. The analysis was focused primarily on the two male patients who shed the virus for up to 158 days after the initial symptoms. ZIKV particles were detected in the spermatozoa cytoplasm and flagella, in immature sperm cells and could also be isolated from semen in cell culture, confirming that the virus is able to preserve integrity and infectivity during replication in the male reproductive system (MRS). Despite the damage caused by ZIKV infection within the MRS, our data showed that ZIKV infection did not result in infertility at least in one of the male patients. This patient was able to conceive a child after the infection. We also detected alterations in the male genital cytokine milieu, which could play an important role in the replication and transmission of the virus which could considerably increase the risk of ZIKV sexual spread. In addition, full genome ZIKV sequences were obtained from several samples (mainly semen), which allowed us to monitor the evolution of the virus within a patient during the infection course. We observed genetic changes over time in consensus sequences and lower frequency intra-host single nucleotide variants (iSNV), that suggested independent compartmentalization of ZIKV populations in the reproductive and urinary systems. Altogether, the present observations confirm the risks associated with the long-term replication and shedding of ZIKV in the MRS and help to elucidate patterns of intra-host genetic evolution during long term replication of the virus.

Keywords: Zika virus; flavivirus; arbovirus; sexual transmission; host genetic variation; immune response

---

1. Introduction

Zika virus (ZIKV) was first identified in 1947 in Africa and subsequently reached Asia and, more recently, the Americas [1,2]. Today, more than 80 countries around the globe have reported cases of active ZIKV transmission and the recent outbreaks have associated the virus with several neurological disorders, including Guillain-Barré syndrome and congenital neurologic birth defects [3–6]. Due to its rapid spread, there is a need to understand how the virus interacts with the human host which includes persistence and shedding in biological fluids in order to improve diagnosis, prevention and treatment.

Reports have shown that ZIKV RNA is present in several body fluids, including urine, blood, saliva, breast milk and secretions from the vaginal tract [7–10], being cleared early from serum but still detected in whole blood, saliva and urine for more than two weeks after symptoms onset [11–14]. ZIKV can also replicate and persist in the male reproductive system and ZIKV RNA has been detected within semen for up to 6 months after initial infection in the male reproductive system (MRS) [15,16]. The potential for persistent ZIKV infections in the MRS raises concerns ranging from the demonstrated sexual transmission of the virus to the damage of germ cells and generation of poor-quality sperm. In fact, ZIKV infection has been shown to cause infertility in mice [17,18]. In addition, since the ZIKV genome is RNA-based, the occurrence of spontaneous mutations may lead to the accumulation of genetic variants during persistent infection, particularly at the MRS, with unpredicted outcomes for the virus–host interactions.

In the present study, we followed the natural course of ZIKV infection in four symptomatic adults (two men and two women) infected with ZIKV in Brazil. The patients were monitored for the presence of the virus in different body fluids, including blood, saliva, urine and semen and for the development of an associated immune response, with emphasis on two male patients who shed the virus for up to 158 days after the initial symptoms. The presence of virus within semen samples, capable of replicating in cell cultures, allowed us to obtain almost full ZIKV genome sequences and evaluate the intra-host virus genetic evolution. These results led us to suggest that ZIKV shows an independent compartmentalization in MRS that may impact the fate of the virus and its interaction with the human host. In addition, we detected alterations in the genital cytokine milieu and a lack of detectable proinflammatory cytokines/chemokines in the blood.

2. Materials and Methods

2.1. Case Definition and Sample Collection

The cases were defined as individuals with ZIKV-like illness (acute onset of rash associated with at least one of the following symptoms: fever, conjunctivitis, pruritus or arthralgia) and the presence of ZIKV RNA in at least one of these clinical samples: serum, saliva, urine and semen. During the outbreak of ZIKV in Brazil, 117 patients with ZIKV illness were tested at the Clinical and Molecular Virology Laboratory in the Institute of Biomedical Sciences at University of São Paulo—USP, São Paulo, Brazil. From the six qRT-PCR positive patients, four of them accepted to be included in this study: ZIKV01, ZIKV17, ZIKV18 and ZIKV19. The study protocol was approved by the Ethics Committee on Research with Human Beings at the University of São Paulo and also evaluated and determined to be exempt by the US Army Medical Research Institute of Infectious Diseases (USAMRIID) Office of Human Use and Ethics. All four patients provided their informed consent for the use of their samples in this study. Following the initial positive result by qRT-PCR, all patients were tested weekly for the presence of ZIKV RNA in urine, serum, saliva and semen (for male patients), until all samples tested negative in at least two consecutive visits. Each patient had the first sample collected between days 3 and 7 after the onset of symptoms and the final sample collected up to a minimum of 78 days and a maximum of 235 days later (ZIKV01, ZIKV17, ZIKV18 and ZIKV19 for 78, 235, 119 and 155 days, respectively). The study timeframe for patient ZIKV01 was between February/2016–May/2016, for patient ZIKV17 between March/2016 until January/2017 and from April/2016 until September/2016 for patients ZIKV18 and ZIKV19.

Clinical Case

Case-ZIKV01 is a 32-year-old woman who presented with a maculopapular rash on her trunk and upper limbs associated with abdominal pain and diarrhea. Two to four days after symptom onset, the exanthema became pruriginous and reached the lower limbs with the appearance of petechiae. She experienced intense epigastralgia that resolved after the fifth day. Arthralgia on ankles and edema of fingers were noticed on day 4 and lasted until day 7. No other symptoms, including fever, were reported. No significant laboratory findings were noted. The patient was subsequently followed for 78 days with no additional complications. The patient, who lives in São Paulo state, reported a trip to Espirito Santo state two weeks before the onset of symptoms.

Case-ZIKV17 is a 33-year-old man who initially reported a fever lasting 2 days, followed by headache and retro-orbital pain (days 2–3). On day 4 he reported a maculopapular rash accompanied by intense itching and diffuse arthralgia. All symptoms cleared up by day 5. The patient was subsequently studied for 298 days. He experienced pain and edema of his right testicle at 25 days post-symptomatic onset. Orchitis due to ZIKV infection was diagnosed after confirmation through serology and qRT-PCR. No other potential agents were identified.

Further monitoring of ZIKV shedding was conducted, with express patient consent, since he was planning to conceive a baby with his partner. During the study period, the patient underwent two prostate ultrasounds (USG prostate) and two spermograms. The patient presented with prostatitis at 71 days post symptoms onset, which normalized by 218 days post symptoms onset. The spermograms were normal at days 100 and 223 post symptoms onset. The couple adopted strict preventive measures with daily use of insect repellent and barrier contraception during sexual intercourse for the entire period of confirmed virus shedding. After the first negative semen sample (day 168), the patient provided weekly samples (day 174) for 2 consecutive weeks, followed by two more biweekly collections (day 200) and finally a monthly collection (day 235), totaling 67 days with negative qRT-PCR results for all tested samples. At 235 days post symptoms onset the patient and his wife began actively trying to conceive. After two months (day 298) the patient's wife confirmed pregnancy. At the time, and further during pregnancy, she was monitored for ZIKV infection by qRT-PCR, IgG and IgM. She remained negative.

Cases-ZIKV18 and **-ZIKV19** are a husband and wife who experienced ZIKV-like illness in close succession. ZIKV19 is a 64-year-old man, who reported lumbar pain, fever and malaise at onset. After 3 days of symptoms a macular rash appeared which resolved after 6 days. The patient was subsequently studied for 155 days.

ZIKV18 is a 68-year-old woman who began experiencing symptoms of malaise five days after her husband. Three days after onset, a macular rash appeared on the face, body and limbs and erythematous plaque in the right leg, accompanied by fever, headache, ocular hyperemia and articular edema. On the fourth day the exanthema became more intense, followed by somnolence, chills and tiredness. The articular edema remained for 5 weeks. The patient was subsequently studied for 108 days. There were no other reports of complications during the study period.

Timelines for all four patients with the principle clinical events and laboratorial results are shown in Figure 1.

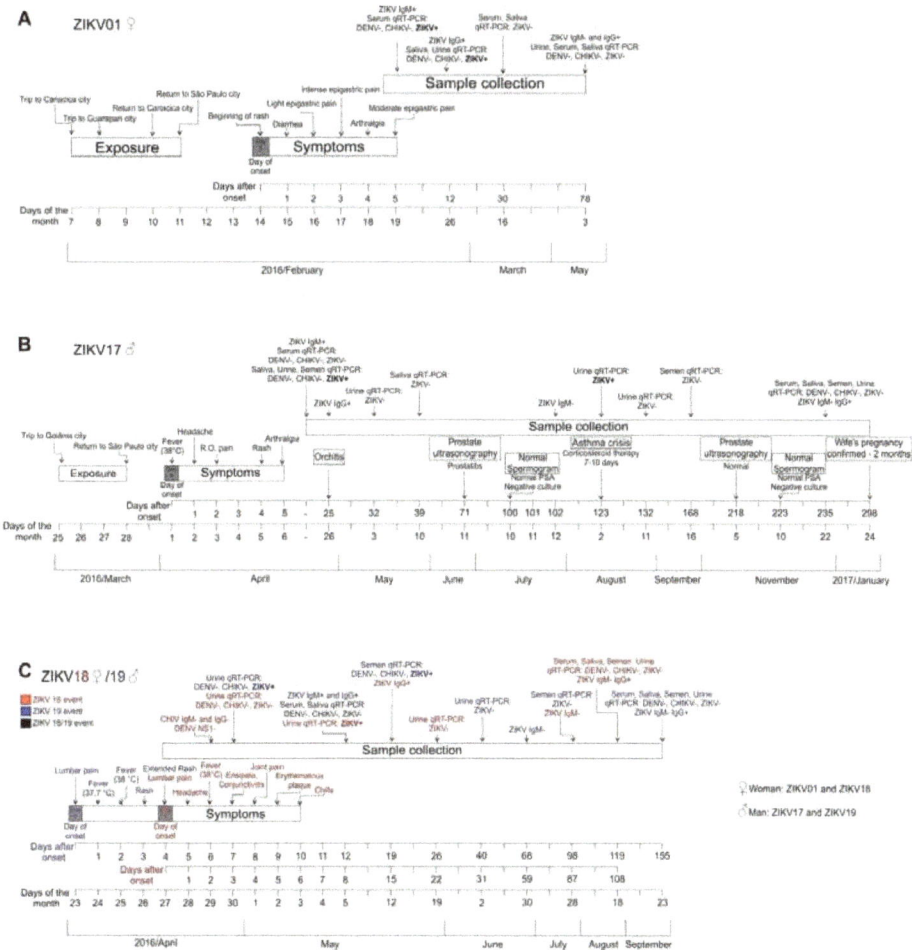

Figure 1. Timelines of ZIKV exposure, symptoms and sample collection in the four subjects enrolled in the present study. Periods of exposure, symptom onset, serology and molecular detection results of ZIKV in the followed subjects are described as: (**A**) case 1—female (ZIKV01), (**B**) case 2—male (ZIKV17), (**C**) case 3—female (ZIKV18) and case 4—male (ZIKV19). Day 0 denotes the onset of symptoms.

2.2. Molecular and Classical Virology

For the serological analysis, ZIKV-specific IgG antibodies were measured using a nonstructural protein ΔNS1-ELISA [19] and ZIKV-specific IgM antibodies were detected using capture ELISA with a specific viral antigen for ZIKV [20]. For the molecular test, quantitative reverse transcription (qRT-PCR) TaqMan assays for detection of ZIKV, Dengue virus (DENV) and Chikungunya virus (CHIKV) RNA were performed. The assays, as well as the RNA extraction methods, are described in the Supplementary Appendix. To ensure RNA integrity and sample quality, all extracts were also tested for the presence of the human RNase P (RNP) gene by qRT-PCR. All extracts showed robust RNP cycle threshold (Ct) values ranging from 16.3 to Ct 33.5 (see Supplementary Appendix for details) demonstrating the integrity of the material collected. Assays for DENV [21] and CHIKV [22] were performed as controls for co-infection, as they have been reported in Brazil during the ZIKV outbreak. To evaluate infectivity, viral isolation was attempted for a subset of positive samples from the two male patients ZIKV17 and ZIKV19. For virus isolation, *Aedes albopictus* mosquito cells (C6/36) were inoculated with 500 μL of saliva, urine or semen. After 8–12 days of incubation, cells were collected and tested for ZIKV RNA presence by qRT-PCR. All samples were passaged in cell culture at least 3 consecutive times before being considered negative for ZIKV presence by qRT-PCR (for details see Supplementary Materials).

2.3. Virus Particle Detection in Semen by Immunofluorescence and Transmission Electron-Microscopy (IFA and TEM, Respectively)

The immunofluorescence assays were conducted using suspensions from semen samples collected on day 39 from patient ZIKV17 and day 40 from patient ZIKV19. The presence of ZIKV particles were also analyzed by TEM in semen from patient ZIKV17 (day 39) and in *Aedes albopictus* mosquito cells (C6/36) inoculated with the ZIKV17 semen sample. Thin sections were stained with uranyl acetate and lead citrate, and observed with a JEOL 1010 transmission electron microscope (for details see Supplementary Materials). C6/36 cells infected with ZIKV isolated from patient ZIKV17 were used as a positive control for both IFA and TEM assays.

2.4. Measurement of Cytokines and Chemokines in Serum and Seminal Plasma

The serum and semen samples from the male patients ZIKV17 and ZIKV19 were analyzed for the presence of the cytokines IL-17, IL-2, IL-4, IL-6, IL-10, TNF-α, IFN-γ and the chemokines CXCL8/IL-8, CCL5/RANTES, CXCL9/MIG, CCL2/MCP-1 and CXCL10/IP-10 using Cytometric Bead Arrays kits (Human Th1/Th2/Th17 and Human Chemokine from Becton Dickinson, CA, USA), according to the manufacturer's instructions. The range of detection for cytokines was 20 to 5000 pg/mL and for chemokines was 10 to 2500 pg/mL. Samples were analyzed using a FACSCanto II flow cytometer, with FCAP Array 3.0 software, version 3.0, both from BD Biosciences. One-way ANOVA with Tukey post-tests were used to evaluate significant differences between groups. For correlation analyses, Pearson coefficient (r) was used. Statistical analysis was performed using GraphPad Prism software. Differences were considered statistically significant when p values were less than 0.05.

2.5. Genome Sequencing and Analysis

For samples that tested positive for ZIKV RNA by qRT-PCR, viral genetic diversity was characterized directly from the clinical specimens using next-generation sequencing. Sequencing libraries were prepared using the TruSeq RNA Access Library Prep kit (Illumina, Menlo Park, CA, USA) with custom ZIKV probes and sequenced using the MiSeq Reagent kit v3 (Illumina, Menlo Park, CA, USA) on an Illumina MiSeq (for details see supplementary appendix). Consensus-level ZIKV genome sequences were assembled for each sample using both de novo and reference-based approaches (for details see Supplementary Materials). These two approaches resulted in nearly identical sequences. However, for several lower coverage samples, contiguous assemblies could only be constructed with the reference-based approach. Consensus genomes were compared using median-joining haplotype networks (PopART v1.7.2) and an approximate maximum-likelihood phylogenetic reconstruction (FastTree v2.1.5). BEAST v1.8.3 [23] was used to estimate dN/dS and the rate of ZIKV evolution within the male reproductive system (MRS), HyPhy v2.3 was used to identify codons with evidence for positive, diversifying selection, and for samples with >50× average coverage, we examined intra host genetic variation using FreeBayes v1.0.2 [24] (for details see Supplementary Materials).

3. Results

3.1. Long Term Monitoring of Four Symptomatic ZIKV-Infected Patients

Four symptomatic ZIKV-infected individuals (two males; patients ZIKV17 and ZIKV19 with 33 and 64 years of age, respectively, and two females; patients ZIKV01 and ZIKV18 with 32 and 68 years) were followed for periods up to 298 days after the onset of symptoms (Figure 1). All patients became serological positive for ZIKV, both for IgM and IgG, during the course of the study. ZIKV IgM was detected in serum of patients ZIKV01, ZIKV17, ZIKV18 and ZIKV19 until day 78, 95, 59 and 54, respectively. All serum samples were positive for ZIKV IgG at the first time point tested, between 12 to 25 days after symptoms onset, and remained positive throughout the study (Figure 1).

In the two females (ZIKV01 and ZIKV18) the ZIKA RNA was detected by qRT-PCR in urine, serum and saliva. ZIKV01 was the only patient in this study that developed viremia, which was detected at day 5 (6.2×10^7 genome equivalents (ge)/mL) and lasted until day 12 (2.2×10^2 ge/mL). ZIKV RNA was also detected in her saliva at day 12 (2×10^2 ge/mL). Both patients had ZIKV RNA detected in urine samples from day 12 (10^2 ge/mL) through day 30 (20 ge/mL) for patient ZIKV01 and at day 8 (5.7×10^4 ge/mL) for patient ZIKV18 (Figure 2A,C).

Both males (ZIKV17 and ZIKV 19) had the virus detected in semen and urine and only one (ZIKV17) had it detected in saliva from day 25 (5.2×10^6 ge/mL) through day 32 (4.2×10^5 ge/mL). This patient also showed high viruria at day 6 (2.5×10^7 ge/mL) which waned by day 32 and persistent viral shedding in semen, which was detected from day 18 (6.5×10^8 ge/mL) through day 158 (15 ge/mL) after symptoms onset (Figure 2B). Similarly to patient ZIKV17, prolonged virusemia was detected as early as day 19 (3.13×10^5 RNA ge/mL) through day 82 (1.33×10^2 RNA ge/mL) in the other male patient (ZIKV19) (Figure 2C). The presence of virus in semen has been directly demonstrated by IFA and TEM, where it was verified in both spermatozoids and immature sperm cells (Figure 3, and Figures S1 and S2). All four patients remained negative for DENV and CHIKV RNA detection throughout the study period.

Replication competent ZIKV particles were successfully isolated from saliva (day 25), urine (days 18, and 25), and semen (days 18, 25, 32, 53, and 117) samples of patient ZIKV17 and from semen samples (days 19, 26 and 40) of patient ZIKV19 (Figure 2B,D). The viral isolation was confirmed by qRT-PCR, IFA and TEM (Figure 3A,B). Although cytokines and chemokines have not been detected in serum by the methodology used, seminal fluids of patients ZIKV17 and ZIKV19 showed enhanced levels of some of them when compared to normal control (semen from a ZIKV-uninfected individual). Patient ZIKV17 showed concentrations of IP-10, MIG, IL-6, IL-10, INF-γ, IL-8, MCP-1and RANTES higher than control, with the highest values found at the beginning of the infection ($p < 0.05$), highlighting a local persistent inflammation in the MRS. Statistical correlation (Pearson's r) between the Zika load and the level of all these chemokines and cytokines were verified, except for IP-10 (Figure 4A and Supplementary Figure S3A). For patient ZIKV19 the same cytokines/chemokines were higher than control, except by IL-10 that remained undetectable. But a statistical correlation was verified only for IFN-γ and IP-10. In addition, an increased concentration of IL-6, IP-10, MCP-1, IL-8 and RANTES in the seminal plasma sample of this patient was also detected after 60 days of the symptoms onset, which was coincident with the period immediately before the viral clearance (Figure 4B and Supplementary Figure S3B). More, IL-2, IL-4, IL17A and TNF−α were not detected in the seminal plasma of both patients.

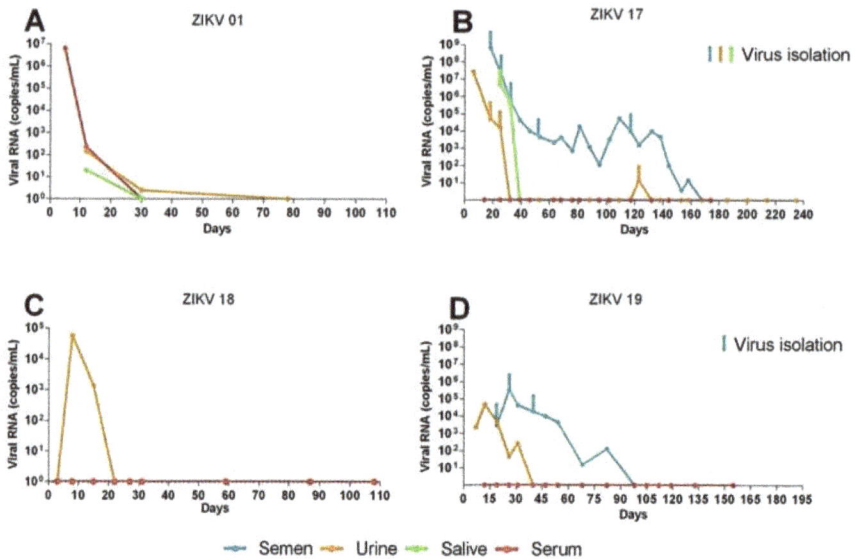

Figure 2. ZIKV RNA load in patient's body fluids and clinical isolates on culture. The graph shows the viral load (genome copies/mL) versus excretion time (days after symptoms onset) of the weekly collection of urine (orange), saliva (green) and serum (red) samples from patients ZIKV01 (**A**), ZIKV17 (**B**), ZIKV18 (**C**) and ZIKV19 (**D**), in addition to the semen (blue) of the two men involved in the study (**C,D**). To confirm the viability of the excreted virus, the urine samples collected from days 18 and 25 after symptoms, saliva from day 25 and the semen from days 18, 25, 32, 53 and 117 for patient ZIKV17 and semen samples from patient ZIKV19 from days 19, 26 and 40 after symptoms onset were tested and the ones with positive results in cell culture are exhibited. All clinical samples and isolated samples were analyzed by qRT-PCR.

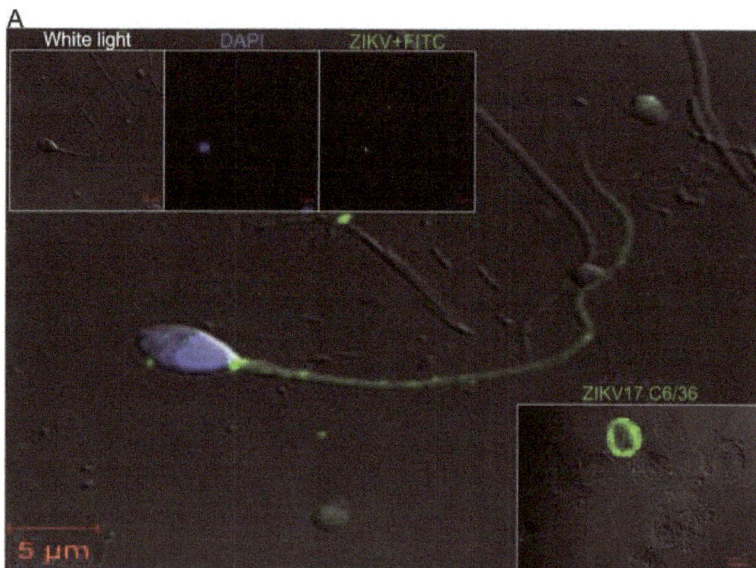

Figure 3. *Cont.*

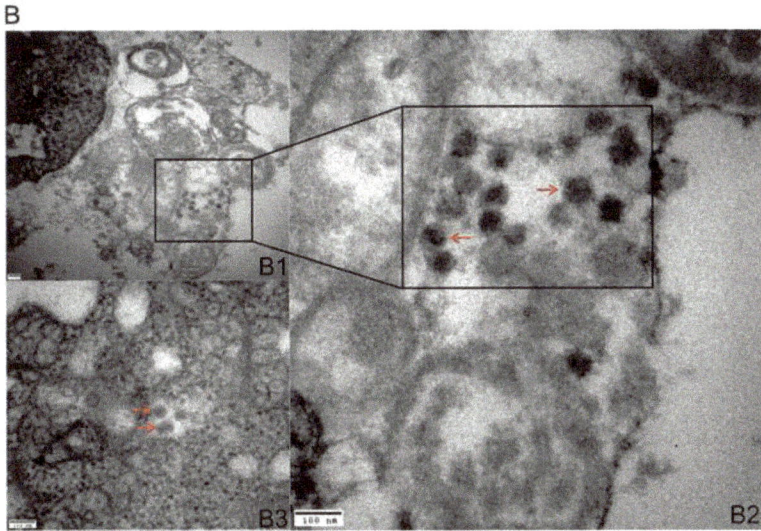

Figure 3. Detection of ZIKV in semen and C636 cells. (**A**) Detection by Indirect Immunofluorescence assay using anti-ZIKV specific antibody. Spermatozoa from semen sample collected from patient ZIKV17 at day 39 stained with FITC conjugate (in green) for virus location and with DAPI for nucleus staining (in blue). The viruses were located in the cytoplasm and flagella. C6/36 cell culture infected with virus from ZIKV17 semen sample. The cell infected presents with a green color (lower right panel). (**B**) Electron Microscopy of ultrathin sections of semen sample. (**B1**) A lower-power view of ZIKV particles inside an infected cell, with the characteristic of an immature sperm cell. (**B2**) Viral particles in a magnified view of the same cell in (**B1**). (**B3**) C6/36 cell infected with a semen sample from patient ZIKV17 with a cluster of dense virions located in the cytoplasm (red arrow).

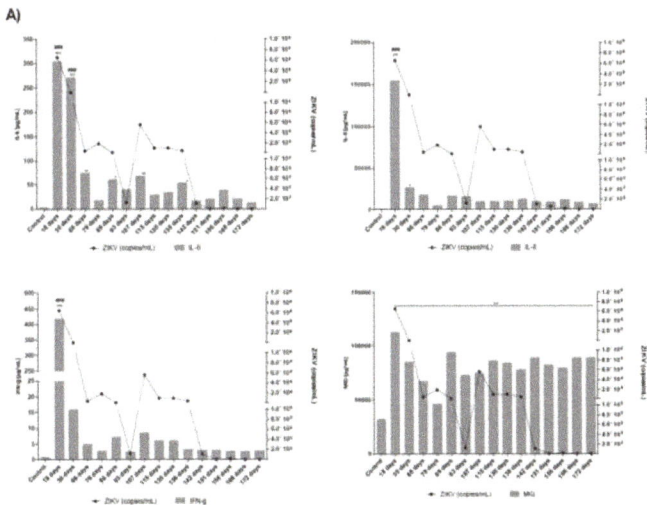

Figure 4. *Cont.*

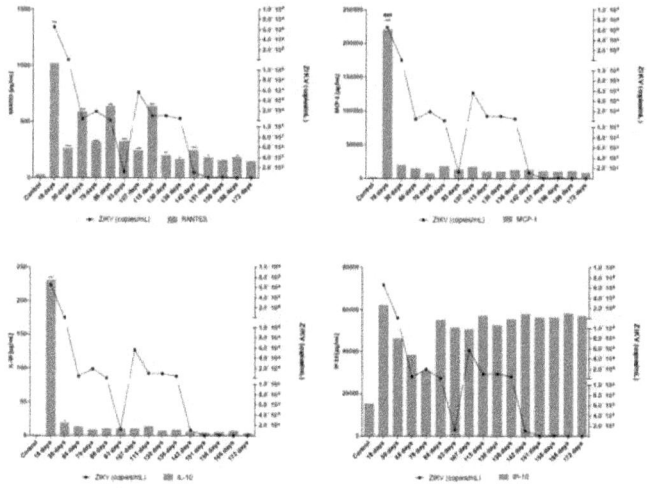

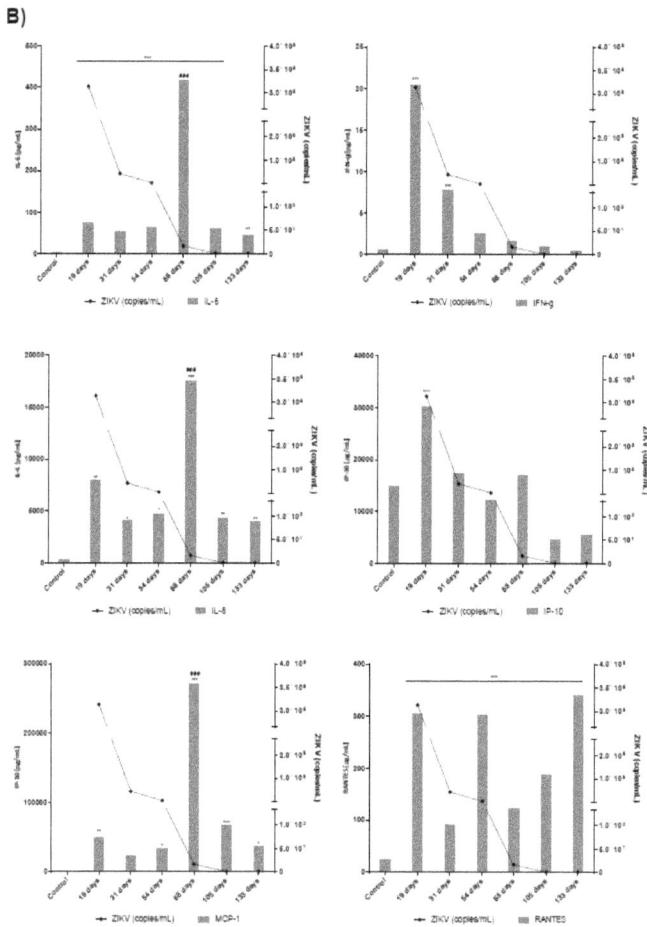

Figure 4. Concentration of cytokines, chemokines and RNA viral load determined on semen of

patients ZIKV17 (**A**) and ZIKV19 (**B**). The levels of the following cytokines and chemokines were measured in blood and seminal plasma—IL-2, IL-4, IL-6, CXCL8 (IL-8), IL-10, IL-17, IFN-γ, TNF–α, CCL2 (MCP-1), CCL5 (RANTES), CXCL9 (MIG), CXCL10 (IP-10). The results are representative of two distinct experiments performed in duplicate. Values of *p* less them 0.05 were considered statistically significant (* $p < 0.05$; ** $p < 0.001$; *** $p < 0.0001$—concentration of cytokines/chemokines in ZIKV patients versus control (semen from Zika—uninfected individual), ### $p < 0.0001$ correlation of concentration of cytokine/chemokines in different days after symptoms onset). IL-2, IL-4, IL17A and TNF–α were not detected in the seminal plasma of both patients. No cytokines or chemokines were detected in serum of both patients—serum results were below the limit of detection of the kit (20 pg/mL for cytokines and 10 pg/mL for chemokines).

3.2. ZIKV Evolution during Prolonged Infection

The isolation of replicative ZIKV particles from different body fluids, mainly seminal fluids, in the same individuals, particularly the two male patients (ZIKV17 and ZIKV19), allowed us to evaluate the extent of genetic variations observed in prolonged persistence of ZIKV in human hosts. With ZIKV17, we obtained near complete genome sequences directly from fourteen sequentially collected semen samples and two urine samples. For patient ZIKV19, five semen and two urine samples yielded near complete genome sequences (Table S2). We also assembled a near complete ZIKV genome from one urine sample of one female patient (ZIKV18, day 15). Phylogenetic inference indicated that all three patients were infected with viruses closely related to those previously circulating in Brazil (Figure S4). As expected from individual prolonged infections, all of the ZIKV genomes obtained from each patient formed well-supported monophyletic clades (Figure S3). Within both patients, we observed ZIKV genetic changes over time both in consensus sequences (Figure 5A,B) and intra-host single nucleotide variant (iSNV) frequencies (Figure 5C,D, Table S3). This is consistent with active viral replication during prolonged ZIKV infections. With the exception of a few low frequency insertions/deletions associated with homopolymer repeats (Table S3), patterns of genetic variation (iSNVs and consensus-level changes) were distinct between urine and semen samples from the same patient (Figure 5; Table S3), consistent with independent compartmentalization of ZIKV populations in the reproductive and urinary systems.

Using time-structured phylogenies, we estimated the rate of evolution during the prolonged infection of the MRS in ZIKV17. Our estimates were highly consistent across multiple models and were indistinguishable from published rates for the entire ZIKV outbreak in the Americas (Figure S3 and Table S4). ZIKV evolution within the MRS was dominated by synonymous substitutions, consistent with strong purifying selection across most of the ZIKV genome. We observed one nonsynonymous and six distinct synonymous substitutions in the MRS of ZIKV17 (dN/dS via robust counting = 0.06) and only a single synonymous substitution in ZIKV19. We also observed a significant difference between the ratio of nonsynonymous:synonymous variants present at different frequencies in samples with a high depth of coverage. Synonymous changes were most prevalent among variants that reached high frequencies (≥50%) during the course of infection, while nonsynonymous changes were more common in variants that were maintained at low frequencies (Figure 5D; Fisher's exact test *p*-value = 0.01). This pattern is consistent with incomplete purifying selection acting on low frequency variants [25].

Despite the overall signal of purifying selection, positive diversifying selection may have affected some regions of the genome. We utilized several phylogenetic-based methods to look for signatures of positive selection at the codon-level. The reconstructed most parsimonious amino acid changes along the ZIKV ML tree topology (Figure 6, Table S5) indicated four synapomorphic changes (K242R, K408R, K985R and I1484V) defining the lineage infecting both patients ZIKV18 and ZIKV19. In addition, the virus in the urine sample of patient ZIKV19 had two additional unique changes in the NS5 peptide (V2650A and R3121K); however, these changes were not observed after the removal of duplicate sequencing reads. Patient ZIKV17 had four defining synapomorphic changes (K1202R, L1298V, A1428V and V1862I). In the urine samples, only one substitution in the NS5 (E2693G) was identified (present in one sample). Semen samples from patient ZIKV17 had a change in the NS5 (R2562H) that was present in genomes reconstructed from eight time points (39, 53, 63, 68, 88, 95, 102 and 109 days after onset symptoms). Interestingly, the consensus genome showed the initial state (2562R) at day 76, which suggests that distinct haplotypes were circulating at varying frequencies over time. Substitutions observed in patients ZIKV17 and ZIKV19 did not alter the conformation of the proteins as measured by homology modeling and structural alignments.

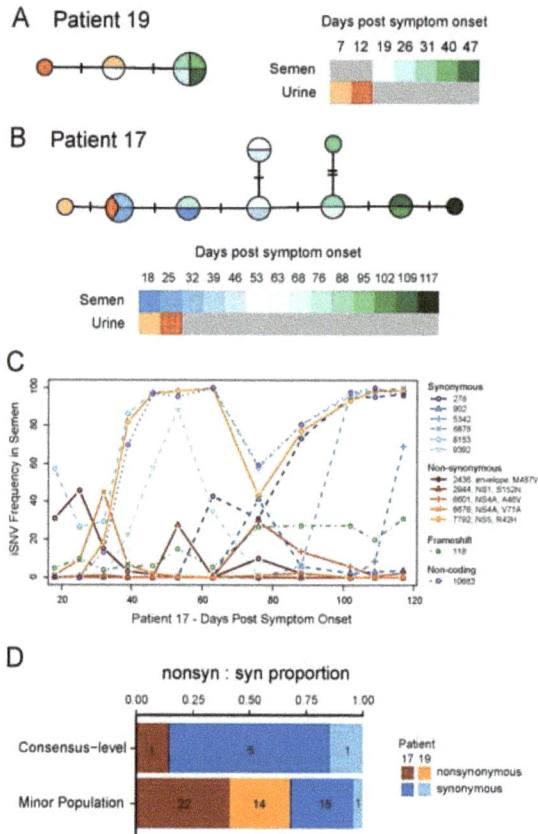

Figure 5. Evolution of ZIKV populations throughout the infection course. Median-joining haplotype networks constructed from full genome alignments of the consensus sequences from patients ZIKV19 (**A**) and ZIKV17 (**B**). Colors indicate sample type and collection date relative to symptoms onset. Each dash represents a single nucleotide substitution differentiating consensus sequences from different samples. (**C**) Intra host single nucleotide variant (iSNV) frequencies over time in semen samples collected from patient ZIKV17. The legend indicates the nucleotide position of each iSNV relative to KX197192.1 (GenBank) and for non-synonymous changes, the affected protein and amino acid change. Only positions with a minimum frequency ≥25% in at least one sample are shown. See Table S3 for details about these mutations and others present at lower frequencies. (**D**) Proportion of nonsynonymous and synonymous ZIKV iSNVs observed in semen samples from patients ZIKV17 and ZIKV19. The relative counts of nonsynonymous and synonymous variants observed above (consensus-level) and below 50% frequency (minor population) in at least one sample were significantly different (Fisher's exact test *p*-value = 0.01).

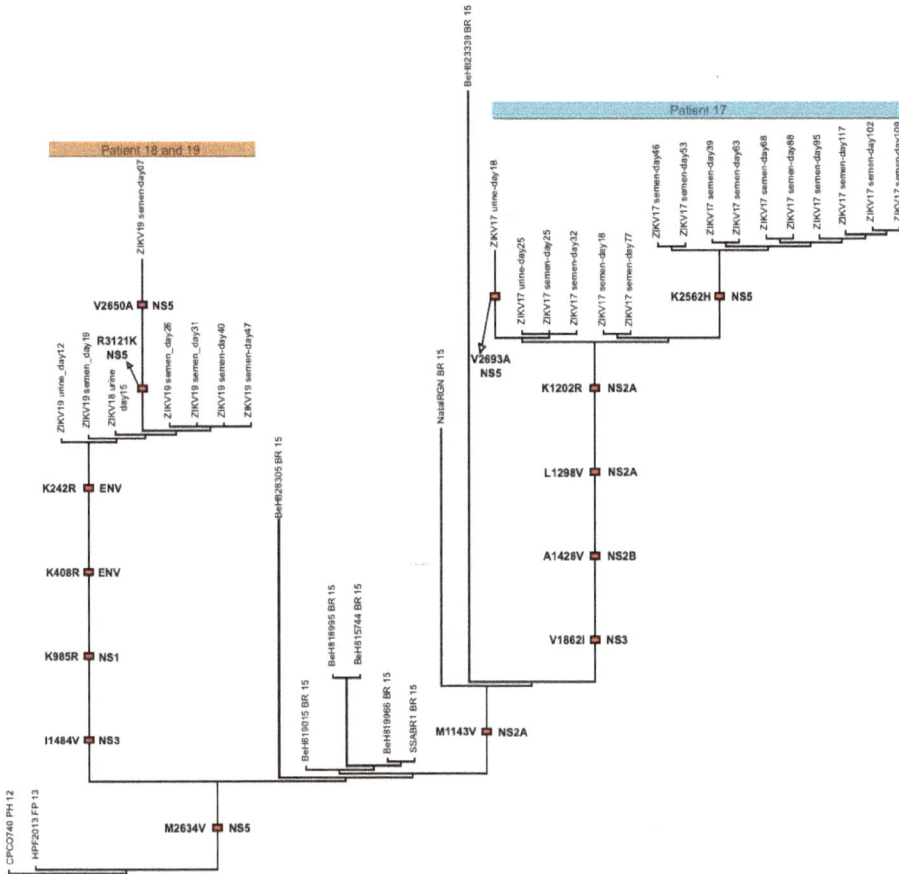

Figure 6. Dendogram showing the most parsimonious unique amino acid changes with high consistency index (CI=1) (black framed red boxes). Reconstructions were made using a set of ZIKV polyproteins from African and Asian lineage viruses. Branch lengths are shown proportional to the number of most parsimonious reconstructions (MPR) of amino acid changes. Amino acid changes that define patient clades are shown as well as the viral proteins affected. Each patient clade (which had 100% support in ML tree shown in Figure S3) was supported by four synapomorphic changes. For both patients ZIKV19 and ZIKV17 changes were observed in the NS5 protein. Although we only show the results for selection detection methods for the three patients, elevated rates of non-synonymous changes were detected for all of the codons containing unique amino acid changes shown. The multiple EM for motif elicitation (MEME) algorithm detected significant positive selection (*p*-value = 0.03) acting on the codons containing the two NS5 changes observed during infection of patient ZIKV17. All MPRs were detected with FUBAR with a Bayes factor >3 and had elevated *dN*. Sites detected by 2-rates FEL had nonsynonymous changes in the absence of detectable synonymous changes. Significant negative, purifying selection was detected by all methods used on several sites of the polyprotein.

4. Discussion

The aim of the present study was to follow the kinetics of ZIKV persistence and secretion in different host compartments and body fluids. The study included four (two males and two females) ZIKV-infected symptomatic adults who were followed for up to 298 days. Our initial conclusions supported previous evidence of prolonged ZIKV shedding in the semen of several different mammalian species, including humans [13,16,17,26,27] and confirmed the importance of semen analyses as a diagnostic tool for males with ZIKV disease. The study also confirmed the presence of ZIKV particles inside spermatic cells and seminal fluids as late as 117 days post the initial onset of symptoms. In contrast to previous reports based on the detection of RNA material, our results confirmed that complete infectious viral particles can be detected in the semen up to 117 days after the onset of symptoms.

On the other hand, the early detection of anti-ZIKV IgG and IgM antibody responses and the rapid clearance of ZIKV from serum strongly suggest that the immune system can easily handle the systemic phase of the infection. The detection of proinflammatory cytokine responses and the presence of infectious virus in seminal fluids long after viral clearance from serum indicate that the local immune system does not efficiently control ZIKV replication in the MRS. Similarly to other flaviviruses, ZIKV may promote some sort of local immunosuppression allowing viral replication despite activation of systemic immune responses. In cases of DENV infection, the virus is capable of antagonizing the innate host responses using multiple strategies including degradation of key proteins, such as STAT2, 2'-O, methylation of adenosine in the viral genome and interfering with RNAi mechanisms [28–30]. It remains to be seen if ZIKV proteins are capable of exerting local negative regulatory effects on the host's immune system, which may contribute to viral persistence. Besides, the alteration in the genital cytokine milieu could play an important role in replication and transmission of the virus as has been seen for other viruses, such as HIV-1 [31], which could considerably increase the risk of ZIKV sexual spread and potentially play a role on the viral spread. In addition, despite, experimental evidence in mice that persistent ZIKV infections can cause infertility in males [17], patient ZIKV17 was able to inseminate his wife approximately two months after virus clearance and the couple had a healthy baby.

The availability of ZIKV-containing semen and urine samples of two patients allowed us to study the genetic evolution of the virus during prolonged replication in the MRS. For the first time, we demonstrated a high level of evolutionary constraint on ZIKV during the prolonged MRS infections. High levels of constraint, as evidenced by low long-term rates of amino acid substitution, have commonly been observed for arthropod-borne viruses like ZIKV [32]. However, the primary source of this constraint is generally thought to be the continual alternation of these viruses between vertebrate and invertebrate hosts, each of which exerts unique selective pressures. By examining ZIKV genetic diversity over time in the semen of patients with prolonged MRS infections, we obtained a rare glimpse into the selective pressures exerted by a single host species. Although a large number of nonsynonymous variants were detected within both patients, few of these mutations ever reached high frequencies (Figure 5). In fact, our estimate of dN/dS from the semen samples of ZIKV17 is very similar to recent long-term dN/dS estimates for ZIKV, which average across the selective pressures from both vertebrate and invertebrate hosts [7]. Our findings, therefore, indicate that the strong evolutionary constraint observed for ZIKV and other arthropod-borne viruses may not simply represent the long term effect of alternating between hosts, but is likely also related to the pressures experienced within individual host species.

Supplementary Materials: The following are available online http://www.mdpi.com/1999-4915/10/11/615/s1: Figure S1: ZIKV characterization by IFI in semen samples, Figure S2: ZIKV detection in semen samples from patient ZIKV17; Figure S3: Concentration of cytokines, chemokines, RNA viral load and laboratorial follow-up of patients ZIKV17 and ZIKV19, Figure S4: Significantly higher proportion of nonsynonymous mutations in low frequency variants; Table S1: qRT-PCR Ct obtained from body fluid samples; Table S2: Zika virus genomes produced in this study; Table S3: Intra-host variant summary; Table S4: Substitution rate estimates for ZIKV during prolonged infection of male reproductive system; Table S5: Probes used for Zika virus targeted enrichment; Table S6: Algorithms for genetic evolution; Table S7: GenBank accessions for the consensus genomes.

Author Contributions: Writing, review, editing and original draft preparation D.B.L.O., G.S.D., E.A.M., J.T.L., L.C.S.F., P.M.A.Z., V.F.B., E.L.D.; Supervision and funding acquisition, G.F.P., P.M.A.Z., E.L.D., L.C.S.F., D.V.T.; Investigation and writing and review D.B.L.O., G.S.D., E.A.M., J.T.L., R.A.S., V.F.B., D.B.A., N.D.P., D.F.L.N., M.P.C., C.T.B., R.P.S.A., M.R.J., L.R.P., S.R.M., F.S.M., V.B.S., L.M.T., S.R.F., F.B.A., R.C.R.M.A., J.M.G., D.V.T., S.F.O., K.P., M.R.W., M.V.S.

Viruses **2018**, *10*, 615

Funding: Funding was granted by Fundação de Amparo à Pesquisa do Estado de São Paulo (FAPESP), projects Nº 2013/07467-1 (DVT); 2014/16333-1 (SRF); 2014/17766-9 (PMAZ); 2016/08727-5 and 2017/50007-2 (DBLO); 2016/20045-7 (LCSF and ELD) and Conselho Nacional de Pesquisa (CNPq) Project 303244/2013-5 (DVT); 440409/2016-0 (LCSF) and Coordenação de Aperfeiçoamento de Pessoal de Nível Superior (CAPES) project 88881.130787/2016-01 (LCSF). Received a FAPESP fellowship: 2014/27228-4 (EAM), 2014/03911-7 (CTB), 2015/25643-7 (FSM), 2016/08204-2 (MPC), 2013/26942-2 (LRP), 2015/02352 (RPSA), 2016/03605-9 (DFLN), 2016/10161-0 (VBS). Received a CAPES fellowship: 88887.131387/2016-00 (DBA); 1522381 (SRM); 1796450 (CTB) and 1473645 (RAS); received CAPES/PRONEX fellowship (JMG), respectively.

Acknowledgments: We thank José Lopes from LVCM-USP for technical support at the diagnosis, Mario Costa Cruz from CEFAP-USP for technical assistance at the Confocal IFA, Gaspar Ferreira de Lima and Roberto Cabado for technical assistance at the Electron Microscopy facilities at USP and Eduardo Gimenes Martins for the administrative and technical support. Our institutional review board approved this study and all biological samples were collected under the approval of the Ethics Committee of the Institute of Biomedical Science (ICB), USP. The authors have no other disclosures. The Center for Genome Sciences at the US Army Medical Research Institute of Infectious Diseases (USAMRIID) was supported for this project by the Defense Advanced Research Projects Agency (DARPA, PI: C. Kane). The content of this publication does not necessarily reflect the views or policies of the US Army.

Conflicts of Interest: The authors declare no conflict of interest.

References

1. Petersen, E.; Wilson, M.E.; Touch, S.; McCloskey, B.; Mwaba, P.; Bates, M.; Dar, O.; Mattes, F.; Kidd, M.; Ippolito, G.; et al. Rapid Spread of Zika Virus in The Americas—Implications for Public Health Preparedness for Mass Gatherings at the 2016 Brazil Olympic Games. *Int. J. Infect. Dis.* **2016**, *44*, 11–15. [CrossRef] [PubMed]

2. Waddell, L.A.; Greig, J.D. Scoping Review of the Zika Virus Literature. *PLoS ONE* **2016**, *11*, e0156376. [CrossRef] [PubMed]

3. Basu, R.; Tumban, E. Zika Virus on a Spreading Spree: What we now know that was unknown in the 1950's. *Virol. J.* **2016**, *13*, 165. [CrossRef] [PubMed]

4. Mlakar, J.; Korva, M.; Tul, N.; Popovic, M.; Poljsak-Prijatelj, M.; Mraz, J.; Kolenc, M.; Resman Rus, K.; Vesnaver Vipotnik, T.; Fabjan Vodusek, V.; et al. Zika Virus Associated with Microcephaly. *N. Engl. J. Med.* **2016**, *374*, 951–958. [CrossRef] [PubMed]

5. Parra, B.; Lizarazo, J.; Jimenez-Arango, J.A.; Zea-Vera, A.F.; Gonzalez-Manrique, G.; Vargas, J.; Angarita, J.A.; Zuniga, G.; Lopez-Gonzalez, R.; Beltran, C.L.; et al. Guillain-Barre Syndrome Associated with Zika Virus Infection in Colombia. *N. Engl. J. Med.* **2016**, *375*, 1513–1523. [CrossRef] [PubMed]

6. USA-CDC: All Countries & Territories with Active Zika Virus Transmission. Available online: https://wwwncdcgov/travel/page/zika-travel-information (accessed on 10 October 2018).

7. Faria, N.R.; Quick, J.; Claro, I.M.; Theze, J.; de Jesus, J.G.; Giovanetti, M.; Kraemer, M.U.G.; Hill, S.C.; Black, A.; da Costa, A.C.; et al. Establishment and cryptic transmission of Zika virus in Brazil and the Americas. *Nature* **2017**, *546*, 406–410. [CrossRef] [PubMed]

8. Giovanetti, M.; Goes de Jesus, J.; Lima de Maia, M.; Junior, J.X.; Castro Amarante, M.F.; Viana, P.; Khouri Barreto, F.; de Cerqueira, E.M.; Pedreira Santos, N.; Barreto Falcao, M.; et al. Genetic evidence of Zika virus in mother's breast milk and body fluids of a newborn with severe congenital defects. *Clin. Microbiol. Infect.* **2018**, *24*, 1111–1112. [CrossRef] [PubMed]

9. Calvet, G.A.; Kara, E.O.; Giozza, S.P.; Botto-Menezes, C.H.A.; Gaillard, P.; de Oliveira Franca, R.F.; de Lacerda, M.V.G.; da Costa Castilho, M.; Brasil, P.; de Sequeira, P.C.; et al. Study on the persistence of Zika virus (ZIKV) in body fluids of patients with ZIKV infection in Brazil. *BMC Infect. Dis.* **2018**, *18*, 49. [CrossRef] [PubMed]

10. Musso, D.; Roche, C.; Nhan, T.X.; Robin, E.; Teissier, A.; Cao-Lormeau, V.M. Detection of Zika virus in saliva. *J. Clin. Virol.* **2015**, *68*, 53–55. [CrossRef] [PubMed]

11. Gourinat, A.C.; O'Connor, O.; Calvez, E.; Goarant, C.; Dupont-Rouzeyrol, M. Detection of Zika virus in urine. *Emerg. Infect. Dis.* **2015**, *21*, 84–86. [CrossRef] [PubMed]

12. Sanchez-Montalva, A.; Pou, D.; Sulleiro, E.; Salvador, F.; Bocanegra, C.; Trevino, B.; Rando, A.; Serre, N.; Pumarola, T.; Almirante, B.; et al. Zika virus dynamics in body fluids and risk of sexual transmission in a non-endemic area. *Trop. Med. Int. Health* **2018**, *23*, 92–100. [CrossRef] [PubMed]

13. Oliveira Souto, I.; Alejo-Cancho, I.; Gascon Brustenga, J.; Peiro Mestres, A.; Munoz Gutierrez, J.; Martinez Yoldi, M.J. Persistence of Zika virus in semen 93 days after the onset of symptoms. *Enferm. Infecc. Microbiol. Clin.* **2018**, *36*, 21–23. [CrossRef] [PubMed]

14. Rossini, G.; Gaibani, P.; Vocale, C.; Cagarelli, R.; Landini, M.P. Comparison of Zika virus (ZIKV) RNA detection in plasma, whole blood and urine—Case series of travel-associated ZIKV infection imported to Italy, 2016. *J. Infect.* **2017**, *75*, 242–245. [CrossRef] [PubMed]

15. Nicastri, E.; Castilletti, C.; Liuzzi, G.; Iannetta, M.; Capobianchi, M.R.; Ippolito, G. Persistent detection of Zika virus RNA in semen for six months after symptom onset in a traveller returning from Haiti to Italy, February 2016. *Eurosurveillance* **2016**, *21*, 30314. [CrossRef] [PubMed]

16. Barzon, L.; Pacenti, M.; Franchin, E.; Lavezzo, E.; Trevisan, M.; Sgarabotto, D.; Palu, G. Infection dynamics in a traveller with persistent shedding of Zika virus RNA in semen for six months after returning from Haiti to Italy, January 2016. *Eurosurveillance* **2016**, *21*, 30316. [CrossRef] [PubMed]

17. Ma, W.; Li, S.; Ma, S.; Jia, L.; Zhang, F.; Zhang, Y.; Zhang, J.; Wong, G.; Zhang, S.; Lu, X.; et al. Zika Virus Causes Testis Damage and Leads to Male Infertility in Mice. *Cell* **2016**, *167*, 1511–1524. [CrossRef] [PubMed]

18. Frank, C.; Cadar, D.; Schlaphof, A.; Neddersen, N.; Gunther, S.; Schmidt-Chanasit, J.; Tappe, D. Sexual transmission of Zika virus in Germany, April 2016. *Eurosurveillance* **2016**, *21*, 30252. [CrossRef] [PubMed]

19. Sow, A.; Loucoubar, C.; Diallo, D.; Faye, O.; Ndiaye, Y.; Senghor, C.S.; Dia, A.T.; Weaver, S.C.; Diallo, M.; Malvy, D.; et al. Concurrent malaria and arbovirus infections in Kedougou, southeastern Senegal. *Malar. J.* **2016**, *15*, 47. [CrossRef] [PubMed]

20. Oliveira, D.B.; Almeida, F.J.; Durigon, E.L.; Mendes, E.A.; Braconi, C.T.; Marchetti, I.; Andreata-Santos, R.; Cunha, M.P.; Alves, R.P.; Pereira, L.R.; et al. Prolonged Shedding of Zika Virus Associated with Congenital Infection. *N. Engl. J. Med.* **2016**, *375*, 1202–1204. [CrossRef] [PubMed]

21. Wagner, D.; de With, K.; Huzly, D.; Hufert, F.; Weidmann, M.; Breisinger, S.; Eppinger, S.; Kern, W.V.; Bauer, T.M. Nosocomial acquisition of dengue. *Emerg. Infect. Dis.* **2004**, *10*, 1872–1873. [CrossRef] [PubMed]

22. Lu, X.; Li, X.; Mo, Z.; Jin, F.; Wang, B.; Zhao, H.; Shan, X.; Shi, L. Rapid identification of Chikungunya and Dengue virus by a real-time reverse transcription-loop-mediated isothermal amplification method. *Am. J. Trop. Med. Hyg.* **2012**, *87*, 947–953. [CrossRef] [PubMed]

23. Drummond, A.J.; Suchard, M.A.; Xie, D.; Rambaut, A. Bayesian phylogenetics with BEAUti and the BEAST 1.7. *Mol. Biol. Evol.* **2012**, *29*, 1969–1973. [CrossRef] [PubMed]

24. Garrison, E.; Marth, G. Haplotype-Based Variant Detection from Short-Read Sequencing. *arXiv* 2012.

25. Park, D.J.; Dudas, G.; Wohl, S.; Goba, A.; Whitmer, S.L.; Andersen, K.G.; Sealfon, R.S.; Ladner, J.T.; Kugelman, J.R.; Matranga, C.B.; et al. Ebola Virus Epidemiology, Transmission, and Evolution during Seven Months in Sierra Leone. *Cell* **2016**, *161*, 1516–1526. [CrossRef] [PubMed]

26. Froeschl, G.; Huber, K.; von Sonnenburg, F.; Nothdurft, H.D.; Bretzel, G.; Hoelscher, M.; Zoeller, L.; Trottmann, M.; Pan-Montojo, F.; Dobler, G.; et al. Long-term kinetics of Zika virus RNA and antibodies in body fluids of a vasectomized traveller returning from Martinique: A. case report. *BMC Infect. Dis.* **2017**, *17*, 55. [CrossRef] [PubMed]

27. Paz-Bailey, G.; Rosenberg, E.S.; Doyle, K.; Munoz-Jordan, J.; Santiago, G.A.; Klein, L.; Perez-Padilla, J.; Medina, F.A.; Waterman, S.H.; Gubern, C.G.; et al. Persistence of Zika Virus in Body Fluids—Final Report. *N. Engl. J. Med.* **2018**, *379*, 1234–1243. [CrossRef] [PubMed]

28. Morrison, J.; Laurent-Rolle, M.; Maestre, A.M.; Rajsbaum, R.; Pisanelli, G.; Simon, V.; Mulder, L.C.; Fernandez-Sesma, A.; Garcia-Sastre, A. Dengue virus co-opts UBR4 to degrade STAT2 and antagonize type I interferon signaling. *PLoS Pathog.* **2013**, *9*, e1003265. [CrossRef] [PubMed]

29. Kakumani, P.K.; Ponia, S.S.; Rajgokul, K.S.; Sood, V.; Chinnappan, M.; Banerjea, A.C.; Medigeshi, G.R.; Malhotra, P.; Mukherjee, S.K.; Bhatnagar, R.K. Role of RNA interference (RNAi) in dengue virus replication and identification of NS4B as an RNAi suppressor. *J. Virol.* **2013**, *87*, 8870–8883. [CrossRef] [PubMed]

30. Dong, H.; Chang, D.C.; Hua, M.H.; Lim, S.P.; Chionh, Y.H.; Hia, F.; Lee, Y.H.; Kukkaro, P.; Lok, S.M.; Dedon, P.C.; et al. 2'-O methylation of internal adenosine by flavivirus NS5 methyltransferase. *PLoS Pathog.* **2012**, *8*, e1002642. [CrossRef] [PubMed]

31. Lisco, A.; Munawwar, A.; Introini, A.; Vanpouille, C.; Saba, E.; Feng, X.; Grivel, J.C.; Singh, S.; Margolis, L. Semen of HIV-1-infected individuals: Local shedding of herpesviruses and reprogrammed cytokine network. *J. Infect. Dis.* **2012**, *205*, 97–105. [CrossRef] [PubMed]

32. Holmes, E.C. Patterns of intra- and interhost nonsynonymous variation reveal strong purifying selection in dengue virus. *J. Virol.* **2003**, *77*, 11296–11298. [CrossRef] [PubMed]

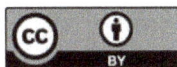

Review

Probing Molecular Insights into Zika Virus–Host Interactions

Ina Lee [1], Sandra Bos [2] , Ge Li [1], Shusheng Wang [1], Gilles Gadea [2] , Philippe Desprès [2] and Richard Y. Zhao [1,3,4,5,*]

[1] Department of Pathology, University of Maryland School of Medicine, Baltimore, MD 21201, USA; ilee1@umm.edu (I.L.); GLi@som.umaryland.edu (G.L.); shushengwang018@gmail.com (S.W.)

[2] Université de la Réunion, INSERM U1187, CNRS UMR 9192, IRD UMR 249, Unité Mixte Processus Infectieux en Milieu Insulaire Tropical, Plateforme Technologique CYROI, 94791 Sainte Clotilde, La Réunion, France; sandrabos.lab@gmail.com (S.B.); gilles.gadea@inserm.fr (G.G.); philippe.despres@univ-reunion.fr (P.D.)

[3] Department of Microbiology and Immunology, University of Maryland School of Medicine, Baltimore, MD 21201, USA

[4] Institute of Global Health, University of Maryland School of Medicine, Baltimore, MD 21201, USA

[5] Institute of Human Virology, University of Maryland School of Medicine, Baltimore, MD 21201, USA

[*] Correspondence: rzhao@som.umaryland.edu; Tel: +1-410-706-6301

Received: 5 April 2018; Accepted: 28 April 2018; Published: 2 May 2018

Abstract: The recent Zika virus (ZIKV) outbreak in the Americas surprised all of us because of its rapid spread and association with neurologic disorders including fetal microcephaly, brain and ocular anomalies, and Guillain–Barré syndrome. In response to this global health crisis, unprecedented and world-wide efforts are taking place to study the ZIKV-related human diseases. Much has been learned about this virus in the areas of epidemiology, genetic diversity, protein structures, and clinical manifestations, such as consequences of ZIKV infection on fetal brain development. However, progress on understanding the molecular mechanism underlying ZIKV-associated neurologic disorders remains elusive. To date, we still lack a good understanding of; (1) what virologic factors are involved in the ZIKV-associated human diseases; (2) which ZIKV protein(s) contributes to the enhanced viral pathogenicity; and (3) how do the newly adapted and pandemic ZIKV strains alter their interactions with the host cells leading to neurologic defects? The goal of this review is to explore the molecular insights into the ZIKV–host interactions with an emphasis on host cell receptor usage for viral entry, cell innate immunity to ZIKV, and the ability of ZIKV to subvert antiviral responses and to cause cytopathic effects. We hope this literature review will inspire additional molecular studies focusing on ZIKV–host Interactions.

Keywords: zika virus; ZIKV–host interactions; viral pathogenesis; cell surface receptors; antiviral responses; viral counteraction; cytopathic effects; microcephaly; ZIKV-associated neurologic disorders

---

1. Introduction

1.1. The Zika Virus (ZIKV): An Emerging Public Health Threat

The 2015 Zika virus (ZIKV) epidemic in the Americas surprised the world because of its rapid global spread and the findings that it associates with various neurologic disorders including microcephaly in newborns and Guillain–Barré syndrome (GBS) in adults. ZIKV was thought to be a mild virus that had little or no threat to humans. Through studies of this new ZIKV pandemic, we have now learned that ZIKV is a rather severe human pathogen that can cause significant neuropathology such as fetal microcephaly, GBS, and various other congenital neurologic and ocular disorders [1–5].

So, it begs the question of what has transformed a benign ZIKV over the past seventy years to generate the contemporary pathogenic ZIKV.

The goal of this article is to review the current literature on ZIKV–host interactions with a focus on molecular aspects. We herein summarize insights on host cell receptor usage for viral entry, cell innate immunity to ZIKV, and the ability of ZIKV to subvert antiviral responses and to cause cytopathic effects. The molecular mechanisms underlying these ZIKV–host interactions, and their potential impacts on ZIKV-induced fetal microcephaly or other neurologic disorders are discussed.

1.2. The Organization of Zika Virus

ZIKV belongs the *flavivirus* genus of the *Flaviviridae* family which includes a number of medically important arboviruses such as Dengue Virus (DENV), Japanese Encephalitis Virus (JEV), and West Nile Virus (WNV). Structurally, ZIKV is similar to other flaviviruses. The nucleocapsid is approximately 25–30 nm in diameter, surrounded by a host membrane-derived lipid bilayer that contains envelope (E) and membrane (M) proteins. The virus particle is approximately 40–65 nm in diameter, with surface projections that measure roughly 5–10 nm [6], leading an overall average size of 45–75 nm. The surface proteins are arranged in an icosahedral-like symmetry [7]. Like its flaviviral siblings, ZIKV contains a positive sense single-stranded RNA [ssRNA(+)] viral genome of approximately 10.7 kilobases (kb) (Figure 1). The genomic RNA is flanked by two terminal non-coding regions (NCR), i.e., the 5' NCR (107 nt) and the 3' NCR (428 nt) [8]. The ZIKV genome includes a single large open reading frame encoding a polyprotein of about 3300 amino acids, which is processed co- and post-translationally by viral and host proteases (PRs) to produce a total of fourteen immature proteins, mature proteins, and small peptides [9]. A total of ten mature viral proteins, i.e., three structural proteins (C, M, and E) and seven nonstructural (NS1, NS2A, NS2B, NS3, NS4A, NS4B, and NS5) proteins are produced after viral processing [6,9,10]. The 2K signal peptide, which is situated between NS4A and NS4B, plays a regulatory role in viral RNA synthesis and viral morphogenesis in other flaviviruses [11,12]. Among the structural proteins, the mature capsid (C) protein is produced by cleavage of the anchor-C (anaC) protein by a viral PR (anaC→C), which in turn triggers the cleavage of the precursor membrane (prM) protein by the host protease Furin. As a result, a mature membrane (M) protein and a Pr protein are produced (PrM→M + Pr) [11,13]. In the case of DENV, noninfectious and immature viral particles contain prM that forms a heterodimer with the E protein [14]. The transition of prM to M by Furin cleavage results in mature and infectious particles [15,16]. The E protein, composing the majority of the virion surface, is involved in binding to the host cell surface and triggering subsequent membrane fusion and endocytosis [8]. Post-translational processing of the non-structural protein region produces four viral enzymes, i.e., PR, helicase, methyl-transferase, and RNA-dependent RNA polymerase (RdRP). A fully active ZIKV PR consists of two protein components, namely the N-terminal domain of NS3 (NS3pro) and a membrane-associated NS2B cofactor [17,18]. The NS3pro is responsible for proteolytic processing of the viral polyprotein, whereas the NS2B cofactor is required for enhancing enzymatic activity and substrate specificity. The C-terminal domain of NS3 protein produces ZIKV helicase, which plays a critical role in NTP-dependent RNA unwinding and translocation during viral replication [19]. The methyl-transferase and RdRP are generated from the N-terminal and C-terminal of NS5, respectively. NS1, NS3, and NS5 are large proteins that are highly-conserved [6]. NS2A, NS2B, NS4A, and NS4B proteins are smaller, hydrophobic proteins [6]. The 3' NCR forms a loop structure that may play a role in translation, RNA packaging, cyclization, genome stabilization and recognition [8]. The 5' NCR allows translation via a methylated nucleotide cap or a genome-linked protein [7]. In addition, ZIKV produces abundant non-coding subgenomic flavivirus RNA (sfRNA) from the 3'UTR in infected cells, which may play a role in the viral life cycle and viral subversion of innate immunity [20].

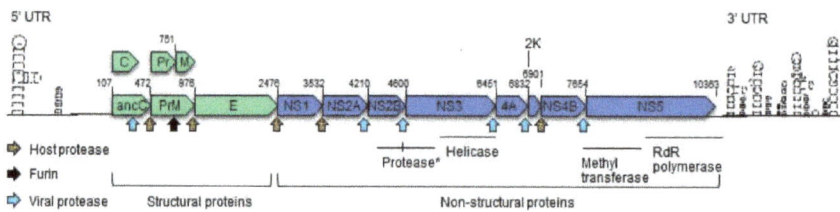

Figure 1. Schematic structure of the Zika virus genome. Each of the viral proteins is drawn based on the relative orientation in the RNA genome. The ZIKV viral protease, host protease and Furin protease are represented by different arrows, as shown. Each arrow points to the specific protease cleavage site. The numbers shown above each protein product indicate the start/end position. Abbreviations: anaC, anchored capsid protein C; C, capsid protein C; prM, precursor membrane protein; M, membrane protein; Pr, protein pr; E, envelope protein; NS, nonstructural protein; *, protease consists of N-terminal of NS3 and C-terminal NS2B as described in the text. C-terminal of NS3 encodes helicase; 2K, signal peptide 2K; NS5 encodes methyltransferase at its N-terminal end and RNA-dependent RNA (RdR) polymerase at its C-terminal end. UTR, untranslated region. The structures of 5′ UTR and 3′ UTR are based on [21]. The information of ZIKV protein products is based on [9].

1.3. The Infectious Cycle of ZIKV and Human Transmission

The ZIKV infectious cycle starts with the virus binding to host cell surface receptors and attachment factors via the E protein, leading to clathrin-dependent endocytosis. Internalized virus particles fuse with the endosomal membrane in a pH-dependent manner, releasing the genomic RNA into the cytoplasm of the host cell. The positive-sense viral genomic ssRNA is translated into a polyprotein that is subsequently cleaved to form structural and non-structural proteins. Viral replication takes place in intracellular membrane-associated compartments located on the surface of the endoplasmic reticulum (ER), resulting in a dsRNA genome synthesized from the genomic ssRNA(+) by viral RdRP. The dsRNA genome is subsequently transcribed and replicated, resulting in additional viral mRNAs/ssRNA(+) genomes. Immature virus particles are assembled within ER. They are then transported through the trans-Golgi network (TGN) where the fully mature infectious virus particles are formed as soon as prM is processed to M by a Furin-like protease. The new virus particles are released into the extracellular environment where they move on to a new infectious life cycle [7].

ZIKV is an arbovirus that is primarily transmitted to mammalian hosts by mosquito vectors from the *Aedes (Ae.)* genus including *Ae. africanus*, *Ae. aegypti*, *Ae. vitattus*, *Ae. furcifer*, *Ae. apicoargenteus*, and *Ae. luteocephalus* [22,23]. The incubation time for ZIKV in mosquito vectors is approximately 10 days [22]. Blood contact via blood transfusion or sexual contact is another route of ZIKV infection [24–26]. Consistent with this notion, human testis has been found to be a reservoir for ZIKV [22,27–29]. In addition, ZIKV can also be transmitted vertically from mother to child via placenta–fetal transmission [30,31]. This has become a main route for the development of fetal microcephaly [32,33].

1.4. A Brief History of ZIKV

The first ZIKV strain was isolated in 1947 from caged monkeys in the Zika forest of Uganda, Africa. A ZIKV strain MR766 (ZIKV$_{MR766}$) from that isolation was established and has been used since for research purpose [34]. Therefore, the ZIKV$_{MR766}$ is often referred to as the historical or ancestral ZIKV strain. Initial characterization of ZIKV$_{MR766}$ showed that it is highly neurotropic in mice, and no virus has been recovered from tissues other than the brains of infected mice [35]. That report further showed that mice at all ages were susceptible to ZIKV$_{MR766}$ by intracerebral inoculations. In contrast, cotton-rats, Guinea pigs, and rabbits showed no sign of ZIKV$_{MR766}$ infection by using the same intracerebral inoculations. Monkeys showed either mild fever (pyrexia) or no signs of infection.

Interestingly, mice younger than two weeks were highly susceptible to intraperitoneal inoculation, whereas mice older than two weeks can rarely be infected by the same route of intraperitoneal injection [35], suggesting established blood-brain barriers in the older mice may prevent ZIKV from accessing the brain.

In a different study, the effect of ZIKV infection on the central nervous system (CNS) of mice was examined by using intracerebral inoculation [36]. Histologic H & E staining showed that ZIKV infects the Ammon's horn (hippocampus proper) area of seven-day-old mouse brain. Detailed examination suggested that ZIKV infected pyriform cells of the Ammon's horn and induced hyperchromatic debris in those cells, suggesting possible DNA or chromosomal aberration. In addition, ZIKV induced gross enlargement (hypertrophy) of astroglial cells of the Ammon's horn, but had little effect on microglial cells of the same area [36]. Ultra-structural studies by electron microscopy (EM) further revealed that ZIKV replicates exclusively in the ER compartment of astroglial cells and neurons, an indication of membrane-associated viral replication [36].

Those early findings in the mouse model suggest that (1) ZIKV is a neurotropic virus with preference to embryonic brains [34,35], (2) ZIKV specifically infect astroglial cells and pyriform cells in the Ammon's horn, and (3) ZIKV primarily replicates in the ER network [36]. At the cellular level, ZIKV appeared to induce gross cell enlargement, chromosomal or DNA aberrations, and mitochondrial dysfunction [36]. Although early data showed that ZIKV was pathogenic to mice, there was no indication that ZIKV was pathogenic to humans [35]. Therefore, some types of virological change are likely to have taken placed during the viral evolution in the past seventy years, leading to pathogenic ZIKV infection of humans.

The first ZIKV infection in human was documented in 1952 [34], and the virus was subsequently isolated from human hosts in Nigeria in 1968 [22]. Since then, multiple studies have confirmed the presence of ZIKV antibodies in human sera from a number of countries in Africa and Asia [22]. However, no severe diseases were clearly linked to those infections. In the recorded history, ZIKV infection appears to have migrated eastward from Africa. A number of outbreaks have taken place over the past seventy years including several minor outbreaks in 1977–1978 in Pakistan, Malaysia, and Indonesia. Two major outbreaks were documented in Yap Island of Micronesia in 2007, and in French Polynesia, New Caledonia, the Cook Islands, and Easter Island in 2013 and 2014 [26,37]. The affected individuals in those outbreaks were in the order of hundreds to thousands. However, in the most recent outbreak, ZIKV infection had been reported in eighty-five countries, territories, or subnational areas with an estimate of over 1.5 million affected individuals according to the World Health Organization (WHO). Brazil was the most affected country, with an estimated 440,000 to 1.3 million cases reported through December of 2015.

Although human ZIKV infection is mostly self-limiting, manifestations of neurological disorders such as GBS became increasingly apparent during the recent outbreaks in French Polynesia and Brazil [32,38]. The number of microcephaly in newborns also increased dramatically, which for the first time indicated a possible link between ZIKV infections and fetal malformations [32,39,40]. More than 4700 suspected cases of microcephaly were reported from mid-2015 through to January 2016 [41], spurring an unprecedented and world-wide effort to unravel this mystery. By March of 2016, the causal relationship between microcephaly in newborn and ZIKV infection was first established [32,39,40]. By April of 2016, a total of 3530 newborns with confirmed microcephaly were reported. In the same year, WHO declared an international public health emergency. In-depth research now shows that ZIKV infection is also associated with a number of other congenital and ocular diseases [1,2].

1.5. What Has Been Learned from the Recent ZIKV Break?

We have learned a great deal about the ZIKV and its etiology through the above described studies. The knowledge we have gained is that fetal microcephaly and other congenital malformations can indeed be caused by ZIKV infection [32,42,43]. Furthermore, those circulating and pathogenic ZIKV strains are most likely derived from the Asian lineage [44,45]. The Asian lineage is likely evolved from the African lineage through viral gene mutations by adaptation of higher cytopathicity that led to enhanced viral pathogenicity. Particular efforts have been put to investigate whether the emergence of new ZIKV epidemic strains was associated with accumulation of specific mutations that would be the leading cause of increased pathogenic effects [44–46]. Also, investigations have been conducted to determine whether pathogenic strains of ZIKV could preferentially infect certain human tissues or cells, especially neural progenitor cells (NPCs) in the brain, or they have acquired greater virulence through accumulated effects of ZIKV gene mutations [47–49]. The antibody-dependent enhancement (ADE) may also contribute to the acquired virulence [50]. This scenario could occur if individuals have previously been exposed to other flaviviruses and have acquired antibodies that partially cross-react with ZIKV. Instead of neutralizing ZIKV, these antibodies could paradoxically argument ZIKV infectivity [50]. As a matter of fact, the opposite scenario has been observed in which pre-exposure of ZIKV was associated with enhanced DENV-2 infection in vitro [51] and in monkeys [52]. Therefore, enhanced ZIKV infection as the result of prior exposure of other flaviviral infection could certainly be feasible [53–56]. However, ADE is less likely to be the predominant mode of enhanced ZIKV pathogenicity in the recent break since ZIKV is known to cause fetal microcephaly in the absence of antibody response to other flaviviruses. We should also be mindful that despite these theories, we cannot exclude another possibility that ZIKV-induced microcephaly may not be the result of ZIKV evolution, but rather a reflection of the advanced technology in disease monitoring and diagnosis. In other words, microcephaly is intrinsic to all ZIKV strains but its evasion from public awareness could be due to the lack of sensitive detection methods in the past. This possibility may not totally be far-fetched, insofar that the very first ZIKV isolate, $ZIKV_{MR766}$, also induced microcephaly in animal and human brain-specific organoid models [40,43,57]. In fact, both African and Asian ZIKV strains (MR766, FSS13025, PF/2013/KD507, SZ01, and various epidemic Brazilian strains, e.g., ZIKV-BR/2015), have been shown to induce microcephaly-like phenotypes in animal and human brain-specific organoid models (Table 1) [40,43,57–59]. Nevertheless, virological activities of the ancestral $ZIKV_{MR766}$ did appear to be different from Asian lineage in embryonic mouse brains [60]. Therefore, as it says that the devil is in the detail. It is very likely that the neurological defects caused by the epidemic Brazilian ZIKV in humans were attributed by subtle but important virological changes. Those newly adapted virological changes could include preferable infection to certain brain and neural cells such as hNPCs, persistent viral replication in host cells, and enduring neuropathic damages that lead to those observed ZIKV-associated neurological disorders. Further and detailed dissections of those virological traits certainly are warranted.

In short, even though we have learned a great deal about the ZIKV etiology, much still remains unknown. Some of the critical questions include; (1) what type of virological changes have taken place to result in increased viral pathogenicity, (2) which ZIKV protein(s) is responsible for the enhanced viral pathogenicity, and (3) how do the newly adapted ZIKV strains alter their interactions with host cells that lead to those neurologic defects? In particular, the specific mechanisms underlying the molecular actions of ZIKV-mediated neurologic disorders such as microcephaly and other neurologic disorders need to be thoroughly investigated.

Table 1. Zika viral strains that are known to cause microcephaly or microcephaly-like phenotypes.

ZIKV Strain	Model Used	Host/Location/Year	Microcephaly-Like Phenotypes	Reference
Human fetal tissue or organoid models				
MR766	Human brain-specific organoids	Rhesus monkey/Uganda/1947	Increased cell death and reduced proliferation, resulting in decreased neuronal cell-layer volume resembling microcephaly.	[40]
MR766	Human neurospheres and organoids	Rhesus monkey/Uganda/1947	Growth impairment of neurospheres and organoids	[43]
MR766	Human cerebral organoids	Rhesus monkey/Uganda/1947	Reduction of organoid growth and volume reminiscent of microcephaly via induction of TLR3	[57]
FSS 13025	Human brain-specific organoids	Human/Cambodia/2010	Increased cell death and reduced proliferation, resulting in decreased neuronal cell-layer volume resembling microcephaly.	[40]
ZIKV(BR)	Human organoids	Human/Brazil/2015	Reduction of proliferative zones and disrupted cortical layers; induction of apoptosis, autophagy and impaired neurodevelopment	[59]
KU527068	Aborted human fetal brain	Human/Brazil/2016	Microcephaly with calcification in the fetal brain and placenta	[32]
FB_GWUH	Aborted human fetal brain	Human/USA/2016	Fetal brain abnormalities with diffuse cerebral cortical thinning	[39]
Mouse models				
PF/2013/KD507	Mouse	Human/French Polynesia/2013	Fetal demise or intrauterine growth restriction	[33]
ZIKV(BR)	Mouse	Human/Brazil/2015	Intrauterine growth restriction, including signs of microcephaly and vertical transmission	[59]
SZ01	Mouse vertical transmission	Human/Samoa/2016	Infection of radial glia cells of dorsal ventricular zone of the fetuses resulting in reduced cavity of lateral ventricles and decreased cortical surface area	[40]
SZ01	Embryonic mouse brain	Human/Samoa/2016	Cell cycle arrest, apoptosis, and inhibition of NPC differentiation, resulting in cortical thinning and microcephaly	[61]
CAM/2010AndVEN/2016	Neonatal mouse brain	Human/Cambodia/2010 Human/Venezuela/2016	Neonatal ZIKV infection of VEN/2016 leads to more severe microcephaly than CAM/2010. VEN/2016 strain infection leads to stronger immune response, more severe calcification, more neuronal death and abolished oligodendrocyte development, but less activation of microglial cells.	[62]

Viral pathogenicity is normally referred to the state of a virus and its ability to cause disease. The attributes of viral pathogenicity are often constituted by the target of organ, tissue, and cells (cell tropism), the level and persistence of viral replication in host cells, and the ability of the virus to cause damage to host cells that is referred to as cytopathic effects (CPEs). Both historical and contemporary ZIKV strains have the capacity to replicate in brain-specific neuronal cells [34]. However, so far, only the epidemic strains were associated to congenital fetal microcephaly and other neurologic disorders, highlighting that viral factors other than the cell tropism are more likely contributing to the increased viral pathogenicity. Furthermore, multifactorial viral functions might have contributed to those ZIKV-associated diseases. Conceivably, it could be the changing balance in ZIKV–host interactions that leads to favorable and persistent ZIKV viral replication in host cells such as hNPCs, increased and lasting CPEs that ultimately contribute to those observed fetal development and neurologic disorders. In the following sections, we will discuss the molecular aspects of ZIKV–host interactions, which include (1) host target cells and cell surface receptors for viral entry, (2) host cellular and immune responses to ZIKV replications, (3) counteracting effects of ZIKV to host antiviral responses, and (4) ZIKV-induced cytopathic effects (restricted cell growth, cell cycle dysregulation, and cell death/apoptosis) that are all known contributing factors to fetal brain development and neurologic impairments [42,57,61].

2. Cellular Targets and Viral Entry

2.1. Cellular Targets

ZIKV primarily infects NPCs in embryonic brains [42,61,63]. In the adult brain, it also infects astroglial and microglial cells, and to lesser extent, neurons [36,42]. In addition, ZIKV infects other tissues such as skin (including dermal fibroblasts and epidermal keratinocytes), testis, and placenta (Table 2). As an arbovirus, ZIKV transmission is predominately through skin by mosquitoes such as *Ae. aegypti* and *Ae. africanus* [22,23]. Consistent with this route of transmission, immature and mature dendritic cells are susceptible to ZIKV infection [64–66]. ZIKV can also be transmitted through sexual contacts [24–26]. Infected Sertoli cells in human testis are known ZIKV reservoirs [27–29]. Several placenta-specific cells have been shown to be prone to ZIKV infection including Hofbauer cells, trophoblasts, and placental endothelial cells, supporting an important role of the placenta in transmitting ZIKV via blood to fetal brains [33,67,68]. In line with the idea that crossing the blood-brain barrier might be required to transmit the virus to the brain compartment [35], ZIKV persistently infects primary human brain microvascular endothelial cells (hBMECs) or established cell lines [69]. Interestingly, a hepatoma cell line Huh-7 appears to be highly permissive to ZIKV infection. However, liver has not yet been documented to be the target organ of ZIKV, even though DENV is well-known to infect liver [70,71].

2.2. The Cellular Receptors for ZIKV Entry

Flaviviruses enter host cells by clathrin-dependent endocytosis, which is initiated when viral particles interact with cell surface receptors. The cell surface receptors bind to the infectious viral particles and direct them to the endocytic pathway. Several cell surface receptors facilitate ZIKV viral entry (Table 2), which include the tyrosine-protein kinase receptor AXL, Tyro3, DC-SIGN, and TIM-1 [64,65]. AXL and Tyro3 are part of the TAM receptor tyrosine kinase family that normally binds to Gas6 and Pros1 ligands. These receptors are known to regulate an array of cellular activities including cell adhesion, migration, proliferation, and survival, as well as the release of inflammatory cytokines, which play pivotal roles in innate immunity [72]. DC-SIGN is an innate immune receptor present on the surface of both macrophages and dendritic cells (DCs). It recognizes a broad range of pathogen-derived ligands and mediates antigen uptake and signaling [73]. The TIM-1 receptor, also known as HAVcr-1 (Hepatitis A virus cellular receptor 1), plays an important role in host response to viral infection.

Even though all of the aforementioned cell surface receptors participate in ZIKV viral entry, they are not unique to ZIKV infection. For example, AXL, Tyro3, and DC-SIGN are used by Lassa virus [74]. The TIM-1 receptor mediates infections of the deadly Ebola virus [75]. In fact, both TAM and TIM families of phosphatidylserine receptors also mediate viral entry of other flaviviruses such as DENV [76] and WNV [77]. For instance, in the case of DENV, TIM receptors facilitate viral entry by directly interacting with virus-associated phosphatidylserine, whereas TAM-mediated infection relies on indirect viral recognition, in which the TAM ligand Gas6 acts as a bridging molecule by binding to phosphatidylserine within the viral particle [76]. Reviews of this topic can be found in [78,79].

Involvement of AXL, Tyro3, DC-SIGN, and, to a lesser extent, TIM-1 was initially described by Hamel et al. when they studied ZIKV entry in skin cells [64]. AXL was subsequently shown to be a prime target receptor for ZIKV viral entry in a variety of cell types including human endothelial cells (hECs) [61], neural stem cells [80], microglia and astrocytes [81], and oligodendrocyte precursor cells [82]. Examination of the AXL expression levels of diverse cell types suggests that AXL is highly expressed on the surface of human radial glial cells, astrocytes, hECs, oligodendrocyte precursor cells, and microglia in the developing human cortex as well as in progenitor cells of the developing retina [80,82]. Other ZIKV permissive and non-neuronal human cell types, which are known to express AXL, Tyro3, and/or TIM1 and likely to mediate viral entry, include placental cells, explants-cytotrophoblasts, endothelial cells, fibroblasts, and Hofbauer cells in chorionic villi as well as amniotic epithelial cells and trophoblast progenitors in amniochorionic membranes [83].

The susceptibility of human ECs to ZIKV positively correlates with the cell surface levels of AXL [61]. Gain- and loss-of-function tests revealed that AXL is required for ZIKV entry at a post-binding step, and small-molecule inhibitors of the AXL kinase significantly reduced ZIKV infection of hECs [61]. In human microglia and astrocytes of the developing brain, like DENV, AXL-mediated ZIKV entry requires the AXL ligand Gas6 to serve as a bridge linking ZIKV particles to glial cells [81]. Following binding, ZIKV is internalized through clathrin-mediated endocytosis and is transported to Rab5+ endosomes to establish productive infection. Downregulation of AXL by an AXL inhibitor R428 or an AXL decoy receptor MYD1 significantly reduced but did not abolish the ZIKV infection, suggesting the AXL receptor might be the primary but not the only receptor that is required for ZIKV infection [81]. Genetic knockdown of AXL in a glial cell line nearly abolished ZIKV infection [82]. It should be mentioned that elimination of any known entry receptor does not result in complete protection from viral infection, as flaviviruses use many different receptors, there is always redundancy and alternatives.

Interestingly, genetic ablation of the AXL receptor by CRISPR/CAS9 did not protect hNPCs and cerebral organoids from ZIKV Infection [84]. In particular, genetic ablation of AXL has no effect on ZIKV entry or ZIKV-mediated cell death in human induced pluripotent stem cell (iPSC)-derived NPCs or cerebral organoids. It is not yet clear what contributes to the observed discrepancy between this and other studies. One possibility is that ZIKV may use different cell surface receptors on iPSC-derived NPCs [84]. For example, TIM-1 plays a more prominent role than AXL in placental cells [83]. Duramycin, a peptide that binds phosphatidylethanolamine in enveloped viral particles and precludes TIM1 binding, reduced ZIKV infection in placental cells and explants. In a mouse study, comparison of homozygous or heterozygous AXL knock-out showed no significant differences in ZIKV viral replication and clinical manifestation, suggesting AXL is dispensable for ZIKV infection in those mice [85].

Table 2. Cellular targets and receptor usages.

Primary Cell	Receptor	References
Brain		
Neural progenitor cells (NPCs)	AXL, TLR3	[80,84,85]
Astroglial cells	AXL	[36,81,86–88]
Microglial cells	AXL	[81]
Placenta		
Hofbauer cells	AXL, Tyro3, TIM1	[67,68,83]
Trophoblasts	AXL, Tyro3, TIM1, TLR3, TLR8	[67,68,83]
Endothelial cells	AXL, Tyro3, TIM1	[33,83]
Skin		
Dermal fibroblasts	AXL, TIM-1, TYRO3, TLR3, RIG-I, MDA5	[64,89]
Epidermal keratinocytes	AXL, TIM-1, TYRO3, TLR3, RIG-I, MDA5	[64]
Immune cells		
Immature dendritic cells	DC-SIGN	[64,65]
Dendritic cells	DC-SIGN	[66]
CD14+ monocytes	Unknown	[90–92]
CD14+CD16+ monocytes	Unknown	[91]
Testis		
Sertoli cell	AXL	[28,93,94]
Spermatozoa	Tyro3	[95,96]
Kidney		
Renal mesangial cell	Unknown	
Glomerular podocytes	Unknown	[97]
Renal Glomerular Endothelial Cell	Unknown	
Retina		
Retinal pericytes	Tyro3, AXL	[1,98]
Retinal microvascular endothelial cells	Tyro3, AXL	

Permissive human cell lines			
Cell line	Origins	Permissiveness	References
SK-N-SH	Brain/Bone marrow	**	[99]
SH-SY5Y	Nerve	**	[100]
SF268	CNS in brain	***	[42,70]
HBMEC	Brain	***	[69,94]
SNB19	CNS in brain	***	[42]
Huh-7	Liver	***	[70]
HFF-1	Skin	***	[64]
A549	Lung	***	[100,101]
HOBIT	Osteoblast-like Cells	***	[102]

Note: **, moderate permissive; ***, highly permissive.

3. Cellular and Immune Responses to ZIKV Infection

Inflammation is one of the first line responses of the cellular immune system to viral infection, which is typically ignited by releasing cytokines including chemokines (Table 3). ZIKV triggers various host cell pro-inflammatory responses (Figure 2) [64,65,101,103]. For example, ZIKV stimulates CD8+ T cell-mediated polyfunctional immune responses to induce NF-κB-mediated production of cytokines such as IL-1β, IL-6, MIP1α, as well as chemokines including IP10 and RANTES [87,103]

(Figure 2, left). These ZIKV-induced T cell immune responses are antiviral because when CD8+ isolates from previously ZIKV infected mice are introduced to naive mice prior to ZIKV infection, viral clearance is enhanced. Conversely, depletion of CD8+ T cells from infected animals compromises viral clearance [65]. ZIKV structural proteins (C, prM, and E) are the major targets of CD8+ T cell and CD4+ T cell responses [104].

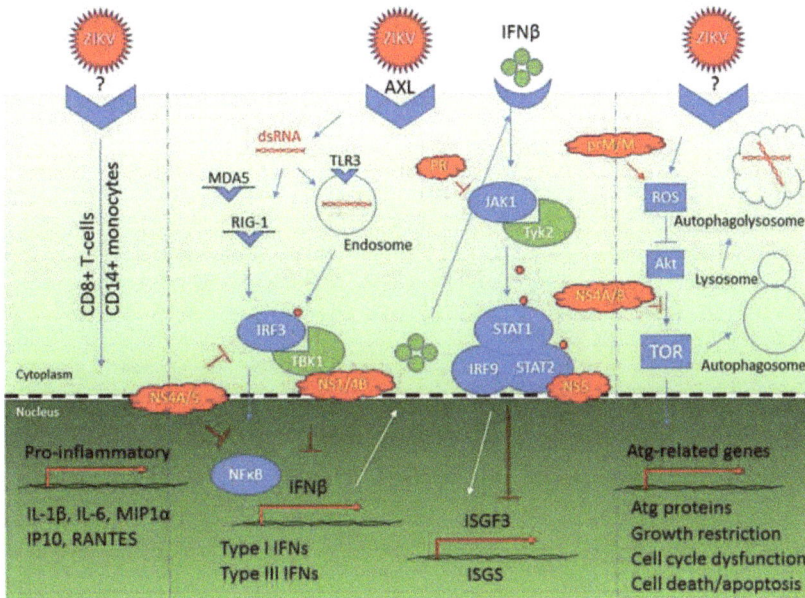

Figure 2. This figure illustrates Zika virus interactions with host cells. The Zika virus or proteins are colored in red. Cellular receptors or proteins that are affected by ZIKV are shown in blue. Cellular proteins shown in green are regulatory proteins such as kinases. Three Zika viruses are used here to show ZIKV-induced T-cell responses (left), ZIKV-mediated type I and type III IFNs productions (middle) and ZIKV-triggered autophagy (right). → indicates a positive interaction. denotes inhibitory action. Small red dots are used to indicate phosphorylation.

ZIKV also elicits humoral immune responses by producing protective and neutralizing antibodies in humans [34,45]. However, this antibody-mediated protection effect against ZIKV could be jeopardized in individuals who have previously been exposed to other flaviviruses such as DENV, which is the closest sibling of ZIKV. Pre-existing neutralizing antibodies against DENV presented in those individuals could, instead of neutralizing ZIKV, actually augment ZIKV infection and lead to more severe diseases [50]. This ADE effect of prior flaviviral infections on ZIKV pathogenicity has been thoroughly reviewed elsewhere [105,106].

Aside from ZIKV-mediated inflammatory and humoral responses, ZIKV also triggers a series of host cell innate immune responses, which are crucial for the recognition of viral invasion, activation of antiviral responses, and determination of the fate of viral infected cells (Figure 2, middle). Generally, primed by the pathogen-associated molecular pattern (PAMP) of different viruses, host cells recognize the invading virus by activating different types of pattern recognition receptors (PRRs), which could be cell surface receptors or endosomal receptors. For example, ZIKV is recognized by an endosomal toll-like receptor 3 (TLR3), which is a PRR that specifically recognizes dsRNA virus [57,64,65]. TLR3 belongs to a class of endosomal receptors that can be found in first line of defense cells such as macrophages or Langerhans cells. TLR3 activation plays a key role in host cell innate immune responses to viral infection. Consistent with the innate immune responses to dsRNA virus, ZIKV-induced TLR3 activation promotes phosphorylation of interferon regulatory factor 3 (IRF3) by TBK1 kinase, leading to induction of type 1 interferon (IFN) signaling pathways [65,107]. This initiates a cascade that further activates cytoplasmic RIG-I-like receptors (RLRs) responses, subsequently inducing transcription of RIG-I, MDA5, and several type I and III IFN-stimulated genes including OAS2, ISG15, and MX1 [64]. Activation of the type I IFN signaling pathway results in production and secretion of IFN-β. Secreted IFN-β binding to IFN-β receptor activates JAK1 and Tyk2 kinases that in turn phosphorylate STAT1 and STAT2 (Figure 2, middle). Upon ZIKV infection, association of the phosphorylated STAT1/STAT2 heterodimer with IRF9 promotes ISRE3-mediated transcription of antiviral interferon stimulated genes (ISGS) [65]. One of the ISGS proteins, viperin (virus-inhibitory protein, endoplasmic reticulum-associated, IFN-inducible), shows strong antiviral activity against ZIKV. Specifically, it restricts ZIKV viral replication by targeting the NS3 protein for proteasomal degradation [108]. Therefore, the production of TLR3- and RIG-1/MDA5-mediated type I IFN production and subsequent activation of the JAK/STAT innate immune pathway confer increased resistance to ZIKV infection [109].

ZIKV is a membrane-associated virus that utilizes host ER for its replication and reproduction along the cellular secretory pathway. Through those cellular membrane interactions, ZIKV can trigger autophagy in a cell-dependent manner (Figure 2, right). This cellular process is normally involved in removal of aggregated or erroneously folded proteins through lysosomal degradation. Activation of cellular autophagy is a hallmark of flavivirus infection, which was thought to be part of the host innate immune response to eliminate invading intracellular pathogens [36,110–112]. Because autophagy activation could halt cellular growth and trigger apoptosis, ZIKV-induced autophagy was implicated in the ZIKV-mediated microcephaly [59,111,112]. Activation of autophagy elicits antiviral activities by removing viral proteins through reticulophagy, a selective form of autophagy that leads to ER degradation, or inclusion of viral proteins in autophagosomes destined for lysosomal degradation [113]. The ER-localized reticulophagy receptor FAM134B serves as a host cell restriction factor to ZIKV and other flaviviruses [114]. However, ZIKV-induced autophagy could be a double edged sword, which shows activities of both pro- and anti-ZIKV infection [113]. Activation of cellular autophagy counteracts ZIKV infection by actively removing viral proteins. As part of the host cell's antiviral responses, type I IFN signaling also limits ZIKV replication by promoting autophagic destruction of the viral NS2B/NS3pro protease in a STAT1-dependent manner [115]. Conversely, ZIKV takes advantage of autophagosome formation, whose presence was associated with enhanced viral replication [64]. ZIKV activates autophagy through the cellular mTOR stress pathway that connects oxidative stress and reactive oxygen species (ROS) production. This virus–host interaction appears to be highly conserved, as in human fetal neural stem cells, ZIKV triggers autophagy through inhibition of the mammalian mTOR pathway via AKT [111]. Similarly, in fission yeast cells, the ZIKV effect on TOR is mediated through a parallel pathway via Tor1 and Tip41, the human equivalents of TSC1 and TIP41 proteins [116,117]. Altogether, ZIKV infection elicits RIG-1/MDA5- and TLR3-mediated innate immune responses leading to releases of type I and type III IFNs to protect cells from viral invasion. ZIKV concurrently triggers cellular activation of the stress TOR signaling pathway that induces autophagy. The balance between pro- and anti-ZIKV activities of autophagy, at least in some cells, determines whether infected cells are protected through viral elimination, or destined to apoptosis as the result of viral propagation in host cells.

Table 3. Cellular antiviral responses and viral counteractions during Zika infection.

Cellular Antiviral Responses to Zika Infection			
Cellular Response	Cellular Protein Involved	Molecular Actions and Consequences	References
Pro-inflammatory CD8+ T-cell immune response	Cytokines: IL-1β, IL-6, MIP1α; chemokines: IP-10, RANTES	T-cell mediated polyfunctional immune responses with releases of antiviral cytokines and chemokines	[65,103,118,119]
CD14+ monocytes and macrophages immune response	CXCL9, CXCL10, CXCL11, CCL5, IL-15	CD14+ monocytes prime NK cell activities during ZIKV infection	[92]
Humoral immune response	IgM, IgG	Production of neutralizing and protective antibodies to ZIKV	[120–122]
Cellular innate immune response: TLR3-mediated response	TLR3, IRF3, TBK1, type I IFNs, and IFNβ	An early response that triggers IRF3 and recognizes ZIKV dsRNA in cytoplasm leading to activation of type I IFNs and IFNβ production	[57,64,65]
Cellular innate immune response: RIG-1/MDA5-mediated response	RIG-1, MDA5, IRF-3, NFkB, type I IFNs, and IFNβ	Late responses that recognize ZIKV dsRNA and contribute to activation of type I IFNs and IFNβ production	[64,65]
Type I and type III interferon activation	OAS2, ISG15, MX1	Production of IFNβ as part of the cellular antiviral responses	[64]
Viral Counteraction			
Viral response	Viral protein involved	Molecular actions and consequences	References
Counteraction to activation of type 1 IFNs and IFNβ production	NS1, NS2A, NS2B, NS4A, NS4B and NS5	Targeting RIG-1 pathway	[123–125]
Inhibition of IFNβ production	NS1, NS4A, NS4B, NS5	NS4A and NS5 inhibit IRF3 and NFkB; NS1 inhibits IRF3 IFNβ production through binding to TBK1	[49]
Inhibition of the JAK/STAT pathway	NS5, PR	NS5 binds to STAT2 for its proteasomal degradation; PR inhibits JAK1 kinase	[115,126,127]
Selective activation of type II IFN signaling	NS5	NS5 promotes the formation of STAT1/STAT1 homodimers and activates type II IFN for viral replication	[123]
Induction of cellular autophagy	prM, M, NS1, NS2A, NS4A	In a yeast study, these ZIKV proteins induced cellular autophagy as indicated by formation of cytoplasmic puncta	[9]
Induction of cellular autophagy	NS4A, NS4B	Inhibit Akt-mediated mTOR pathway through Tor1/TSC1 and Tip41	[9,111]

4. Viral Counteraction to Host Antiviral Responses and ZIKV-Induced Cytopathic Effects

4.1. Viral Counteraction to Host Antiviral Responses

To establish successful viral infection, ZIKV has adopted various strategies to counteract host antiviral responses (Table 3). The final infection outcome depends on the balance between the host antiviral responses and the viral counteracting actions. A number of ZIKV-mediated counteracting actions are known. For example, once ZIKV infection is successfully established, it becomes resistant to IFN treatment, suggesting ZIKV might have deployed effective counteractive measures against host innate immune responses [101,125]. Resultant to this finding, no secreted type I and type III IFNs were detectable from ZIKV-infected cells [65]. Indeed, ZIKV impairs the induction of type I IFN by binding to IRF3, a member of the IRF family [49,125,128]. These ZIKV-mediated counteracting effects are achieved through multiple non-structural ZIKV proteins (NS1, NS2A, NS2B, NS4A, NS4B, and NS5). All of these ZIKV proteins suppress, to various degrees, IFN-β production by targeting distinct components of the RIG-I pathway [49]. For instance, the NS1, NS4A, and NS5 proteins specifically inhibit IRF3 and NFkB [125], and the NS1 and NS4B proteins block IRF3 activation [49,115]. Interestingly, an A188V mutated NS1, which was found during the ZIKV epidemic starting in 2012, showed enhanced ability to block IFN-β induction, and facilitated mosquito-mediated virus transmission [49]. This acquired mutation enables NS1 binding to TBK1 and reduces TBK1 phosphorylation. Reversion of this mutation to the pre-epidemic genotype weakens the ability of ZIKV to counteract IFN-β production. Consistent with the idea that ZIKV blocks the IFN-β production through IRF3, IRF3 knockout cells lost this ZIKV effect [48,49].

ZIKV has also developed mechanisms to block the JAK/STAT pathway [65] (Figure 2, middle). For example, it blocks JAK1/Tyk2-mediated STAT1 and STAT2 phosphorylation resulting in ISGF3 transcription and ISGS translation shutdown [65]. On one hand, ZIKV utilizes its PR to inhibit JAK1 kinase [115]. On the other, ZIKV uses NS5 protein through direct binding to promote STAT2 proteasome-mediated degradation [125,126,128].

4.2. ZIKV-Induced Cytopathic Effects

Persistent viral replication and propagation inevitably confer adverse CPEs to host cells (Table 4). Like many other viruses, ZIKV encodes a limited number of proteins and, conceivably, has to rely on host cell resources to ensure its successful viral reproduction. Thus, a variety of devious approaches are utilized in order to commandeer host cell resources to create an environment for its own benefit. One common viral strategy is to deter host cell growth, or to subvert the host cell cycle into a specific phase whereby the virus gains optimal benefit by maximizing availability of cellular resources for its transcription, translation and assembly. This indeed is true for ZIKV in that ZIKV infection of hNPCs restricts cell growth and induces cell cycle dysfunction and apoptosis [42,61,63]. Further, these ZIKV-mediated CPEs appear to be associated with clinical neurological manifestations such as microcephaly [42,129]. For instance, ZIKV-induced CPEs correlate with the decrease of neuronal cell-layer volume of the brain organoids reminiscent of processes resulting in microcephaly, supporting that ZIKV-induced microcephaly is likely the result of ZIKV-mediated increase of CPEs [40,43,57,59].

Table 4. ZIKV proteins and associated cytopathic effects.

Protein	Primary Function	Main Phenotypes	References
		Structural Proteins	
anaC	Anchored capsid protein	In the fission yeast cells, it restricts cellular growth and affects cell cycling. It also induces cellular oxidative stress leading to cell death.	[9]
C	Capsid protein	In the fission yeast cells, it restricts cellular growth. It also induces cellular oxidative stress leading to cell death; in hNPCs, it induces ribosomal stress and apoptosis.	[9,130]
prM	Precursor membrane protein	In the fission yeast cells, it restricts cellular growth and affects cell cycling. It also induces cellular oxidative stress and autophagy leading to cell death; a single prM mutation contributes to fetal microcephaly	[9,131]
M	Membrane protein	In the fission yeast cells, it restricts cellular growth and affects cell cycling. It also induces cellular oxidative stress and autophagy, leading to cell death.	[9]
Pr	Cleaved product from prM	Unknown	
E	Envelope protein	A putative cytopathic factor based on a yeast study. E protein facilitates viral entry. A single residue in the αB helix of the E protein is critical for Zika virus thermostability, and interaction with the host cell membrane.	[9,132]
		Non-structural Proteins	
NS1	Viral replication, pathogenesis and immune evasion	In the fission yeast cells, it induces cellular oxidative stress and autophagy leading to cell death; An essential role in viral replication and immune evasion. It presents on the cell surface and presents as a dimer within cells, and as a hexamer once being secreted. NS1-mediated CPEs in mammalian cells have not yet been established.	[47–49,133]
NS2A	Unknown	In the fission yeast cells, it induces cellular oxidative stress and autophagy leading to cell death; ZIKV-encoded NS2A disrupts mammalian cortical neurogenesis by degrading adherens junction (AJ) proteins, leading to reduced proliferation and premature differentiation of radial glial cells and aberrant positioning of newborn neurons.	[131]
NS2B	Protease cofactor	In fission yeast cells, it restricts cellular growth. Forms a protease complex with NS3; a putative cytopathic factor based on a yeast study	[9,134]
NS3	Protease and helicase	NS3-mediated CPEs in mammalian cells have not yet been established.	[131]
NS4A	Viral RNA synthesis and viral morphogenesis	In the fission yeast cells, it restricts cellular growth and affects cell cycling. It also induces cellular oxidative stress and autophagy leading to cell death. It induces autophagy by inhibiting Atk-mediated TOR pathway through Tor1/TSC1 and Tip41 in both yeast and mammalian cells.	[9,111]
2K	A signal peptide	Viral RNA synthesis and viral morphogenesis. 2K-mediated CPEs have not yet been established.	[9,11,12]
NS4B	Viral RNA synthesis and viral morphogenesis	Synergistic to NS4A on inhibiting Akt-mediated TOR pathway	[111]
NS5	Methyltrasferase; RNA-dependent polymerase	NS5-mediated CPEs in mammalian cells have not yet been established.	[128]

Although ZIKV confers various CPEs as described above, the identity of which ZIKV protein(s) is responsible, and the mechanism by which ZIKV mediates those effects, remains elusive. To assist in identifying which ZIKV viral protein(s) is responsible for those observed CPEs, we performed a genome-wide analysis of ZIKV proteins by using fission yeast (*Schizosaccharomyces pombe*) as a surrogate system [9,135]. Fission yeast is particularly useful here because the aforementioned ZIKV-mediated CPEs affect highly conserved cellular activities among all eukaryotes [136–139]. Each of the fourteen ZIKV viral cDNA encoding a specific protein or a small peptide was cloned into previously described fission yeast gene expression systems [140,141]. All of the ZIKV viral activities were measured simultaneously under the same inducible conditions, thus allowing concurrent functional characterization of each ZIKV protein. Consistent with the idea that ZIKV is a cell membrane-associated virus, and that the ER is the major "viral factory" [36,110,142], nine of the fourteen ZIKV proteins and peptides were found to associate with the ER network, including the nuclear membrane, ER, and Golgi [36,142,143]. Seven ZIKV proteins, including five mature and immature structural proteins (anaC/C, prM/M, and E), and two non-structural proteins (NS2B and NS4A), conferred a number of the same CPEs as reported in the ZIKV-infected mammalian cells infected by ZIKV [9,36,40,42,43]. Specifically, the ZIKV protein-producing yeast cells displayed restricted cellular growth, cellular autophagy, cell hypertrophy, cell cycle dysfunction, and cell death [9]. As described below, some of the same ZIKV protein-mediated CPEs have also been reported in mammalian cells.

4.3. The Structural Proteins

Cytopathic effects induced by ZIKV structural proteins are summarized in Table 4. Briefly, the yeast study showed that both the anaC and C proteins localize to the nuclei, triggering cellular oxidative stress leading to cell death [9]. Consistently, C protein is known to localize in the nucleus for other flaviviruses [144,145]. ZIKV C protein is present in human NPC nucleoli, sub-nuclear structures where ribosome biogenesis takes place, and also plays a role in cellular response to stress [130]. The presence of C protein in nucleoli was associated with activation of ribosomal stress and apoptosis [130]. Deleting part of the C protein prevented nucleolar localization, ribosomal stress, and apoptosis [130].

The E protein is a major viral surface protein that is responsible for the viral entry. Thus, it is a crucial viral determinant for initiating the ZIKV–host interaction. Comparison of E protein sequence and structure with that of other flaviviruses suggest ZIKV E protein is unique among flaviviruses, although some portions of it resemble its counterparts in WNV, JEV, and DENV [146,147]. During flaviviral assembly, E interacts with prM to form the prM-E heterodimers that protrude from the viral surface in the non-infectious and immature viral particles [14]. It is also involved in fusing the viral membrane with the host endosome membrane. As with other flaviviruses, the ZIKV E protein is glycosylated at amino acid N154. The E glycosylation appears to be critical for ZIKV infection of mammalian and mosquito cells, because a glycosylation mutant N154Q diminished oral infectivity by *Ae. aegypti* vector and showed reduced viremia and diminished mortality in mouse models [148]. Interestingly, knockout of E glycosylation does not significantly affect neurovirulence in mouse models [148]. While ZIKV encoding non-glycosylated E protein displayed attenuated and defective neuroinvasion when delivered subcutaneously, it replicated well following intracranial inoculation, suggesting possible involvement of E in passing through the blood-brain barrier [149]. Furthermore, ZIKV viral particles lacking the E protein glycan were still able to infect Raji cells expressing the lectin DC-SIGN receptor, indicating the prM glycan of partially mature particles can facilitate the viral entry [150]. The E protein, specifically its extended CD-loop, may confer viral stability, cell cycle-dependent viral replication, and in vivo pathogenesis, as shortening the CD-loop destabilizes the virus, and Δ346 mutation in this loop disrupts thermal stability of the virus [151].

In DENV, the prM protein forms a heterodimer with the E protein and affects viral particle formation and secretion [14]. The resultant non-infectious and immature viral particles are transported through the TGN, where prM is cleaved by a host protease Furin, resulting in mature infectious particles [15,16]. The transition from prM to M via the cleavage of host protease Furin is required for viral infectivity [11,13]. Therefore, both prM and M play important roles in viral pathogenesis. Consistent with the prM/M activities in host cells, in the yeast study, we showed that both prM and M proteins localize in ER [9]. Similarly, prM also localizes in ER in Vero cells [47]. In addition, the prM protein restricts cellular growth, and affects cell cycling leading to cell death in the yeast [9]. At the time of this writing, no description has yet been reported on the effect of individual prM or M protein on those basic cellular functions in mammalian cells. However, mutational analysis shows that the activity of prM protein contributes to fetal microcephaly [152]. Specifically, evolutionary analysis shows that a S139N substitution in the prM protein has persisted in the circulating ZIKV strains since the 2013 outbreak in French Polynesia to the subsequent spread to the Americas. A single serine(S)-to-asparagine(N) substitution (S139N) in the viral polyprotein of a presumably less neurovirulent Cambodian ZIKV$_{FSS13025}$ strain [153], substantially increased ZIKV infectivity in both human and mouse NPCs, and led to more severe microcephaly in the mouse fetus, as well as higher mortality rates in neonatal mice [152]. Results of this study underscore the important contribution of prM to fetal microcephaly. However, the manner in which prM contributes to microcephaly, and the impact of S139N mutation on the prM function, are presently unknown. It is intriguing to note that residue 139 is actually located in the Pr region of the prM protein. Since neither prM nor Pr are present in the mature and infectious viral particles [15,16], it would be interesting to learn the molecular mechanism underlying the effect of the S139N mutation causing increased viral infectivity.

4.4. The Non-Structural Proteins

ZIKV PR, which consists of forty residues of the NS2B cofactor and the NS3pro domain of the NS3 [154], has been actively investigated for its PR activities (Table 4) [134,155,156]. In addition to ZIKV PR-mediated proteolysis for its own replication, ZIKV PR also cleaves the ER-localized reticulophagy receptor FAM134B to counteract host cell restriction through a selective form of autophagy known as reticulophagy [114]. Indeed, depletion of FAM134B by RNAi significantly enhanced ZIKV replication [114]. The production of the same PRs by other flaviviruses causes cell death by apoptosis [157,158]. However, whether ZIKV PR causes apoptosis is presently unknown. The yeast study showed that expression of the *NS2B* gene, which encodes the co-factor of the ZIKV PR, does induces cellular autophagy and cell death [9]. It would be of interest to test if fully active ZIKV PR can induce cell death in yeast and mammalian cells.

The NS4A protein, in conjunction with NS4B, activates cellular autophagy through inhibition of the mammalian TOR pathway via AKT [111]. Similarly, NS4A also inhibits the Tor1 pathway in the fission yeast. Furthermore, the yeast study showed that the inhibitory NS4A effect on TOR was mediated through Tor1 and Tip41, which are the human equivalents of TSC1 and TIP41 proteins [116,117].

Expression of NS2A reduces cell proliferation and causes premature differentiation of radial glial cells in the developing mouse brain [131]. In addition, NS2A interacts with adherens junction (AJ) proteins that are present at the epithelial–endothelial cell junctions, resulting in degradation and malformation of the AJ complex [131]. These NS2A-induced growth defect in the embryonic mouse cortex are unique to ZIKV, as the same effects were not seen in DENV. These NS2A effects could pay a role in the pathogenic mechanism underlying ZIKV infection in the developing mammalian brain [131].

NS1 is a highly conserved protein among flaviviruses. It is an essential viral glycoprotein that plays a major role in virus–host interaction as it participates in viral replication, pathogenesis, and immune evasion [159]. As with other flaviviruses, NS1 is expressed at the cell surface and exists in diverse forms. Intracellular NS1 exists as a dimer that is required for viral replication, whereas the secreted NS1 hexamer interacts with host factors and plays a role in immune evasion [159,160]. Freire et al. [161] first revealed adaptation of the NS1 codon to human housekeeping genes in ZIKV Asian lineage, which could facilitate viral replication in humans. Indeed, an alanine(A)-to-valine(V) amino acid substitution at residue 188 (A188V) of the NS1 protein was acquired by the ancient ZIKV strain since the turning of the century in Southeastern Asia. This A188V-carrying ZIKV strain circulated in that region before dissemination to Southern Pacific islands and the Americas [162]. Residue 188 is located within the interface of two NS1 monomers. However, this A188V substitution does not affect NS1 dimerization, instead increasing its secretability [48]. Strikingly, the A188V-carrying ZIKV epidemic strains were much more infectious in mosquitoes (*Ae. aegypti*) than the earlier Cambodia ZIKV$_{FSS13025}$ strain, resulting in increased NS1 antigenemia. Enhancement of NS1 antigenemia in infected hosts promotes ZIKV infectivity and prevalence in mosquitoes, which could have facilitated transmission during the recent ZIKV epidemics [48]. Consistent with this idea, acquisition of the A188V substitution also correlates with enhanced ZIKV evasion of host interferon induction [49].

Interestingly, another pathogenic mutation T233A was isolated from the brain tissue of a ZIKV infected fetus with neonatal microcephaly [47]. The ZIKV NS1 T233A mutation, also located at the dimer interface, was not found in any other flaviviruses. This finding could potentially be significant because wildtype T233 organizes a central hydrogen bonding network at the NS1 dimer interface, while the T233A mutation disrupts this network and destabilizes the NS1 dimeric assembly in vitro [47]. However, the pathogenic potential of this mechanism has not yet been tested. Together, these studies on the NS1 protein suggest that ZIKV has acquired specific mutation(s) that increases its ability to evade host immune responses, and favors persistent viral replication, leading to enhanced viral pathogenicity.

5. Concluding Remarks

Since the global ZIKV pandemic in 2015, an unprecedented world-wide effort is being made to understand the ZIKV etiology and its associated human diseases. We have learned a great deal about its epidemiology, genetic diversity, viral pathogenicity, and clinical manifestations that are linked to ZIKV-associated human neurological diseases. In this article, we describe molecular interactions of ZIKV with its host cells. In particular, we briefly outline different cell types and receptors utilized by ZIKV for viral entry and infection. We then describe host cellular and immune responses to fight against ZIKV invasion. In response, ZIKV has adopted various counteracting strategies to defeat those host antiviral responses. The overall balance between host antiviral defenses and viral countermeasures determine the outcome of host cells, and the success of viral propagation and survival. Persistent viral replication and propagation inevitably damage human host cells, tissues, and organs, ultimately resulting in fetal microcephaly and a number of other neurologic disorders. Yet, we have only just begun to understand the molecular mechanisms underlying ZIKV interactions with host cells, and how those interactions relate to the observed neurological disorders caused by those newly adopted pathogenic ZIKVs. Much work is still needed to answer some of those same questions as we asked at the beginning, e.g., (1) what specific virological changes have taken place that transformed the ZIKV from a benign virus to a highly pathogenic virus, (2) how could viral mutations, such as those described in this review, alter the viral pathogenicity enabling recently observed neurological disorders, and (3) what specific changes in ZIKV–host interactions ultimately tilt the balance in favor of enhanced CPEs and viral pathogenicity? Ongoing and future research will no doubt continue to strive to provide answers to these questions. We hope this review will serve as a helpful reference to those who study ZIKV–host interactions, and that the information described herein will encourage additional studies focusing on the molecular mechanisms of this virus.

Acknowledgments: We want to thank all of those who have contributed our understanding of the emerging Zika virus especially those studies molecular mechanism underlying Zika virus–host interactions. We also want to apologize in advance if we have missed any important references that we should have included in this review. This work was supported in part by funding from the National Institute of Health (NIH R21 AI129369) and University of Maryland Medical Center (to R.Y.Z). This work was also supported by the ZIKAlert project (European Union-Région Réunion programme under grant agreement n° SYNERGY: RÉ0001902). S.B. has PhD degree scholarship from La Réunion Island University (Ecole Doctorale STS), funded by the French ministry MEESR.

Conflicts of Interest: The authors declare that there is no conflict of interest of any kind. The opinions expressed by the authors contributing to this journal do not necessarily reflect the opinions of the institutions with which the authors are affiliated.

Abbreviations

ADE	Antibody-dependent enhancement
CPE	Cytotoxic effect
CNS	Central nerve system
DC	Dendritic cell
DENV	Dengue virus
dsRNA	Double stranded RNA
ER	Endoplasmic reticulum
HAVcr-1	Hepatitis A virus cellular receptor 1
hEC	Human epithelial cell
hNPC	Human neural progenitor cell
hBMEC	Human brain microvascular endothelial cell
GBS	Guillain–Barré syndrome
IFN	Interferon
iPSC	Induced pluripotent stem cell
IRF3	Interferon regulatory factor 3
ISGS	Interferon stimulated genes
JEV	Japanese Encephalitis Virus
NPCs	Neural progenitor stem cells
PAMP	Pathogen-associated molecular pattern
PR	Protease
PRRs	Pattern recognition receptors
RdRP	RNA-dependent RNA polymerase
RLRs	RIG-I like receptors
sfRNA	Subgenomic flavivirus RNA
TGN	Trans-Golgi network
TLR3	Toll-like receptor 3
TOR	Target of rapamycin
WHO	World health organization
WNV	West Nile Virus
ZIKV	Zika virus

References

1. Zhao, Z.; Yang, M.; Azar, S.R.; Soong, L.; Weaver, S.C.; Sun, J.; Chen, Y.; Rossi, S.L.; Cai, J. Viral retinopathy in experimental models of zika infection. *Investig. Ophthalmol. Vis. Sci.* **2017**, *58*, 4355–4365. [CrossRef] [PubMed]
2. Sahiner, F.; Sig, A.K.; Savasci, U.; Tekin, K.; Akay, F. Zika virus-associated ocular and neurologic disorders: The emergence of new evidence. *Pediatr. Infect. Dis. J.* **2017**, *36*, e341–e346. [CrossRef] [PubMed]
3. Smith, D.W.; Mackenzie, J. Zika virus and Guillain-Barre syndrome: Another viral cause to add to the list. *Lancet* **2016**, *387*, 1486–1488. [CrossRef]
4. Wen, Z.; Song, H.; Ming, G.L. How does Zika virus cause microcephaly? *Genes Dev.* **2017**, *31*, 849–861. [CrossRef] [PubMed]
5. Carod-Artal, F.J. Neurological complications of Zika virus infection. *Expert Rev. Anti-Infect. Ther.* **2018**. [CrossRef] [PubMed]
6. Chambers, T.J.; Hahn, C.S.; Galler, R.; Rice, C.M. Flavivirus genome organization, expression, and replication. *Annu. Rev. Microbiol.* **1990**, *44*, 649–688. [CrossRef] [PubMed]
7. De Paula Freitas, B.; de Oliveira Dias, J.R.; Prazeres, J.; Sacramento, G.A.; Ko, A.I.; Maia, M.; Belfort, R., Jr. Ocular findings in infants with microcephaly associated with presumed Zika virus congenital infection in salvador, Brazil. *JAMA Ophthalmol.* **2016**, *134*, 529–535. [CrossRef] [PubMed]

8. Faye, O.; Freire, C.C.; Iamarino, A.; Faye, O.; de Oliveira, J.V.; Diallo, M.; Zanotto, P.M.; Sall, A.A. Molecular evolution of Zika virus during its emergence in the 20th century. *PLoS Negl. Trop. Dis.* **2014**, *8*, e2636. [CrossRef] [PubMed]

9. Li, G.; Poulsen, M.; Fenyvuesvolgyi, C.; Yashiroda, Y.; Yoshida, M.; Simard, J.M.; Gallo, R.C.; Zhao, R.Y. Characterization of cytopathic factors through genome-wide analysis of the zika viral proteins in fission yeast. *Proc. Natl. Acad. Sci. USA* **2017**, *114*, E376–E385. [CrossRef] [PubMed]

10. Harris, E.; Holden, K.L.; Edgil, D.; Polacek, C.; Clyde, K. Molecular biology of flaviviruses. *Novartis Found. Symp.* **2006**, *277*, 23–39, discussion 40, 71–23, 251–253. [PubMed]

11. Lobigs, M.; Lee, E.; Ng, M.L.; Pavy, M.; Lobigs, P. A flavivirus signal peptide balances the catalytic activity of two proteases and thereby facilitates virus morphogenesis. *Virology* **2010**, *401*, 80–89. [CrossRef] [PubMed]

12. Miller, S.; Kastner, S.; Krijnse-Locker, J.; Buhler, S.; Bartenschlager, R. The non-structural protein 4A of dengue virus is an integral membrane protein inducing membrane alterations in a 2K-regulated manner. *J. Biol. Chem.* **2007**, *282*, 8873–8882. [CrossRef] [PubMed]

13. Amberg, S.M.; Nestorowicz, A.; McCourt, D.W.; Rice, C.M. NS2B-3 proteinase-mediated processing in the yellow fever virus structural region: In vitro and in vivo studies. *J. Virol.* **1994**, *68*, 3794–3802. [PubMed]

14. Lin, J.C.; Lin, S.C.; Chen, W.Y.; Yen, Y.T.; Lai, C.W.; Tao, M.H.; Lin, Y.L.; Miaw, S.C.; Wu-Hsieh, B.A. Dengue viral protease interaction with NF-κB inhibitor α/β results in endothelial cell apoptosis and hemorrhage development. *J. Immunol.* **2014**, *193*, 1258–1267. [CrossRef] [PubMed]

15. Stadler, K.; Allison, S.L.; Schalich, J.; Heinz, F.X. Proteolytic activation of tick-borne encephalitis virus by furin. *J. Virol.* **1997**, *71*, 8475–8481. [PubMed]

16. Elshuber, S.; Allison, S.L.; Heinz, F.X.; Mandl, C.W. Cleavage of protein prM is necessary for infection of BHK-21 cells by tick-borne encephalitis virus. *J. Gen. Virol.* **2003**, *84*, 183–191. [CrossRef] [PubMed]

17. Li, L.; Li, H.S.; Pauza, C.D.; Bukrinsky, M.; Zhao, R.Y. Roles of HIV-1 auxiliary proteins in viral pathogenesis and host-pathogen interactions. *Cell Res.* **2005**, *15*, 923–934. [CrossRef] [PubMed]

18. Melino, S.; Fucito, S.; Campagna, A.; Wrubl, F.; Gamarnik, A.; Cicero, D.O.; Paci, M. The active essential CFNS3d protein complex. *FEBS J.* **2006**, *273*, 3650–3662. [CrossRef] [PubMed]

19. Cao-Lormeau, V.M.; Blake, A.; Mons, S.; Lastere, S.; Roche, C.; Vanhomwegen, J.; Dub, T.; Baudouin, L.; Teissier, A.; Larre, P.; et al. Guillain-Barre syndrome outbreak associated with Zika virus infection in French polynesia: A case-control study. *Lancet* **2016**, *387*, 1531–1539. [CrossRef]

20. Goertz, G.P.; Abbo, S.R.; Fros, J.J.; Pijlman, G.P. Functional RNA during Zika virus infection. *Virus Res.* **2017**. [CrossRef] [PubMed]

21. Zhu, Z.; Chan, J.F.; Tee, K.M.; Choi, G.K.; Lau, S.K.; Woo, P.C.; Tse, H.; Yuen, K.Y. Comparative genomic analysis of pre-epidemic and epidemic zika virus strains for virological factors potentially associated with the rapidly expanding epidemic. *Emerg. Microbes Infect.* **2016**, *5*, e22. [CrossRef] [PubMed]

22. Hayes, E.B. Zika virus outside Africa. *Emerg. Infect. Dis.* **2009**, *15*, 1347–1350. [CrossRef] [PubMed]

23. Huang, Y.J.; Higgs, S.; Horne, K.M.; Vanlandingham, D.L. Flavivirus-mosquito interactions. *Viruses* **2014**, *6*, 4703–4730. [CrossRef] [PubMed]

24. Foy, B.D.; Kobylinski, K.C.; Chilson Foy, J.L.; Blitvich, B.J.; Travassos da Rosa, A.; Haddow, A.D.; Lanciotti, R.S.; Tesh, R.B. Probable non-vector-borne transmission of zika virus, Colorado, USA. *Emerg. Infect. Dis.* **2011**, *17*, 880–882. [CrossRef] [PubMed]

25. Mead, P.S.; Hills, S.L.; Brooks, J.T. Zika virus as a sexually transmitted pathogen. *Curr. Opin. Infect. Dis.* **2018**, *31*, 39–44. [CrossRef] [PubMed]

26. Musso, D.; Nhan, T.; Robin, E.; Roche, C.; Bierlaire, D.; Zisou, K.; Shan Yan, A.; Cao-Lormeau, V.M.; Broult, J. Potential for Zika virus transmission through blood transfusion demonstrated during an outbreak in French Polynesia, November 2013 to February 2014. *Eurosurveillance* **2014**, *19*. [CrossRef]

27. Govero, J.; Esakky, P.; Scheaffer, S.M.; Fernandez, E.; Drury, A.; Platt, D.J.; Gorman, M.J.; Richner, J.M.; Caine, E.A.; Salazar, V.; et al. Zika virus infection damages the testes in mice. *Nature* **2016**, *540*, 438–442. [CrossRef] [PubMed]

28. Ma, W.; Li, S.; Ma, S.; Jia, L.; Zhang, F.; Zhang, Y.; Zhang, J.; Wong, G.; Zhang, S.; Lu, X.; et al. Zika virus causes testis damage and leads to male infertility in mice. *Cell* **2017**, *168*, 542. [CrossRef] [PubMed]

29. Joguet, G.; Mansuy, J.M.; Matusali, G.; Hamdi, S.; Walschaerts, M.; Pavili, L.; Guyomard, S.; Prisant, N.; Lamarre, P.; Dejucq-Rainsford, N.; et al. Effect of acute Zika virus infection on sperm and virus clearance in body fluids: A prospective observational study. *Lancet Infect. Dis.* **2017**, *17*, 1200–1208. [CrossRef]

30. Cao, B.; Diamond, M.S.; Mysorekar, I.U. Maternal-fetal transmission of zika virus: Routes and signals for infection. *J. Interferon Cytokine Res.* **2017**, *37*, 287–294. [CrossRef] [PubMed]

31. Zanluca, C.; de Noronha, L.; Duarte Dos Santos, C.N. Maternal-fetal transmission of the zika virus: An intriguing interplay. *Tissue Barriers* **2018**, *6*, e1402143. [CrossRef] [PubMed]

32. Mlakar, J.; Korva, M.; Tul, N.; Popovic, M.; Poljsak-Prijatelj, M.; Mraz, J.; Kolenc, M.; Resman Rus, K.; Vesnaver Vipotnik, T.; Fabjan Vodusek, V.; et al. Zika virus associated with microcephaly. *N. Engl. J. Med.* **2016**, *374*, 951–958. [CrossRef] [PubMed]

33. Miner, J.J.; Cao, B.; Govero, J.; Smith, A.M.; Fernandez, E.; Cabrera, O.H.; Garber, C.; Noll, M.; Klein, R.S.; Noguchi, K.K.; et al. Zika virus infection during pregnancy in mice causes placental damage and fetal demise. *Cell* **2016**, *165*, 1081–1091. [CrossRef] [PubMed]

34. Dick, G.W.; Kitchen, S.F.; Haddow, A.J. Zika virus. I. Isolations and serological specificity. *Trans. R. Soc. Trop. Med. Hyg.* **1952**, *46*, 509–520. [CrossRef]

35. Dick, G.W. Zika virus. II. Pathogenicity and physical properties. *Trans. R. Soc. Trop. Med. Hyg.* **1952**, *46*, 521–534. [CrossRef]

36. Bell, T.M.; Field, E.J.; Narang, H.K. Zika virus infection of the central nervous system of mice. *Arch. Gesamte Virusforsch.* **1971**, *35*, 183–193. [CrossRef] [PubMed]

37. Duffy, M.R.; Chen, T.H.; Hancock, W.T.; Powers, A.M.; Kool, J.L.; Lanciotti, R.S.; Pretrick, M.; Marfel, M.; Holzbauer, S.; Dubray, C.; et al. Zika virus outbreak on Yap Island, federated states of Micronesia. *N. Engl. J. Med.* **2009**, *360*, 2536–2543. [CrossRef] [PubMed]

38. Ioos, S.; Mallet, H.P.; Leparc Goffart, I.; Gauthier, V.; Cardoso, T.; Herida, M. Current Zika virus epidemiology and recent epidemics. *Med. Mal. Infect.* **2014**, *44*, 302–307. [CrossRef] [PubMed]

39. Driggers, R.W.; Ho, C.Y.; Korhonen, E.M.; Kuivanen, S.; Jaaskelainen, A.J.; Smura, T.; Rosenberg, A.; Hill, D.A.; DeBiasi, R.L.; Vezina, G.; et al. Zika virus infection with prolonged maternal viremia and fetal brain abnormalities. *N. Engl. J. Med.* **2016**, *374*, 2142–2151. [CrossRef] [PubMed]

40. Qian, X.; Nguyen, H.N.; Song, M.M.; Hadiono, C.; Ogden, S.C.; Hammack, C.; Yao, B.; Hamersky, G.R.; Jacob, F.; Zhong, C.; et al. Brain-region-specific organoids using mini-bioreactors for modeling ZIKV exposure. *Cell* **2016**, *165*, 1238–1254. [CrossRef] [PubMed]

41. Victora, C.G.; Schuler-Faccini, L.; Matijasevich, A.; Ribeiro, E.; Pessoa, A.; Barros, F.C. Microcephaly in Brazil: How to interpret reported numbers? *Lancet* **2016**, *387*, 621–624. [CrossRef]

42. Tang, H.; Hammack, C.; Ogden, S.C.; Wen, Z.; Qian, X.; Li, Y.; Yao, B.; Shin, J.; Zhang, F.; Lee, E.M.; et al. Zika virus infects human cortical neural progenitors and attenuates their growth. *Cell Stem Cell* **2016**, *18*, 587–590. [CrossRef] [PubMed]

43. Garcez, P.P.; Loiola, E.C.; Madeiro da Costa, R.; Higa, L.M.; Trindade, P.; Delvecchio, R.; Nascimento, J.M.; Brindeiro, R.; Tanuri, A.; Rehen, S.K. Zika virus impairs growth in human neurospheres and brain organoids. *Science* **2016**, *352*, 816–818. [CrossRef] [PubMed]

44. Haddow, A.D.; Schuh, A.J.; Yasuda, C.Y.; Kasper, M.R.; Heang, V.; Huy, R.; Guzman, H.; Tesh, R.B.; Weaver, S.C. Genetic characterization of Zika virus strains: Geographic expansion of the Asian lineage. *PLoS Negl. Trop. Dis.* **2012**, *6*, e1477. [CrossRef] [PubMed]

45. Dowd, K.A.; DeMaso, C.R.; Pelc, R.S.; Speer, S.D.; Smith, A.R.Y.; Goo, L.; Platt, D.J.; Mascola, J.R.; Graham, B.S.; Mulligan, M.J.; et al. Broadly neutralizing activity of Zika virus-immune sera identifies a single viral serotype. *Cell Rep.* **2016**, *16*, 1485–1491. [CrossRef] [PubMed]

46. Anfasa, F.; Siegers, J.Y.; van der Kroeg, M.; Mumtaz, N.; Stalin Raj, V.; de Vrij, F.M.S.; Widagdo, W.; Gabriel, G.; Salinas, S.; Simonin, Y.; et al. Phenotypic differences between Asian and African lineage Zika viruses in human neural progenitor cells. *MSphere* **2017**, *2*. [CrossRef] [PubMed]

47. Wang, D.; Chen, C.; Liu, S.; Zhou, H.; Yang, K.; Zhao, Q.; Ji, X.; Chen, C.; Xie, W.; Wang, Z.; et al. A mutation identified in neonatal microcephaly destabilizes Zika virus NS1 assembly in vitro. *Sci Rep.* **2017**, *7*, 42580. [CrossRef] [PubMed]

48. Liu, Y.; Liu, J.; Du, S.; Shan, C.; Nie, K.; Zhang, R.; Li, X.F.; Zhang, R.; Wang, T.; Qin, C.F.; et al. Evolutionary enhancement of Zika virus infectivity in *Aedes aegypti* mosquitoes. *Nature* **2017**, *545*, 482–486. [CrossRef] [PubMed]

49. Xia, H.; Luo, H.; Shan, C.; Muruato, A.E.; Nunes, B.T.D.; Medeiros, D.B.A.; Zou, J.; Xie, X.; Giraldo, M.I.; Vasconcelos, P.F.C.; et al. An evolutionary NS1 mutation enhances Zika virus evasion of host interferon induction. *Nat. Commun.* **2018**, *9*, 414. [CrossRef] [PubMed]

50. Sariol, C.A.; Nogueira, M.L.; Vasilakis, N. A tale of two viruses: Does heterologous flavivirus immunity enhance Zika disease? *Trends Microbiol.* **2018**, *26*, 186–190. [CrossRef] [PubMed]

51. Kawiecki, A.B.; Christofferson, R.C. Zika virus-induced antibody response enhances dengue virus serotype 2 replication in vitro. *J. Infect. Dis.* **2016**, *214*, 1357–1360. [CrossRef] [PubMed]

52. George, J.; Valiant, W.G.; Mattapallil, M.J.; Walker, M.; Huang, Y.S.; Vanlandingham, D.L.; Misamore, J.; Greenhouse, J.; Weiss, D.E.; Verthelyi, D.; et al. Prior exposure to Zika virus significantly enhances peak Dengue-2 viremia in Rhesus macaques. *Sci. Rep.* **2017**, *7*, 10498. [CrossRef] [PubMed]

53. Dejnirattisai, W.; Supasa, P.; Wongwiwat, W.; Rouvinski, A.; Barba-Spaeth, G.; Duangchinda, T.; Sakuntabhai, A.; Cao-Lormeau, V.M.; Malasit, P.; Rey, F.A.; et al. Dengue virus sero-cross-reactivity drives antibody-dependent enhancement of infection with Zika virus. *Nat. Immunol.* **2016**, *17*, 1102–1108. [CrossRef] [PubMed]

54. Paul, L.M.; Carlin, E.R.; Jenkins, M.M.; Tan, A.L.; Barcellona, C.M.; Nicholson, C.O.; Michael, S.F.; Isern, S. Dengue virus antibodies enhance Zika virus infection. *Clin. Transl. Immunol.* **2016**, *5*, e117. [CrossRef] [PubMed]

55. Londono-Renteria, B.; Troupin, A.; Cardenas, J.C.; Hall, A.; Perez, O.G.; Cardenas, L.; Hartstone-Rose, A.; Halstead, S.B.; Colpitts, T.M. A relevant in vitro human model for the study of Zika virus antibody-dependent enhancement. *J. Gen. Virol.* **2017**, *98*, 1702–1712. [CrossRef] [PubMed]

56. Cohen, J. Dengue may bring out the worst in Zika. *Science* **2017**, *355*, 1362. [CrossRef] [PubMed]

57. Dang, J.; Tiwari, S.K.; Lichinchi, G.; Qin, Y.; Patil, V.S.; Eroshkin, A.M.; Rana, T.M. Zika virus depletes neural progenitors in human cerebral organoids through activation of the innate immune receptor TLR3. *Cell Stem Cell* **2016**, *19*, 258–265. [CrossRef] [PubMed]

58. Hasan, S.S.; Miller, A.; Sapparapu, G.; Fernandez, E.; Klose, T.; Long, F.; Fokine, A.; Porta, J.C.; Jiang, W.; Diamond, M.S.; et al. A human antibody against Zika virus crosslinks the e protein to prevent infection. *Nat. Commun.* **2017**, *8*, 14722. [CrossRef] [PubMed]

59. Cugola, F.R.; Fernandes, I.R.; Russo, F.B.; Freitas, B.C.; Dias, J.L.; Guimaraes, K.P.; Benazzato, C.; Almeida, N.; Pignatari, G.C.; Romero, S.; et al. The Brazilian Zika virus strain causes birth defects in experimental models. *Nature* **2016**, *534*, 267–271. [CrossRef] [PubMed]

60. Shao, Q.; Herrlinger, S.; Zhu, Y.N.; Yang, M.; Goodfellow, F.; Stice, S.L.; Qi, X.P.; Brindley, M.A.; Chen, J.F. The African Zika virus MR-766 is more virulent and causes more severe brain damage than current Asian lineage and dengue virus. *Development* **2017**, *144*, 4114–4124. [CrossRef] [PubMed]

61. Li, C.; Xu, D.; Ye, Q.; Hong, S.; Jiang, Y.; Liu, X.; Zhang, N.; Shi, L.; Qin, C.F.; Xu, Z. Zika virus disrupts neural progenitor development and leads to microcephaly in mice. *Cell Stem Cell* **2016**, *19*, 120–126. [CrossRef] [PubMed]

62. Zhang, F.; Wang, H.J.; Wang, Q.; Liu, Z.Y.; Yuan, L.; Huang, X.Y.; Li, G.; Ye, Q.; Yang, H.; Shi, L.; et al. American strain of Zika virus causes more severe microcephaly than an old Asian strain in neonatal mice. *EBioMedicine* **2017**, *25*, 95–105. [CrossRef] [PubMed]

63. Shao, Q.; Herrlinger, S.; Yang, S.L.; Lai, F.; Moore, J.M.; Brindley, M.A.; Chen, J.F. Zika virus infection disrupts neurovascular development and results in postnatal microcephaly with brain damage. *Development* **2016**, *143*, 4127–4136. [CrossRef] [PubMed]

64. Hamel, R.; Dejarnac, O.; Wichit, S.; Ekchariyawat, P.; Neyret, A.; Luplertlop, N.; Perera-Lecoin, M.; Surasombatpattana, P.; Talignani, L.; Thomas, F.; et al. Biology of Zika virus infection in human skin cells. *J. Virol.* **2015**, *89*, 8880–8896. [CrossRef] [PubMed]

65. Bowen, J.R.; Zimmerman, M.G.; Suthar, M.S. Taking the defensive: Immune control of Zika virus infection. *Virus Res.* **2017**. [CrossRef] [PubMed]

66. Sun, X.; Hua, S.; Chen, H.R.; Ouyang, Z.; Einkauf, K.; Tse, S.; Ard, K.; Ciaranello, A.; Yawetz, S.; Sax, P.; et al. Transcriptional changes during naturally acquired Zika virus infection render dendritic cells highly conducive to viral replication. *Cell Rep.* **2017**, *21*, 3471–3482. [CrossRef] [PubMed]

67. Bayer, A.; Lennemann, N.J.; Ouyang, Y.; Bramley, J.C.; Morosky, S.; Marques, E.T., Jr.; Cherry, S.; Sadovsky, Y.; Coyne, C.B. Type III interferons produced by human placental trophoblasts confer protection against Zika virus infection. *Cell Host Microbe* **2016**, *19*, 705–712. [CrossRef] [PubMed]

68. Quicke, K.M.; Bowen, J.R.; Johnson, E.L.; McDonald, C.E.; Ma, H.; O'Neal, J.T.; Rajakumar, A.; Wrammert, J.; Rimawi, B.H.; Pulendran, B.; et al. Zika virus infects human placental macrophages. *Cell Host Microbe* **2016**, *20*, 83–90. [CrossRef] [PubMed]

69. Mladinich, M.C.; Schwedes, J.; Mackow, E.R. Zika virus persistently infects and is basolaterally released from primary human brain microvascular endothelial cells. *MBio* **2017**, *8*. [CrossRef] [PubMed]

70. Chan, J.F.; Yip, C.C.; Tsang, J.O.; Tee, K.M.; Cai, J.P.; Chik, K.K.; Zhu, Z.; Chan, C.C.; Choi, G.K.; Sridhar, S.; et al. Differential cell line susceptibility to the emerging Zika virus: Implications for disease pathogenesis, non-vector-borne human transmission and animal reservoirs. *Emerg. Microbes Infect.* **2016**, *5*, e93. [CrossRef] [PubMed]

71. Thepparit, C.; Smith, D.R. Serotype-specific entry of dengue virus into liver cells: Identification of the 37-kilodalton/67-kilodalton high-affinity laminin receptor as a dengue virus serotype 1 receptor. *J. Virol.* **2004**, *78*, 12647–12656. [CrossRef] [PubMed]

72. Lemke, G.; Burstyn-Cohen, T. Tam receptors and the clearance of apoptotic cells. *Ann. N. Y. Acad. Sci.* **2010**, *1209*, 23–29. [CrossRef] [PubMed]

73. Garcia-Vallejo, J.J.; Ambrosini, M.; Overbeek, A.; van Riel, W.E.; Bloem, K.; Unger, W.W.; Chiodo, F.; Bolscher, J.G.; Nazmi, K.; Kalay, H.; et al. Multivalent glycopeptide dendrimers for the targeted delivery of antigens to dendritic cells. *Mol. Immunol.* **2013**, *53*, 387–397. [CrossRef] [PubMed]

74. Shimojima, M.; Stroher, U.; Ebihara, H.; Feldmann, H.; Kawaoka, Y. Identification of cell surface molecules involved in dystroglycan-independent Lassa virus cell entry. *J. Virol.* **2012**, *86*, 2067–2078. [CrossRef] [PubMed]

75. Kondratowicz, A.S.; Lennemann, N.J.; Sinn, P.L.; Davey, R.A.; Hunt, C.L.; Moller-Tank, S.; Meyerholz, D.K.; Rennert, P.; Mullins, R.F.; Brindley, M.; et al. T-cell immunoglobulin and mucin domain 1 (TIM-1) is a receptor for zaire ebolavirus and lake victoria marburgvirus. *Proc. Natl. Acad. Sci. USA* **2011**, *108*, 8426–8431. [CrossRef] [PubMed]

76. Meertens, L.; Carnec, X.; Lecoin, M.P.; Ramdasi, R.; Guivel-Benhassine, F.; Lew, E.; Lemke, G.; Schwartz, O.; Amara, A. The TIM and TAM families of phosphatidylserine receptors mediate dengue virus entry. *Cell Host Microbe* **2012**, *12*, 544–557. [CrossRef] [PubMed]

77. Morizono, K.; Chen, I.S. Role of phosphatidylserine receptors in enveloped virus infection. *J. Virol.* **2014**, *88*, 4275–4290. [CrossRef] [PubMed]

78. Perera-Lecoin, M.; Meertens, L.; Carnec, X.; Amara, A. Flavivirus entry receptors: An update. *Viruses* **2013**, *6*, 69–88. [CrossRef] [PubMed]

79. Smit, J.M.; Moesker, B.; Rodenhuis-Zybert, I.; Wilschut, J. Flavivirus cell entry and membrane fusion. *Viruses* **2011**, *3*, 160–171. [CrossRef] [PubMed]

80. Nowakowski, T.J.; Pollen, A.A.; Di Lullo, E.; Sandoval-Espinosa, C.; Bershteyn, M.; Kriegstein, A.R. Expression analysis highlights AXL as a candidate Zika virus entry receptor in neural stem cells. *Cell Stem Cell* **2016**, *18*, 591–596. [CrossRef] [PubMed]

81. Meertens, L.; Labeau, A.; Dejarnac, O.; Cipriani, S.; Sinigaglia, L.; Bonnet-Madin, L.; Le Charpentier, T.; Hafirassou, M.L.; Zamborlini, A.; Cao-Lormeau, V.M.; et al. AXL mediates Zika virus entry in human glial cells and modulates innate immune responses. *Cell Rep.* **2017**, *18*, 324–333. [CrossRef] [PubMed]

82. Retallack, H.; Di Lullo, E.; Arias, C.; Knopp, K.A.; Laurie, M.T.; Sandoval-Espinosa, C.; Mancia Leon, W.R.; Krencik, R.; Ullian, E.M.; Spatazza, J.; et al. Zika virus cell tropism in the developing human brain and inhibition by azithromycin. *Proc. Natl. Acad. Sci. USA* **2016**, *113*, 14408–14413. [CrossRef] [PubMed]

83. Tabata, T.; Petitt, M.; Puerta-Guardo, H.; Michlmayr, D.; Wang, C.; Fang-Hoover, J.; Harris, E.; Pereira, L. Zika virus targets different primary human placental cells, suggesting two routes for vertical transmission. *Cell Host Microbe* **2016**, *20*, 155–166. [CrossRef] [PubMed]

84. Wells, M.F.; Salick, M.R.; Wiskow, O.; Ho, D.J.; Worringer, K.A.; Ihry, R.J.; Kommineni, S.; Bilican, B.; Klim, J.R.; Hill, E.J.; et al. Genetic ablation of AXL does not protect human neural progenitor cells and cerebral organoids from Zika virus infection. *Cell Stem Cell* **2016**, *19*, 703–708. [CrossRef] [PubMed]

85. Wang, Z.Y.; Wang, Z.; Zhen, Z.D.; Feng, K.H.; Guo, J.; Gao, N.; Fan, D.Y.; Han, D.S.; Wang, P.G.; An, J. AXL is not an indispensable factor for Zika virus infection in mice. *J. Gen. Virol.* **2017**, *98*, 2061–2068. [CrossRef] [PubMed]

86. Hamel, R.; Ferraris, P.; Wichit, S.; Diop, F.; Talignani, L.; Pompon, J.; Garcia, D.; Liegeois, F.; Sall, A.A.; Yssel, H.; et al. African and Asian Zika virus strains differentially induce early antiviral responses in primary human astrocytes. *Infect. Genet. Evol.* **2017**, *49*, 134–137. [CrossRef] [PubMed]

87. Stefanik, M.; Formanova, P.; Bily, T.; Vancova, M.; Eyer, L.; Palus, M.; Salat, J.; Braconi, C.T.; Zanotto, P.M.A.; Gould, E.A.; et al. Characterisation of Zika virus infection in primary human astrocytes. *BMC Neurosci* **2018**, *19*, 5. [CrossRef] [PubMed]

88. Chen, J.; Yang, Y.F.; Yang, Y.; Zou, P.; Chen, J.; He, Y.; Shui, S.L.; Cui, Y.R.; Bai, R.; Liang, Y.J.; et al. AXL promotes Zika virus infection in astrocytes by antagonizing type i interferon signalling. *Nat. Microbiol.* **2018**, *3*, 302–309. [CrossRef] [PubMed]

89. Persaud, M.; Martinez-Lopez, A.; Buffone, C.; Porcelli, S.A.; Diaz-Griffero, F. Infection by zika viruses requires the transmembrane protein AXL, endocytosis and low ph. *Virology* **2018**, *518*, 301–312. [CrossRef] [PubMed]

90. Foo, S.S.; Chen, W.; Chan, Y.; Bowman, J.W.; Chang, L.C.; Choi, Y.; Yoo, J.S.; Ge, J.; Cheng, G.; Bonnin, A.; et al. Asian Zika virus strains target CD14$^+$ blood monocytes and induce M2-skewed immunosuppression during pregnancy. *Nat. Microbiol.* **2017**, *2*, 1558–1570. [CrossRef] [PubMed]

91. Michlmayr, D.; Andrade, P.; Gonzalez, K.; Balmaseda, A.; Harris, E. CD14$^+$ CD16$^+$ monocytes are the main target of Zika virus infection in peripheral blood mononuclear cells in a paediatric study in Nicaragua. *Nat. Microbiol.* **2017**, *2*, 1462–1470. [CrossRef] [PubMed]

92. Lum, F.M.; Lee, D.; Chua, T.K.; Tan, J.J.L.; Lee, C.Y.P.; Liu, X.; Fang, Y.; Lee, B.; Yee, W.X.; Rickett, N.Y.; et al. Zika virus infection preferentially counterbalances human peripheral monocyte and/or NK cell activity. *MSphere* **2018**, *3*. [CrossRef] [PubMed]

93. Sheng, Z.Y.; Gao, N.; Wang, Z.Y.; Cui, X.Y.; Zhou, D.S.; Fan, D.Y.; Chen, H.; Wang, P.G.; An, J. Sertoli cells are susceptible to zikv infection in mouse testis. *Front. Cell. Infect. Microbiol.* **2017**, *7*, 272. [CrossRef] [PubMed]

94. Siemann, D.N.; Strange, D.P.; Maharaj, P.N.; Shi, P.Y.; Verma, S. Zika virus infects human sertoli cells and modulates the integrity of the in vitro blood-testis barrier model. *J. Virol.* **2017**, *91*. [CrossRef] [PubMed]

95. Salam, A.P.; Horby, P. Isolation of viable Zika virus from spermatozoa. *Lancet Infect. Dis.* **2018**, *18*, 144. [CrossRef]

96. Bagasra, O.; Addanki, K.C.; Goodwin, G.R.; Hughes, B.W.; Pandey, P.; McLean, E. Cellular targets and receptor of sexual transmission of zika virus. *Appl. Immunohistochem. Mol. Morphol.* **2017**, *25*, 679–686. [CrossRef] [PubMed]

97. Alcendor, D.J. Zika virus infection of the human glomerular cells: Implications for viral reservoirs and renal pathogenesis. *J. Infect. Dis.* **2017**, *216*, 162–171. [CrossRef] [PubMed]

98. Roach, T.; Alcendor, D.J. Zika virus infection of cellular components of the blood-retinal barriers: Implications for viral associated congenital ocular disease. *J. Neuroinflamm.* **2017**, *14*, 43. [CrossRef] [PubMed]

99. Offerdahl, D.K.; Dorward, D.W.; Hansen, B.T.; Bloom, M.E. Cytoarchitecture of Zika virus infection in human neuroblastoma and aedes albopictus cell lines. *Virology* **2017**, *501*, 54–62. [CrossRef] [PubMed]

100. Bos, S.; Viranaicken, W.; Turpin, J.; El-Kalamouni, C.; Roche, M.; Krejbich-Trotot, P.; Despres, P.; Gadea, G. The structural proteins of epidemic and historical strains of Zika virus differ in their ability to initiate viral infection in human host cells. *Virology* **2018**, *516*, 265–273. [CrossRef] [PubMed]

101. Frumence, E.; Roche, M.; Krejbich-Trotot, P.; El-Kalamouni, C.; Nativel, B.; Rondeau, P.; Misse, D.; Gadea, G.; Viranaicken, W.; Despres, P. The south pacific epidemic strain of Zika virus replicates efficiently in human epithelial A549 cells leading to IFN-β production and apoptosis induction. *Virology* **2016**, *493*, 217–226. [CrossRef] [PubMed]

102. Colavita, F.; Musumeci, G.; Caglioti, C. Human osteoblast-like cells are permissive for Zika virus replication. *J. Rheumatol.* **2018**, *45*, 443. [CrossRef] [PubMed]

103. Tappe, D.; Perez-Giron, J.V.; Zammarchi, L.; Rissland, J.; Ferreira, D.F.; Jaenisch, T.; Gomez-Medina, S.; Gunther, S.; Bartoloni, A.; Munoz-Fontela, C.; et al. Cytokine kinetics of zika virus-infected patients from acute to reconvalescent phase. *Med. Microbiol. Immunol.* **2016**, *205*, 269–273. [CrossRef] [PubMed]

104. Grifoni, A.; Pham, J.; Sidney, J.; O'Rourke, P.H.; Paul, S.; Peters, B.; Martini, S.R.; de Silva, A.D.; Ricciardi, M.J.; Magnani, D.M.; et al. Prior dengue virus exposure shapes t cell immunity to Zika virus in humans. *J. Virol.* **2017**, *91*. [CrossRef] [PubMed]

105. Elong Ngono, A.; Shresta, S. Immune response to dengue and zika. *Annu. Rev. Immunol.* **2018**. [CrossRef] [PubMed]

106. Rey, F.A.; Stiasny, K.; Vaney, M.C.; Dellarole, M.; Heinz, F.X. The bright and the dark side of human antibody responses to flaviviruses: Lessons for vaccine design. *EMBO Rep.* **2018**, *19*, 206–224. [CrossRef] [PubMed]

107. Smith, J.L.; Jeng, S.; McWeeney, S.K.; Hirsch, A.J. A microrna screen identifies the wnt signaling pathway as a regulator of the interferon response during flavivirus infection. *J. Virol.* **2017**, *91*. [CrossRef] [PubMed]

108. Panayiotou, C.; Lindqvist, R.; Kurhade, C.; Vonderstein, K.; Pasto, J.; Edlund, K.; Upadhyay, A.S.; Overby, A.K. Viperin restricts Zika virus and tick-borne encephalitis virus replication by targeting NS3 for proteasomal degradation. *J. Virol.* **2018**, *92*. [CrossRef] [PubMed]

109. Anglero-Rodriguez, Y.I.; MacLeod, H.J.; Kang, S.; Carlson, J.S.; Jupatanakul, N.; Dimopoulos, G. Aedes aegypti molecular responses to Zika virus: Modulation of infection by the toll and Jak/Stat immune pathways and virus host factors. *Front. Microbiol.* **2017**, *8*, 2050. [CrossRef] [PubMed]

110. Moran, M.; Delmiro, A.; Blazquez, A.; Ugalde, C.; Arenas, J.; Martin, M.A. Bulk autophagy, but not mitophagy, is increased in cellular model of mitochondrial disease. *Biochim. Biophys. Acta* **2014**, *1842*, 1059–1070. [CrossRef] [PubMed]

111. Liang, Q.; Luo, Z.; Zeng, J.; Chen, W.; Foo, S.S.; Lee, S.A.; Ge, J.; Wang, S.; Goldman, S.A.; Zlokovic, B.V.; et al. Zika virus NS4A and NS4B proteins deregulate Akt-mTOR signaling in human fetal neural stem cells to inhibit neurogenesis and induce autophagy. *Cell Stem Cell* **2016**, *19*, 663–671. [CrossRef] [PubMed]

112. Tetro, J.A. Zika and microcephaly: Causation, correlation, or coincidence? *Microbes Infect.* **2016**, *18*, 167–168. [CrossRef] [PubMed]

113. Chiramel, A.I.; Best, S.M. Role of autophagy in Zika virus infection and pathogenesis. *Virus Res.* **2017**. [CrossRef] [PubMed]

114. Lennemann, N.J.; Coyne, C.B. Dengue and zika viruses subvert reticulophagy by NS2B3-mediated cleavage of FAM134B. *Autophagy* **2017**, *13*, 322–332. [CrossRef] [PubMed]

115. Wu, Y.; Liu, Q.; Zhou, J.; Xie, W.; Chen, C.; Wang, Z.; Yang, H.; Cui, J. Zika virus evades interferon-mediated antiviral response through the co-operation of multiple nonstructural proteins in vitro. *Cell Discov.* **2017**, *3*, 17006. [CrossRef] [PubMed]

116. Weisman, R.; Roitburg, I.; Schonbrun, M.; Harari, R.; Kupiec, M. Opposite effects of TOR1 and TOR2 on nitrogen starvation responses in fission yeast. *Genetics* **2007**, *175*, 1153–1162. [CrossRef] [PubMed]

117. Fenyvuesvolgyi, C.; Elder, R.T.; Benko, Z.; Liang, D.; Zhao, R.Y. Fission yeast homologue of Tip41-like proteins regulates type 2A phosphatases and responses to nitrogen sources. *Biochim. Biophys. Acta* **2005**, *1746*, 155–162. [CrossRef] [PubMed]

118. Elong Ngono, A.; Vizcarra, E.A.; Tang, W.W.; Sheets, N.; Joo, Y.; Kim, K.; Gorman, M.J.; Diamond, M.S.; Shresta, S. Mapping and role of the CD8$^+$ T cell response during primary Zika virus infection in mice. *Cell Host Microbe* **2017**, *21*, 35–46. [CrossRef] [PubMed]

119. Zammarchi, L.; Tappe, D.; Fortuna, C.; Remoli, M.E.; Gunther, S.; Venturi, G.; Bartoloni, A.; Schmidt-Chanasit, J. Zika virus infection in a traveller returning to Europe from Brazil, March 2015. *Eurosurveillance* **2015**, *20*, 21153. [CrossRef] [PubMed]

120. Andrade, D.V.; Harris, E. Recent advances in understanding the adaptive immune response to Zika virus and the effect of previous flavivirus exposure. *Virus Res.* **2017**. [CrossRef] [PubMed]

121. Bardina, S.V.; Bunduc, P.; Tripathi, S.; Duehr, J.; Frere, J.J.; Brown, J.A.; Nachbagauer, R.; Foster, G.A.; Krysztof, D.; Tortorella, D.; et al. Enhancement of Zika virus pathogenesis by preexisting antiflavivirus immunity. *Science* **2017**, *356*, 175–180. [CrossRef] [PubMed]

122. Priyamvada, L.; Quicke, K.M.; Hudson, W.H.; Onlamoon, N.; Sewatanon, J.; Edupuganti, S.; Pattanapanyasat, K.; Chokephaibulkit, K.; Mulligan, M.J.; Wilson, P.C.; et al. Human antibody responses after dengue virus infection are highly cross-reactive to zika virus. *Proc. Natl. Acad. Sci. USA* **2016**, *113*, 7852–7857. [CrossRef] [PubMed]

123. Lazear, H.M.; Govero, J.; Smith, A.M.; Platt, D.J.; Fernandez, E.; Miner, J.J.; Diamond, M.S. A mouse model of zika virus pathogenesis. *Cell Host Microbe* **2016**, *19*, 720–730. [CrossRef] [PubMed]

124. Rossi, S.L.; Tesh, R.B.; Azar, S.R.; Muruato, A.E.; Hanley, K.A.; Auguste, A.J.; Langsjoen, R.M.; Paessler, S.; Vasilakis, N.; Weaver, S.C. Characterization of a novel murine model to study zika virus. *Am. J. Trop. Med. Hyg.* **2016**, *94*, 1362–1369. [CrossRef] [PubMed]

125. Kumar, A.; Hou, S.; Airo, A.M.; Limonta, D.; Mancinelli, V.; Branton, W.; Power, C.; Hobman, T.C. Zika virus inhibits type-I interferon production and downstream signaling. *EMBO Rep.* **2016**, *17*, 1766–1775. [CrossRef] [PubMed]

126. Grant, A.; Ponia, S.S.; Tripathi, S.; Balasubramaniam, V.; Miorin, L.; Sourisseau, M.; Schwarz, M.C.; Sanchez-Seco, M.P.; Evans, M.J.; Best, S.M.; et al. Zika virus targets human Stat2 to inhibit type I interferon signaling. *Cell Host Microbe* **2016**, *19*, 882–890. [CrossRef] [PubMed]

127. Hertzog, J.; Dias Junior, A.G.; Rigby, R.E.; Donald, C.L.; Mayer, A.; Sezgin, E.; Song, C.; Jin, B.; Hublitz, P.; Eggeling, C.; et al. Infection with a Brazilian isolate of Zika virus generates RIG-I stimulatory RNA and the viral NS5 protein blocks type I IFN induction and signaling. *Eur. J. Immunol.* **2018**. [CrossRef] [PubMed]

128. Chaudhary, V.; Yuen, K.S.; Chan, J.F.; Chan, C.P.; Wang, P.H.; Cai, J.P.; Zhang, S.; Liang, M.; Kok, K.H.; Chan, C.P.; et al. Selective activation of type ii interferon signaling by Zika virus NS5 protein. *J. Virol.* **2017**, *91*. [CrossRef] [PubMed]

129. Nguyen, H.N.; Qian, X.; Song, H.; Ming, G.L. Neural stem cells attacked by zika virus. *Cell Res.* **2016**, *26*, 753–754. [CrossRef] [PubMed]

130. Slomnicki, L.P.; Chung, D.H.; Parker, A.; Hermann, T.; Boyd, N.L.; Hetman, M. Ribosomal stress and Tp53-mediated neuronal apoptosis in response to capsid protein of the Zika virus. *Sci. Rep.* **2017**, *7*, 16652. [CrossRef] [PubMed]

131. Yoon, K.J.; Song, G.; Qian, X.; Pan, J.; Xu, D.; Rho, H.S.; Kim, N.S.; Habela, C.; Zheng, L.; Jacob, F.; et al. Zika-virus-encoded NS2A disrupts mammalian cortical neurogenesis by degrading adherens junction proteins. *Cell Stem Cell* **2017**, *21*, 349–358 e346. [CrossRef] [PubMed]

132. Xie, D.Y.; Liu, Z.Y.; Nian, Q.G.; Zhu, L.; Wang, N.; Deng, Y.Q.; Zhao, H.; Ji, X.; Li, X.F.; Wang, X.; et al. A single residue in the alphab helix of the e protein is critical for Zika virus thermostability. *Emerg. Microbes Infect.* **2018**, *7*, 5. [CrossRef] [PubMed]

133. Brault, A.C.; Domi, A.; McDonald, E.M.; Talmi-Frank, D.; McCurley, N.; Basu, R.; Robinson, H.L.; Hellerstein, M.; Duggal, N.K.; Bowen, R.A.; et al. A zika vaccine targeting NS1 protein protects immunocompetent adult mice in a lethal challenge model. *Sci. Rep.* **2017**, *7*, 14769. [CrossRef] [PubMed]

134. Lei, J.; Hansen, G.; Nitsche, C.; Klein, C.D.; Zhang, L.; Hilgenfeld, R. Crystal structure of Zika virus NS2B-NS3 protease in complex with a boronate inhibitor. *Science* **2016**, *353*, 503–505. [CrossRef] [PubMed]

135. Bukrinsky, M. Yeast help identify cytopathic factors of zika virus. *Cell Biosci.* **2017**, *7*, 12. [CrossRef] [PubMed]

136. Nasmyth, K. A prize for proliferation. *Cell* **2001**, *107*, 689–701. [CrossRef]

137. Nurse, P. Cyclin dependent kinases and cell cycle control (nobel lecture). *Chembiochem* **2002**, *3*, 596–603. [CrossRef]

138. Tooze, S.A.; Dikic, I. Autophagy captures the Nobel Prize. *Cell* **2016**, *167*, 1433–1435. [CrossRef] [PubMed]

139. Zhao, R.Y. Yeast for virus research. *Microb. Cell* **2017**, *4*, 311–330. [CrossRef] [PubMed]

140. Zhao, Y.; Elder, R.T.; Chen, M.; Cao, J. Fission yeast expression vectors adapted for positive identification of gene insertion and green fluorescent protein fusion. *Biotechniques* **1998**, *25*, 438–440, 442, 444. [PubMed]

141. Li, G.; Zhao, R.Y. Molecular cloning and characterization of small viral genome in fission yeast. *Methods Mol. Biol.* **2018**, *1721*, 47–61. [PubMed]

142. Romero-Brey, I.; Bartenschlager, R. Endoplasmic reticulum: The favorite intracellular niche for viral replication and assembly. *Viruses* **2016**, *8*, 160. [CrossRef] [PubMed]

143. Kaufusi, P.H.; Kelley, J.F.; Yanagihara, R.; Nerurkar, V.R. Induction of endoplasmic reticulum-derived replication-competent membrane structures by West Nile virus non-structural protein 4B. *PLoS ONE* **2014**, *9*, e84040. [CrossRef] [PubMed]

144. Sangiambut, S.; Keelapang, P.; Aaskov, J.; Puttikhunt, C.; Kasinrerk, W.; Malasit, P.; Sittisombut, N. Multiple regions in dengue virus capsid protein contribute to nuclear localization during virus infection. *J. Gen. Virol.* **2008**, *89*, 1254–1264. [CrossRef] [PubMed]

145. Stock, N.K.; Escadafal, C.; Achazi, K.; Cisse, M.; Niedrig, M. Development and characterization of polyclonal peptide antibodies for the detection of yellow fever virus proteins. *J. Virol. Methods* **2015**, *222*, 110–116. [CrossRef] [PubMed]

146. Cox, B.D.; Stanton, R.A.; Schinazi, R.F. Predicting Zika virus structural biology: Challenges and opportunities for intervention. *Antivir. Chem. Chemother.* **2015**, *24*, 118–126. [CrossRef] [PubMed]

147. Kostyuchenko, V.A.; Lim, E.X.; Zhang, S.; Fibriansah, G.; Ng, T.S.; Ooi, J.S.; Shi, J.; Lok, S.M. Structure of the thermally stable zika virus. *Nature* **2016**, *533*, 425–428. [CrossRef] [PubMed]

148. Fontes-Garfias, C.R.; Shan, C.; Luo, H.; Muruato, A.E.; Medeiros, D.B.A.; Mays, E.; Xie, X.; Zou, J.; Roundy, C.M.; Wakamiya, M.; et al. Functional analysis of glycosylation of Zika virus envelope protein. *Cell Rep.* **2017**, *21*, 1180–1190. [CrossRef] [PubMed]

149. Annamalai, A.S.; Pattnaik, A.; Sahoo, B.R.; Muthukrishnan, E.; Natarajan, S.K.; Steffen, D.; Vu, H.L.X.; Delhon, G.; Osorio, F.A.; Petro, T.M.; et al. Zika virus encoding non-glycosylated envelope protein is attenuated and defective in neuroinvasion. *J. Virol.* **2017**, *91*. [CrossRef] [PubMed]

150. Goo, L.; DeMaso, C.R.; Pelc, R.S.; Ledgerwood, J.E.; Graham, B.S.; Kuhn, R.J.; Pierson, T.C. The Zika virus envelope protein glycan loop regulates virion antigenicity. *Virology* **2018**, *515*, 191–202. [CrossRef] [PubMed]

151. Gallichotte, E.N.; Dinnon, K.H., 3rd; Lim, X.N.; Ng, T.S.; Lim, E.X.Y.; Menachery, V.D.; Lok, S.M.; Baric, R.S. CD-loop extension in Zika virus envelope protein key for stability and pathogenesis. *J. Infect. Dis.* **2017**, *216*, 1196–1204. [CrossRef] [PubMed]

152. Yuan, L.; Huang, X.Y.; Liu, Z.Y.; Zhang, F.; Zhu, X.L.; Yu, J.Y.; Ji, X.; Xu, Y.P.; Li, G.; Li, C.; et al. A single mutation in the prm protein of Zika virus contributes to fetal microcephaly. *Science* **2017**, *358*, 933–936. [CrossRef] [PubMed]

153. Shan, C.; Xie, X.; Muruato, A.E.; Rossi, S.L.; Roundy, C.M.; Azar, S.R.; Yang, Y.; Tesh, R.B.; Bourne, N.; Barrett, A.D.; et al. An infectious cdna clone of Zika virus to study viral virulence, mosquito transmission, and antiviral inhibitors. *Cell Host Microbe* **2016**, *19*, 891–900. [CrossRef] [PubMed]

154. Mahawaththa, M.C.; Pearce, B.J.G.; Szabo, M.; Graham, B.; Klein, C.D.; Nitsche, C.; Otting, G. Solution conformations of a linked construct of the Zika virus NS2B-NS3 protease. *Antiviral Res.* **2017**, *142*, 141–147. [CrossRef] [PubMed]

155. Phoo, W.W.; Li, Y.; Zhang, Z.; Lee, M.Y.; Loh, Y.R.; Tan, Y.B.; Ng, E.Y.; Lescar, J.; Kang, C.; Luo, D. Structure of the NS2B-NS3 protease from Zika virus after self-cleavage. *Nat. Commun.* **2016**, *7*, 13410. [CrossRef] [PubMed]

156. Lee, H.; Ren, J.; Nocadello, S.; Rice, A.J.; Ojeda, I.; Light, S.; Minasov, G.; Vargas, J.; Nagarathnam, D.; Anderson, W.F.; et al. Identification of novel small molecule inhibitors against NS2B/NS3 serine protease from zika virus. *Antiviral Res.* **2017**, *139*, 49–58. [CrossRef] [PubMed]

157. Shafee, N.; AbuBakar, S. Dengue virus type 2 NS3 protease and NS2B-NS3 protease precursor induce apoptosis. *J. Gen. Virol.* **2003**, *84*, 2191–2195. [CrossRef] [PubMed]

158. Yang, T.C.; Shiu, S.L.; Chuang, P.H.; Lin, Y.J.; Wan, L.; Lan, Y.C.; Lin, C.W. Japanese encephalitis virus NS2B-NS3 protease induces caspase 3 activation and mitochondria-mediated apoptosis in human medulloblastoma cells. *Virus Res.* **2009**, *143*, 77–85. [CrossRef] [PubMed]

159. Rastogi, M.; Sharma, N.; Singh, S.K. Flavivirus ns1: A multifaceted enigmatic viral protein. *Virol. J.* **2016**, *13*, 131. [CrossRef] [PubMed]

160. Viranaicken, W.; Ndebo, A.; Bos, S.; Souque, P.; Gadea, G.; El-Kalamouni, C.; Krejbich-Trotot, P.; Charneau, P.; Despres, P.; Roche, M. Recombinant zika ns1 protein secreted from vero cells is efficient for inducing production of immune serum directed against NS1 dimer. *Int. J. Mol. Sci.* **2017**, *19*, 38. [CrossRef] [PubMed]

161. Freire, C.C.M.; Lamarino, A.; Neto, D.F.L.N.; Sall, A.A.; Zanotto, P.M.A. Spread of the pandemic Zika virus lineage is associated with NS1 codon usage adaptation in humans. *BioRxiv* **2015**. [CrossRef]

162. Delatorre, E.; Mir, D.; Bello, G. Tracing the origin of the NS1 A188V substitution responsible for recent enhancement of Zika virus Asian genotype infectivity. *Mem. Inst. Oswaldo Cruz* **2017**, *112*, 793–795. [CrossRef] [PubMed]

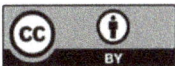

Review

Suppression of Type I Interferon Signaling by *Flavivirus* NS5

Stephanie Thurmond [1,2], Boxiao Wang [3], Jikui Song [3,*] and Rong Hai [1,2,*]

[1] Department of Microbiology and Plant Pathology, University of California, Riverside, Riverside, CA 92521, USA; sthur002@ucr.edu

[2] Graduate Program in Cell, Molecular and Developmental Biology, University of California, Riverside, Riverside, CA 92521, USA

[3] Department of Biochemistry, University of California, Riverside, Riverside, CA 92521, USA; bwang030@ucr.edu

* Correspondence: jikui.song@ucr.edu (J.S.); ronghai@ucr.edu (R.H.)

Received: 21 November 2018; Accepted: 9 December 2018; Published: 14 December 2018

Abstract: Type I interferon (IFN-I) is the first line of mammalian host defense against viral infection. To counteract this, the flaviviruses, like other viruses, have encoded a variety of antagonists, and use a multi-layered molecular defense strategy to establish their infections. Among the most potent antagonists is non-structural protein 5 (NS5), which has been shown for all disease-causing flaviviruses to target different steps and players of the type I IFN signaling pathway. Here, we summarize the type I IFN antagonist mechanisms used by flaviviruses with a focus on the role of NS5 in regulating one key regulator of type I IFN, signal transducer and activator of transcription 2 (STAT2).

Keywords: *flavivirus*; ZIKV; NS5; type I IFN antagonist

1. Introduction

Flaviviruses are globally significant arthropod-borne viruses that cause disease in hundreds of millions of people each year. The *Flavivirus* genus is part of the *Flaviviridae* family and comprises over 70 species, including dengue, Zika, yellow fever, West Nile, Japanese encephalitis, and tick-borne encephalitis viruses. Facilitated by the warming climate, urbanization, and increasing travel to endemic areas, many of these pathogens have expanded into new territories, and flaviviral infections have increased worldwide [1]. Despite the enormous burden on public health posed by flaviviruses, there are currently no antiviral therapies available and limited vaccines.

To establish successful infection in vertebrates, flaviviruses must first overcome the host antiviral response, which is primarily mediated by type I interferons (IFN-I) [2]. IFN-I stimulates expression of hundreds of genes that disrupt various stages of the viral life cycle. The power and importance of this host defense is demonstrated by the fact that all flaviviruses have evolved elaborate mechanisms to antagonize and evade the type I IFN response. The ability of individual viruses to suppress this pathway determines host and tissue tropisms and severity of disease [3,4]. Therefore, understanding the interaction between the host immune response and viral antagonism of this defense at the molecular level elucidates mechanisms of pathogenesis and facilitates the development of safe and effective antiviral therapies and vaccines.

Flaviviruses employ diverse strategies to subvert the host immune system. To avoid being recognized as "non-self," which triggers IFN-I production, flaviviruses mask their genome with RNA caps that mimic that of the host and the intermediate RNAs are hidden from cytoplasmic sensors by membranes hijacked by viral replication proteins [5]. Flaviviruses also actively antagonize proteins that function within the IFN-I signaling pathway by inhibiting their post-translational modifications, competing for protein–protein interactions, or targeting them for degradation [2]. These diverse mechanisms of IFN antagonism are typically carried out by flavivirus non-structural proteins.

Non-structural protein 5 (NS5) is the largest and most conserved flavivirus protein [6]. It is responsible for replicating and capping the viral genome, but is also a potent innate immune antagonist in all flaviviruses studied thus far [7]. However, the mechanisms utilized by the NS5 proteins from related viruses have been shown to diverge significantly. This review discusses the IFN-I-mediated defense mounted by flavivirus-infected hosts and the various mechanisms employed by flaviviruses to counteract this defense, with special emphasis given to NS5-mediated suppression of human signal transducer and activator of transcription 2 (hSTAT2)-dependent IFN signaling. Three of the major disease-causing flaviviruses' NS5 proteins interact with and inhibit hSTAT2, a central regulator of the type I IFN response. We discuss the ways in which this interaction diverges among the highly related flaviviruses and the impact of hSTAT2 inhibition on viral pathogenesis.

2. *Flavivirus* Disease and Transmission

Disease caused by flaviviruses ranges from mild symptoms such as fever, rash, and joint pain to more severe illness that includes hemorrhagic fever, encephalitis, and neurological sequelae. However, very few infected individuals experience serious illness, and most are entirely asymptomatic. It is currently not possible to predict an individual's disease outcome due to our inadequate understanding of the molecular basis of the pathogenesis of severe disease. There are no vaccines available for dengue, Zika, or West Nile viruses. Even for flaviviruses with effective vaccines, such as yellow fever, Japanese encephalitis, and tick-borne encephalitis viruses, outbreaks still occur from time to time in developing countries.

Dengue virus (DENV) is responsible for the highest incidence of disease among the flaviviruses ($\approx$400 million annually) [8]. There are four genetically distinct serotypes of DENV and infection with one serotype confers long-lasting immunity against only the infecting serotype. Primary infections are frequently asymptomatic but can result in fever and rash, whereas secondary infections, especially with a heterologous serotype, can cause dengue hemorrhagic fever and shock syndrome, likely due to antibody-dependent enhancement (ADE) [9]. Zika virus (ZIKV), which emerged recently in several major epidemics in Asia and the Americas, causes similar symptoms to dengue fever and has additionally been causally linked to congenital microcephaly and Guillain-Barré syndrome [10]. West Nile virus (WNV) is common in Africa, the Middle East, and Europe, and appeared in North America in 1999 [11]. In addition to febrile illness, WNV is a major cause of viral encephalitis [12].

The human pathogen flaviviruses are vector-borne, although different tick and mosquito species are utilized by different viruses. Yellow fever virus (YFV), DENV, and ZIKV are transmitted primarily by *Aedes* mosquitoes [13], whereas WNV and Japanese encephalitis virus (JEV) are transmitted through the *Culex* species [14,15]. Flaviviruses are also zoonotic and rely on non-human animal vectors for widespread circulation. For example, pigs and birds are amplifying hosts for JEV [16], and non-human primates are ZIKV amplification hosts [17]. Flaviviruses alternate between two distinct transmission cycles: sylvatic and urban. The sylvatic transmission cycle refers to the transmission of the virus between the arboreal vector and non-human animal hosts, and the urban cycle consists of circulation between arthropods and humans [18]. The recent ZIKV epidemics have revealed additional mechanisms of transmission that may be unique to Zika, such as sexual contact and perinatal transmission [19,20].

Because of the necessity of alternating between vertebrate and arthropod hosts, flaviviruses have adapted their immune restriction mechanisms for distinct species. For example, DENV proteins can cleave the human immune factors stimulator of interferon genes (STING) and STAT2 (discussed below) but not non-human primate STING or murine STAT2 [3,21,22]. Similarly, ZIKV causes the degradation of human but not murine STAT2 [3]. These species-specific immune suppression mechanisms help to explain in part why DENV fails to reach high titers non-human primate models [23,24], and why immunocompetent mice are poor disease models for many flaviviruses, including ZIKV and DENV [25, 26].

3. *Flavivirus* Genome and Life Cycle

Flavivirus genomes are 10-11 kb single-stranded positive-sense RNA molecules flanked by structured 5′ and 3′ UTRs. A recent study demonstrated pervasive higher-order structures throughout the ZIKV [27] and DENV2 RNA genomes, spanning at least eight distinct regions [28]. A virally encoded methyltransferase provides a ^{m7}GpppN cap structure to the 5′ end of the genome similar to mammalian mRNA caps [29], but the flaviviral genome lacks a 3′ polyadenylation tail. The genome is translated as a single polyprotein, which is then proteolytically processed by host and viral proteases to generate three structural proteins (capsid (C), pre-membrane (prM), and envelope (E)), and seven non-structural proteins (NS1, NS2A, NS2B, NS3, NS4A, NS4B, and NS5). The non-structural (NS) proteins are responsible for replication of the viral genome, polyprotein processing, and host immune response antagonism. Mature virions are ≈50 μm in diameter and consist of the RNA genome encapsulated by a lipid envelope and the three structural proteins C, prM, and E [6].

Flaviviruses enter the cell via endocytosis and traffic to endosomes where the envelope protein undergoes a low pH-induced conformational change to induce fusion of the endosomal membrane with the viral membrane. This fusion event allows the nucleocapsid to be released from the endosome, and the genome is rapidly translated at the surface of the endoplasmic reticulum (ER) [30]. The viral NS proteins facilitate the formation of replication complexes by hijacking host cytoplasmic membranes. These compartments coordinate the replication and translation of the viral genome and help to shield viral components from host recognition. The NS proteins form a replication complex that generates negative-sense RNAs that function as templates for positive-sense genome RNA. Newly synthesized viral RNA is packaged, and the immature virion is transported through the host secretory pathway where it is further processed by host proteases to generate a mature virion that is released from the infected cell by exocytosis [6].

4. Host Innate Immune Response to *Flavivirus* Infection

The type I IFN signaling pathway is one of the first lines of defense against flavivirus infection of mammals. Type I IFNs are produced by mammalian cells in response to viral infection and play a pivotal role in counteracting viral pathogenesis [31]. Flavivirus-infected individuals have elevated levels of immune-related gene transcripts and serum IFN [32–36]. In mouse and cell models, similar elevations have been reported [37–39] and production has been shown to play a protective role [10–13]. Several proteins that function within this signaling pathway have been identified with direct and specific antiviral roles during flavivirus infection [37,38,40,41]. IFN-I has even been tested as a treatment for clinical flavivirus disease, but has not been successful [42,43]. This may be explained by the universal ability of flaviviruses to inhibit the Janus kinase-signal transducer and activator of transcription (JAK-STAT) pathway. As discussed below, the NS proteins are the primary actors in this suppression, and understanding the molecular mechanisms mediating this suppression would contribute to the development of effective antiviral therapies.

The innate immune response against flaviviruses is triggered by sensing the pathogen-associated molecular patterns (PAMPs) via the cytosolic and endosomal pattern recognition receptors (PRRs) retinoic acid-inducible gene-1 (RIG-I), melanoma differentiation-associated protein 5 (MDA5), Toll-like receptor (TLR) 7/8, or TLR3 [44–46]. PAMP sensing PRRs activate various kinases including inhibitor of nuclear factor kappa-B (NF-κB) kinase subunit epsilon (IKKε), tumor necrosis factor (TNF) receptor-associated factor (TRAF) family member-associated NF-κB (TANK)-binding kinase-1 (TBK-1), and TRAF3, which ultimately result in the phosphorylation of NF-κB and interferon regulatory factor 3 (IRF3) [45,47]. Activated NF-κB and IRF3 translocate to the nucleus to stimulate the production of type I IFNs.

The type I IFNs consist primarily of two secreted cytokines, IFN-α and IFN-ß. Upon secretion, IFN-α/ß bind to their cognate receptor IFNAR on infected and neighboring cells. IFNAR consists of two subunits (IFNAR1 and IFNAR2) whose intracellular domains are constitutively associated with the Janus kinases JAK1 and Tyk2. IFN binding to IFNAR activates JAK1 and Tyk2 to phosphorylate the latent cytoplasmic signal transducers of activation 1 and 2 (STAT1 and STAT2). Tyrosine phosphorylated STAT1 and STAT2 dimerize and then associate with a third protein, interferon regulatory factor 9 (IRF9). This trimeric complex, known as interferon-stimulated gene factor 3 (ISGF3), translocates into the nucleus where it binds to interferon stimulated response elements (ISRE) to drive transcription of over 300 interferon stimulated genes (ISGs) that directly or indirectly counter flavivirus infection. IRF9 binds to the ISRE, STAT2 contributes a potent transactivation domain, and STAT1 stabilizes the complex through additional DNA interactions [48,49].

The components of ISGF3 are constitutively expressed at a low level and reside in the cytoplasm in their latent forms. Upon IFN stimulation and tyrosine phosphorylation of STATs 1 and 2, ISGF3 rapidly assembles and directs a robust, transient antiviral response that includes the upregulation of ISGF3 components themselves. This response, however, additionally increases the expression of pro-apoptotic and anti-proliferative genes that can be damaging to the host cell, so downregulation of these genes occurs quickly after IFN stimulation. This response is mediated by several negative feedback mechanisms, such as the suppressor of cytokine signaling (SOCS) proteins, which are also induced by type I IFN [50]. In contrast, a subset of the antiviral ISGs upregulated by the initial IFN stimulation, including STAT1, STAT2, and IRF9, are sustained for several days, resulting in increased levels of the unphosphorylated forms of these proteins [51]. These proteins interact to form the trimeric unphosphorylated ISGF (U-ISGF3), which is responsible for the sustained ISG transcription, allowing for extended resistance to viral infection [52].

Recently, evidence has emerged for the existence of STAT1-independent complexes that can drive IFN-I-stimulated ISG expression [53]. For example, STAT2 can interact with IRF9 to form an "ISGF3-like" complex that activates ISRE-promoted genes in response to type I IFN [54]. This complex can direct a similar but prolonged ISGF3-like transcriptome in the absence of STAT1. However, some STAT2/IRF9-specific ISGF3-independent ISGs have been identified, including *CCL8* and *CX3CL1*. The promoter regions of these genes do not contain the classical ISRE sequences, suggesting that a DNA sequence distinct from ISRE may be involved in STAT2/IRF9-specific gene regulation. Additionally it has been demonstrated that this alternative pathway can mediate antiviral responses to several viruses including dengue, vesicular stomatitis, encephalomyocarditis, measles, Crimean-Congo hemorrhagic fever, and lymphocytic choriomeningitis viruses [55–59]. The cyclic guanosine monophosphate (GMP)–adenosine monophosphate (AMP) synthase (cGAS) is a cytosolic DNA sensor that directs the synthesis of cyclic GMP-AMP (cGAMP) upon binding to DNA. cGAMP activates the stimulator of the IFN gene (STING), which promotes type I IFN production via IRF3 activation [60]. It was recently demonstrated that the cGAS/STING pathway becomes activated during DENV infection, even in the absence of viral DNA intermediates [21]. DENV infection induces mitochondrial swelling, causing the release of mitochondrial DNA, which activates cGAS [61]. The involvement of the cGAS/STING pathway in other flavivirus infections has yet to be determined.

Although type I IFNs are produced by nearly all cells in the body and are essential for restricting viral replication, two additional IFN signaling pathways exist and have been shown to respond to viral infection. The type III IFNs (IFN-λ1-4) are the primary antiviral IFNs generated by epithelial cells and have similar functions and signaling pathways as IFN-I, but the cellular receptor is not ubiquitously expressed [62]. An antiviral effect for IFN-λ has been demonstrated for West Nile and Zika viruses. Mice deficient in the IFN-λ receptor exhibited increased blood–brain barrier (BBB) permeability after WNV infection [63], suggesting type III IFN signaling is involved in WNV neurotropism. Primary human trophoblast cells from human placenta were found to release type III IFN constitutively, conferring resistance to ZIKV infection [64]. The ability of ZIKV to be vertically transmitted from mother to fetus suggests the existence of a viral factor that may be able to overcome the type III IFN response in placental cells. The NS5 protein from ZIKV is a likely candidate as it was shown to inhibit the type III response in HEK293T cells [65].

While ZIKV NS5 was shown to suppress both the type I and III IFN responses, it was also able to activate type II IFN signaling [65]. The type II IFNs (IFN-γ) are generated mainly by immune cells and have some antiviral functions. ZIKV infection, however, is enhanced by type II IFN signaling, which generates proinflammatory cytokines that can facilitate viral spread and exacerbate Zika disease [66]. The concurrent NS5-mediated suppression of type I and III pathways and activation of the type II pathway was suggested to occur through increased homodimerization of STAT1, which upregulates gene expression at γ-activated sites (GAS). Because ZIKV NS5 induces the degradation of STAT2 (discussed below), which is required for the formation of transcription complexes involved in type I and III IFN signaling, the intracellular balance of STAT-containing complexes shifts to STAT1-STAT1 dimers, resulting in increased IFN-γ-induced gene expression. To date, ZIKV NS5 is the only viral protein known to concurrently suppress type I and III IFN pathways while activating type II [65].

5. *Flavivirus* Antagonism of Host Type I IFN Response

Just as hosts have evolved multiple mechanisms for inhibiting viral infection, viral proteins have gained the ability to antagonize the host IFN response over time. One mechanism by which the type I IFN response is passively avoided by flaviviruses is evasion of the host PRRs, described above. Flaviviruses encode their own methyltransferase that caps the RNA genome to mimic the RNAs present in the host cell. The cap structure hides the viral genome from members of the interferon-induced tetratricopeptide repeats (IFIT) protein family, which binds to and sequesters viral RNA, and prevents recognition by the RIG-I [67]. Flaviviruses also shield their genome from host sensing by enclosing their replication complex (RC) in membranes on the ER surface, a mechanism that has been observed in the early stages of DENV, WNV, and tick-borne encephalitis virus (TBEV) infections [68,69]. However, late in the infection, newly synthesized viral RNA is abundant, and the RC loses some integrity, which may lead to the release of RNA intermediates that could activate RIG-I or MDA5 signaling [70].

Flaviviruses have also been demonstrated to actively abrogate the activity of protein functioning within the type I IFN signaling pathway. One common mechanism is interference with post-translational modifications of these proteins. For example, the DENV, WNV, and YFV NS4B inhibit STAT1 phosphorylation [71,72]. WNV NS4B is additionally implicated in preventing the phosphorylation of JAK1 and Tyk2 [27,28], and NS2A, NS2B, NS3, NS4A, and NS4B from Kunjin virus (KUN), a close relative to WNV, are all implicated in JAK-STAT inhibition [73]. This mechanism is not always mediated by NS proteins, however. Flaviviruses produce small RNAs called subgenomic flavivirus RNAs (sfRNAs) that are generated by the incomplete degradation of the viral genome by the host endonuclease XrnI [74]. In DENV, this sfRNA binds to TRIM25, which normally interacts with RIG-I to promote its ubiquitination and interaction with mitochondrial antiviral signaling protein (MAVS) [75]. The DENV sfRNA prevents the deubiquitination of TRIM25, an essential upstream activator for RIG-I activation [76].

Another mechanism of active interference with the type I IFN system is competitive binding. DENV and WNV NS3 proteins compete with RIG-I for 14-3-3ε binding, a chaperone responsible for trafficking RNA-bound RIG-I to the mitochondrial membrane [77]. Additionally, the DENV NS4A protein sequesters MAVS, preventing RIG-I-MAVS interaction, IRF3 activation, and IFN-I production [78].

Finally, many flavivirus NS proteins have evolved mechanisms to degrade host immune proteins, or to induce the degradation of these proteins by hijacking the host proteasome system. For example, the DENV NS2B/NS3 viral protease suppresses the DNA sensing pathway and RIG-I sensing by cleaving STING, resulting in reduced type I IFN production [21]. Additionally, NS2B by itself promotes the autophagy-lysosome-dependent degradation of cGAS [21].

6. NS5 Structure and Function

NS5 is the most conserved flavivirus protein, with less than 45% amino acid difference reported among the vector-borne flaviviruses [3]. The N-terminus encodes the viral methyltransferase (MTase), while the C-terminus encodes the RNA-dependent RNA polymerase (RdRp) [79]. The RdRp generates positive- and negative-sense RNAs from the RNA genome de novo [80,81], and the replication process is thought to involve three different conformational states: pre-initiation, initiation, and elongation [82,83]. The MTase domain caps the RNA genome via a two-step reaction and also serves as the guanylyltransferase [29].

To date, structures of full-length NS5 from JEV [84], DENV3 [85], and ZIKV [79,86,87] have been reported. The ZIKV and JEV NS5 conformations exhibit a high degree of similarity, suggesting structural conservation among the flaviviruses [79]. In contrast, the domain orientations of ZIKV and DENV NS5s differ significantly, although the residues at the domain interface are highly conserved among ZIKV, DENV, and JEV [79]. These observations support an earlier observation that the flavivirus NS5 exhibits a high degree of flexibility in solution and can adopt a compact or extended conformation [88], which may impact on the diverse functions of NS5. Indeed, mutagenesis of the conserved interface residues of the DENV3 NS5 caused enhanced RdRp activity, but inhibited viral infectivity [85]. Furthermore, recent structural evidence suggests that the two subdomains cooperate in the execution of the sequential replication and capping functions, although the mechanism remains unknown [84,89]. Taken together, these reports suggest that the flexibility and distinct conformations of the flavivirus NS5 may be linked to the various steps involved in RNA capping and replication. More experiments are needed to clarify the potential role of the conformational changes in regulating NS5 activities.

Several post-translational modifications of flavivirus NS5s have also been documented with potential regulatory roles. Serine/threonine phosphorylation appears to be conserved throughout the *Flaviviridae* family [90,91], but the function of this modification and the identity of the host kinases involved are largely unknown. The DENV NS5 protein is phosphorylated by both mammalian and mosquito protein kinase G at a conserved Thr449 in the RdRp domain [92,93]. The differential phosphorylation of DENV NS5 was shown to affect its interaction with the viral helicase, NS3, which is required for genome replication [94]. The WNV NS5 MTase domain is also phosphorylated by, and interacts with, protein kinase G, and abolishing this interaction inhibits viral replication [95]. SUMOylation of the DENV NS5 was shown to be important for DENV replication [96]. In addition, glutathionylation of the DENV and ZIKV NS5s has been reported [97].

Replication of the flavivirus genome occurs exclusively in the cytoplasm [69,98]. However, a significant portion of the NS5 protein is observed within the nucleus during YFV [99], JEV [100], ZIKV [3], WNV [101], and DENV [102] infections. Inhibiting the nuclear localization of DENV and WNV NS5 significantly decreases viral titers [101,103]. Inversely, inhibiting the nuclear export of DENV NS5 decreased the induction of IL-8, which plays a role in induction of inflammation [104], suggesting nuclear localization of NS5 may be important for immune modulation [105]. This observation is further supported by a study showing that interaction of NS5 with host spliceosome components leads to changes in mRNA isoform abundance of antiviral factors [106]. There are differences, however, in the level of NS5 nuclear localization among the different DENV serotypes. NS5 from serotypes 2 and 3 accumulate in the nucleus, while DENV1 and 4 NS5 reside in the cytoplasm [107]. For serotype 4, cytoplasmic localization is likely due to the lack of a functional nuclear localization signal (NLS) [107]. Levels of IL-8 did not change with the different serotypes, and the function of the differential localization is still unknown [107].

7. IFN Suppressor Function of *Flavivirus* NS5 Protein

While multiple proteins capable of IFN antagonism have been described for the major disease-causing flaviviruses, NS5 is the most potent and direct antagonist [3]. This is significant because NS5-mediated IFN antagonism is required for counteraction of IFN in cell culture [108] and for virulence in mouse models [109]. Remarkably, even though this protein utilizes similar MTase and RdRp mechanisms no matter the flavivirus species to replicate and cap their RNA genomes, the mechanism of NS5-mediated IFN suppression diverges within the genus. The evolution and divergence of this role for NS5 may have been facilitated by the strategy of expression of flaviviral proteins from a single open reading frame. This results in excess expression of NS5, while only small amounts are needed for RdRp and MTase functions. Due to the lack of high-resolution structures for the complexes of various NS5s and their interacting host partners, how NS5 is able to retain its roles as MTase and RdRp while evolving divergent IFN suppression mechanisms remains elusive.

NS5 frequently employs multiple strategies to suppress the JAK-STAT signaling pathway not only among different species of *Flavivirus*, but also within the same species. For example, the ZIKV NS5 protein has been shown to both inhibit the phosphorylation of STAT1 and induce the degradation of STAT2. The JEV, DENV, and WNV NS5 proteins have similarly been shown to antagonize this pathway at multiple steps. STAT2 is a common target for NS5-mediated IFN suppression, and at least two flavivirus NS5 proteins have been demonstrated to target this protein for degradation. The mechanisms by which the DENV and ZIKV NS5s degrade STAT2 diverge, however, and the molecular details of these mechanisms are still being elucidated.

7.1. Dengue Virus

DENV NS5 binds to human STAT2 and inhibits its phosphorylation, resulting in reduced ISG transcription. The mechanism of this inhibition has not been elucidated, but the IFN suppression activity was mapped to the RdRp domain [110]. Expression of NS5 also reduces IFN-α-, but not IFN-γ-, mediated STAT1 phosphorylation, although NS5 does not directly interact with STAT1 [110].

Ashour et al. demonstrated STAT2 degradation as an additional mechanism of DENV NS5-mediated IFN antagonism [111,112]. However, while this study also found that binding of NS5 to STAT2 is sufficient to prevent IFN signaling, STAT2 degradation is detected only when the N-terminus of NS5 is proteolytically processed, as it would be in the context of viral infection. NS5 is separated from NS4B during polyprotein processing by the viral NS2B/NS3 protease, and co-expression of NS5 with NS2B/NS3 induces STAT2 degradation. Replacement of the viral cleavage site at the N-terminus of NS5 with a host protease cleavage site, however, also allows for the efficient degradation of STAT2, suggesting the cleavage does not need to be mediated by the viral protease. Additionally, the identity of the N-terminal residue of NS5 does not appear to be important to this processing event, as replacing the glycine residue at position 1 of NS5 with methionine resulted in efficient STAT2 degradation [112]. This study also demonstrated that NS5-mediated STAT2 degradation is dependent on the ubiquitin-proteasome pathway, implying the involvement of a host E3 ligase. In a follow-up study, the García-Sastre group identified this protein as UBR box N-recognin-4 (UBR4), which is part of the N-recognin family [113]. Members of this family target proteins that undergo conformational changes to expose a destabilizing N-terminal residue for degradation, a mechanism for the N-end rule pathway [114]. UBR4 binds to the first five amino acids of NS5; deleting the first ten amino acids of NS5 eliminates its ability to induce STAT2 degradation [112,113]. The binding domain for STAT2, however, was mapped to residues 202–306 [112], suggesting that the DENV NS5 central and N terminal regions together serve as a bridge between STAT2 and UBR4. In this scenario, it is possible that NS5 and STAT2 are both targeted by UBR4 and similarly degraded [7]. Experimental evidence, however, is still needed for verification of the role of the N-end rule pathway in DENV NS5-mediated STAT2 degradation.

7.2. Zika Virus

Similar to DENV NS5, ZIKV NS5 binds to human STAT2, triggering its degradation. However, unlike what was observed for DENV NS5, ZIKV NS5 does not need to undergo proteolytic processing for depletion of STAT2 [3]. Additionally, it was demonstrated that the first ten amino acids of NS5 are dispensable for depletion of STAT2, suggesting that the N-end rule does not apply to ZIKV NS5 [115]. STAT2 is ubiquitinated prior to degradation, and proteasome inhibitors rescue STAT2 protein levels in the presence of NS5 [65]. However, unlike that occurs for DENV NS5, UBR4 is not involved in mediating STAT2 degradation [3]. This suggests that ZIKV NS5-mediated STAT2 degradation utilizes the host ubiquitin proteasome system and the participating host E3 ligase has yet to be identified.

Chaudhary et al. demonstrated an additional consequence of ZIVK NS5-mediated STAT2 degradation, aside from decreased ISG induction. In an uninfected cell, unphosphorylated STAT2 can bind to both unphosphorylated and phosphorylated STAT1 to prevent translocation of STAT1 and activation of the type II IFN response [116]. In ZIKV-infected and NS5-transfected cells, however, an increase in STAT1 homodimerization is observed, concurrent with an increase in type II IFN and a decrease in type I IFN signaling. In this model, the degradation of STAT2 frees up STAT1 proteins to homodimerize and translocate to the nucleus to selectively activate ISGs controlled by gamma activated sites (GAS) [65].

7.3. Yellow Fever Virus

The YFV NS5 also targets STAT2 as part of its IFN-I suppression mechanism. YFV NS5 binds to STAT2, but this interaction is uniquely dependent on host cell stimulation with type I or III IFNs. This stimulation induces several intracellular events required for NS5 association with STAT2. First, as in an uninfected cell, stimulation with IFN induces the phosphorylation and heterodimerization of STAT1 and STAT2. STAT2 does not need to be phosphorylated for NS5 interaction. Instead, the association of STAT1 and STAT2 induces a conformational change within STAT2 that allows for NS5 binding. Second, IFN stimulation promotes the ubiquitination of YFV NS5 by TRIM23; non-ubiquitinated NS5 cannot interact with STAT2. Unlike the DENV and ZIKV NS5s, YFV NS5 does not induce the degradation of STAT2, and is able to bind STAT2 both in the cytoplasm and in the nucleus. YFV NS5 blocks IFN production either by directly interfering with ISGF3 binding to ISRE promoter elements in the nucleus, or by preventing IRF9 association with STAT1/2 heterodimers in the cytoplasm. A domain mapping study identified the first ten amino acids of the YFV NS5 as essential for both STAT2 interaction and IFN-I inhibition, consistent with the requirement of TRIM23 ubiquitinating K6 of NS5 [117].

8. Other NS5 Interactions

8.1. Spondweni Virus

Spondweni virus (SPOV) is the closest known relative of ZIKV [118], and their NS5 proteins share 77% amino acid identity [3]. While SPOV NS5 does not directly interact with STAT2 as the ZIKV NS5 does, it is an inhibitor of JAK-STAT signaling, as SPOV NS5-transfected cells inhibit ISRE-dependent gene expression [3]. The STATs are also phosphorylated and translocated to the nucleus upon IFN stimulation. SPOV NS5 is localized primarily to the nucleus of the cell, so it is possible the mechanism of ISG suppression occurs inside the nucleus [3].

8.2. Japanese Encephalitis Virus

The JEV NS5 protein alone can inhibit Tyk2 and STAT1 phosphorylation via protein tyrosine phosphatase (PTP) activity, as PTP inhibitors rescue phosphorylation, but specific NS5 interactions with innate immune proteins have not yet been implicated in this suppression mechanism [119]. The region of NS5 required for suppression of STAT1 activation was mapped to the N terminus [119]. JEV NS5 has also been shown to inhibit the nuclear translocation of IRF3 and NF-κB by competitively interacting with importin-α4 and importin-α3 [120]. These interactions are mediated by the NLS of JEV NS5 and mutagenesis of key residues in this region restored ISG expression [120].

8.3. Tick-Borne Encephalitis, Langat, and West Nile Viruses

Langat virus (LGTV) is a member of the tick-borne encephalitis virus (TBEV) serogroup. Both LGTV and TBEV NS5s suppress phosphorylation of STAT1, STAT2, Tyk2, and JAK1 [121].

The region of LGTV NS5 responsible for this suppression mechanism was mapped to the RdRp domain of NS5 [122]. The minimal linear sequence required was mapped to residues 355–735 which overlap with the finger region and the eight conserved RdRp motifs [122]. The specific amino acids required lay within two noncontiguous stretches of amino acids: 374–380 within the finger domain and 624–647 within the palm domain [122]. When modeled on the crystal structure of the WNV RdRp, these two amino acid stretches are adjacent to one another, suggesting cooperative action [122].

It was later determined that LGTV and TBEV NS5s also interact with prolidase (PEPD), a host protein that is required for IFNAR1 maturation [109]. This interaction was mapped to the same region as that required for LGTV NS5-mediated STAT1 phosphorylation inhibition [121]. STAT1, STAT2, Tyk2, and JAK1 phosphorylation occur downstream of IFNAR1, so this NS5 interaction elucidated the mechanism of NS5-mediated IFN suppression in addition to the mechanism of IFNAR1 downregulation. LGTV and TBEV NS5s are also known to interact with IFNAR2 and IFNGR1, but the function of these interactions is still unknown [121].

TBEV NS5 has also been shown to interact with the mammalian membrane protein Scribble which has been implicated in T cell activation [123]. The interaction was mapped to the MTase domain of TBEV NS5 and the PSD-95, Discs-large, ZO-1 domain 4 (PDZ4) of Scribble [123]. In IFN-stimulated cells depleted for Scribble, phosphorylation and nuclear localization of STAT1 was restored [123].

WNV NS5, like LGTV and TBEV, was also shown to interact with PEPD to downregulate IFNAR expression [110]. This interaction may be the mechanism by which WNV NS5 inhibits STAT1 and STAT2 phosphorylation, but further investigation is required for this conclusion [3,108].

9. Summary

Effective inhibition of type I IFN production is necessary for flaviviruses to establish infection in mammalian hosts. The viral non-structural proteins have evolved to be multi-functional, encoding diverse IFN suppression mechanisms in addition to their essential roles in the viral life cycle. NS5 is one of the most important IFN-I antagonists. Three of the most pervasive disease-causing flaviviruses—YFV, ZIKV, and DENV—inhibit human STAT2 through NS5-hSTAT2 interaction. Detailed mechanistic understanding of these interactions provides at least two opportunities for translational research. First, recombinant viruses that incorporate loss-of-function mutations in NS5 are attractive candidates for live-attenuated vaccine strains. Second, antivirals that target the NS5-hSTAT2 interaction would inhibit an early step common to these flaviviruses, despite divergent downstream mechanisms employed by the NS5s. These applications require deeper mechanistic understandings of the interaction between NS5 and hSTAT2.

Acknowledgments: We apologize to those with relevant work who could not be discussed/cited due to space limitations. This research was supported by UCR Regent Fellowships to R.H. and J.S. and provided in part by the National Institutes of Health grant 1R35GM11972 to J.S.

Conflicts of Interest: The authors declare no conflict of interest.

References

1. Daep, C.A.; Muñoz-Jordán, J.L.; Eugenin, E.A. Flaviviruses, an expanding threat in public health: Focus on dengue, West Nile, and Japanese encephalitis virus. *J. Neurovirol.* **2014**, *20*, 539–560. [CrossRef] [PubMed]
2. Miorin, L.; Maestre, A.M.; Fernandez-Sesma, A.; García-Sastre, A. Antagonism of type I interferon by flaviviruses. *Biochem. Biophys. Res. Commun.* **2017**, *492*, 587–596. [CrossRef] [PubMed]
3. Grant, A.; Ponia, S.S.; Tripathi, S.; Balasubramaniam, V.; Miorin, L.; Sourisseau, M.; Schwarz, M.C.; Sánchez-Seco, M.P.; Evans, M.J.; Best, S.M.; et al. Zika Virus Targets Human STAT2 to Inhibit Type I Interferon Signaling. *Cell Host and Microbe* **2016**, 1–10. [CrossRef] [PubMed]
4. Keller, B.C.; Fredericksen, B.L.; Samuel, M.A.; Mock, R.E.; Mason, P.W.; Diamond, M.S.; Gale, M. Resistance to alpha/beta interferon is a determinant of West Nile virus replication fitness and virulence. *J. Virol.* **2006**, *80*, 9424–9434. [CrossRef] [PubMed]

5. Bradrick, S.S. Causes and Consequences of Flavivirus RNA Methylation. *Front. Microbiol.* **2017**, *8*, 2374. [CrossRef] [PubMed]
6. Chambers, T.J.; Hahn, C.S.; Galler, R.; Rice, C.M. Flavivirus genome organization, expression, and replication. *Annu. Rev. Microbiol.* **1990**, *44*, 649–688. [CrossRef] [PubMed]
7. Best, S.M. The Many Faces of the Flavivirus NS5 Protein in Antagonism of Type I Interferon Signaling. *J. Virol.* **2017**, *91*, e01970-16. [CrossRef]
8. Gaunt, M.W.; Sall, A.A.; de Lamballerie, X.; Falconar, A.K.; Dzhivanian, T.I.; Gould, E.A. Phylogenetic relationships of flaviviruses correlate with their epidemiology, disease association and biogeography. *J. Gen. Virol.* **2001**, *82*, 1867–1876. [CrossRef]
9. Screaton, G.; Mongkolsapaya, J.; Yacoub, S.; Roberts, C. New insights into the immunopathology and control of dengue virus infection. *Nat. Rev. Microbiol.* **2015**, *15*, 745–759. [CrossRef]
10. Krauer, F.; Riesen, M.; Reveiz, L.; Oladapo, O.T.; Martínez-Vega, R.; Porgo, T.V.; Haefliger, A.; Broutet, N.J.; Low, N.; WHO. Zika Virus Infection as a Cause of Congenital Brain Abnormalities and Guillain-Barré Syndrome: Systematic Review. *PLoS Med.* **2017**, *14*, e1002203. [CrossRef]
11. Nash, D.; Mostashari, F.; Fine, A.; Miller, J.; O'Leary, D.; Murray, K.; Huang, A.; Rosenberg, A.; Greenberg, A.; Sherman, M.; et al. The outbreak of West Nile virus infection in the New York City area in 1999. *N. Engl. J. Med.* **2001**, *344*, 1807–1814. [CrossRef] [PubMed]
12. Petersen, L.R.; Brault, A.C.; Nasci, R.S. West Nile virus: Review of the literature. *JAMA* **2013**, *310*, 308–315. [CrossRef] [PubMed]
13. Nene, V.; Wortman, J.R.; Lawson, D.; Haas, B.; Kodira, C.; Tu, Z.J.; Loftus, B.; Xi, Z.; Megy, K.; Grabherr, M. Genome sequence of Aedes aegypti, a major arbovirus vector. *Science* **2007**, *316*, 1718–1723. [CrossRef] [PubMed]
14. Rosen, L. The natural history of Japanese encephalitis virus. *Annu. Rev. Microbiol.* **1986**, *40*, 395–414. [CrossRef] [PubMed]
15. Hayes, E.B.; Komar, N.; Nasci, R.S.; Montgomery, S.P.; O'Leary, D.R.; Campbell, G.L. Epidemiology and transmission dynamics of West Nile virus disease. *Emerg. Infect. Dis.* **2005**, *11*, 1167–1173. [CrossRef] [PubMed]
16. Solomon, T.; Dung, N.M.; Kneen, R.; Gainsborough, M.; Vaughn, D.W.; Khanh, V.T. Japanese encephalitis. *J. Neurol. Neurosurg. Psychiatry* **2000**, *68*, 405–415. [CrossRef] [PubMed]
17. Duffy, M.R.; Chen, T.-H.; Hancock, W.T.; Powers, A.M.; Kool, J.L.; Lanciotti, R.S.; Pretrick, M.; Marfel, M.; Holzbauer, S.; Dubray, C. Zika virus outbreak on Yap Island, Federated States of Micronesia. *N. Engl. J. Med.* **2009**, *360*, 2536–2543. [CrossRef]
18. Vasilakis, N.; Weaver, S.C. Flavivirus transmission focusing on Zika. *Curr. Opin. Virol.* **2017**, *22*, 30–35. [CrossRef]
19. Foy, B.D.; Kobylinski, K.C.; Chilson Foy, J.L.; Blitvich, B.J.; Travassos da Rosa, A.; Haddow, A.D.; Lanciotti, R.S.; Tesh, R.B. Probable non-vector-borne transmission of Zika virus, Colorado, USA. *Emerg. Infect. Dis.* **2011**, *17*, 880–882. [CrossRef]
20. Petersen, E.E.; Staples, J.E.; Meaney-Delman, D.; Fischer, M.; Ellington, S.R.; Callaghan, W.M.; Jamieson, D.J. Interim Guidelines for Pregnant Women during a Zika Virus Outbreak—United States, 2016. *Morb. Mortal. Wkly. Rep.* **2016**, *65*, 30–33. [CrossRef]
21. Aguirre, S.; Luthra, P.; Sánchez-Aparicio, M.T.; Maestre, A.M.; Patel, J.; Lamothe, F.; Fredericks, A.C.; Tripathi, S.; Zhu, T.; Pintado-Silva, J. Dengue virus NS2B protein targets cGAS for degradation and prevents mitochondrial DNA sensing during infection. *Nat. Microbiol.* **2017**, *2*, 17037. [CrossRef] [PubMed]
22. Stabell, A.C.; Meyerson, N.R.; Gullberg, R.C.; Gilchrist, A.R.; Webb, K.J.; Old, W.M.; Perera, R.; Sawyer, S.L. Dengue viruses cleave STING in humans but not in nonhuman primates, their presumed natural reservoir. *Elife* **2018**, *7*, e31919. [CrossRef] [PubMed]
23. Cassetti, M.C.; Durbin, A.; Harris, E.; Rico-Hesse, R.; Roehrig, J.; Rothman, A.; Whitehead, S.; Natarajan, R.; Laughlin, C. Report of an NIAID workshop on dengue animal models. *Vaccine* **2010**, *28*, 4229–4234. [CrossRef] [PubMed]
24. Zompi, S.; Harris, E. Animal Models of Dengue Virus Infection. *Viruses* **2012**, *4*, 62–82. [CrossRef] [PubMed]
25. Ashour, J.; Morrison, J.; Laurent-Rolle, M.; Belicha-Villanueva, A.; Plumlee, C.R.; Bernal-Rubio, D.; Williams, K.L.; Harris, E.; Fernandez-Sesma, A.; Schindler, C. Mouse STAT2 Restricts Early Dengue Virus Replication. *Cell Host Microbe* **2010**, *8*, 410–421. [CrossRef] [PubMed]

26. Dowall, S.D.; Graham, V.A.; Rayner, E.; Atkinson, B.; Hall, G.; Watson, R.J.; Bosworth, A.; Bonney, L.C.; Kitchen, S.; Hewson, R. A Susceptible Mouse Model for Zika Virus Infection. *PLoS Negl. Trop. Dis.* **2016**, *10*, e0004658. [CrossRef] [PubMed]

27. Ziv, O.; Gabryelska, M.M.; Lun, A.T.L.; Gebert, L.F.R.; Sheu-Gruttadauria, J.; Meredith, L.W.; Liu, Z.-Y.; Kwok, C.K.; Qin, C.-F.; MacRae, I.J.; et al. COMRADES determines in vivo RNA structures and interactions. *Nat. Methods* **2018**, *15*, 785–788. [CrossRef]

28. Dethoff, E.A.; Boerneke, M.A.; Gokhale, N.S.; Muhire, B.M.; Martin, D.P.; Sacco, M.T.; McFadden, M.J.; Weinstein, J.B.; Messer, W.B.; Horner, S.M.; et al. Pervasive tertiary structure in the dengue virus RNA genome. *Proc. Natl. Acad. Sci. USA* **2018**, *115*, 11513–11518. [CrossRef]

29. Issur, M.; Geiss, B.J.; Bougie, I.; Picard-Jean, F.; Despins, S.; Mayette, J.; Hobdey, S.E.; Bisaillon, M. The flavivirus NS5 protein is a true RNA guanylyltransferase that catalyzes a two-step reaction to form the RNA cap structure. *RNA* **2009**, *15*, 2340–2350. [CrossRef]

30. Smit, J.M.; Moesker, B.; Rodenhuis-Zybert, I.; Wilschut, J. Flavivirus cell entry and membrane fusion. *Viruses* **2011**, *3*, 160–171. [CrossRef]

31. Fensterl, V.; Chattopadhyay, S.; Sen, G.C. No Love Lost Between Viruses and Interferons. *Annu. Rev. Virol.* **2015**, *2*, 549–572. [CrossRef] [PubMed]

32. Kurane, I.; Innis, B.L.; Nimmannitya, S.; Nisalak, A.; Meager, A.; Ennis, F.A. High levels of interferon alpha in the sera of children with dengue virus infection. *Am. J. Trop. Med. Hyg.* **1993**, *48*, 222–229. [CrossRef] [PubMed]

33. Simmons, C.P.; Popper, S.; Dolocek, C.; Chau, T.N.B.; Griffiths, M.; Dung, N.T.P.; Long, T.H.; Hoang, D.M.; Chau, N.V.; Thao, L.T.T.; et al. Patterns of host genome-wide gene transcript abundance in the peripheral blood of patients with acute dengue hemorrhagic fever. *J. Infect. Dis.* **2007**, *195*, 1097–1107. [CrossRef] [PubMed]

34. Becquart, P.; Wauquier, N.; Nkoghe, D.; Ndjoyi-Mbiguino, A.; Padilla, C.; Souris, M.; Leroy, E.M. Acute dengue virus 2 infection in Gabonese patients is associated with an early innate immune response, including strong interferon alpha production. *BMC Infect. Dis.* **2010**, *10*, 356. [CrossRef]

35. Tolfvenstam, T.; Lindblom, A.; Schreiber, M.J.; Ling, L.; Chow, A.; Ooi, E.E.; Hibberd, M.L. Characterization of early host responses in adults with dengue disease. *BMC Infect. Dis.* **2011**, *11*, 209. [CrossRef] [PubMed]

36. Sun, P.; García, J.; Comach, G.; Vahey, M.T.; Wang, Z.; Forshey, B.M.; Morrison, A.C.; Sierra, G.; Bazan, I.; Rocha, C.; Vilcarromero, S.; et al. Sequential waves of gene expression in patients with clinically defined dengue illnesses reveal subtle disease phases and predict disease severity. *PLoS Negl. Trop. Dis.* **2013**, *7*, e2298. [CrossRef]

37. Jiang, D.; Weidner, J.M.; Qing, M.; Pan, X.-B.; Guo, H.; Xu, C.; Zhang, X.; Birk, A.; Chang, J.; Shi, P.-Y.; et al. Identification of Five Interferon-Induced Cellular Proteins That Inhibit West Nile Virus and Dengue Virus Infections. *J. Virol.* **2010**, *84*, 8332–8341. [CrossRef]

38. Helbig, K.J.; Carr, J.M.; Calvert, J.K.; Wati, S.; Clarke, J.N.; Eyre, N.S.; Narayana, S.K.; Fiches, G.N.; McCartney, E.M.; Beard, M.R. Viperin is induced following dengue virus type-2 (DENV-2) infection and has anti-viral actions requiring the C-terminal end of viperin. *PLoS Negl. Trop. Dis.* **2013**, *7*, e2178. [CrossRef]

39. Chang, T.-H.; Liao, C.-L.; Lin, Y.-L. Flavivirus induces interferon-beta gene expression through a pathway involving RIG-I-dependent IRF-3 and PI3K-dependent NF-kappaB activation. *Microbes Infect.* **2006**, *8*, 157–171. [CrossRef]

40. Brass, A.L.; Huang, I.-C.; Benita, Y.; John, S.P.; Krishnan, M.N.; Feeley, E.M.; Ryan, B.J.; Weyer, J.L.; van der Weyden, L.; Fikrig, E.; et al. The IFITM proteins mediate cellular resistance to influenza A H1N1 virus, West Nile virus, and dengue virus. *Cell* **2009**, *139*, 1243–1254. [CrossRef]

41. Lin, R.-J.; Yu, H.-P.; Chang, B.-L.; Tang, W.-C.; Liao, C.-L.; Lin, Y.-L. Distinct antiviral roles for human 2′,5′-oligoadenylate synthetase family members against dengue virus infection. *J. Immunol.* **2009**, *183*, 8035–8043. [CrossRef] [PubMed]

42. Manns, M.P.; McHutchison, J.G.; Gordon, S.C.; Rustgi, V.K.; Shiffman, M.; Reindollar, R.; Goodman, Z.D.; Koury, K.; Ling, M.-H.; Albrecht, J.K. Peginterferon alfa-2b plus ribavirin compared with interferon alfa-2b plus ribavirin for initial treatment of chronic hepatitis C: A randomised trial. *Lancet* **2001**, *358*, 958–965. [CrossRef]

43. Solomon, T.; Dung, N.M.; Wills, B.; Kneen, R.; Gainsborough, M.; Diet, T.V.; Thuy, T.T.N.; Loan, H.T.; Khanh, V.C.; Vaughn, D.W.; et al. Interferon alfa-2a in Japanese encephalitis: A randomised double-blind placebo-controlled trial. *Lancet* **2003**, *361*, 821–826. [CrossRef]

44. Nasirudeen, A.M.A.; Wong, H.H.; Thien, P.; Xu, S.; Lam, K.-P.; Liu, D.X. RIG-I, MDA5 and TLR3 synergistically play an important role in restriction of dengue virus infection. *PLoS Negl. Trop. Dis.* **2011**, *5*, e926. [CrossRef]

45. Wang, J.P.; Liu, P.; Latz, E.; Golenbock, D.T.; Finberg, R.W.; Libraty, D.H. Flavivirus Activation of Plasmacytoid Dendritic Cells Delineates Key Elements of TLR7 Signaling beyond Endosomal Recognition. *J. Immunol.* **2006**, *177*, 7114–7121. [CrossRef]

46. Suthar, M.S.; Aguirre, S.; Fernandez-Sesma, A. Innate immune sensing of flaviviruses. *PLoS Pathog.* **2013**, *9*, e1003541. [CrossRef]

47. Seth, R.B.; Sun, L.; Ea, C.-K.; Chen, Z.J. Identification and characterization of MAVS, a mitochondrial antiviral signaling protein that activates NF-kappaB and IRF 3. *Cell* **2005**, *122*, 669–682. [CrossRef]

48. Bhattacharya, S.; Eckner, R.; Grossman, S.; Oldread, E.; Arany, Z.; D'Andrea, A.; Livingston, D.M. Cooperation of Stat2 and p300/CBP in signalling induced by interferon-α. *Nature* **1996**, *383*, 344–347. [CrossRef]

49. Martinez-Moczygemba, M.; Gutch, M.J.; French, D.L.; Reich, N.C. Distinct STAT Structure Promotes Interaction of STAT2 with the p48 Subunit of the Interferon-α-stimulated Transcription Factor ISGF3. *J. Biol. Chem.* **1997**, *272*, 20070–20076. [CrossRef]

50. Yoshimura, A.; Naka, T.; Kubo, M. SOCS proteins, cytokine signalling and immune regulation. *Nat. Rev. Immunol.* **2007**, *7*, 454–465. [CrossRef]

51. Cheon, H.; Stark, G.R. Unphosphorylated STAT1 prolongs the expression of interferon-induced immune regulatory genes. *Proc. Natl. Acad. Sci. USA* **2009**, *106*, 9373–9378. [CrossRef] [PubMed]

52. Cheon, H.; Holvey-Bates, E.G.; Schoggins, J.W.; Forster, S.; Hertzog, P.; Imanaka, N.; Rice, C.M.; Jackson, M.W.; Junk, D.J.; Stark, G.R. IFNβ-dependent increases in STAT1, STAT2, and IRF9 mediate resistance to viruses and DNA damage. *EMBO J.* **2013**, *32*, 2751–2763. [CrossRef] [PubMed]

53. Blaszczyk, K.; Nowicka, H.; Kostyrko, K.; Antonczyk, A.; Wesoly, J.; Bluyssen, H.A.R. The unique role of STAT2 in constitutive and IFN-induced transcription and antiviral responses. *Cytokine Growth Factor Rev.* **2016**, *29*, 71–81. [CrossRef] [PubMed]

54. Bluyssen, H.A.R.; Levy, D.E. Stat2 Is a Transcriptional Activator That Requires Sequence-specific Contacts Provided by Stat1 and p48 for Stable Interaction with DNA. *J. Biol. Chem.* **1997**, *272*, 4600–4605. [CrossRef] [PubMed]

55. Blaszczyk, K.; Olejnik, A.; Nowicka, H.; Ozgyin, L.; Chen, Y.-L.; Chmielewski, S.; Kostyrko, K.; Wesoly, J.; Balint, B.L.; Lee, C.-K.; et al. STAT2/IRF9 directs a prolonged ISGF3-like transcriptional response and antiviral activity in the absence of STAT1. *Biochem. J.* **2015**, *466*, 511–524. [CrossRef]

56. Hahm, B.; Trifilo, M.J.; Zuniga, E.I.; Oldstone, M.B.A. Viruses evade the immune system through type I interferon-mediated STAT2-dependent, but STAT1-independent, signaling. *Immunity* **2005**, *22*, 247–257. [CrossRef]

57. Ousman, S.S.; Wang, J.; Campbell, I.L. Differential regulation of interferon regulatory factor (IRF)-7 and IRF-9 gene expression in the central nervous system during viral infection. *J. Virol.* **2005**, *79*, 7514–7527. [CrossRef]

58. Perry, S.T.; Buck, M.D.; Lada, S.M.; Schindler, C.; Shresta, S. STAT2 mediates innate immunity to Dengue virus in the absence of STAT1 via the type I interferon receptor. *PLoS Pathog.* **2011**, *7*, e1001297. [CrossRef]

59. Bowick, G.C.; Airo, A.M.; Bente, D.A. Expression of interferon-induced antiviral genes is delayed in a STAT1 knockout mouse model of Crimean-Congo hemorrhagic fever. *Virol. J.* **2012**, *9*, 122. [CrossRef]

60. Sun, L.; Wu, J.; Du, F.; Chen, X.; Chen, Z.J. Cyclic GMP-AMP synthase is a cytosolic DNA sensor that activates the type I interferon pathway. *Science* **2013**, *339*, 786–791. [CrossRef]

61. Sun, B.; Sundström, K.B.; Chew, J.J.; Bist, P.; Gan, E.S.; Tan, H.C.; Goh, K.C.; Chawla, T.; Tang, C.K.; Ooi, E.E. Dengue virus activates cGAS through the release of mitochondrial DNA. *Sci. Rep.* **2017**, *7*, 3594. [CrossRef] [PubMed]

62. Lazear, H.M.; Nice, T.J.; Diamond, M.S. Interferon-λ: Immune Functions at Barrier Surfaces and Beyond. *Immunity* **2015**, *43*, 15–28. [CrossRef] [PubMed]

63. Lazear, H.M.; Daniels, B.P.; Pinto, A.K.; Huang, A.C.; Vick, S.C.; Doyle, S.E.; Gale, M.; Klein, R.S.; Diamond, M.S. Interferon-λ restricts West Nile virus neuroinvasion by tightening the blood-brain barrier. *Sci. Transl. Med.* **2015**, *7*, 284ra59. [CrossRef] [PubMed]

64. Bayer, A.; Lennemann, N.J.; Ouyang, Y.; Bramley, J.C.; Morosky, S.; De Azeved Marques, E.T., Jr.; Cherry, S.; Sadovsky, Y.; Coyne, C.B. Type III Interferons Produced by Human Placental Trophoblasts Confer Protection against Zika Virus Infection. *Cell Host Microbe* **2016**, *19*, 705–712. [CrossRef] [PubMed]

65. Chaudhary, V.; Yuen, K.-S.; Chan, J.F.-W.; Chan, C.-P.; Wang, P.-H.; Cai, J.-P.; Zhang, S.; Liang, M.; Kok, K.-H.; Chan, C.-P.; et al. Selective Activation of Type II Interferon Signaling by Zika Virus NS5 Protein. *J. Virol.* **2017**, *91*, e00163-17. [CrossRef]

66. Pingen, M.; Bryden, S.R.; Pondeville, E.; Schnettler, E.; Kohl, A.; Merits, A.; Fazakerley, J.K.; Graham, G.J.; McKimmie, C.S. Host Inflammatory Response to Mosquito Bites Enhances the Severity of Arbovirus Infection. *Immunity* **2016**, *44*, 1455–1469. [CrossRef]

67. Diamond, M.S.; Farzan, M. The broad-spectrum antiviral functions of IFIT and IFITM proteins. *Nat. Rev. Immunol.* **2013**, *13*, 46–57. [CrossRef]

68. Welsch, S.; Miller, S.; Romero-Brey, I.; Merz, A.; Bleck, C.K.E.; Walther, P.; Fuller, S.D.; Antony, C.; Krijnse-Locker, J.; Bartenschlager, R. Composition and three-dimensional architecture of the dengue virus replication and assembly sites. *Cell Host Microbe* **2009**, *5*, 365–375. [CrossRef]

69. Gillespie, L.K.; Hoenen, A.; Morgan, G.; Mackenzie, J.M. The endoplasmic reticulum provides the membrane platform for biogenesis of the flavivirus replication complex. *J. Virol.* **2010**, *84*, 10438–10447. [CrossRef]

70. Fredericksen, B.L.; Gale, M. West Nile virus evades activation of interferon regulatory factor 3 through RIG-I-dependent and -independent pathways without antagonizing host defense signaling. *J. Virol.* **2006**, *80*, 2913–2923. [CrossRef]

71. Muñoz-Jordán, J.L.; Sánchez-Burgos, G.G.; Laurent-Rolle, M.; García-Sastre, A. Inhibition of interferon signaling by dengue virus. *Proc. Natl. Acad. Sci. USA* **2003**, *100*, 14333–14338. [CrossRef] [PubMed]

72. Muñoz-Jordán, J.L.; Laurent-Rolle, M.; Ashour, J.; Martínez-Sobrido, L.; Ashok, M.; Lipkin, W.I.; García-Sastre, A. Inhibition of alpha/beta interferon signaling by the NS4B protein of flaviviruses. *J. Virol.* **2005**, *79*, 8004–8013. [CrossRef] [PubMed]

73. Liu, W.J.; Wang, X.J.; Mokhonov, V.V.; Shi, P.Y.; Randall, R.; Khromykh, A.A. Inhibition of Interferon Signaling by the New York 99 Strain and Kunjin Subtype of West Nile Virus Involves Blockage of STAT1 and STAT2 Activation by Nonstructural Proteins. *J. Virol.* **2005**, *79*, 1934–1942. [CrossRef] [PubMed]

74. Slonchak, A.; Khromykh, A.A. Subgenomic flaviviral RNAs: What do we know after the first decade of research. *Antivir. Res.* **2018**, *159*, 13–25. [CrossRef] [PubMed]

75. Gack, M.U.; Shin, Y.C.; Joo, C.-H.; Urano, T.; Liang, C.; Sun, L.; Takeuchi, O.; Akira, S.; Chen, Z.; Inoue, S.; et al. TRIM25 RING-finger E3 ubiquitin ligase is essential for RIG-I-mediated antiviral activity. *Nature* **2007**, *446*, 916–920. [CrossRef] [PubMed]

76. Manokaran, G.; Finol, E.; Wang, C.; Gunaratne, J.; Bahl, J.; Ong, E.Z.; Tan, H.C.; Sessions, O.M.; Ward, A.M.; Gubler, D.J.; et al. Dengue subgenomic RNA binds TRIM25 to inhibit interferon expression for epidemiological fitness. *Science* **2015**, *350*, 217–221. [CrossRef]

77. Chan, Y.K.; Gack, M.U. A phosphomimetic-based mechanism of dengue virus to antagonize innate immunity. *Nat. Immunol.* **2016**, *17*, 523–530. [CrossRef]

78. He, Z.; Zhu, X.; Wen, W.; Yuan, J.; Hu, Y.; Chen, J.; An, S.; Dong, X.; Lin, C.; Yu, J.; et al. Dengue Virus Subverts Host Innate Immunity by Targeting Adaptor Protein MAVS. *J. Virol.* **2016**, *90*, 7219–7230. [CrossRef]

79. Wang, B.; Tan, X.-F.; Thurmond, S.; Zhang, Z.-M.; Lin, A.; Hai, R.; Song, J. The structure of Zika virus NS5 reveals a conserved domain conformation. *Nat. Commun.* **2017**, *8*, 14763. [CrossRef]

80. Ackermann, M.; Padmanabhan, R. De novo synthesis of RNA by the dengue virus RNA-dependent RNA polymerase exhibits temperature dependence at the initiation but not elongation phase. *J. Biol. Chem.* **2001**, *276*, 39926–39937. [CrossRef]

81. Kao, C.C.; Singh, P.; Ecker, D.J. De Novo Initiation of Viral RNA-Dependent RNA Synthesis. *Virology* **2001**, *287*, 251–260. [CrossRef] [PubMed]

82. Malet, H.; Massé, N.; Selisko, B.; Romette, J.-L.; Alvarez, K.; Guillemot, J.C.; Tolou, H.; Yap, T.L.; Vasudevan, S.; Lescar, J.; et al. The flavivirus polymerase as a target for drug discovery. *Antivir. Res.* **2008**, *80*, 23–35. [CrossRef] [PubMed]

83. Selisko, B.; Potisopon, S.; Agred, R.; Priet, S.; Varlet, I.; Thillier, Y.; Sallamand, C.; Debart, F.; Vasseur, J.-J.; Canard, B. Molecular basis for nucleotide conservation at the ends of the dengue virus genome. *PLoS Pathog.* **2012**, *8*, e1002912. [CrossRef]

84. Lu, G.; Gong, P. Crystal Structure of the full-length Japanese encephalitis virus NS5 reveals a conserved methyltransferase-polymerase interface. *PLoS Pathog.* **2013**, *9*, e1003549. [CrossRef]

85. Zhao, Y.; Soh, T.S.; Zheng, J.; Chan, K.W.K.; Phoo, W.W.; Lee, C.C.; Tay, M.Y.F.; Swaminathan, K.; Cornvik, T.C.; Lim, S.P.; et al. A crystal structure of the Dengue virus NS5 protein reveals a novel inter-domain interface essential for protein flexibility and virus replication. *PLoS Pathog.* **2015**, *11*, e1004682. [CrossRef] [PubMed]

86. Upadhyay, A.K.; Cyr, M.; Longenecker, K.; Tripathi, R.; Sun, C.; Kempf, D.J. Crystal structure of full-length Zika virus NS5 protein reveals a conformation similar to Japanese encephalitis virus NS5. *Acta Crystallogr. F Struct. Biol. Commun.* **2017**, *73*, 116–122. [CrossRef]

87. Zhao, B.; Yi, G.; Du, F.; Chuang, Y.-C.; Vaughan, R.C.; Sankaran, B.; Kao, C.C.; Li, P. Structure and function of the Zika virus full-length NS5 protein. *Nat. Commun.* **2017**, *8*, 14762. [CrossRef] [PubMed]

88. Bussetta, C.; Choi, K.H. Dengue virus nonstructural protein 5 adopts multiple conformations in solution. *Biochemistry* **2012**, *51*, 5921–5931. [CrossRef] [PubMed]

89. Potisopon, S.; Priet, S.; Collet, A.; Decroly, E.; Canard, B.; Selisko, B. The methyltransferase domain of dengue virus protein NS5 ensures efficient RNA synthesis initiation and elongation by the polymerase domain. *Nucleic Acids Res.* **2014**, *42*, 11642–11656. [CrossRef]

90. Morozova, O.V.; Tsekhanovskaya, N.A.; Maksimova, T.G.; Bachvalova, V.N.; Matveeva, V.A.; Kit, Y.Y. Phosphorylation of tick-borne encephalitis virus NS5 protein. *Virus Res.* **1997**, *49*, 9–15. [CrossRef]

91. Reed, K.E.; Gorbalenya, A.E.; Rice, C.M. The NS5A/NS5 proteins of viruses from three genera of the family flaviviridae are phosphorylated by associated serine/threonine kinases. *J. Virol.* **1998**, *72*, 6199–6206.

92. Bhattacharya, D.; Mayuri; Best, S.M.; Perera, R.; Kuhn, R.J.; Striker, R. Protein kinase G phosphorylates mosquito-borne flavivirus NS5. *J. Virol.* **2009**, *83*, 9195–9205. [CrossRef] [PubMed]

93. Keating, J.A.; Bhattacharya, D.; Rund, S.S.C.; Hoover, S.; Dasgupta, R.; Lee, S.J.; Duffield, G.E.; Striker, R. Mosquito protein kinase G phosphorylates flavivirus NS5 and alters flight behavior in Aedes aegypti and Anopheles gambiae. *Vector Borne Zoonotic Dis.* **2013**, *13*, 590–600. [CrossRef] [PubMed]

94. Kapoor, M.; Zhang, L.; Ramachandra, M.; Kusukawa, J.; Ebner, K.E.; Padmanabhan, R. Association between NS3 and NS5 Proteins of Dengue Virus Type 2 in the Putative RNA Replicase Is Linked to Differential Phosphorylation of NS5. *J. Biol. Chem.* **1995**, *270*, 19100–19106. [CrossRef]

95. Keating, J.A.; Bhattacharya, D.; Lim, P.-Y.; Falk, S.; Weisblum, B.; Bernard, K.A.; Sharma, M.; Kuhn, R.J.; Striker, R. West Nile virus methyltransferase domain interacts with protein kinase G. *Virol. J.* **2013**, *10*, 242. [CrossRef] [PubMed]

96. Su, C.-I.; Tseng, C.-H.; Yu, C.-Y.; Lai, M.M.C. SUMO Modification Stabilizes Dengue Virus Nonstructural Protein 5 to Support Virus Replication. *J. Virol.* **2016**, *90*, 4308–4319. [CrossRef]

97. Saisawang, C.; Kuadkitkan, A.; Auewarakul, P.; Smith, D.R.; Ketterman, A.J. Glutathionylation of dengue and Zika NS5 proteins affects guanylyltransferase and RNA dependent RNA polymerase activities. *PLoS ONE* **2018**, *13*, e0193133. [CrossRef]

98. Westaway, E.G.; Brinton, M.A.; Gaidamovich, S.Y.; Horzinek, M.C.; Igarashi, A.; Kääriäinen, L.; Lvov, D.K.; Porterfield, J.S.; Russell, P.K.; Trent, D.W. Flaviviridae. *Intervirology* **1985**, *24*, 183–192. [CrossRef]

99. Buckley, A.; Gaidamovich, S.; Turchinskaya, A.; Gould, E.A. Monoclonal antibodies identify the NS5 yellow fever virus non-structural protein in the nuclei of infected cells. *J. Gen. Virol.* **1992**, *73 Pt 5*, 1125–1130. [CrossRef]

100. Uchil, P.D.; Kumar, A.V.A.; Satchidanandam, V. Nuclear localization of flavivirus RNA synthesis in infected cells. *J. Virol.* **2006**, *80*, 5451–5464. [CrossRef]

101. Lopez-Denman, A.J.; Russo, A.; Wagstaff, K.M.; White, P.A.; Jans, D.A.; Mackenzie, J.M. Nucleocytoplasmic shuttling of the West Nile virus RNA-dependent RNA polymerase NS5 is critical to infection. *Cell Microbiol.* **2018**, *20*, e12848. [CrossRef] [PubMed]

102. Pryor, M.J.; Rawlinson, S.M.; Butcher, R.E.; Barton, C.L.; Waterhouse, T.A.; Vasudevan, S.G.; Bardin, P.G.; Wright, P.J.; Jans, D.A.; Davidson, A.D. Nuclear localization of dengue virus nonstructural protein 5 through its importin alpha/beta-recognized nuclear localization sequences is integral to viral infection. *Traffic* **2007**, *8*, 795–807. [CrossRef] [PubMed]

103. Wagstaff, K.M.; Sivakumaran, H.; Heaton, S.M.; Harrich, D.; Jans, D.A. Ivermectin is a specific inhibitor of importin α/β-mediated nuclear import able to inhibit replication of HIV-1 and dengue virus. *Biochem. J.* **2012**, *443*, 851–856. [CrossRef] [PubMed]

104. Petering, H.; Götze, O.; Kimmig, D.; Smolarski, R.; Kapp, A.; Elsner, J. The biologic role of interleukin-8: Functional analysis and expression of CXCR1 and CXCR2 on human eosinophils. *Blood* **1999**, *93*, 694–702. [PubMed]

105. Rawlinson, S.M.; Pryor, M.J.; Wright, P.J.; Jans, D.A. CRM1-mediated Nuclear Export of Dengue Virus RNA Polymerase NS5 Modulates Interleukin-8 Induction and Virus Production. *J. Biol. Chem.* **2009**, *284*, 15589–15597. [CrossRef] [PubMed]

106. De Maio, F.A.; Risso, G.; Iglesias, N.G.; Shah, P.; Pozzi, B.; Gebhard, L.G.; Mammi, P.; Mancini, E.; Yanovsky, M.J.; Andino, R.; et al. The Dengue Virus NS5 Protein Intrudes in the Cellular Spliceosome and Modulates Splicing. *PLoS Pathog.* **2016**, *12*, e1005841. [CrossRef] [PubMed]

107. Hannemann, H.; Sung, P.-Y.; Chiu, H.-C.; Yousuf, A.; Bird, J.; Lim, S.P.; Davidson, A.D. Serotype-specific differences in dengue virus non-structural protein 5 nuclear localization. *J. Biol. Chem.* **2013**, *288*, 22621–22635. [CrossRef] [PubMed]

108. Laurent-Rolle, M.; Boer, E.F.; Lubick, K.J.; Wolfinbarger, J.B.; Carmody, A.B.; Rockx, B.; Liu, W.; Ashour, J.; Shupert, W.L.; Holbrook, M.R.; et al. The NS5 Protein of the Virulent West Nile Virus NY99 Strain Is a Potent Antagonist of Type I Interferon-Mediated JAK-STAT Signaling. *J. Virol.* **2010**, *84*, 3503–3515. [CrossRef] [PubMed]

109. Lubick, K.J.; Robertson, S.J.; McNally, K.L.; Freedman, B.A.; Rasmussen, A.L.; Taylor, R.T.; Walts, A.D.; Tsuruda, S.; Sakai, M.; Ishizuka, M.; et al. Flavivirus Antagonism of Type I Interferon Signaling Reveals Prolidase as a Regulator of IFNAR1 Surface Expression. *Cell Host Microbe* **2015**, *18*, 61–74. [CrossRef] [PubMed]

110. Mazzon, M.; Jones, M.; Davidson, A.; Chain, B.; Jacobs, M. Dengue virus NS5 inhibits interferon-alpha signaling by blocking signal transducer and activator of transcription 2 phosphorylation. *J. Infect. Dis.* **2009**, *200*, 1261–1270. [CrossRef] [PubMed]

111. Jones, M.; Davidson, A.; Hibbert, L.; Gruenwald, P.; Schlaak, J.; Ball, S.; Foster, G.R.; Jacobs, M. Dengue Virus Inhibits Alpha Interferon Signaling by Reducing STAT2 Expression. *J. Virol.* **2005**, *79*, 5414–5420. [CrossRef] [PubMed]

112. Ashour, J.; Laurent-Rolle, M.; Shi, P.-Y.; García-Sastre, A. NS5 of dengue virus mediates STAT2 binding and degradation. *J. Virol.* **2009**, *83*, 5408–5418. [CrossRef] [PubMed]

113. Morrison, J.; Laurent-Rolle, M.; Maestre, A.M.; Rajsbaum, R.; Pisanelli, G.; Simon, V.; Mulder, L.C.F.; Fernandez-Sesma, A.; García-Sastre, A. Dengue virus co-opts UBR4 to degrade STAT2 and antagonize type I interferon signaling. *PLoS Pathog.* **2013**, *9*, e1003265. [CrossRef] [PubMed]

114. Gibbs, D.J.; Bacardit, J.; Bachmair, A.; Holdsworth, M.J. The eukaryotic N-end rule pathway: Conserved mechanisms and diverse functions. *Trends Cell Biol.* **2014**, *24*, 603–611. [CrossRef] [PubMed]

115. Kumar, A.; Hou, S.; Airo, A.M.; Limonta, D.; Mancinelli, V.; Branton, W.; Power, C.; Hobman, T.C. Zika virus inhibits type-I interferon production and downstream signaling. *EMBO Rep.* **2016**, *17*, 1766–1775. [CrossRef] [PubMed]

116. Ho, J.; Pelzel, C.; Begitt, A.; Mee, M.; Elsheikha, H.M.; Scott, D.J.; Vinkemeier, U. STAT2 Is a Pervasive Cytokine Regulator due to Its Inhibition of STAT1 in Multiple Signaling Pathways. *PLoS Biol.* **2016**, *14*, e2000117. [CrossRef] [PubMed]

117. Laurent-Rolle, M.; Morrison, J.; Rajsbaum, R.; Macleod, J.M.L.; Pisanelli, G.; Pham, A.; Ayllon, J.; Miorin, L.; Martinez, C.; tenOever, B.R.; García-Sastre, A. The interferon signaling antagonist function of yellow fever virus NS5 protein is activated by type I interferon. *Cell Host Microbe* **2014**, *16*, 314–327. [CrossRef] [PubMed]

118. Grard, G.; Moureau, G.; Charrel, R.N.; Holmes, E.C.; Gould, E.A.; de Lamballerie, X. Genomics and evolution of Aedes-borne flaviviruses. *J. Gen. Virol.* **2010**, *91*, 87–94. [CrossRef] [PubMed]

119. Lin, R.J.; Chang, B.L.; Yu, H.P.; Liao, C.L.; Lin, Y.L. Blocking of Interferon-Induced Jak-Stat Signaling by Japanese Encephalitis Virus NS5 through a Protein Tyrosine Phosphatase-Mediated Mechanism. *J. Virol.* **2006**, *80*, 5908–5918. [CrossRef]

120. Ye, J.; Chen, Z.; Li, Y.; Zhao, Z.; He, W.; Zohaib, A.; Song, Y.; Deng, C.; Zhang, B.; Chen, H.; et al. Japanese Encephalitis Virus NS5 Inhibits Type I Interferon (IFN) Production by Blocking the Nuclear Translocation of IFN Regulatory Factor 3 and NF-κB. *J. Virol.* **2017**, *91*, e00039-17. [CrossRef]

121. Best, S.M.; Morris, K.L.; Shannon, J.G.; Robertson, S.J.; Mitzel, D.N.; Park, G.S.; Boer, E.; Wolfinbarger, J.B.; Bloom, M.E. Inhibition of interferon-stimulated JAK-STAT signaling by a tick-borne flavivirus and identification of NS5 as an interferon antagonist. *J. Virol.* **2005**, *79*, 12828–12839. [CrossRef] [PubMed]
122. Park, G.S.; Morris, K.L.; Hallett, R.G.; Bloom, M.E.; Best, S.M. Identification of residues critical for the interferon antagonist function of Langat virus NS5 reveals a role for the RNA-dependent RNA polymerase domain. *J. Virol.* **2007**, *81*, 6936–6946. [CrossRef] [PubMed]
123. Werme, K.; Wigerius, M.; Johansson, M. Tick-borne encephalitis virus NS5 associates with membrane protein scribble and impairs interferon-stimulated JAK-STAT signalling. *Cell Microbiol.* **2008**, *10*, 696–712. [CrossRef] [PubMed]

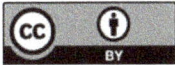

MDPI

Article

Functional Genomics and Immunologic Tools: The Impact of Viral and Host Genetic Variations on the Outcome of Zika Virus Infection

Sang-Im Yun [1,†], **Byung-Hak Song** [1,†], **Jordan C. Frank** [1,†], **Justin G. Julander** [1,2],
Aaron L. Olsen [1], **Irina A. Polejaeva** [1,3], **Christopher J. Davies** [1,3], **Kenneth L. White** [1,3]
and Young-Min Lee [1,3,*]

1   Department of Animal Dairy and Veterinary Sciences, College of Agriculture and Applied Sciences,
    Utah State University, Logan, UT 84322, USA; sangim.yun@usu.edu (S.-I.Y.);
    byunghak.song@aggiemail.usu.edu (B.-H.S.); jc.frank@aggiemail.usu.edu (J.C.F);
    justin.julander@usu.edu (J.G.J); aaron.olsen@usu.edu (A.L.O.); irina.polejaeva@usu.edu (I.A.P.);
    chris.davies@usu.edu (C.J.D.); ken.white@usu.edu (K.L.W.)
2   Institute for Antiviral Research, Utah State University, Logan, UT 84322, USA
3   Veterinary Diagnostics and Infectious Diseases, Utah Science Technology and Research,
    Utah State University, Logan, UT 84341, USA
*   Correspondence: youngmin.lee@usu.edu; Tel.: +1-435-797-9667
†   These authors contributed equally to this work.

Received: 30 June 2018; Accepted: 2 August 2018; Published: 11 August 2018

Abstract: Zika virus (ZIKV) causes no-to-mild symptoms or severe neurological disorders.
To investigate the importance of viral and host genetic variations in determining ZIKV infection
outcomes, we created three full-length infectious cDNA clones as bacterial artificial chromosomes
for each of three spatiotemporally distinct and genetically divergent ZIKVs: MR-766 (Uganda,
1947), P6-740 (Malaysia, 1966), and PRVABC-59 (Puerto Rico, 2015). Using the three molecularly
cloned ZIKVs, together with 13 ZIKV region-specific polyclonal antibodies covering nearly the entire
viral protein-coding region, we made three conceptual advances: (i) We created a comprehensive
genome-wide portrait of ZIKV gene products and their related species, with several previously
undescribed gene products identified in the case of all three molecularly cloned ZIKVs. (ii) We found
that ZIKV has a broad cell tropism in vitro, being capable of establishing productive infection in 16 of
17 animal cell lines from 12 different species, although its growth kinetics varied depending on both
the specific virus strain and host cell line. More importantly, we identified one ZIKV-non-susceptible
bovine cell line that has a block in viral entry but fully supports the subsequent post-entry steps.
(iii) We showed that in mice, the three molecularly cloned ZIKVs differ in their neuropathogenicity,
depending on the particular combination of viral and host genetic backgrounds, as well as in the
presence or absence of type I/II interferon signaling. Overall, our findings demonstrate the impact
of viral and host genetic variations on the replication kinetics and neuropathogenicity of ZIKV and
provide multiple avenues for developing and testing medical countermeasures against ZIKV.

Keywords: Zika virus; flavivirus; infectious cDNA; replication; gene expression; neuropathogenesis;
viral genetic variation; host genetic variation

---

1. Introduction

Discovered in Uganda in 1947 in a febrile rhesus macaque [1], Zika virus (ZIKV) is a medically
important flavivirus [2] related to Japanese encephalitis (JEV), West Nile (WNV), dengue, and yellow
fever viruses [3]. Originally, it was confined within an equatorial belt running from Africa to Asia,
with only about a dozen cases of human illness reported [4]. In 2007, however, it caused a major

outbreak of mild illness characterized by fever, rash, arthralgia, and conjunctivitis on the western Pacific Island of Yap [5,6]. Since then, it has spread eastward across the Pacific Ocean, invading French Polynesia and other Pacific Islands in 2013–2014 [7], reaching the Americas and Caribbean in 2015–2016 [8,9], and now threatening much of the world [10,11]. ZIKV is spread to humans mainly through the bite of an infected *Aedes* species mosquito, e.g., *Aedes aegypti* or *Aedes albopictus* [12], but it can also be transmitted from a mother to her child during pregnancy [13,14] or through sexual contact [15,16]. Serious concerns have been raised over links to congenital neurological malformations (e.g., microcephaly) and severe neurological complications (e.g., Guillain–Barré syndrome) [17,18]. Despite its continuous rapid spread and high pandemic potential, no vaccine or drug is available to prevent or treat ZIKV infection.

ZIKV is an enveloped RNA virus with a nucleocapsid core comprising an ~11 kb plus-strand RNA genome and multiple copies of the C protein; this core is surrounded by a lipid bilayer bearing the anchored M and E proteins [19,20]. With regard to the molecular events that occur during ZIKV infection, our current understanding of the molecular biology of closely related flaviviruses offers a promising starting point for ZIKV research [21]. As the first step in flavivirus replication, the virion binds to one or more cellular proteins on the surface of a host cell, and is then internalized via clathrin-mediated endocytosis in a viral glycoprotein E-dependent manner [22–24]. Within endosomes, the E glycoprotein undergoes low pH-induced conformational changes, followed by fusion of the viral and host cell membranes [25–27]. In the cytoplasm, the viral genomic RNA functions initially as an mRNA for the translation of a single long open reading frame (ORF) flanked by 5′ and 3′ non-coding regions (NCRs) [28,29]; the resulting polyprotein is cleaved by viral and cellular proteases to generate at least 10 mature proteins [30,31]: three structural (C, prM, and E) and seven nonstructural (NS1, 2A, 2B, 3, 4A, 4B, and 5). In JEV and WNV, ribosomal frameshifting is also used for the expression of NS1′, a C-terminally extended form of NS1 [32–34]. A complex of the seven nonstructural proteins directs viral RNA replication on the distinct virus-induced membranous compartments derived from endoplasmic reticulum (ER) [35,36]. This replication process is catalyzed by two main viral components: (i) NS3, with serine protease (and its cofactor, NS2B) and RNA helicase/NTPase/RTPase activity, and (ii) NS5, with methyltransferase/guanylyltransferase and RNA-dependent RNA polymerase activity [37]. Virus assembly begins with budding of the C proteins, complexed with a newly made viral genomic RNA, into the ER lumen, and acquisition of the viral prM and E proteins. The prM-containing immature virions travel through the secretory pathway; in the trans-Golgi network, a cellular furin-like protease cleaves prM to yield the mature M protein, converting the immature particle to a mature virion [38].

The clinical presentation of ZIKV infection is highly variable, ranging from no apparent symptoms or mild self-limiting illness, to severe neurological disorders, such as microcephaly and Guillain–Barré syndrome [10,17]. Fundamentally, the varied outcomes after infection with a pathogen depend on the specific combination of pathogen and host genotypes [39]. On the virus side, a limited but significant number of ZIKVs have been isolated from Africa, Asia, and the Americas during the past 70 years. Recent phylogenetic analyses based on complete or near-complete viral genome sequences have revealed that the spatiotemporally distinct ZIKV strains are grouped into two major genetic lineages, African and Asian, with the 2015–2016 American epidemic strains originating from a common ancestor of the Asian lineage [40–42]. Despite the continuous expansion of its genetic diversity, little is known about the effect of viral genetic variation on the pathogenicity of ZIKV between the two lineages or between different strains within a particular lineage. On the host side, much progress has recently been made in developing murine models for ZIKV infection [43], including mice genetically engineered to lack one or more components of the innate and adaptive immune systems that affect the development, severity, and progression of ZIKV-induced disease [44–49]. However, the influence of host genetic variation on susceptibility to ZIKV infection is largely unknown.

To assess, experimentally, the impact of viral and host genetic variations on the outcome of ZIKV infection, we have now generated (i) a unique panel of three functional bacterial artificial chromosomes

(BACs), each containing a full-length infectious cDNA for one of three genetically divergent ZIKV strains, and (ii) an exclusive collection of 13 rabbit antisera capable of detecting almost all of the ZIKV gene products and their related species. Using these functional genomics and immunologic tools, together with various cell culture and mouse infection model systems, we show that the three molecularly defined cDNA-derived ZIKVs have a similar viral protein expression profile, but display biologically significant differences in in vitro growth properties and in vivo neuropathogenic potential that depend on both viral and host genetic traits. Our study not only provides a powerful system for the functional study of viral and host genetics in ZIKV replication and pathogenesis, but also offers a valuable platform for the rational design of vaccines and therapeutics against ZIKV.

2. Materials and Methods

2.1. Cells and Viruses

Details of the 17 cell lines used in this study, including their growth medium and culture conditions, are presented in Table 1. ZIKV MR-766 and P6-740 were obtained from the World Reference Center for Emerging Viruses and Arboviruses, University of Texas Medical Branch (Galveston, TX, USA), and ZIKV PRVABC-59 was provided by the Centers for Disease Control and Prevention (Fort Collins, CO, USA). In the case of all three ZIKVs, viral stocks were amplified once in Vero cells at a multiplicity of infection (MOI) of 1.

Table 1. Cells used in this study.

Organism	Cell	Tissue	Growth Medium [a]	Culture Condition	Source (Catalog Number) [b]
Human	HEK	Embryo, kidney	MEM supplemented with 10% FBS, 2 mM L-glutamine, 0.1 mM NEAA, 1.0 mM SP, and PS	37°C, 5% CO_2	ATCC (CRL-1573)
Human	Huh-7	Liver	DMEM supplemented with 10% FBS, 0.1 mM NEAA, and PS	37°C, 5% CO_2	Charles M. Rice, RU
Human	SH-SY5Y	Bone marrow	A 1:1 mixture of MEM and Ham's F-12 nutrient medium supplemented with 10% FBS, 0.1 mM NEAA, and PS	37°C, 5% CO_2	ATCC (CRL-2266)
Mouse	MEF	Embryo (C57BL/6), fibroblast	DMEM supplemented with 10% FBS and PS	37°C, 5% CO_2	ATCC (SCRC-1008)
Mouse	NIH/3T3	Embryo (NIH/Swiss), fibroblast	DMEM supplemented with 10% FBS and PS	37°C, 5% CO_2	ATCC (CRL-1658)
Mouse	NSC-34	Motor neuron-like hybrid	DMEM (without SP) supplemented with 10% FBS and PS	37°C, 5% CO_2	Cedarlane (CLU140)
Monkey	Vero	Kidney	α-MEM supplemented with 10% FBS and PS	37°C, 5% CO_2	ATCC (WHO-Vero)
Cow	BT	Turbinate	DMEM (without SP) supplemented with 10% HS and PS	37°C, 5% CO_2	ATCC (CRL-1390)
Cow	MDBK	Kidney	DMEM (without SP) supplemented with 10% HS and PS	37°C, 5% CO_2	ATCC (CCL-22)
Pig	ST	Testis	α-MEM supplemented with 10% FBS and PS	37°C, 5% CO_2	ATCC (CRL-1746)
Sheep	SFF-6	Fetus, fibroblast	DMEM supplemented with 15% FBS and PS	37°C, 5% CO_2	Irina A. Polejaeva, USU
Goat	GFF-4	Fetus, fibroblast	DMEM supplemented with 15% FBS and PS	37°C, 5% CO_2	Irina A. Polejaeva, USU
Horse	NBL-6	Skin, dermis	EMEM supplemented with 10% FBS and PS	37°C, 5% CO_2	ATCC (CCL-57)
Dog	MDCK	Kidney	MEM supplemented with EBSS, 10% FBS, 0.1 mM NEAA, 1.0 mM SP, and PS	37°C, 5% CO_2	ATCC (CCL-34)
Cat	CRFK	Kidney, cortex	MEM supplemented with EBSS, 10% HS, 0.1 mM NEAA, 1.0 mM SP, and PS	37°C, 5% CO_2	ATCC (CCL-94)
Chicken	CEF	Embryo, fibroblast	DMEM supplemented with 10% FBS and PS	37°C, 5% CO_2	Sung-June Byun, KNIAS
Mosquito	C6/36	Larva (*Aedes albopictus*)	MEM supplemented with EBSS, 10% FBS, 2 mM L-glutamine, 0.1 mM NEAA, 1.0 mM SP, and PS	28°C, 5% CO_2	ATCC (CRL-1660)

[a] MEM, minimum essential medium; α-MEM, alpha minimum essential medium; DMEM, Dulbecco's modified eagle medium; EMEM, Eagle's minimum essential medium; EBSS, Earle's balanced salt solution; FBS, fetal bovine serum; HS, horse serum; NEAA, nonessential amino acids; SP, sodium pyruvate; PS, penicillin-streptomycin. [b] ATCC, American Type Culture Collection; RU, Rockefeller University; USU, Utah State University; KNIAS, Korea National Institute of Animal Science.

2.2. Sequence Alignment and Phylogenetic Analysis

Multiple sequence alignments were performed via ClustalX, and the phylogenetic tree was constructed using MEGA and visualized via TreeView, as described [50]. Sequence identities between aligned nucleotide and amino acid sequences were calculated using ClustalX.

2.3. Cloning

Standard molecular cloning techniques were used to create three full-length ZIKV cDNAs [51], one each for MR-766, P6-740, and PRVABC-59 in the BAC plasmid pBeloBAC11 [52], designated pBac/MR-766, pBac/P6-740, and pBac/PRVABC-59. The same cloning strategy was used to construct all three full-length ZIKV cDNAs with the appropriate primer sets listed in Table 2. Essentially, each full-length ZIKV cDNA flanked by the 5′ SP6 promoter and the 3′ *PsrI/BarI* restriction enzyme site was created by joining five overlapping RT-PCR-generated cDNA fragments at four natural restriction enzyme sites found in the viral genome (see below for detailed description of cloning strategy). The cloned cDNAs were checked by restriction enzyme mapping and sequencing.

Table 2. Oligonucleotides used in this study.

Oligonucleotide	Sequence [a] (5′ to 3′)	Position [b]	Direction
Z1RT	GCTATTGGGTTCATGCCACAGATGGTCATCA	4531–4561	Reverse
Z1F	tatgtttaaacAGTTGTTGATCTGTGTGAATCAGACTGCGA	1–30	Forward
Z1R	tatggcgcgccAGGACCACCTTGAGTATGATCTCTCTCATG	4502–4531	Reverse
Z2RT	ATTGTCATTGTGTCAATGTCAGTCACCACTA	7369–7399	Reverse
Z2F	tatgtttaaacTCATTGTTTGGAGGAATGTCCTGGTTCTCA	2340–2369	Forward
Z2R	tatggcgcgccTCAATGTCAGTCACCACTATTCCATCCACA	7358–7387	Reverse
Z3RT	CTCCAGTTCAGGCCCCAGATTGAAGGGTGGGG	10603–10634	Reverse
Z3F	tatgtttaaacGGAAGTCCCAGAGAGAGCCTGGAGCTCAGG	5627–5656	Forward
Z3R	tatggcgcgccAAGGGTGGGGAAGGTCGCCACCTTCTTTTC	10583–10612	Reverse
S123-5sp1F	ctaggatccttaattaacctgcaggggggctgtta		Forward
S123-5sp1R	GATCAACAACTctatagtgtcccctaaatc	1–11	Reverse
S1-5sp2F	ggacactatagAGTTGTTGATCTGTGTGAGTC	1–21	Forward
S1-5sp2R	tatccgcggTAGCGCAAACCCGGGGTTCCTGAAT	860–884	Reverse
S1-3roF	tatccgcggGGAAAAAGGGAGGACTTATGGTGTG	10191–10215	Forward
S1-3roR	agggcggccgcgtatgtcgcgttccgtacgttctagAGAAACCATGGATTTCCCCACACC	10785–10807	Reverse
S23-5sp2F	ggacactatagAGTTGTTGATCTGTGTGAATC	1–21	Forward
S23-5sp2R	tatccgcggAACGCAAAGCCAGGGTTCCTGAATA	859–883	Reverse
S23-3roF	tatccgcggGGGAAAAAGGGAAGACTTATGGTGT	10190–10214	Forward
S23-3roR	agggcggccgcgtatgtcgccttccgtacgttctagAGACCCATGGATTTCCCCACACCG	10784–10807	Reverse
ZikaC-F	tttgaattcGGTCTCATCAATAGATGGGGT	297–317	Forward
ZikaC-R	tttctcgagctattaTCGTCTCTTCTTCTTCTCCTTCCT	399–419	Reverse
ZikaM-F	tttgaattcGCTGTGACGCTCCCCTCCCAT	753–773	Forward
ZikaM-R	tttctcgagctattaGACTCTAATCAAGTGCTTTGT	828–848	Reverse
ZikaE-F	tttgaattcCAGCACAGTGGGGATGATCGTT	1416–1436	Forward
ZikaE-R	tttctcgagctattaTCCTAGGCTTCCAAAACCCCC	1518–1538	Reverse
ZikaNS4A-F	tttgaattcGGAGCGGCTTTTGGAGTGATG	6465–6485	Forward
ZikaNS4A-R	tttctcgagctattaGGTCTCCGGCAATTGGGCCGC	6597–6617	Reverse
ZikaNS4B-F	tttgaattcGTGACTGACATTGACACAATG	7374–7394	Forward
ZikaNS4B-R	tttctcgagctattaGGAAGTTGCGGCTGTGATCAG	7506–7526	Reverse
ZikaF	GAAGTGGAAGTCCCAGAGAG	5622–5641	Forward
ZikaR	TGCTGAGCTGTATGACCCG	5757–5775	Reverse
ZikaProbe	FAM-TGGAGCTCAGGCTTTGATTGGGTGAC-BHQ1	5646–5671	Forward
VeroF	*AGCGGGAAATCGTGCGTGAC*	624–643	Forward
VeroR	*CAATGGTGATGACCTGGCCA*	742–761	Reverse
VeroProbe	HEX-*CACGGCGGCTTCTAGCTCCTCCC*-BHQ2	694–716	Forward

[a] ZIKV-specific sequences are indicated in uppercase normal letters, and Vero β-actin-specific sequences are shown in uppercase italic letters. Other nonviral sequences are indicated in lowercase letters. Restriction enzyme sites used for cDNA cloning are underlined. FAM, 6-Carboxyfluorescein; HEX, Hexachlorofluorescein; BHQ, Black hole quencher. [b] Nucleotide position refers to the complete genome sequence of ZIKV PRVABC-59 (GenBank accession number KX377337) or to the mRNA sequence of Vero β-actin (GenBank accession number AB004047).

(1) pBac/MR-766: The genomic RNA of ZIKV MR-766 (GenBank accession no. KX377335) was used as a template for the synthesis of three overlapping cDNA fragments by RT-PCR with the following primer sets: Frag-A[MR-766] (4552 bp), Z1RT, and Z1F + Z1R; Frag-B[MR-766] (5070 bp), Z2RT, and Z2F + Z2R; and Frag-C[MR-766] (5008 bp), Z3RT, and Z3F + Z3R. Each of the three cDNA amplicons was subcloned into pBAC[SP6]/JVFLx/XbaI [53], a derivative of the pBeloBAC11 plasmid,

by ligating the 8381 bp *PmeI-MluI* fragment of pBAC^{SP6}/JVFLx/XbaI with the 4538, 5056, and 4994 bp *PmeI-AscI* fragments of the Frag-A^{MR-766}, Frag-B^{MR-766}, and Frag-C^{MR-766} amplicons, respectively. This generated pBac/Frag-A^{MR-766} to -C^{MR-766}. To introduce an SP6 promoter immediately upstream of the first adenine residue of the viral genome, two cDNA fragments were first amplified individually by (i) PCR of pBAC^{SP6}/JVFLx/XbaI with a pair of primers, S123-5sp1F + S123-5sp1R (S123-5sp1R contains the antisense sequence of the SP6 promoter) and (ii) PCR of pRs/5′NCR^{MR-766} [54] with another pair of primers, S1-5sp2F + S1-5sp2R. Subsequently, these two fragments were fused by a second round of PCR with the outer forward and reverse primers S123-5sp1F + S1-5sp2R. The 1025 bp *BamHI-SacII* fragment of the fused PCR amplicons was ligated with the 2718 bp *BamHI-SacII* fragment of pRs2, creating pRs/5′SP^{MR-766}. To engineer a unique *PsrI* run-off site just downstream of the last thymine residue of the viral genome, one cDNA fragment was amplified by PCR of pRs/3′NCR^{MR-766} [54] with primers S1-3roF + S1-3roR (S1-3roR contains the antisense sequence of the *PsrI* and *NotI* recognition sites in a row). The 649 bp *SacII-NotI* fragment of the resulting amplicons was ligated with the 2667 bp *SacII-NotI* fragment of pRs2, creating pRs/3′RO^{MR-766}. The full-length MR-766 cDNA clone pBac/MR-766 was then assembled by sequentially joining the 7456 bp *PacI-NotI* fragment of pBAC^{SP6}/JVFLx/XbaI with the following five DNA fragments: (i) the 1004 bp *PacI-XmaI* fragment of pRs/5′SP^{MR-766}, (ii) the 3160 bp *XmaI-XhoI* fragment of pBac/Frag-A^{MR-766}, (iii) the 3144 bp *XhoI-NsiI* fragment of pBac/Frag-B^{MR-766}, (iv) the 3041 bp *NsiI-BamHI* fragment of pBac/Frag-C^{MR-766}, and (v) the 619 bp *BamHI-NotI* fragment of pRs/3′RO^{MR-766}.

(2) pBac/P6-740: The genomic RNA of ZIKV P6-740 (GenBank accession no. KX377336) was used as a template for the synthesis of three overlapping cDNA fragments by RT-PCR with the following primer sets: Frag-A^{P6-740} (4553 bp), Z1RT, and Z1F + Z1R; Frag-B^{P6-740} (5070 bp), Z2RT, and Z2F + Z2R; and Frag-C^{P6-740} (5008 bp), Z3RT, and Z3F + Z3R. Each of the three cDNA amplicons was subcloned into pBAC^{SP6}/JVFLx/XbaI, by ligating the 8381 bp *PmeI-MluI* fragment of pBAC^{SP6}/JVFLx/XbaI with the 4539, 5056, and 4994 bp *PmeI-AscI* fragments of the Frag-A^{P6-740}, Frag-B^{P6-740}, and Frag-C^{P6-740} amplicons, respectively. This generated pBac/Frag-A^{P6-740} to -C^{P6-740}. To introduce an SP6 promoter immediately upstream of the first adenine residue of the viral genome, two cDNA fragments were first amplified individually by (i) PCR of pBAC^{SP6}/JVFLx/XbaI with a pair of primers, S123-5sp1F + S123-5sp1R (S123-5sp1R contains the antisense sequence of the SP6 promoter) and (ii) PCR of pRs/5′NCR^{P6-740} [54] with another pair of primers, S23-5sp2F + S23-5sp2R. Subsequently, these two fragments were fused by a second round of PCR with the outer forward and reverse primers S123-5sp1F + S23-5sp2R. The 1025 bp *BamHI-SacII* fragment of the fused PCR amplicons was ligated with the 2718 bp *BamHI-SacII* fragment of pRs2, creating pRs/5′SP^{P6-740}. To engineer a unique *BarI* run-off site just downstream of the last thymine residue of the viral genome, one cDNA fragment was amplified by PCR of pRs/3′NCR^{P6-740} [54] with primers S23-3roF + S23-3roR (S23-3roR contains the antisense sequence of the *BarI* and *NotI* recognition sites in a row). The 649 bp *SacII-NotI* fragment of the resulting amplicons was ligated with the 2667 bp *SacII-NotI* fragment of pRs2, creating pRs/3′RO^{P6-740}. The full-length P6-740 cDNA clone pBac/P6-740 was then assembled by sequentially joining the 7456 bp *PacI-NotI* fragment of pBAC^{SP6}/JVFLx/XbaI with the following five DNA fragments: (i) the 187 bp *PacI-NheI* fragment of pRs/5′SP^{P6-740}, (ii) the 2930 bp *NheI-SpeI* fragment of pBac/Frag-A^{P6-740}, (iii) the 3359 bp *SpeI-NgoMIV* fragment of pBac/Frag-B^{P6-740}, (iv) the 4059 bp *NgoMIV-StuI* fragment of pBac/Frag-C^{P6-740}, and (v) the 433 bp *StuI-NotI* fragment of pRs/3′RO^{P6-740}.

(3) pBac/PRVABC-59: The genomic RNA of ZIKV PRVABC-59 (GenBank accession no. KX377337) was used as a template for the synthesis of three overlapping cDNA fragments by RT-PCR with the following primer sets: Frag-A$^{PRVABC-59}$ (4553 bp), Z1RT, and Z1F + Z1R; Frag-B$^{PRVABC-59}$ (5070 bp), Z2RT, and Z2F + Z2R; and Frag-C$^{PRVABC-59}$ (5008 bp), Z3RT, and Z3F + Z3R. Each of the three cDNA amplicons was subcloned into pBAC^{SP6}/JVFLx/XbaI, by ligating the 8381 bp *PmeI-MluI* fragment of pBAC^{SP6}/JVFLx/XbaI with the 4539, 5056, and 4994 bp *PmeI-AscI* fragments of the Frag-A$^{PRVABC-59}$, Frag-B$^{PRVABC-59}$, and Frag-C$^{PRVABC-59}$ amplicons, respectively. This generated pBac/Frag-A$^{PRVABC-59}$ to -C$^{PRVABC-59}$. To introduce an SP6 promoter immediately upstream of the first

adenine residue of the viral genome, two cDNA fragments were first amplified individually by (i) PCR of pBAC^{SP6}/JVFLx/XbaI with a pair of primers, S123-5sp1F + S123-5sp1R (S123-5sp1R contains the antisense sequence of the SP6 promoter) and (ii) PCR of pRs/5′NCR^{PRVABC-59} [54] with another pair of primers, S23-5sp2F + S23-5sp2R. Subsequently, these two fragments were fused by a second round of PCR with the outer forward and reverse primers S123-5sp1F + S23-5sp2R. The 1025 bp *Bam*HI-*Sac*II fragment of the fused PCR amplicons was ligated with the 2718 bp *Bam*HI-*Sac*II fragment of pRs2, creating pRs/5′SP^{PRVABC-59}. To engineer a unique *Bar*I run-off site just downstream of the last thymine residue of the viral genome, one cDNA fragment was amplified by PCR of pRs/3′NCR^{PRVABC-59} [54] with primers S23-3roF + S23-3roR (S23-3roR contains the antisense sequence of the *Bar*I and *Not*I recognition sites in a row). The 649 bp *Sac*II-*Not*I fragment of the resulting amplicons was ligated with the 2667 bp *Sac*II-*Not*I fragment of pRs2, creating pRs/3′RO^{PRVABC-59}. The full-length PRVABC-59 cDNA clone pBac/PRVABC-59 was then assembled by sequentially joining the 7456 bp *Pac*I-*Not*I fragment of pBAC^{SP6}/JVFLx/XbaI with the following five DNA fragments: (i) the 187 bp *Pac*I-*Nhe*I fragment of pRs/5′SP^{PRVABC-59}, (ii) the 4426 bp *Nhe*I-*Eco*NI fragment of pBac/Frag-A^{PRVABC-59}, (iii) the 2114 bp *Eco*NI-*Sac*II fragment of pBac/Frag-B^{PRVABC-59}, (iv) the 3808 bp *Sac*II-*Stu*I fragment of pBac/Frag-C^{PRVABC-59}, and (v) the 433 bp *Stu*I-*Not*I fragment of pRs/3′RO^{PRVABC-59}.

A total of five bacterial expression plasmids were constructed, each of which was used to express a 32 to 51 aa non-hydrophobic region of the ZIKV polyprotein as a glutathione *S*-transferase (GST) fusion protein. In all cases, a defined region of the ZIKV ORF was amplified by PCR using pBac/PRVABC-59 as a template and the appropriate pair of primers listed in Table 2: (i) Frag-zC (147 bp), ZikaC-F + ZikaC-R; (ii) Frag-zM (120 bp), ZikaM-F + ZikaM-R; (iii) Frag-zE (147 bp), ZikaE-F + ZikaE-R; (iv) Frag-zNS4A (177 bp), ZikaNS4A-F + ZikaNS4A-R; and (v) Frag-zNS4B (177 bp), ZikaNS4B-F + ZikaNS4B-R. Each of the resulting amplicons was cloned into pGex-4T-1 (GE Healthcare, Piscataway, NJ, USA) by ligating the 4954 bp *Eco*RI-*Xho*I fragment of the pGex-4T-1 vector with 135, 108, 135, 165, and 165 bp *Eco*RI-*Xho*I fragments of the Frag-zC, -zM, -zE, -zNS4A, and -zNS4B amplicons, respectively. This created pGex-zC, -zM, -zE, -zNS4A, and -zNS4B.

2.4. Transcription and Transfection

Infectious transcripts were synthesized from *Psr*I/*Bar*I-linearized BAC plasmid DNA with SP6 RNA polymerase as described [53] in reactions containing m⁷GpppA (New England Biolabs, Ipswich, MA, USA). RNA integrity was examined by agarose gel electrophoresis. RNA was transfected into Vero cells by electroporation using the BTX ECM 830 electroporator with a 2-mm-gap cuvette under optimized conditions (980 V, 99 μs pulse length, and 3 pulses); RNA infectivity was quantified by infectious center assay [55,56]. The infectious centers of plaques/foci formed on the monolayer of Vero cells were visualized at 5 days after transfection either nonspecifically by counterstaining of uninfected cells with crystal violet [55] or specifically by immunostaining of ZIKV-infected cells with rabbit anti-ZIKV NS1 (α-ZNS1) antiserum and horseradish peroxidase-conjugated goat α-rabbit IgG (Jackson ImmunoResearch, West Grove, PA, USA), followed by developing with 3,3′-diaminobenzidine [56].

2.5. Growth Kinetics and Cytopathogenicity

Viral growth kinetics and cytopathogenicity were analyzed in 17 animal cell lines from 12 different species. In each case, naïve cells were seeded into 35 mm culture dishes at a density of 3×10^5 cells/dish for 12 h, and then mock-infected or infected with viruses at an MOI of 1 for 1 h at 37 °C. Following incubation, cell monolayers were washed and incubated with complete medium. At 6, 12, 18, 24, 36, 48, 60, 72, and 96 h post-infection (hpi), ZIKV-infected cells were examined morphologically under a light-inverted microscope (Primo Vert, Carl Zeiss, Jena, Germany) to assess the degree of ZIKV-induced cytopathic effect (CPE) as compared to mock-infected cells, and culture supernatants were collected to evaluate the levels of virus production by plaque assays on Vero cells, as described [57]. The infectious centers of plaques were visualized at 5 days after infection by counterstaining of uninfected cells with crystal violet [55].

2.6. Real-Time RT-PCR

ZIKV RNA levels in infected Vero cells were quantified as described [57] by real-time RT-PCR with the primer pairs and fluorogenic probes listed in Table 2: the ZikaF + ZikaR and ZikaProbe specific for the ZIKV NS3-coding region that has the identical sequences in all three ZIKVs, and the VeroF + VeroR and VeroProbe specific for the Vero β-actin coding region. Each ZIKV RNA level was normalized to the corresponding β-actin mRNA level as an internal control.

2.7. Immunoblotting, Confocal Microscopy, and Flow Cytometry

Individual ZIKV proteins were identified by immunoblotting [31] using each of our six previously characterized JEV region-specific rabbit antisera that cross-react with their ZIKV counterparts, or seven newly generated ZIKV region-specific rabbit antisera. The rabbit antibody was detected using alkaline phosphatase (AP)-conjugated goat α-rabbit IgG (Jackson ImmunoResearch, West Grove, PA, USA), and the AP enzyme was visualized using colorimetric detection with 5-bromo-4-chloro-3-indolyl phosphate and nitro blue tetrazolium (Sigma, St. Louis, MO, USA). ZIKV E proteins were visualized by confocal microscopy [57] with rabbit α-ZE antiserum, followed by secondary labeling with fluorescein isothiocyanate-conjugated goat α-rabbit IgG (Jackson ImmunoResearch). ZIKV NS4A proteins were detected by flow cytometry [58] with rabbit α-ZNS4A antiserum, followed by secondary labeling with Alexa 488-conjugated goat α-rabbit IgG (Invitrogen, Carlsbad, CA, USA).

2.8. Mouse Studies

ZIKV neuropathogenicity was examined in male and female mice of four strains: CD-1 (1, 2, and 4 weeks, Charles River, Wilmington, MA, USA), C57BL/6J (4 weeks, the Jackson Laboratory, Bar Harbor, ME, USA), A129 (4 weeks, bred in-house), and AG129 (4 weeks, bred in-house). Groups of mice were inoculated via the intramuscular (im, 50 μL) or intracerebral (ic, 20 μL) route with 10-fold serial dilutions of virus stock in α-minimal essential medium and monitored for any ZIKV-induced clinical signs, weight loss, or death daily for 20 days. The im and ic lethal dose 50% (LD_{50}) values for each virus were calculated from the respective dose-dependent survival curves of the infected mice, as described [57].

2.9. Ethics Statement

All mouse studies were conducted in strict accordance with the Guide for the Care and Use of Laboratory Animals of the National Institutes of Health, United States of America. The animal protocol was approved by the Institutional Animal Care and Use Committee (IACUC) of Utah State University (approved IACUC protocol #2505, 30/03/2016). Discomfort, distress, pain, and injury were minimized as much as possible through limited handling and euthanization of mice when they were moribund.

3. Results

3.1. Characterization of Three Spatiotemporally Distinct and Genetically Divergent ZIKV Strains

As an initial step in examining the genetic diversity of ZIKV and its biological significance for viral replication and pathogenesis, we selected three historically important strains of distinct geographical and temporal origins: (i) MR-766, the first ZIKV identified from the blood of a rhesus macaque monkey in Uganda in 1947 [1]; (ii) P6-740, the first non-African strain, isolated from a pool of *A. aegypti* mosquitoes in Malaysia in 1966 [59]; and (iii) PRVABC-59, the recent American strain recovered from the blood of a human patient in Puerto Rico in 2015 [60]. To compare the genome sequence and composition of these three ZIKVs, we determined the consensus nucleotide sequence for each of their full-length genomic RNAs [54]. In all three strains of ZIKV, we found that the genomic RNA is 10,807 nt long, with a single ORF of 10,272 nt flanked by a 106 or 107 nt 5′NCR and a 428 or 429 nt 3′NCR (Figure 1A). Also, the three genomic RNAs all begin with the dinucleotide 5′-AG and end with the dinucleotide CU-3′, both of which are conserved among all mosquito- and tick-borne flaviviruses. However, pairwise sequence comparisons of the three complete genomes showed a considerable degree of genetic diversity, with a range in sequence identity of 89.1–95.6% at the nucleotide level and 96.8–98.8% at the amino acid level over the 3423 aa polyprotein encoded by the single ORF of the genomic RNA (Figure 1B).

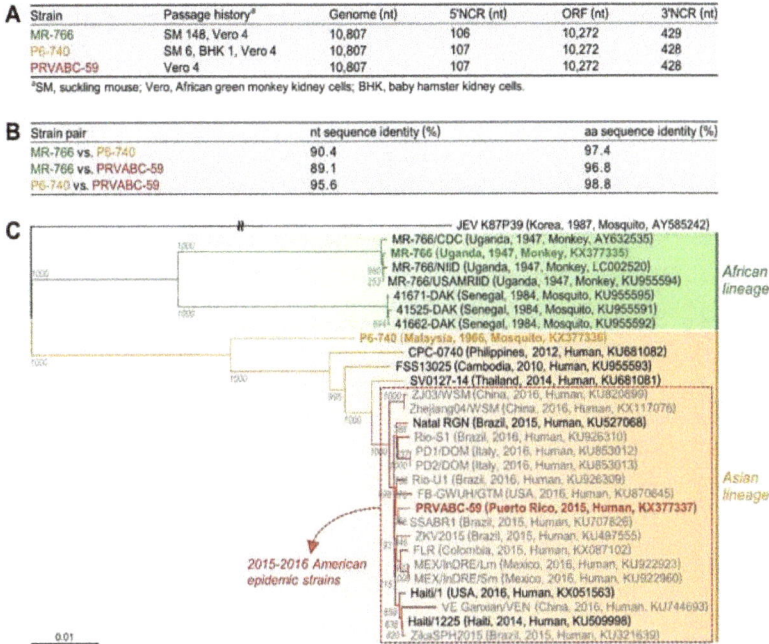

Figure 1. A spectrum of ZIKV genetic diversity is represented by three historically important and spatiotemporally distinct strains: MR-766, P6-740, and PRVABC-59. The consensus nucleotide sequence for each of their full-length genomic RNAs was determined by sequencing three overlapping uncloned cDNA amplicons collectively representing the entire genomic RNA, except for the 5′ and 3′ termini, which were subsequently defined by performing both 5′- and 3′-rapid amplification of cDNA ends (RACE); each of these RACEs was followed by cDNA cloning and sequencing of ~20 randomly picked clones. (**A**) Genomic organization of the three ZIKV strains; (**B**) Pairwise comparison of the complete nucleotide (nt) and deduced amino acid (aa) sequences of the three ZIKV genomes; (**C**) Phylogenetic tree based on the nucleotide sequence of 29 ZIKV genomes, including the 15 complete (MR-766, green; P6-740, orange; PRVABC-59, red; and 12 others, black) and 14 near-complete (gray) genomes, with Japanese encephalitis virus (JEV) K87P39 included as an outgroup. Bootstrap values from 1000 replicates are shown at each node of the tree. The scale bar represents the number of nucleotide substitutions per site. The strain name is followed by a description in parenthesis of the country, year, and host of isolation and the GenBank accession numbers. Note that MR-766 has been fully sequenced in this study and by three other groups (designated MR-766/CDC, MR-766/NIID, and MR-766/USAMRIID).

To examine the genetic relationship between the three spatiotemporally distinct ZIKVs and their associations with other strains, we performed a multiple sequence alignment for phylogenetic analysis using the nucleotide sequence of all 29 ZIKV genomes (15 complete, 14 near-complete) in GenBank at the time of analysis (June 2016), including our complete nucleotide sequence of the genomes of MR-766, P6-740, and PRVABC-59. Construction of a genome-based rooted phylogenetic tree using JEV K87P39 as an outgroup revealed two distinct phylogenetic groups (Figure 1C), in agreement with previous ORF-based phylogenetic studies that classified 10–40 ZIKV isolates into two major genetic lineages, African and Asian [40–42]. The African lineage branches into two clusters, one including four different versions of the Ugandan MR-766 strain (1947) that are not identical in genome sequence, mainly because of a variation in the passage history of the virus, and the other including the three Senegalese isolates 41671-DAK, 41525-DAK, and 41662-DAK, all isolated in 1984. On the other hand, the Asian lineage contains a single cluster of the Malaysian P6-740 (1966), Cambodian FSS13025 (2010), Philippine CPC-0740 (2012), and Thai SV0127-14 (2014) strains, as well as 18 other isolates collected during the 2015–2016 American epidemic, including the Puerto Rican PRVABC-59 strain (2015). Notably, the four pre-epidemic Asian strains (P6-740, FSS13025, CPC-0740, and SV0127-14) are closely related to the 2015–2016 American epidemic strains, but each forms a single minor branch. Overall, our data indicate that MR-766 belongs to the African lineage, whereas both P6-740 and PRVABC-59 belong to the Asian lineage, with PRVABC-59 being derived from an ancestor of the Asian lineage.

3.2. Development of Genetically Stable Full-Length Infectious cDNA Clones for the Three ZIKV Strains

We constructed three full-length infectious ZIKV cDNAs for the MR-766, P6-740, and PRVABC-59 strains, each capable of serving as a template for the rescue of molecularly cloned ZIKVs (Figure 2). In each strain, five overlapping cDNA fragments representing the 10,807 nt genomic RNA were sequentially assembled into a full-length cDNA in the single-copy BAC vector pBeloBAC11, in order to ensure the stable maintenance of the cloned cDNA during propagation in *Escherichia coli*, with an SP6 promoter sequence positioned immediately upstream of the viral 5′-end and a unique restriction endonuclease recognition site (*Psr*I for MR-766, *Bar*I for P6-740 and PRVABC-59) placed just downstream of the viral 3′-end. Both the SP6 promoter and the unique restriction site were engineered so that in vitro run-off transcription could be used to produce m^7G-capped synthetic RNAs bearing authentic 5′ and 3′ ends of the viral genomic RNA. Using this BAC-based cloning strategy, we thus created a panel of three full-length ZIKV cDNAs, designated pBac/MR-766, pBac/P6-740, and pBac/PRVABC-59 (Figure 2A).

To evaluate the functionality of the three full-length ZIKV BACs, we determined the viability of the synthetic RNAs transcribed in vitro from each BAC by measuring their specific infectivity after RNA transfection into a ZIKV-susceptible African green monkey kidney (Vero) cell line. To prepare a DNA template for in vitro run-off transcription, the three full-length ZIKV BACs were first linearized by digestion with *Psr*I (for pBac/MR-766) or *Bar*I (for pBac/P6-740 and pBac/PRVABC-59). Each was then used as a template for a run-off transcription reaction using SP6 RNA polymerase in the presence of the m^7GpppA cap structure analog. After removal of the DNA template by DNase I digestion, we transfected Vero cells with the RNA transcripts, quantifying their infectivity as the number of plaque-forming units (PFU) per μg of transfected RNA. In all three BACs, the RNA transcripts invariably had a high infectivity of $8.1–8.6 \times 10^5$ PFU/μg and were capable of producing a high-titer stock of infectious ZIKVs in culture medium that reached $1.3–5.0 \times 10^6$ PFU/mL at 36 h after transfection (Figure 2B). Each of the three recombinant BAC-derived ZIKVs (designated by the prefix "r") formed a homogeneous population of plaques that differed from the others in size, with mean diameters of 5.7 (rMR-766), 1.6 (rP6-740), and 5.2 (rPRVABC-59) mm (Figure 2C). We also demonstrated that using pBac/P6-740, the infectivity of its RNA transcripts was decreased by ~4 logs to a barely detectable level (55–105 PFU/μg), with a single $C^{9804} \rightarrow U$ substitution (an unintended mutation introduced during the overlapping cDNA synthesis by RT-PCR) replacing a His with Tyr at position 713 of the viral NS5 protein (Figure S1A,B). On the crystal structure of ZIKV NS5 [61,62], the His-713 residue is located within the conserved structural motif E region near the priming loop in the RNA-dependent RNA polymerase domain (Figure S1C), suggesting a critical role for His-713 in the polymerase function of ZIKV NS5.

Next, we examined the genetic stability of the three full-length ZIKV BACs that are important for reliable and efficient recovery of infectious viruses from the cloned cDNAs. A single colony of

E. coli DH10B carrying each of the three full-length ZIKV BACs was grown in liquid medium and serially passaged for 4 days by diluting it 10^6-fold daily, such that each passage represented ~20 generations, as we described previously [53]. In all three cases, we found no differences in specific infectivity of the RNA transcripts made from the BAC plasmids even after 80 generations, indicating that the three full-length ZIKV BACs are stable during propagation in bacteria (Figure S2). In sum, we have established genetically stable BAC-based reverse genetics platforms for the recovery of three molecularly cloned, genetically distinct ZIKVs.

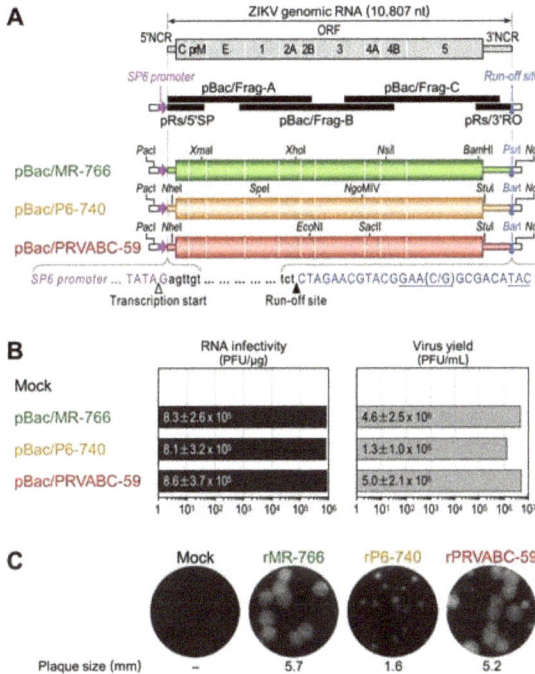

Figure 2. A trio of functional ZIKV cDNAs was created for the rescue of three molecularly cloned genetically divergent strains: rMR-766, rP6-740, and rPRVABC-59. (**A**) Construction of three full-length ZIKV cDNAs as BACs for MR-766, P6-740, and PRVABC-59. In all three cases, each genomic RNA (top panel) was first subcloned into five overlapping cDNAs (middle panel), which were then joined at four shared restriction sites as indicated to assemble its full-length cDNA without introducing any point mutations for cloning (bottom panel). Presented below the three full-length cDNAs are the sequences corresponding to the 5′ and 3′ termini conserved in all three ZIKVs (black lowercase), an SP6 promoter placed just upstream of the viral genome (magenta uppercase), and a run-off site positioned immediately downstream of the viral genome (*Psr*I or *Bar*I, blue uppercase). Marked below the sequences are the transcription start (white arrowhead) and run-off (black arrowhead) sites; (**B**) Functionality of the three full-length ZIKV cDNAs. After linearization with *Psr*I or *Bar*I, as appropriate, each full-length cDNA was used as a template for in vitro transcription with SP6 RNA polymerase in the presence of the dinucleotide cap analog m^7GpppA. Capped RNA transcripts were transfected into Vero cells to determine the number of infectious centers (plaques) counterstained with crystal violet at 5 days after transfection (RNA infectivity). At 36 h post-transfection, culture supernatants from RNA-transfected cells were harvested to estimate the level of virus production by plaque assays on Vero cells (Virus yield). Means and standard deviations from three independent experiments are shown; (**C**) Plaque morphology. The average plaque sizes were estimated by measuring 20 representative plaques.

3.3. Differential Replication Kinetics and Cytopathogenicity among Three Molecularly Cloned ZIKVs in Human, Mosquito, and Animal Cell Lines

To test whether the genetic variation in ZIKV can have differential effects on its replication kinetics and cytopathogenicity, we infected monkey kidney-derived Vero cells at an MOI of 1, then examined the replicative and cytopathic properties of the three cloned cDNA-derived ZIKVs (rMR-766, rP6-740, and rPRVABC-59) as compared to those of the uncloned parental ZIKVs (MR-766, P6-740, and PRVABC-59) used for cDNA construction. In all three strains, we saw no noticeable differences between the cloned and uncloned viruses in the accumulation of viral genomic RNA over the first 24 hpi (Figure 3A), paralleling not only the kinetics of viral growth and CPE development over the first 3 days post-infection (Figure 3B) but also the average sizes of the α-ZNS1 antibody-reactive foci immunostained at 5 days post-infection (Figure 3C). However, we did observe clear differences between the three strains, regardless of whether they were cloned or uncloned viruses, with respect to their replication kinetics and cytopathogenicity (Figure 3A–C). Our specific findings are as follows: (i) rMR-766/MR-766 displayed the fastest rate of RNA replication, induced complete lysis of the infected cells by 36 hpi, achieved the highest virus titer of 2.0–3.3×10^7 PFU/mL at 36–48 hpi, and formed the largest foci of 6.3 mm diameter. (ii) rP6-740/P6-740 had the slowest rate of RNA replication, did not cause complete CPE until 72 hpi, reached its maximal virus titer of 1.1–1.2×10^7 PFU/mL at 60–72 hpi, and generated the smallest foci of 2.4 mm diameter. (iii) rPRVABC-59/PRVABC-59 had a rate of RNA replication slightly slower than rMR-766/MR-766 but much faster than that of rP6-740/P6-740; it caused complete CPE by 48 hpi, with a peak virus titer of 0.9–1.4×10^7 PFU/mL at 36–48 hpi, and produced foci of 5.9 mm diameter.

We further analyzed the replicative and cytopathic potential of the three cDNA-derived ZIKVs in 16 other animal cell lines from 11 different species, over the first 4 days after infection of the cells with each virus at an MOI of 1. Our data revealed seven distinct patterns of viral growth kinetics and cytopathogenesis, depending on a combination of the viral strain and host cell line (Figure 3D and Figure S3): (1) In all three human cell types (embryonic kidney HEK, hepatocarcinoma Huh-7, and neuroblastoma SH-SY5Y), rMR-766 and rP6-740 grew equally well, to maximum titers of 10^7–10^8 PFU/mL at 48–72 hpi, but rPRVABC-59 always grew at a slower rate, attaining a peak titer 1–2 logs lower than that of the other two strains at 72–96 hpi (HEK and SH-SY5Y) or reaching a peak titer similar to that of the other two strains only at 96 hpi (Huh-7); all three ZIKVs induced cell death, with a correlation between the degree of CPE and the magnitude of viral replication. (2) In swine testis (ST) and equine skin (NBL-6) cells, the three ZIKVs replicated to their peak titers of 10^6–10^7 PFU/mL at 48 hpi, with differential growth rates similar to those seen in Vero cells (rMR-766, fastest; rP6-740, slowest; rPRVABC-59, intermediate) that paralleled the kinetics of CPE development. (3) In sheep fetal fibroblast (SFF-6) and *A. albopictus* (C6/36) cells, the three ZIKVs shared a superimposable growth curve, characterized by a steady increase in virus titers up to ~10^7 PFU/mL by 96 hpi, except for rP6-740, which had an exponential growth during 24–48 hpi in C6/36, but not SFF-6 cells. None of the three ZIKVs produced any visible CPE. (4) In goat fetal fibroblast (GFF-4), canine kidney (MDCK), and feline kidney (CRFK) cells and in all three mouse cell types (C57BL/6-derived embryonic fibroblast MEF, NIH/Swiss-derived embryonic fibroblast NIH/3T3, and motor neuron-like hybrid NSC-34), rMR-766 was the fastest-growing, reaching its highest titer of 10^6–10^7 PFU/mL at 48–96 hpi; rPRVABC-59 was the slowest-growing, gaining a maximum titer of only 10^3–10^4 PFU/mL during the same period; and rP6-740 was intermediate in growth rate. However, none of these viruses produced visible CPE. (5) In chicken embryo fibroblast (CEF) cells, both rMR-766 and rP6-740 had a relatively long lag period of 36 h, followed by a gradual increase in virus titer up to 10^5–10^6 PFU/mL by 96 hpi; in contrast, rPRVABC-59 grew extremely poorly, resulting in a slow decrease in virus titer to 45 PFU/mL by 96 hpi. No CPE was observed for any of the three ZIKV-infected CEF cells. (6) In bovine turbinate (BT) cells, the three ZIKVs showed substantial differences in growth kinetics, reaching a plateau at 96 hpi, with peak titers of 4.4×10^5 (rMR-766), 5.0×10^4 (rPRVABC-59), and 8.8×10^2 (rP6-740) PFU/mL. However, no visible CPE was induced in any of the ZIKV-infected cells. (7) In bovine kidney (MDBK) cells, the titers of all three ZIKVs declined to undetectable levels at 60–96 hpi, with no overt signs of viral replication.

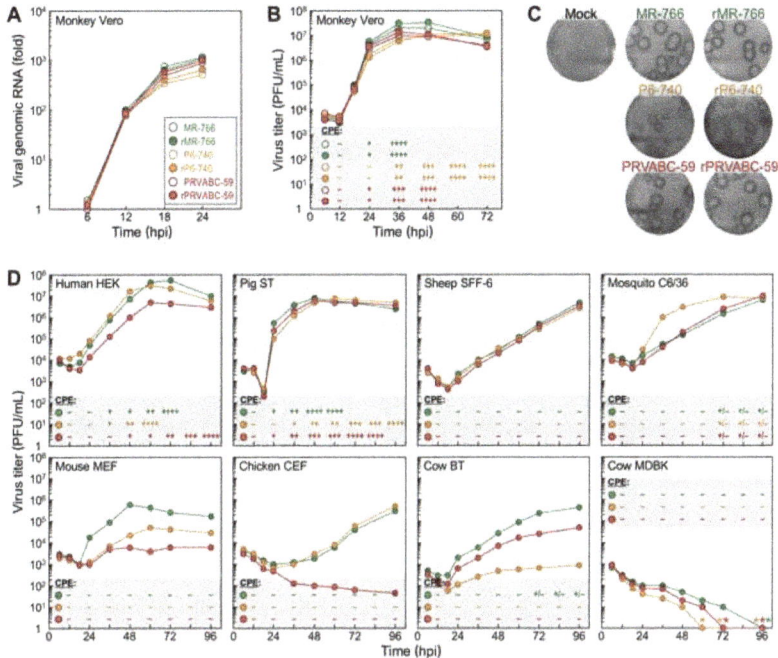

Figure 3. ZIKV replication kinetics and cytopathogenicity in cell cultures depend on the particular combination of virus strain and host cells. (**A–C**) Replicative and cytopathic properties of three cloned cDNA-derived ZIKVs (rMR-766, rP6-740, and rPRVABC-59) and their uncloned parental ZIKVs (MR-766, P6-740, and PRVABC-59) in Vero cells. Cells were infected with each of the six ZIKVs (MOI = 1). At the time points indicated after infection, cells were lysed to examine the accumulation levels of viral genomic RNA by real-time RT-PCR with a ZIKV-specific fluorogenic probe (**A**), and supernatants were collected to analyze the production levels of progeny virions by plaque assays on Vero cells (**B**). At 5 days post-infection, cell monolayers maintained under a semisolid overlay medium were immunostained with rabbit α-ZNS1 antiserum to visualize the infectious foci (**C**). (**D**) Growth kinetics and cytopathogenicity of the three cloned cDNA-derived ZIKVs in a wide range of animal cells (see also Figure S3). Each virus was used to infect the cell lines (MOI = 1) specified in the figure. At the indicated time points, cells were examined microscopically for the degree of ZIKV-induced cytopathic effect (CPE) (−, 0%; +, 0–25%; ++, 25–50%; +++, 50–75%; ++++, 75–100% cell death), and supernatants were assayed for virus production by plaque assays on Vero cells. hpi, hours post-infection.

Subsequently, we showed that MDBK cells are not susceptible to ZIKV infection, but instead are permissive for ZIKV RNA replication, by using (i) single cell-based immunofluorescence (Figure 4A) and flow cytometry (Figure 4B) assays to determine the number of cells expressing ZIKV proteins (E or NS4A), when MDBK cells were either infected with each of the three cDNA-derived ZIKVs or transfected with each of the three infectious RNAs transcribed in vitro from their corresponding cDNAs; and (ii) total cell lysate-based immunoblot analyses to assess the accumulation levels of ZIKV NS1 protein in the virus-infected vs RNA-transfected MDBK cells (Figure 4C). In all these experiments, we used Vero cells, a ZIKV-susceptible cell line, as a control. Our results led us to postulate that MDBK cells might lack one or more host factors required for ZIKV entry; alternatively, they might have a general defect in the clathrin-dependent endocytic pathway that ZIKV utilizes for internalization [63]. We thus investigated the functional integrity of the clathrin-dependent endocytic pathway in MDBK cells, by analyzing the susceptibility of these cells to infection by two other enveloped RNA viruses whose entry depends on clathrin-mediated endocytosis: bovine viral diarrhea virus (BVDV) and vesicular stomatitis virus (VSV). In contrast to their resistance to ZIKV infection, we found that MDBK cells were highly susceptible to infection with both BVDV and VSV, as demonstrated by their plaque formation and high level of progeny virion production (Figure S4A,B). These results indicate that the cellular machinery associated with the clathrin-dependent endocytic pathway is functional in MDBK cells, and they support our hypothesis that MDBK cells lack a host factor(s) promoting ZIKV entry.

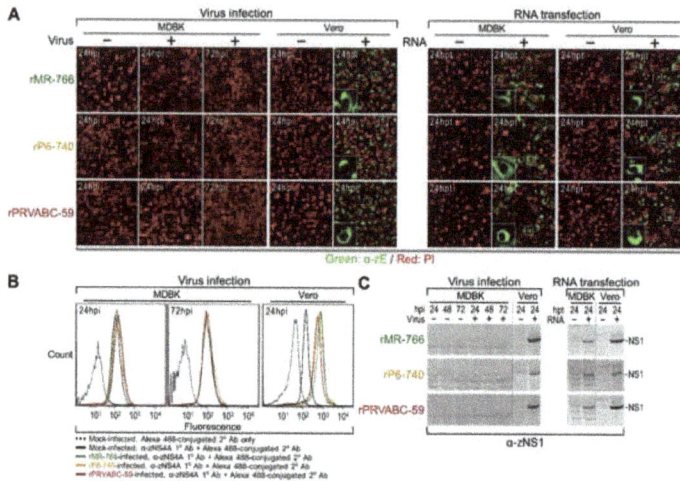

Figure 4. MDBK cells are permissive for ZIKV RNA replication but are not susceptible to infection with the virus. MDBK cells were mock-infected or infected with rMR-766, rP6-740, or rPRVABC-59 at an MOI of 3 (for virus infection experiments), or mock-transfected or transfected with 3 μg of synthetic RNAs transcribed in vitro from their respective infectious cDNAs (for RNA transfection experiments). At the indicated time points, the expression of three ZIKV proteins (E, NS1, and NS4A) within the cells was analyzed by confocal microscopy for E (**A**), flow cytometry for NS4A (**B**), and immunoblotting for NS1 (**C**). The insets in panel A show enlarged views of the boxed areas with the fluorescence of propidium iodide (PI)-stained nuclei excluded. In all experiments, ZIKV-susceptible Vero cells were included in parallel. hpi, hours post-infection; hpt, hours post-transfection.

3.4. Genome-Wide Landscape of the Viral Gene Products and Their Related Species Produced by the Molecularly Cloned ZIKVs

To identify all the viral proteins produced by rMR-766, rP6-740, and rPRVABC-59, we examined total cell lysates of mock- and ZIKV-infected Vero cells in two series of immunoblotting experiments. In the first series, we probed with each of our 15 JEV region-specific rabbit antisera (Figure S5), originally produced to detect all JEV gene products [31], which we estimated to have the potential for cross-reactivity with their ZIKV counterparts, given the relatively high levels (35–71%) of amino acid sequence identity between their antigenic regions (Figure 5A). Indeed, six (α-JE^{N-term}, α-JNS1^{C-term}, α-JNS2B, α-JNS3^{C-term}, α-JNS5^{N-term}, and α-JNS5^{C-term}) of the 15 antisera showed moderate-to-strong cross-reactivity with their respective ZIKV gene products, but the remaining nine had no reactivity (Figure 5B). To cover the remaining undetected parts of ZIKV ORF, we then generated seven ZIKV region-specific rabbit antisera, using rPRVABC-59 as the viral strain of choice, immunizing the rabbits with five bacterially expressed GST fusion proteins (α-ZC, α-ZM, α-ZE, α-ZNS4A, and α-ZNS4B) or two chemically synthesized oligopeptides (α-ZNS1 and α-ZNS2B) (Figure S6A,B). In all cases, the 19 to 51 aa antigenic regions of ZIKV were selected to have relatively low levels (16–42%) of amino acid sequence identity with those of JEV (Figure 6A). The resulting seven ZIKV region-specific antisera were used for a second series of immunoblots, in which we detected their respective ZIKV gene products (Figure 6B). In all immunoblots, we included two additional cell lysates (as a reference for JEV proteins) extracted from Vero cells infected with the virulent JEV strain SA_{14} or its attenuated strain SA_{14}-14-2; both JEVs share the same genome-wide viral protein expression profile, except that the NS1' protein is expressed only by SA_{14} [57].

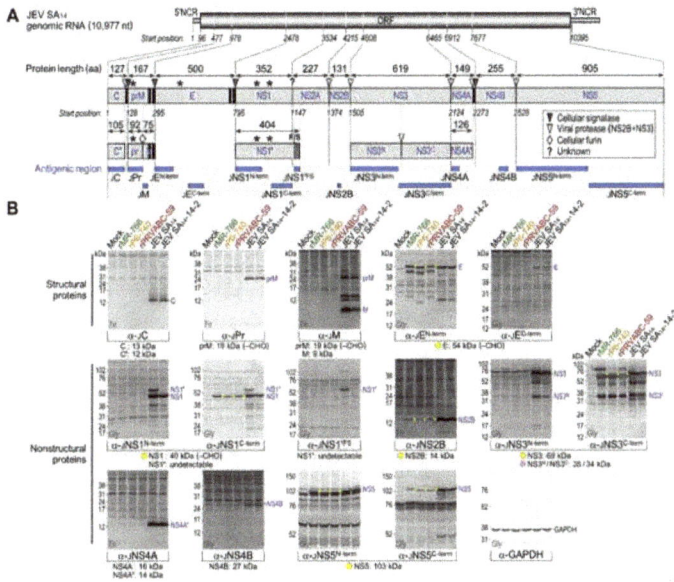

Figure 5. A subset of 15 JEV region-specific polyclonal antibodies detects the cross-reactive ZIKV E, NS1, NS2B, NS3, NS5, and their related species in ZIKV-infected cells. (**A**) Schematic illustration showing the antigenic regions recognized by 15 JEV region-specific rabbit antisera. The 10,977 nt genomic RNA of JEV SA_{14} has a 95 nt 5'NCR, a 10,299 nt ORF, and a 583 nt 3'NCR (top panel). The ORF encodes a 3432 aa polyprotein that is processed by viral and cellular proteases into at least 10 mature proteins (middle panel). Marked on the polyprotein are one or two transmembrane domains (vertical black bar) at the C-termini of three structural proteins (C, prM, and E) and at the junction of NS4A/NS4B, as well as four *N*-glycosylation sites (asterisk) in the pr portion of prM (^{15}NNT), E (^{154}NYS), and NS1 (^{130}NST and ^{207}NDT). During viral morphogenesis, prM is cleaved by furin protease into a soluble pr peptide and a virion-associated M protein. NS1' is the product of a −1 ribosomal frameshift (F/S) event that occurs at codons 8–9 of NS2A, adding a 52 aa C-terminal extension to the NS1 protein. The bottom panel displays the antigenic regions (horizontal blue bar) recognized by 15 JEV region-specific rabbit antisera. (**B**) Identification of viral proteins in ZIKV-infected cells by immunoblotting. Vero cells were mock-infected or infected at MOI 1 with each of three ZIKVs (rMR-766, rP6-740, and rPRVABC-59) or two JEVs (SA_{14} and SA_{14}-14-2, for reference). At 20 h post-infection, total cell lysates were separated by SDS-PAGE on a glycine (Gly) or tricine (Tri) gel and analyzed by immunoblotting with each of the 15 JEV region-specific rabbit antisera or α-GAPDH rabbit antiserum as a loading and transfer control. Molecular size markers are given on the left of each blot, and major JEV proteins for reference are labeled on the right. Provided below each blot are the estimated molecular sizes of the predicted ZIKV proteins, and marked on the blot are the predicted proteins (yellow or pink dot) and presumed cleavage intermediates or further cleavage/degradation products (white circle). CHO, *N*-glycosylation.

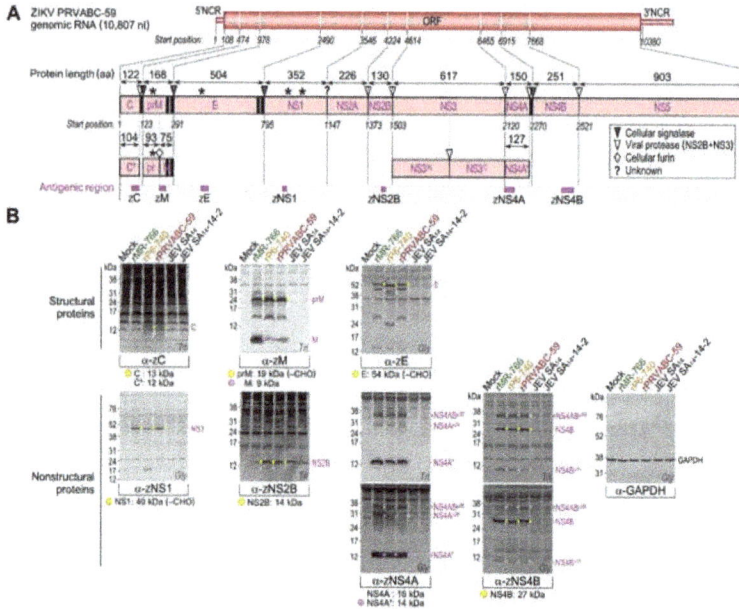

Figure 6. A panel of seven ZIKV region-specific polyclonal antibodies identifies ZIKV C, prM/M, E, NS1, NS2B, NS4A', NS4B, and their related species in ZIKV-infected cells. (**A**) Schematic illustration showing the antigenic regions recognized by seven ZIKV region-specific rabbit antisera. The 10,807 nt genomic RNA of ZIKV PRVABC-59 consists of a 107 nt 5'NCR, a 10,272 nt ORF, and a 428 nt 3'NCR (top panel). The ORF encodes a 3423 aa polyprotein that is predicted to be cleaved by viral and cellular proteases into at least 10 mature proteins (middle panel). Marked on the polyprotein and its products are one or two transmembrane domains (vertical black bar) at the C-termini of three structural proteins (C, prM, and E) and at the junction of NS4A/NS4B, as well as four *N*-glycosylation sites (asterisk) in the pr portion of prM (^{70}NTT), E (^{154}NDT), and NS1 (^{130}NNS and ^{207}NDT). The bottom panel shows the antigenic regions (horizontal magenta bar) recognized by seven ZIKV region-specific rabbit antisera. (**B**) Identification of viral proteins in ZIKV-infected cells by immunoblotting. Vero cells were mock-infected or infected at MOI 1 with each of three ZIKVs (rMR-766, rP6-740, and rPRVABC-59) or two JEVs (SA$_{14}$ and SA$_{14}$-14-2, for comparison). At 20 h post-infection, total cell lysates were separated by SDS-PAGE on a glycine (Gly) or tricine (Tri) gel and analyzed by immunoblotting with each of the seven ZIKV region-specific rabbit antisera or α-GAPDH rabbit antiserum as a loading and transfer control. Molecular size markers are given on the left of each blot, and major ZIKV proteins are labeled on the right. Provided below each blot are the estimated molecular sizes of predicted ZIKV proteins, and marked on the blot are the predicted proteins (yellow or pink dot) and presumed cleavage intermediates or further cleavage/degradation products (white circle). CHO, *N*-glycosylation.

Our immunoblot analysis using a collection of 13 ZIKV antigen-reactive region-specific rabbit antisera allowed us to create a full catalog of viral gene products and their related species, except for the predicted 24 kDa NS2A (Figures 5 and 6): (1) α-ZC recognized the 13 kDa C protein, with no accumulation of the further-processed 12 kDa C' (see below for description of virion-associated proteins), but with appearance of one or two cleavage products of 10–11 kDa in rPRVABC-59- or rP6-740-infected cells, respectively; however, this antiserum did not react with any of the C-related proteins of rMR-766. (2) α-ZM reacted strongly with the 9 kDa M protein and its 24 kDa precursor prM, with the ratio of M:prM varying in the presence of equal amounts of the loading control GAPDH protein, depending on the viral strain; the observed size of prM was 5 kDa larger than its predicted size, consistent with an addition of *N*-glycans at Asn-70 (^{70}NTT) to its pr domain [64] that is conserved in all three ZIKVs. Also, the α-ZM reacted weakly with at least two minor proteins of 15 and 19 kDa. (3) α-JE$^{N\text{-term}}$/α-ZE detected four E-related proteins (of 54/56, 43/45, 24/26, and 14 kDa). Among these, the first three proteins from rP6-740 were all 2 kDa smaller than those from rMR-766 and rPRVABC-59, in agreement with a missense mutation of the *N*-glycosylation site at Asn-154 (^{154}NDT→NDI) in the E protein of rP6-740 relative to that of rMR-766 and rPRVABC-59 [19,20]. Indeed, the three 2 kDa smaller proteins from rP6-740 became similar in size to those from rMR-766 and rPRVABC-59, when the mutated *N*-glycosylation motif in rP6-740 was restored by changing ^{154}NDI into ^{154}NDT, but not by changing ^{154}NDI into ^{154}QDT (Figure S7A–C). (4) Both α-JNS1$^{C\text{-term}}$ and α-ZNS1 identified the 45 kDa NS1 exclusively. This protein was 5 kDa larger than predicted by its amino acid sequence because of the addition of *N*-glycans at Asn-130 (^{130}NNS) and Asn-207 (^{207}NDT), both of which are conserved in all three ZIKVs [65,66]. As expected, these data also showed that only NS1, and not its frameshift product NS1', was produced by all three ZIKVs. (5) α-JNS2B/α-ZNS2B revealed the 14 kDa NS2B, together with a minor protein of 11 kDa at a barely detectable level. (6) α-JNS3$^{C\text{-term}}$ recognized the 69 kDa NS3; it also reacted more strongly with a major cleavage product of 34 kDa, representing the C-terminal half of the full-length NS3 [31], and less intensely with at least seven minor proteins of 33–60 kDa. Intriguingly, α-JNS3$^{C\text{-term}}$ detected a species with a mass of 85 kDa, corresponding to the calculated size of an NS2B-3 or NS3-4A/4A' processing intermediate. (7) α-ZNS4A did not detect the predicted 16 kDa NS4A, but did predominantly recognize its further-processed 14 kDa NS4A', which ran as a single species in tricine–SDS-PAGE but migrated as a doublet in glycine–SDS-PAGE. Unexpectedly, this antiserum also identified two clusters of multiple protein bands, one at 29 kDa (NS4A^{P29}) and the other at 35 kDa (NS4AB^{P35}, which also reacted with α-ZNS4B; Figure S8A,B). (8) α-ZNS4B stained the predicted major 27 kDa NS4B, along with two minor proteins at 11 kDa (NS4B^{P11}) and 35 kDa (NS4AB^{P35}, which again reacted with α-ZNS4A; Figures S8A,B). (9) α-JNS5$^{N\text{-term}}$ and α-JNS5$^{C\text{-term}}$ reacted with the predicted 103 kDa NS5.

In addition to the three full-length structural proteins (C, prM/M, and E) of ZIKV, their multiple smaller products were accumulated to lower but still significant amounts in Vero cells infected with each of the three ZIKVs, with nearly the same protein expression profile (Figure 6). To define the actual viral structural proteins incorporated into ZIKV particles, rPRVABC-59 was used to profile all the structural proteins associated with extracellular virions, which were purified by pelleting through a 20% sucrose cushion. We then compared them with their cell-associated counterparts by immunoblotting with α-ZC, α-ZM, and α-ZE (Figure 7). The purified ZIKV particles were shown to contain (i) the 12 kDa C' protein, which appeared as a closely spaced doublet with the lower band being more prominent than the upper band and migrating in a gel marginally faster than one cell-associated major 13 kDa C protein, but slower than the other cell-associated minor 10 kDa C-derived cleavage product; (ii) the 9 kDa M protein and a trace amount of its glycosylated precursor prM, which appeared as two bands, the slightly less intense and faster one migrating with a mass of 23–24 kDa and the slightly more intense and slower one at 25–26 kDa, reflecting the trimming of high mannose and the addition of more complex sugars to the cell-associated 24 kDa prM protein during virus release through the cellular secretory pathway [67]; and (iii) the glycosylated 58 kDa E protein, which ran slightly slower than the cell-associated 56 kDa E protein, again reflecting the difference in its glycosylation status. Collectively, we have demonstrated that the extracellular ZIKVs are composed of three post-translationally modified full-length structural proteins, excluding their smaller species.

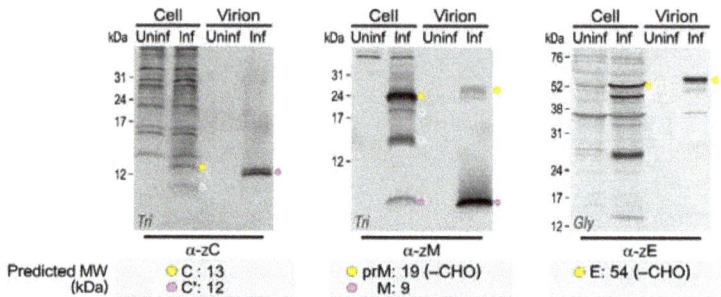

Figure 7. Profiling of virion-associated ZIKV proteins compared to their cell-associated counterparts. Vero cells were left uninfected (Uninf) or infected (Inf) with ZIKV rPRVABC-59 at an MOI of 1. For cell-associated viral proteins, total cell lysates were prepared by lysing the cell monolayers at 20 h post-infection. For virion-associated viral proteins, cell culture supernatants were collected at the same time point, and extracellular virions were pelleted by ultracentrifugation through a 20% sucrose cushion. Equivalent portions of total cell lysates and pelleted virions were resolved by SDS-PAGE on a glycine (Gly) or tricine (Tri) gel and analyzed by immunoblotting with α-ZC, α-ZM, or α-ZE. Molecular weight markers are shown on the left of each blot. The molecular weights of predicted C, C', prM, M, and E proteins are indicated below each blot. Marked on each blot are the predicted proteins (yellow or pink dot) and presumed further cleavage/degradation products (white circle). CHO, N-glycosylation.

3.5. Wide Range of Differences in Age-Dependent Neuropathogenicity among Three Molecularly Cloned ZIKVs in Outbred CD-1 Mice

We compared the virulence of rMR-766, rP6-740, and rPRVABC-59 in CD-1 mice at three different ages (1, 2, and 4 weeks) by examining two neuropathogenic properties: (i) neuroinvasiveness (the ability to penetrate the central nervous system from a peripheral site), quantified by generating the dose-dependent survival curve and determining the LD_{50} after an im inoculation; and (ii) neurovirulence (the ability to establish a lethal infection within the central nervous system), quantified by creating the dose-dependent survival curve and measuring the LD_{50} after an ic inoculation. For both im and ic inoculations, we first determined the appropriate dose ranges for calculating the LD_{50} values, and we optimized the study designs prior to the performance of full-scale experiments. For these pilot experiments, we injected all three age groups of the mice with a maximum dose of each virus: 1.2×10^5 PFU/mouse for im inoculations and 3.6×10^4 PFU/mouse for ic inoculations. If necessary, we then performed a series of large-scale dose-response studies, inoculating groups of the mice at 1, 2, and 4 weeks of age via the im or ic route with serial 10-fold dilutions of the virus. Following infection, the mice were monitored daily for mortality, weight loss, and other clinical signs of illness over 20 days.

The comparative assessments of our dose-dependent survival curves and LD_{50} values revealed the following (Figure 8A): (i) rMR-766 exhibited age-dependent neuroinvasiveness, as evidenced by an im LD_{50} of 90.2 PFU for 1-week-old mice and $>1.2 \times 10^5$ PFU for 2- and 4-week-old mice, yet it displayed a high level of neurovirulence at all three ages, as evidenced by an ic LD_{50} of <3.6, 3.6, and 5.7 PFU for 1-, 2-, and 4-week-old mice, respectively. (ii) rP6-740 showed barely detectable neuroinvasiveness in 1-week-old mice, with only 1 or 3 of 10 infected mice dying when inoculated with the two highest doses, 3.6×10^3 or 3.6×10^4 PFU/mouse, respectively (im LD_{50}, $>3.6 \times 10^4$ PFU). Similarly, it had no detectable neuroinvasiveness in 2- and 4-week-old mice, with no infected mice dying even when inoculated with the highest dose, 1.2×10^5 PFU/mouse (im LD_{50}, $>1.2 \times 10^5$ PFU). However, rP6-740 showed age-dependent neurovirulence, as it was highly neurovirulent in 1-week-old mice (ic LD_{50}, <3.6 PFU) but non-neurovirulent in 2- and 4-week-old mice (ic LD_{50}, $>3.6 \times 10^4$ PFU). (iii) rPRVABC-59 was essentially non-neuroinvasive and non-neurovirulent, regardless of the mouse age, with its im and ic LD$_{50}$ values estimated to be greater than the highest dose used for each route of infection, without a single death. Of the three ZIKVs, therefore, rMR-766 was the most virulent, rPRVABC-59 was the least virulent, and rP6-740 showed intermediate virulence. The observed differences in virulence are correlated with the variations in viral passage history in mice (Figure 1A).

Moreover, we recognized not only the lethal virulence displayed by rMR-766 and rP6-740 but also the non-lethal virulence exhibited by all of the three ZIKVs, including rPRVABC-59. This effect was most prominent in 1-week-old mice (Figure 8B). The lethal virulence was invariably associated with a sharp drop in the body weight of infected mice that began ~3 days prior to death, in conjunction with clinical signs. It began with decreased activity, ruffled fur, and hunched posture, and often progressed to tremors and hind limb paralysis. Various viral loads were detected postmortem in the brains of all mice that died (8.0×10^3–3.9×10^8 PFU/brain). Non-lethal virulence, in contrast, was characterized by an initial weight loss of various degrees, albeit without obvious clinical signs, and a subsequent recovery, to some extent, that was not complete. At the end of the study, no infectious ZIKV was detected in the brains of any of the mice that survived. In both the lethal and non-lethal virulent cases, no changes in body temperature were observed. Altogether, we found that in CD-1 mice, the three ZIKVs had a wide range of virulence, depending on the virus strain, mouse age, and route of infection.

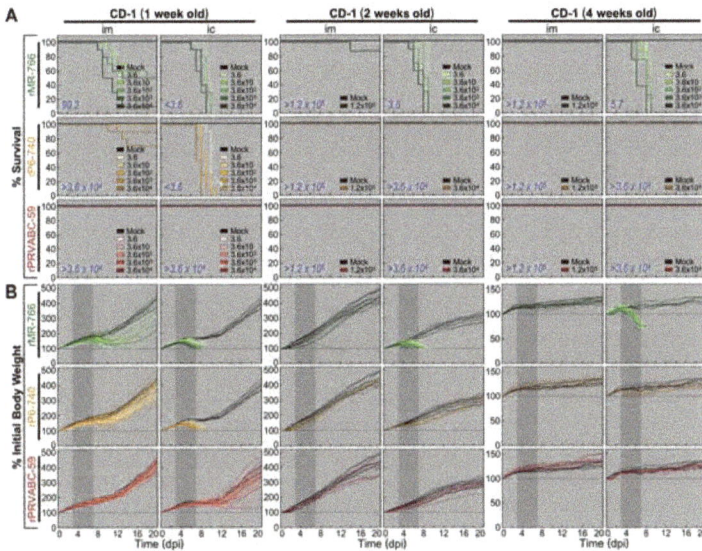

Figure 8. Three molecularly cloned ZIKVs display a full range of variation in neuropathogenicity for outbred CD-1 mice in an age-dependent manner. Groups of CD-1 mice (*n* = 8–10, half male, half female) were mock-inoculated or inoculated at 1, 2, and 4 weeks of age via the intramuscular (im) or intracerebral (ic) route with a maximum dose of 3.6×10^4 or 1.2×10^5 PFU, or serial 10-fold dilutions of rMR-766, rP6-740, or rPRVABC-59. (**A**) Survival curves were generated by the Kaplan–Meier method, and LD$_{50}$ values were determined by the Reed–Muench method and are presented in the bottom left corner of each curve. (**B**) Weight changes are plotted, with each mouse represented by one color-coded line. dpi, days post-infection.

3.6. High Degree of Variation in Interferon (IFN) Sensitivity among Three Molecularly Cloned ZIKVs in Mice Lacking Type I (IFNAR$^{-/-}$) or Both Type I and II IFN (IFNAR$^{-/-}$/IFNGR$^{-/-}$) Receptors

To compare the contributions of the host IFN response to the virulence of rMR-766, rP6-740, and rPRVABC-59, we examined their neuroinvasiveness and neurovirulence by using groups of 4-week-old A129 (IFNAR$^{-/-}$) mice and groups of age-matched wild-type inbred C57BL/6J mice as a control (Figure 9A). In the control mice, rMR-766 was non-neuroinvasive (im LD_{50}, $>1.2 \times 10^5$ PFU) but neurovirulent (ic LD_{50}, 7.8 PFU). In contrast, both rP6-740 and rPRVABC-59 were non-neuroinvasive (im LD_{50}, $>1.2 \times 10^5$ PFU) as well as non-neurovirulent (ic LD_{50}, $>3.6 \times 10^4$ PFU), in agreement with the data obtained in age-matched outbred CD-1 mice (Figure 8A). In A129 mice, however, the neurovirulence of all three ZIKVs was increased sharply, and they became highly neurovirulent (ic LD_{50}, <3.6 PFU), with median survival times estimated to be 4 (rMR-766), 5 (rP6-740), and 7 (rPRVABC-59) days, with a lethal dose of 3.6×10^2 PFU/mouse. Similarly, the neuroinvasiveness of the three ZIKVs was also elevated but to different degrees, as evidenced by the estimated im LD_{50} of <1.2 (rMR-766), 576.1 (rP6-740), and $>1.2 \times 10^5$ (rPRVABC-59) PFU. Noticeably, rPRVABC-59 was nearly non-neuroinvasive in A129 mice. This finding prompted us to further test the neuroinvasiveness of rPRVABC-59, as compared to that of the other two ZIKVs, in 4-week-old AG129 (IFNAR$^{-/-}$/IFNGR$^{-/-}$) mice (Figure 9A). In AG129 mice, all three ZIKVs were highly neuroinvasive (im LD_{50}, <1.2 PFU), although the median survival times for the three viruses varied from 7 (rMR-766) to 12 (rP6-740) and 13 (rPRVABC-59) days, with a lethal dose of 1.2×10^2 PFU/mouse. Furthermore, in all three mouse strains (C57BL/6J, A129, and AG129), the two LD_{50}-based neuropathogenic properties of the three ZIKVs were always corroborated by the decreases in body weight (Figure 9B), accompanied by the typical clinical signs seen in CD-1 mice. In all the mice that died, various viral loads were detected in their brains postmortem, with higher loads being found in the absence of IFN signaling, i.e., 4.7×10^4–2.0×10^8 PFU/brain for C57BL/6J, 1.3×10^6–1.0×10^9 PFU/brain for A129, and 8.5×10^6–3.6×10^9 PFU/brain for AG129. In the case of all mice that survived, however, we detected no infectious ZIKV in the brain at the end of the study. Taken together, these data show a full range of variation in IFN sensitivity among the three cloned ZIKVs in mice.

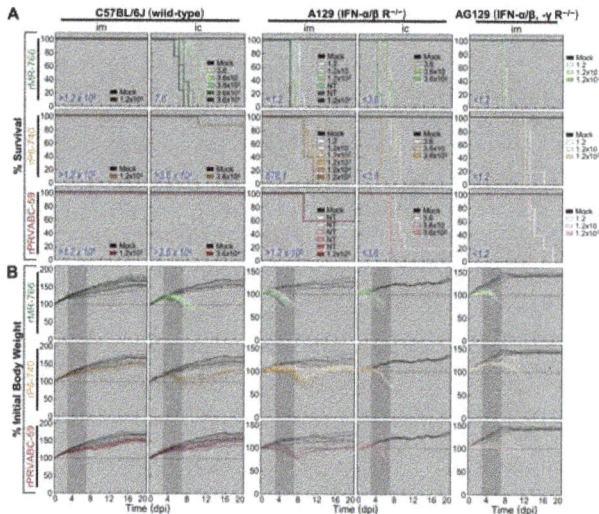

Figure 9. Three molecularly cloned ZIKVs show a full spectrum of variation in IFN sensitivity in mice lacking type I or both type I and II IFN receptors. Groups of 4-week-old C57BL/6J ($n = 8$), A129 ($n = 5$), or AG129 ($n = 5$) mice, approximately half of each sex, were mock-inoculated or inoculated through the intramuscular (im) or intracerebral (ic) route with a maximum dose of 3.6×10^4 or 1.2×10^5 PFU, or serial 10-fold dilutions of rMR-766, rP6-740, or rPRVABC-59. (**A**) Survival curves were created by the Kaplan–Meier method, and LD_{50} values were calculated by the Reed–Muench method and are given in the bottom left corner of each curve; (**B**) Weight changes are plotted, with each mouse indicated by one color-coded line. NT, not tested; dpi, days post-infection.

4. Discussion

Here, we report the first development of three full-length infectious ZIKV cDNAs as BACs for each of three spatiotemporally distinct and genetically divergent ZIKV strains [54]: MR-766 (Uganda, 1947), P6-740 (Malaysia, 1966), and PRVABC-59 (Puerto Rico, 2015). We have also produced 13 ZIKV region-specific polyclonal rabbit antisera capable of identifying all the viral structural and nonstructural proteins and their related species, except for NS2A. Using our functional cDNAs and antibodies in combination with various cell culture and murine model systems, we have demonstrated that the three molecularly cloned cDNA-derived ZIKVs have the nearly same genome-wide viral protein expression profile but differ in their replication kinetics and neuropathogenicity (neuroinvasiveness and neurovirulence), depending on the particular combination of viral and host genetic backgrounds, as well as in the presence or absence of type I/II IFN signaling. In particular, our results demonstrate that type I IFN regulates ZIKV neuroinvasiveness in a virus strain-dependent manner. In all, these reagents offer a new toolbox for viral genome engineering and protein analysis. Together with a roster of in vitro and in vivo infection models, these tools will not only provide an ideal platform for defining the viral and host genetic factors that contribute to ZIKV replication and pathogenesis at the cellular and organismic levels, but also offer promising new avenues for developing and testing an effective, critically needed vaccine against ZIKV.

The advent of functional cDNA-based reverse genetics has revamped the field of RNA viruses [68]. For flaviviruses, however, the cloned cDNAs are commonly unstable because of the toxicity of their prM-E genes in host cells, posing a major technical challenge to functional cDNA construction [69]. In the present study, we cloned a complete cDNA copy of the ZIKV genomic RNA into a BAC vector that is capable of stably housing a DNA fragment of >300 kb in bacteria [70], as we have already done for JEV [53,58]. In the case of all three ZIKVs (MR-766, P6-740, and PRVABC-59), we showed that the structural and functional integrity of their full-length BACs remained stable for at least 80 generations of growth in *E. coli*. To date, the BAC cloning technology has been applied to constructing full-length infectious cDNAs for ~10 members of three plus-strand RNA virus families (*Flaviviridae*, *Arteriviridae*, and *Coronaviridae*), all of which have a large genome size of 11–31 kb [52]. Moreover, we performed site-directed mutagenesis to introduce a point mutation(s) into the full-length infectious cDNA BAC clone of ZIKV P6-740, which demonstrated (i) the functional importance of His-713 within the conserved structural motif E region in the RNA-dependent RNA polymerase domain of ZIKV NS5 for viral RNA replication and (ii) the functional significance of the *N*-glycosylation site at Asn-154 in the viral E protein for its biogenesis. These results indicate that targeted mutations can be engineered by manipulating the infectious ZIKV BACs in *E. coli*. Thus, our BAC-based reverse genetics for ZIKV will facilitate genetic studies of both viral RNA elements and gene products associated with all aspects of ZIKV biology.

We formulated a strategy to assemble three full-length infectious ZIKV cDNAs, each capable of generating m^7G-capped in vitro-transcribed RNAs identical in nucleotide sequence to their respective genomic RNAs, particularly regarding the 5'- and 3'-end sequences. On the 5' side, we positioned an SP6 promoter sequence (5'-ATTTAGGGGACACTATA<u>G</u>, with transcription starting at the underlined G) upstream of the first adenine nucleotide of the viral genome to incorporate the dinucleotide cap analog m^7GpppA in SP6 RNA polymerase-driven in vitro transcription reactions. The importance of an m^7G cap at the 5'-end of transcribed RNAs in maximizing RNA infectivity was shown by our finding that uncapped RNAs derived from each of the three functional ZIKV cDNAs always had an infectivity >3-logs lower than that of their m^7G-capped counterparts. On the 3' side, we placed a unique restriction endonuclease recognition site, *Psr*I [$(N_7\downarrow N_{12})GAACN_6TAC(N_{12}\downarrow N_7)$] or *Bar*I [$(N_7\downarrow N_{12})GAAGN_6TAC(N_{12}\downarrow N_7)$], downstream of the last thymine nucleotide of the viral genome. The use of *Psr*I/*Bar*I for cDNA linearization is particularly advantageous because both are extremely rare-cutting endonucleases that cut out their recognition sequences after any nucleotide, which makes this approach applicable for all plus-strand RNA viruses, regardless of the identity of the nucleotide at the 3' end of the viral genome. We found that RNA transcripts with 11 ZIKV-unrelated nucleotides hanging on their 3′ ends were ~1-log less infectious than those with authentic 3′ ends, indicating the importance of the authentic 3′ end for the production of infectious ZIKV RNAs.

Several functional cDNAs for ZIKV have hitherto been made using two different strategies, depending on the vector adopted to clone its full-length cDNA and the method applied to create the viral 5′ and 3′ ends: (i) The low-copy plasmid pACYC177 (~15 copies/cell) has been utilized to house a complete cDNA flanked by a 5′ bacteriophage T7 promoter and a 3′ hepatitis delta virus ribozyme (HDVr). This T7-HDVr system, analogous to our SP6-*PsrI*/*BarI* system, requires an in vitro transcription and transfection of transcribed RNAs into cells for virus recovery. This "RNA-initiated" approach has been implemented to clone the viral genomic RNA of the 2010 Cambodian FSS13025 strain [71]. To circumvent the need for a single plasmid containing a full-length cDNA, in vitro ligation of two or four cDNA fragments pre-cloned individually into the low-copy pACYC177 or high-copy pUC57 (500–700 copies/cell) plasmid, although relatively inefficient, has been done to generate a full-length cDNA template prior to in vitro transcription using the T7-HDVr system for the Ugandan MR-766 (1947), French Polynesian H/PF/2013 (2013), Puerto Rican PRVABC-59 (2015), and Brazilian SPH2015 (2015) and BeH819015 (2015) strains [49,72]. (ii) The low-copy pACNR1811 (10–20 copies/cell) or high-copy pcDNA6.2 (500–700 copies/cell) plasmid is used to house a full-length cDNA containing one or two artificial introns to restrict its instability during propagation in *E. coli*. In this case, a eukaryotic RNA polymerase (RNAP) II-dependent cytomegalovirus (CMV) promoter is positioned before the viral 5′ end, and a pair of HDVr and an SV40 poly(A) signal/RNAP II terminator are placed after the viral 3′ end. Unlike our SP6-*PsrI*/*BarI* system, the CMV-HDVr system requires transfection of cells with a plasmid carrying the intron-bearing full-length cDNA. This "DNA-initiated" approach has been applied to clone the viral genomic RNA of the Ugandan MR-766 (1947) and Brazilian Paraiba (2015) strains [73,74]. Alternatively, a circular form of the intronless full-length cDNA for the 2015 Brazilian Natal strain has been generated by PCR-mediated joining of eight overlapping cDNA fragments that are pre-cloned individually into the high-copy pUC plasmid [75]. Although far less efficient, a similar PCR-based method has also been reported that uses three overlapping cDNA fragments covering the viral genomic RNA with no joining of these fragments into a circular cDNA [76]. In the present study, we developed a single plasmid-based RNA-initiated reverse genetics system for ZIKV that not only maximizes the genetic stability of its cloned cDNA using a single-copy BAC as a vector, but also optimizes the synthesis of infectious RNAs in vitro using the SP6-*PsrI*/*BarI* system.

ZIKV circulates in a sylvatic cycle between nonhuman primates (NHPs) and forest-dwelling mosquitoes, as well as in an urban cycle between humans and town-dwelling mosquitoes [12]. Apart from NHPs, however, information is scarce on any potential animal hosts or reservoirs for ZIKV transmission. Using our three cDNA-derived genetically distinct ZIKVs, we evaluated their ability to infect and replicate in 17 animal cell lines from 12 different species (monkeys, humans, mosquitoes, mice, cows, pigs, sheep, goats, horses, dogs, cats, and chickens). Our data showed that ZIKV has a broad cell tropism in vitro, being capable of establishing productive infection in 16 of the 17 cell lines we tested, although its growth rate and ability to induce CPE varied widely depending on both the specific virus strain and host cell line. Of particular note, all three ZIKVs grew readily in both porcine ST and equine NBL-6 cells, with their growth kinetics similar to those observed in simian Vero cells; generally, they also replicated and spread equally well in ovine SFF-6 cells and in aedine C6/36 cells. These results raise a question as to whether several agriculturally important domestic animals (e.g., pigs, sheep, and horses) are susceptible to ZIKV infection, particularly when young. With respect to this question, two recent studies have reported that fetal and neonatal piglets are susceptible to experimental infection with ZIKV [77,78]. Another pilot study has suggested that a range of adult animals, including rabbits, goats, pigs, cattle, chickens, and ducks, are less likely to act as animal hosts for ZIKV, based on the levels of viremia and neutralizing antibody titer induced following ZIKV infection; of these animals, however, rabbits and pigs are proposed to be able to serve as sentinels for ZIKV surveillance [79]. Clearly, further investigation is needed to elucidate the susceptibility of these animals to ZIKV infection, preferentially in the presence or absence of type I IFN signaling, and might provide new opportunities to increase our understanding of ZIKV biology and to develop a non-murine model for ZIKV research. Moreover, we discovered a nonsusceptible bovine MDBK cell line that has a block in ZIKV entry but fully supports the subsequent post-entry steps; however, this cell line remained highly susceptible to infection by two other enveloped RNA viruses, BVDV [80] and VSV [81], which like ZIKV [63], enter the cells through clathrin-dependent endocytic pathway. This ZIKV-nonsusceptible bovine cell line thus offers a unique opportunity to identify the host factors involved in ZIKV entry.

To our knowledge, this work is the first to generate such a large panel of 13 ZIKV region-specific antibodies that can identify experimentally nearly all the viral gene products and their related species in ZIKV-infected Vero cells and define all three structural proteins associated with extracellular virions. Our data are in overall good agreement with the current model for flavivirus polyprotein processing [21], but they have also revealed a considerable number of previously undescribed, presumed cleavage intermediates or further cleavage/degradation products. The main findings from our study are as follows: (1) While the full-length 13 kDa C and its one or two processed 10 to 11 kDa proteins were accumulated intracellularly, the extracellular virion-associated C' protein appeared as a tightly spaced 12 kDa doublet. (2) For each of the two viral surface glycoproteins (24 kDa prM and 54/56 kDa E), two or three smaller products were also cell-associated but not virion-associated. (3) Only the 45 kDa NS1, and not its theoretically frameshift-derived product NS1', was expressed. (4) In addition to the intact 14 kDa NS2B, its processed 11 kDa product was also stained, although weakly. (5) The full-length 69 kDa NS3 was processed to yield multiple truncated species of 33–60 kDa, of which the C-terminal 34 kDa fragment was the most prominent species. (6) The predicted 16 kDa NS4A was completely undetectable, but three unpredicted NS4A-related proteins were readily identified, i.e., a major doublet at 14 kDa (NS4A') and two minor protein clusters at 29 kDa (NS4AP^{29}) and 35 kDa (NS4ABP^{35}). (7) Not only the predicted 27 kDa NS4B but also two unpredicted NS4B-related proteins were observed, one at 11 kDa (NS4BP^{11}) and the other at 35 kDa (NS4ABP^{35}). However, the functional importance of the previously undescribed cleavage intermediates or further cleavage/degradation products in ZIKV biology remains to be determined.

Much progress has been made over the past year in developing animal models (i.e., mice and NHPs) for ZIKV [43]. To date, the mouse is the most feasible small animal that mimics aspects of ZIKV infection in humans, albeit with some limitations resulting from species differences in innate immunity, reproductive system, and fetal development. Previously, no productive infection was detected when several strains of immunocompetent adult mice were inoculated peripherally with diverse ZIKVs, but robust peripheral ZIKV infection causing substantial morbidity and mortality was observed in both immunocompromised adult and immunocompetent neonatal mice [44,46,82–89]. We call attention, however, to the large variation in ZIKV pathogenicity among the previous studies, which were conducted by inoculating a variety of ZIKVs into different strains of mice via various routes. In the current report, we have shown in immunocompetent CD-1 mice at 1, 2, and 4 weeks of age that ZIKV neuropathogenicity can only be defined in the context of a virus-host combination, particularly depending on both viral strain and mouse age, as evidenced by comparison of the neuroinvasiveness and neurovirulence of our three molecularly cloned, genetically distinct ZIKVs: (i) rMR-766 exhibited neonate-specific age-dependent neuroinvasiveness but displayed a high level of neurovirulence at all three ages. (ii) rP6-740 had little-to-no neuroinvasiveness at all three ages but possessed neonate-specific age-dependent neurovirulence. (iii) rPRVABC-59 was non-neuroinvasive and non-neurovirulent at all three ages. Also, we showed marked differences in IFN sensitivity among the three ZIKVs: In 4-week-old A129 (IFNAR$^{-/-}$) mice, the three ZIKVs were uniformly neurovirulent but varied in neuroinvasiveness (rMR-766, neuroinvasive; rP6-740, intermediate; and rPRVABC-59, almost non-neuroinvasive); however, all three ZIKVs, including rPRVABC-59, were neuroinvasive in age-matched AG129 (IFNAR$^{-/-}$/IFNGR$^{-/-}$) mice. Consistent with previous work, we noted a greater susceptibility and more severe disease in AG129 mice than in A129 mice [44–49]. In all fatal cases, the mortality was related to the productive infection in the brain, coupled with tremors, ataxia, and hind limb paralysis.

In conclusion, use of our newly developed comparative functional genomics and immunologic tools, combined with various cell culture and mouse infection model systems, will facilitate further research leading to ZIKV disease prevention and therapy, as well as an in-depth understanding of ZIKV biology.

Supplementary Materials: The following are available online at http://www.mdpi.com/1999-4915/10/8/422/s1, Figure S1: A single $C^{9804} \rightarrow U$ substitution essentially eliminates the specific infectivity of RNA transcripts derived from a full-length infectious cDNA clone of ZIKV P6-740, Figure S2: Three functional ZIKV cDNA clones are stably propagated in bacteria as BACs, Figure S3: ZIKV growth kinetics and cytopathogenicity in cell cultures depend on the particular combination of virus strain and host cells, Figure S4: MDBK cells are highly susceptible to infection with both BVDV and VSV, Figure S5: Details of the 15 JEV region-specific rabbit antisera used to detect their antigenically cross-reactive ZIKV counterparts, Figure S6: Details of the seven ZIKV region-specific rabbit antisera used to identify ZIKV gene products and their related species, Figure S7: A missense mutation eliminating the N-glycosylation site at Asn-154 in the viral protein E of rP6-740 is responsible for the observed lower molecular weights of the E and its two related proteins, Figure S8: Multiple NS4A- and NS4B-related proteins are accumulated in ZIKV-infected cells.

Author Contributions: S.-I.Y. and Y.-M.L. conceived and designed the experiments; S.-I.Y., B.-H.S. and J.C.F. performed the experiments; J.G.J., A.L.O., I.A.P., C.J.D. and K.L.W. contributed with reagents and materials/analysis tools; S.-I.Y., B.-H.S., J.C.F., I.A.P., C.J.D. and Y.-M.L. analyzed the data; S.-I.Y. and Y.-M.L. wrote the paper with contributions from all authors.

Funding: This work was funded in part by grants from the Utah Science Technology and Research (A34637 and A36815) and by a grant from the American Board of Obstetrics and Gynecology, the American College of Obstetricians and Gynecologists, the American Society for Reproductive Medicine, and the Society for Reproductive Endocrinology and Infertility (200784-00001). This research was also supported by the Utah Agricultural Experiment Station (UTA01345) and approved as journal paper number #8929.

Acknowledgments: We thank Robert Tesh for providing ZIKV MR-766 and P6-740, Barbara Johnson for providing ZIKV PRVABC-59, Heidi Julander and Lynnette Potter for outstanding animal care, and Deborah McClellan for critical reading of the manuscript. Also, we thank Emily Robb, Jackeline Wilkinson, and Michael Berentzen for producing GST-tagged fusion proteins.

Conflicts of Interest: The authors declare no conflicts of interest. The founding sponsors had no role in the design of the study; in the collection, analyses, or interpretation of data; in the writing of the manuscript; or in the decision to publish the results.

References

1. Dick, G.W.; Kitchen, S.F.; Haddow, A.J. Zika virus. I. Isolations and serological specificity. *Trans. R. Soc. Trop. Med. Hyg.* **1952**, *46*, 509–520. [CrossRef]
2. Petersen, L.R.; Jamieson, D.J.; Powers, A.M.; Honein, M.A. Zika virus. *N. Engl. J. Med.* **2016**, *374*, 1552–1563. [CrossRef] [PubMed]
3. Yun, S.I.; Lee, Y.M. Zika virus: An emerging flavivirus. *J. Microbiol.* **2017**, *55*, 204–219. [CrossRef] [PubMed]
4. Musso, D.; Gubler, D.J. Zika virus. *Clin. Microbiol. Rev.* **2016**, *29*, 487–524. [CrossRef] [PubMed]
5. Lanciotti, R.S.; Kosoy, O.L.; Laven, J.J.; Velez, J.O.; Lambert, A.J.; Johnson, A.J.; Stanfield, S.M.; Duffy, M.R. Genetic and serologic properties of Zika virus associated with an epidemic, Yap State, Micronesia, 2007. *Emerg. Infect. Dis.* **2008**, *14*, 1232–1239. [CrossRef] [PubMed]
6. Duffy, M.R.; Chen, T.H.; Hancock, W.T.; Powers, A.M.; Kool, J.L.; Lanciotti, R.S.; Pretrick, M.; Marfel, M.; Holzbauer, S.; Dubray, C.; et al. Zika virus outbreak on Yap Island, Federated States of Micronesia. *N. Engl. J. Med.* **2009**, *360*, 2536–2543. [CrossRef] [PubMed]
7. Cao-Lormeau, V.M.; Musso, D. Emerging arboviruses in the Pacific. *Lancet* **2014**, *384*, 1571–1572. [CrossRef]
8. Campos, G.S.; Bandeira, A.C.; Sardi, S.I. Zika virus outbreak, Bahia, Brazil. *Emerg. Infect. Dis.* **2015**, *21*, 1885–1886. [CrossRef] [PubMed]
9. Zanluca, C.; Melo, V.C.; Mosimann, A.L.; Santos, G.I.; Santos, C.N.; Luz, K. First report of autochthonous transmission of Zika virus in Brazil. *Mem. Inst. Oswaldo Cruz* **2015**, *110*, 569–572. [CrossRef] [PubMed]
10. Lessler, J.; Chaisson, L.H.; Kucirka, L.M.; Bi, Q.; Grantz, K.; Salje, H.; Carcelen, A.C.; Ott, C.T.; Sheffield, J.S.; Ferguson, N.M.; et al. Assessing the global threat from Zika virus. *Science* **2016**, *353*, aaf8160. [CrossRef] [PubMed]

11. Song, B.H.; Yun, S.I.; Woolley, M.; Lee, Y.M. Zika virus: History, epidemiology, transmission, and clinical presentation. *J. Neuroimmunol.* **2017**, *308*, 50–64. [CrossRef] [PubMed]

12. Weaver, S.C.; Costa, F.; Garcia-Blanco, M.A.; Ko, A.I.; Ribeiro, G.S.; Saade, G.; Shi, P.Y.; Vasilakis, N. Zika virus: History, emergence, biology, and prospects for control. *Antiviral Res.* **2016**, *130*, 69–80. [CrossRef] [PubMed]

13. Calvet, G.; Aguiar, R.S.; Melo, A.S.; Sampaio, S.A.; de Filippis, I.; Fabri, A.; Araujo, E.S.; de Sequeira, P.C.; de Mendonca, M.C.; de Oliveira, L.; et al. Detection and sequencing of Zika virus from amniotic fluid of fetuses with microcephaly in Brazil: A case study. *Lancet Infect. Dis.* **2016**, *16*, 653–660. [CrossRef]

14. Mlakar, J.; Korva, M.; Tul, N.; Popovic, M.; Poljsak-Prijatelj, M.; Mraz, J.; Kolenc, M.; Resman Rus, K.; Vesnaver Vipotnik, T.; Fabjan Vodusek, V.; et al. Zika virus associated with microcephaly. *N. Engl. J. Med.* **2016**, *374*, 951–958. [CrossRef] [PubMed]

15. Foy, B.D.; Kobylinski, K.C.; Chilson Foy, J.L.; Blitvich, B.J.; Travassos da Rosa, A.; Haddow, A.D.; Lanciotti, R.S.; Tesh, R.B. Probable non-vector-borne transmission of Zika virus, Colorado, USA. *Emerg. Infect. Dis.* **2011**, *17*, 880–882. [CrossRef] [PubMed]

16. Musso, D.; Roche, C.; Robin, E.; Nhan, T.; Teissier, A.; Cao-Lormeau, V.M. Potential sexual transmission of Zika virus. *Emerg. Infect. Dis.* **2015**, *21*, 359–361. [CrossRef] [PubMed]

17. Lazear, H.M.; Diamond, M.S. Zika virus: New clinical syndromes and its emergence in the Western Hemisphere. *J. Virol.* **2016**, *90*, 4864–4875. [CrossRef] [PubMed]

18. Panchaud, A.; Stojanov, M.; Ammerdorffer, A.; Vouga, M.; Baud, D. Emerging role of Zika virus in adverse fetal and neonatal outcomes. *Clin. Microbiol. Rev.* **2016**, *29*, 659–694. [CrossRef] [PubMed]

19. Kostyuchenko, V.A.; Lim, E.X.; Zhang, S.; Fibriansah, G.; Ng, T.S.; Ooi, J.S.; Shi, J.; Lok, S.M. Structure of the thermally stable Zika virus. *Nature* **2016**, *533*, 425–428. [CrossRef] [PubMed]

20. Sirohi, D.; Chen, Z.; Sun, L.; Klose, T.; Pierson, T.C.; Rossmann, M.G.; Kuhn, R.J. The 3.8 A resolution cryo-EM structure of Zika virus. *Science* **2016**, *352*, 467–470. [CrossRef] [PubMed]

21. Lindenbach, B.D.; Murray, C.L.; Thiel, H.J.; Rice, C.M. Flaviviridae. In *Fields Virology*, 6th ed.; Knipe, D.M., Howley, P.M., Cohen, J.I., Griffin, D.E., Lamb, R.A., Martin, M.A., Racaniello, V.R., Roizman, B., Eds.; Wolters Kluwer Health: Philadelphia, PA, USA, 2013; pp. 712–746.

22. Perera-Lecoin, M.; Meertens, L.; Carnec, X.; Amara, A. Flavivirus entry receptors: An update. *Viruses* **2014**, *6*, 69–88. [CrossRef] [PubMed]

23. Pierson, T.C.; Kielian, M. Flaviviruses: Braking the entering. *Curr. Opin. Virol.* **2013**, *3*, 3–12. [CrossRef] [PubMed]

24. Sirohi, D.; Kuhn, R.J. Zika virus structure, maturation, and receptors. *J. Infect. Dis.* **2017**, *216* (Suppl. 10), S935–S944. [CrossRef] [PubMed]

25. Kaufmann, B.; Rossmann, M.G. Molecular mechanisms involved in the early steps of flavivirus cell entry. *Microbes Infect.* **2011**, *13*, 1–9. [CrossRef] [PubMed]

26. Smit, J.M.; Moesker, B.; Rodenhuis-Zybert, I.; Wilschut, J. Flavivirus cell entry and membrane fusion. *Viruses* **2011**, *3*, 160–171. [CrossRef] [PubMed]

27. Harrison, S.C. Viral membrane fusion. *Nat. Struct. Mol. Biol.* **2008**, *15*, 690–698. [CrossRef] [PubMed]

28. Paranjape, S.M.; Harris, E. Control of dengue virus translation and replication. *Curr. Top. Microbiol. Immunol.* **2010**, *338*, 15–34. [CrossRef] [PubMed]

29. Gebhard, L.G.; Filomatori, C.V.; Gamarnik, A.V. Functional RNA elements in the dengue virus genome. *Viruses* **2011**, *3*, 1739–1756. [CrossRef] [PubMed]

30. Brinton, M.A. Replication cycle and molecular biology of the West Nile virus. *Viruses* **2014**, *6*, 13–53. [CrossRef] [PubMed]

31. Kim, J.K.; Kim, J.M.; Song, B.H.; Yun, S.I.; Yun, G.N.; Byun, S.J.; Lee, Y.M. Profiling of viral proteins expressed from the genomic RNA of Japanese encephalitis virus using a panel of 15 region-specific polyclonal rabbit antisera: Implications for viral gene expression. *PLoS ONE* **2015**, *10*, e0124318. [CrossRef] [PubMed]

32. Ye, Q.; Li, X.F.; Zhao, H.; Li, S.H.; Deng, Y.Q.; Cao, R.Y.; Song, K.Y.; Wang, H.J.; Hua, R.H.; Yu, Y.X.; et al. A single nucleotide mutation in NS2A of Japanese encephalitis-live vaccine virus (SA$_{14}$-14-2) ablates NS1′ formation and contributes to attenuation. *J. Gen. Virol.* **2012**, *93*, 1959–1964. [CrossRef] [PubMed]

33. Melian, E.B.; Hinzman, E.; Nagasaki, T.; Firth, A.E.; Wills, N.M.; Nouwens, A.S.; Blitvich, B.J.; Leung, J.; Funk, A.; Atkins, J.F.; et al. NS1' of flaviviruses in the Japanese encephalitis virus serogroup is a product of ribosomal frameshifting and plays a role in viral neuroinvasiveness. *J. Virol.* **2010**, *84*, 1641–1647. [CrossRef] [PubMed]

34. Firth, A.E.; Atkins, J.F. A conserved predicted pseudoknot in the NS2A-encoding sequence of West Nile and Japanese encephalitis flaviviruses suggests NS1' may derive from ribosomal frameshifting. *Virol. J.* **2009**, *6*, 14. [CrossRef] [PubMed]

35. Welsch, S.; Miller, S.; Romero-Brey, I.; Merz, A.; Bleck, C.K.; Walther, P.; Fuller, S.D.; Antony, C.; Krijnse-Locker, J.; Bartenschlager, R. Composition and three-dimensional architecture of the dengue virus replication and assembly sites. *Cell Host Microbe* **2009**, *5*, 365–375. [CrossRef] [PubMed]

36. Gillespie, L.K.; Hoenen, A.; Morgan, G.; Mackenzie, J.M. The endoplasmic reticulum provides the membrane platform for biogenesis of the flavivirus replication complex. *J. Virol.* **2010**, *84*, 10438–10447. [CrossRef] [PubMed]

37. Bollati, M.; Alvarez, K.; Assenberg, R.; Baronti, C.; Canard, B.; Cook, S.; Coutard, B.; Decroly, E.; de Lamballerie, X.; Gould, E.A.; et al. Structure and functionality in flavivirus NS-proteins: Perspectives for drug design. *Antiviral Res.* **2010**, *87*, 125–148. [CrossRef] [PubMed]

38. Pierson, T.C.; Diamond, M.S. Degrees of maturity: The complex structure and biology of flaviviruses. *Curr. Opin. Virol.* **2012**, *2*, 168–175. [CrossRef] [PubMed]

39. Methot, P.O.; Alizon, S. What is a pathogen? Toward a process view of host-parasite interactions. *Virulence* **2014**, *5*, 775–785. [CrossRef] [PubMed]

40. Haddow, A.D.; Schuh, A.J.; Yasuda, C.Y.; Kasper, M.R.; Heang, V.; Huy, R.; Guzman, H.; Tesh, R.B.; Weaver, S.C. Genetic characterization of Zika virus strains: Geographic expansion of the Asian lineage. *PLoS Negl. Trop. Dis.* **2012**, *6*, e1477. [CrossRef] [PubMed]

41. Faria, N.R.; Azevedo Rdo, S.; Kraemer, M.U.; Souza, R.; Cunha, M.S.; Hill, S.C.; Theze, J.; Bonsall, M.B.; Bowden, T.A.; Rissanen, I.; et al. Zika virus in the Americas: Early epidemiological and genetic findings. *Science* **2016**, *352*, 345–349. [CrossRef] [PubMed]

42. Wang, L.; Valderramos, S.G.; Wu, A.; Ouyang, S.; Li, C.; Brasil, P.; Bonaldo, M.; Coates, T.; Nielsen-Saines, K.; Jiang, T.; et al. From mosquitos to humans: Genetic evolution of Zika virus. *Cell Host Microbe* **2016**, *19*, 561–565. [CrossRef] [PubMed]

43. Morrison, T.E.; Diamond, M.S. Animal models of Zika virus infection, pathogenesis, and immunity. *J. Virol.* **2017**, *91*, e00009-17. [CrossRef] [PubMed]

44. Rossi, S.L.; Tesh, R.B.; Azar, S.R.; Muruato, A.E.; Hanley, K.A.; Auguste, A.J.; Langsjoen, R.M.; Paessler, S.; Vasilakis, N.; Weaver, S.C. Characterization of a novel murine model to study Zika virus. *Am. J. Trop. Med. Hyg.* **2016**, *94*, 1362–1369. [CrossRef] [PubMed]

45. Aliota, M.T.; Caine, E.A.; Walker, E.C.; Larkin, K.E.; Camacho, E.; Osorio, J.E. Characterization of lethal Zika virus infection in AG129 mice. *PLoS Negl. Trop. Dis.* **2016**, *10*, e0004682. [CrossRef] [PubMed]

46. Miner, J.J.; Sene, A.; Richner, J.M.; Smith, A.M.; Santeford, A.; Ban, N.; Weger-Lucarelli, J.; Manzella, F.; Ruckert, C.; Govero, J.; et al. Zika virus infection in mice causes panuveitis with shedding of virus in tears. *Cell Rep.* **2016**, *16*, 3208–3218. [CrossRef] [PubMed]

47. Julander, J.G.; Siddharthan, V.; Evans, J.; Taylor, R.; Tolbert, K.; Apuli, C.; Stewart, J.; Collins, P.; Gebre, M.; Neilson, S.; et al. Efficacy of the broad-spectrum antiviral compound BCX4430 against Zika virus in cell culture and in a mouse model. *Antiviral Res.* **2017**, *137*, 14–22. [CrossRef] [PubMed]

48. Zmurko, J.; Marques, R.E.; Schols, D.; Verbeken, E.; Kaptein, S.J.; Neyts, J. The viral polymerase inhibitor 7-deaza-2'-C-methyladenosine is a potent inhibitor of in vitro Zika virus replication and delays disease progression in a robust mouse infection model. *PLoS Negl. Trop. Dis.* **2016**, *10*, e0004695. [CrossRef] [PubMed]

49. Weger-Lucarelli, J.; Duggal, N.K.; Bullard-Feibelman, K.; Veselinovic, M.; Romo, H.; Nguyen, C.; Ruckert, C.; Brault, A.C.; Bowen, R.A.; Stenglein, M.; et al. Development and characterization of recombinant virus generated from a New World Zika virus infectious clone. *J. Virol.* **2017**, *91*, e01765-16. [CrossRef] [PubMed]

50. Yun, S.I.; Kim, S.Y.; Choi, W.Y.; Nam, J.H.; Ju, Y.R.; Park, K.Y.; Cho, H.W.; Lee, Y.M. Molecular characterization of the full-length genome of the Japanese encephalitis viral strain K87P39. *Virus Res.* **2003**, *96*, 129–140. [CrossRef]

51. Sambrook, J.; Fritsch, E.F.; Maniatis, T. *Molecular Cloning: A Laboratory Manual*, 2nd ed.; Cold Spring Harbor Laboratory: Cold Spring Harbor, NY, USA, 1989.

52. Yun, S.I.; Song, B.H.; Kim, J.K.; Lee, Y.M. Bacterial artificial chromosomes: A functional genomics tool for the study of positive-strand RNA viruses. *J. Vis. Exp.* **2015**, *106*, e53164. [CrossRef] [PubMed]

53. Yun, S.I.; Kim, S.Y.; Rice, C.M.; Lee, Y.M. Development and application of a reverse genetics system for Japanese encephalitis virus. *J. Virol.* **2003**, *77*, 6450–6465. [CrossRef] [PubMed]

54. Yun, S.I.; Song, B.H.; Frank, J.C.; Julander, J.G.; Polejaeva, I.A.; Davies, C.J.; White, K.L.; Lee, Y.M. Complete genome sequences of three historically important, spatiotemporally distinct, and genetically divergent strains of Zika virus: MR-766, P6-740, and PRVABC-59. *Genome Announc.* **2016**, *4*, e00800-16. [CrossRef] [PubMed]

55. Kim, J.M.; Yun, S.I.; Song, B.H.; Hahn, Y.S.; Lee, C.H.; Oh, H.W.; Lee, Y.M. A single *N*-linked glycosylation site in the Japanese encephalitis virus prM protein is critical for cell type-specific prM protein biogenesis, virus particle release, and pathogenicity in mice. *J. Virol.* **2008**, *82*, 7846–7862. [CrossRef] [PubMed]

56. Yun, S.I.; Choi, Y.J.; Song, B.H.; Lee, Y.M. 3′ *cis*-acting elements that contribute to the competence and efficiency of Japanese encephalitis virus genome replication: Functional importance of sequence duplications, deletions, and substitutions. *J. Virol.* **2009**, *83*, 7909–7930. [CrossRef] [PubMed]

57. Yun, S.I.; Song, B.H.; Polejaeva, I.A.; Davies, C.J.; White, K.L.; Lee, Y.M. Comparison of the live-attenuated Japanese encephalitis vaccine SA$_{14}$-14-2 strain with its pre-attenuated virulent parent SA$_{14}$ strain: Similarities and differences in vitro and in vivo. *J. Gen. Virol.* **2016**, *97*, 2575–2591. [CrossRef] [PubMed]

58. Yun, S.I.; Song, B.H.; Kim, J.K.; Yun, G.N.; Lee, E.Y.; Li, L.; Kuhn, R.J.; Rossmann, M.G.; Morrey, J.D.; Lee, Y.M. A molecularly cloned, live-attenuated Japanese encephalitis vaccine SA$_{14}$-14-2 virus: A conserved single amino acid in the *ij* hairpin of the viral E glycoprotein determines neurovirulence in mice. *PLoS Pathog.* **2014**, *10*, e1004290. [CrossRef] [PubMed]

59. Marchette, N.J.; Garcia, R.; Rudnick, A. Isolation of Zika virus from *Aedes aegypti* mosquitoes in Malaysia. *Am. J. Trop. Med. Hyg.* **1969**, *18*, 411–415. [CrossRef] [PubMed]

60. Lanciotti, R.S.; Lambert, A.J.; Holodniy, M.; Saavedra, S.; Signor Ldel, C. Phylogeny of Zika virus in Western Hemisphere, 2015. *Emerg. Infect. Dis.* **2016**, *22*, 933–935. [CrossRef] [PubMed]

61. Zhao, B.; Yi, G.; Du, F.; Chuang, Y.C.; Vaughan, R.C.; Sankaran, B.; Kao, C.C.; Li, P. Structure and function of the Zika virus full-length NS5 protein. *Nat. Commun.* **2017**, *8*, 14762. [CrossRef] [PubMed]

62. Wang, B.; Tan, X.F.; Thurmond, S.; Zhang, Z.M.; Lin, A.; Hai, R.; Song, J. The structure of Zika virus NS5 reveals a conserved domain conformation. *Nat. Commun.* **2017**, *8*, 14763. [CrossRef] [PubMed]

63. Meertens, L.; Labeau, A.; Dejarnac, O.; Cipriani, S.; Sinigaglia, L.; Bonnet-Madin, L.; Le Charpentier, T.; Hafirassou, M.L.; Zamborlini, A.; Cao-Lormeau, V.M.; et al. Axl mediates Zika virus entry in human glial cells and modulates innate immune responses. *Cell Rep.* **2017**, *18*, 324–333. [CrossRef] [PubMed]

64. Prasad, V.M.; Miller, A.S.; Klose, T.; Sirohi, D.; Buda, G.; Jiang, W.; Kuhn, R.J.; Rossmann, M.G. Structure of the immature Zika virus at 9 A resolution. *Nat. Struct. Mol. Biol.* **2017**, *24*, 184–186. [CrossRef] [PubMed]

65. Brown, W.C.; Akey, D.L.; Konwerski, J.R.; Tarrasch, J.T.; Skiniotis, G.; Kuhn, R.J.; Smith, J.L. Extended surface for membrane association in Zika virus NS1 structure. *Nat. Struct. Mol. Biol.* **2016**, *23*, 865–867. [CrossRef] [PubMed]

66. Xu, X.; Song, H.; Qi, J.; Liu, Y.; Wang, H.; Su, C.; Shi, Y.; Gao, G.F. Contribution of intertwined loop to membrane association revealed by Zika virus full-length NS1 structure. *EMBO J.* **2016**, *35*, 2170–2178. [CrossRef] [PubMed]

67. Roby, J.A.; Setoh, Y.X.; Hall, R.A.; Khromykh, A.A. Post-Translational regulation and modifications of flavivirus structural proteins. *J. Gen. Virol.* **2015**, *96*, 1551–1569. [CrossRef] [PubMed]

68. Stobart, C.C.; Moore, M.L. RNA virus reverse genetics and vaccine design. *Viruses* **2014**, *6*, 2531–2550. [CrossRef] [PubMed]

69. Aubry, F.; Nougairede, A.; Gould, E.A.; de Lamballerie, X. Flavivirus reverse genetic systems, construction techniques and applications: A historical perspective. *Antiviral Res.* **2015**, *114*, 67–85. [CrossRef] [PubMed]

70. Shizuya, H.; Birren, B.; Kim, U.J.; Mancino, V.; Slepak, T.; Tachiiri, Y.; Simon, M. Cloning and stable maintenance of 300-kilobase-pair fragments of human DNA in *Escherichia coli* using an F-factor-based vector. *Proc. Natl. Acad. Sci. USA* **1992**, *89*, 8794–8797. [CrossRef] [PubMed]

71. Shan, C.; Xie, X.; Muruato, A.E.; Rossi, S.L.; Roundy, C.M.; Azar, S.R.; Yang, Y.; Tesh, R.B.; Bourne, N.; Barrett, A.D.; et al. An infectious cDNA clone of Zika virus to study viral virulence, mosquito transmission, and antiviral inhibitors. *Cell Host Microbe* **2016**, *19*, 891–900. [CrossRef] [PubMed]

72. Widman, D.G.; Young, E.; Yount, B.L.; Plante, K.S.; Gallichotte, E.N.; Carbaugh, D.L.; Peck, K.M.; Plante, J.; Swanstrom, J.; Heise, M.T.; et al. A reverse genetics platform that spans the Zika virus family tree. *mBio* **2017**, *8*, e02014-16. [CrossRef] [PubMed]

73. Tsetsarkin, K.A.; Kenney, H.; Chen, R.; Liu, G.; Manukyan, H.; Whitehead, S.S.; Laassri, M.; Chumakov, K.; Pletnev, A.G. A full-length infectious cDNA clone of Zika virus from the 2015 epidemic in Brazil as a genetic platform for studies of virus-host interactions and vaccine development. *mBio* **2016**, *7*, e01114-16. [CrossRef] [PubMed]

74. Schwarz, M.C.; Sourisseau, M.; Espino, M.M.; Gray, E.S.; Chambers, M.T.; Tortorella, D.; Evans, M.J. Rescue of the 1947 Zika virus prototype strain with a cytomegalovirus promoter-driven cDNA clone. *mSphere* **2016**, *1*, e00246-16. [CrossRef] [PubMed]

75. Setoh, Y.X.; Prow, N.A.; Peng, N.; Hugo, L.E.; Devine, G.; Hazlewood, J.E.; Suhrbier, A.; Khromykh, A.A. *De Novo* generation and characterization of new Zika virus isolate using sequence data from a microcephaly case. *mSphere* **2017**, *2*, e00190-17. [CrossRef] [PubMed]

76. Atieh, T.; Baronti, C.; de Lamballerie, X.; Nougairede, A. Simple reverse genetics systems for Asian and African Zika viruses. *Sci. Rep.* **2016**, *6*, 39384. [CrossRef] [PubMed]

77. Wichgers Schreur, P.J.; van Keulen, L.; Anjema, D.; Kant, J.; Kortekaas, J. Microencephaly in fetal piglets following in utero inoculation of Zika virus. *Emerg. Microbes Infect.* **2018**, *7*, 42. [CrossRef] [PubMed]

78. Darbellay, J.; Lai, K.; Babiuk, S.; Berhane, Y.; Ambagala, A.; Wheler, C.; Wilson, D.; Walker, S.; Potter, A.; Gilmour, M.; et al. Neonatal pigs are susceptible to experimental Zika virus infection. *Emerg. Microbes Infect.* **2017**, *6*, e6. [CrossRef] [PubMed]

79. Ragan, I.K.; Blizzard, E.L.; Gordy, P.; Bowen, R.A. Investigating the potential role of North American animals as hosts for Zika virus. *Vector Borne Zoonotic Dis.* **2017**, *17*, 161–164. [CrossRef] [PubMed]

80. Lecot, S.; Belouzard, S.; Dubuisson, J.; Rouille, Y. Bovine viral diarrhea virus entry is dependent on clathrin-mediated endocytosis. *J. Virol.* **2005**, *79*, 10826–10829. [CrossRef] [PubMed]

81. Cureton, D.K.; Massol, R.H.; Whelan, S.P.; Kirchhausen, T. The length of vesicular stomatitis virus particles dictates a need for actin assembly during clathrin-dependent endocytosis. *PLoS Pathog.* **2010**, *6*, e1001127. [CrossRef] [PubMed]

82. Lazear, H.M.; Govero, J.; Smith, A.M.; Platt, D.J.; Fernandez, E.; Miner, J.J.; Diamond, M.S. A mouse model of Zika virus pathogenesis. *Cell Host Microbe* **2016**, *19*, 720–730. [CrossRef] [PubMed]

83. Dowall, S.D.; Graham, V.A.; Rayner, E.; Atkinson, B.; Hall, G.; Watson, R.J.; Bosworth, A.; Bonney, L.C.; Kitchen, S.; Hewson, R. A susceptible mouse model for Zika virus infection. *PLoS Negl. Trop. Dis.* **2016**, *10*, e0004658. [CrossRef] [PubMed]

84. Li, H.; Saucedo-Cuevas, L.; Regla-Nava, J.A.; Chai, G.; Sheets, N.; Tang, W.; Terskikh, A.V.; Shresta, S.; Gleeson, J.G. Zika virus infects neural progenitors in the adult mouse brain and alters proliferation. *Cell Stem Cell* **2016**, *19*, 593–598. [CrossRef] [PubMed]

85. Smith, D.R.; Hollidge, B.; Daye, S.; Zeng, X.; Blancett, C.; Kuszpit, K.; Bocan, T.; Koehler, J.W.; Coyne, S.; Minogue, T.; et al. Neuropathogenesis of Zika virus in a highly susceptible immunocompetent mouse model after antibody blockade of type I interferon. *PLoS Negl. Trop. Dis.* **2017**, *11*, e0005296. [CrossRef] [PubMed]

86. Larocca, R.A.; Abbink, P.; Peron, J.P.; Zanotto, P.M.; Iampietro, M.J.; Badamchi-Zadeh, A.; Boyd, M.; Ng'ang'a, D.; Kirilova, M.; Nityanandam, R.; et al. Vaccine protection against Zika virus from Brazil. *Nature* **2016**, *536*, 474–478. [CrossRef] [PubMed]

87. Manangeeswaran, M.; Ireland, D.D.; Verthelyi, D. Zika (PRVABC59) infection is associated with T cell infiltration and neurodegeneration in CNS of immunocompetent neonatal C57BL/6 mice. *PLoS Pathog.* **2016**, *12*, e1006004. [CrossRef] [PubMed]

88. Fernandes, N.C.; Nogueira, J.S.; Ressio, R.A.; Cirqueira, C.S.; Kimura, L.M.; Fernandes, K.R.; Cunha, M.S.; Souza, R.P.; Guerra, J.M. Experimental Zika virus infection induces spinal cord injury and encephalitis in newborn Swiss mice. *Exp. Toxicol. Pathol.* **2017**, *69*, 63–71. [CrossRef] [PubMed]

89. Chan, J.F.; Zhang, A.J.; Chan, C.C.; Yip, C.C.; Mak, W.W.; Zhu, H.; Poon, V.K.; Tee, K.M.; Zhu, Z.; Cai, J.P.; et al. Zika virus infection in dexamethasone-immunosuppressed mice demonstrating disseminated infection with multi-organ involvement including orchitis effectively treated by recombinant type I interferons. *EBioMedicine* **2016**, *14*, 112–122. [CrossRef] [PubMed]

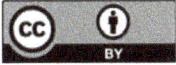

Article

Subversion of the Heme Oxygenase-1 Antiviral Activity by Zika Virus

Chaker El Kalamouni [1,†], Etienne Frumence [1,†], Sandra Bos [1], Jonathan Turpin [1], Brice Nativel [2], Wissal Harrabi [1], David A. Wilkinson [1], Olivier Meilhac [2,3], Gilles Gadea [1], Philippe Desprès [1], Pascale Krejbich-Trotot [1,*] and Wildriss Viranaïcken [1,*]

[1] Université de La Réunion, INSERM UMR 1187, CNRS 9192, IRD 249 UMR PIMIT, Processus Infectieux en Milieu Insulaire Tropical, Plateforme CYROI, 2, rue Maxime Rivière, F-97490 Sainte-Clotilde, France; chaker.el-kalamouni@univ-reunion.fr (C.E.K.); etienne.frumence@univ-reunion.fr (E.F.); sandrabos.lab@gmail.com (S.B.); jonas97480@live.fr (J.T.); wissalharrabi500@yahoo.fr (W.H.); dwilkin799@gmail.com (D.A.W.); gilles.gadea@inserm.fr (G.G.); philippe.despres@univ-reunion.fr (P.D.)
[2] Université de la Réunion, Inserm, UMR 1188 Diabète Athérothrombose Thérapies Réunion Océan Indien (DéTROI), F-97490 Sainte-Clotilde, France; brice.nativel@gmail.com (B.N.); olivier.meilhac@inserm.fr (O.M.)
[3] CHU de La Réunion, Saint-Denis de La Réunion, F-97400 Bellepierre, France
[*] Correspondence: pascale.krejbich@univ-reunion.fr (P.K.-T.); wildriss.viranaicken@univ-reunion.fr (W.V.); Tel.: +33-262938829 (P.K.-T. & W.V.)
[†] These authors contributed equally to this work.

Received: 15 October 2018; Accepted: 18 December 2018; Published: 20 December 2018

Abstract: Heme oxygenase-1 (HO-1), a rate-limiting enzyme involved in the degradation of heme, is induced in response to a wide range of stress conditions. HO-1 exerts antiviral activity against a broad range of viruses, including the Hepatitis C virus, the human immunodeficiency virus, and the dengue virus by inhibiting viral growth. It has been reported that HO-1 displays antiviral activity against the Zika virus (ZIKV) but the mechanisms of viral inhibition remain largely unknown. Using a ZIKV RNA replicon with the Green Fluorescent Protein (GFP) as a reporter protein, we were able to show that HO-1 expression resulted in the inhibition of viral RNA replication. Conversely, we observed a decrease in HO-1 expression in cells replicating the ZIKV RNA replicon. The study of human cells infected with ZIKV showed that the HO-1 expression level was significantly lower once viral replication was established, thereby limiting the antiviral effect of HO-1. Our work highlights the capacity of ZIKV to thwart the anti-replicative activity of HO-1 in human cells. Therefore, the modulation of HO-1 as a novel therapeutic strategy against ZIKV infection may display limited effect.

Keywords: antiviral; heme-oxygenase 1; Zika virus; viral replication

1. Introduction

Zika virus (ZIKV) is an emerging mosquito-borne flavivirus (family Flaviviridae), which has become a major medical problem worldwide. In 2007, the first documented outbreak of ZIKV occurred on Yap Island, affecting more than 70% of the population. Subsequently, ZIKV continued to spread in the South Pacific Islands and has largely emerged in the Americas since 2015 [1]. Phylogenetic analysis of viral sequences has identified two main virus lineages, African and Asian, the latter being the main cause of large, current epidemics with millions of cases of infection [2,3].

Classically, the human disease known as Zika fever is characterized by mild flu-like symptoms with fever, maculopapular rash, headache and sometimes conjunctivitis, arthralgia, and myalgia. Epidemiological studies from the recent epidemics have shown that infection due to ZIKV can also cause serious complications in humans such as microcephaly in newborns or Guillain–Barré Syndrome (GBS) in adults [4,5]. Once ZIKV has entered the human body, most commonly through the bite of a mosquito, it targets many types of cells, such as epithelial cells, in order to replicate and produce a viral progeny. Similar to other flaviviruses, the life cycle of ZIKV leads to the release of its single-strand positive sense genomic RNA in the cell cytoplasm where it is translated into a single polyprotein. The polyprotein is cleaved by host and viral proteases into three structural proteins (C, prM/M and E), and seven nonstructural proteins (NS) (NS1, NS2A, NS2B, NS3, NS4A, NS4B and NS5) [6]. The NS proteins initiate the replication process. The viral cycle continues with the production and maturation of envelope proteins, encapsidation, budding, and the release of the virions by exocytosis.

HO-1 is an ubiquitously expressed, stress-inducible enzyme that catabolizes heme into biliverdin, carbon monoxide, and ferrous iron [7]. These products contribute to the cytoprotective effect of HO-1 by acting as anti-oxidant, anti-inflammatory, and immunomodulatory molecules [7]. In addition, it has been shown that HO-1 can display antiviral activity. The upregulation of HO-1 was shown to limit infection by Hepatitis C and B virus (HCV and HBV), Ebola virus (EBOV), human immunodeficiency virus (HIV), and Dengue virus (DENV) [8].

Even if no therapeutic ZIKV control strategy is available to date, it has been previously proposed that the FDA approved drug Hemin could be used for its anti-viral activity, based on its action on HO-1 [9]. However, the direct effect of HO-1 on ZIKV replication has not yet been demonstrated. Here, using cells expressing a molecular ZIKV replicon, we provide evidence that cobalt protoporphyrin (CoPP), an inducer of HO-1, or direct overexpression of HO-1 inhibits ZIKV replication. Unexpectedly, we observe that ZIKV is able to downregulate HO-1 expression as a result of its own replication. Based on these observations, we conclude that the induction of HO-1 to limit ZIKV infection is likely to be ineffective as a therapeutic strategy.

2. Materials and Methods

2.1. Virus and Cell Lines

The clinical isolate PF-25013-18 (PF13) of ZIKV has been previously described [10]. Cell lines used in this study included the A549-Dual™cell line (InvivoGen, a549d-nfis), referred to hereafter as "A549 cells", and the HEK-Blue™ IFN-α/β cell line (InvivoGen, San Diego, CA, USA) which possesses the HEK-293A backbone and is referred to hereafter as "HEK-293A cells". Both cell lines were cultured at 37 °C with 5% CO_2 in MEM Eagle medium, supplemented with 10% heat inactivated fetal bovine serum and 2 mmol·L^{-1} L-Glutamine, 1 mmol·L^{-1} sodium pyruvate, 100 U·mL^{-1} of penicillin, 0.1 mg·mL^{-1} of streptomycin and 0.5 µg·mL^{-1} of fungizone (PAN Biotech, Aidenbach, Germany). Additionally, A549 cellular growth medium was supplemented with 10 µg·mL^{-1} blasticidin and 100 µg·mL^{-1} zeocin (InvivoGen) and HEK-293A cell growth medium was supplemented with 30 µg·mL^{-1} blasticidin and 100 µg·mL^{-1} zeocin (InvivoGen). Cells were harvested and stored as frozen pellets for further protein or mRNA analysis.

2.2. Generation of ZIKV Replicon by the ISA Method

The production of a ZIKV RNA replicon with GFP as a reporter protein, named ZIKV replicon in the study, was based on the sequence of ZIKV strain MR766 Uganda 47-NIID (Genbank access # LC002520) using the ISA (Infectious Subgenomic Amplicons) method [11]. The design of the viral genome, without the structural protein region, into four viral genomic fragments Z1-PURO, Z2, Z3, and Z4-IRES-eGFP (Figure 1A) was chosen to mimic those used to construct the molecular clone MR766^MC [11]. Compared to the conventional method based on the in vitro transcription from a T7 promoter, our construction was designed to allow the in cellulo transcription of recombinant DNA obtained from the four viral genomic fragments Z, by replacing the T7 promoter with a CytoMegaloVirus (CMV) promoter [12]. The fragment Z1-PURO contains the CMV promoter immediately adjacent to the 5′ non-coding region of MR766 followed by the puromycin resistance

(PAC) cassette fused in frame to the first 33 amino acids of the ZIKV C protein. It is ended by the porcine teschovirus-1 2A protease and the nucleotide sequence coding for the last 95 C-terminal amino acids of the E protein. The fragments Z2, Z3, and Z4 have been previously described [11]. The fragment Z4-IRES-eGFP contains a cassette containing the Interne Ribosomal Entry Site IRES2 sequence from Clontech followed by the eGFP sequence between the NS5 gene and the 3′NTR from Z4. HEK-293A cells were electroporated with the four fragments Z1-PURO to Z4-IRES-eGFP, using a gene pulser II according to manufacturer protocol (BioRad, Hercules, CA, USA). Cells harboring the ZIKV replicon were selected with puromycin (1 µg·mL^{-1}) for at least five days (Figure 1A). The selected cells were kept in culture throughout the experiment (passage 1 to 5). GFP expression was checked periodically by RT-PCR (Figure 1B), cytometry (Figure 1C), as well as by microscopy (Figure 1D). The replicon maintenance was followed by RT-PCR (Figure 1B) and the immunodetection of double-stranded RNA (Figure 1D). Viral protein expression was verified during the different passages by immunodetection (Supplemental Figure S1).

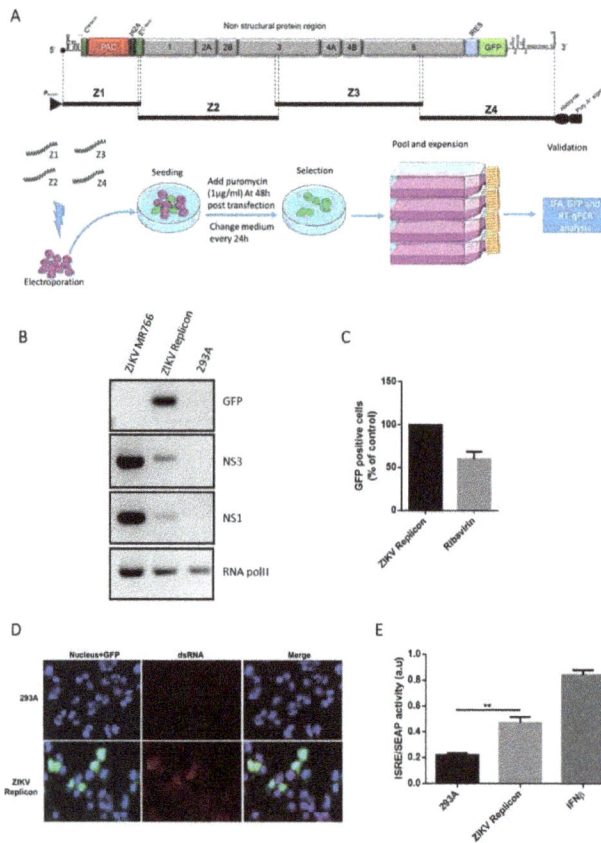

Figure 1. Generation and validation of ZIKA Virus (ZIKV) replicon in HEK-293A cells. (**A**) Schematic representation of overlapping fragments Z1 to Z4 covering of ZIKV replicon. Below, the flow chart representing the design of the experiment. (**B**) GFP, ZIKV NS3, ZIKV NS1 and RNA pol-II mRNA expression assessed by RT-PCR in ZIKV-infected A549 cells, ZIKV replicon cells and HEK 293A cells. (**C**) Cytometry monitoring of GFP after ribavirin treatment. (**D**) Fluorescence microscopy images of ZIKV replicon cells (GFP positive) after immunostaining of dsRNA with J2 antibody (red). (**E**) ISRE/SEAP activity evaluated in HEK 293A cells and ZIKV replicon cells. As positive control, cells were treated for 24 h with recombinant IFN-β (10,000 UI·mL^{-1}). ** $p < 0.01$.

2.3. RNA Isolation and RT-PCR

Total RNA was extracted from cells seeded in 60 mm Petri dishes with the RNeasy Mini Kit (Qiagen, Venlo, Netherlands). RT-PCR was performed using M-MLV Reverse Transcriptase (Invitrogen, Carlsbad, CA, USA) using 500 ng of total RNA and the GoTaq®enzyme (Promega, Madison, WI, USA) according to manufacturer's recommended procedures [13]. The primers used for RT-PCR were GFP F: 5′-AAGGCTACGTCCAGGAGCGC-3′, R: 5′-CTTGTGCCCCAGGATGTTGC-3′; NS1: F 5′-AGAGGACCATCTCTGAGATC-3′, R 5′-GGCCTTATCTCCATTCCATACC-3′; NS3: F 5′-ATGC ACACTGGCTTGAAGC-3′, R 5′-CAGATGCAACCTGATAGGC-3′; RNA PolII: F 5′-GCACCACGTCCAATG-3′, R 5′-GTGCGGCTGCTTCCA-3′; GAPDH: F 5′-GGGAGCCAAAAG GGTCATCA-3′, R 5′-TGATGGCATGGACTGTGGTC-3′. RT-PCR products were visualized by agarose gel electrophoresis. qPCR was performed using the GoTaq® qPCR Master Mix (Promega). All steps were conducted according to the manufacturer's instructions. The qPCR data were analyzed using the $\Delta\Delta Ct$ method and results were normalized to GAPDH, which was used as an internal control.

2.4. Western Blot Analysis

Cells seeded in 6-well plates were harvested after two washes with Phosphate buffered saline (PBS) containing phosphatase and protease inhibitors (Thermo Fischer Scientific, Waltham, MA, USA) and lyzed with RIPA lysis Buffer (Sigma-Aldrich, St. Louis, MS, USA). Proteins were separated by 12% SDS-PAGE and transferred onto nitrocellulose membranes [14]. The membranes were first blocked with 5% milk in TBS-Tween for 1 h, then incubated with appropriate dilutions of primary antibody at 1:1000 for 2 h. Anti-rabbit immunoglobulin-horseradish peroxidase and anti-mouse immunoglobulin-horseradish peroxidase conjugates were used as secondary antibodies (dilution 1:2000, Vectors). The membranes were incubated with Amersham *ECL Select* or *prime* Western Blotting Detection Reagent (GE Healthcare, Chicago, IL, USA) and exposed to a film or on an Amersham imager 600 (GE Healthcare) or GeneGnome imager (Syngene, Cambridge, UK). Horseradish peroxidase-conjugated anti-rabbit and anti-mouse antibodies were purchased from Vector Labs. The mouse anti-pan flavivirus envelope E protein mAb 4G2 was produced by RD Biotech. Mouse antibody against HO-1was from Abcam and the mouse antibody against α-tubulin, β-tubulin and M2 FLAG were from Sigma–Aldrich. All Western-blot data are representative of three independent experiments.

2.5. ISRE/SEAP Activity Quantification

Interferon-sensitive response element (ISRE) promoter activation was evaluated in supernatant of HEK-293A cells expressing the ZIKV replicon using the substrate Quanti-blue (Invivogen) according to the manufacturer's recommendations to measured secreted embryonic alkaline phosphatase (SEAP) activity. As a positive control, HEK-293A cells were treated for 24 h with recombinant IFN-β $(10,000 \text{ UI·mL}^{-1}, \text{Peprotech})$.

2.6. Flow Cytometry Assay

To detect GFP-expressing cells, cells were harvest after trypsinization and fixed with 3.7% PFA in PBS at room temperature for 10 min. Fixed cells were subjected to a flow cytometric analysis using FACScan flow cytometer (Becton Dickinson, Franklin Lakes, NJ, USA). The percentage of GFP-positive cells was determined using the FlowJo software package.

2.7. Cell Immunofluorescence Staining

HEK-293A cells expressing the ZIKV replicon were grown on glass coverslips, fixed and permeabilized for further incubation in monoclonal mouse anti-double-stranded RNA, clone J2 (English & Scientific Consulting Kft, Szirák, Hungary, J2-1104) (1:200) in 1% PBS-BSA and then with Alexa594-conjugated anti-mouse Ig (1:1000). Nuclei were revealed by DAPI staining (final concentration 100 ng/mL). Coverslips were mounted in Vectashield (Vector Labs; Clinisciences, Nanterre, France), and fluorescence was observed using a Nikon Eclipse E2000-U microscope (Nikon, Tokyo, Japan). Images were obtained using the Nikon Digital sight PS-U1 camera system and the imaging software NIS-Element AR (Nikon).

2.8. HO-1 Overexpression

HEK-293A cells expressing the ZIKV replicon were seeded on 6-well plates and transfected with the expression plasmid pcDNA3.1-Neo or pcDNA3.1-HO-1-Flag-Neo encoding the human HO-1 protein using Lipofectamine 3000 (Invitrogen) according to the manufacturer's instructions. Transfected cells were cultivated in media with G418 to enforce the expression of HO-1. For preparation of pcDNA3.1-HO-1-Flag-Neo, the human HO-1 open reading frame was synthesized and cloned between the KpnI and XhoI restriction sites of the pcDNA3.1-Neo plasmid (Invitrogen) by GeneCust (Ellange, Luxembourg).

2.9. Crystal Violet Assay

To assess cell viability, we used the crystal violet staining assay (adapted from Saotome et al. [15]). Briefly, cells seeded in 6-well plates were washed with PBS and then stained with 0.1% crystal violet in PBS for 15 min. The plates were carefully washed with water. Then, 500 μL of 1% sodium dodecyl sulfate was added to each well to solubilize the stain and absorbance was read at 590 nm.

2.10. Statistical Analysis

All values are expressed as mean ± SD and represent at least three independent experiments. Comparisons between different treatments were analyzed using a one-way ANOVA test. Values of $p < 0.05$ were considered statistically significant for a post-hoc Tukey–Kramer test in order to compare treated versus non-treated. RT-qPCR statistical analysis was carried out by the Student's *t*-test. All statistical tests were performed using the software Graph-Pad Prism version 5.01 (San Diego, CA, USA). Degrees of significance are indicated in the figure captions as follow: * $p < 0.05$; ** $p < 0.01$; *** $p < 0.001$, ns = not significant.

3. Results

3.1. Generation of a ZIKV Replicon in HEK-293A Cells by the ISA Method.

For enveloped viruses, most antiviral therapies consist of drugs which target a specific viral protein or cellular cofactor that mediates important steps in the viral life cycle, including viral entry, fusion, replication or egress. Antiviral activity of HO-1 against flaviviruses results in the inhibition of replication [9,16]. To address the effect of HO-1 on ZIKV replication in epithelial cells, independently of other steps in the viral life cycle, we produced HEK-293A cells stably expressing and replicating an RNA molecule acting as a ZIKV replication reporter, i.e., a ZIKV replicon (Figure 1A).

To validate the maintenance of a ZIKV replicon in the puromycin selected cells, we checked the presence of RNA molecules encoding for NS1, NS3 and the GFP reporter gene by RT-PCR (Figure 1B). These observations were further supported by the expression of NS1 protein (Supplemental Figure S1). The presence of the GFP reporter gene in the construct allowed us to follow the ZIKV replicon expressing cells by flow cytometry. To ensure that the replicon was maintained in cells, we used Ribavirin, a synthetic nucleoside that inhibits RNA virus replication and blocks their nucleic acid synthesis [17]. The decrease of the GFP signal observed with ribavirin likely corresponds to the effect on self-replication of the replicon (Figure 1C) and has been used elsewhere as direct evidence previously used to validate the function of viral replicons [12,18]. We then confirmed the presence of double-stranded RNA (dsRNA), which corresponds to the active replication of the ZIKV replicon, by immunodetection with the J2 antibody (Figure 1D). Cells expressing the GFP reporter gene were also positive for the J2 staining. Lastly, the presence of dsRNA should trigger an antiviral response through type I interferon production. Since ZIKV replicon cells provide a reporter gene with an ISRE fused to secreted embryonic alkaline phosphatase (SEAP), we were able to confirm the IFN-β response by the measure of SEAP activity in the cell media (Figure 1E). This is additional evidence that the self-replicating system specific to the viral replicon is maintained. The ZIKV replicon was able to assemble and replicate autonomously in the ZIKV replicon cells.

3.2. HO-1 Reduces ZIKV RNA Replication

To investigate the effect of HO-1 on ZIKV replication, we first treated HEK-293A cells expressing ZIKV replicon with CoPP, an inducer of HO-1. We verified the upregulation of HO-1 in a dose-dependent manner with increasing concentrations of CoPP (Figure 2A). Under these conditions, no cytotoxic effects were observed using neutral red assay (data not shown).

We then assessed the replication efficiency of the ZIKV replicon by measuring the percentage of GFP-positive cells by flow cytometry analysis (Figure 2B). We found that CoPP treatment significantly reduced the percentage of GFP-expressing cells at all tested doses and noted that CoPP was able to inhibit ZIKV replicon replication as efficiently as ribavirin.

CoPP is known to upregulate the expression of genes that are under the control of the Antioxidant Response Element (ARE-driven gene) including HO-1 and NQO1 [19]. To investigate a direct involvement of HO-1 in the CoPP-induced inhibition of ZIKV replicon, we quantified the effect of an overexpression of HO-1 in our system. HEK-293A cells with ZIKV replicon were transfected with a plasmid pcDNA3.1-HO-1-Flag-Neo and checked for HO-1 overexpression (Figure 2C). As previously seen with CoPP treatment, the percentage of GFP-positive cells decreased upon HO-1 overexpression (Figure 2D).

Given that the system used to generate the replicon requires the use of the CMV promoter and since it cannot be excluded that the initial DNA fragments may provide constitutive expression of the GFP, we verified that the effect of HO-1 was specific to the replicon and could not be exerted on a CMV dependent transcription. To support an effect of HO-1 induction or overexpression on the replicon and not on such a phenomenon, we confirmed that there was no change in the constitutive expression of GFP under CMV promoter (Supplemental Figure S2A and S2B).

To further characterize the effect of HO-1 on the ZIKV replicon, the transfected cells were continuously cultured in media containing G418 and puromycin for 7 days to enforce the expression of HO-1 and ZIKV replicon, respectively. The puromycin N-acetyltransferase (PAC) expression is directly linked to replication of ZIKV replicon. If HO-1 had a negative effect on the upkeep of the ZIKV replicon, we expected a progressive reduction of the puromycin resistance, leading to a growth defect (Figure 2E). Using the crystal violet assay, we observed a massive cell death in the HO-1 overexpressing cell, which is related to a capacity of the enzyme to downregulate the replication of the ZIKV replicon (Figure 2F). Notably, co-expression of a plasmid carrying the PAC gene (pSilencer-puro) and the plasmid pcDNA3.1-HO-1-Flag-Neo does not induce cell death upon selection with puromycin and G418 (Supplemental Figure S2C).

The results are consistent with available data on the protective effect of HO-1 on ZIKV [9]. In order to be sure that HO-1 was also able to reduce the ZIKV RNA replication during infection in the same assay system as the ZIKV-replicon, i.e., the HEK-293A cells. These backbone cells overexpressing HO-1 were infected with the recombinant ZIKV-GFP [11]. We did notice a reduction in the number of infected cells and a similar reduction was observed in cells treated with CoPP (Supplemental Figure S2D).

Taken together, all of these observations support the inhibition of ZIKV replication by the action of HO-1.

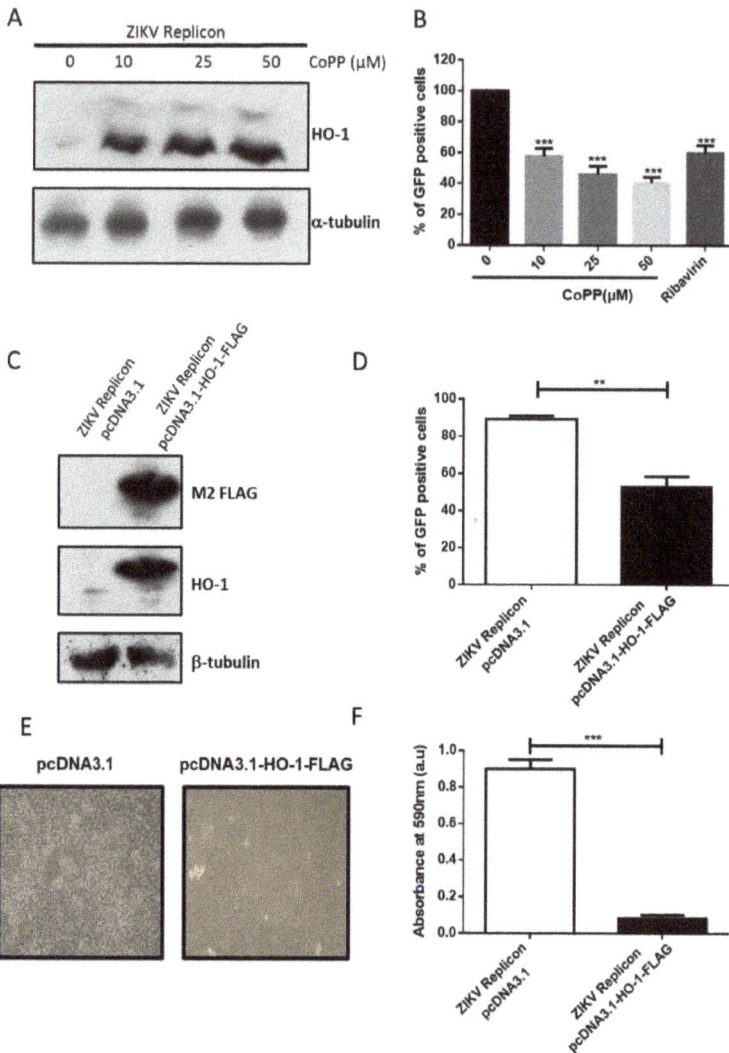

Figure 2. ZIKV replicon expression is inhibited by HO-1 induction or overexpression. (**A**) HO-1 protein expression was assessed by Western blot in HEK-293A cells expressing ZIKV replicon after treatment with several doses of CoPP for 20 h. Antibody against α-tubulin served as the protein loading control. (**B**) The percentage of GFP-expressing cells was analyzed by flow cytometry assay in ZIKV replicon cells after treatment with different concentrations of CoPP for 20 h. As positive control, cells were treated for 24 h with 40 μg·mL^{-1} (164 μM) of ribavirin. *** $p < 0.001$. (**C**) Overexpression of HO-1 in ZIKV replicon cells transfected with pcDNA3.1-HO-1-FLAG-Neo was assessed by Western blot using the anti-FLAG M2 and antibody against HO-1. Antibody against β-tubulin served as protein loading control. (**D**) The percentage of GFP-expressing cells was analyzed by flow cytometry assay in ZIKV replicon cells after transfection with pcDNA3.1-HO-1-FLAG encoding the human HO-1 protein or with pcDNA3.1. ** $p < 0.01$. In (**E**) and (**F**), cell viability was observed by optical microscopy or crystal violet staining respectively in ZIKV replicon cells transfected with pcDNA3.1 or pcDNA3.1-HO-1-FLAG after 7 days of treatment with G418 and puromycin to respectively allow the expression of HO-1 and the expression of ZIKV replicon. *** $p < 0.001$.

3.3. *ZIKV Inhibits HO-1 Expression*

HO-1 is known to be rapidly induced for cellular protection under various stresses, including many types of viral infection. Classical swine fever virus (CSFV) or human cytomegalovirus (HMCV) induces an increase in HO-1 expression [20,21]. Conversely, HIV, HCV and Bovine viral diarrhea virus infections are associated with a down-regulation in HO-1 expression [19,22,23]. To determine whether ZIKV interferes with the expression of HO-1, we analyzed whether the level of HO-1 protein was modulated in HEK-293A cells expressing the ZIKV replicon. We found that HO-1 was no longer detectable at the protein level (Figure 3A) and was reduced at the mRNA level (Figure 3B). qPCR values indicate approximately a halving in the number of transcripts (Figure 3C). This suggests that the regulation of HO-1 expression may take place at both transcriptional and post-transcriptional levels upon replication of the ZIKV replicon and/or expression of NS proteins. To confirm that the observed deregulation of HO-1 was indeed a property of ZIKV, A549 cells that are more susceptible to ZIKV than HEK 293A were chosen to be infected with a clinical isolate of ZIKV (ZIKV-PF13) [10] and assessed for HO-1 expression at different times post-infection. HO-1 protein was markedly reduced 24 h post-infection (Figure 3D). It should be noted that molecular clones representing viruses of the African ancestral strain (MR766) or the Brazilian epidemic strain (BR15) were also able to decrease HO-1 expression in another cell line model (Supplemental Figure S3). In addition, we could confirm a slight significant decrease in HO-1 expression at the level of quantified transcripts in ZIKV-infected A549 cells (Figure 3E,F).

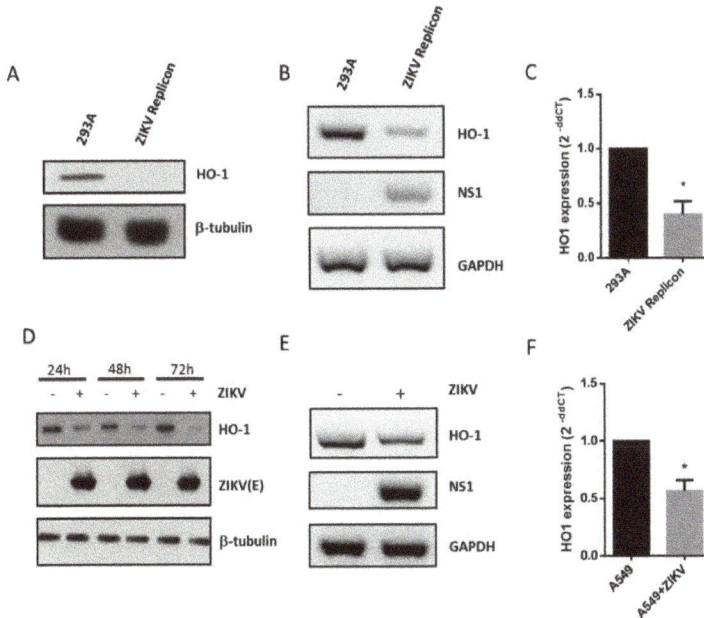

Figure 3. ZIKV replication and ZIKV infection decrease HO-1 protein and mRNA levels. (**A**) Western blot analysis of HO-1 protein expression in HEK 293A cells and ZIKV replicon cells using anti-HO-1. (**B**) RT-PCR analysis of HO-1, ZIKV NS1 and GAPDH mRNA expression in HEK 293A cells and ZIKV replicon cells. (**C**) RT-qPCR analysis of HO-1 expression in HEK 293A cells and ZIKV replicon cells. A549 cells were infected with ZIKV-PF13 at multiplicity of infection (MOI) of 5. In (**D**), HO-1 and ZIKV-E protein expression were analyzed by Western blot using anti-HO-1 and anti-ZIKV-E 4G2 antibody. Antibody against β-tubulin served as protein loading control. In (**E**), HO-1, ZIKV NS1 and GAPDH mRNA expression were analyzed by RT-PCR 24-h post infection. In (**F**) RT-qPCR analysis of HO-1 expression in A549 cells infected with ZIKV-PF13 24-h post-infection. * $p < 0.05$.

3.4. Inhibition of HO-1 Induction During ZIKV Infection

The inhibiting effect of ZIKV on HO-1 expression may be a limitation in the use of an HO-1 inducer for antiviral purposes [9]. We first tested whether HO-1-induction by CoPP was able to inhibit viral growth of the epidemic ZIKV-PF13 strain. The effect of HO-1 induction by CoPP on viral growth was followed by adding CoPP 2-h post-infection with ZIKV-PF13 at multiplicity of infection (MOI) of 0.1 or 1 (Supplemental Figure S4). In this experiment, induction of HO-1 with CoPP only decreased the viral progeny production of ZIKV-PF13 at lower MOI. This observation and the down-regulation of HO-1 upon ZIKV infection observed above suggest that the inhibition of HO-1-induction depends on the viral load. To test this hypothesis, we evaluated whether ZIKV was able to counteract the induction of HO-1 by CoPP. We infected A549 cells for 2 h with ZIKV-PF13 at different MOIs and then induced HO-1 expression with CoPP for an additional 16 h. We can see that, despite the presence of CoPP, ZIKV inhibited HO-1 protein level in an MOI-dependent manner (Figure 4A). The ability of ZIKV to inhibit HO-1 induction in response to CoPP at the protein level was not correlated to a significant decreased in HO-1 at the mRNA level (Figure 4B,C). Indeed, ZIKV induces a more robust translational or post-translational downregulation of HO-1 than a transcriptional or post-transcriptional regulation of HO-1 expression.

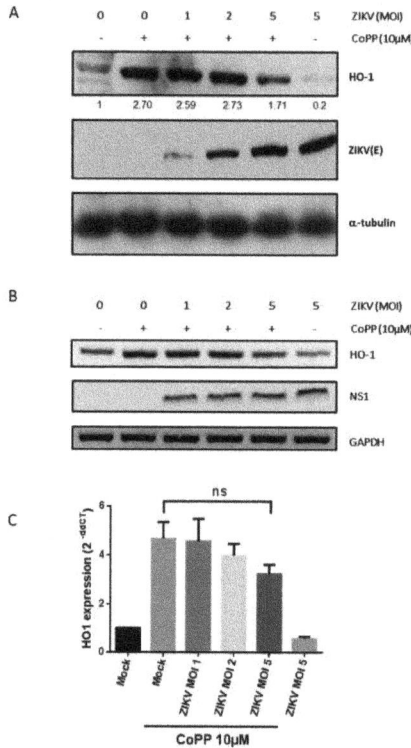

Figure 4. ZIKV infection decreases HO-1 induction mediated by CoPP at the protein and the mRNA levels. A549 cells were infected with ZIKV-PF13 at several multiplicity of infection (MOI) and then treated 2 h post-infection with CoPP for 16 h. In (**A**), HO-1 and ZIKV-E protein expression were analyzed by Western blot using anti-HO-1 and anti-ZIKV-E 4G2 antibody. Antibody against α-tubulin served as protein loading control. Quantification was done with the ImageJ software. In (**B**), HO-1, ZIKV NS1 and GAPDH mRNA expression were analyzed by RT-PCR. In (**C**) RT-qPCR analysis of HO-1 expression. ns = not significant.

4. Discussion and Conclusions

In the recent years, HO-1 has gained increasing interest as a potential "super cytoprotective agent". Much work has been done to provide a therapeutic value for HO-1 and to find ways to activate or modulate its expression and activity. Research in this field shows a strong interest in molecules capable of inducing HO-1, including various natural substances such as curcumin [24,25]. Numerous observations have also supported a major role of HO-1 in the control of viral infections, notably through the direct inhibition of viral replication. A role of HO-1 has been described in the case of Dengue after induction by lucidone, a plant extract [26], and the use of HO-1 induction by Hemin has been proposed as a novel modality for developing new therapeutic strategies against ZIKV infection [9].

In the present study we provide evidence that HO-1 induction by CoPP or its direct overexpression is able to inhibit ZIKV replication (Figure 2, Figure S2C and S2D). Our results, therefore, support a beneficial effect of HO-1 in the context of ZIKA pathology which would justify renewed efforts to find effective HO-1 inducers for therapeutic purposes. The modulation of ZIKV growth by HO-1 is related to an effect on replication (Figure 2). It has been previously shown that biliverdin, a product of heme degradation by HO-1, is able to inhibit DENV replication through an interaction with NS2B/NS3 protease activity [16]. This mechanism can be conserved during ZIKV infection and needs to be confirmed by an in vitro assay of ZIKV NS2B/NS3 protease activity.

To our knowledge, this is the first report showing that ZIKV infection modulates HO-1 expression (Figures 3 and 4) in order to limit the antiviral effect of this cytoprotective protein (Figure 5). This result appears to be inconsistent with the effect recently observed with the FDA-approved formulation of Hemin which, by inducing HO-1, inhibits viral growth during ZIKV infection [9]. However, in this report, the formulation of Hemin was added at 100 μM, 24 h before the infection with ZIKV at low MOI (0.01). We therefore assume that under these drastic conditions the virus is not able to counteract the effect of HO-1 by blocking its translation or post-translational regulations. These differences would rather suggest that HO-1 targeting can only work in a preventive but not curative way for the control of ZIKV infection.

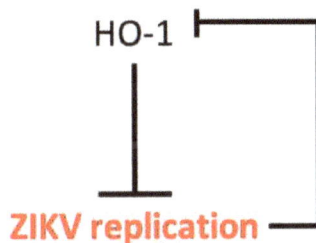

Figure 5. The model of the crosstalk between HO-1 and ZIKV. HO-1 induction inhibits ZIKV at the replication level. ZIKV growth downregulates HO-1 level through its own replication.

While our study confirms that HO-1 induction could be an effective cell-based strategy to control ZIKV infection, it highlights the ability of the virus to target and counteract this antiviral response (Figure 5). Therefore, if HO-1 induction is to be maintained as a promising strategy in the fight against ZIKV infection, it will be necessary to understand at what level ZIKV interferes with HO-1 expression. Nrf2 (the nuclear factor erythroid-related factor 2) is an important transcription factor that activates HO-1 expression through ARE elements located in the HO-1 promoter gene [27]. HO-1 down-regulation during ZIKV replication could occur through the modulation of Nrf2 transcription factor activity or expression. To the best of our knowledge, several viruses (HBV, HCV, DENV, HIV, Respiratory syncytial virus, Marburg virus) induce Nrf2 activation and the subsequent upregulation of the antioxidant responses genes such as NQO1, GSPT2 and HO-1 [28]. The control of HO-1 expression by ZIKV seems quite outstanding and therefore necessitates an understanding of its mechanism of action for the inhibition of the Nrf2/ARE pathway, which results in decreased host defenses against viral infection. This may be extremely important in the case of viruses' co-circulation (such as DENV during ZIKV outbreak in Brazil in 2015), as ZIKA virus infection may lower cell antiviral defense resulting in exacerbated viremia of the second infecting virus.

In addition, during the induction of HO-1, the effect of ZIKV on HO-1 expression is more pronounced on the level of the protein than of mRNA. This last point therefore suggests that the virus may interfere with the translation of the HO-1 messenger or the degradation of the the HO-1 protein. As it has been previously shown that ZIKV infection can trigger Endoplasmic-Reticulum stress (ER stress) [29] and that HO-1 can be degraded through the Endoplasmic-Reticulum-Associated protein Degradation (ERAD), a proteasome pathway induced during ER stress [30,31], it will be of interest to test if ZIKV downregulation of HO-1 is a combination of the ERAD pathway during ZIKV infection and an interference of ZIKV with Nrf2 transactivation of ARE elements in the HO-1 promoter. While many unanswered questions remain, these observations suggest that a better understanding of ZIKV pathogenicity (such as that associated with the Brazilian epidemic in 2015) may be achieved through a mechanistic understanding of HO-1 inhibition. Here we have established a cellular system to conduct such studies and have observed a crosstalk between HO-1 expression and ZIKV replication (Figure 5), suggesting that HO-1 targeting treatments may be of limited therapeutic efficacy against ZIKV infection.

Supplementary Materials: The following are available online at http://www.mdpi.com/1999-4915/11/1/2/s1.

Author Contributions: W.V., E.F, P.K.-T. and P.D. designed the research; P.K.-T., E.F, C.E.K, J.T., B.N., W.H., W.V., performed the research; P.K.-T., B.N, S.B., C.E.K., G.G, P.D., W.V. contributed new reagents/analytic tools; all authors analyzed the data; P.K.-T, E.F, W.V., DA.W. wrote, revised and edited the manuscript.

Funding: This work was supported by the Federation BioST from Reunion Island University, the ZIKAlliance project (European Union-Horizon 2020 program under grant agreement n°735548) and the ZIKAlert project (European Union-Région Réunion program under grant agreement n° SYNERGY: RE0001902). E.F. holds a fellowship from the Regional Council of Reunion Island (European Union-Région Réunion program under grant agreement n° SYNERGY: RE0012406). B.N. holds a fellowship (DIRED 20131515) from the Regional Council of Reunion Island. S.B. has a PhD degree scholarship from La Réunion Island University (Ecole Doctorale STS), funded by the French ministry MEESR.

Acknowledgments: We thank the members of PIMIT and DéTROI laboratories for helpful discussions. Servier Medical art provided the icons used in Figure 1.

Conflicts of Interest: The authors declare no conflict of interest.

References

1. Gatherer, D.; Kohl, A. Zika virus: A previously slow pandemic spreads rapidly through the Americas. *J. Gen. Virol.* **2016**, *97*, 269–273. [CrossRef] [PubMed]

2. Giovanetti, M.; Faria, N.R.; Nunes, M.R.T.; de Vasconcelos, J.M.; Lourenço, J.; Rodrigues, S.G.; Vianez, J.L.; da Silva, S.P.; Lemos, P.S.; Tavares, F.N.; et al. Zika virus complete genome from Salvador, Bahia, Brazil. *Infect. Genet. Evol.* **2016**, *41*, 142–145. [CrossRef]

3. Beaver, J.T.; Lelutiu, N.; Habib, R.; Skountzou, I. Evolution of Two Major Zika Virus Lineages: Implications for Pathology, Immune Response, and Vaccine Development. *Front. Immunol.* **2018**, *9*, 1640. [CrossRef] [PubMed]

4. Cao-Lormeau, V.M.; Blake, A.; Mons, S.; Lastere, S.; Roche, C.; Vanhomwegen, J.; Dub, T.; Baudouin, L.; Teissier, A.; Larre, P.; et al. Guillain-Barré Syndrome outbreak associated with Zika virus infection in French Polynesia: A case-control study. *Lancet* **2016**, *387*, 1531–1539. [CrossRef]

5. Morris, G.; Barichello, T.; Stubbs, B.; Köhler, C.A.; Carvalho, A.F.; Maes, M. Zika Virus as an Emerging Neuropathogen: Mechanisms of Neurovirulence and Neuro-Immune Interactions. *Mol. Neurobiol.* **2018**, *55*, 4160–4184. [CrossRef] [PubMed]

6. Apte-Sengupta, S.; Sirohi, D.; Kuhn, R.J. Coupling of replication and assembly in flaviviruses. *Curr. Opin. Virol.* **2014**, *9*, 134–142. [CrossRef] [PubMed]

7. Waza, A.A.; Hamid, Z.; Ali, S.; Bhat, S.A.; Bhat, M.A. A review on heme oxygenase-1 induction: Is it a necessary evil. *Inflamm. Res.* **2018**, *67*, 579–588. [CrossRef] [PubMed]
8. Espinoza, J.A.; León, M.A.; Céspedes, P.F.; Gómez, R.S.; Canedo-Marroquín, G.; Riquelme, S.A.; Salazar-Echegarai, F.J.; Blancou, P.; Simon, T.; Anegon, I.; et al. Heme Oxygenase-1 Modulates Human Respiratory Syncytial Virus Replication and Lung Pathogenesis during Infection. *J. Immunol.* **2017**, *199*, 212–223. [CrossRef] [PubMed]
9. Huang, H.; Falgout, B.; Takeda, K.; Yamada, K.M.; Dhawan, S. Nrf2-dependent induction of innate host defense via heme oxygenase-1 inhibits Zika virus replication. *Virology* **2017**, *503*, 1–5. [CrossRef] [PubMed]
10. Frumence, E.; Roche, M.; Krejbich-Trotot, P.; El-Kalamouni, C.; Nativel, B.; Rondeau, P.; Missé, D.; Gadea, G.; Viranaicken, W.; Desprès, P. The South Pacific epidemic strain of Zika virus replicates efficiently in human epithelial A549 cells leading to IFN-β production and apoptosis induction. *Virology* **2016**, *493*, 217–226. [CrossRef] [PubMed]
11. Gadea, G.; Bos, S.; Krejbich-Trotot, P.; Clain, E.; Viranaicken, W.; El-Kalamouni, C.; Mavingui, P.; Desprès, P. A robust method for the rapid generation of recombinant Zika virus expressing the GFP reporter gene. *Virology* **2016**, *497*, 157–162. [CrossRef] [PubMed]
12. Xie, X.; Zou, J.; Shan, C.; Yang, Y.; Kum, D.B.; Dallmeier, K.; Neyts, J.; Shi, P.-Y. Zika Virus Replicons for Drug Discovery. *EBioMedicine* **2016**, *12*, 156–160. [CrossRef]
13. Bos, S.; Viranaicken, W.; Turpin, J.; El-Kalamouni, C.; Roche, M.; Krejbich-Trotot, P.; Desprès, P.; Gadea, G. The structural proteins of epidemic and historical strains of Zika virus differ in their ability to initiate viral infection in human host cells. *Virology* **2018**, *516*, 265–273. [CrossRef] [PubMed]
14. Viranaicken, W.; Gasmi, L.; Chaumet, A.; Durieux, C.; Georget, V.; Denoulet, P.; Larcher, J.-C. L-Ilf3 and L-NF90 traffic to the nucleolus granular component: Alternatively-spliced exon 3 encodes a nucleolar localization motif. *PLoS ONE* **2011**, *6*, e22296. [CrossRef] [PubMed]
15. Saotome, K.; Morita, H.; Umeda, M. Cytotoxicity test with simplified crystal violet staining method using microtitre plates and its application to injection drugs. *Toxicol. In Vitro* **1989**, *3*, 317–321. [CrossRef]
16. Tseng, C.-K.; Lin, C.-K.; Wu, Y.-H.; Chen, Y.-H.; Chen, W.-C.; Young, K.-C.; Lee, J.-C. Human heme oxygenase 1 is a potential host cell factor against dengue virus replication. *Sci. Rep.* **2016**, *6*, 32176. [CrossRef]
17. Parker, W.B. Metabolism and antiviral activity of ribavirin. *Virus Res.* **2005**, *107*, 165–171. [CrossRef]
18. Li, J.-Q.; Deng, C.-L.; Gu, D.; Li, X.; Shi, L.; He, J.; Zhang, Q.-Y.; Zhang, B.; Ye, H.-Q. Development of a replicon cell line-based high throughput antiviral assay for screening inhibitors of Zika virus. *Antivir. Res.* **2018**, *150*, 148–154. [CrossRef]
19. Zhang, C.; Pu, F.; Zhang, A.; Xu, L.; Li, N.; Yan, Y.; Gao, J.; Liu, H.; Zhang, G.; Goodfellow, I.G.; et al. Heme Oxygenase-1 Suppresses Bovine Viral Diarrhoea Virus Replication in vitro. *Sci. Rep.* **2015**, *5*, 15575. [CrossRef]
20. Shi, Z.; Sun, J.; Guo, H.; Yang, Z.; Ma, Z.; Tu, C. Down-regulation of cellular protein heme oxygenase 1 inhibits proliferation of classical swine fever virus in PK-15 cells. *Virus Res.* **2013**, *173*, 315–320. [CrossRef]
21. Lee, J.; Koh, K.; Kim, Y.-E.; Ahn, J.-H.; Kim, S. Upregulation of Nrf2 expression by human cytomegalovirus infection protects host cells from oxidative stress. *J. Gen. Virol.* **2013**, *94*, 1658–1668. [CrossRef] [PubMed]
22. Abdalla, M.Y.; Britigan, B.E.; Wen, F.; Icardi, M.; McCormick, M.L.; LaBrecque, D.R.; Voigt, M.; Brown, K.E.; Schmidt, W.N. Down-regulation of heme oxygenase-1 by hepatitis C virus infection in vivo and by the in vitro expression of hepatitis C core protein. *J. Infect. Dis.* **2004**, *190*, 1109–1118. [CrossRef] [PubMed]
23. Gill, A.J.; Kovacsics, C.E.; Cross, S.A.; Vance, P.J.; Kolson, L.L.; Jordan-Sciutto, K.L.; Gelman, B.B.; Kolson, D.L. Heme oxygenase-1 deficiency accompanies neuropathogenesis of HIV-associated neurocognitive disorders. *J. Clin. Investig.* **2014**, *124*, 4459–4472. [CrossRef] [PubMed]
24. Pae, H.-O.; Jeong, G.-S.; Jeong, S.-O.; Kim, H.S.; Kim, S.-A.; Kim, Y.-C.; Yoo, S.-J.; Kim, H.-D.; Chung, H.-T. Roles of heme oxygenase-1 in curcumin-induced growth inhibition in rat smooth muscle cells. *Exp. Mol. Med.* **2007**, *39*, 267–277. [CrossRef] [PubMed]
25. Son, Y.; Lee, J.H.; Chung, H.-T.; Pae, H.-O. Therapeutic roles of heme oxygenase-1 in metabolic diseases: Curcumin and resveratrol analogues as possible inducers of heme oxygenase-1. *Oxid. Med. Cell. Longev.* **2013**, *2013*, 639541. [CrossRef] [PubMed]
26. Chen, W.-C.; Tseng, C.-K.; Lin, C.-K.; Wang, S.-N.; Wang, W.-H.; Hsu, S.-H.; Wu, Y.-H.; Hung, L.-C.; Chen, Y.-H.; Lee, J.-C. Lucidone suppresses dengue viral replication through the induction of heme oxygenase-1. *Virulence* **2018**, *9*, 588–603. [CrossRef]

27. Li, L.; Dong, H.; Song, E.; Xu, X.; Liu, L.; Song, Y. Nrf2/ARE pathway activation, HO-1 and NQO1 induction by polychlorinated biphenyl quinone is associated with reactive oxygen species and PI3K/AKT signaling. *Chem. Biol. Interact.* **2014**, *209*, 56–67. [CrossRef]

28. Ramezani, A.; Nahad, M.P.; Faghihloo, E. The role of Nrf2 transcription factor in viral infection. *J. Cell. Biochem.* **2018**, *119*, 6366–6382. [CrossRef]

29. Monel, B.; Compton, A.A.; Bruel, T.; Amraoui, S.; Burlaud-Gaillard, J.; Roy, N.; Guivel-Benhassine, F.; Porrot, F.; Génin, P.; Meertens, L.; et al. Zika virus induces massive cytoplasmic vacuolization and paraptosis-like death in infected cells. *EMBO J.* **2017**, *36*, 1653–1668. [CrossRef]

30. Lin, P.-H.; Chiang, M.-T.; Chau, L.-Y. Ubiquitin-proteasome system mediates heme oxygenase-1 degradation through endoplasmic reticulum-associated degradation pathway. *Biochim. Biophys. Acta* **2008**, *1783*, 1826–1834. [CrossRef]

31. Zimmermann, K.; Baldinger, J.; Mayerhofer, B.; Atanasov, A.G.; Dirsch, V.M.; Heiss, E.H. Activated AMPK boosts the Nrf2/HO-1 signaling axis—A role for the unfolded protein response. *Free Radic. Biol. Med.* **2015**, *88*, 417–426. [CrossRef] [PubMed]

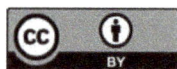

viruses

MDPI

Article

Characterizing the Different Effects of Zika Virus Infection in Placenta and Microglia Cells

Maria del Pilar Martinez Viedma [1] and Brett E. Pickett [2,*]

[1] J. Craig Venter Institute, 4120 Capricorn Lane, La Jolla, CA 92037, USA; pviedma@jcvi.org
[2] J. Craig Venter Institute, 9605 Medical Center Drive, Rockville, MD 20850, USA
* Correspondence: bpickett@jcvi.org; Tel.: +1-301-795-7000

Received: 26 September 2018; Accepted: 16 November 2018; Published: 18 November 2018

Abstract: Zika virus (ZIKV) is a neuropathic virus that causes serious neurological abnormalities such as Guillain-Barre syndrome in adults and congenital Zika syndrome (CZS) in fetuses, which makes it an important concern for global human health. A catalogue of cells that support ZIKV replication, pathogenesis, and/or the persistence of the virus still remains unknown. Here, we studied the behavior of the virus in human placenta (JEG-3) and human microglia (HMC3) cell lines in order to better understand how different host tissues respond during infection. We quantified the host transcriptional response to ZIKV infection in both types of cells at 24 and 72 h post-infection. A panel of 84 genes that are involved in the innate or adaptive immune responses was used to quantify differential expression in both cell lines. HMC3 cells showed a unique set of significant differentially expressed genes (DEGs) compared with JEG-3 cells at both time points. Subsequent analysis of these data using modern pathway analysis methods revealed that the TLR7/8 pathway was strongly inhibited in HMC3 cells, while it was activated in JEG-3 cells during virus infection. The disruption of these pathways was subsequently confirmed with specific small interfering RNA (siRNA) experiments that characterize their role in the viral life cycle, and may partially explain why ZIKV infection in placental tissue contributes to extreme neurological problems in a developing fetus.

Keywords: zika virus; placenta cells; microglia cells; siRNA; TLR7/8

1. Introduction

Zika virus (ZIKV) is an enveloped positive-sense, single-stranded RNA virus that belongs to the *Flavivirus* genus of the *Flaviviridae* family. Viruses belonging to this taxon include several human pathogens, such as yellow fever (YFV), dengue (DENV), Japanese encephalitis (JEV), tick-borne encephalitis (TBEV), and West Nile (WNV) viruses. ZIKV is transmitted mainly by *Aedes* spp. mosquitoes, and was originally discovered in 1947 in the blood of a febrile Rhesus monkey in Uganda's Zika forest [1].

Most ZIKV infections were associated with mild symptoms characterized by fever, rash, joint pain, and conjunctivitis. However, the recent worldwide epidemic has demonstrated that ZIKV can exhibit neurotropism that causes serious neurological abnormalities in humans. Specifically, Guillain-Barre syndrome has been observed in adults after infection, and congenital Zika syndrome (CZS) has been observed in the fetuses of infected mothers, with microcephaly being one of the most devastating consequences of this infection [2,3]. After a surge in microcephaly cases was associated with the recent severe Zika virus outbreak in Brazil [4], the World Health Organization declared ZIKV to be a Public Health Emergency of International Concern on 1 February 2016.

A marked difference between Zika and other flaviviruses is that ZIKV can be sexually transmitted [5–8] and is part of the "TORCH" pathogens, which include *Toxoplasma gondii*, *Listeria monocytogenes*, human immunodeficiency virus (HIV), varicella zoster virus, and other infectious agents that are associated with congenital anomalies [9]. The most recent studies have demonstrated that ZIKV is highly neurotropic; it infects and crosses the placenta in pregnant women, can be vertically transmitted from the infected mother to the fetus, and can produce CZS [10].

Despite a large effort by researchers, the molecular mechanism(s) of the vertical transmission of infection across the placenta barrier is still unknown [10]. Various cell types in the placenta are susceptible to infection with Zika virus [11]. Specifically, observations of hydropic and hyperplastic chorionic villi, as well as the proliferation of Hofbauer cells, have been reported during infection with Zika virus [12]. However, these cellular effects have not been shown to significantly impact placental function [12,13]. It is difficult to establish accurate laboratory models, since there are substantial anatomical differences between the placenta in humans versus other animals. Although human cell lines cannot currently replicate all of the gestational stages or the inherent structure of the human placenta, they are a useful initial tool to better understand the mechanism of action of teratogenic pathogens. Recognizing both the practicality and the limitations of these cell lines will help researchers better interpret experimental results.

Recent studies have described the cellular innate immune response against ZIKV infection, specifically, the role of Toll-like receptors [14,15], as well as specific molecules involved in this response such as STAT2 [16,17]. In this work, we better characterize the role of the intracellular immune response during Zika virus infection. To do so, we infected either human placenta or human microglia cell lines with ZIKV, and studied their innate immune response against ZIKV infection across multiple time points. Specifically, we studied the role of TLR7, TLR8, and STAT2 during ZIKV infection, since they are key molecules in the cellular antiviral and IFN-mediated responses. This work improves our understanding of how the virus is able to cross the placental barrier and the role of microglia cells during infection of the fetal brain. We demonstrate that the intracellular response of specific immunological pathways against ZIKV infection differs depending on the type of cells being infected.

2. Materials and Methods

2.1. Cells and Virus

Microglia HMC3 (CRL-3344), epithelial placenta JEG-3 (HTB-36), and epithelial Vero (CCL-81) cells were purchased from the American Type Culture Collection (ATCC, Bethesda, MD, USA) and maintained in high-glucose Dulbecco's modified Eagle's medium (DMEM), containing 10% fetal bovine serum (FBS; HyClone Laboratories, South Logan, UT, USA) and 1% penicillin/streptomycin at 37 °C in a 5% CO_2 incubator. ZIKV Puerto Rican strain (PRVABC59) was obtained through Biodefense and Emerging Infections (BEI) research resources (Zika Virus, PRVABC59, NR-50240).

2.2. Cell Infection

Cells were plated one day prior to infection in complete DMEM at 37 °C in a 5% CO_2 incubation chamber. ZIKV stock was diluted in DMEM with 2% FBS to obtain an inoculum with a multiplicity of infection (MOI) of 0.01, which was then incubated with the cells at 37 °C in a 5% CO_2 incubation chamber for one hour and rocked every 15 min. The inoculum was removed after one hour, complete DMEM was added, and cells were incubated at 37 °C in a 5% CO_2 incubation chamber until the collection time point.

2.3. LIVE/DEAD Cellular Assay

The cytopathic effects (CPE) of ZIKV infection on the different cells was measured by using the LIVE/DEAD Cell Imaging Kit (ThermoFisher, R37601, Waltham, MA, USA), based on a cell-permeable dye for staining live cells and a cell-impermeable dye for staining dead and dying cells, which are characterized by compromised cell membranes. For this assay, cells were plated and ZIKV-infected at a MOI of 0.01 and incubated for five days. Supernatants were collected at each time point and saved for viral titering. In parallel, cells were exposed to the staining reagent included in the LIVE/DEAD Cell

Imaging Kit for 15 min. The image data were captured using a Celigo Imaging Cytometer (Nexcelom Bioscience, Lawrence, MA, USA) at different times of infection, identifying healthy cells in green and damaged cells in red.

2.4. RNA Extraction, cDNA, RT-qPCR, qPCR Arrays, and Standard Curve

RNA from mock or ZIKV-infected cells was extracted from samples using the RNeasy mini kit from Qiagen (Hilden, Germany). Subsequent cDNA synthesis was performed with the SuperScript™ III First-Strand Synthesis SuperMix (ThermoFisher 18080400, Waltham, MA, USA). RT-qPCR was performed using specific primers for gene expression experiments (IDT; Supplementary Table S1) and PowerUp™ SYBR® Green Master Mix (ThermoFisher A25778, Waltham, MA, USA). The RT^2 Profiler PCR Array Human Innate and Adaptive Immune Responses (Qiagen, Hilden, Germany) was used following the manufacturer's protocol (Supplementary Table S2) for pathway-focused gene expression analysis.

The ZIKV standard curve was established using custom TaqMan Primers and Probe (IDT; Supplementary Table S3). Briefly, 10-fold serial dilutions of ZIKV genetic material from BEI resources (NR-50244) were used to establish the correlation between the cycle threshold (Ct) value and the number of molecules/µL of viral RNA. The RNA copy number (number of molecules/µL) was calculated as: [RNA concentration (g/mL)]/[RNA transcript length (nucleotides) × molecular weight of a nucleotide (330 g/mol) × Avogadro's number (6.023×10^{23}). In the same way, RNA from ZIKV stock (BEI, NR-50240) was serially diluted to establish the correlation between Ct and PFU/mL.

Separate primers and probes were designed for the Asian and African lineages, with the African lineage used as a negative control in these sets of experiments. Specifically, bioinformatics analysis was performed to identify the best sequences for primers and probes. This workflow consisted of: (1) collecting available Asian and African ZIKV complete genomes from the Virus Pathogen Resource (ViPR) database [18], (2) generating a multiple sequence alignment with MAFFT [19], (3) performing a statistical analysis to identify nucleotide positions that significantly differed between Asian and African lineages [20], and (4) confirming the specificity of the reagents using BLAST [21].

2.5. Plaque Assays

Viral titers were determined by plaque assay on Vero cells, which were plated one day before the assay at 90% of confluency in complete DMEM at 37 °C in a 5% CO_2 incubation chamber. Supernatants collected at various time points after infection were serially diluted and inoculated on the cells for one hour, with rocking every 15 min, at 37 °C in a 5% CO_2 incubation chamber. After that, a 1:1 mixture of 0.6% agarose and DMEM with 2% FBS was added and incubated at 37 °C in a 5% CO_2 incubation chamber. The overlay was removed after three days, cells were washed with phosphate-buffered saline (PBS), and stained and fixed with a crystal violet solution (2 g crystal violet + 60 mL 100% Ethanol + 40 mL 37% Formaldehyde + 100 mL PBS) for 30 min at room temperature in the dark. The excess crystal violet solution was removed by washing with water. After the plates were dry, plaques were visualized, and the number of plaque-forming units (PFU)/mL was determined. All of the experiments were performed in triplicate.

2.6. siRNA Experiments

ON-TARGET plus SMARTpool siRNA for human TLR7, TLR8, and STAT2 together with positive and negative controls were purchased from Dharmacon (51284, 51311,6773, D-001830-10-05, D-001810-10-05 respectively) and transfected into the cells with the transfection reagent Lipofectamine™ RNAiMAX (ThermoFisher 13778030, Waltham, MA, USA) following the manufacturer's protocol. Cells were infected with virus eight hours after transfection, once the effect of the siRNA was corroborated. Efficiency controls for the siRNA experiments were included (Supplementary Figure S1), and were used as the negative control to normalize the gene expression data. Supernatants from cell cultures were collected for viral titering at one day or three days post-transfection in each cell type, and at one day or three days post-transfection and subsequent viral infection in each cell type. Cells were washed with PBS and collected at the same time points for RNA extraction.

2.7. Signaling Pathway Analysis

The R implementation of the signaling pathway impact analysis algorithm (SPIA) was used to predict activated or inhibited pathways. Specifically, pathway data from five publicly available databases were used to generate a null distribution of the genes in each signal cascade pathway (1000 bootstrap replicates) and calculate a Bonferroni-corrected *p*-value in order to account for multiple hypothesis testing. The total net accumulated perturbation in each pathway was calculated by using the differential expression values and pathway topology. Positive perturbation values indicate pathway activation, while negative values represent pathway inhibition. Pathways that contained a statistically significant number of detected differentially expressed genes in the different cell types at each time point were categorized as either "activated" or "inhibited" in the algorithm output and subsequently ranked by *p*-value [22].

2.8. Statistical Analysis

Data analysis was performed using Prism (GraphPad Software, La Jolla, CA, USA) for statistical analysis. All of the experiments were carried out in triplicate, and values were presented as means ± SEM. *p*-values of these experiments were calculated with a non-paired Student's *t*-test. Statistical significance was accepted at $p < 0.05$.

3. Results

3.1. ZIKV Production, Titer, Cell Infection, and Cytopathic Effects (CPE)

After infecting different cell lines with ZIKV at 0.01 MOI, we showed that ZIKV was able to replicate in both cell lines (HMC3, JEG-3) as well as in the control cells (VERO), increasing its replication along the time of infection (Figure 1A). A standard curve was generated to establish the correlation between Ct values and the number of molecules/µL of viral RNA (Figure 1A upper panel) using a ZIKV-specific TaqMan probe. It is of note that the rate of ZIKV replication was at least 10-fold lower in placenta cells than in microglia or VERO cells when quantified by qPCR (Figure 1A lower panel) as well as through plaque assays (Figure 1B, lower panel). When we performed a live/dead assay, we observed CPE in ZIKV-infected placenta and microglia cells starting to appear at four days post-infection. Compared with the mock-infected cells, the images captured immediately after the assay showed a steady number of healthy cells (green) over time in mock-infected samples, and a decrease in the number of cells in ZIKV-infected samples (Figure 1B). This decrease is due to the increased detachment and loss of dead cells, as well as an increase in damaged cells (red) (Figure 1B, upper panel). In order to quantify the levels of infection in each time point, we performed plaque assays to determine the viral particles released to the media along the time (Figure 1B, lower panel). Based on these initial results, we chose one day post-infection (dpi) and three dpi as the optimal time points for further experiments, with the aim of studying the kinetics of the intracellular transcriptional response during viral infection before transcription associated with the cytopathic effects overcomes the virus-specific transcriptional signal.

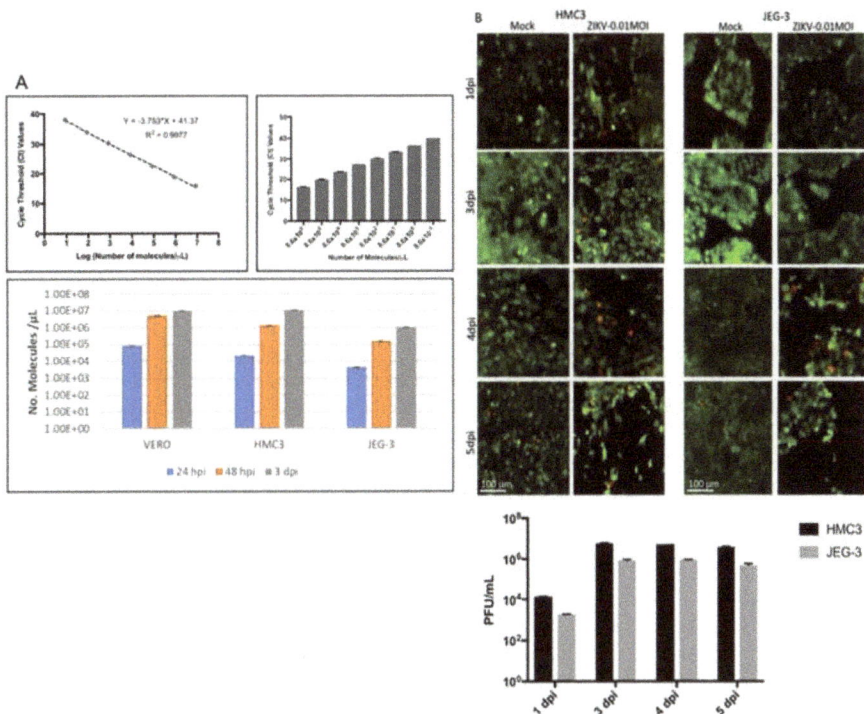

Figure 1. Quantification of Zika virus (ZIKV) titer, replication, and cytopathic effects (CPE) over time. (**A**) RT-qPCR standard curve to measure the number of virus genomes (upper panels); RT-qPCR to quantify ZIKV molecules in VERO, HMC3 and JEG-3 cells after one, two, and three days of infection. (**B**) CPE induced by ZIKV infection in HMC3 and JEG-3 cells at one, three, four, and five days post-infection, with the green stain representing healthy cells and the red stain indicating unhealthy and/or dying cells and the scale bar representing 100 micrometers. The lower panel shows the results from plaque assays performed in triplicate to quantify the ZIKV particles released to the media at each time point. Error bars represent standard deviation.

3.2. Host Intracellular Innate Immune Response and Differentially Affected Signaling Pathways

ZIKV is able to cross the placenta in pregnant women and infect the fetal brain; however, the mechanism by which this occurs has not been fully elucidated. To better understand the intracellular transcriptional response in placenta and microglia cell lines during ZIKV infection, we used RT-qPCR to evaluate an unbiased panel of 84 genes involved in the human innate and adaptive immune response (Supplementary Table S2). The results of this analysis are shown in Figure 2, where each dot or square represents a single transcript. When we compared the differentially expressed transcripts at one dpi versus three dpi (Figure 2A), there was a significant difference in the transcriptional regulation in infected cells compared with uninfected cells in microglia cells, but there was not a difference in placenta cells. Also, when we checked infected (I) cells versus uninfected (UI), a significant difference in differentially expressed genes from microglia cells compared with placenta cells at both time points one dpi and three dpi was observed (Figure 2B).

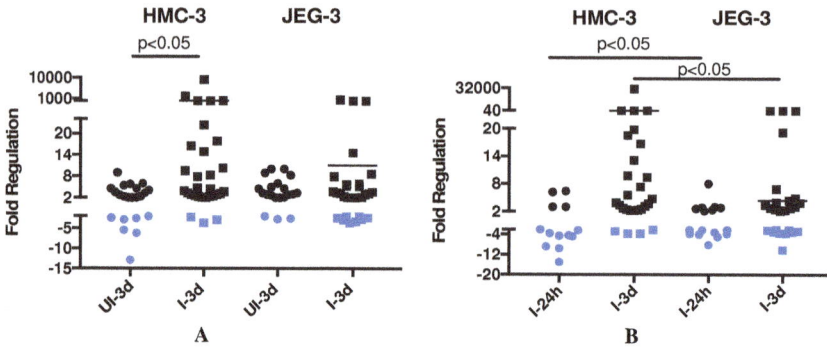

Figure 2. Results from an intracellular innate immune response RT-qPCR array. Each circle or square represents an individual gene that was either upregulated (black) or downregulated (blue). (**A**) Differentially expressed genes at one dpi versus three dpi in human microglia and placenta cells. (**B**) Differentially expressed genes of ZIKV-infected (I) samples versus time-matched mock-infected (UI) samples at 24 h and three days post infection with ZIKV. The numerical values on the Y-axis have been collapsed in regions that had no differentially expressed genes in order to improve visibility.

The significant differences observed in the RT-qPCR data led us to hypothesize that genes in specific signaling pathways were differently affected in each cell type within three days after ZIKV infection. Therefore, we analyzed these data using the signaling pathway impact analysis algorithm (SPIA) to identify the signaling pathways (i.e., networks of genes flowing from receptors to transcription factors) that were either significantly activated or inhibited in the different cells and at the different time points (Table 1). The summarized results from this analysis displayed several pathways that consistently differed between both cells lines. The predicted results for the TLR7/8 cascade appeared interesting, since they showed opposite phenotypes (e.g., activation or inhibition) in each cell line. Specifically, these pathways were predicted to be inhibited in infected microglia cells (blue), but activated in infected placenta cells (orange) when comparing the three dpi and one dpi time points in ZIKV-infected cells. This pattern was repeated in all of the pathways involving TLR7/8.

Table 1. Bonferroni-corrected *p*-values of differentially affected signaling pathways detected with the signaling pathway impact analysis (SPIA) algorithm in: ZIKV-infected (I) or time-matched mock-infected (UI) cells at each of two time points in each cell type.

	HMC3 (Human Microglia)				JEG3 (Human Placenta)			
	1 dpi (I vs. UI)	3 dpi (I vs. UI)	Infected (3 dpi vs. 1 dpi)	Uninfected (3 dpi vs. 1 dpi)	1 dpi (I vs. UI)	3 dpi (I vs, UI)	Infected (3 dpi vs. 1 dpi)	Uninfected (3 dpi vs. 1 dpi)
Jak-STAT signaling pathway	7.88×10^{-6}	6.85×10^{-8}	2.77×10^{-8}	6.58×10^{-8}	7.90×10^{-4}	1.26×10^{-7}	1.06×10^{-13}	2.05×10^{-7}
NF-kappa B signaling pathway	2.05×10^{-3}	2.13×10^{-11}	6.23×10^{-10}	5.13×10^{-10}	8.00×10^{-8}	2.12×10^{-9}	2.16×10^{-9}	1.02×10^{-11}
Toll-like receptor signaling pathway	9.21×10^{-12}	1.44×10^{-29}	5.48×10^{-28}	2.87×10^{-20}	1.25×10^{-23}	1.02×10^{-31}	3.44×10^{-33}	1.22×10^{-27}
Toll-like receptor TLR1:TLR2 cascade	N.S.	1.55×10^{-5}	1.43×10^{-7}	1.04×10^{-5}	4.89×10^{-3}	9.80×10^{-11}	1.20×10^{-8}	7.44×10^{-4}
Toll-like receptor TLR6:TLR2 cascade	N.S.	1.36×10^{-5}	1.54×10^{-7}	1.17×10^{-5}	4.92×10^{-3}	9.00×10^{-11}	1.24×10^{-8}	7.25×10^{-4}
TRIF-mediated TLR3/TLR4 signaling	N.S.	7.07×10^{-7}	3.30×10^{-7}	4.47×10^{-7}	5.53×10^{-3}	1.11×10^{-8}	2.12×10^{-3}	4.70×10^{-7}
TRAF6-mediated IRF7 activation in TLR7/8 or 9 signaling	2.23×10^{-2}	2.20×10^{-3}	6.63×10^{-9}	9.52×10^{-6}	N.S.	N.S.	1.98×10^{-3}	1.69×10^{-8}
Caspase activation via extrinsic apoptotic signaling pathway	N.S.	N.S.	N.S.	2.53×10^{-2}	8.02×10^{-3}	2.24×10^{-8}	4.23×10^{-4}	2.34×10^{-4}
IFN-alpha signaling pathway	N.S.	3.34×10^{-3}	2.63×10^{-3}	7.99×10^{-3}	N.S.	1.07×10^{-5}	2.40×10^{-7}	N.S.
PI3K-Akt signaling pathway	N.S.	2.34×10^{-3}	1.50×10^{-3}	N.S.	2.86×10^{-2}	4.47×10^{-5}	4.66×10^{-6}	N.S.
Toll-like receptor 7/8 (TLR7/8) cascade	N.S.	7.57×10^{-6}	5.30×10^{-10}	8.80×10^{-6}	N.S.	N.S.	3.18×10^{-2}	1.00×10^{-5}
Toll-like receptor 9 (TLR9) cascade	N.S.	9.55×10^{-6}	6.03×10^{-10}	1.17×10^{-5}	N.S.	N.S.	3.77×10^{-2}	1.28×10^{-5}
TRAF6-mediated induction of NFkB and MAP kinases upon TLR7/8 or 9 activation	N.S.	5.13×10^{-4}	5.82×10^{-8}	1.97×10^{-4}	N.S.	N.S.	2.74×10^{-2}	5.23×10^{-4}
TRAF6-mediated IRF7 activation	N.S.	4.14×10^{-4}	2.92×10^{-4}	3.78×10^{-6}	N.S.	N.S.	5.97×10^{-4}	9.19×10^{-3}
Regulation of nuclear SMAD2/3 signaling	N.S.	7.12×10^{-5}	1.93×10^{-3}	N.S.	N.S.	N.S.	N.S.	4.02×10^{-2}
TRAF3-dependent IRF activation pathway	N.S.	2.58×10^{-3}	2.02×10^{-3}	3.55×10^{-3}	N.S.	N.S.	N.S.	N.S.
TRIF-mediated programmed cell death	N.S.	N.S.	N.S.	N.S.	N.S.	1.59×10^{-8}	1.94×10^{-3}	8.05×10^{-4}
Apoptosis	N.S.	2.53×10^{-2}	N.S.	3.22×10^{-2}	N.S.	N.S.	N.S.	N.S.
Regulation of IFNA signaling	N.S.	N.S.	N.S.	N.S.	N.S.	1.85×10^{-2}	2.23×10^{-4}	N.S.

N.S.: Not Significant; Blue: inhibited pathway; Orange: activated pathway.

3.3. Effect of siRNA against TLR7, TLR8, or Both

We then tested the role of TLR7 and TLR8 in the host–pathogen interaction network. To do so, we used pools of siRNAs that specifically target these receptors, and measured the impact on viral replication (Figure 3) and the level of expression of a group of well-known genes involved in intracellular antiviral and innate immune responses (toll-like receptors, transcription factors, and interferon-stimulated genes) (Figures 4 and 5).

3.3.1. Viral Replication

We quantified viral replication by measuring the number of whole infectious viral particles released to the media through plaque assays after knocking down TLR7 and/or TLR8 (Figure 3A). We compared these numbers to the Ct values that were obtained from ZIKV RT-qPCR, and saw that they corresponded with each other (Figure 3B). We observed that siRNA against TLR7 and/or TLR8 had no effect on viral replication three dpi when compared with the siRNA control in microglia cells (HMC3). However, when the same transcripts were knocked down in placenta cells (JEG-3), ZIKV replication was significantly increased three dpi compared with the control. These assays confirmed the previous results in each of our selected cell lines.

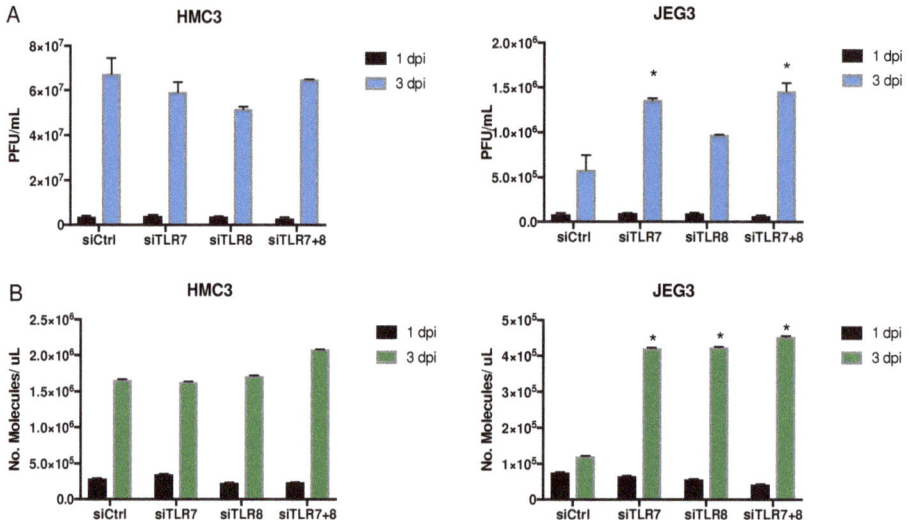

Figure 3. Viral and transcriptional effects of siRNAs targeting TLR7, TLR8, or TLR7 + TLR8 on ZIKV virus replication in different cell types over time. (**A**) Plaque-forming units (PFU) per mL of supernatant were measured to quantify infectious virus production at each time point in each cell type. (**B**) The number of ZIKV RNA molecules from the same samples was measured with RT-qPCR to quantify viral genome replication at both time points in each cell type ($* p < 0.05$). Error bars represent standard deviation.

3.3.2. Innate Immune Response in Microglia and Placenta Cells

In order to determine whether other intracellular factors contributed to ZIKV replication, we quantified the level of expression of other components in the innate immune system. Specifically, we evaluated: transcription factors STAT1, STAT2, IRF3, IRF7, and IRF9; as well as the interferon-stimulated genes (ISGs) CXCL10, IFIT1, and MX1 in mock-infected (UI) and ZIKV-infected (I) placenta cells (Figure 4, left panel) and microglia cells (Figure 4, right panel). Placenta cells showed a strong induction of the ISGs at two and three days after Zika infection, but no noticeable induction of the remaining studied genes. Conversely, the microglial cells showed induction of almost the entire panel of transcripts three days after infection.

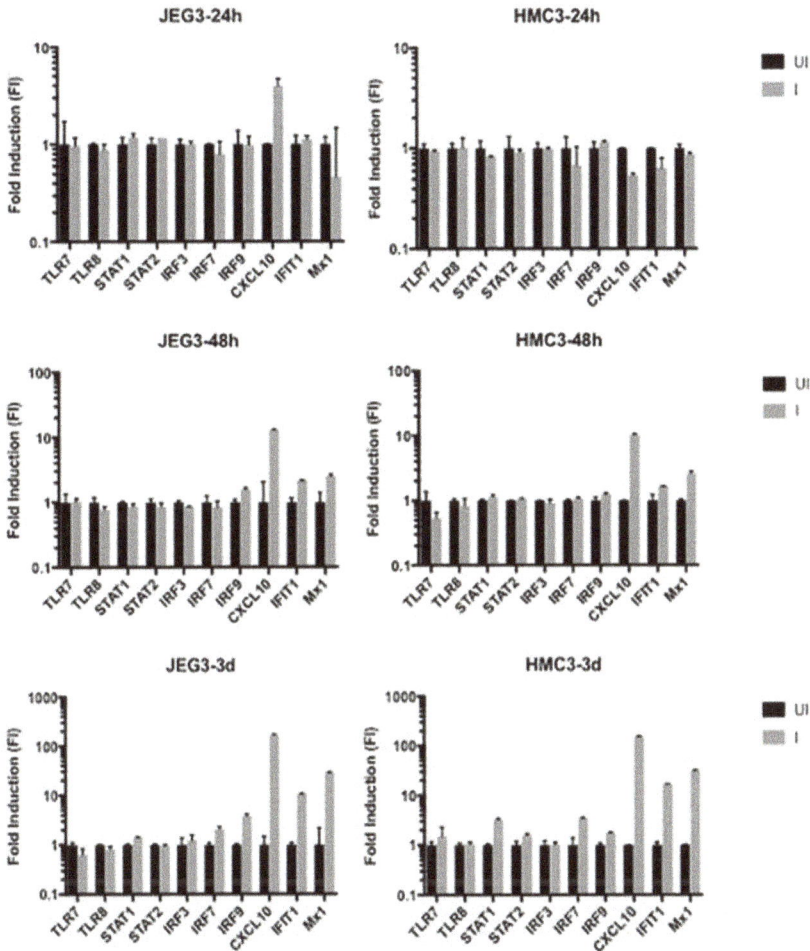

Figure 4. Fold induction values for genes involved in the innate immune response of time-matched mock-infected (UI) versus ZIKV-infected (I) HMC3 and JEG-3 cells at 24 h post infection (hpi), 48 hpi, and three dpi. Values were determined by calculating the fold induction (FI) using the delta-delta cycle threshold ($\Delta\Delta$Ct) method for each gene, normalizing the values for each gene to the UI results.

We next wanted to understand how the differential expression of these transcripts was affected after blocking TLR7, TLR8, or both (Figure 5, Supplementary Figure S2). In microglia cells (Figure 5A), after siRNA transfections, there was an initial response from some of the transcription factors at day one and three. However, that induction returned to normal when the transfection was followed by ZIKV infection. At three dpi, the ZIKV-infected microglia cells showed sporadic induction compared with uninfected cells (Figure 4), but not with cells that were ZIKV-infected and previously transfected with the specific siRNAs (Figure 5A, right lower plot). Similar results were observed in placenta cells (Figure 5B), where cells transfected with siRNAs against TLR7 and/or TLR8 showed a strong upregulation of a subset of genes (Figure 5B, left plots) that mostly disappeared when these cells were transfected and infected with ZIKV (Figure 5B, right plots). In addition, the observed upregulation of cytokines in infected placenta and microglia cells (Figure 4) was not as strong when the cells were transfected with siRNAs, or transfected and infected.

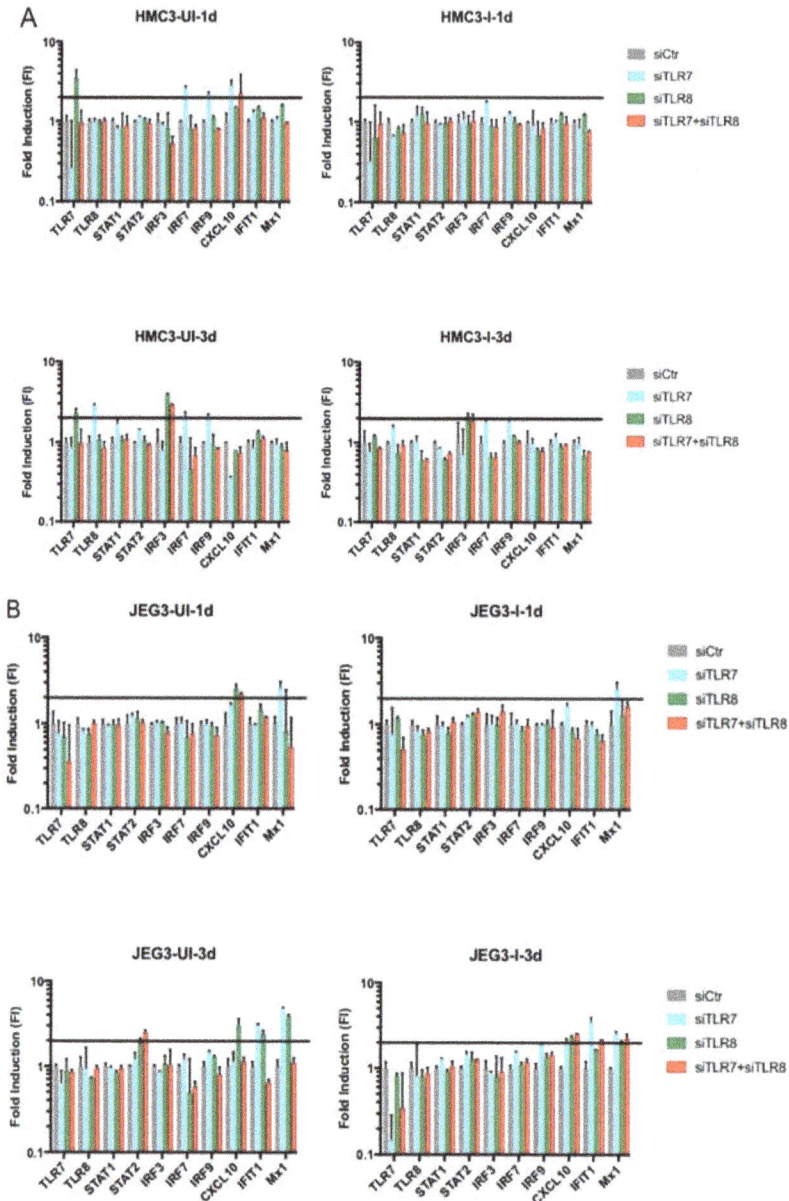

Figure 5. A comparison of the effects of a panel of siRNAs including TLR7, TLR8, TLR7 + TLR8, or scramble (control) on the expression of selected innate immune response factors. (**A**) HMC3 cells transfected with siRNA and either time-matched mock-infected (UI) or infected with ZIKV (I) at one dpi and three dpi. (**B**) JEG3 cells transfected with siRNA and either time-matched mock-infected (UI) or infected with ZIKV (I) at one dpi and three dpi. The horizontal black line marks the two-fold induction (FI) threshold in each plot.

3.4. Role of STAT2 in Host Intracellular Response after ZIKV Infection

We next decided to study the role of STAT2 in the intracellular transcriptional response after ZIKV infection. This decision was partially dependent on the results from the previous experiments performed in this study, and also based on previous reports that showed that ZIKV can degrade STAT2 in specific cells [16]. We first observed a significant upregulation of STAT2 after three days of infection in microglia cells; however, this upregulation was absent in placenta cells (Figure 6A). Transfecting cells with pools of STAT2-specific siRNAs to knockdown STAT2 transcript levels resulted in a dramatic reduction in the expression levels for genes involved in the intracellular innate immune response in both cell lines at both time points. The only exception to this trend was found for CXCL10 in placenta cells, which was upregulated after STAT2 knockdown; however, this upregulation decreased somewhat after ZIKV infection (Figure 6B). We then quantified the number of ZIKV RNA molecules in each cell type as a measure of viral replication after STAT2 knockdown. This experiment showed an increase in the ZIKV RNA molecules in microglia cells compared to the siRNA control, but no changes were observed in placenta cells (Figure 6C).

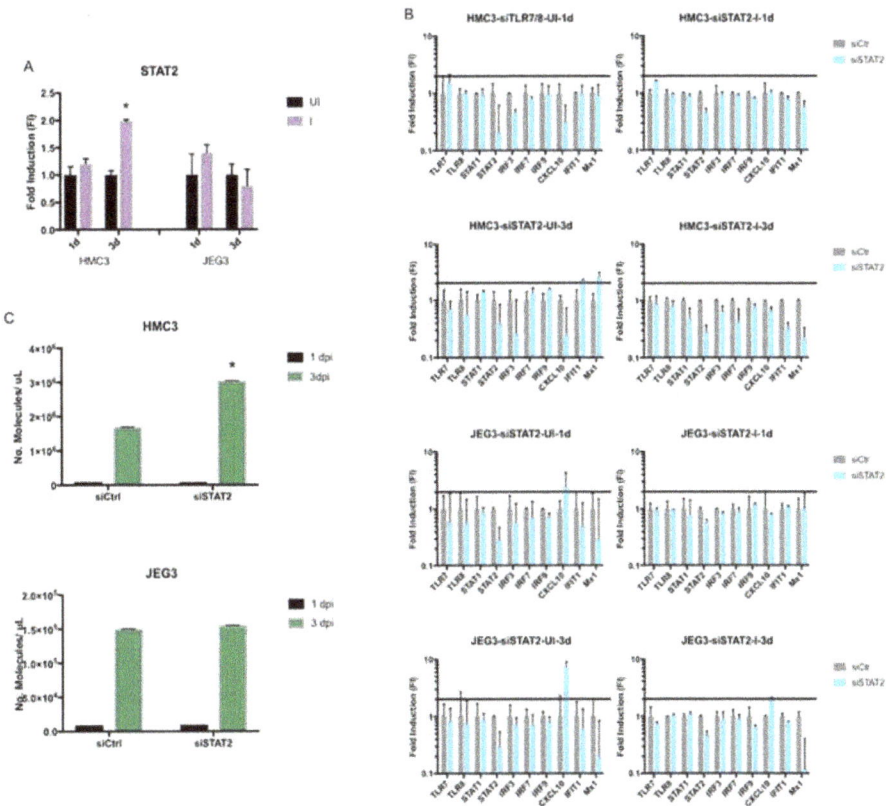

Figure 6. Role of STAT2 in ZIKV replication and in the intracellular response to infection. (**A**) STAT2 expression in time-matched mock-infected (UI) and ZIKV-infected (I) HMC3 and JEG-3 cells at one dpi and three dpi. (**B**) Effect of STAT2 knockdown on selected innate immune genes in time-matched mock-infected (UI) and infected (I) HMC3 and JEG-3 cells at one dpi and three dpi. The horizontal black line represents the two-fold induction (FI) threshold in each plot. (**C**) Number of ZIKV RNA molecules detected from the total RNA collected from cells treated with siRNAs against STAT2. (* $p < 0.05$).

3.5. Role of Viral Receptor AXL in Microglia and Placenta Cells

The AXL gene encodes a tyrosine protein kinase receptor that has been shown to be a cellular receptor used by the Zika virus to gain entry into host cells [23]. When we studied this receptor, AXL showed a significantly higher expression one day after infection in placenta cells when compared to uninfected cells; however, those expression levels returned to normal within three days after infection. In contrast, there was no differential-expression of AXL in infected microglia cells when compared to the uninfected cells (Figure 7A). Therefore, we wanted to test the effect of siRNAs against STAT2, TLR7, and/or TLR8 on AXL expression in these two cell lines. We observed that AXL maintained relatively normal levels of expression in microglia cells after blocking TLR7, TLR8, TLR7/8, and STAT2. However, in placenta cells, we saw that siRNA against TLR8 significantly decreased AXL expression after three days, with a similar downregulation also observed after TLR7 knockdown three days after infection. In contrast, siRNA against STAT2 in infected placenta cells significantly induced AXL expression after three days of infection when compared to control cells (Figure 7B).

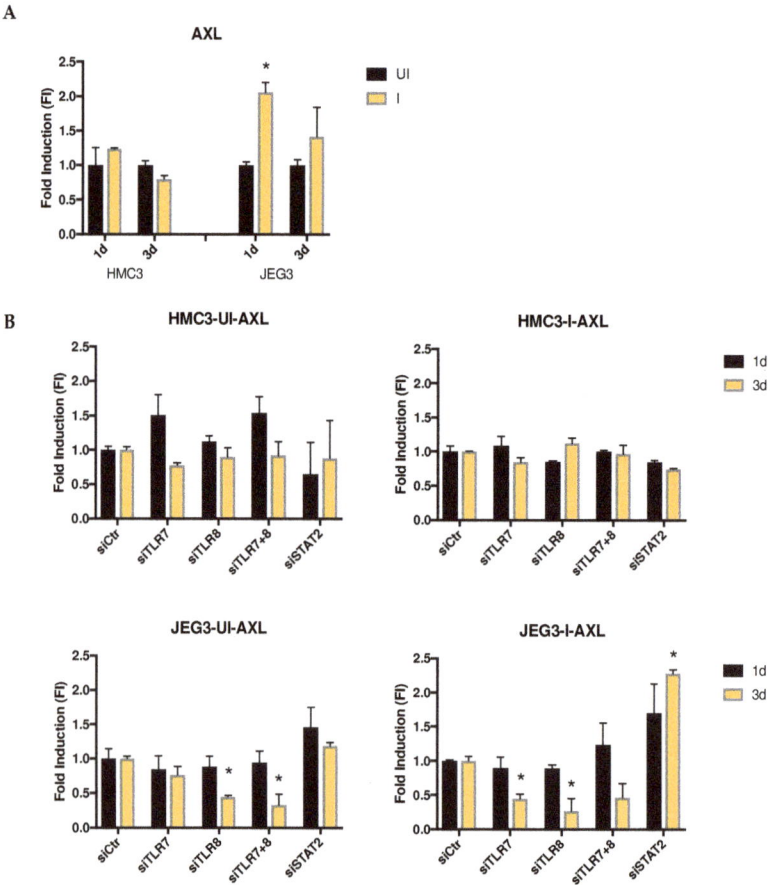

Figure 7. Role of AXL in ZIKV infection. (**A**) AXL fold induction ZIKV-infected (I) relative to time-matched mock-infected (UI) HMC3 and JEG-3 cells at one dpi and three dpi. (**B**) Effect of siRNAs targeting TLR7, TLR8, TLR7 + TLR8, or STAT2 on AXL expression in time-matched mock-infected (UI) and ZIKV-infected (I) HMC3 and JEG-3 cells at one dpi and three dpi. (* $p < 0.05$). Error bars represent standard deviation.

4. Discussion

Defining the mechanisms by which ZIKV causes neuropathic effects is critical to predict future risks as well as establish control measures against the disease. In this study, we evaluated the behavior of ZIKV in two target cell lines, placenta and microglia, with the aim of understanding how the virus counteracts the intracellular antiviral response in these two cell lines during infection. Several studies have demonstrated that ZIKV infection can result in different interferon (IFN) responses depending on the cell type [24–27]. In concordance with these studies, we first demonstrated that Zika is able to replicate in both cell lines, placenta (JEG-3) and microglia (HMC3), causing cytopathic effects after four days of infection. Interestingly, the host intracellular response to ZIKV infection was different in each of the cell lines that we tested. Not only did we identify sets of significant differentially expressed genes that are involved in the intracellular innate immune response when we compared the two cell types, but we also observed differences in the activation and/or inhibition of immunological signaling pathways. Due to the different function of each cell type, we expected to observe a higher immune activation in microglia cells, which are known as the "macrophages of the brain", to fight against any pathogen that could compromise this tissue. In contrast, the placenta cells function as a barrier to protect the fetus from any disturbance such as inflammation or immune activation that could affect its stability and development, which led us to expect an active but more subdued antiviral response.

Assuming these functional differences and based on immunological pathways analysis results, we demonstrated that knocking down the expression of TLR7 and/or TLR8 had different consequences for viral replication in each cell line. We demonstrated that TLR7/8 inhibits viral replication in placenta cells but not in microglia, as this pathway is already inhibited by the virus. Prior studies carried out with the TLR7/8 agonist R848 demonstrated that this molecule blocks ZIKV replication in monocytes and macrophages by inducing the antiviral protein Viperin [15]. Follow-up experiments will be needed to test whether Viperin is also involved in the inhibition of virus replication in placenta cells. The stronger inhibitory response after ZIKV infection on a selected group of genes when the TLR7/8 signaling pathway was blocked in both cell lines demonstrates its role in the intracellular innate immune response. It has been recently shown that the inhibition of TLR8 in ZIKV-infected trophoblasts abrogated the inflammatory cytokine responses, which is in accordance with our findings [14].

Previous investigations to determine the mechanism causing a reduction in the intracellular IFN response showed that the ZIKV NS5 protein is able to degrade STAT2, which is an IFN pathway precursor molecule [16]. However, this mechanism is not expanded to other cell types such as dendritic cells, where ZIKV is able to antagonize IFN type I response by impeding STAT1 and STAT2 phosphorylation [28]. In this study, we demonstrate that STAT2 is significantly upregulated in infected microglia cells when compared with uninfected cells, but its levels do not change during the infection of placenta cells. We validated that the virus behaves differently in each cell line to counteract the unique intracellular antiviral response, which likely reflects the functions of their respective tissues. In addition, ZIKV showed a significantly higher replication rate when STAT2 was knocked down in microglia cells compared with the control; however, no significant differences were observed in placenta cells under similar conditions. As observed when we knocked down TLR7/8, after reducing STAT2 transcript abundance, we observed a stronger inhibition of the set of genes involved in the intracellular innate immune response. These data justify performing more in-depth studies into the pathogenic mechanism(s) of Zika virus in these and other cell types that are susceptible to ZIKV infection. We expect that such experiments would greatly contribute to the discovery of specific targets for antiviral drug development.

Another controversial molecule in ZIKV infection is the cellular receptor AXL. While in some cell types it acts as a ZIKV viral entry receptor [24,29], it has been demonstrated that AXL does not always perform this role during ZIKV infection [30,31]. In accordance with these publications, our study demonstrates that AXL gene expression is different in these two cell lines. Interestingly, AXL is associated with viral infection, TLR7/8 transcript abundance, and STAT2 transcript abundance in placenta cells, since their levels vary both when these cells are infected as well as when TLR7/8

Viruses **2018**, *10*, 649

or STAT2 are knocked down. Global transcriptomic methods, such as RNAseq could be used in future experiments in order to decipher this relationship during ZIKV infection and its implications in viral pathogenesis. Such an approach would give us much more information about host–pathogen interactions and the relevant molecules and pathways involved in ZIKV pathogenesis in placenta, microglia, and/or other cells. Confirmation of these findings at the protein level will also be important to better define the mechanism of action of Zika pathogenesis and neurotropism in different cell types.

In this manuscript, we have demonstrated that the antiviral response during ZIKV infection is highly dependent on the type of host cell being infected. Based on the results presented here, we propose a Zika virus–host cell interaction molecular model for placenta and microglia cells involving TLR7/8, STAT2, and AXL (Figure 8). This model will enable better understanding of the mechanism of action of the virus and as well as the design and development of specific antiviral drugs.

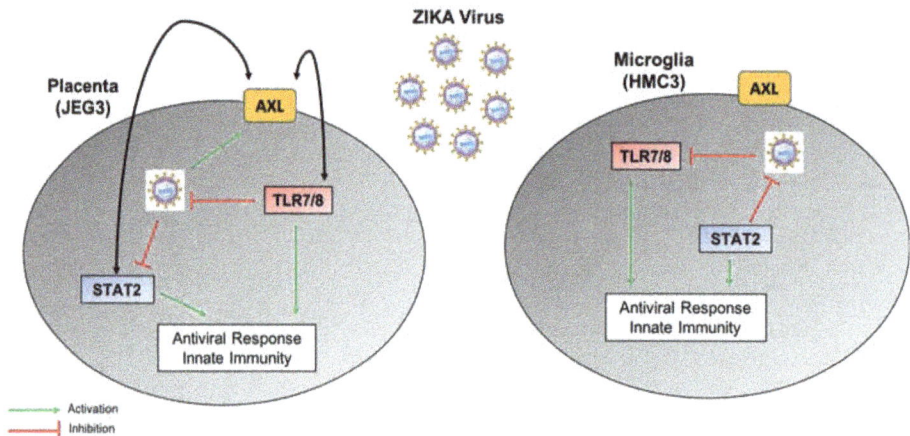

Figure 8. A potential schematic molecular model depicting the differing relationships between the expression of STAT2, TLR7, TLR8, and AXL during ZIKV infection in human placenta (JEG-3) and microglia (HMC3) cells.

Supplementary Materials: The following are available online at http://www.mdpi.com/1999-4915/10/11/649/s1, Figure S1: Fold-induction values of control siRNAs in untreated (UT) or positive control (PSC) samples at 1dpi and 3dpi following siRNA transfection in each HMC3 and JEG3 cells. Figure S2: Fold-induction values for each cell type at time-matched mock-infected cells after only siRNA-control transfection (UI), siRNA-control transfection plus virus infection (I), or transfected with either siRNAs targeting TLR8 or TLR7 + TLR8 (upper panel), TLR7 or TLR7 + TLR8 (middle panel) or STAT2 (lower panel) prior to infection with ZIKV at 1dpi and 3dpi in each of two human cell types. Table S1: set of primers used for measuring transcriptional expression levels through RT-PCR. Table S2: Innate and Adaptive Immune Responses RT^2 Profiler PCR Array list of genes. Table S3: Zika virus TaqMan primers and Probe for RT-qPCR.

Author Contributions: Conceptualization, M.d.P.M.V. and B.E.P.; Methodology, M.d.P.M.V. and B.E.P.; Software, M.d.P.M.V. and B.E.P.; Validation, M.d.P.M.V. and B.E.P.; Formal Analysis, M.d.P.M.V. and B.E.P.; Writing—Original Draft Preparation, M.d.P.M.V. and B.E.P.; Writing—Review & Editing, M.d.P.M.V. and B.E.P.; Visualization, M.d.P.M.V. and B.E.P.; Supervision, B.E.P.; Project Administration, B.E.P.; Funding Acquisition, B.E.P.

Funding: This research received no external funding.

Acknowledgments: We gratefully acknowledge the technical and administrative support provided by the J. Craig Venter Institute for their assistance in making this study possible.

Conflicts of Interest: The authors declare no conflict of interest

References

1. Dick, G.W.; Kitchen, S.F.; Haddow, A.J. Zika virus. I. Isolations and serological specificity. *Trans. R. Soc. Trop. Med. Hyg.* **1952**, *46*, 509–520. [CrossRef]

2. White, M.K.; Wollebo, H.S.; David Beckham, J.; Tyler, K.L.; Khalili, K. Zika virus: An emergent neuropathological agent. *Ann. Neurol.* **2016**, *80*, 479–489. [CrossRef] [PubMed]

3. Russo, F.B.; Jungmann, P.; Beltrao-Braga, P.C.B. Zika infection and the development of neurological defects. *Cell. Microbiol.* **2017**, *19*. [CrossRef] [PubMed]

4. Musso, D. Zika Virus Transmission from French Polynesia to Brazil. *Emerg. Infect. Dis.* **2015**, *21*, 1887. [CrossRef] [PubMed]

5. D'Ortenzio, E.; Matheron, S.; Yazdanpanah, Y.; de Lamballerie, X.; Hubert, B.; Piorkowski, G.; Maquart, M.; Descamps, D.; Damond, F.; Leparc-Goffart, I. Evidence of Sexual Transmission of Zika Virus. *N. Engl. J. Med.* **2016**, *374*, 2193–2195. [CrossRef] [PubMed]

6. Moreira, J.; Lamas, C.C.; Siqueira, A. Sexual Transmission of Zika Virus: Implications for Clinical Care and Public Health Policy. *Clin. Infect. Dis.* **2016**, *63*, 141–142. [CrossRef] [PubMed]

7. McDonald, E.M.; Duggal, N.K.; Brault, A.C. Pathogenesis and sexual transmission of Spondweni and Zika viruses. *PLoS Negl. Trop. Dis.* **2017**, *11*, e0005990. [CrossRef] [PubMed]

8. Musso, D.; Richard, V.; Teissier, A.; Stone, M.; Lanteri, M.C.; Latoni, G.; Alsina, J.; Reik, R.; Busch, M.P.; Recipient, E.; et al. Detection of Zika virus RNA in semen of asymptomatic blood donors. *Clin. Microbiol. Infect.* **2017**, *23*. [CrossRef] [PubMed]

9. Schwartz, D.A. The Origins and Emergence of Zika Virus, the Newest TORCH Infection: What's Old Is New Again. *Arch. Pathol. Lab. Med.* **2017**, *141*, 18–25. [CrossRef] [PubMed]

10. Arora, N.; Sadovsky, Y.; Dermody, T.S.; Coyne, C.B. Microbial Vertical Transmission during Human Pregnancy. *Cell Host Microbe* **2017**, *21*, 561–567. [CrossRef] [PubMed]

11. Jurado, K.A.; Simoni, M.K.; Tang, Z.; Uraki, R.; Hwang, J.; Householder, S.; Wu, M.; Lindenbach, B.D.; Abrahams, V.M.; Guller, S.; et al. Zika virus productively infects primary human placenta-specific macrophages. *JCI Insight* **2016**, *1*. [CrossRef] [PubMed]

12. Rosenberg, A.Z.; Yu, W.; Hill, D.A.; Reyes, C.A.; Schwartz, D.A. Placental Pathology of Zika Virus: Viral Infection of the Placenta Induces Villous Stromal Macrophage (Hofbauer Cell) Proliferation and Hyperplasia. *Arch. Pathol. Lab. Med.* **2017**, *141*, 43–48. [CrossRef] [PubMed]

13. Adibi, J.J.; Marques, E.T., Jr.; Cartus, A.; Beigi, R.H. Teratogenic effects of the Zika virus and the role of the placenta. *Lancet* **2016**, *387*, 1587–1590. [CrossRef]

14. Luo, H.; Winkelmann, E.R.; Fernandez-Salas, I.; Li, L.; Mayer, S.V.; Danis-Lozano, R.; Sanchez-Casas, R.M.; Vasilakis, N.; Tesh, R.; Barrett, A.D.; Weaver, S.C.; et al. Zika, dengue and yellow fever viruses induce differential anti-viral immune responses in human monocytic and first trimester trophoblast cells. *Antiviral Res.* **2018**, *151*, 55–62. [CrossRef] [PubMed]

15. Vanwalscappel, B.; Tada, T.; Landau, N.R. Toll-like receptor agonist R848 blocks Zika virus replication by inducing the antiviral protein viperin. *Virology* **2018**, *522*, 199–208. [CrossRef] [PubMed]

16. Grant, A.; Ponia, S.S.; Tripathi, S.; Balasubramaniam, V.; Miorin, L.; Sourisseau, M.; Schwarz, M.C.; Sanchez-Seco, M.P.; Evans, M.J.; Best, S.M.; et al. Zika Virus Targets Human STAT2 to Inhibit Type I Interferon Signaling. *Cell Host Microbe* **2016**, *19*, 882–890. [CrossRef] [PubMed]

17. Hertzog, J.; Dias Junior, A.G.; Rigby, R.E.; Donald, C.L.; Mayer, A.; Sezgin, E.; Song, C.; Jin, B.; Hublitz, P.; Eggeling, C.; et al. Infection with a Brazilian isolate of Zika virus generates RIG-I stimulatory RNA and the viral NS5 protein blocks type I IFN induction and signaling. *Eur. J. Immunol.* **2018**, *48*, 1120–1136. [CrossRef] [PubMed]

18. Pickett, B.E.; Sadat, E.L.; Zhang, Y.; Noronha, J.M.; Squires, R.B.; Hunt, V.; Liu, M.; Kumar, S.; Zaremba, S.; Gu, Z.; et al. ViPR: An open bioinformatics database and analysis resource for virology research. *Nucleic Acids Res.* **2012**, *40*, D593–D598. [CrossRef] [PubMed]

19. Nakamura, T.; Yamada, K.D.; Tomii, K.; Katoh, K. Parallelization of MAFFT for large-scale multiple sequence alignments. *Bioinformatics* **2018**, *34*, 2490–2492. [CrossRef] [PubMed]

20. Pickett, B.E.; Liu, M.; Sadat, E.L.; Squires, R.B.; Noronha, J.M.; He, S.; Jen, W.; Zaremba, S.; Gu, Z.; Zhou, L.; et al. Metadata-driven comparative analysis tool for sequences (meta-CATS): An automated process for identifying significant sequence variations that correlate with virus attributes. *Virology* **2013**, *447*, 45–51. [CrossRef] [PubMed]

21. Altschul, S.F.; Gish, W.; Miller, W.; Myers, E.W.; Lipman, D.J. Basic local alignment search tool. *J. Mol. Biol.* **1990**, *215*, 403–410. [CrossRef]

22. Tarca, A.L.; Draghici, S.; Khatri, P.; Hassan, S.S.; Mittal, P.; Kim, J.S.; Kim, C.J.; Kusanovic, J.P.; Romero, R. A novel signaling pathway impact analysis. *Bioinformatics* **2009**, *25*, 75–82. [CrossRef] [PubMed]

23. Nowakowski, T.J.; Pollen, A.A.; Di Lullo, E.; Sandoval-Espinosa, C.; Bershteyn, M.; Kriegstein, A.R. Expression Analysis Highlights AXL as a Candidate Zika Virus Entry Receptor in Neural Stem Cells. *Cell Stem Cell* **2016**, *18*, 591–596. [CrossRef] [PubMed]

24. Hamel, R.; Dejarnac, O.; Wichit, S.; Ekchariyawat, P.; Neyret, A.; Luplertlop, N.; Perera-Lecoin, M.; Surasombatpattana, P.; Talignani, L.; Thomas, F.; et al. Biology of Zika Virus Infection in Human Skin Cells. *J. Virol.* **2015**, *89*, 8880–8896. [CrossRef] [PubMed]

25. Bayer, A.; Lennemann, N.J.; Ouyang, Y.; Bramley, J.C.; Morosky, S.; Marques, E.T., Jr.; Cherry, S.; Sadovsky, Y.; Coyne, C.B. Type III Interferons Produced by Human Placental Trophoblasts Confer Protection against Zika Virus Infection. *Cell Host Microbe* **2016**, *19*, 705–712. [CrossRef] [PubMed]

26. Quicke, K.M.; Bowen, J.R.; Johnson, E.L.; McDonald, C.E.; Ma, H.; O'Neal, J.T.; Rajakumar, A.; Wrammert, J.; Rimawi, B.H.; Pulendran, B.; et al. Zika Virus Infects Human Placental Macrophages. *Cell Host Microbe* **2016**, *20*, 83–90. [CrossRef] [PubMed]

27. Chaudhary, V.; Yuen, K.S.; Chan, J.F.; Chan, C.P.; Wang, P.H.; Cai, J.P.; Zhang, S.; Liang, M.; Kok, K.H.; Chan, C.P.; et al. Selective Activation of Type II Interferon Signaling by Zika Virus NS5 Protein. *J. Virol.* **2017**, *91*. [CrossRef] [PubMed]

28. Bowen, J.R.; Quicke, K.M.; Maddur, M.S.; O'Neal, J.T.; McDonald, C.E.; Fedorova, N.B.; Puri, V.; Shabman, R.S.; Pulendran, B.; Suthar, M.S. Zika Virus Antagonizes Type I Interferon Responses during Infection of Human Dendritic Cells. *PLoS Pathog.* **2017**, *13*, e1006164. [CrossRef] [PubMed]

29. Meertens, L.; Labeau, A.; Dejarnac, O.; Cipriani, S.; Sinigaglia, L.; Bonnet-Madin, L.; Le Charpentier, T.; Hafirassou, M.L.; Zamborlini, A.; Cao-Lormeau, V.M.; et al. Axl Mediates ZIKA Virus Entry in Human Glial Cells and Modulates Innate Immune Responses. *Cell Rep.* **2017**, *18*, 324–333. [CrossRef] [PubMed]

30. Wells, M.F.; Salick, M.R.; Wiskow, O.; Ho, D.J.; Worringer, K.A.; Ihry, R.J.; Kommineni, S.; Bilican, B.; Klim, J.R.; Hill, E.J.; et al. Genetic Ablation of AXL Does Not Protect Human Neural Progenitor Cells and Cerebral Organoids from Zika Virus Infection. *Cell Stem Cell* **2016**, *19*, 703–708. [CrossRef] [PubMed]

31. Chen, J.; Yang, Y.F.; Yang, Y.; Zou, P.; Chen, J.; He, Y.; Shui, S.L.; Cui, Y.R.; Bai, R.; Liang, Y.J.; et al. AXL promotes Zika virus infection in astrocytes by antagonizing type I interferon signalling. *Nat. Microbiol.* **2018**, *3*, 302–309. [CrossRef] [PubMed]

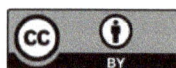

viruses

MDPI

Article

The Effect of Permethrin Resistance on *Aedes aegypti* Transcriptome Following Ingestion of Zika Virus Infected Blood

Liming Zhao [1,*] , Barry W. Alto [1], Dongyoung Shin [1] and Fahong Yu [2]

[1] Florida Medical Entomology Laboratory, University of Florida, 200 9th Street South East, Vero Beach, FL 32962, USA; bwalto@ufl.edu (B.W.A.); dshin@ufl.edu (D.S.)
[2] Interdisciplinary Center for Biotechnology Research, University of Florida, 2033 Mowry Road, Gainesville, FL 32611, USA; fyu@ufl.edu
* Correspondence: lmzhao@ufl.edu; Tel.: +1-772-778-7200

Received: 11 July 2018; Accepted: 26 August 2018; Published: 1 September 2018

Abstract: *Aedes aegypti* (L.) is the primary vector of many emerging arboviruses. Insecticide resistance among mosquito populations is a consequence of the application of insecticides for mosquito control. We used RNA-sequencing to compare transcriptomes between permethrin resistant and susceptible strains of Florida *Ae. aegypti* in response to Zika virus infection. A total of 2459 transcripts were expressed at significantly different levels between resistant and susceptible *Ae. aegypti*. Gene ontology analysis placed these genes into seven categories of biological processes. The 863 transcripts were expressed at significantly different levels between the two mosquito strains (up/down regulated) more than 2-fold. Quantitative real-time PCR analysis was used to validate the Zika-infection response. Our results suggested a highly overexpressed P450, with AAEL014617 and AAEL006798 as potential candidates for the molecular mechanism of permethrin resistance in *Ae. aegypti*. Our findings indicated that most detoxification enzymes and immune system enzymes altered their gene expression between the two strains of *Ae. aegypti* in response to Zika virus infection. Understanding the interactions of arboviruses with resistant mosquito vectors at the molecular level allows for the possible development of new approaches in mitigating arbovirus transmission. This information sheds light on Zika-induced changes in insecticide resistant *Ae. aegypti* with implications for mosquito control strategies.

Keywords: *Aedes aegypti*; RNA-seq; insecticide resistance; Zika virus; detoxification and immune system responses

---

1. Introduction

Aedes aegypti (L.) is the primary vector of emergent mosquito-borne viruses, including yellow fever, dengue, chikungunya, and Zika [1,2]. Zika fever is an emerging viral disease (family Flaviviridae, genus *Flavivirus*) that is transmitted to humans by infected female mosquitoes, primarily *Ae. aegypti* and *Ae. albopictus*. Zika virus (ZIKV) consists of three lineages, one from Asia and two from Africa [3]. Molecular analyses indicate that ZIKV originated in Uganda and spread to Central and West Africa through two introductions occurring in 1935 and 1940 [3]. Zika spread eastward to Asia around 1945 [3]. The Asian lineage of ZIKV was responsible for the first epidemic on Yap Island, Micronesia in 2007 followed by another outbreak in French Polynesia during 2013 [4]. Zika was detected in northeastern Brazil in early 2015 resulting in 1.5 million human cases [5,6]. Since the arrival of Zika in Brazil, the mosquito-borne pathogen has spread throughout the Americas and local transmission in the U.S. is a major public health risk among parts of the Gulf Coast. Symptoms associated with Zika infection are only observed in 20% of cases, and symptoms are often mild including fever, rash, joint pain, conjunctivitis, headache, and muscle pain. However, ZIKV is strongly associated with more severe outcomes including birth defects, such as microcephaly [7], and neurological complications, such as Guillain–Barré syndrome [8].

Recurrent use of insecticides in mosquito control and agricultural pest control has selected for insecticide resistance in mosquito populations [9–15]. Permethrin resistance is widespread in *Ae. aegypti* which compromises mosquito control and disease prevention efforts [11,13]. There are several modes that mosquito populations have become resistant to insecticides in nature. Insecticide resistance mechanisms can be divided into penetration resistance, behavioral resistance, target-site insensitivity, and metabolic detoxification of insecticides [16,17]. Penetration resistance occurs when insects absorb an insecticide more slowly than susceptible insects attributable to cuticle barriers. Behavioral resistance occurs when insects recognize and alter their behavior (feeding and movement) in the presence of an insecticide. Target-site insensitivity results from modifications (e.g., point mutations in genes encoding target proteins) to sites where the insecticide binds to reduce the detrimental effects of an insecticide. Metabolic detoxification of insecticides results when resistant insects detoxify or destroy insecticides more effectively than susceptible insects. Metabolic detoxification of insecticides is one of the most common mechanisms of resistance. Detoxification of insecticides in mosquitoes include three major gene families: Cytochrome P450s, esterases, and glutathion S-transferases (GSTs) [18,19].

Pyrethroid/permethrin resistant mosquitoes exhibit insecticide resistance through elevated levels of multiple detoxification enzymes, including GSTs [14,20–22], ATP-binding cassette (ABC) transporters [21,23], carboxylesterase [14,24,25], and cytochrome P450 [14,26–33]. Penetration resistance occurs through modifications in cuticular proteins [14,34]; metabolic resistance occurs by detoxification enzymes and G-protein-coupled receptor [26], UDP glucuronosyltransferase, and glucosyl/glucuronosyl transferase [32,35]; and target site insensitivity is mediated by changes in the voltage-gated sodium channel gene [11,15,36,37], and transcription factor Maf-S [38].

Multigene expression in response to arbovirus infection has been reported in *Ae. aegypti* and other species of mosquitoes [39–43]. Many genes are involved in the mosquito's antiviral immunity, such as antimicrobial peptide (AMP)-coding genes [44]. Immune responses and several arthropod immunity pathways such as Toll, Imd, JAK/STAT, and RNAi also play important roles during mosquito arboviral infection [39,41,42,45]. In addition to antiviral responses, several studies have reported changes in expression levels of multiple categories of biological processes in response to ingestion of arbovirus infected blood. An infection study showed that trypsins, metalloproteinases, and serine-type endopeptidases were significantly upregulated in mosquitoes following ingestion of chikungunya virus infected blood [39]. Along the same lines, another study reported that dengue virus infection induced upregulation of gene expression associated with lipogenesis, lipolysis and fatty acid β-oxidation, and lipid metabolism [46].

The unprecedented global spread of ZIKV has created a need to improve our understanding of host–microbe interactions in this mosquito–arbovirus system [43,45,47,48]. Understanding the mechanism(s) of insecticide resistance may provide insight into novel molecular strategies that may be used to improve control of Zika vector. To understand mechanisms by which pyrethroid/permethrin resistant *Ae. aegypti* populations alter their gene expression in response to ZIKV infection, we used RNA-sequencing (RNA-seq) and functional analysis to explore the difference between a permethrin resistant *Ae. aegypti* population (Key West, FL, USA) and a permethrin susceptible population (Orlando, FL, USA). Zika infection activated metabolic pathways (e.g., drug metabolism) in which some transcripts were putatively linked to insecticide resistance. Our observations provide a global picture of gene expression associated with metabolic detoxification among permethrin resistant and susceptible populations of *Ae. aegypti*, including antiviral responses following ingestion of ZIKV. This study aims to improve our understanding of the entomological components of ZIKV epidemiology in context of insecticide-based control through a combination of traditional genetic and biochemical approaches to address issues related to mosquito vector control.

2. Materials and Methods

2.1. Mosquito Strains

Ae. aegypti larvae were collected from Key West (24.55° N, 81.78° W), Florida, USA and maintained at the Florida Medical Entomological Laboratory (FMEL) in Vero Beach, FL since 2011. The parental collection of *Ae. aegypti* from the field was initially tested for permethrin resistance, then subjected to permethrin selection for 15 generations (see below) and again assayed for resistance (referred to as the resistant strain). Assays for resistance followed WHO protocols for mortality thresholds using the permethrin CDC bottle bioassay with a diagnostic dose and mortality rate (>90%) in laboratory bioassays using modified WHO bottle bioassay (WHO 2016). Bottles used in the assays were coated with a known amount of permethrin (diagnostic dose, 47 µg/bottle), after which adult *Ae. aegypti* mosquitoes were placed in the bottle and observed for 2 h and mortality was recorded.

The Orlando strain of *Ae. aegypti* was collected from Orlando (28.53° N, 81.37° W), Florida, USA and reared in the Mosquito and Fly Research Unit, Center for Medical, Agricultural and Veterinary Entomology, ARS-USDA in Gainesville, FL since 1952. The Orlando strain is recognized as a permethrin susceptible strain of *Ae. aegypti* [9].

2.2. Zika Virus Infection

Four-day-old female adults were fed defibrinated bovine blood containing either ZIKV (treatment) or blood lacking virus (control). The method utilized in this study was as previously described by Zhao et al. [48]. Mosquitoes were deprived of sucrose, but not water, 24 h before blood feeding trials performed in a biosafety level-3 laboratory at the FMEL. Isolates of the Asian lineage of ZIKV (strain PRVABC59, GenBank accession # KU501215.1) from Puerto Rico were prepared in African green monkey (Vero) cells and used in the mosquito infection study. Monolayers of Vero cells were inoculated with 500 µL of diluted stock virus (multiplicity of infection, 0.1) and incubated for 1 h at 37 °C and 5% CO_2 atmosphere, after which 24 mL media (M199 medium supplemented with 10% fetal bovine serum, penicillin/streptomycin, and mycostatin) were added to each tissue culture flask and incubated for six days for propagation of ZIKV. Freshly harvested media from infected cell cultures were combined with defibrinated bovine blood and ATP (0.005 M) and presented to mosquitoes using a membrane feeding system (Hemotek, Lancashire, UK) for one hour feeding trials. Control blood meals were prepared similarly except that monolayers of Vero cells were inoculated with media only. Samples of infected blood were collected at the time of the feedings and stored at −80 °C for later determination of virus titer. Mosquitoes were fed 6.4 log10 plaque forming units (pfu)/mL of ZIKV (Table 1). The experiments were replicated three times. The ZIKV infected and control mosquitoes from two *Ae. aegypti* strains were harvested for a time course study. Individual mosquitoes were dissected into body and legs and tested to confirm susceptibility to infection and disseminated infection rates, respectively. Ten mosquitoes (12 h and 7 days post ZIKV infection) were pooled for each sample for RNA sequencing.

Table 1. Transcription profiles of detoxification enzymes associated with permethrin resistance. (A) Genes related to detoxification significant upregulated in the Zika infection in the permethrin resistant (KW) strain compared with susceptible (OR) strain *Aedes aegypti* 7-days post infection. (B) Detoxification related gene significant upregulated/downregulated in the Control in the permethrin resistant (KW) strain compared with the susceptible (OR) strain *Aedes aegypti* 7-days post injection.

Gene ID	logFC	p-adj	Gene Description	Gene Name	Publications
			A		
AAEL012457	2.2934	3.09×10^{-10}	alcohol dehydrogenase		Faucon et al., 2015 [32]
AAEL009044	2.5174	4.04×10^{-11}	amine oxidase		Faucon et al., 2015 [32]
AAEL002385	2.0902	2.33×10^{-3}	Carboxy/choline esterase	CCEAE3B	Dusfour, 2015 [49]

Table 1. *Cont.*

Gene ID	logFC	p-adj	Gene Description	Gene Name	Publications
			A		
AAEL001960	2.1283	7.7×10^{-7}	cytochrome P450	CYP6M9	Faucon et al., 2015 [32]
AAEL002031	1.837	1.37×10^{-19}	cytochrome P450	CYP12F7	Faucon et al., 2015 [32]
AAEL006798	2.8656	8.05×10^{-3}	cytochrome P450	CYPJ10	Faucon et al., 2017 [31]
AAEL006805	2.6907	6.0×10^{-18}	cytochrome P450	CYP9J2	Faucon et al., 2015 [32]
AAEL006815	2.4201	6.0×10^{-17}	cytochrome P450	CYP9J16	Faucon et al., [31,32]
AAEL007473	2.1909	5.5×10^{-15}	cytochrome P450	CYP6AH1	Faucon et al., 2015 [32]
AAEL009018	2.5349	4.5×10^{-8}	cytochrome P450	CYP6CB1	Faucon et al., 2015 [32]
AAEL009123	2.4747	7.8×10^{-9}	cytochrome P450	CYP6Z6	Faucon et al., 2017 [31]
AAEL009125	2.6551	7.0×10^{-13}	cytochrome P450	CYP6M10	Faucon et al., 2017 [31]
AAEL009129	2.4377	2.6×10^{-34}	cytochrome P450	CYP6Z9	Faucon et al., 2017 [31]
AAEL014603	2.4789	2.24×10^{-3}	cytochrome P450	CYP9J30	Faucon et al., [31,32]
AAEL014607	2.1961	4.6×10^{-4}	cytochrome P450	CYP9J?	Faucon et al., 2015 [32]
AAEL014608	1.9517	8.2×10^{-3}	cytochrome P450	CYP9J?	Faucon et al., 2017 [31]
AAEL014609	2.4159	1.1×10^{-12}	cytochrome P450	CYP9J26	Faucon et al., [31,32]
AAEL014614	3.9363	4.1×10^{-8}	cytochrome P450	CYP9J?	Faucon et al., 2015 [32]
AAEL014617	2.3975	5.7×10^{-4}	cytochrome P450	CYP9J28	Faucon et al., 2015 [32]
AAEL014893	2.2053	2.1×10^{-8}	cytochrome P450	CYP6BB2	Faucon et al., 2015 [32]
AAEL015663	4.0198	9.0×10^{-6}	cytochrome P450	CYP25?	Faucon et al., 2015 [32]
AAEL017297	3.2113	1.7×10^{-6}	cytochrome P450	CYP6M9	Faucon et al., [31,32]
AAEL003099	3.0651	1.4×10^{-4}	glucosyl/glucuronosyl transferases		Faucon et al., 2015 [32]
			B		
AAEL001312	2.0651	2.5×10^{-4}	cytochrome P450	CYP9M6	Faucon et al., 2017 [31]
AAEL006798	3.6029	5.1×10^{-4}	cytochrome P450	CYP9J10	Faucon et al., 2015 [32]
AAEL006811	2.5971	2.37×10^{-3}	cytochrome P450	CYP9J8	Faucon et al., [31,32]
AAEL014606	1.9372	1.49×10^{-6}	cytochrome P450	CYPJ7	Faucon et al., 2015 [32]
AAEL014617	2.2615	3.35×10^{-3}	cytochrome P450	CYPJ28	Faucon et al., 2015 [32]
AAEL014891	−2.8122	3.8×10^{-4}	cytochrome P450	CYP6P12	Faucon et al., 2017 [31]
AAEL007947	2.5390	8.31×10^{-32}	glutathione transferase	GSTE	Faucon et al., 2017 [31]

2.3. RNA Extraction

All samples (10 mosquitoes per pool) were homogenized with a plastic pestle in the 1 mL TRIzol reagent (Ambion, Life Technologies, Carlsbad, CA, USA). Total RNAs were isolated using TRIzol reagent according to the manufacturer's instruction and followed a standard protocol (Ambion, Life Technologies). To avoid genomic DNA contamination, the RNA samples were processed by DNase I (RNase-free) following the manufacturer's instructions (Thermo Scientific, Wilmington, DE, USA). The RNA samples were quantitated by NANODROP 2000 Spectrophotometer (Thermo Scientific, Wilmington, DE, USA).

2.4. RNA-Seq Library Preparation and Sequencing

Preparation and sequencing libraries were carried out in the Interdisciplinary Center for Biotechnology Research (ICBR), at the University of Florida following the manufacturer's protocol (Illumina, Inc., San Diego, CA, USA). The TruSeq DNA Library Preparation Kit (Illumina, Inc., San Diego, CA, USA) was used to prepare DNA libraries with insert sizes from 300–500 bp for high-throughput sequencing. For the Illumina NextSeq 500 run, the NCS v1.2 control software was used. The libraries were pooled at equimolar concentrations to yield a 4 nM stock solution, containing 0.33 nM of each library. The library pool was prepared for sequencing following the manufacturer protocol. The Illumina® NextSeq® 500 sequencing platform was used to create paired-end reads using Illumina's sequencing-by-synthesis approach (Illumina®, San Diego, CA, USA) using 2 × 150 cycles.

2.5. Data Mining and RNA-Seq Analysis

Reads acquired from the sequencing platform were cleaned up with the Cutadapt program (Martin 2011) to trim off sequencing adaptors, low quality bases, and potential errors introduced during sequencing or library preparation. Reads with a quality phred-like score <20 and read length <40 bases were excluded from RNA-seq analysis.

The transcripts of *Ae. aegypti* (18,840 sequences) were retrieved from the VectorBase (https://www.vectorbase.org/organisms/aedes-aegypti/liverpool) and used as reference sequences for

RNA-seq analysis. The cleaned reads of each sample were mapped independently to the reference sequences using the bowtie2 mapper (version. 2.2.3) with a "3 mismatches a read" allowance [50]. The mapping results were processed with the samtools and scripts developed in house at ICBR to remove potential PCR duplicates and to choose uniquely mapped reads for gene expression analysis. Gene expression was assessed by counting the number of mapped reads for each transcript [51]. Significant up- and downregulated genes were selected using the adjusted *p*-value (p-adj), log2 fold-change (log2FC), or both for the analysis. The RNA-seq data have been deposited to NCBI (Accession number: GSE118858, https://www.ncbi.nlm.nih.gov/gds/?term=GSE118858).

2.6. Assignments of Gene Ontology (GO) Terms and Pathway Analyses

All genes with p-adj ≤ 0.01 were selected for the GO enrichment analysis (http://amigo. geneontology.org/amigo). The GO terms of *Ae. aegypti* genes were retrieved from the VectorBase and assigned to GO hierarchies and functional groups. The genes matched to the functional categories of immune system process (GO:0002376), response to stimulus (GO:0050896), developmental process (GO:0032502), cellular process (GO:0009987), signal transducer activity (GO:0004871), biological regulation (GO:0065007), electron carrier activity (GO:0009055), transporter activity (GO:0005215), catalytic activity (GO:0003824), and metabolic process (GO:0008152) were divided into two pools: the downregulated and upregulated gene pools based on the log2 transformed-fold-change of the RNA-seq results. The selected genes that were not assigned GO terms or categorized to other functional groups were treated as the unknown group.

2.7. C-DNA Synthesized and qPCR Amplification

C-DNA synthesis was performed using methods described by Zhao 2017 et al. [48]. The qPCR assay for confirming genes in *Ae. aegypti* was performed using Platinum® SYBR® Green qPCR SuperMix-UDG with ROX (Invitrogen, Carlsbad, CA, USA) in a volume of 15 µL on a BIO-RAD C1000 Touch Thermal Cycler, CFX 96™ Real-Time System ("Bio-Rad"). The primers were designed using Primer3 program https://sourceforge.net/projects/primer3 (Table S1).

3. Results

3.1. Global Changes in Transcriptome of the Aedes Aegypti Female Adult in Response to ZIKV Infection

To understand the molecular interactions of the arbovirus with permethrin resistant *Ae. aegypti* from Florida, RNA-seq was conducted to explore the global changes in the *Ae. aegypti* (Key West and Orlando strains) transcriptome in response to oral ingestion of ZIKV infected blood and ZIKV infection. In this study, four-day-old female *Ae. aegypti* adults were fed a blood meal containing 6.4 log10 pfu/mL of ZIKV (Figure 1). Fresh fed mosquitoes ingested 4.2 to 4.3 log10 pfu/mL of ZIKV. By 7 days post infection (dpi), ZIKV titer in mosquito bodies were 4.1 ± 1.7 log10 pfu/mL and 3.6 ± 1.2 log10 pfu/mL for the permethrin resistant and susceptible strains of *Ae. aegypti*, respectively. A two-tailed *t*-test showed no significant differences in ZIKV titer in the bodies of the two strains of *Ae. aegypti* (t17 = 0.77, *p* = 0.44). By 10 dpi, ZIKV titer in permethrin resistant strain mosquito bodies were 6.5 ± 0.05 log10 pfu/mL, which was 100-fold higher (t4 = 8.12, *p* = 0.001) than the titer of the susceptible strain (4.5 ± 0.34 log10 pfu/mL). This result demonstrated that the ZIKV replication rates were higher at this point in the infection process for the permethrin resistant strain than the susceptible strain.

Twelve hours post infection and 7 dpi, RNAs from female *Ae. aegypti* were extracted. A total of 24 RNA-seq libraries were created from *Ae. aegypti* infected by ZIKV (12 h and 7 dpi) and control (fed uninfected blood, 12 h and 7 dpi). Three replicates of each group were prepared and sequenced. A total of 706,051,842 raw reads were generated from the permethrin resistant and susceptible strains. The cleanup resulted in 705,983,440 cleaned reads, which mapped to 18,840 transcripts of *Ae. aegypti* (Table

S2). The qPCR of the selected 13 genes showed significantly different expression levels between the two *Ae. aegypti* strains in response to ZIKV at 7 dpi, supporting the RNA seq data analysis (Figure 2).

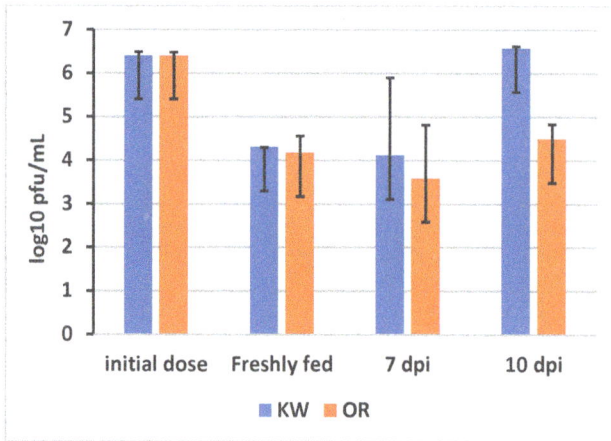

Figure 1. Zika virus titers in infectious blood meals and blood fed mosquitoes for permethrin resistant (KW) and susceptible (OR) strains of *Aedes aegypti*, including initial dose in bloodmeal, freshly fed, 7 days post infection (7 dpi), and 10 days post infection (10 dpi). Zika virus (strain PRVABC59, GenBank accession # KU501215.1) isolated from a human infected in Puerto Rico in 2015.

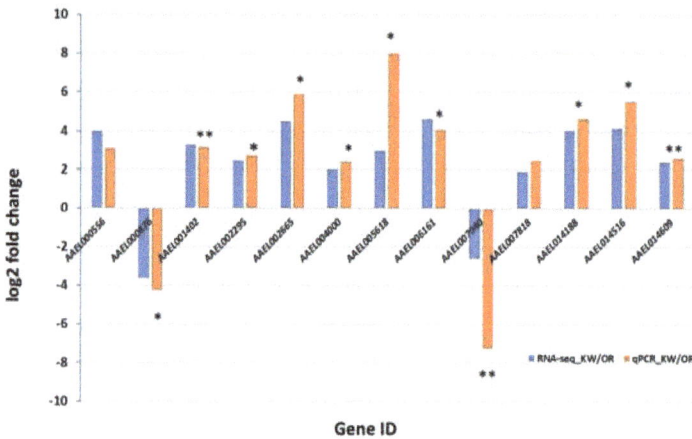

Figure 2. Validation of the expression of transcripts between the permethrin resistant (KW) and susceptible (OR) strains of *Aedes aegypti* by qRT-PCR. * $p < 0.05$. ** $p < 0.01$.

3.1.1. Expression Profiles of Differentially Expressed (DE) Transcripts in Response to Blood Feeding (Control) between Two *Aedes aegypti* Strains, Resistant Versus Susceptible Strains

Functional analysis based on Gene Ontology were conducted on the significant differentially expressed (DE) transcripts between the permethrin resistant and susceptible strains of *Ae. aegypti*. Comparison of the transcriptome profiles showed a relatively low number of DE transcripts 12 h after blood-feeding. There were 90 DE transcripts at 12 h post blood-feeding (p-adj $\leq$ 0.01), of which 35 were upregulated and 55 were downregulated (Figure 3A and Figure S1A). The largest proportion of total number of DE genes (38.9%) had unknown functions (Figure 3A and Figure S1A). Other DE transcripts mainly belonged to the functional categories of Binding (23.3%), Catalytic activity (14.4%), Cellular process (12.2%), Response to stimulus (5.6%), and Transporter activity (4.4%). All other categories were less than 1%. After 7-days post blood-feeding, 631 DE genes were significantly different, (p-adj $\leq$ 0.01; 291 upregulated and 340 downregulated) (Figure 3E and Figure S1E). Of those 631 transcripts, 36.8% of those genes were assigned to an unknown function (Figure 3E and Figure S1E). Other DE genes were mainly placed in functional categories of Binding (20.0%), Catalytic activity (13.9%), Cellular process (14.1%), Response to stimulus (7.9%), and Transporter activity (4.8%).

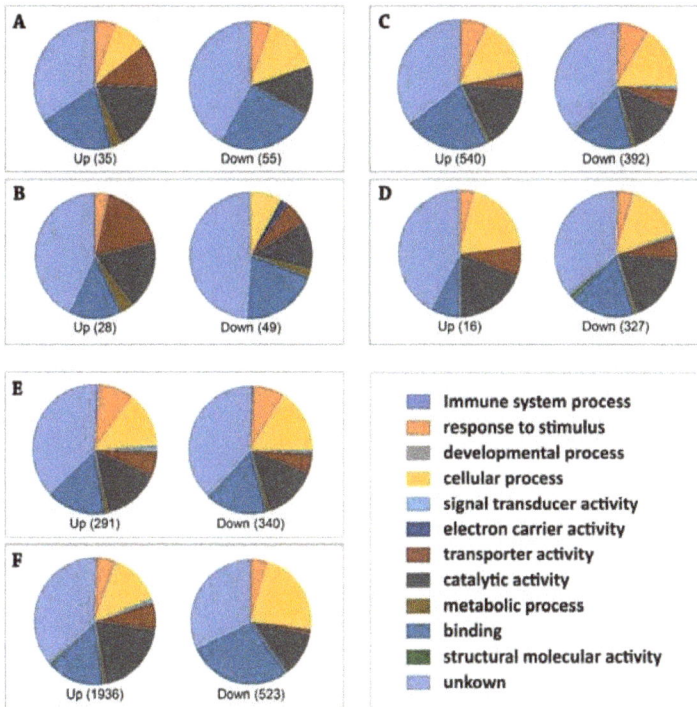

Figure 3. Overview of the functional categories of differentially expressed (DE) transcripts in response to ZIKV infection and between the permethrin resistant (KW) and susceptible (OR) strains of *Aedes aegypti* blood-feeding control. DE transcripts were determined based on statistical analysis by DESeq package. The total number of DE transcripts for each comparison is shown in parentheses in each figure. Gene ontology analysis of DE genes was performed based on the database of AmiGO 2 (http://amigo.geneontology.org/amigo), and pie charts were generated using Excel. Up, upregulated DE genes; Down, downregulated DE genes. Please also notice the details in the Supplementary Figure S1. GO analyses for RNA-seq data. (**A**) 12 h post injection KW-Control compared with OR-Control; (**B**) 12 h post infection, KW-ZIKV compared with OR-ZIKV; (**C**) 7 dpi, KW-ZIKV compared with KW-Control; (**D**) 7 dpi, OR-ZIKV compared with OR-Control; (**E**) 7 dpi, KW-Control compared with OR-Control; (**F**) 7 dpi, KW-ZIKV compared with OR-ZIKV.

3.1.2. Expression Profiles of DE Transcripts in *Aedes Aegypti*, Resistant and Susceptible Strains, in Response to ZIKV

Analysis of mRNA expression profiles of *Ae. aegypti* mosquitoes at different time points of ZIKV infection revealed a relatively low number of DE transcripts 12-h after blood-feeding. Only five DE transcripts were identified in the susceptible strain and none in the resistant strain. However, there were 932 DE genes (p-adj $\leq$ 0.01; 540 upregulated and 392 downregulated) in the resistant strain of *Ae. aegypti* at 7 dpi with ZIKV (Figure 3C and Figure S1C). Most of these transcripts (36.2% in the total: 35.0% in the Up; 37.8% in the Down) had unknown functions. The remaining of the DE transcripts matched to the functional categories of Binding (19.5% in the total: 22.0% in the Up; 16.1% in the Down), Catalytic activity (15.0% in the total: 15.7% in the Up; 14.1% in the Down), Cellular process (14.95 in the total: 14.3% in the Up; 15.8% in the Down), Response to stimulus (7.5% in the total: 7.0% in the Up; 8.2% in the Down), and Transporter activity (4.4% in the total: 4.1% in the Up; 4.8% in the Down). All other categories were lower than 1%. About 57.9% of 932 DE transcripts were upregulated in the *Ae. aegypti* resistant strain in response to the ZIKV infection at 7 dpi.

Functional analysis based on the significant DE transcripts between the ZIKV exposed susceptible strain and control susceptible at 7 dpi showed that most of the transcripts were downregulated (p-adj $\leq$ 0.01; 26 upregulated and 327 downregulated) (Figure 3D and Figure S1D). Approximately 36.8% of the DE transcripts (42.3% in the Up; 36.4% in the Down) had unknown functions. The other DE transcripts were categorized into the functional groups of Binding (16.4% in the total: 7.7% in the Up; 16.5% in the Down), Catalytic activity (18.1% in the total: 19.2% in the Up; 18.0% in the Down), Cellular process (15.3% in the total: 19.2% in the Up; 15.0% in the Down), Response to stimulus (4.2% in the total: 3.8% in the Up; 4.3% in the Down), and Transporter activity (5.6% in the total: 7.7% in the Up; 5.5% in the Down). All other categories were lower than 1%. Most of the DE transcripts (92.6% of 353 transcripts) were downregulated in the susceptible strain in response to the ZIKV infection at 7 dpi.

3.1.3. Expression Profiles of DE Transcripts in Response to ZIKV Infection between Two Strains *Aedes Aegypti*, Resistant Versus Susceptible Strains

Analysis and comparison of mRNA expression profiles of *Ae. aegypti* at different strains following ZIKV infection revealed that ZIKV induced a relatively low number of DE transcripts 12 h after blood-feeding. We observed 77 DE transcripts (p-adj $\leq$ 0.01), of which 28 were upregulated and 49 were downregulated (Figure 3B and Figure S1B) at 12 h post infection. Among those DE transcripts, 46.8% in total (42.9% in the UP; 49% in the Down) had unknown functions. The other DE transcripts mainly belonged to the functional categories of Binding (18.2% in the total: 14.3% in the Up; 20.4% in the Down), Catalytic activity (14.2% in the total: 17.9% in the Up; 12.2% in the Down), Cellular process (5.2% in the total: 0% in the Up; 8.2% in the Down), and Transporter activity (10.4% in the total: 17.9% in the Up; 6.1% in the Down). All other categories were lower than 1%. Most of the DE genes (63.6%) were downregulated in the *Ae. aegypti* resistant strain compared to the susceptible strain at the 12 h post infection.

Comparison of the transcriptome profiles of two *Ae. aegypti* strains in response to ZIKV 7 dpi revealed 2459 DE transcripts (p-adj $\leq$ 0.01; 1936 upregulated and 523 downregulated, Figure 3F and Figure S1F). Most of those DE transcripts (35.5% in the total) had unknown functions (Figure 3F and Figure S1F). Of the DE transcripts that were up regulated in the resistant strain, 36.6% had unknown functions; while 31.7% of the downregulated DE transcripts were of unknown function. The remaining DE transcripts matched the functional categories of Catalytic activity (18.2% in the total: 19.8% in the Up; 12.0% in the Down), Cellular process (15.0% in the total: 13.7% in the Up; 22.0% in the Down), Response to stimulus (5.0% in the total: 5.1% in the Up; 4.5% in the Down), and Transporter activity (5.5% in the total: 6.6% in the Up; 1.3% in the Down). All other categories were lower than 1%. Most of the DE transcripts (78.7%) were upregulated in the *Ae. aegypti* resistant strain compared to the susceptible strain at the 7 dpi. The data showed global changes in the two strains of *Ae. aegypti* female adult transcriptome in response to ZIKV infection.

3.1.4. DE Transcripts Related to Immunity in Response to ZIKV Infection

When *Ae. aegypti* were infected with ZIKV at 7 dpi, a total of 863 transcripts had 2-fold or more changes (p-adj $\leq$ 0.01; log2 fold change > $\pm$2.0). Seventy-one immunity-related DE transcripts were significantly upregulated in response to ZIKV 7 dpi between the two strains. These results suggest that ingestion of ZIKV can induce an immune response in the permethrin resistant Key West strain (Table S3A). These upregulated immunity related genes encoded two allergens, one caspase-1, eleven Clip-domain serine protease family B and D, four C-type lectins, two C-type lysozymes, one cysteine-rich protein, one cysteine-rich venom protein (AAEL005098, 5.77 log2 fold change), one environmental stress-induced protein, five fibrinogen and fibronectins, two Gram-negative binding proteins (GNBP), one granzyme A precursor, one lachesin, thirteen leucine-rich immune proteins, one M protein, one neuroendocrine protein, one p37NB protein, one peptidoglycan recognition protein (AAEL012380), one prophenoloxidase (AAEL011763), one rh antigen, SEC14, SEC15, SEC16, one thioester-containing protein (tep2), one toll protein and four Toll-like receptors, eight trypsins, and three venom allergens (Table S3A).

Compared with the control group, more immune related enzymes at 7 dpi infected with ZIKV were detected and most of them were upregulated significantly (Table S3A,B). The comparison between *Ae. aegypti* infected with ZIKV and the control at the 7-dpi in the resistant strain revealed that 318 transcripts had changes of 2-fold or more in either direction. Fifteen DE transcripts related to immunity were significantly dysregulated more than 2-fold (seven upregulated and eight downregulated, Table S3C). These transcripts encoded two Class C Scavenger Receptors, two Clip-domain serine proteases family B, two C-type lectins, one cysteine-rich venom protein (AAEL005098, 2.71 log2 fold change), one Gram-negative binding protein, one lachesin, three leucine-rich transmembrane proteins, a shoc2, one venom allergen, and one Wnt10a protein (Table S3C). In the Orlando strains infected with ZIKV at 7 dpi, a total 128 transcripts had changes of 2-fold or more, but only one was upregulated. All 14 DE transcripts related to immunity between ZIKV infected and the control group at 7 dpi were significantly downregulated (Table S3D). These transcripts encoded six Clip-domain serine proteases family B, one C-type lectin, five leucine-rich immune proteins, one Trypsin 3A1 precursor, and one tyrosine kinase receptor (Table S3D). Both the *Ae. aegypti* resistant and susceptible strains infected with ZIKV at the 7 dpi shown regulated with Clip-domain serine protease family B, C-type lectin, and some leucine-rich proteins.

Some important immunity transcripts were significantly upregulated (more than 4-fold) in the permethrin resistant than the susceptible strains, such as prophenoloxidase and M protein. The prophenoloxidase (AAEL011763) is a modified form of the complement response found in insects, and a major innate defense system in invertebrates that controls the melanization of pathogens and damaged tissues [52]. M protein (AAEL011747), a strongly antiphagocytic and a major virulence factor in viruses, parasites, and bacteria aids in entering by counteracting the mosquito's defenses [53,54]. In addition, two lachesins, a novel immunoglobulin superfamily protein required for morphogenesis of the Drosophila tracheal system, were also significantly upregulated [55]. The peptidoglycan recognition protein (AAEL012380), an important role in the innate immune response, was correspondingly upregulated significantly in the Key West strain [56].

3.1.5. DE Transcripts Related to Detoxification in Response to ZIKV Infection

The RNAseq study between two *Ae. aegypti* strains infected with ZIKV at 7 dpi showed that 62 DE transcripts related to detoxifications were upregulated more than 2-fold in response to ZIKV. These transcripts encoded one alcohol dehydrogenase, two aldehyde oxidases, one aldo-keto reductase, two Carboxy/choline esterases, one core 1 UDP-galactose galactosyltransferase, 33 cytochrome P450, one d-amino acid oxidase, one epoxide hydrolase, seven glucosyl/glucuronosyl transferases, one glutamate semialdehyde dehydrogenase, three n-acetylgalactosaminyltransferases, one prophenoloxidase, four short-chain dehydrogenases, one sterol desaturase, and one thioredoxin peroxidase (Table S4A).

Four cytochrome P450 (AAEL009018, AAEL014609, AAEL014617, and AAEL014893) were reported as associated with insecticide resistance in several populations of *Ae. aegypti* [31,32,57]. Compared with the control, between the Key West strain and the Orlando strain at 7 dpi infected with

ZIKV, more detoxification enzymes were detected and most of them were upregulated significantly more than 2-fold (Table S4A,B), suggesting those genes might associate with insecticide resistance.

Comparing the Key West *Ae. aegypti* infected with ZIKV with the Key West control at the 7 dpi, 19 DE transcripts related to detoxification were significantly regulated (11 upregulated and eight downregulated, Table S4C). Nevertheless, all 14 DE transcripts related to detoxification were significantly downregulated between the Orlando *Ae. aegypti* infected with ZIKV and the Orlando control at the 7 dpi (Table S4D).

According to previous studies [31,32,57], 23 transcriptions of detoxification enzymes associated with permethrin resistance were significantly upregulated at 7 dpi between the Key West strain and the Orlando strain in response to ZIKV infection (Table 1A). They encoded an alcohol dehydrogenase (AAEL012457), an amine oxidase (AAEL009044), Carboxy/choline esterase (AAEL002385), 19 Cytochrome P450, and a glucosyl/glucuronosyl transferase (AAEL003099). In the control at 7 dpi, we observed six cytochromes and a glutathione transferase (AAEL007964) that were significantly expressed between the Key West and Orlando Controls fed uninfected blood (Table 1B). Nineteen Cytochrome P450 included, CYP6CB1 (AAEL009018), CYP9M10 (AAEL009125), and P450s of the CYP9J subfamily such as CYP9J10 (AAEL006798) and CYP9J28 (AAEL014617), from which several members were shown to contribute to deltamethrin metabolism [31,32,58,59]. The glucosyl/glucuronosyl transferases (AAEL003099) were reported as differentially expressed in pyrethroid resistant populations relative to the susceptible strain [32,59].

3.1.6. DE Transcripts Likely Related to Permethrin resistance in Response to ZIKV Infection

Except detoxification enzymes, many other enzymes related to insecticide resistance have been reported. We analyzed the DE transcripts possible related to permethrin resistance in response to ZIKV infection. Most of the fifty-five DE transcripts likely related to permethrin resistance were upregulated in response to ZIKV 7 dpi in the Key West strain compared with the Orlando strain, but only one zinc finger protein (AAEL002388) was downregulated (Table S5A). These transcripts encoded one acetylcholine receptor, two adenylate cyclases, four alkaline phosphatases, one ATP-binding cassette transporter, three ATP-dependent bile acid permeases, two brain chitinase and chias, two bumetanide-sensitive Na-K-Cl cotransport proteins, two cgmp-dependent protein kinases, one glutamate decarboxylase, three glutamate receptors, one glutamate transporter, one glutamate-gated chloride channel, five GPCR related genes, two guanine nucleotide-binding proteins, two matrix metalloproteinases, one metalloproteinase, two prolylcarboxypeptidases, eight protease m1 zinc metalloproteases, two voltage-gated potassium channels, five zinc carboxypeptidases, four zinc finger proteins, and one zinc metalloprotease (Table S5A).

Nineteen DE transcripts likely related to permethrin resistance, except some detoxification enzymes, were regulated (14 upregulated and five downregulated) in response blood feeding control in the Key West strain compared with the Orlando strain (Table S5B). The voltage-gated sodium channel (AAEL006019) was only upregulated 1.4-fold, which may play an important role in the Key West *Ae. aegypti* strain. Between Key West *Ae. aegypti* infected with ZIKV and the Key West control at the 7 dpi, 14 DE transcripts possibly related to permethrin resistance were significantly regulated (six upregulated and eight downregulated) in response to ZIKV infection (Table S5C). Nonetheless, all 16 DE transcripts related to detoxification were significantly downregulated between the Orlando *Ae. aegypti* infected with ZIKV and the Orlando control at the 7 dpi (Table S5D).

3.1.7. DE Transcripts Related to Cytoskeleton in Response to ZIKV Infection

A cytoskeleton with multitude of functions is present in all cells of all domains of life, including archaea, bacteria, and eukaryotes. The cytoskeleton assists the cell move in its environment and controls the movement of the cell's interior workings. Our RNAseq study of two strains of *Ae. aegypti* following ZIKV infection at 7 dpi revealed that all 56 DE transcripts related to the cytoskeleton were upregulated in response to ZIKV 7 dpi in the Key West strain compared with the Orlando strain

(Table S6A). These genes encoded four actin, one ca-activated cl channel protein, one cadherin, one calcium-binding protein, two calcium-transporting ATPases, one calmin, two calponin/transgelins, one calsyntenin-1 precursor, one coronin, one dynein heavy chain, one flagellar radial spoke protein, one gelsolin precursor, one gliotactin, three innexins, one integrin alpha-ps, one jnk interacting protein, one laminin, one leucokinins precursor, one mitogen activated protein kinase, one muscle lim protein, one myo inositol monophosphatase, one myoinositol oxygenase, nine myosins, one myosin regulatory light chain, one nuclear lamin L1 alpha, one nucleosome assembly protein, one otopetrin, one paramyosin, one pyrokinin, one talin, one testisin precursor, one titin protein, one tropomyosin invertebrate, five troponins, one unconventional myosin 95e isoform, and one vesamicol binding protein (Table S6A).

According to RNA-seq analysis, 21 cytoskeletons related to DE transcripts were significantly regulated (12 upregulated and nine downregulated) in response to blood feeding control in the Key West strain compared with the Orlando strain (Table S6B). Nineteen DE cytoskeleton transcripts were regulated (nine upregulated and 10 downregulated) in the ZIKV infected group of the Key West strain at the 7 dpi (Table S6C). However, all six DE transcripts related to the cytoskeleton were significantly downregulated in the ZIKV infected group of the Orlando strain at the 7 dpi (Table S6D).

We found that most genes were downregulated in the *Ae. aegypti* Orlando susceptible strain at 7 dpi following ZIKV infection. In contract, most genes were upregulated in the *Ae. aegypti* Key West permethrin resistant strain (Tables S3–S6). Compared with the *Ae. aegypti* Orlando susceptible strain at 7 dpi following ZIKV infection, *Ae. aegypti* Key West permethrin resistant strain showed a global upregulation of endogenous genes, many of which encode proteins specifically involved in immunity, detoxification, pesticide resistance, and cytoskeleton movement related genes.

4. Discussion

Arbovirus–mosquito interactions alter global gene expression in *Ae. aegypti* and other mosquitoes [39,40,43,48,60,61]. Although Zika infection had been reported to change transcript levels in *Ae. aegypti* [43], the mechanism(s) of insecticide resistance in *Ae. aegypti*-ZIKV remains unknown. Since insecticide-resistance monitoring is the key to controlling arboviruses, we need to improve our understanding of mosquito–virus interactions in both resistant and susceptible strains to facilitate surveillance and monitoring of Zika vector populations under control.

Many reports have been shown that the upregulated genes contained multiple detoxification genes and several immune-related genes in insecticide resistant mosquitoes, including *Ae. aegypti*, *Anopheles gambiae*, *An. sinesis*, *An. stephensi*, and *Culex quinquefasciatus* [23,31,33,62–65]. To the best of our knowledge, this is one of the first documentations showing an association between insecticide resistance and altered mosquito–arbovirus interactions. However, we are unable to rule out the possibility that inherent genetic differences between the two strains of *Ae. aegypti*, in part, contribute to differences in ZIKV infection. Although the mechanism(s) responsible for altered interactions between mosquitoes and pathogens is not fully understood, changes in oxidative stress and vector immunity have been proposed as potential sources [66]. Our observed results are consistent with Alout et al. 2013 [67] showing higher *Plasmodium falciparum* prevalence at both the oocyst and sporozoite stages, in *Anopheles gambiae* s.s. resistant to pyrethroids and DDT than in a susceptible strain. In contrast, insecticide-resistant (organophosphate) *Culex quinquefasciatus* mosquitoes were less capable of transmitting the filarial parasite *Wuchereria bancrofti* than insecticide-susceptible conspecifics, mediated by disrupted development of the parasite [68,69]. It is likely that the biological processes in response to mosquito infection of arboviruses differs from that of parasites such as filarial worms and *Plasmodium*. Regardless, taken together, these observations suggest a connection between insecticide resistance and altered physiology that translates to changes in interactions between mosquitoes and the disease agents they transmit.

To obtain a global view of changes in gene expression between *Ae. aegypti* Key West permethrin resistant strain and *Ae. aegypti* Orlando susceptible strains, we analyzed RNA-seq data and identified at least 23 detoxification enzymes linked to insecticide resistance that were significantly upregulated in response to ZIKV infection [31,32]. Our current study showed that the *Ae. aegypti* Key West permethrin resistant strain and the *Ae. aegypti* Orlando susceptible strain differentially altered their gene expression in response to ZIKV infection.

To survive in a world full of pathogens, insects have developed a powerful defense mechanism that recognizes and removes microbial threats [70]. Insects depend on innate immunity for their survival. The immune system accommodates host colonization by the virus, maintains virus–host homeostasis and defends against pathogens. Viral infections are detected by innate antiviral responses [71]. Pathogen receptors in the innate immune system play a role in the detection of viral nucleic acids in different ways [71]. Toll-like receptors detected viral DNA or RNA in endosomal compartments in immune cells [45,72], while retinoic acid inducible gene-I-like receptors recognized viral RNA in the cytoplasm and DNA sensors detected cytoplasmic viral DNA [71]. The Toll pathways have previously been shown to suppress arbovirus infection in *Ae. aegypti* midgut tissue [45]. Peptidoglycan recognition proteins, conserved from insects to mammals, are pattern recognition molecules that recognize microbes and their unique cell wall component, peptidoglycan [73]. Our transcriptomic study revealed that five Toll-like receptors and three peptidoglycan recognition proteins were significantly upregulated in the Key West permethrin resistant strain *Ae. aegypti* at 7 dpi following ZIKV infection compared with the Orlando susceptible *Ae. aegypti* (Table S3A,B). Clip-domain serine proteases are the essential components of extracellular signaling cascades in various biological processes and function in developmental processes and innate immune responses [74,75]. Twelve Clip-domain serine proteases were upregulated between the Key West permethrin resistant and the Orlando susceptible strains of *Ae. aegypti*. CLIP proteases are found in insect hemolymph and participate in cascade pathways that activate prophenoloxidase in the melanization response and synthesis of antimicrobial peptides [74], including immune signaling in *Ae. aegypti* [76,77].

Other immune related enzymes, such as cecropin antimicrobial peptide, Class B scavenger receptor, defensin antimicrobial peptide, fibrinogen and fibronectin, and leucine-rich immune proteins were also upregulated between the Key West permethrin resistant strain *Ae. aegypti* and the Orlando susceptible *Ae. aegypti*. Cysteine-rich venom proteins, found in the fluids of animal venoms, inhibit both smooth muscle contraction and cyclic nucleotide-gated ion channels [78]. Previous studies displayed that cysteine-rich venom proteins were changed in yellow fever and ZIKV-infected mosquitoes and silencing the gene led to an increase in replication of dengue viruses, which indicated their possible importance in replication of these viruses [43,79]. The current study showed that cysteine-rich venom proteins (AAEL005098) were upregulated 2.71 log2 fold change in the Key West strain ZIKV compared with Key West control, and upregulated 5.77 log2 fold change when compared with the Orlando strain *Ae. aegypti* in response to ZIKV. Further studies may need to demonstrate the role of cysteine-rich venom proteins play in response to Zika infection. These data indicated the permethrin resistant Key West *Ae. aegypti* mosquitoes altered immune system in response to ZIKV infection, differently from the susceptible Orlando *Ae. aegypti* strain.

The activation of multiple signaling pathways following virus infection, the detoxification genes implicated in the establishment of the antiviral state, and the strategies used by viruses and their specific viral products to antagonize and evade the host antiviral response. Recent studies have utilized [31] deep targeted DNA sequencing for identification of increases in gene copy number in the genome associated with pyrethroid resistance in populations of *Ae. aegypti* and subsequently identified novel genomic resistance markers potentially associated with their cis-regulation and modifications of their protein structure confirmation [31,32]. The current RNA-seq study also confirmed 23 over expression of detoxification enzymes associated with insecticide resistance in Key West *Ae. aegypti* in response to ZIKV 7 dpi compared with Orlando *Ae. aegypti* susceptible strain. CYP6CB1-like AAEL009018, considerably favor the binding of an HNF-3 element and overexpression of this gene in resistant populations has frequently been associated with the regulation of drug-metabolizing P450s [31,49]. CYP9M10, AAEL009125, was not only demonstrated in the *Ae. aegypti* mosquito but also reported in the resistant strain of *Culex quinquefasciatus* [31,80,81]. The current study also confirmed that detoxification enzymes, such as carboxy/choline esterase and glucosyl/glucuronosyl transferases, were associated with resistance mosquitoes in response to ZIKV infection [31,32,82,83]. The mechanisms for regulation of detoxification enzymes in response to ZIKV and their relevance to insecticide resistance are unclear. It has been proposed that regulation in some metabolic detoxification genes may result from responses to various endogenous and exogenous compounds, or to pathophysiological signals [33,63,64,84,85].

The actin and microtubule cytoskeleton play important roles in the life cycle of viruses. Viruses succeed as intracellular parasites and interact with the actin cytoskeleton at various stages of the host cell throughout their life cycles to facilitate the infection process [86,87]. Many animal viruses interact with cytoskeleton elements inside infected cells at different stages of replication and cytoskeleton involvement in virus budding [88]. The microfilament signal pathway is involved in DENV infection through regulation of actin reorganization in EAhy926 cells [89]. Viral interaction with the host microtubule (MT) cytoskeleton is critical to infection by many viruses, with modifying MT dynamics and functions that affect processes beyond virion transport [90]. Myosin protein enforced track selection on the microtubule and actin networks in vitro, depending on the active transport of diverse intracellular cargo on the ubiquitous actin and microtubule networks [91]. Some studies showed that the manipulation of host actin cytoskeleton is essential for viral pathogens to invade the host cells [92]. Our current data show that 56 DE transcripts related to cytoskeleton, including four actin and 10 myosin proteins, were significantly upregulated in the Zika infected Key West strain compared with the Orlando strain *Ae. aegypti* 7-day post infection. The overexpression of actin cytoskeleton genes in the permethrin resistance strain of *Ae. aegypti* might be associated with higher viral loads later during the infection process, although the precise functional importance of these interactions and their roles in pathogenesis remain largely unresolved.

Our observations provide an overview of gene expression associated with metabolic detoxification among permethrin resistant and susceptible populations of *Ae. aegypti*, including antiviral responses following ingestion of ZIKV. Our understanding of host–virus interactions in mosquito systems combining traditional genetic and biochemical approaches with "omics" based approaches in both laboratory and natural environmental studies is key to improving the surveillance and monitoring of Zika vector populations under control. One of the limitations of this approach is that it falls short of providing an in-depth analysis of any one specific mechanism, or collection of mechanisms. Rather, our broad approach is aimed at providing a global view to identify candidate genes and functional categories for subsequent studies using other methods (e.g., reverse genetics) that target candidate genes for elucidating molecular mechanisms of insecticide resistance and the development of novel molecular mechanisms to circumvent resistance.

Supplementary Materials: The following are available online at http://www.mdpi.com/1999-4915/10/9/470/s1, Figure S1: GO analyses for RNA-seq data. Table S1: Primers for validation of the expression of transcripts between two strains of *Aedes aegypti*. Table S2. Summary of RNA-seq analysis based on the *Aedes aegypti* transcriptomes. Tables S3–S6: Related gene significant upregulated/downregulated.

Author Contributions: Conceptualization, L.Z., B.W.A., and D.S.; Methodology, L.Z., B.W.A., D.S., and F.Y.; Software, F.Y. and L.Z.; Validation, L.Z., B.W.A., D.S., and F.Y.; Formal Analysis, L.Z., B.W.A., D.S., and F.Y.; Investigation, L.Z., B.W.A., D.S., and F.Y.; Resources, L.Z., B.W.A., and D.S.; Data Curation, F.Y. and L.Z.; Writing-Original Draft Preparation, L.Z.; Writing-Review & Editing, L.Z., B.W.A., D.S., and F.Y.; Visualization, L.Z., B.W.A., D.S., and F.Y.; Supervision, L.Z.; Project Administration, L.Z.; Funding Acquisition, L.Z. and B.W.A.

Funding: This research was funded by the Florida Department of Agriculture and Consumer Services: Contract Numbers 024246 and 023557 to Jorge Rey and Contract Number 020180 to Walter Tabachnick, Contract Numbers 021803 and 022399 to Liming Zhao and Barry Alto.

Acknowledgments: We thank Melissa Williams, Bradley Eastmond, Ayse Civana, and Keenan Wiggins of the Florida Medical Entomology Laboratory, University of Florida for their excellent technical support. We would also like to thank Walter Tabachnick and Jorge Rey for their support. The isolate of Zika virus was graciously provided by the Centers for Disease Control and Prevention. We thank Mosquito and Fly Research Unit, Center for Medical, Agricultural, and Veterinary Entomology, ARS-USDA for providing us with *Ae. aegypti* from Orlando, FL.

Conflicts of Interest: All authors declare no conflict of interest.

References

1. Mousson, L.; Dauga, C.; Garrigues, T.; Schaffner, F.; Vazeille, M.; Failloux, A.B. Phylogeography of *Aedes (Stegomyia) aegypti* (L.) and *Aedes (Stegomyia) albopictus* (Skuse) (Diptera: Culicidae) based on mitochondrial DNA variations. *Genet. Res.* **2005**, *86*, 1–11. [CrossRef] [PubMed]
2. Goindin, D.; Delannay, C.; Ramdini, C.; Gustave, J.; Fouque, F. Parity and longevity of *Aedes aegypti* according to temperatures in controlled conditions and consequences on dengue transmission risks. *PLoS ONE* **2015**, *10*, e0135489. [CrossRef] [PubMed]
3. Faye, O.; Freire, C.C.; Iamarino, A.; de Oliveira, J.V.; Diallo, M.; Zanotto, P.M.; Sall, A.A. Molecular evolution of Zika virus during its emergence in the 20(th) century. *PLoS Negl. Trop. Dis.* **2014**, *8*, e2636. [CrossRef] [PubMed]
4. Cao-Lormeau, V.M.; Roche, C.; Teissier, A.; Robin, E.; Berry, A.L.; Mallet, H.P.; Sall, A.A.; Musso, D. Zika virus, French polynesia, South pacific, 2013. *Emerg. Infect. Dis.* **2014**, *20*, 1085–1086. [CrossRef] [PubMed]
5. Campos, G.S.; Bandeira, A.C.; Sardi, S.I. Zika Virus Outbreak, Bahia, Brazil. *Emerg. Infect. Dis.* **2015**, *21*, 1885–1886. [CrossRef] [PubMed]
6. Sacramento, C.Q.; de Melo, G.R.; de Freitas, C.S.; Rocha, N.; Hoelz, L.V.; Miranda, M.; Fintelman-Rodrigues, N.; Marttorelli, A.; Ferreira, A.C.; Barbosa-Lima, G.; et al. The clinically approved antiviral drug sofosbuvir inhibits Zika virus replication. *Sci. Rep.* **2017**, *7*, 40920. [CrossRef] [PubMed]
7. Cuevas, E.L.; Tong, V.T.; Rozo, N.; Valencia, D.; Pacheco, O.; Gilboa, S.M.; Mercado, M.; Renquist, C.M.; González, M.; Ailes, E.C.; et al. Preliminary Report of Microcephaly Potentially Associated with Zika Virus Infection During Pregnancy—Colombia, January–November 2016. *MMWR Morb. Mortal. Wkly. Rep.* **2016**, *65*, 1409–1413. [CrossRef] [PubMed]
8. Pinto-Díaz, C.A.; Rodríguez, Y.; Monsalve, D.M.; Acosta-Ampudia, Y.; Molano-González, N.; Anaya, J.M.; Ramírez-Santana, C. Autoimmunity in Guillain-Barré syndrome associated with Zika virus infection and beyond. *Autoimmun. Rev.* **2017**, *16*, 327–334. [CrossRef] [PubMed]
9. Estep, A.S.; Sanscrainte, N.D.; Waits, C.M.; Louton, J.E.; Becnel, J.J. Resistance Status and Resistance Mechanisms in a Strain of *Aedes aegypti* (Diptera: Culicidae) From Puerto Rico. *J. Med. Entomol.* **2017**, *54*, 1643–1648. [CrossRef] [PubMed]
10. Antonio-Nkondjio, C.; Sonhafouo-Chiana, N.; Ngadjeu, C.S.; Doumbe-Belisse, P.; Talipouo, A.; Djamouko-Djonkam, L.; Kopya, E.; Bamou, R.; Awono-Ambene, P.; Wondji, C.S. Review of the evolution of insecticide resistance in main malaria vectors in Cameroon from 1990 to 2017. *Parasit. Vectors* **2017**, *10*, 472. [CrossRef] [PubMed]
11. Ponce-García, G.; Del Río-Galvan, S.; Barrera, R.; Saavedra-Rodriguez, K.; Villanueva-Segura, K.; Felix, G.; Amador, M.; Flores, A.E. Knockdown Resistance Mutations in *Aedes aegypti* (Diptera: Culicidae) From Puerto Rico. *J. Med. Entomol.* **2016**, *53*, 1410–1414. [CrossRef] [PubMed]
12. Wu, Z.M.; Chu, H.L.; Wang, G.; Zhu, X.J.; Guo, X.X.; Zhang, Y.M.; Xing, D.; Yan, T.; Zhao, M.H.; Dong, Y.D.; et al. Multiple-Insecticide Resistance and Classic Gene Mutations to Japanese Encephalitis Vector *Culex tritaeniorhynchus* from China. *J. Am. Mosq. Control Assoc.* **2016**, *32*, 144–151. [CrossRef] [PubMed]
13. Francis, S.; Saavedra-Rodriguez, K.; Perera, R.; Paine, M.; Black, W.C.; Delgoda, R. Insecticide resistance to permethrin and malathion and associated mechanisms in *Aedes aegypti* mosquitoes from St. Andrew Jamaica. *PLoS ONE* **2017**, *12*, e0179673.
14. Seixas, G.; Grigoraki, L.; Weetman, D.; Vicente, J.L.; Silva, A.C.; Pinto, J.; Vontas, J.; Sousa, C.A. Insecticide resistance is mediated by multiple mechanisms in recently introduced *Aedes aegypti* from Madeira Island (Portugal). *PLoS Negl. Trop. Dis.* **2017**, *11*, e0005799. [CrossRef] [PubMed]
15. Aguirre-Obando, O.A.; Martins, A.J.; Navarro-Silva, M.A. First report of the Phe1534Cys kdr mutation in natural populations of *Aedes albopictus* from Brazil. *Parasit. Vectors* **2017**, *10*, 160. [CrossRef] [PubMed]
16. Liu, N. Insecticide resistance in mosquitoes: Impact, mechanisms, and research directions. *Annu. Rev. Entomol.* **2015**, *60*, 537–559. [CrossRef] [PubMed]
17. Dang, K.; Doggett, S.L.; Veera Singham, G.; Lee, C.Y. Insecticide resistance and resistance mechanisms in bed bugs, *Cimex* spp. (Hemiptera: Cimicidae). *Parasit. Vectors* **2017**, *10*, 318. [CrossRef] [PubMed]
18. Liu, H.; Cupp, E.W.; Guo, A.; Liu, N. Insecticide resistance in Alabama and Florida mosquito strains of *Aedes albopictus*. *J. Med. Entomol.* **2004**, *41*, 946–952. [CrossRef] [PubMed]

19. Hemingway, J.; Hawkes, N.J.; McCarroll, L.; Ranson, H. The molecular basis of insecticide resistance in mosquitoes. *Insect. Biochem. Mol. Biol.* **2004**, *34*, 653–665. [CrossRef] [PubMed]

20. Alemayehu, E.; Asale, A.; Eba, K.; Getahun, K.; Tushune, K.; Bryon, A.; Morou, E.; Vontas, J.; van Leeuwen, T.; Duchateau, L.; et al. Mapping insecticide resistance and characterization of resistance mechanisms in *Anopheles arabiensis* (Diptera: Culicidae) in Ethiopia. *Parasit. Vectors* **2017**, *10*, 407. [CrossRef] [PubMed]

21. Pignatelli, P.; Ingham, V.A.; Balabanidou, V.; Vontas, J.; Lycett, G.; Ranson, H. The *Anopheles gambiae* ATP-binding cassette transporter family: Phylogenetic analysis and tissue localization provide clues on function and role in insecticide resistance. *Insect. Mol. Biol.* **2017**, *27*, 110–122. [CrossRef] [PubMed]

22. Zhong, D.; Chang, X.; Zhou, G.; He, Z.; Fu, F.; Yan, Z.; Zhu, G.; Xu, T.; Bonizzoni, M.; Wang, M.H.; et al. Relationship between knockdown resistance, metabolic detoxification and organismal resistance to pyrethroids in *Anopheles sinensis*. *PLoS ONE* **2013**, *8*, e55475. [CrossRef] [PubMed]

23. Mastrantonio, V.; Ferrari, M.; Epis, S.; Negri, A.; Scuccimarra, G.; Montagna, M.; Favia, G.; Porretta, D.; Urbanelli, S.; Bandi, C. Gene expression modulation of ABC transporter genes in response to permethrin in adults of the mosquito malaria vector *Anopheles stephensi*. *Acta Trop.* **2017**, *171*, 37–43. [CrossRef] [PubMed]

24. Grigoraki, L.; Pipini, D.; Labbé, P.; Chaskopoulou, A.; Weill, M.; Vontas, J. Carboxylesterase gene amplifications associated with insecticide resistance in *Aedes albopictus*: Geographical distribution and evolutionary origin. *PLoS Negl. Trop. Dis.* **2017**, *11*, e0005533. [CrossRef] [PubMed]

25. Grigoraki, L.; Lagnel, J.; Kioulos, I.; Kampouraki, A.; Morou, E.; Labbé, P.; Weill, M.; Vontas, J. Transcriptome Profiling and Genetic Study Reveal Amplified Carboxylesterase Genes Implicated in Temephos Resistance, in the Asian Tiger Mosquito *Aedes albopictus*. *PLoS Negl. Trop. Dis.* **2015**, *9*, e0003771. [CrossRef] [PubMed]

26. Li, T.; Liu, N. Regulation of P450-mediated permethrin resistance in *Culex quinquefasciatus* by the GPCR/Gαs/AC/cAMP/PKA signaling cascade. *Biochem. Biophys. Rep.* **2017**, *12*, 12–19. [CrossRef] [PubMed]

27. Guo, Q.; Huang, Y.; Zou, F.; Liu, B.; Tian, M.; Ye, W.; Guo, J.; Sun, X.; Zhou, D.; Sun, Y.; et al. The role of miR-2∼13∼71 cluster in resistance to deltamethrin in *Culex pipiens pallens*. *Insect. Biochem. Mol. Biol.* **2017**, *84*, 15–22. [CrossRef] [PubMed]

28. Al Nazawi, A.M.; Aqili, J.; Alzahrani, M.; McCall, P.J.; Weetman, D. Combined target site (kdr) mutations play a primary role in highly pyrethroid resistant phenotypes of *Aedes aegypti* from Saudi Arabia. *Parasit. Vectors* **2017**, *10*, 161. [CrossRef] [PubMed]

29. Gong, Y.; Li, T.; Feng, Y.; Liu, N. The function of two P450s, CYP9M10 and CYP6AA7, in the permethrin resistance of *Culex quinquefasciatus*. *Sci. Rep.* **2017**, *7*, 587. [CrossRef] [PubMed]

30. Chang, K.S.; Kim, H.C.; Klein, T.A.; Ju, Y.R. Insecticide resistance and cytochrome-P450 activation in unfed and blood-fed laboratory and field populations of *Culex pipiens pallens*. *J. Pest. Sci.* **2017**, *90*, 759–771. [CrossRef] [PubMed]

31. Faucon, F.; Gaude, T.; Dusfour, I.; Navratil, V.; Corbel, V.; Juntarajumnong, W.; Girod, R.; Poupardin, R.; Boyer, F.; Reynaud, S.; et al. In the hunt for genomic markers of metabolic resistance to pyrethroids in the mosquito *Aedes aegypti*: An integrated next-generation sequencing approach. *PLoS Negl. Trop. Dis.* **2017**, *11*, e0005526. [CrossRef] [PubMed]

32. Faucon, F.; Dusfour, I.; Gaude, T.; Navratil, V.; Boyer, F.; Chandre, F.; Sirisopa, P.; Thanispong, K.; Juntarajumnong, W.; Poupardin, R.; et al. Identifying genomic changes associated with insecticide resistance in the dengue mosquito *Aedes aegypti* by deep targeted sequencing. *Genome. Res.* **2015**, *25*, 1347–1359. [CrossRef] [PubMed]

33. Reid, W.R.; Zhang, L.; Gong, Y.; Li, T.; Liu, N. Gene expression profiles of the Southern house mosquito *Culex quinquefasciatus* during exposure to permethrin. *Insect Sci.* **2018**, *25*, 439–453. [CrossRef] [PubMed]

34. Sun, X.; Guo, J.; Ye, W.; Guo, Q.; Huang, Y.; Ma, L.; Zhou, D.; Shen, B.; Sun, Y.; Zhu, C. Cuticle genes CpCPR63 and CpCPR47 may confer resistance to deltamethrin in *Culex pipiens pallens*. *Parasitol. Res.* **2017**, *116*, 2175–2179. [CrossRef] [PubMed]

35. Ishak, I.H.; Riveron, J.M.; Ibrahim, S.S.; Stott, R.; Longbottom, J.; Irving, H.; Wondji, C.S. The Cytochrome P450 gene CYP6P12 confers pyrethroid resistance in kdr-free Malaysian populations of the dengue vector *Aedes albopictus*. *Sci. Rep.* **2016**, *6*, 24707. [CrossRef] [PubMed]

36. Smith, L.B.; Kasai, S.; Scott, J.G. Voltage-sensitive sodium channel mutations S989P + V1016G in *Aedes aegypti* confer variable resistance to pyrethroids, DDT and oxadiazines. *Pest. Manag. Sci.* **2017**, *74*, 737–745. [CrossRef] [PubMed]

37. Hamid, P.H.; Prastowo, J.; Widyasari, A.; Taubert, A.; Hermosilla, C. Knockdown resistance (kdr) of the voltage-gated sodium channel gene of *Aedes aegypti* population in Denpasar, Bali, Indonesia. *Parasit. Vectors* **2017**, *10*, 283. [CrossRef] [PubMed]

38. Ingham, V.A.; Pignatelli, P.; Moore, J.D.; Wagstaff, S.; Ranson, H. The transcription factor Maf-S regulates metabolic resistance to insecticides in the malaria vector *Anopheles gambiae*. *BMC Genom.* **2017**, *18*, 669. [CrossRef] [PubMed]

39. Dong, S.; Behura, S.K.; Franz, A.W.E. The midgut transcriptome of *Aedes aegypti* fed with saline or protein meals containing chikungunya virus reveals genes potentially involved in viral midgut escape. *BMC Genom.* **2017**, *18*, 382. [CrossRef] [PubMed]

40. Shin, D.; Civana, A.; Acevedo, C.; Smartt, C.T. Transcriptomics of differential vector competence: West Nile virus infection in two populations of *Culex pipiens quinquefasciatus* linked to ovary development. *BMC Genom.* **2014**, *15*, 513. [CrossRef] [PubMed]

41. Shrinet, J.; Srivastava, P.; Sunil, S. Transcriptome analysis of *Aedes aegypti* in response to mono-infections and co-infections of dengue virus-2 and chikungunya virus. *Biochem. Biophys. Res. Commun.* **2017**, *492*, 617–623. [CrossRef] [PubMed]

42. Shrinet, J.; Jain, S.; Jain, J.; Bhatnagar, R.K.; Sunil, S. Next generation sequencing reveals regulation of distinct *Aedes* microRNAs during chikungunya virus development. *PLoS Negl. Trop. Dis.* **2014**, *8*, e2616. [CrossRef] [PubMed]

43. Etebari, K.; Hegde, S.; Saldaña, M.A.; Widen, S.G.; Wood, T.G.; Asgari, S.; Hughes, G.L. Global Transcriptome Analysis of *Aedes aegypti* Mosquitoes in Response to Zika Virus Infection. *mSphere* **2017**, *2*, e00456-17. [CrossRef] [PubMed]

44. Wang, H.; Smagghe, G.; Meeus, I. The role of a single gene encoding the Single von Willebrand factor C-domain protein (SVC) in bumblebee immunity extends beyond antiviral defense. *Insect Biochem. Mol. Biol.* **2017**, *91*, 10–20. [CrossRef] [PubMed]

45. Angleró-Rodríguez, Y.I.; MacLeod, H.J.; Kang, S.; Carlson, J.S.; Jupatanakul, N.; Dimopoulos, G. Molecular Responses to Zika Virus: Modulation of Infection by the Toll and Jak/Stat Immune Pathways and Virus Host Factors. *Front. Microbiol.* **2017**, *8*, 2050. [CrossRef] [PubMed]

46. Tongluan, N.; Ramphan, S.; Wintachai, P.; Jaresitthikunchai, J.; Khongwichit, S.; Wikan, N.; Rajakam, S.; Yoksan, S.; Wongsiriroj, N.; Roytrakul, S.; et al. Involvement of fatty acid synthase in dengue virus infection. *Virol. J.* **2017**, *14*, 28. [CrossRef] [PubMed]

47. Saldaña, M.A.; Etebari, K.; Hart, C.E.; Widen, S.G.; Wood, T.G.; Thangamani, S.; Asgari, S.; Hughes, G.L. Zika virus alters the microRNA expression profile and elicits an RNAi response in *Aedes aegypti* mosquitoes. *PLoS Negl. Trop. Dis.* **2017**, *11*, e0005760. [CrossRef] [PubMed]

48. Zhao, L.; Alto, B.W.; Smartt, C.T.; Shin, D. Transcription Profiling for Defensins of *Aedes aegypti* (Diptera: Culicidae) During Development and in Response to Infection With Chikungunya and Zika Viruses. *J. Med. Entomol.* **2017**, *55*, 78–89.

49. Dusfour, I.; Zorrilla, P.; Guidez, A.; Issaly, J.; Girod, R.; Guillaumot, L.; Robello, C.; Strode, C. Deltamethrin Resistance Mechanisms in *Aedes aegypti* Populations from Three French Overseas Territories Worldwide. *PLoS Negl. Trop. Dis.* **2015**, *9*, e0004226. [CrossRef] [PubMed]

50. Langmead, B.; Salzberg, S.L. Fast gapped-read alignment with Bowtie 2. *Nat. Methods* **2012**, *9*, 357–359. [CrossRef] [PubMed]

51. Yao, J.Q.; Yu, F. DEB: A web interface for RNA-seq digital gene expression analysis. *Bioinformation* **2011**, *7*, 44–45. [CrossRef] [PubMed]

52. Cerenius, L.; Söderhäll, K. The prophenoloxidase-activating system in invertebrates. *Immunol. Rev.* **2004**, *198*, 116–126. [CrossRef] [PubMed]

53. Fischetti, V.A. Streptococcal M protein: Molecular design and biological behavior. *Clin. Microbiol. Rev.* **1989**, *2*, 285–314. [CrossRef] [PubMed]

54. Glinton, K.; Beck, J.; Liang, Z.; Qiu, C.; Lee, S.W.; Ploplis, V.A.; Castellino, F.J. Variable region in streptococcal M-proteins provides stable binding with host fibrinogen for plasminogen-mediated bacterial invasion. *J. Biol. Chem.* **2017**, *292*, 6775–6785. [CrossRef] [PubMed]

55. Llimargas, M.; Strigini, M.; Katidou, M.; Karagogeos, D.; Casanova, J. Lachesin is a component of a septate junction-based mechanism that controls tube size and epithelial integrity in the *Drosophila* tracheal system. *Development* **2004**, *131*, 181–190. [CrossRef] [PubMed]

56. Ghosh, A.; Lee, S.; Dziarski, R.; Chakravarti, S. A novel antimicrobial peptidoglycan recognition protein in the cornea. *Invest. Ophthalmol. Vis. Sci.* **2009**, *50*, 4185–4191. [CrossRef] [PubMed]

57. Moyes, C.L.; Vontas, J.; Martins, A.J.; Ng, L.C.; Koou, S.Y.; Dusfour, I.; Raghavendra, K.; Pinto, J.; Corbel, V.; David, J.P.; et al. Contemporary status of insecticide resistance in the major *Aedes* vectors of arboviruses infecting humans. *PLoS Negl. Trop. Dis.* **2017**, *11*, e0005625. [CrossRef] [PubMed]

58. Stevenson, B.J.; Pignatelli, P.; Nikou, D.; Paine, M.J. Pinpointing P450s associated with pyrethroid metabolism in the dengue vector, *Aedes aegypti*: Developing new tools to combat insecticide resistance. *PLoS Negl. Trop. Dis.* **2012**, *6*, e1595. [CrossRef] [PubMed]

59. Bariami, V.; Jones, C.M.; Poupardin, R.; Vontas, J.; Ranson, H. Gene amplification, ABC transporters and cytochrome P450s: Unraveling the molecular basis of pyrethroid resistance in the dengue vector, *Aedes aegypti*. *PLoS Negl. Trop. Dis.* **2012**, *6*, e1692. [CrossRef] [PubMed]

60. Etebari, K.; Osei-Amo, S.; Blomberg, S.P.; Asgari, S. Dengue virus infection alters post-transcriptional modification of microRNAs in the mosquito vector *Aedes aegypti*. *Sci. Rep.* **2015**, *5*, 15968. [CrossRef] [PubMed]

61. Acharya, D.; Paul, A.M.; Anderson, J.F.; Huang, F.; Bai, F. Loss of Glycosaminoglycan Receptor Binding after Mosquito Cell Passage Reduces Chikungunya Virus Infectivity. *PLoS Negl. Trop. Dis.* **2015**, *9*, e0004139. [CrossRef] [PubMed]

62. Yan, Z.W.; He, Z.B.; Yan, Z.T.; Si, F.L.; Zhou, Y.; Chen, B. Genome-wide and expression-profiling analyses suggest the main cytochrome P450 genes related to pyrethroid resistance in the malaria vector, *Anopheles sinensis* (Diptera Culicidae). *Pest. Manag. Sci.* **2018**, *74*, 1810–1820. [CrossRef] [PubMed]

63. Bonizzoni, M.; Ochomo, E.; Dunn, W.A.; Britton, M.; Afrane, Y.; Zhou, G.; Hartsel, J.; Lee, M.C.; Xu, J.; Githeko, A.; et al. RNA-seq analyses of changes in the *Anopheles gambiae* transcriptome associated with resistance to pyrethroids in Kenya: Identification of candidate-resistance genes and candidate-resistance SNPs. *Parasit. Vectors* **2015**, *8*, 474. [CrossRef] [PubMed]

64. Lv, Y.; Wang, W.; Hong, S.; Lei, Z.; Fang, F.; Guo, Q.; Hu, S.; Tian, M.; Liu, B.; Zhang, D.; et al. Comparative transcriptome analyses of deltamethrin-susceptible and -resistant *Culex pipiens pallens* by RNA-seq. *Mol. Genet. Genom.* **2016**, *291*, 309–321. [CrossRef] [PubMed]

65. Bonizzoni, M.; Afrane, Y.; Dunn, W.A.; Atieli, F.K.; Zhou, G.; Zhong, D.; Li, J.; Githeko, A.; Yan, G. Comparative transcriptome analyses of deltamethrin-resistant and -susceptible *Anopheles gambiae* mosquitoes from Kenya by RNA-Seq. *PLoS ONE* **2012**, *7*, e44607. [CrossRef] [PubMed]

66. Rivero, A.; Vézilier, J.; Weill, M.; Read, A.F.; Gandon, S. Insecticide control of vector-borne diseases: When is insecticide resistance a problem? *PLoS Pathog.* **2010**, *6*, e1001000. [CrossRef] [PubMed]

67. Alout, H.; Ndam, N.T.; Sandeu, M.M.; Djégbe, I.; Chandre, F.; Dabiré, R.K.; Djogbénou, L.S.; Corbel, V.; Cohuet, A. Insecticide resistance alleles affect vector competence of *Anopheles gambiae* s.s. for *Plasmodium falciparum* field isolates. *PLoS ONE* **2013**, *8*, e63849. [CrossRef] [PubMed]

68. McCarroll, L.; Hemingway, J. Can insecticide resistance status affect parasite transmission in mosquitoes? *Insect. Biochem. Mol. Biol.* **2002**, *32*, 1345–1351. [CrossRef]

69. McCarroll, L.; Paton, M.G.; Karunaratne, S.H.; Jayasuryia, H.T.; Kalpage, K.S.; Hemingway, J. Insecticides and mosquito-borne disease. *Nature.* **2000**, *407*, 961–962. [CrossRef] [PubMed]

70. Mondotte, J.A.; Saleh, M.C. Antiviral Immune Response and the Route of Infection in *Drosophila melanogaster*. *Adv. Virus Res.* **2018**, *100*, 247–278. [PubMed]

71. Yoneyama, M.; Fujita, T. Recognition of viral nucleic acids in innate immunity. *Rev. Med. Virol.* **2010**, *20*, 4–22. [CrossRef] [PubMed]

72. Onomoto, K.; Yoneyama, M.; Fujita, T. Recognition of viral nucleic acids and regulation of type I. IFN expression. *Nihon Rinsho* **2006**, *64*, 1236–1243. [PubMed]

73. Dziarski, R. Peptidoglycan recognition proteins (PGRPs). *Mol. Immunol.* **2004**, *40*, 877–886. [CrossRef] [PubMed]

74. Kanost, M.R.; Jiang, H. Clip-domain serine proteases as immune factors in insect hemolymph. *Curr. Opin. Insect Sci.* **2015**, *11*, 47–55. [CrossRef] [PubMed]

75. Conway, M.J.; Watson, A.M.; Colpitts, T.M.; Dragovic, S.M.; Li, Z.; Wang, P.; Feitosa, F.; Shepherd, D.T.; Ryman, K.D.; Klimstra, W.B.; et al. Mosquito saliva serine protease enhances dissemination of dengue virus into the mammalian host. *J. Virol.* **2014**, *88*, 164–175. [CrossRef] [PubMed]

76. Shin, S.W.; Bian, G.; Raikhel, A.S. A toll receptor and a cytokine, Toll5A and Spz1C, are involved in toll antifungal immune signaling in the mosquito *Aedes aegypti*. *J. Biol. Chem.* **2006**, *281*, 39388–39395. [CrossRef] [PubMed]

77. Zou, Z.; Shin, S.W.; Alvarez, K.S.; Kokoza, V.; Raikhel, A.S. Distinct melanization pathways in the mosquito *Aedes aegypti*. *Immunity* **2010**, *32*, 41–53. [CrossRef] [PubMed]

78. Yamazaki, Y.; Morita, T. Structure and function of snake venom cysteine-rich secretory proteins. *Toxicon* **2004**, *44*, 227–231. [CrossRef] [PubMed]

79. Londono-Renteria, B.; Troupin, A.; Conway, M.J.; Vesely, D.; Ledizet, M.; Roundy, C.M.; Cloherty, E.; Jameson, S.; Vanlandingham, D.; Higgs, S.; et al. Dengue Virus Infection of *Aedes aegypti* Requires a Putative Cysteine Rich Venom Protein. *PLoS Pathog.* **2015**, *11*, e1005202. [CrossRef] [PubMed]

80. Itokawa, K.; Komagata, O.; Kasai, S.; Kawada, H.; Mwatele, C.; Dida, G.O.; Njenga, S.M.; Mwandawiro, C.; Tomita, T. Global spread and genetic variants of the two CYP9M10 haplotype forms associated with insecticide resistance in *Culex quinquefasciatus* Say. *Heredity (Edinb)* **2013**, *111*, 216–226. [CrossRef] [PubMed]

81. Itokawa, K.; Komagata, O.; Kasai, S.; Ogawa, K.; Tomita, T. Testing the causality between CYP9M10 and pyrethroid resistance using the TALEN and CRISPR/Cas9 technologies. *Sci. Rep.* **2016**, *6*, 24652. [CrossRef] [PubMed]

82. David, J.P.; Faucon, F.; Chandor-Proust, A.; Poupardin, R.; Riaz, M.A.; Bonin, A.; Navratil, V.; Reynaud, S. Comparative analysis of response to selection with three insecticides in the dengue mosquito *Aedes aegypti* using mRNA sequencing. *BMC Genom.* **2014**, *15*, 174. [CrossRef] [PubMed]

83. Riaz, M.A.; Chandor-Proust, A.; Dauphin-Villemant, C.; Poupardin, R.; Jones, C.M.; Strode, C.; Régent-Kloeckner, M.; David, J.P.; Reynaud, S. Molecular mechanisms associated with increased tolerance to the neonicotinoid insecticide imidacloprid in the dengue vector *Aedes aegypti*. *Aquat. Toxicol.* **2013**, *126*, 326–337. [CrossRef] [PubMed]

84. Yang, T.; Liu, N. Genome analysis of cytochrome P450s and their expression profiles in insecticide resistant mosquitoes, *Culex quinquefasciatus*. *PLoS ONE* **2011**, *6*, e29418. [CrossRef] [PubMed]

85. Zhu, G.; Zhong, D.; Cao, J.; Zhou, H.; Li, J.; Liu, Y.; Bai, L.; Xu, S.; Wang, M.H.; Zhou, G.; et al. Transcriptome profiling of pyrethroid resistant and susceptible mosquitoes in the malaria vector, *Anopheles sinensis*. *BMC Genom.* **2014**, *15*, 448. [CrossRef] [PubMed]

86. Cudmore, S.; Reckmann, I.; Way, M. Viral manipulations of the actin cytoskeleton. *Trends Microbiol.* **1997**, *5*, 142–148. [CrossRef]

87. Sanders, M.C.; Theriot, J.A. Tails from the hall of infection: Actin-based motility of pathogens. *Trends Microbiol.* **1996**, *4*, 211–213. [CrossRef]

88. Luftig, R.B.; Lupo, L.D. Viral interactions with the host-cell cytoskeleton: The role of retroviral proteases. *Trends Microbiol.* **1994**, *2*, 178–182. [CrossRef]

89. Zhang, J.; Wu, N.; Gao, N.; Yan, W.; Sheng, Z.; Fan, D.; An, J. Small G Rac1 is involved in replication cycle of dengue serotype 2 virus in EAhy926 cells via the regulation of actin cytoskeleton. *Sci. China Life Sci.* **2016**, *59*, 487–494. [CrossRef] [PubMed]

90. Brice, A.; Whelan, D.R.; Ito, N.; Shimizu, K.; Wiltzer-Bach, L.; Lo, C.Y.; Blondel, D.; Jans, D.A.; Bell, T.D.; Moseley, G.W. Quantitative Analysis of the Microtubule Interaction of Rabies Virus P3 Protein: Roles in Immune Evasion and Pathogenesis. *Sci. Rep.* **2016**, *6*, 33493. [CrossRef] [PubMed]

91. Oberhofer, A.; Spieler, P.; Rosenfeld, Y.; Stepp, W.L.; Cleetus, A.; Hume, A.N.; Mueller-Planitz, F.; Ökten, Z. Myosin Va's adaptor protein melanophilin enforces track selection on the microtubule and actin networks in vitro. *Proc. Natl. Acad. Sci. USA* **2017**, *114*, E4714–E4723. [CrossRef] [PubMed]

92. Yang, G.; Xiao, X.; Yin, D.; Zhang, X. The interaction between viral protein and host actin facilitates the virus infection to host. *Gene* **2012**, *507*, 139–145. [CrossRef] [PubMed]

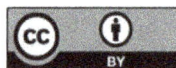

viruses

MDPI

Article

Integrated MicroRNA and mRNA Profiling in Zika Virus-Infected Neurons

Francine Azouz [1,†], Komal Arora [2,†], Keeton Krause [1], Vivek R. Nerurkar [1]
and Mukesh Kumar [2,*]

[1]   Department of Tropical Medicine, Medical Microbiology and Pharmacology, Pacific Center for Emerging
     Infectious Diseases Research, John A. Burns School of Medicine, University of Hawai'i at Mānoa, Honolulu,
     HI 96813, USA; azouzf@hawaii.edu (F.A.); krausek@hawaii.edu (K.K.); nerurkar@hawaii.edu (V.R.N.)
[2]   Department of Biology, College of Arts and Sciences, Georgia State University, Atlanta, GA 30303, USA;
     karora@gsu.edu
*   Correspondence: mkumar8@gsu.edu
†   These authors contributed equally to this work.

Received: 10 January 2019; Accepted: 14 February 2019; Published: 16 February 2019

Abstract: Zika virus (ZIKV) infections have caused a wide spectrum of neurological diseases, such as
Guillain-Barré syndrome, myelitis, meningoencephalitis, and congenital microcephaly. No effective
therapies currently exist for treating patients infected with ZIKV. MicroRNAs (miRNAs) are a
group of small RNAs involved in the regulation of a wide variety of cellular and physiological
processes. In this study, we analyzed digital miRNA and mRNA profiles in ZIKV-infected primary
mouse neurons using the nCounter technology. A total of 599 miRNAs and 770 mRNAs were
examined. We demonstrate that ZIKV infection causes global downregulation of miRNAs with
only few upregulated miRNAs. ZIKV-modulated miRNAs including miR-155, miR-203, miR-29a,
and miR-124-3p are known to play critical role in flavivirus infection, anti-viral immunity and brain
injury. ZIKV infection also results in downregulation of miRNA processing enzymes. In contrast,
ZIKV infection induces dramatic upregulation of anti-viral, inflammatory and apoptotic genes.
Furthermore, our data demonstrate an inverse correlation between ZIKV-modulated miRNAs and
target host mRNAs induced by ZIKV. Biofunctional analysis revealed that ZIKV-modulated miRNAs
and mRNAs regulate the pathways related to neurological development and neuroinflammatory
responses. Functional studies targeting specific miRNA are warranted to develop therapeutics for
the management of ZIKV neurological disease.

Keywords: Zika virus; flavivirus; microRNAs; neurons; neuroinflammation; anti-viral immunity

1. Introduction

Zika virus (ZIKV) is an emerging mosquito-borne pathogen that is part of the Spondweni
serocomplex of the genus Flavivirus, family *Flaviviridae*. ZIKV is closely related to other pathogens
of public health importance including yellow fever virus (YFV), dengue virus (DENV), Japanese
encephalitis virus (JEV), and West Nile virus (WNV). The ZIKV genome is comprised of a
single-stranded, positive-sense 11-kb RNA that contains three structural and seven nonstructural
genes [1,2]. ZIKV is highly neurotropic in human fetal infections and has been linked to
the development of severe fetal abnormalities that include spontaneous abortion, stillbirth,
hydranencephaly, microcephaly, and placental insufficiency that may cause intrauterine growth
restriction [1]. An increased incidence of Guillain-Barré syndrome (GBS), neuropathy of the peripheral
nervous system, has also been reported in ZIKV-infected patients [3]. No effective therapies currently
exist for treating patients infected with ZIKV.

ZIKV has been shown to replicate and induce cell death in neuronal cells of fetal mice as well as in human neural progenitor cells and brain organoids, a mechanism thought to play an important role in the pathogenesis of ZIKV neurological disease [4–7]. It is known that immunocompetent adult mice are resistant to subcutaneous or intraperitoneal inoculation of ZIKV [8,9]. However, it has been demonstrated that intracerebral inoculation of ZIKV in adult immunocompetent mice results in neurological disease [10]. Additionally, several studies have reported that neonatal immunocompetent mice inoculated with ZIKV via subcutaneously or intracerebral route develop ZIKV disease, and ZIKV infection can be detected in the neurons [11–13]. It has also been demonstrated that ZIKV infection during the period of maximal brain growth causes microcephaly and corticospinal neuron apoptosis in wild-type mice [14]. However, to date the effect of ZIKV infection on microRNAs (miRNAs) expression in primary mouse neurons has not been examined.

miRNAs are a group of small RNAs involved in the regulation of a wide variety of cellular and physiological processes. miRNAs are considered novel diagnostic and interventional candidates due to their biochemical structure [15]. They function by directly binding to the 3' untranslated regions (3'UTRs) of specific target mRNA, causing a block of translation or degradation of the target mRNA. miRNAs have been demonstrated to play a crucial regulatory role in neurodegenerative diseases such as Alzheimer and Parkinson [16]. miRNAs also play a critical role in the regulation of immune response; including differentiation, proliferation, cell fate determination, function of immune cells, and inflammatory mediator release as well as the intracellular signaling pathways [17,18].

miRNAs of infected cells can influence the ability of a virus to replicate or spread. It is known that endogenous miRNAs inhibit replication of a number of RNA viruses including HIV-1, Ebola virus and vesicular stomatitis virus [19–23]. For example, miR-28, miR-125b, miR-150, miR- 223, miR-198, and miR-382 inhibit HIV replication in CD4 T cells by directly targeting HIV RNA or by modulating cellular factors responsible for its replication [24]. Furthermore, miR-122 supports HCV replication by enhancing colony formation efficiency of HCV [25], whereas miR-196 and miR-296 substantially attenuate virus replication through type I interferon (IFN)-associated pathways in liver cells [26]. Over-expression of miRNA-30e, let-7c, and miRNA-126-5p inhibits DENV replication [27–29]. Cellular miR-532-5p inhibits WNV replication via suppression of host genes SESTD1 and TAB3 required for virus replication [30]. miRNA HS_154 contributes to WNV-mediated apoptosis in vitro in the human neuronal cell line, SK-N-MC [31]. Moreover, incorporation of a target sequence for cellular microRNAs expressed in the central nervous system (CNS) into the flavivirus genome alters the neurovirulence of the virus and prevents the development of lethal encephalitis in mice [32].

We have previously demonstrated the role of cellular miRNAs in the pathogenesis of WNV encephalitis [33,34]. In this study, we analyzed miRNA and mRNA profiles in ZIKV-infected neurons using the nCounter system. Unlike other platforms (such as microarray and next generation sequencing), the nCounter platform enables high throughput, sensitive, quantitative, and reproducible gene expression analysis without the need of enzymatic target amplification. This technology utilizes 100 nucleotide molecular bar codes which measure gene quantities without an amplification step [35]. To our knowledge, this is the first study to evaluate the modulation of miRNAs following ZIKV infection using relevant cells, primary neurons.

2. Materials and Methods

2.1. Neuronal Cultures

Mouse cortical neuron cultures were prepared from one-day old pups of either gender (approximately equivalent numbers) obtained from established colonies of wild-type C57BL/6J mice as described previously [36]. The neurons were plated onto poly-D-lysine-coated 6-well or 24-well plates in serum Neurobasal A medium. The cultures were maintained in serum-free Neurobasal A medium supplemented with B27 for seven days prior to infection [36,37]. This study was carried out in accordance with the recommendations of the National Institutes of Health and the Institutional

Animal Care and Use Committee (IACUC). The protocol was approved by the University of Hawaii IACUC (protocol number 17-2721) and Georgia State University (protocol number A19005).

2.2. ZIKV Infection and Plaque Assay

In this study, we used a low cell-culture-passaged and sequence-verified ZIKV strain, PRVABC59 (BEI Resources, NR-50240). Virus strain was amplified once in Vero E6 cells and had titers of 5×10^6 plaque-forming units (PFU)/mL. Cells were infected with ZIKV or PBS (Mock) at multiplicity of infection (MOI)-1 and supernatants and cell lysates were harvested at 12, 24, 48, and 72 h after infection [38]. ZIKV titers were measured in cell supernatants using plaque assay [38,39]. Experiments were repeated to obtain four biological replicates of mock- and ZIKV-infected neurons at each time point for the NanoString analysis (*n* = 4 per group per time point).

2.3. Indirect-Immunofluorescence Microscopy

Neuronal cell monolayers were grown on coverslips in 24-well plates and infected with ZIKV or PBS at MOI-1. Cells were fixed in 4% paraformaldehyde (PFA) and immunostained using mouse anti-dsRNA (1:1000) antibody followed by secondary antibody conjugated with Alexa Fluor 555 (Millipore, Burlington, MA, USA) as described previously [40].

2.4. NanoString nCounter® Gene Expression

Total RNA was isolated using miRNeasy Mini Kit (Qiagen, Hilden, Germany) as described previously [33]. Genomic DNA contamination was eliminated by digesting the RNA with RNase-free DNase (Ambion, Cambridge, MA, USA). RNA was quantitated using Nanodrop (Thermo Scientific, Waltham, MA, USA), and the 28S/18S RNA ratios of all RNA samples were between 1.8 and 2.0. RNA quality was analyzed using the Bioanalyzer [33,41]. For miRNA analysis, we used the nCounter® Mouse miRNA Expression Panel (NanoString, Seattle, WA, USA, Cat: CSO-MMIR15-12). Raw data was normalized using the geometric mean values of the top 100 expressed miRNA in each sample using the nSolver Analysis Software (NanoString), according to the manufacturer's guidelines. For mRNA analysis, we utilized the nCounter® Mouse PanCancer Immune Profiling Panel to count 770 immune-related genes (NanoString, Cat: XT-CSO-MIP1-12). Raw data was normalized with a set of housekeeping genes and analyzed using the nSolver Analysis Software (NanoString), according to the manufacturer's guidelines.

2.5. qRT-PCR

Total RNA was isolated using miRNeasy Mini Kit, and cDNA prepared using a miScript II RT Kit (Qiagen) [33,34]. qRT-PCR was performed using specific miRNA primer (Qiagen), and the miScript SYBR green PCR kit (containing Universal reverse primer) [33]. For mRNA analysis, cDNA was prepared using iScript™ cDNA Synthesis Kit (Bio-Rad, Hercules, CA, USA), and qRT-PCR was conducted as described previously [41,42]. The primer sequences used for qRT-PCR are listed in Table 1.

Table 1. Primer sequences used for qRT-PCR.

Gene (Accession No.)	Primer Sequence (5′-3′)
IFIT1 (NM_008331)	
Forward	GTTGTTGTTGTTGTTCGT
Reverse	CAGCAGGAATCAGTTGTG
IL6 (NM_031168)	
Forward	ATCCAGTTGCCTTCTTGGGACTGA
Reverse	TAAGCCTCCGACTTGTGAAGTGGT

Table 1. *Cont.*

Gene (Accession No.)	Primer Sequence (5'-3')
IFIT3 (NM_010501)	
Forward	GTCCTCTCTACTCTTTGG
Reverse	CATCCTCTGTCTTCTCTC
Caspase1 (NM_009807)	
Forward	GGAAGCAATTTATCAACTCAGTG
Reverse	GCCTTGTCCATAGCAGTAATG
Dicer-1 (NM_148948)	
Forward	TGTCATCTTGCGATTCTA
Reverse	TCTCTTCCAATTCCTCTG
DROSHA (NM_001130149)	
Forward	CTTCAACAGTTACCAGAAC
Reverse	CCTTTGGGAGTGAGTATG
AGO1 (NM_001317174)	
Forward	CCTGTGTATGATGGAAAGA
Reverse	CACTTGATGGAGACCTTAA
AGO2 (NM_153178)	
Forward	GGAGAACAATCAAACTACAG
Reverse	CAGATTCTTCCTTCCATCA
DGCR8 (NM_033324)	
Forward	CAGATAAGAAGGATGAGGAA
Reverse	GCTCCAAATTGTCAGTAAA
miR-155 (MIMAT0000165)	
Forward	UUAAUGCUAAUUGUGAUAGGGGUA
miR-203 (MIMAT0000236)	
Forward	GUGAAAUGUUUAGGACCACUAG
miR-29a (MIMAT0000535)	
Forward	UAGCACCAUCUGAAAUCGGUUA
miR-124-3p (MIMAT0000134)	
Forward	UAAGGCACGCGGUGAAUGCC

2.6. Measurement of Cytokines and Chemokines

The levels of cytokines and chemokines were measured in the cell supernatants by multiplex immunoassay using MILLIPLEX MAP mouse Cytokine/Chemokine magnetic panel as per manufacturer's instructions (Millipore) [43,44].

2.7. Ingenuity Pathways Analysis (IPA)

Target prediction and pathway analysis were conducted using IPA (Ingenuity Systems Inc., Redwood City, CA, USA) as described previously [33,34,41]. Fisher's exact test, using IPA, was used to calculate the cut-off point of significance. $p < 0.05$ is considered significant. We also conducted correlation pairing with mRNA expression data and significantly modulated miRNAs using IPA. For multiplex immunoassay analysis, unpaired Student's *t*-test using Graph Pad was used to calculate *p* values.

3. Results

3.1. ZIKV Can Infect Primary Mouse Cortical Neurons

ZIKV infection of neuronal cells plays an important role in the pathogenesis of ZIKV neurological disease. Therefore, we used primary neurons for our experiments. We first determined ZIKV infection and replication kinetics in primary mouse cortical neurons by plaque assay. Mouse cortical neuron cultures were infected with ZIKV (PRVABC59 strain) or PBS (Mock) at MOI-1 and supernatants were collected at 12, 24, 48, and 72 h after infection. High ZIKV replication was observed as early as 12 h after infection. Viral titers peaked at 48 h (log 7–8 PFU/mL) followed by a slight decline at 72 h after infection (Figure 1A). Immunofluorescence staining of ZIKV-infected neurons demonstrated robust dsRNA staining in the cytoplasm. Based on a total of 5,000 cells counted in 10 independent fields, dsRNA was detected in approximately 60% of cells at 48 h after infection (Figure 1B,C).

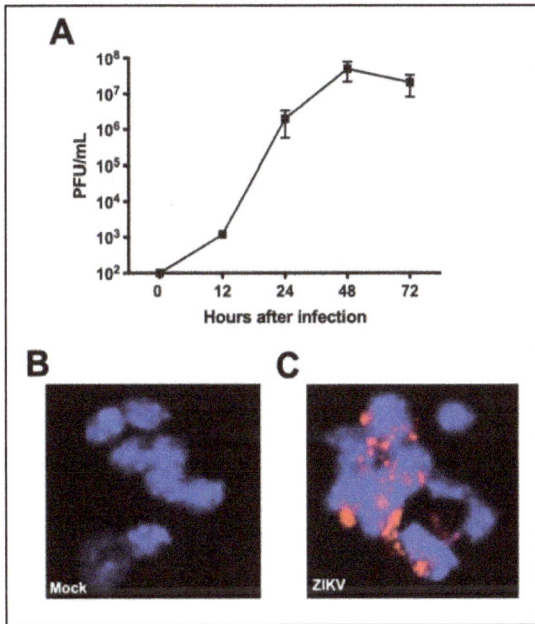

Figure 1. Zika virus (ZIKV) infection of the primary mouse neurons. Mouse cortical neuron cultures were prepared from one-day old pups. Neurons were infected with ZIKV (PRVABC59 strain) or PBS (Mock) at multiplicity of infection (MOI)-1. (**A**) ZIKV titers in culture supernatant were determined by plaque assay. Viral titers are expressed as plaque forming units (PFU)/mL of supernatant. Data represents the mean ± SEM. Neurons grown and fixed on coverslips at 48 h after infection were stained with anti-dsRNA antibody (red) and counterstained with DAPI (blue). (**B**) Mock-infected cells. 20× magnification. (**C**) ZIKV-infected cells demonstrate robust virus staining in the cytoplasm. 20× magnification.

3.2. ZIKV Infection Modulates Cellular miRNA Expression

Neurons were infected with ZIKV (PRVABC59 strain) or PBS (Mock) at MOI-1 and cell lysates were harvested at 24 and 48 h after infection. We used nCounter® Technology (NanoString) to evaluate the global miRNA expression profiles in the mock-and ZIKV-infected neurons at 24 and 48 h after infection (n = 4 per group per time point). Among 599 miRNAs present on the array, 67 and 45 miRNAs were significantly modulated at 24 and 48 h, respectively. miRNAs that were altered at least 2-fold were considered significant. While 62 miRNAs were significantly downregulated (between 2- to

4-fold), only five miRNAs were upregulated (between 2 to 18-fold) in ZIKV-infected neurons when compared to mock-infected neurons at 24 h (Tables 2 and 3). Similarly, 40 miRNAs were significantly downregulated (between 2- to 6-fold), and only five were upregulated (between 2 to 10-fold) at 48 h (Tables 2 and 4). As depicted in the Venn diagram (Figure 2A), three upregulated and 26 downregulated miRNAs were common in both 24 and 48 h-infected neurons. Among upregulated miRNAs; miR-155, miR-29a, and miR-29b were induced at both 24 and 48 h. miR-3471 and miR-2145 were upregulated only at 24 h, and miR-203 and miR-1902 were upregulated only at 48 h. The miRNAs with the highest induction during the course of infection were miR-155 (18.2-fold), miR-3471 (4.9-fold), and miR-203 (4.6-fold) (Table 2). Among downregulated miRNAs, miR-124-3p was the highest downregulated miRNA at both 24 (4-fold) and 48 (6.6-fold) h. Other miRNAs with high downregulation were miR-883a-3p (3.9-fold) and miR-2137 (2.9-fold). We also conducted qRT-PCR to confirm the expression changes of a selected number of differentially expressed miRNAs. Similar to the NanoString data, miR-155, miR-29a, and miR-203 were significantly upregulated, and miR-124-3p was downregulated in ZIKV-infected neurons (Figure 2B).

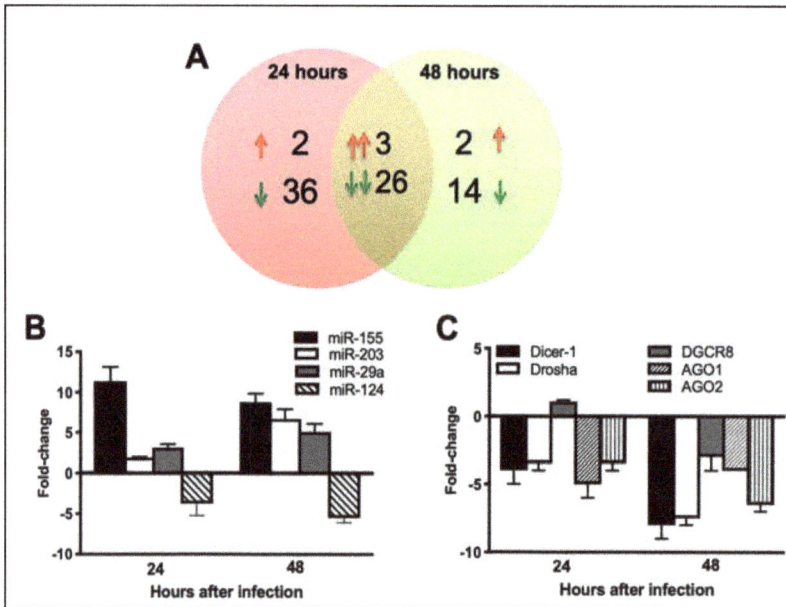

Figure 2. ZIKV infection of the primary mouse neurons causes changes in cellular miRNA expression. Neurons were infected with ZIKV (PRVABC59 strain) or PBS (Mock) at MOI-1. (**A**) Venn diagram showing the number of differentially expressed miRNAs at 24 and 48 h after infection. Sets of upregulated miRNAs are represented by upward red arrows and sets of downregulated miRNAs are represented by downward green arrows. Pairs of arrows in the intersection refer to the number of miRNAs upregulated (double red arrows) or down regulated (double green arrows) at both 24 and 48 h after infection. (**B**) qRT-PCR was conducted on RNA extracted from mock and ZIKV-infected neurons to determine fold-change in miR-155, miR-203, miR-29a, and miR-124-3p expression. Changes in the levels of each miRNA were first normalized to the snoRNA and then the fold-change in ZIKV-infected cells was calculated in comparison to corresponding mock-infected cells. Data represents the mean ± SEM. (**C**) qRT-PCR was conducted on RNA extracted from mock and ZIKV-infected neurons to determine fold-change in Dicer-1, Drosha, DGCR8, AGO1, and AGO2 expression. Changes in the levels of each mRNA were first normalized to the β-actin and then the fold-change in ZIKV-infected cells was calculated in comparison to corresponding mock-infected cells. Data represents the mean ± SEM.

Table 2. Upregulated miRNAs in Zika virus (ZIKV)-infected neurons at 24 h and 48 h.

miRNA	Fold-change (24 h)	miRNA	Fold-change (48 h)
miR-155	18.29	miR-155	10.61
miR-3471	4.96	miR-203	4.61
miR-2145	2.33	miR-1902	2.95
miR-29a	2.09	miR-29b	2.1
miR-29b	2.05	miR-29a	2.08

Table 3. Downregulated miRNAs at 24 h.

miRNA	Fold-change	miRNA	Fold-change
miR-124-3p	−4.02	miR-144	−2.15
miR-M1-1	−2.97	miR-201	−2.15
miR-1892	−2.85	miR-764-5p	−2.15
miR-883a-3p	−2.7	miR-1895	−2.13
miR-879	−2.69	miR-871	−2.12
miR-669g	−2.65	miR-m108-1	−2.12
miR-654-3p	−2.62	miR-1928	−2.11
miR-339-3p	−2.52	miR-1941-5p	−2.11
miR-1960	−2.51	miR-759	−2.11
miR-207	−2.51	miR-1187	−2.1
miR-2861	−2.51	miR-666-3p	−2.1
miR-412	−2.48	miR-1966	−2.09
miR-741	−2.47	miR-1942	−2.08
miR-770-5p	−2.41	miR-1946a	−2.08
miR-673-5p	−2.38	miR-1967	−2.08
miR-1941-3p	−2.37	miR-m01-1	−2.07
miR-493	−2.33	miR-383	−2.06
miR-465a-3p	−2.31	miR-186	−2.05
miR-1956	−2.26	miR-323-5p	−2.05
miR-1194	−2.25	miR-M1-3	−2.05
miR-709	−2.25	miR-433	−2.04
miR-m107-1-5p	−2.25	miR-767	−2.04
miR-877	−2.23	miR-1188	−2.03
miR-331-5p	−2.22	miR-694	−2.03
miR-483	−2.22	miR-665	−2.02
miR-675-5p	−2.2	miR-2139	−2.02
miR-1957	−2.19	miR-883a-5p	−2.02
miR-M23-1-3p	−2.19	miR-1943	−2
miR-1898	−2.18	miR-346	−2
miR-1940	−2.17	miR-764-3p	−2
miR-1894-5p	−2.16	miR-710	−2

Table 4. Downregulated miRNAs at 48 h.

miRNA	Fold-change	miRNA	Fold-change
miR-124-3p	−6.68	miR-m21-1	−2.15
miR-883a-3p	−3.93	miR-335-3p	−2.14
miR-2137	−2.92	miR-1957	−2.12
miR-2133	−2.74	miR-764-5p	−2.11
miR-714	−2.56	miR-1194	−2.08
miR-669g	−2.54	miR-683	−2.08
miR-467g	−2.5	miR-509-5p	−2.07
miR-1188	−2.41	miR-463	−2.06
miR-879	−2.33	miR-741	−2.06
miR-760	−2.25	miR-761	−2.05
miR-298	−2.21	miR-710	−2.03
miR-m01-3	−2.21	miR-346	−2.01
miR-764-3p	−-2.2	miR-882	−2.01
miR-370	−2.18	miR-1898	−2.01
miR-1892	−2.16	miR-759	−2
miR-m01-2	−2.16	miR-433	−2
miR-133b	−2.15	miR-709	−2
miR-1894-5p	−2.15	miR-1956	−2
miR-666-3p	−2.15	miR-483	−2
miR-877	−2.15	miR-1941-5p	−2

3.3. ZIKV Infection Results in Downregulation of miRNA Processing Enzymes

Flaviviruses have been shown to induce downregulation in the expression of cellular miRNAs by targeting miRNA processing enzymes [45–48]. Our data also demonstrated a trend toward decrease in miRNA expression in ZIKA-infected cells. Therefore, we next evaluated the expression of miRNA processing enzymes in ZIKV-infected neurons. mRNA expression levels of Dicer-1, Drosha, AGO1, and AGO2 were downregulated in ZIKV-infected neurons as compared to mock-infected neurons at both 24 and 48 h (Figure 2C). mRNA expression of DGCR8 increased slightly at 24 h followed by a decrease in the expression at 48 h.

3.4. Functional Analysis of ZIKV-Modulated miRNAs and Their Predicted Targets

Biofunctional analysis of ZIKV-modulated miRNAs and their targets revealed organismal injury and abnormalities, immunological disease, inflammatory response, neurological disease, and nervous system development and function as the top pathways in signaling pathways category (Table 5). Since ZIKV infection is associated with a wide spectrum of neurological and immunological diseases, these miRNAs may play an important role in the development of brain abnormalities following ZIKV infection.

Table 5. Top biological functions regulated by significantly modulated miRNAs.

Biological Process/Pathway	*p*-Value	Number of miRNAs
Cancer	4.02×10^{-10}	18
Organismal Injury and Abnormalities	4.02×10^{-10}	23
Reproductive System Disease	4.02×10^{-10}	18

Table 5. *Cont.*

Biological Process/Pathway	*p*-Value	Number of miRNAs
Immunological Disease	6.98×10^{-10}	13
Inflammatory Disease	6.98×10^{-10}	13
Inflammatory Response	6.98×10^{-10}	11
Neurological Disease	6.98×10^{-10}	10
Connective Tissue Disorders	1.46×10^{-8}	10
Respiratory Disease	1.46×10^{-8}	7
Nervous System Development and Function	7.20×10^{-7}	6

3.5. ZIKV Infection Induces Dramatic Upregulation of Anti-Viral, Inflammatory, and Apoptotic Genes in Neurons

We next analyzed the mRNA expression of key anti-viral, inflammatory, and apoptotic genes in the ZIKV-infected neurons to examine whether differentially expressed miRNAs could regulate their target mRNAs. Mouse cortical neuron cultures were infected with ZIKV (PRVABC59 strain) or PBS (Mock) at MOI-1 and cell lysates were harvested at 24 h and 48 h after infection. We utilized the nCounter® Mouse PanCancer Immune Profiling Panel to count 770 immune-related genes. mRNA expression profiles for ZIKV-infected neurons were compared with mock-infected neurons. Only mRNAs that were altered at least 2-fold were considered significant. Figure 3A demonstrates total numbers of up- and downregulated differentially expressed mRNAs in ZIKV-infected neurons at 24 and 48 h. The number of differentially expressed mRNAs was higher at 48 h after infection, which correlates with significantly higher viral load observed at 48 h as compared to 24 h (Figure 1A). At 24 h, 65 mRNAs were upregulated with fold change values ranging from 2.0 to 26 (Table 6). mRNAs were not downregulated at 24 h. At 48 h, 116 mRNAs were upregulated with fold change values ranging from 2.0 to 244 (Tables 6 and 7) and 12 mRNAs were downregulated (Table 8). 62 upregulated mRNAs were common in both 24 and 48 h- infected neurons (Table 6). MMP9, SOCS3 and IFI27 were upregulated only at 24 h. 54 mRNAs were upregulated only at 48 h (Table 7).

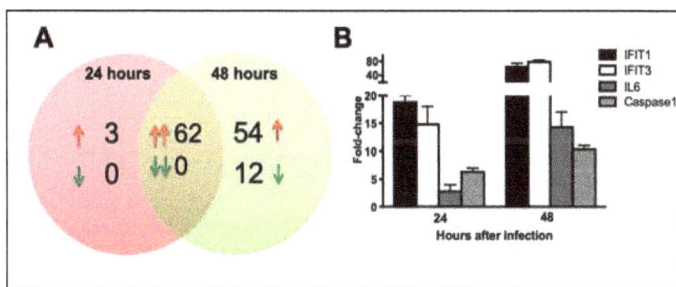

Figure 3. ZIKV infection of the primary mouse neurons causes changes in cellular mRNA expression. Neurons were infected with ZIKV (PRVABC59 strain) or PBS (Mock) at MOI-1. (**A**) Venn diagram showing the number of differentially expressed mRNAs at 24 and 48 h after infection. Sets of upregulated mRNAs are represented by upward red arrows and sets of downregulated mRNAs are represented by downward green arrows. Pairs of arrows in the intersection refer to the number of mRNAs upregulated (double red arrows) or down regulated (double green arrows) at both 24 and 48 h after infection. (**B**) qRT-PCR was conducted on RNA extracted from mock and ZIKV-infected neurons to determine fold-change in IFIT1, IFIT3, IL6, and Caspase1 expression. Changes in the levels of each mRNA were first normalized to the β-actin and then the fold-change in ZIKV-infected cells was calculated in comparison to corresponding mock-infected cells. Data represents the mean ± SEM.

Table 6. Upregulated mRNAs in ZIKV-infected neurons at 24 and 48 h.

mRNA	Fold-Change (24 h)	Fold-Change (48 h)	mRNA	Fold-Change (24 h)	Fold-Change (48 h)
Rsad2	26.44	244.24	Ccl2	3.91	14.32
Cxcl10	22.31	113.73	Ifna4	2.85	14.02
Ifit3	21.63	103.85	Nlrc5	3.42	13.39
Ifi44	18.36	103.12	Psmb10	3.13	12.78
Irf7	12.53	96.42	Stat2	5.55	12.37
Ifit1	24.52	75.06	H2-K1	2	12.34
Isg15	20.58	69.08	Cfb	2.04	12.04
Lcn2	27.07	68.88	Ifi35	4.05	11.3
Zbp1	13.57	55.1	Ddx58	3.84	10.56
Gbp5	12.51	44.43	Psmb9	2.4	10.03
Ifit2	2.53	41.91	Tap1	2.77	9.85
Ccl5	24.11	37.65	C3	3.29	9.22
Oas2	10.64	37.13	Casp1	2.76	7.63
Oasl1	5.15	34.55	Socs1	2.13	6.63
Usp18	9.7	32.04	H2-Ab1	2.21	5.82
Isg20	5.57	30.07	Cxcl1	3.49	5.5
H2-T23	3.61	28.33	Ifitm1	3.94	5.39
Ifih1	6.11	25.37	Ccl12	3.68	5.38
Ddx60	7.87	23.88	Pml	2	5.38
Stat1	6.92	21.99	Vcam1	2.23	5.24
Bst2	4.92	21.62	Myd88	2.38	4.87
Mx2	7.55	20.85	Cxcl9	2.83	4.7
Psmb8	4.31	20.39	Il6	2.07	3.63
Ccl7	2.71	19.98	Ptgs2	2.02	3.32
Cd274	4.02	19.34	Cxcl2	2.68	3.27
Cmpk2	4.01	18.95	Sbno2	3.05	2.86
Xaf1	8.02	18.06	Ccl4	2.52	2.84
Herc6	3.68	17.33	Lif	2.75	2.47
Ifnb1	2.97	16.75	Il13ra1	2.01	2.33
Tlr3	3.84	16.4	Runx1	2	2.15
Irgm2	6.29	15.13	Litaf	2	2.01

Table 7. Upregulated mRNAs in ZIKV-infected neurons at 48 h only.

mRNA	Fold-Change	mRNA	Fold-Change
Cxcl11	17.69	Slamf7	2.81
C2	9.88	Tnfrsf14	2.76
Tnfsf10	9.53	Fcgr4	2.6
Cxcl13	9.29	Mill2	2.59
Cd74	8.49	Ptprc	2.59
C1ra	7.96	H2-Dma	2.57
H2-D1	7.64	Nfkbia	2.52
H2-Aa	7.35	Tnfaip3	2.51
Tap2	6.53	Cxcl5	2.47
Ccl11	5.49	A2m	2.46
Fcgr1	5.32	Ifna1	2.38
H2-M3	5.25	Il3ra	2.36
Ccrl2	4.9	Ctss	2.34
Cd47	4.2	Ripk2	2.34
Tapbp	3.97	H2-DMb1	2.28
C4b	3.96	Lck	2.27
Ifna2	3.96	Cd80	2.26
Irf1	3.88	Cxcl16	2.19
Tlr2	3.87	Cybb	2.19
C1s1	3.56	Icosl	2.18
Lbp	3.44	Cfi	2.14
Il7	3.3	Irf2	2.1
Irf5	3.03	Nod1	2.02
Cd69	2.99	Atm	2
Serping1	2.91	Axl	2
Flt3l	2.87	H2-Eb1	2
Bid	2.85	Relb	2

Table 8. Downregulated mRNAs in ZIKV-infected neurons.

mRNA	Fold-Change (48 h)	mRNA	Fold-Change (48 h)
Cd36	−2	Cd207	−2.19
Elane	−2	Timd4	−2.22
Il17f	−2	Xcl1	−2.31
Ticam2	−2	Card9	−2.65
Pax5	−2.02	Sh2d1b1	−2.76
Il1rapl2	−2.15	Mpped1	−2.87

Genes associated with virus sensing and type 1 IFN signaling were the most upregulated genes after ZIKV infection. ZIKV infection also induced a strong upregulation of multiple cytokines and chemokines in the neurons. Most of the chemokines and cytokines were significantly upregulated after ZIKV infection, including CXCL10, CCL5, CCL7, CCL2, CXCL1, CCL12, CXCL9, CXCL2, CCL4,

CXCL11, CXCL13, CCL11, CXCL5, IL6, IL7, PTGS2, and LIF. Several genes involved in cell death (CASP1, TNFSF10, RIPK2, and BID) were also activated upon ZIKV infection (Tables 6 and 7). We also validated the expression of selected upregulated mRNAs using qRT-PCR. Similar to the NanoString data, IFIT1, IFIT3, IL6, and Caspase1 were significantly upregulated in the ZIKV-infected neurons as compared to mock-infected neurons at both 24 and 48 h (Figure 3B). To examine that this increase in mRNA expression also lead to increased protein levels, we measured protein levels of key chemokines and cytokines in the cell culture supernatants using multiplex immunoassay. Similar to the mRNA expression, protein levels of the key chemokines such as CCL2, CCL4, CCL5, CCL11, CXCL1, CXCL2, CXCL9, and CXCL10, and cytokines such as IL6 and LIF were significantly increased in ZIKV-infected neurons as compared to mock-infected neurons (Figure 4).

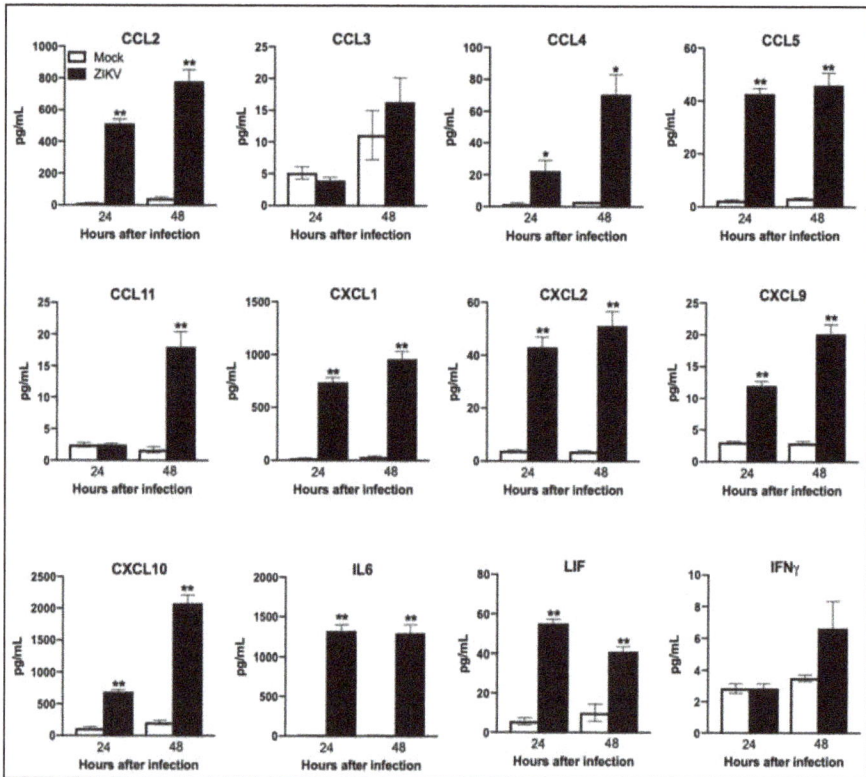

Figure 4. Enhanced production of cytokines and chemokines in ZIKV-infected neurons. Mouse cortical neuron cultures were infected with ZIKV (PRVABC59 strain) or PBS (Mock) at MOI-1 and supernatants were collected at 24 and 48 h after infection. Levels of chemokines and cytokines as noted in the figure were measured in cell supernatants using multiplex immunoassay and are expressed as the mean concentration (pg/mL) ± SEM. *$p < 0.05$, **$p < 0.001$.

3.6. Functional Analysis of ZIKV-Modulated mRNAs

To investigate the biological interactions of differentially expressed mRNAs and identify important functional networks, significantly modulated mRNAs were imported into the IPA tool. The highest activated networks (high z-score) were identified using IPA. Figure 5 depicts the top 10 activated canonical pathways after ZIKV infection. The topmost activated canonical pathway after ZIKV infection was 'Neuroinflammation Signaling'. In addition, key players in inflammation and innate immunity, such as 'Activation of IRFs by Cytosolic Pattern Recognition Receptors (PRR)', 'Role of PRR in Recognition of Viruses and Bacteria', and 'IFN Signaling' were also highly activated (positive z-score). To further understand the role of these differentially activated canonical pathways, we generated the network maps of 'PRR in Recognition of Viruses and Bacteria' and 'IFN Signaling'.

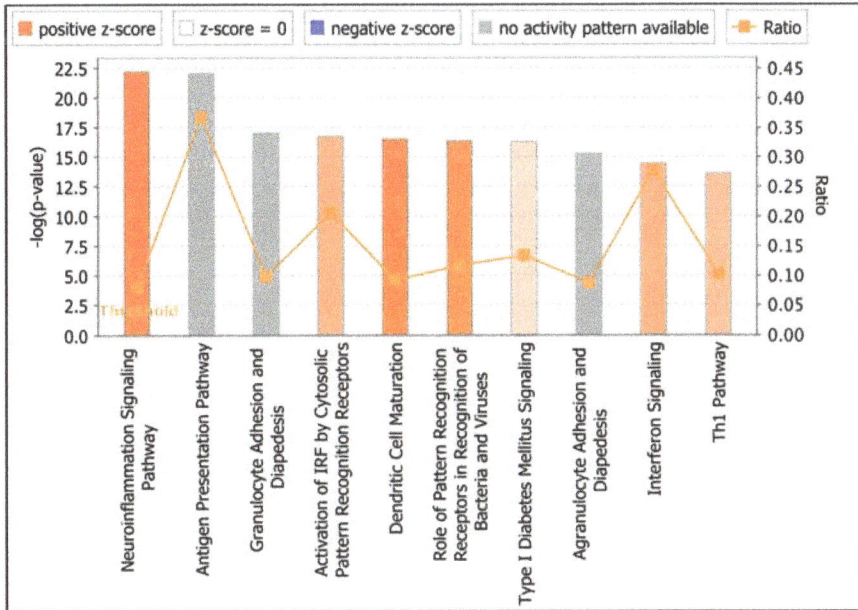

Figure 5. Core functional pathway analysis of ZIKV-modulated mRNAs using IPA. Top canonical signaling pathways regulated by significantly modulated mRNAs. Threshold bar indicates cut-off point of significance $p < 0.05$, using Fisher's exact test. Range of activation z-score is also depicted in the figure. The color of the bars indicates predicted pathway activation based on z-score (orange = activation; blue = inhibition; gray = no prediction can be made; white = z-score close to 0). Orange line represents the ratio = number of genes in dataset/total number of genes that compose that pathway.

3.6.1. Pattern Recognition Receptors

Our data demonstrate that ZIKV infection induces the expression of all three major PRR; retinoic-acid-inducible gene-I (RIG-I)-like receptors (RLR), toll-like receptors (TLR), and the nucleotide oligomerization domain (Nod)-like receptors (NLR) (Figure 6A). The RLR are a family of cytosolic RNA helicase proteins comprised of three members: RIG-I, myeloma differentiation antigen 5 (MDA5), and LGP2 [49]. Both RIG-I and MDA5 were upregulated after ZIKV infection. The importance of the RLR signaling pathway in protection against flaviviruses has been validated by several studies in vivo [49–51]. The TLR family is composed of more than 10 members, with each acting as a sensor of conserved microbial component, that drive the induction of immune response [52]. Our data show that ZIKV infection induces the expression of TLR2, TLR3, and adaptor molecule MYD88. NLR are soluble or cytosolic receptors in the mammalian cell cytoplasm [53]. Activation of NOD1 and NLRC5 was observed following ZIKV infection. In addition to RLR, TLR, and NLR; PKR and OAS are classes of IFN-inducible PRR that can recognize dsRNA and restrict a number of viruses. Our data demonstrate the activation of OAS after infection with ZIKV. Furthermore, we observed increased levels of type 1 interferons and several pro-inflammatory mediators after ZIKV infection in neurons, which correlate with PRR activation in these cells.

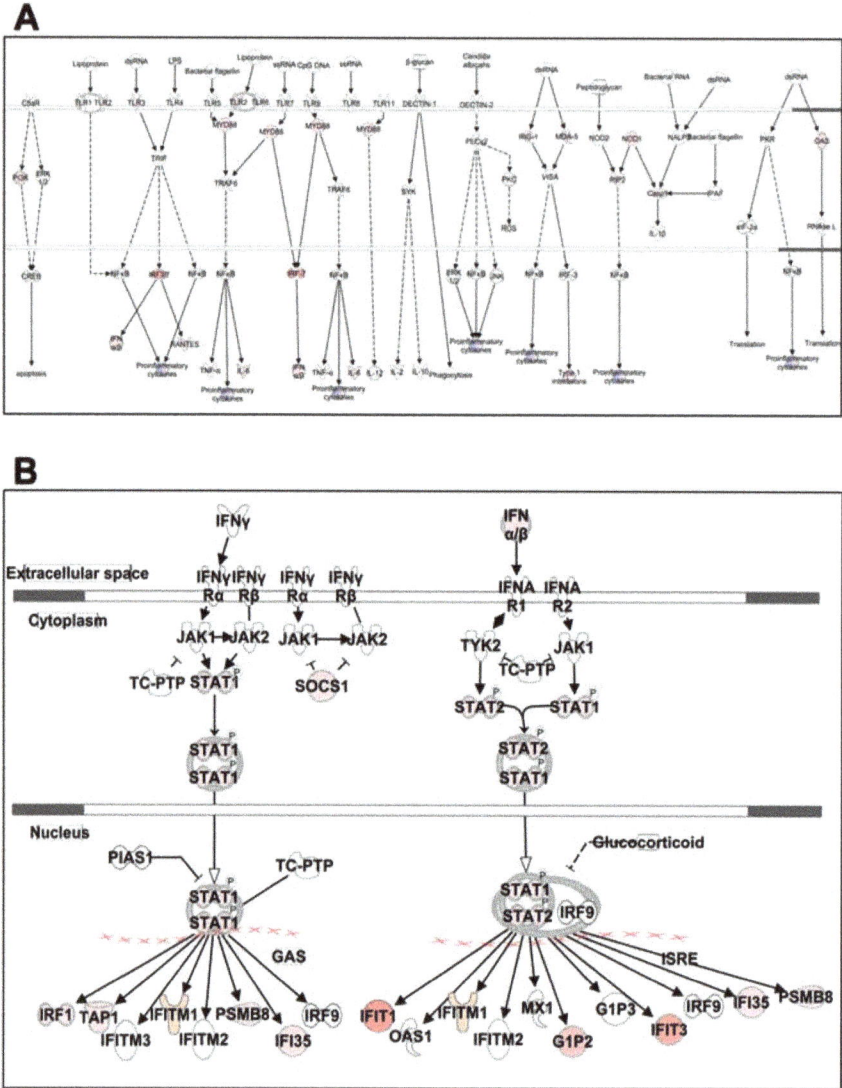

Figure 6. Pathway analysis for PRR and IFN signaling. Genes associated with (**A**) PRR and (**B**) IFN signaling activated by ZIKV infection are shown. Differentially expressed mRNAs are highlighted in color. Color intensity indicates the degree of upregulation (red) relative to the mock-infected neurons. Solid lines represent direct interactions and dashed lines indirect interactions. Shading intensity indicates the degree that each mRNA was upregulated.

3.6.2. IFN Signaling

ZIKV infection induced strong upregulation of genes associated with IFN signaling such as IFNα, IFNβ, STAT1, and STAT2 (Figure 6B). Interferon-stimulated genes (ISG) such as MX2, IFIT1, IFIT3, IFITM1, IFI35, and RSAD2 (Viperin) were significantly upregulated after ZIKV infection. The IFN response is central to the innate defense mechanisms of the host against flavivirus infection.

The paracrine and autocrine secretion of IFN creates an anti-viral state by inducing several genes including ISG [49,54].

3.7. Network Analysis of Expression of miRNAs and mRNAs From ZIKV-Infected Neurons

We next sought to determine whether mRNA expression changes might be influenced by the differential expression of cellular miRNAs during ZIKV infection. To analyze the direct and indirect miRNA–mRNA interactions, we conducted IPA expression pairing analysis with mRNA expression data and significantly modulated miRNAs. Several miRNAs were found to directly or indirectly target multiple mRNAs analyzed in our study and demonstrated an inverse correlation with mRNA expression induced by ZIKV. These targets are predicted by TargetScan. miR-124-3p was the highest downregulated miRNA. Our data demonstrated increased expression of all the predicted targets of miR-124-3p including IL7, CCL2, LITAF, IRF1, and SBNO2 in ZIKV-infected neurons (Figure 7A). Other known targets of miR-124 includes SOCS5, TLR6, STAT3, TNF, and NF-kB [55]. Similarly, miR-654-3p was downregulated and its predicted targets—CD69, FLT3LG, IFIT1, TLR2, ZBP1, LITAF—were upregulated in ZIKV-infected neurons (Figure 7B). These targets involve genes belonging to anti-viral and inflammatory response signaling pathways. Furthermore, downregulation of miR-331-5p and miR-509-5p was inversely correlated to their predicted targets IL7, CD274, HLA-DRB5, XAF1, IL13RA1, TAP1, and CD80 (Figure 7C,D). Our data further indicate that miR-335-3p may play an important role in regulating inflammatory and apoptotic genes in the neurons following ZIKV infection. miR-335-3p targets Caspase1, CCL5, CXCL3, PTPRC, and GBP5. These genes play significant roles in mediating inflammation and cell death (Figure 7E). We also show an increase in the protein levels of the target genes such as CCL2, CCL5, and CXCL10 (Figure 4). It is interesting to see the correlation between ZIKV-modulated miRNAs and target genes at both mRNA and protein level, which is consistent with the miRNA–mRNA–protein triad and demonstrate the functional importance of our results.

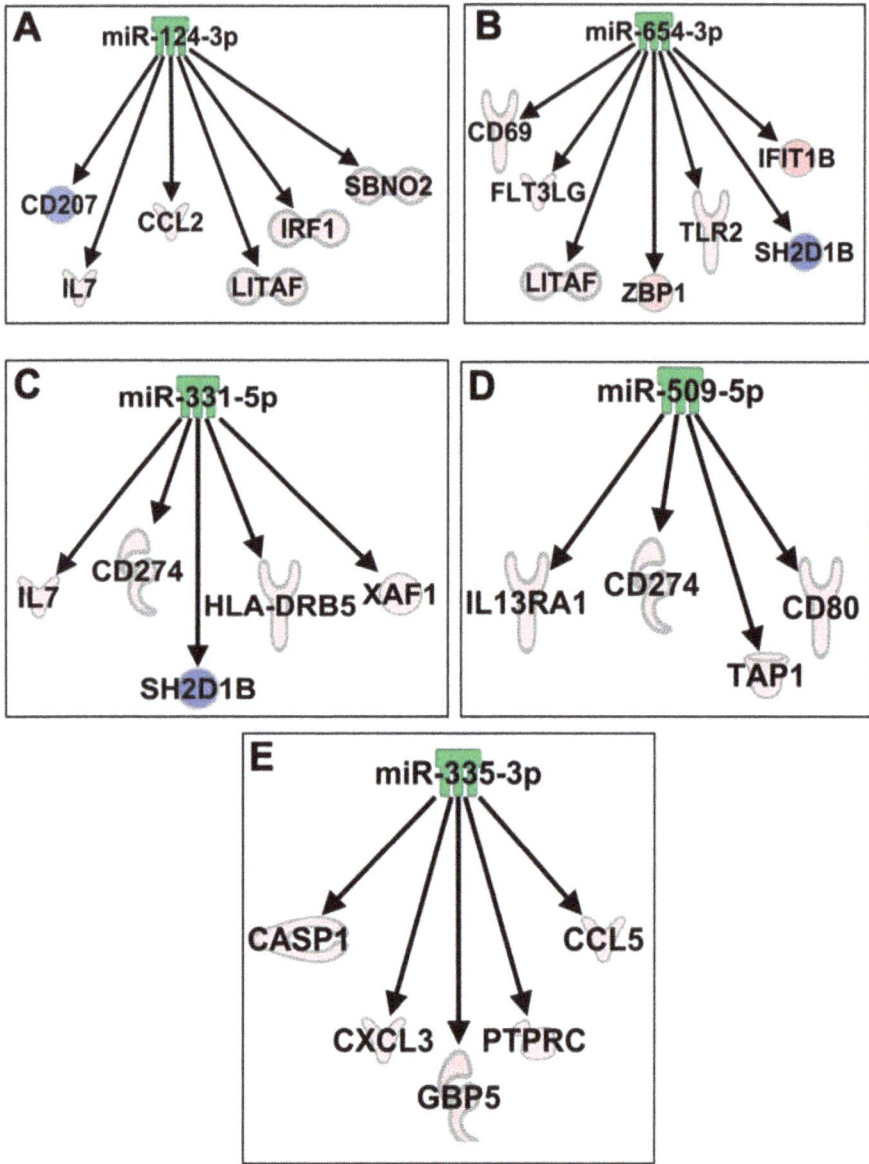

Figure 7. Networks of the interactions of the miRNA target genes. IPA tool was used to generate the miRNA-mRNA interaction network of (**A**) miR-124-3p, (**B**) miR-654-3p, (**C**) miR-331-5p, (**D**) miR-509-5p, and (**E**) miR-335-3p and mRNAs significantly modulated in neurons after ZIKV infection. Red (increased expression) and green (decreased expression).

4. Discussion

In this study, we used nCounter technology to identify miRNAs and mRNAs modulated by ZIKV infection in neurons. Our data demonstrate that ZIKV infection causes global downregulation of miRNAs with only few upregulated miRNAs. ZIKV infection also results in downregulation of miRNA processing enzymes. Upregulated miRNAs including miR-155, miR-203, and miR-29a have been previously shown to play critical role in flavivirus infection and anti-viral immunity [22,56–60]. ZIKV infection in the neurons significantly induced the expression of anti-viral, inflammatory and apoptotic genes. Biofunctional analysis revealed that ZIKV-modulated miRNAs and their target genes regulate the pathways related to neurological development and neuroinflammatory responses. Furthermore, our data show an inverse correlation between ZIKV-modulated miRNAs and target host immune mRNAs induced by ZIKV infection.

Flaviviruses have been shown to induce downregulation in the expression of cellular miRNAs by targeting miRNA processing enzymes [33,45–48,61]. It has been reported that depletion of Dicer and Drosha by siRNA-mediated silencing results in increase in flavivirus replication [46,47,61]. We also observed a trend towards decrease in miRNAs expression in ZIKA-infected cells. Similar to our data, ZIKV infection in human astrocytes induces global downregulation of miRNAs [62]. It has been demonstrated that ZIKV infection in *Aedes aegypti* mosquitoes downregulates expression of host miRNAs [63]. In this study, we also show that ZIKV infection results in downregulation of miRNA processing enzymes. Downregulation of genes involved in miRNA processing enzymes including Dicer-1 was also reported in ZIKV-infected astrocytes [62]. Similarly, ZIKV infection in HepG2 cells led to a decrease in DGCR8, Ago1, and Ago3 expression [64]. It is known that non-coding, subgenomic RNA (sfRNA) of WNV and DENV can interfere with miRNA biogenesis pathway. WNV sfRNA is processed by Dicer and suppresses RNAi [33,45–48,61]. Future experiments are warranted to elucidate whether this sfRNA function holds for all flaviviruses including ZIKV. Since miRNAs negatively regulate mRNA expression, decrease in cellular miRNA expression results in increase in apoptotic and inflammatory genes associated with flavivirus infection [27,30,31,33,41]. Our data also demonstrate that ZIKV infection is associated with dramatic upregulation of several anti-viral, apoptotic and inflammatory genes.

We observed significant upregulation of miR-155, miR-203, miR-29a, and miR-29b in ZIKV-infected neurons. These miRNAs have been shown to play an important role in viral infection [19–21,65,66]. miR-155 is multifunctional and widely reported to modulate different stages of innate immune response during inflammation and infection [21,22,56]. miR-155 not only modulates TLR-mediated innate immune response, but also targets complement regulatory proteins and facilitate complement activation [56,57]. This phenomenon is critical to eliminate the virus from infected cells. Several published studies have demonstrated the essential role of miR-155 in viral infections caused by Epstein–Barr, Borna disease, and reticuloendotheliosis viruses [19,20,56,65]. For example, overexpression of miR-155 significantly suppressed human HIV infection in activated macrophages [21]. Similarly, miR-155 suppresses JEV replication in microglial cells and regulates JEV-induced inflammatory response in mice brain [22,67]. Studies have shown that miR-203 is also involved in regulating the anti-viral immune response [59,60]. It has been demonstrated that miR-29b regulates JEV-induced neuroinflammation [58]. Since these miRNAs are known to have a role in anti-viral immunity, upregulation of these miRNAs might play a role in controlling ZIKV infection and associated neurotoxicity. A recent study identified upregulation of miR-30e-3p, miR-30e-5p, and miR-17-5p in ZIKV infection of human astrocytes [62]. However, we did not observe upregulation of these miRNAs in ZIKV-infected mouse neurons. This could be due to the difference in the neural cell type and species studied.

In our study, miRNAs with the highest downregulation were miR-124-3p, miR-883a-5p and miR-2137. miR-124 is the most abundant miRNA in the brain and affects a broad spectrum of biological functions in the CNS [55,68–70]. miR-124 has been reported to participate in chronic stress, neurodegeneration, alcohol/cocaine neuroadaptation, synapse morphology, neurotransmission, long-term potentiation, neurodevelopment, myeloid cell function, and hematopoiesis. In mammalian neurons, miR-124 suppresses the levels of many non-neural genes, which contributes to the acquisition and maintenance of neuronal identity [69]. Furthermore, when miR-124 is aberrantly expressed, it contributes to pathological conditions involving the CNS [68–70]. It has also been shown to be useful as a diagnostic and prognostic indicator of CNS disorders, such as brain tumors and stroke [68].

miR-883a has been demonstrated to be involved in inflammatory pathways, and target genes belonging to the TLR signaling pathway as well as the VEGF and chemokine signaling pathways [71]. miR-2137 is involved in the pathogenesis of traumatic brain injury [72]. IPA analysis also revealed that individual miRNA including miR-124a-3p, miR-654-3p, miR-331-5p, miR-335-3p, and miR-509-5p can modulate multiple upstream regulatory genes. There was an inverse correlation between these miRNAs and target host immune mRNAs induced by ZIKV infection. Since these miRNAs are known to have a role in brain injury and inflammatory responses, downregulation of these miRNAs following ZIKV infection possibly resulted in upregulation of neuroinflammatory and apoptotic genes. However, further experiments are required to validate their biological functions in ZIKV infection.

This study has few limitations. First, we only analyzed the mRNA expression of genes primarily involved in immune response, which introduce a bias in the analysis towards anti-viral response. Second, additional experimental studies are warranted to validate the interplay between miRNA, mRNA, and ZIKV replication, which includes knockdown of individual miRNA and its effect on the expression levels of its target mRNAs and virus titers.

In conclusion, this is the first study to evaluate the modulation of miRNAs following ZIKV infection in neurons. ZIKV-modulated miRNAs in neurons are also known to play a role in the pathogenesis of other flaviviruses and anti-viral immune response. In this study, the utility of the nCounter system enabling rapid miRNA and mRNA expression analysis was also demonstrated. Collectively, these data suggest that miRNAs regulate downstream gene expression, important in ZIKV disease pathogenesis, and can be targeted in the future to develop therapeutics for the management of ZIKV neurological disease.

Author Contributions: Conceptualization, M.K. and V.R.N.; Methodology, M.K., K.A., F.A., and K.K.; Software, M.K., F.A., and K.A.; Validation, F.A. and K.A.; Formal analysis, M.K., K.A., F.A., and V.R.N.; Writing—original draft preparation, M.K. and K.A.; Writing—review and editing, M.K., K.A., F.A., K.K., and V.R.N.; Funding acquisition, M.K.

Funding: This work was supported by a grant (P30GM114737) from the Centers of Biomedical Research Excellence, National Institute of General Medical Sciences, grant (R21NS099838) from National Institute of Neurological Disorders and Stroke, grant (R21OD024896) from the Office of the Director, National Institutes of Health, and grant (18CON-90812) from Hawaii Community Foundation.

Conflicts of Interest: The authors declare no conflict of interest.

References

1. Musso, D.; Gubler, D.J. Zika virus. *Clin. Microbiol. Rev.* **2016**, *29*, 487–524. [CrossRef] [PubMed]
2. Klase, Z.A.; Khakhina, S.; Schneider Ade, B.; Callahan, M.V.; Glasspool-Malone, J.; Malone, R. Zika fetal neuropathogenesis: Etiology of a viral syndrome. *PLoS Negl. Trop. Dis.* **2016**, *10*, e0004877. [CrossRef] [PubMed]
3. Cao-Lormeau, V.M.; Blake, A.; Mons, S.; Lastere, S.; Roche, C.; Vanhomwegen, J.; Dub, T.; Baudouin, L.; Teissier, A.; Larre, P.; et al. Guillain-Barré syndrome outbreak associated with zika virus infection in french polynesia: A case-control study. *Lancet* **2016**, *387*, 1531–1539. [CrossRef]
4. Tang, H.; Hammack, C.; Ogden, S.C.; Wen, Z.; Qian, X.; Li, Y.; Yao, B.; Shin, J.; Zhang, F.; Lee, E.M.; et al. Zika virus infects human cortical neural progenitors and attenuates their growth. *Cell Stem Cell* **2016**, *18*, 587–590. [CrossRef] [PubMed]
5. Anfasa, F.; Siegers, J.Y.; van der Kroeg, M.; Mumtaz, N.; Stalin Raj, V.; de Vrij, F.M.S.; Widagdo, W.; Gabriel, G.; Salinas, S.; Simonin, Y.; et al. Phenotypic differences between asian and african lineage zika viruses in human neural progenitor cells. *mSphere* **2017**, *2*. [CrossRef] [PubMed]
6. Gaburro, J.; Bhatti, A.; Sundaramoorthy, V.; Dearnley, M.; Green, D.; Nahavandi, S.; Paradkar, P.N.; Duchemin, J.B. Zika virus-induced hyper excitation precedes death of mouse primary neuron. *Virol. J.* **2018**, *15*, 79. [CrossRef]
7. Rosenfeld, A.B.; Doobin, D.J.; Warren, A.L.; Racaniello, V.R.; Vallee, R.B. Replication of early and recent zika virus isolates throughout mouse brain development. *Proc. Natl. Acad. Sci. USA* **2017**, *114*, 12273–12278. [CrossRef]

8. Lazear, H.M.; Govero, J.; Smith, A.M.; Platt, D.J.; Fernandez, E.; Miner, J.J.; Diamond, M.S. A mouse model of zika virus pathogenesis. *Cell host microbe* **2016**, *19*, 720–730. [CrossRef]

9. Rossi, S.L.; Tesh, R.B.; Azar, S.R.; Muruato, A.E.; Hanley, K.A.; Auguste, A.J.; Langsjoen, R.M.; Paessler, S.; Vasilakis, N.; Weaver, S.C. Characterization of a novel murine model to study zika virus. *Am. J. Trop Med. Hyg.* **2016**, *94*, 1362–1369. [CrossRef]

10. Duggal, N.K.; Ritter, J.M.; McDonald, E.M.; Romo, H.; Guirakhoo, F.; Davis, B.S.; Chang, G.J.; Brault, A.C. Differential neurovirulence of african and asian genotype zika virus isolates in outbred immunocompetent mice. *Am. J. Trop Med. Hyg.* **2017**, *97*, 1410–1417. [CrossRef]

11. Manangeeswaran, M.; Ireland, D.D.; Verthelyi, D. Zika (prvabc59) infection is associated with t cell infiltration and neurodegeneration in cns of immunocompetent neonatal c57bl/6 mice. *PLoS pathog.* **2016**, *12*, e1006004. [CrossRef] [PubMed]

12. Van den Pol, A.N.; Mao, G.; Yang, Y.; Ornaghi, S.; Davis, J.N. Zika virus targeting in the developing brain. *J. Neurosci.* **2017**, *37*, 2161–2175. [CrossRef] [PubMed]

13. Fernandes, N.C.; Nogueira, J.S.; Ressio, R.A.; Cirqueira, C.S.; Kimura, L.M.; Fernandes, K.R.; Cunha, M.S.; Souza, R.P.; Guerra, J.M. Experimental zika virus infection induces spinal cord injury and encephalitis in newborn swiss mice. *Exp. Toxicol. Pathol.* **2017**, *69*, 63–71. [CrossRef] [PubMed]

14. Huang, W.C.; Abraham, R.; Shim, B.S.; Choe, H.; Page, D.T. Zika virus infection during the period of maximal brain growth causes microcephaly and corticospinal neuron apoptosis in wild type mice. *Sci. Rep.* **2016**, *6*, 34793. [CrossRef] [PubMed]

15. Garofalo, M.; Condorelli, G.; Croce, C.M. Micrornas in diseases and drug response. *Curr. Opin. Pharmacol.* **2008**, *8*, 661–667. [CrossRef] [PubMed]

16. Junn, E.; Mouradian, M.M. Micrornas in neurodegenerative diseases and their therapeutic potential. *Pharmacol. Ther.* **2012**, *133*, 142–150. [CrossRef] [PubMed]

17. Pauley, K.M.; Chan, E.K. Micrornas and their emerging roles in immunology. *Ann. NY Acad. Sci.* **2008**, *1143*, 226–239. [CrossRef]

18. O'Connell, R.M.; Rao, D.S.; Baltimore, D. Microrna regulation of inflammatory responses. *Annu. Rev. Immunol.* **2012**, *30*, 295–312. [CrossRef]

19. Zhai, A.; Qian, J.; Kao, W.; Li, A.; Li, Y.; He, J.; Zhang, Q.; Song, W.; Fu, Y.; Wu, J.; et al. Borna disease virus encoded phosphoprotein inhibits host innate immunity by regulating mir-155. *Antiviral Res.* **2013**, *98*, 66–75. [CrossRef]

20. Bolisetty, M.T.; Dy, G.; Tam, W.; Beemon, K.L. Reticuloendotheliosis virus strain t induces Mir-155, which targets JARID2 and promotes cell survival. *J. Virol.* **2009**, *83*, 12009–12017. [CrossRef]

21. Swaminathan, G.; Rossi, F.; Sierra, L.J.; Gupta, A.; Navas-Martin, S.; Martin-Garcia, J. A role for microrna-155 modulation in the anti-HIV-1 effects of toll-like receptor 3 stimulation in macrophages. *PLoS Pathog.* **2012**, *8*, e1002937. [CrossRef] [PubMed]

22. Pareek, S.; Roy, S.; Kumari, B.; Jain, P.; Banerjee, A.; Vrati, S. Mir-155 induction in microglial cells suppresses japanese encephalitis virus replication and negatively modulates innate immune responses. *J. Neuroinflammation* **2014**, *11*, 97. [CrossRef] [PubMed]

23. Fabozzi, G.; Nabel, C.S.; Dolan, M.A.; Sullivan, N.J. Ebolavirus proteins suppress the effects of small interfering rna by direct interaction with the mammalian rna interference pathway. *J. Virol.* **2011**, *85*, 2512–2523. [CrossRef]

24. Huang, J.; Wang, F.; Argyris, E.; Chen, K.; Liang, Z.; Tian, H.; Huang, W.; Squires, K.; Verlinghieri, G.; Zhang, H. Cellular micrornas contribute to hiv-1 latency in resting primary CD4+ T lymphocytes. *Nat. Med.* **2007**, *13*, 1241–1247. [CrossRef] [PubMed]

25. Jopling, C.L.; Yi, M.; Lancaster, A.M.; Lemon, S.M.; Sarnow, P. Modulation of hepatitis c virus rna abundance by a liver-specific microrna. *Science* **2005**, *309*, 1577–1581. [CrossRef] [PubMed]

26. Pedersen, I.M.; Cheng, G.; Wieland, S.; Volinia, S.; Croce, C.M.; Chisari, F.V.; David, M. Interferon modulation of cellular micrornas as an antiviral mechanism. *Nature* **2007**, *449*, 919–922. [CrossRef] [PubMed]

27. Bavia, L.; Mosimann, A.L.; Aoki, M.N.; Duarte Dos Santos, C.N. A glance at subgenomic flavivirus rnas and micrornas in flavivirus infections. *Virol. J.* **2016**, *13*, 84. [CrossRef] [PubMed]

28. Zhu, X.; He, Z.; Hu, Y.; Wen, W.; Lin, C.; Yu, J.; Pan, J.; Li, R.; Deng, H.; Liao, S.; et al. MicroRNA-30e* suppresses dengue virus replication by promoting NF-κB -dependent IFN production. *PLoS Negl. Trop Dis.* **2014**, *8*, e3088. [CrossRef]

29. Escalera-Cueto, M.; Medina-Martinez, I.; del Angel, R.M.; Berumen-Campos, J.; Gutierrez-Escolano, A.L.; Yocupicio-Monroy, M. Let-7c overexpression inhibits dengue virus replication in human hepatoma Huh-7 cells. *Virus Res.* **2015**, *196*, 105–112. [CrossRef]

30. Slonchak, A.; Shannon, R.P.; Pali, G.; Khromykh, A.A. Human microrna MiR-532-5p exhibits antiviral activity against west nile virus via suppression of host genes SESTD1 and TAB3 required for virus replication. *J. Virol.* **2015**, *90*, 2388–2402. [CrossRef]

31. Smith, J.L.; Grey, F.E.; Uhrlaub, J.L.; Nikolich-Zugich, J.; Hirsch, A.J. Induction of the cellular microrna, hs_154, by west nile virus contributes to virus-mediated apoptosis through repression of antiapoptotic factors. *J. Virol.* **2012**, *86*, 5278–5287. [CrossRef] [PubMed]

32. Heiss, B.L.; Maximova, O.A.; Pletnev, A.G. Insertion of microrna targets into the flavivirus genome alters its highly neurovirulent phenotype. *J. virol.* **2011**, *85*, 1464–1472. [CrossRef] [PubMed]

33. Kumar, M.; Nerurkar, V.R. Integrated analysis of micrornas and their disease related targets in the brain of mice infected with west nile virus. *Virology* **2014**, *452–453*, 143–151. [CrossRef] [PubMed]

34. Shin, O.S.; Kumar, M.; Yanagihara, R.; Song, J.W. Hantaviruses induce cell type- and viral species-specific host microrna expression signatures. *Virology* **2013**, *446*, 217–224. [CrossRef] [PubMed]

35. Geiss, G.K.; Bumgarner, R.E.; Birditt, B.; Dahl, T.; Dowidar, N.; Dunaway, D.L.; Fell, H.P.; Ferree, S.; George, R.D.; Grogan, T.; et al. Direct multiplexed measurement of gene expression with color-coded probe pairs. *Nat. Biotechnol.* **2008**, *26*, 317–325. [CrossRef] [PubMed]

36. Wakayama, I.; Song, K.J.; Nerurkar, V.R.; Yoshida, S.; Garruto, R.M. Slow dendritic transport of dissociated mouse hippocampal neurons exposed to aluminum. *Brain Res.* **1997**, *748*, 237–240. [CrossRef]

37. Forest, K.H.; Alfulaij, N.; Arora, K.; Taketa, R.; Sherrin, T.; Todorovic, C.; Lawrence, J.L.M.; Yoshikawa, G.T.; Ng, H.L.; Hruby, V.J.; et al. Protection against beta-amyloid neurotoxicity by a non-toxic endogenous n-terminal beta-amyloid fragment and its active hexapeptide core sequence. *J. Neurochem.* **2018**, *144*, 201–217. [CrossRef] [PubMed]

38. Kim, J.A.; Seong, R.K.; Kumar, M.; Shin, O.S. Favipiravir and ribavirin inhibit replication of asian and african strains of zika virus in different cell models. *Viruses* **2018**, *10*, 72. [CrossRef] [PubMed]

39. Kumar, M.; Krause, K.K.; Azouz, F.; Nakano, E.; Nerurkar, V.R. A guinea pig model of zika virus infection. *Virol. J.* **2017**, *14*, 75. [CrossRef] [PubMed]

40. Verma, S.; Lo, Y.; Chapagain, M.; Lum, S.; Kumar, M.; Gurjav, U.; Luo, H.; Nakatsuka, A.; Nerurkar, V.R. West nile virus infection modulates human brain microvascular endothelial cells tight junction proteins and cell adhesion molecules: Transmigration across the in vitro blood-brain barrier. *Virology* **2009**, *385*, 425–433. [CrossRef]

41. Kumar, M.; Belcaid, M.; Nerurkar, V.R. Identification of host genes leading to west nile virus encephalitis in mice brain using RNA-Seq analysis. *Sci. Rep.* **2016**, *6*, 26350. [CrossRef] [PubMed]

42. Kumar, M.; Verma, S.; Nerurkar, V.R. Pro-inflammatory cytokines derived from west nile virus (WNV)-infected SK-N-SH cells mediate neuroinflammatory markers and neuronal death. *J. Neuroinflammation* **2010**, *7*, 73. [CrossRef] [PubMed]

43. Kumar, M.; Roe, K.; Nerurkar, P.V.; Namekar, M.; Orillo, B.; Verma, S.; Nerurkar, V.R. Impaired virus clearance, compromised immune response and increased mortality in type 2 diabetic mice infected with west nile virus. *PLoS ONE* **2012**, *7*, e44682. [CrossRef] [PubMed]

44. Kumar, M.; Roe, K.; Orillo, B.; Muruve, D.A.; Nerurkar, V.R.; Gale, M., Jr.; Verma, S. Inflammasome adaptor protein apoptosis-associated speck-like protein containing card (ASC) is critical for the immune response and survival in west nile virus encephalitis. *J. Virol.* **2013**, *87*, 3655–3667. [CrossRef] [PubMed]

45. Pijlman, G.P. Flavivirus rnai suppression: Decoding non-coding rna. *Curr. Opin. Virol.* **2014**, *7*, 55–60. [CrossRef]

46. Schnettler, E.; Sterken, M.G.; Leung, J.Y.; Metz, S.W.; Geertsema, C.; Goldbach, R.W.; Vlak, J.M.; Kohl, A.; Khromykh, A.A.; Pijlman, G.P. Noncoding flavivirus rna displays rna interference suppressor activity in insect and mammalian cells. *J. Virol.* **2012**, *86*, 13486–13500. [CrossRef]

47. Kakumani, P.K.; Ponia, S.S.; S., R.K.; Sood, V.; Chinnappan, M.; Banerjea, A.C.; Medigeshi, G.R.; Malhotra, P.; Mukherjee, S.K.; Bhatnagar, R.K. Role of RNA interference (RNAi) in dengue virus replication and identification of ns4b as an rnai suppressor. *J. Virol.* **2013**, *87*, 8870–8883. [CrossRef]

48. Moon, S.L.; Dodd, B.J.; Brackney, D.E.; Wilusz, C.J.; Ebel, G.D.; Wilusz, J. Flavivirus sfrna suppresses antiviral rna interference in cultured cells and mosquitoes and directly interacts with the rnai machinery. *Virology* **2015**, *485*, 322–329. [CrossRef]

49. Fredericksen, B.L. The neuroimmune response to west nile virus. *J. Neurovirol.* **2014**, *20*, 113–121. [CrossRef]

50. Fredericksen, B.L.; Keller, B.C.; Fornek, J.; Katze, M.G.; Gale, M., Jr. Establishment and maintenance of the innate antiviral response to west nile virus involves both rig-i and mda5 signaling through IPS-1. *J. Virol.* **2008**, *82*, 609–616. [CrossRef]

51. Errett, J.S.; Suthar, M.S.; McMillan, A.; Diamond, M.S.; Gale, M., Jr. The essential, nonredundant roles of rig-i and mda5 in detecting and controlling west nile virus infection. *J. Virol.* **2013**, *87*, 11416–11425. [CrossRef] [PubMed]

52. Akira, S.; Uematsu, S.; Takeuchi, O. Pathogen recognition and innate immunity. *Cell* **2006**, *124*, 783–801. [CrossRef] [PubMed]

53. Kaushik, D.K.; Gupta, M.; Kumawat, K.L.; Basu, A. Nlrp3 inflammasome: Key mediator of neuroinflammation in murine japanese encephalitis. *PLoS ONE* **2012**, *7*, e32270. [CrossRef] [PubMed]

54. Diamond, M.S.; Gale, M., Jr. Cell-intrinsic innate immune control of west nile virus infection. *Trends Immunol.* **2012**, *33*, 522–530. [CrossRef] [PubMed]

55. Qin, Z.; Wang, P.Y.; Su, D.F.; Liu, X. Mirna-124 in immune system and immune disorders. *Front. Immunol.* **2016**, *7*, 406. [CrossRef] [PubMed]

56. Jiang, M.; Broering, R.; Trippler, M.; Wu, J.; Zhang, E.; Zhang, X.; Gerken, G.; Lu, M.; Schlaak, J.F. Microrna-155 controls toll-like receptor 3- and hepatitis C virus-induced immune responses in the liver. *J. Viral. Hepat.* **2014**, *21*, 99–110. [CrossRef] [PubMed]

57. Dickey, L.L.; Hanley, T.M.; Huffaker, T.B.; Ramstead, A.G.; O'Connell, R.M.; Lane, T.E. MicroRNA 155 and viral-induced neuroinflammation. *J. Neuroimmunol.* **2017**, *308*, 17–24. [CrossRef]

58. Thounaojam, M.C.; Kaushik, D.K.; Kundu, K.; Basu, A. MicroRNA-29b modulates japanese encephalitis virus-induced microglia activation by targeting tumor necrosis factor alpha-induced protein 3. *J. Neurochem.* **2014**, *129*, 143–154. [CrossRef] [PubMed]

59. Buggele, W.A.; Horvath, C.M. Microrna profiling of sendai virus-infected a549 cells identifies MiR-203 as an interferon-inducible regulator of IFIT1/ISG56. *J. Virol.* **2013**, *87*, 9260–9270. [CrossRef] [PubMed]

60. Zhang, S.; Li, J.; Li, J.; Yang, Y.; Kang, X.; Li, Y.; Wu, X.; Zhu, Q.; Zhou, Y.; Hu, Y. Upregulation of microrna-203 in influenza A virus infection inhibits viral replication by targeting dr1. *Sci. Rep.* **2018**, *8*, 6797. [CrossRef]

61. Song, M.S.; Rossi, J.J. Molecular mechanisms of dicer: Endonuclease and enzymatic activity. *Biochem. J.* **2017**, *474*, 1603–1618. [CrossRef] [PubMed]

62. Kozak, R.A.; Majer, A.; Biondi, M.J.; Medina, S.J.; Goneau, L.W.; Sajesh, B.V.; Slota, J.A.; Zubach, V.; Severini, A.; Safronetz, D.; et al. MicroRNA and mRNA dysregulation in astrocytes infected with zika virus. *Viruses* **2017**, *9*, 297. [CrossRef] [PubMed]

63. Saldana, M.A.; Etebari, K.; Hart, C.E.; Widen, S.G.; Wood, T.G.; Thangamani, S.; Asgari, S.; Hughes, G.L. Zika virus alters the microrna expression profile and elicits an rnai response in aedes aegypti mosquitoes. *PLoS Negl. Trop Dis.* **2017**, *11*, e0005760. [CrossRef] [PubMed]

64. Ferreira, R.N.; Holanda, G.M.; Pinto Silva, E.V.; Casseb, S.M.M.; Melo, K.F.L.; Carvalho, C.A.M.; Lima, J.A.; Vasconcelos, P.F.C.; Cruz, A.C.R. Zika virus alters the expression profile of microrna-related genes in liver, lung, and kidney cell lineages. *Viral. Immunol.* **2018**, *31*, 583–588. [CrossRef] [PubMed]

65. Lu, F.; Weidmer, A.; Liu, C.G.; Volinia, S.; Croce, C.M.; Lieberman, P.M. Epstein–Barr virus-induced mir-155 attenuates NF-KB signaling and stabilizes latent virus persistence. *J.Virol.* **2008**, *82*, 10436–10443. [CrossRef] [PubMed]

66. Tili, E.; Croce, C.M.; Michaille, J.J. Mir-155: On the crosstalk between inflammation and cancer. *Int. Rev. Immunol.* **2009**, *28*, 264–284. [CrossRef] [PubMed]

67. Thounaojam, M.C.; Kundu, K.; Kaushik, D.K.; Swaroop, S.; Mahadevan, A.; Shankar, S.K.; Basu, A. MicroRNA 155 regulates Japanese encephalitis virus-induced inflammatory response by targeting src homology 2-containing inositol phosphatase 1. *J. Virol.* **2014**, *88*, 4798–4810. [CrossRef] [PubMed]

68. Sun, Y.; Luo, Z.M.; Guo, X.M.; Su, D.F.; Liu, X. An updated role of microrna-124 in central nervous system disorders: A review. *Front. Cell Neurosci.* **2015**, *9*, 193. [CrossRef] [PubMed]

69. Papagiannakopoulos, T.; Kosik, K.S. MicroRNA-124: Micromanager of neurogenesis. *Cell Stem Cell* **2009**, *4*, 375–376. [CrossRef]

70. Roy, B.; Dunbar, M.; Shelton, R.C.; Dwivedi, Y. Identification of microRNA-124-3p as a putative epigenetic signature of major depressive disorder. *Neuropsychopharmacology* **2017**, *42*, 864–875. [CrossRef]
71. Ge, Q.; Gerard, J.; Noel, L.; Scroyen, I.; Brichard, S.M. MicroRNAs regulated by adiponectin as novel targets for controlling adipose tissue inflammation. *Endocrinology* **2012**, *153*, 5285–5296. [CrossRef] [PubMed]
72. Meissner, L.; Gallozzi, M.; Balbi, M.; Schwarzmaier, S.; Tiedt, S.; Terpolilli, N.A.; Plesnila, N. Temporal profile of microRNA expression in contused cortex after traumatic brain injury in mice. *J. Neurotrauma.* **2016**, *33*, 713–720. [CrossRef] [PubMed]

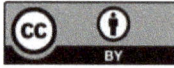

![viruses logo] *viruses*

MDPI

Review

Zika Virus in the Male Reproductive Tract

Liesel Stassen [iD], Charles W. Armitage, David J. van der Heide, Kenneth W. Beagley
and Francesca D. Frentiu * [iD]

Institute of Health and Biomedical Innovation, and School of Biomedical Sciences,
Queensland University of Technology, Brisbane 4006, Queensland, Australia; liesel.stassen@qut.edu.au (L.S.);
charles.armitage@qut.edu.au (C.W.A.); d.vanderheide@qut.edu.au (D.J.v.d.H.); k2.beagley@qut.edu.au (K.W.B.)
* Correspondence: francesca.frentiu@qut.edu.au; Tel.: +61-731-386-185

Received: 19 March 2018; Accepted: 13 April 2018; Published: 16 April 2018

Abstract: Arthropod-borne viruses (arboviruses) are resurging across the globe. Zika virus (ZIKV) has caused significant concern in recent years because it can lead to congenital malformations in babies and Guillain-Barré syndrome in adults. Unlike other arboviruses, ZIKV can be sexually transmitted and may persist in the male reproductive tract. There is limited information regarding the impact of ZIKV on male reproductive health and fertility. Understanding the mechanisms that underlie persistent ZIKV infections in men is critical to developing effective vaccines and therapies. Mouse and macaque models have begun to unravel the pathogenesis of ZIKV infection in the male reproductive tract, with the testes and prostate gland implicated as potential reservoirs for persistent ZIKV infection. Here, we summarize current knowledge regarding the pathogenesis of ZIKV in the male reproductive tract, the development of animal models to study ZIKV infection at this site, and prospects for vaccines and therapeutics against persistent ZIKV infection.

Keywords: flavivirus; arbovirus; Zika; sexual transmission; testis; prostate

---

1. Emergence of Zika Virus

Zika virus (ZIKV), a previously obscure and scientifically neglected virus, became a serious public health concern in 2015 due to an association with microcephaly (refer to Glossary) in Brazil [1]. ZIKV is a positive-sense, nonsegmented, enveloped, single-stranded RNA virus that belongs to the *flavivirus* genus within the *Flaviviridae* family [2,3]. The genus also includes other medically important flaviviruses such as dengue, yellow fever, West Nile, and Japanese encephalitis viruses [2,4]. The virion is spherical with an icosahedral symmetry and approximately 50 nm in diameter [2,3]. The C protein comprises the viral capsid which is surrounded by a lipid bilayer derived from the host, and the M and E proteins are anchored in the outer surface membrane. The 10.8 Kb ssRNA genome comprises a 5′ untranslated region (UTR), a single open reading frame, and a 3′ UTR. The open reading frame encodes a single polyprotein which is cleaved into the structural (C, prM and E) and nonstructural (NS1, NS2A, NS2B, NS3, NS4A, NS4B, and NS5) proteins [2,3]. ZIKV is an arthropod-borne virus (arbovirus) that is mainly transmitted to humans through the bite of mosquitoes [5,6], specifically *Aedes aegypti* and *Aedes albopictus* species [4]. ZIKV was first isolated from sentinel monkeys in Uganda in 1947 [7], and thereafter several ZIKV isolates were sampled from *Aedes africanus* mosquitoes [5]. Since the first reported human cases in 1952 [8], ZIKV has been sporadically detected in equatorial Africa and Asia over the next five decades [9,10]. Prior to 2007, only 14 human cases had ever been reported and ZIKV had been regarded as an arbovirus with mild clinical symptoms and inconsequential sequelae [11,12] that typically involved headache, fever, rash, conjunctivitis, arthralgia, and myalgia [2,11,13]. Fifty to 80% of infections remain asymptomatic [11,14,15]. Three genotypes of the virus have been identified: East African, West African, and Asian [13].

The first large outbreaks of ZIKV occurred in 2007 on the island of Yap in Micronesia, as the virus moved from Asia to the Pacific. The Yap outbreak is estimated to have affected ~73% of Yap residents older than three years of age [11,13]. The Yap outbreak was followed by a second large outbreak, this time in French Polynesia, during 2013–2014 [16,17]. During the French Polynesian outbreak, Guillain-Barré syndrome (GBS) was linked to ZIKV infection for the first time [18]. In May 2015, the World Health Organization (WHO) received the first reports of locally-transmitted ZIKV in Brazil [19]. In February 2016, due to the rapid expansion of ZIKV and a suspected causal relationship between the virus and microcephaly in Brazil, the WHO declared ZIKV a public health emergency of international concern. The epidemics in the Pacific and the Americas have seen increased rates of congenital neural abnormalities such as microcephaly, malformations of cortical development, brain calcifications, and hearing and vision loss [1,17,20–22], with infection often resulting in fetal demise during pregnancy [22,23]. Retrospective investigations of the 2013–2014 French Polynesian outbreak have linked microcephaly in newborns to ZIKV [17]. In adults, infection may lead to GBS [24,25], encephalitis [26], thrombocytopenia [27], and ocular and auditory disturbances [28]. To date, 84 countries have been affected, with almost one million cases, and at least 23 countries have reported a surge in the incidence of GBS (WHO, 10 March 2017).

2. Sexual Transmission of ZIKV

Probable sexual transmission of ZIKV was first reported in 2011 when a scientist, who had contracted the virus while working in Senegal in 2008, infected his wife after returning home [29]. This was the first report of sexual transmission for any arbovirus to date. Since then, at least 14 countries outside the endemic range of ZIKV have reported person-to-person transmission of the virus (Figure 1). Both Asian and African genotypes of ZIKV have been reported to be sexually transmitted [29,30], suggesting that this mode of transmission appeared early in the evolution of the virus and prior to the divergence of genotypes [31]. Male-to-male [32], female-to-male [33], and male-to-female [29,30,34,35] cases of sexual transmission have been documented, with the latter being the most common [36]. Sexual transmission from men with no obvious symptoms has also been reported [37,38], although the prevalence is unclear since asymptomatic cases are inherently difficult to identify. Mathematical models predict the contribution of sexual transmission to the spread of ZIKV to be 3–4.8% [39,40]. However, one recent study suggests the risk of sustained sexual transmission may be much higher [41]. Differences in the age- and sex-specific attack rates of ZIKV have been observed, with women of childbearing age having the highest incidence of infection [36,42]. However, reporting bias may partially account for this pattern, as more women than men may have sought diagnosis due to increased fear of infection during pregnancy [39]. Although sexual transmission is unlikely to lead to sustained cycles of infection in areas without mosquito vectors, it could increase the likelihood of outbreaks occurring, and the size and duration of epidemics [39–41,43,44].

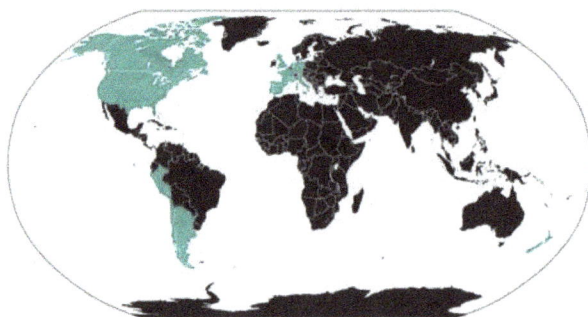

Figure 1. Countries outside of the endemic range of ZIKV that have reported cases of sexual transmission, 2011–2018 (shown in green).

3. Persistent Shedding of ZIKV in Semen

ZIKV RNA has been detected in the semen of symptomatically [35,45–49] and asymptomatically-infected [50,51] men, sometimes for many months post onset of infection. Very high concentrations of ZIKV RNA can be found in semen during the clinically symptomatic phase of the infection [30]. One study has shown that up to 73% of infected men have detectable ZIKV RNA in their semen over the short term [48]. ZIKV has also been found attached to sperm [48,49,52,53], in particular to the mid-piece of mature spermatozoa [53], suggesting this could be a route of infection in addition to semen. The infectivity and longevity of ZIKV in semen varies [51]. The risk of sexual transmission by men is particularly high in the first few weeks of infection [54], with the median time between sexual contact and onset of symptoms in women estimated to be 9.5 days [43]. Persistent viral replication and shedding of infectious virus could, however, prolong this risk. Viral RNA and infectious virus have been detected in semen for up to 6 months [47] and 69 days [51,54] post-infection, respectively. Most studies have reported the presence of viral RNA in semen rather than infectious titers, possibly due to the difficulty of culturing viable virus from this fluid. How long infectious ZIKV persists in semen is therefore unclear. Nonetheless, the longevity of infectious ZIKV in semen, compared to vaginal fluids [55], indicates viral seeding and local replication occur in the genital organs and cells of the male reproductive tract (MRT). Persistently infected males may therefore be acting as potential reservoirs of ZIKV, which could account for some of the observed asymmetry in sexual transmission [36,41].

4. The MRT and Immune Privilege

Persistent viral replication and shedding of infectious virus from organs of the male reproductive tract (Figure 2A) could prolong the risk of sexual transmission [56]. Some regions of the MRT offer an immune-privileged environment that may lead to lowered fertility if disrupted by infection. Maintenance of immune privilege in the testis, the major organ where sperm are produced and androgens synthesized, is essential for healthy spermatogenesis. Within the testis, developing sperm are also protected from autoimmune attack by a physical blood-testis-barrier (BTB) formed by tight junctions between adjacent Sertoli cells that prevent immunoglobulin entry into the lumen (Figure 2B). An immune-privileged environment is also achieved through the suppression of normal immune responses that could lead to inflammation [57–60]. During male adolescence and throughout adult life, germ cells in the testes divide and differentiate to produce spermatogonia that are released into the lumen of the seminiferous tubules (Figure 2B). Immature sperm then travel to the epididymis and vas deferens where they mature and remain until ejaculation. Spermatozoa in the testes and regions of the epididymis are isolated from the host adaptive immune system to prevent the development of anti-sperm lymphocytes and, importantly, the production of anti-sperm antibodies (ASA). This immunosuppressive environment is enabled by the sequestration of antigens in phagocytosing Sertoli cells and testicular macrophages, downregulation of antigen presentation by macrophages and dendritic cells in the draining lymphatics, and the tight barrier formation between adjacent Sertoli cells preventing permeability of immunoglobulin [60]. Disruption of key cells involved in spermatogenesis, such as Sertoli and Leydig cells (Figure 2B), through infection and loss of immune privilege, could lead to autoimmune attack of spermatozoa and development of ASA, thereby lowering fertility.

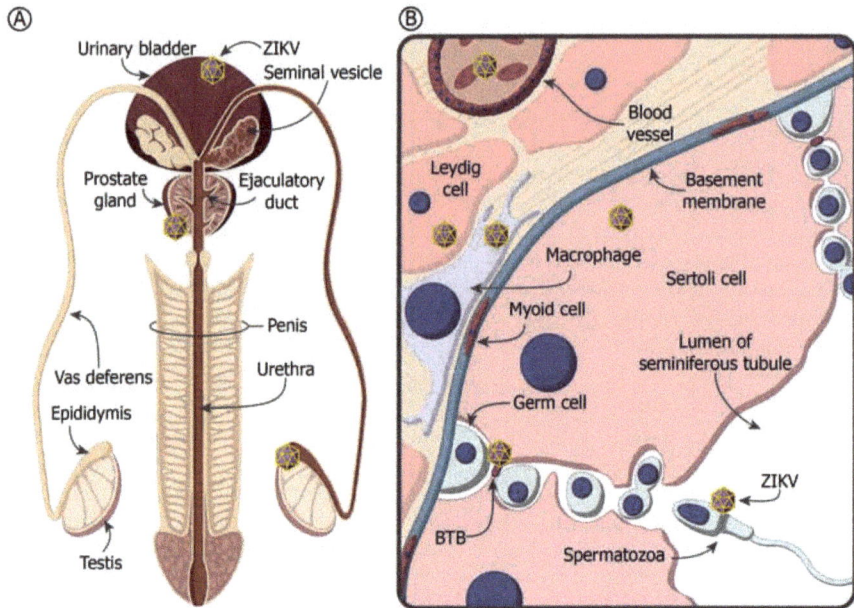

Figure 2. (**A**) Schematic representation of the male reproductive tract indicating potential ZIKV reservoirs. (**B**) Cross section of a portion of the seminiferous tubule within the testis. The seminiferous tubules contain the developing sperm cells and their supporting Sertoli cells. Sertoli cells form the lumen of the seminiferous tubules for release and transport of spermatozoa into the epididymis. Surrounding the seminiferous tubules are one or more continuous layers of peritubular myoid cells that function in the expulsion of spermatozoa out of the tubules and into the epididymis. The basement membranes of the seminiferous tubules are linked by tight junctions that, coupled with the myoid cells, form the blood-testis barrier (BTB). The interstitial compartment located between the tubules contains the Leydig cells, which are also essential for normal sperm development, maintenance of the blood-testis barrier, immune privilege, and Sertoli-germ cell junction assembly and disassembly.

5. ZIKV in the Testis and Prostate Gland

Prostatitis, hematospermia, and microhematospermia have been reported in ZIKV-infected men [29,34,61,62], as well as the presence of leukocytes in semen that is suggestive of inflammation in the MRT [62]. ZIKV may be breaching the BTB, disrupting immune privilege in the testes and replicating at these sites. ZIKV-infected human Sertoli cells show enhanced expression of cytokines and cell-adhesion molecules, increasing the adhesion of leukocytes and permeability of the BTB [63]. Inflammatory mediators released by ZIKV-infected testicular macrophages could also compromise the integrity of the BTB [63]. Low sperm counts have been observed in ZIKV-infected men [48,49,62], indicating that infection in the testis may be affecting sperm production. The lack of a correlation between the highest ZIKV loads in semen and serum [64] suggests that localized ZIKV replication occurs in the testicles and/or seminal glands [49]. The receptors used by ZIKV to enter the different cell types present in the MRT remain to be elucidated. However, the tyrosin kinase Axl is a major candidate entry receptor for ZIKV [65–68] and is expressed throughout the MRT, including the testes (particularly in Sertoli cells), the epididymis, and the prostate [69]. Axl is also an essential regulator in spermatogenesis [69]. Imaging of ZIKV-infected semen samples found that the virus colocalized to the Tyro3 receptor expressed at the mid-piece of mature spermatozoa, suggesting a role in ZIKV binding and entry [53]. Interestingly, Tyro3 receptors serve as entry ligands for Ebola and Marburg viruses [70], which have also been isolated from human semen and can be sexually transmitted [71].

Other as yet unidentified cell surface receptors may exist that could account for the tropism and sexual transmission of ZIKV.

The immunochemical detection of ZIKV inside the spermatozoa of a patient [49], as well as virus detection, isolation, and sexual transmission in the absence of spermatozoa [38,72,73], indicate that ZIKV could be present in semen as free virus particles or associated with cells. In the latter case, ZIKV could be transmitted to sperm by infected Sertoli cells, or virus particles could adsorb or penetrate spermatozoa during epididymal transit. The length of time required for sperm development in the seminiferous tubule (~2 months), relative to sperm maturation in the epididymis (~2 weeks), suggests most infectious virus could be acquired during the latter phase. However, additional studies are needed to determine the exact fate of ZIKV virions in the MRT.

Virus may also be present in semen as a result of viral replication in the male accessory glands [71]. Sexual transmission of ZIKV from a vasectomized male to his female partner has recently been reported [72]. The presence of ZIKV in the semen of vasectomized men [72,73] has strongly implicated the prostate and seminal vesicles as potential reservoirs facilitating sexual transmission. Recently, in vitro infection of human prostate stromal, epithelial cells, and organoids demonstrated that ZIKV, but not dengue virus, actively infects and replicates in these cells, producing infectious virus in significant quantities [74]. The prostate is a strong candidate organ for prolonged viral shedding because it can host chronic infections with a variety of pathogens [56] and contributes a large proportion of seminal fluid during ejaculation [75].

6. Mouse Models of ZIKV in the MRT

Mice have proved the most tractable model to investigate ZIKV in the MRT, with a plethora of recent studies (Table 1) [31,52,76–90]. However, as ZIKV does not naturally replicate and cause disease in wild-type mice, studies of ZIKV pathogenesis have primarily utilized immunodeficient mice (Table 1). In such mouse models, the antiviral immune response is impaired, allowing replication and dissemination of ZIKV into different organs and tissues. Mouse models of sexual transmission have indicated the presence of infectious virus in 60–70% of ejaculates [31,79,84], and male-to-female sexual transmission in 50% of all matings [84]. Additionally, sexual transmission resulted in significantly greater morbidity and mortality and higher ZIKV titers in the female reproductive tract than subcutaneous or intravaginal inoculation [91]. A study using vasectomized mice showed that sexual transmission of ZIKV still occurred, despite semen containing significantly lower levels of infectious virus [84]. Overall, studies of pathogenesis in the MRT of mice have detected ZIKV in the testes [31,52,76–86,88–90] of all animals tested and the epididymis [31,52,76–78,80,84,86–89] of most mice (Table 1). ZIKV was also detected in the seminal fluid inside the lumen of the vas deferens [80] and the seminal vesicles [31,84,89] of some infected mice (Table 1). Although most studies did not investigate prostate tissues, one team reported negative results for ZIKV in the prostate [77], whereas two others did detect virus in this gland [88,89].

Androgen levels were altered in infected mice [79], concordant with ZIKV-induced reproductive hormone changes reported in men [48]. Inhibin B [76] and testosterone levels [76–78] were significantly decreased in mice, likely due to Leydig cell infection and apoptosis [76,78]. Furthermore, mouse ZIKV infection typically results in disruption of the BTB [77,86], breakdown of the epithelium and seminiferous tubules [76,77,79,86–88,90], inflammation and tissue injury to the epididymis and testis [76,77,80,83,84,87,89], and testicular atrophy [31,76–78,81,82,87]. Cytokine production within the testis, as well as infiltration of inflammatory cells, immune cells, and macrophages into this organ, seminiferous and epididymal tubules were observed [76,77,84,86–88]. ZIKV infection in mouse models also resulted in altered sperm morphology and motility, an absence of spermatozoa or reduction in total sperm counts, and a measurable reduction in fertility [52,76–79,81,87].

Testicular cells contribute much of the infectious virus shed in the seminal fluid of mice [84], however, mouse studies offer conflicting evidence regarding which exact cell types are targeted. In agreement with reports that human primary Sertoli cells support persistent ZIKV replication for at least six weeks [63,68], some mouse studies report Sertoli cells to be the major targets for ZIKV in testes [76,79,87,89,92]. Other studies report Leydig and myoid cells to be completely destroyed, resulting in the reduction in testosterone production and testicular atrophy in mice [77,78]. Virions attached to developing and mature sperm in the testes and epididymis, respectively, have been observed by transmission electron microscopy [52]. Some mouse models suggest that ZIKV infected cells are likely to be germinal spermatogonia or primary spermatocytes [76,77,83,84]. However, the detection of virus in epididymal spermatozoa 7 days post-infection strongly suggests that ZIKV directly infects spermatozoa in the epididymal lumen [76]. Sperm may therefore serve as a vehicle to transmit ZIKV in addition to semen.

The observed difference in disease manifestation and severity between different mouse models could, in part, be explained by the use of varying mouse strains and ages at infection [89], ZIKV genotype, and virus dose and inoculation routes [76,85,86]. Although some of the key phenotypes observed in humans are recapitulated in immunodeficient mice, there are inherent limitations to using mouse models for the study of persistent ZIKV infection in the MRT. Compared to ZIKV-infected men [48,49], the injury to the MRT observed in mice is much more severe, and spermatogenesis more drastically affected [76,77]. Furthermore, the role of human immunity in ZIKV pathogenesis cannot be fully captured in immunodeficient mouse models. Using nonlethal mouse models [80,89] that allow for the long-term study of ZIKV infection kinetics and pathological progression, with an antibody response similar to macaques [85], could offer a way forward.

7. Primate Models of ZIKV Pathogenesis in the MRT

Rhesus, cynomolgus, and pig-tailed macaques have been shown to be susceptible to a variety of ZIKV strains [93–98] and have been used to study ZIKV tropism and test ZIKV vaccine platforms [44,94,97–99]. Macaque models have been suggested as an alternative to mice because they develop clinical symptoms, viremia, widespread tissue infection, and a robust adaptive immune response comparable to human infection [93,95,98,100,101]. Clinical symptoms in infected macaques are generally mild [93,98,102], with plasma viremia peaking 2 to 6 days after infection and resolving within 10 to 14 days [93,95,97,102]. Infected rhesus macaques developed ZIKV-specific humoral and cell-mediated immune responses [93–95,102], protecting them from re-challenge with either homologous or heterologous ZIKV strains [97,102]. Both vector [93,95–97] and sexual [44] transmission routes have been studied in macaques. Asymmetry in ZIKV infectivity between males and females has also been observed in macaques [44]. Using in situ hybridization and quantitative reverse transcription PCR (RT-PCR) analysis to detect viral RNA, ZIKV dissemination into many tissues has been observed in macaques, including to the urogenital tract and shedding into mucosal secretions [94,95,98,100]. ZIKV persistence in the testes [95,100] and shedding of infectious virus in the semen [95] have been demonstrated. Importantly, the high viral load present in the testes of macaques, long after the systemic viral load has resolved [95,100], indicates that virus might be replicating at these anatomical sites. Immunohistochemistry of infected testes has shown virus localizing to Sertoli cells [95]. In addition, ZIKV has been detected in the seminal vesicles and prostate of rhesus and cynomolgus macaques for up to 35 days post infection [95,98]. However, not all studies using rhesus macaques have been able to detect ZIKV RNA in the testes [98], epididymis, and prostate [94]. Interestingly, pathogenesis studies have also detected ZIKV RNA in the kidney, bladder and urine [95,98], suggesting that ZIKV may also seed into semen from the urethra. The impact of ZIKV infection seems much less pronounced in immunocompetent macaque models versus mice. Although none of these macaque studies report the impact of ZIKV infection on testis structure and integrity and fertility, they clearly show that viral shedding continues unabated in the MRT.

Table 1. ZIKV localization in mouse models of MRT pathogenesis.

Mouse Genotype (Background)	ZIKV Genotype (Strain)	Inoculation Route	Testis (Infected Cells)	Epididymis	Seminal Vesicles	Vas Deferens	Prostate	Ref.
Wild Type (BALB/c) Dexamethasone Tx	Asian (PRVABC59)	IP	+ (ND)	+	ND	ND	+	[88]
Wild Type (C57BL/6) + anti-IFNαβR mAb	Asian (H/FP/2013)	SC	+ (SG, PS, ST, LC)	+	ND	ND	ND	[76]
	Afr (Dakar 41519)	SC	+ (SG, PS, ST, LC)	+	ND	ND	ND	[76]
Rag1−/− (C57BL/6) + anti-IFNαβR mAb	Asian (Paraiba_01/2015)	IP	+ (SG, PS)	ND	ND	ND	ND	[83]
Ifnar1−/− (C57BL/6)	Asian (ZIKV_SMGC-1)	IP	+ (LC, GC, PMC, SG)	+	−	ND	−	[77]
	Asian (Mex2-81)	SC	+ (LC)	+	ND	ND	ND	[78]
	Asian (PRVABC59)	SC	+ (ND)	ND	ND	ND	ND	[82]
	Asian (PRVABC59)	SC	+ (ST, MSC)	+	ND	ND	ND	[87]
	Asian (H/FP/2013)	SC	+ (ND)	ND	ND	ND	ND	[85]
	Asian (PRVABC59)	SC	+ (ST)	+	−	ND	+	[89]
	Asian (Mex2-81)	SC	+ (SG)	+	ND	ND	ND	[52]
	Asian (ZIKV_Natal)	SC	+(ND)	ND	ND	ND	ND	[90]
(A129)	Asian (PRVABC59)	SC	+ (ND)	−	ND	ND	ND	[86]
	Asian (PRVABC59)	IP	+ (ND)	ND	ND	ND	ND	[51]
	African (MP1751)	SC	+ (ND)	+	ND	ND	ND	[86]
Ifnar1−/− × Ifngr−/− (AG129)	Asian (PRVABC59)	SC	+ (LC)	+	+	ND	+	[89]
	Asian (PRVABC59/FSS13025/P6-740)	SC	+ (ND)	+	+	ND	ND	[31]
	Asian (PRVABC59)	IP	+ (SG)	+	+	ND	ND	[84]
	African (Dakar 41524)	SC	+ (ND)	+	+	ND	ND	[31]
(AG6)	Asian (CAS-ZK01)	SC	+ (ST, MC)	ND	ND	ND	ND	[79]
Irf3−/− × Irf7−/− (C57BL/6)	African (MR766)	SC	+ (GC)	+	ND	+	ND	[80]

Abbreviations: Afr, African; mAb, monoclonal antibodies; SC, subcutaneous; IP, intraperitoneally; ND, not determined; SG, spermatogonia; PS, primary spermatocyte; ST, Sertoli cells; LC, Leydig cells; GC, germ cells; PMC, peritubular-myoid cells; MSC, maturing spermatogenic cells; MC, macrophage cells; + and −, detected and not detected, respectively. ZIKV Strains: PRVABC59 (Puerto Rico, 2015); H/FP/2013 (French Polynesia, 2013); Dakar 41519 (Senegal, 1984); Paraiba_01/2015 (Paraiba, 2015); ZIKV_SMGC-1 (Fiji and Samoa, 2016); Mex2-81 (Mexico, 2016); ZIKV_Natal (Brazil, 2015); MP1751 (Uganda, 1962); Dakar 41524 (Senegal, 1984); FSS13025 (Cambodia, 2010); P6-740 (Malaysia, 1966); CAS-ZK01 (Institute of Microbiology, Chinese Academy of Sciences, Beijing, China); MR766 (Uganda, 1947).

8. Implications for the Development of Therapeutics and Vaccines

Reservoirs of persistent infection in the MRT could complicate the development of vaccines, antivirals, and/or other therapeutics for ZIKV. Proposed interventions and vaccines [103] need to be evaluated in their ability to clear persistent infection in the immune-privileged sites such as the male gonad. Evidence from HIV suggests that the testes may represent a distinctive virus sanctuary site in patients receiving suppressive antiviral therapy, with lingering virus detected in the testicles despite the virus been cleared from the bloodstream [104]. In this regard, although the antiviral Ribavirin was recently shown to suppress viremia in ZIKV-infected STAT1-deficient mice [105], it failed to suppress viral load in the brain, another immune-privileged site. Several compounds have shown promise as ZIKV prophylactic and therapeutic agents in vitro [66,68]. The antibiotic azithromycin has been shown to reduce ZIKV proliferation and cytopathic effects in vitro in glial cell lines, human astrocytes, and Sertoli cells [66,68]. Further studies are needed to investigate their effectiveness in vivo. Recently, the basic fibroblast growth factor (FGF2) was shown to be significantly upregulated in ZIKV-infected human Sertoli cells and to enhance viral replication and persistence [68]. Pre-treatment of Sertoli cells with either a neutralizing antibody to FGF2 or a FGF receptor inhibitor significantly inhibited ZIKV replication without affecting cell viability [68], thus indicating the therapeutic potential of FGF receptor antagonists.

A successful vaccine must provoke a subclass of immunoglobulin (IgG) inside the seminiferous tubules, as it has been proposed that only certain subclasses of IgG (i.e., IgG4) can cross the BTB [53]. Antibody treatments have shown promise in providing protection against persistent ZIKV infection. Human antibodies to the dengue virus E-dimer epitope (EDE1-B10), in addition to their inhibitory effects against dengue virus, have shown therapeutic potential against ZIKV [106]. EDE1-B10 treatment administered 1 to 3 days post infection was able to reduce viral persistence in the brain and testis, protect against ZIKV-induced inflammation, and damage to the seminiferous tubules, and preserve sperm counts [106]. The treatment, however, failed when administered 5 days after ZIKV infection. Polyclonal antibody treatment given 1 day prior to challenge [82], as well as live-attenuated and DNA-based vaccines [81,87], have protected mice against testicular atrophy and damage. In addition, DNA-based vaccines have been shown to induce sterilizing immunity against ZIKV challenge [99,107,108]. A vaccinia-based single vector construct, multi-pathogen vaccine, which encodes the structural polyprotein cassettes of both Zika and chikungunya (CHIKV) viruses, has recently been developed [90]. A single vaccination of *Ifnar1*$^{-/-}$ mice induced neutralizing antibodies to both viruses and protected mice from CHIKV and ZIKV infection and disease, including testicular infection and pathology in males [90]. Vaccination resulted in complete clearance of ZIKV RNA in the testes from challenged male *Ifnar1*$^{-/-}$ mice [90]. Initial murine studies have rapidly translated to clinical trials and have demonstrated that humans also develop neutralizing antibodies to the vaccine, which can provide passive immunity to mice during lethal ZIKV challenge [109]. Whilst a prophylactic ZIKV vaccine is achievable, the efficacy of current candidates as a therapeutic vaccine for chronically infected males remains unknown. The limited amount of immunoglobulin and lymphocytic infiltrate in the testes during infection may impede the success of current approaches.

9. Concluding Remarks and Future Prospects

Numerous questions regarding ZIKV infection in the MRT remain as yet unanswered (Box 1). The long-term effects of persistent ZIKV infection on male reproductive function, as well as on sperm production and fertility, including those exposed in utero, remain to be investigated. Of note, cryptorchidia, hypospadias, and micropenis have been described in newborns from infected mothers [110], but their prevalence is unknown. Although questions regarding pathogenesis can be answered using functional studies in animals, any effect of ZIKV infection on male fertility will only be detected with long-term epidemiological studies. Asymptomatic, persistent ZIKV replication in men and cryptic sexual transmission remain a risk to conception, given the large number of ZIKV infections that are silent. ZIKV-infected reproductive tissue (e.g., infected sperm) could pose a threat to patients seeking fertility services. Prospective studies of infected men are starting to reveal how long travelers from ZIKV-endemic areas should wait before trying to conceive naturally, donate gametes, or proceed with fertility treatments. Such data will aid in formulating appropriate public health guidelines to mitigate the risk of ZIKV infection through sexual transmission.

Box 1. Key questions remaining to be answered regarding ZIKV in the MRT.

- What are the cellular and molecular mechanisms of ZIKV persistence in the MRT?
- What is the origin of ZIKV in semen?
- What is the ZIKV entry receptor in the MRT?
- Which cells in the MRT are primarily infected following ZIKV attachment and entry?
- What are the viral and host characteristics that influence the infectivity and longevity of ZIKV in semen?

Acknowledgments: This collaborative review was facilitated by a Queensland University of Technology Institute for Health and Biomedical Innovation Mid-Career Researcher Development grant awarded to Francesca D. Frentiu in 2017.

Conflicts of Interest: The authors declare no conflict of interest.

Glossary

Arthralgia	Non-inflammatory joint pain.
Blood-testis-barrier	Physical barrier between blood vessels and the Sertoli cells of the seminiferous tubules in the mammalian testes.
Conjunctivitis	Inflammation of the outer layer of the eye and inside of the eyelid that causes the eye to turn pink.
Cryptorchidia	Condition in which one or both of the testes fail to descend from the abdomen into the scrotum.
Encephalitis	Inflammation of the brain.
Epididymis	Highly convoluted duct behind the testis, along which sperm passes to the vas deferens.
Guillain-Barré syndrome (GBS)	Autoimmune disease where antibodies and lymphocytes attack and damage the peripheral nerves causing weakness/paralysis and/or abnormal sensations and pain.
Hematospermia	Blood in the semen.
Hypospadias	A congenital condition in males in which the opening of the urethra is on the underside of the penis.
$Ifnar1^{-/-} \times Ifngr^{-/-}$ (AG129) mice	Interferon alpha, beta and gamma receptor deficient mice on a 129 background.
$Ifnar1^{-/-}$ mice	Interferon alpha and beta receptor deficient mice.
Immune-privileged site	Sites that are able to tolerate the introduction of antigens without eliciting an inflammatory immune response. Immune-privileged sites include the central nervous system, the brain, the eye, and regions of the male reproductive tract.
$Irf3^{-/-} \times Irf7^{-/-}$ mice	Interferon 3 and 7 double knockout mice.
Leydig cells	Testosterone-producing cells located in the connective tissue surrounding the seminiferous tubules in the testicle.
Male accessory glands	In humans, these are the seminal vesicles, prostate gland, and the bulbourethral glands.
Microcephaly	Medical condition in which the brain does not develop properly resulting in a smaller than normal head.
Microhematospermia	Hematospermia not evident by macroscopic examinations of the semen, but detected by tests for occult blood.
Micropenis	An unusually small penis.
Myalgia	Pain in a muscle or group of muscles.
Organoids	Three-dimensional cell cultures that incorporate some of the key features of the represented organ.
Prostatitis	Inflammation of the prostate gland.
$Rag1^{-/-}$ mice	Recombination activating gene 1 (Rag1) deficient mice.
Seminal glands	Accessory glands of the MRT, located between the bladder and the rectum that contribute approximately 60–70% of the ejaculate.
Seminiferous tubules	The site of the germination, maturation, and transportation of the sperm cells within the male testis.
Sertoli cells	Somatic cells of the testis that are part of a seminiferous tubule and facilitate the nourishment and progression of germ cells to spermatozoa.
Spermatocytes	Diploid cells formed through the process of spermatogenesis.

Spermatogenesis	The origin and development of the sperm cells within the male reproductive organs.
Spermatogonia	Undifferentiated male germ cell, formed in the wall of a seminiferous tubule and giving rise by mitosis to spermatocytes.
Spermatozoa	The mature motile male sex cell.
Testicular atrophy	Medical condition in which the testes diminish in size and may be accompanied by loss of function.
Testicular macrophages	Antigen-presenting cells, the most prevalent cell type in the testicular interstitium. They are in close morphological association and functional interaction with Leydig cells.
The male reproductive tract (MRT)	The male gonads, associated ducts and glands, and external genitalia that function during procreation.
Thrombocytopenia	Condition characterized by abnormally low levels of thrombocytes, also known as platelets, in the blood. This causes bleeding into the tissues, bruising, and slow blood clotting after injury.
Vas deferens	Tiny muscular tube in the MRT that carries sperm from the epididymis to the ejaculatory duct.

References

1. Mlakar, J.; Korva, M.; Tul, N.; Popovic, M.; Poljsak-Prijatelj, M.; Mraz, J.; Kolenc, M.; Rus, K.R.; Vipotnik, T.V.; Vodusek, V.F.; et al. Zika virus associated with microcephaly. *N. Engl. J. Med.* **2016**, *374*, 951–958. [CrossRef] [PubMed]
2. Wang, A.; Thurmond, S.; Islas, L.; Hui, K.; Hai, R. Zika virus genome biology and molecular pathogenesis. *Emerg. Microbes Infect.* **2017**, *6*, e13. [CrossRef] [PubMed]
3. Yun, S.I.; Lee, Y.M. Zika virus: An emerging flavivirus. *J. Microbiol.* **2017**, *55*, 204–219. [CrossRef] [PubMed]
4. Holbrook, M.R. Historical perspectives on Flavivirus research. *Viruses* **2017**, *9*, 97. [CrossRef] [PubMed]
5. Weinbren, M.P.; Williams, M.C. Zika virus: Further isolations in the Zika area, and some studies on the strains isolated. *Trans. R. Soc. Trop. Med. Hyg.* **1958**, *52*, 263–268. [CrossRef]
6. Valderrama, A.; Díaz, Y.; López-Vergès, S. Interaction of Flavivirus with their mosquito vectors and their impact on the human health in the Americas. *Biochem. Biophys. Res. Commun.* **2017**, *492*, 541–547. [CrossRef] [PubMed]
7. Dick, G.W.A.; Kitchen, S.F.; Haddow, A.J. Zika virus. 1. Isolations and serological specificity. *Trans. R. Soc. Trop. Med. Hyg.* **1952**, *46*, 509–520. [CrossRef]
8. Smithburn, K.C. Neutralizing antibodies against certain recently isolated viruses in the sera of human beings residing in East Africa. *J. Immunol.* **1952**, *69*, 223–234. [PubMed]
9. Waggoner, J.J.; Pinsky, B.A. Zika virus: Diagnostics for an emerging pandemic threat. *J. Clin. Microbiol.* **2016**, *54*, 860–867. [CrossRef] [PubMed]
10. Kindhauser, M.K.; Allen, T.; Frank, V.; Santhana, R.S.; Dye, C. Zika: The origin and spread of a mosquito-borne virus. *Bull. World Health Organ.* **2016**, *94*, 675–686. [CrossRef] [PubMed]
11. Duffy, M.R.; Chen, T.H.; Hancock, W.T.; Powers, A.M.; Kool, J.L.; Lanciotti, R.S.; Pretrick, M.; Marfel, M.; Holzbauer, S.; Dubray, C.; et al. Zika virus outbreak on Yap Island, Federated States of Micronesia. *N. Engl. J. Med.* **2009**, *360*, 2536–2543. [CrossRef] [PubMed]
12. Chan, J.F.W.; Choi, G.K.Y.; Yip, C.C.Y.; Cheng, V.C.C.; Yuen, K.Y. Zika fever and congenital Zika syndrome: An unexpected emerging arboviral disease. *J. Infect.* **2016**, *72*, 507–524. [CrossRef] [PubMed]
13. Lanciotti, R.S.; Kosoy, O.L.; Laven, J.J.; Velez, J.O.; Lambert, A.J.; Johnson, A.J.; Stanfield, S.M.; Duffy, M.R. Genetic and serologic properties of Zika virus associated with an epidemic, Yap State, Micronesia, 2007. *Emerg. Infect. Dis.* **2008**, *14*, 1232–1239. [CrossRef] [PubMed]
14. Aubry, M.; Teissier, A.; Huart, M.; Merceron, S.; Vanhomwegen, J.; Roche, C.; Vial, A.L.; Teururai, S.; Sicard, S.; Paulous, S.; et al. Zika virus seroprevalence, French Polynesia, 2014–2015. *Emerg. Infect. Dis.* **2017**, *23*, 669–672. [CrossRef] [PubMed]
15. Ioos, S.; Mallet, H.P.; Goffart, I.L.; Gauthier, V.; Cardoso, T.; Herida, M. Current Zika virus epidemiology and recent epidemics. *Med. Mal. Infect.* **2014**, *44*, 302–307. [CrossRef] [PubMed]
16. Musso, D.; Nilles, E.J.; Cao-Lormeau, V.M. Rapid spread of emerging Zika virus in the Pacific area. *Clin. Microbiol. Infect.* **2014**, *20*, O595–O596. [CrossRef] [PubMed]
17. Cauchemez, S.; Besnard, M.; Bompard, P.; Dub, T.; Guillemette-Artur, P.; Eyrolle-Guignot, D.; Salje, H.; Van Kerkhove, M.D.; Abadie, V.; Garel, C.; et al. Association between Zika virus and microcephaly in French Polynesia, 2013-15: A retrospective study. *Lancet* **2016**, *387*, 2125–2132. [CrossRef]
18. Watrin, L.; Ghawche, F.; Larre, P.; Neau, J.P.; Mathis, S.; Fournier, E. Guillain-Barre syndrome (42 cases) occurring during a Zika virus outbreak in French Polynesia. *Medicine* **2016**, *95*, e3257. [CrossRef] [PubMed]

19. Hennessey, M.; Fischer, M.; Staples, J.E. Zika virus spreads to new areas—Region of the Americas, May 2015–January 2016. *MMWR Morb. Mortal. Wkly. Rep.* **2016**, *65*, 55–58. [CrossRef] [PubMed]

20. Faria, N.R.; Azevedo, R.D.D.; Kraemer, M.U.G.; Souza, R.; Cunha, M.S.; Hill, S.C.; Theze, J.; Bonsall, M.B.; Bowden, T.A.; Rissanen, I.; et al. Zika virus in the Americas: Early epidemiological and genetic findings. *Science* **2016**, *352*, 345–349. [CrossRef] [PubMed]

21. Brasil, P.; Pereira, J.P.; Moreira, M.E.; Nogueira, R.M.R.; Damasceno, L.; Wakimoto, M.; Rabello, R.S.; Valderramos, S.G.; Halai, U.A.; Salles, T.S.; et al. Zika virus infection in pregnant women in Rio de Janeiro. *N. Engl. J. Med.* **2016**, *375*, 2321–2334. [CrossRef] [PubMed]

22. Pomar, L.; Malinger, G.; Benoist, G.; Carles, G.; Ville, Y.; Rousset, D.; Hcini, N.; Pomar, C.; Jolivet, A.; Lambert, V. Association between Zika virus and fetopathy: A prospective cohort study in French Guiana. *Ultrasound Obstet. Gynecol.* **2017**, *49*, 729–736. [CrossRef] [PubMed]

23. Bhatnagar, J.; Rabeneck, D.B.; Martines, R.B.; Reagan-Steiner, S.; Ermias, Y.; Estetter, L.B.C.; Suzuki, T.; Ritter, J.; Keating, M.K.; Hale, G.; et al. Zika virus RNA replication and persistence in brain and placental tissue. *Emerg. Infect. Dis.* **2017**, *23*, 405–414. [CrossRef] [PubMed]

24. Cao-Lormeau, V.M.; Blake, A.; Mons, S.; Lastere, S.; Roche, C.; Vanhomwegen, J.; Dub, T.; Baudouin, L.; Teissier, A.; Larre, P.; et al. Guillain-Barre syndrome outbreak associated with Zika virus infection in French Polynesia: A case-control study. *Lancet* **2016**, *387*, 1531–1539. [CrossRef]

25. Willison, H.J.; Jacobs, B.C.; van Doorn, P.A. Guillain-Barre syndrome. *Lancet* **2016**, *388*, 717–727. [CrossRef]

26. Soares, C.N.; Brasil, P.; Carrera, R.M.; Sequeira, P.; De Filippis, A.B.; Borges, V.A.; Theophilo, F.; Ellul, M.A.; Solomon, T. Fatal encephalitis associated with Zika virus infection in an adult. *J. Clin. Virol.* **2016**, *83*, 63–65. [CrossRef] [PubMed]

27. Chammard, T.B.; Schepers, K.; Breurec, S.; Messiaen, T.; Destrem, A.L.; Mahevas, M.; Souillou, A.; Janaud, L.; Curlier, E.; Hermann-Storck, C. Severe thrombocytopenia after Zika virus infection, Guadeloupe, 2016. *Emerg. Infect. Dis.* **2017**, *23*, 696–698. [CrossRef] [PubMed]

28. Vinhaes, E.S.; Santos, L.A.; Dias, L.; Andrade, N.A.; Bezerra, V.H.; de Carvalho, A.T.; de Moraes, L.; Henriques, D.F.; Azar, S.R.; Vasilakis, N.; et al. Transient hearing loss in adults associated with Zika virus infection. *Clin. Infect. Dis.* **2017**, *64*, 675–677. [CrossRef] [PubMed]

29. Foy, B.D.; Kobylinski, K.C.; Foy, J.L.C.; Blitvich, B.J.; da Rosa, A.T.; Haddow, A.D.; Lanciotti, R.S.; Tesh, R.B. Probable non-vector-borne transmission of Zika virus, Colorado, USA. *Emerg. Infect. Dis.* **2011**, *17*, 880–882. [CrossRef] [PubMed]

30. D'Ortenzio, E.; Matheron, S.; Yazdanpanah, Y. Evidence of sexual transmission of Zika virus. *N. Engl. J. Med.* **2016**, *374*, 2195–2198. [CrossRef] [PubMed]

31. McDonald, E.M.; Duggal, N.K.; Brault, A.C. Pathogenesis and sexual transmission of Spondweni and Zika viruses. *PLoS Negl. Trop. Dis.* **2017**, *11*, e0005990. [CrossRef] [PubMed]

32. Deckard, D.T.; Chung, W.M.; Brooks, J.T.; Smith, J.C.; Woldai, S.; Hennessey, M.; Kwit, N.; Mead, P. Male-to-male sexual transmission of Zika virus—Texas, January 2016. *MMWR Morb. Mortal. Wkly. Rep.* **2016**, *65*, 372–374. [CrossRef] [PubMed]

33. Davidson, A.; Slavinski, S.; Komoto, K.; Rakeman, J.; Weiss, D. Suspected female-to-male sexual transmission of Zika virus—New York City, 2016. *MMWR Morb. Mortal. Wkly. Rep.* **2016**, *65*, 716–717. [CrossRef] [PubMed]

34. Musso, D.; Roche, C.; Robin, E.; Nhan, T.; Teissier, A.; Cao-Lormeau, V. Potential sexual transmission of Zika virus. *Emerg. Infect. Dis.* **2015**, *21*, 359–361. [CrossRef] [PubMed]

35. Turmel, J.M.; Abgueguen, P.; Hubert, B.; Vandamme, Y.M.; Maquart, M.; Le Guillou-Guillemette, H.; Leparc-Goffart, I. Late sexual transmission of Zika virus related to persistence in the semen. *Lancet* **2016**, *387*, 2501. [CrossRef]

36. Coelho, F.C.; Durovni, B.; Saraceni, V.; Lemos, C.; Codeco, C.T.; Camargo, S.; de Carvalho, L.M.; Bastos, L.; Arduini, D.; Villela, D.A.M.; et al. Higher incidence of Zika in adult women than adult men in Rio de Janeiro suggests a significant contribution of sexual transmission from men to women. *Int. J. Infect. Dis.* **2016**, *51*, 128–132. [CrossRef] [PubMed]

37. Brooks, R.B.; Carlos, M.P.; Myers, R.A.; White, M.G.; Bobo-Lenoci, T.; Aplan, D.; Blythe, D.; Feldman, K.A. Likely sexual transmission of Zika virus from a man with no symptoms of infection—Maryland, 2016. *MMWR Morb. Mortal. Wkly. Rep.* **2016**, *65*, 915–916. [CrossRef] [PubMed]

38. Freour, T.; Mirallie, S.; Hubert, B.; Splingart, C.; Barriere, P.; Maquart, M.; Leparc-Goffart, I. Sexual transmission of Zika virus in an entirely asymptomatic couple returning from a Zika epidemic area, France, April 2016. *Euro Surveill.* **2016**, *21*, 10–12. [CrossRef] [PubMed]

39. Maxian, O.; Neufeld, A.; Talis, E.J.; Childs, L.M.; Blackwood, J.C. Zika virus dynamics: When does sexual transmission matter? *Epidemics* **2017**, *21*, 48–55. [CrossRef] [PubMed]

40. Gao, D.Z.; Lou, Y.J.; He, D.H.; Porco, T.C.; Kuang, Y.; Chowell, G.; Ruan, S.G. Prevention and control of Zika as a mosquito-borne and sexually transmitted disease: A mathematical modeling analysis. *Sci. Rep.* **2016**, *6*, 28070. [CrossRef] [PubMed]

41. Allard, A.; Althouse, B.M.; Hebert-Dufresne, L.; Scarpino, S.V. The risk of sustained sexual transmission of Zika is underestimated. *PLoS Pathog.* **2017**, *13*, e1006633. [CrossRef] [PubMed]

42. Pacheco, O.; Beltrán, M.; Nelson, C.A.; Valencia, D.; Tolosa, N.; Farr, S.L.; Padilla, A.V.; Tong, V.T.; Cuevas, E.L.; Espinosa-Bode, A. Zika virus disease in Colombia—Preliminary report. *N. Engl. J. Med.* **2016**. [CrossRef] [PubMed]

43. Yakob, L.; Kucharski, A.; Hue, S.; Edmunds, W.J. Low risk of a sexually-transmitted Zika virus outbreak. *Lancet Infect. Dis.* **2016**, *16*, 1100–1102. [CrossRef]

44. Haddow, A.D.; Nalca, A.; Rossi, F.D.; Miller, L.J.; Wiley, M.R.; Perez-Sautu, U.; Washington, S.C.; Norris, S.L.; Wollen-Roberts, S.E.; Shamblin, J.D.; et al. High infection rates for adult macaques after intravaginal or intrarectal inoculation with Zika virus. *Emerg. Infect. Dis.* **2017**, *23*, 1274–1281. [CrossRef] [PubMed]

45. Mansuy, J.M.; Pasquier, C.; Daudin, M.; Chapuy-Regaud, S.; Moinard, N.; Chevreau, C.; Izopet, J.; Mengelle, C.; Bujan, L. Zika virus in semen of a patient returning from a non-epidemic area. *Lancet Infect. Dis.* **2016**, *16*, 894–895. [CrossRef]

46. Matheron, S.; d'Ortenzio, E.; Leparc-Goffart, I.; Hubert, B.; de Lamballerie, X.; Yazdanpanah, Y. Long-lasting persistence of Zika virus in semen. *Clin. Infect. Dis.* **2016**, *63*, 1264. [CrossRef] [PubMed]

47. Nicastri, E.; Castilletti, C.; Liuzzi, G.; Iannetta, M.; Capobianchi, M.R.; Ippolito, G. Persistent detection of Zika virus RNA in semen for six months after symptom onset in a traveller returning from Haiti to Italy, February 2016. *Euro Surveill.* **2016**, *21*, 6–9. [CrossRef] [PubMed]

48. Joguet, G.; Mansuy, J.M.; Matusali, G.; Hamdi, S.; Walschaerts, M.; Pavili, L.; Guyomard, S.; Prisant, N.; Lamarre, P.; Dejucq-Rainsford, N.; et al. Effect of acute Zika virus infection on sperm and virus clearance in body fluids: A prospective observational study. *Lancet Infect. Dis.* **2017**, *17*, 1200–1208. [CrossRef]

49. Mansuy, J.M.; Suberbielle, E.; Chapuy-Regaud, S.; Mengelle, C.; Bujan, L.; Marchou, B.; Delobel, P.; Gonzalez-Dunia, D.; Malnou, C.E.; Izopet, J.; et al. Zika virus in semen and spermatozoa. *Lancet Infect. Dis.* **2016**, *16*, 1106–1107. [CrossRef]

50. Musso, D.; Richard, V.; Teissier, A.; Stone, M.; Lanteri, M.C.; Lantoni, G.; Alsina, J.; Reik, R.; Busch, M. Detection of ZIKV RNA in semen of asymptomatic blood donors. *Clin. Microbiol. Infect.* **2017**, *23*, 1001.e1–1001.e3. [CrossRef] [PubMed]

51. Garcia-Bujalance, S.; Gutierrez-Arroyo, A.; De la Calle, F.; Diaz-Menendez, M.; Arribas, J.R.; Garcia-Rodriguez, J.; Arsuaga, M. Persistence and infectivity of Zika virus in semen after returning from endemic areas: Report of 5 cases. *J. Clin. Virol.* **2017**, *96*, 110–115. [CrossRef] [PubMed]

52. Uraki, R.; Jurado, K.A.; Hwang, J.; Szigeti-Buck, K.; Horvath, T.L.; Iwasaki, A.; Fikrig, E. Fetal growth restriction caused by sexual transmission of Zika virus in mice. *J. Infect. Dis.* **2017**, *215*, 1720–1724. [CrossRef] [PubMed]

53. Bagasra, O.; Addanki, K.C.; Goodwin, G.R.; Hughes, B.W.; Pandey, P.; McLean, E. Cellular targets and receptor of sexual transmission of Zika virus. *Appl. Immunohistochem. Mol. Morphol.* **2017**, *25*, 679–686. [CrossRef] [PubMed]

54. Atkinson, B.; Thorburn, F.; Petridou, C.; Bailey, D.; Hewson, R.; Simpson, A.J.H.; Brooks, T.J.G.; Aarons, E.J. Presence and persistence of Zika virus RNA in semen, United Kingdom, 2016. *Emerg. Infect. Dis.* **2017**, *23*, 611–615. [CrossRef] [PubMed]

55. Visseaux, B.; Mortier, E.; Houhou-Fidouh, N.; Brichler, S.; Collin, G.; Larrouy, L.; Charpentier, C.; Descamps, D. Zika virus in the female genital tract. *Lancet Infect. Dis.* **2016**, *16*, 1220. [CrossRef]

56. Dejucq-Rainsford, N.; Jegou, B. Viruses in semen and male genital tissues—Consequences for the reproductive system and therapeutic perspectives. *Curr. Pharm. Des.* **2004**, *10*, 557–575. [CrossRef] [PubMed]

57. Fijak, M.; Meinhardt, A. The testis in immune privilege. *Immunol. Rev.* **2006**, *213*, 66–81. [CrossRef] [PubMed]

58. Hedger, M.P.; Hales, D.B. Immunophysiology of the male reproductive tract. In *Knobil and Neill's Physiology of Reproduction*, 3rd ed.; Neil, J.D., Ed.; Elsevier Academic Press: St. Louis, MO, USA, 2006; Volume 1, 2, pp. 1195–1286. ISBN 9780125154000.

59. Mruk, D.D.; Cheng, C.Y. The mammalian blood-testis barrier: Its biology and regulation. *Endocr. Rev.* **2015**, *36*, 564–591. [CrossRef] [PubMed]

60. Hedger, M.P. Macrophages and the immune responsiveness of the testis. *J. Reprod. Immunol.* **2002**, *57*, 19–34. [CrossRef]

61. Torres, J.R.; Martinez, N.; Moros, Z. Microhematospermia in acute Zika virus infection. *Int. J. Infect. Dis.* **2016**, *51*, 127. [CrossRef] [PubMed]

62. Huits, R.M.H.G.; De Smet, B.; Ariën, K.K.; Van Esbroeck, M.; de Jong, B.C.; Bottieau, E.; Cnops, L. Kinetics of Zika virus persistence in semen. *Bull. World Health Organ.* **2016**. [CrossRef]

63. Siemann, D.N.; Strange, D.P.; Maharaj, P.N.; Shi, P.Y.; Verma, S. Zika virus infects human Sertoli cells and modulates the integrity of the in vitro blood-testis barrier model. *J. Virol.* **2017**, *91*, e00623-17. [CrossRef] [PubMed]

64. De Laval, F.; Matheus, S.; Briolant, S. Kinetics of Zika viral load in semen. *N. Engl. J. Med.* **2017**, *377*, 697–699. [CrossRef] [PubMed]

65. Hamel, R.; Dejarnac, O.; Wichit, S.; Ekchariyawat, P.; Neyret, A.; Luplertlop, N.; Perera-Lecoin, M.; Surasombatpattana, P.; Talignani, L.; Thomas, F.; et al. Biology of Zika virus infection in human skin cells. *J. Virol.* **2015**, *89*, 8880–8896. [CrossRef] [PubMed]

66. Retallack, H.; Di Lullo, E.; Arias, C.; Knopp, K.A.; Laurie, M.T.; Sandoval-Espinosa, C.; Leon, W.R.M.; Krencik, R.; Ullian, E.M.; Spatazza, J.; et al. Zika virus cell tropism in the developing human brain and inhibition by azithromycin. *Proc. Natl. Acad. Sci. USA* **2016**, *113*, 14408–14413. [CrossRef] [PubMed]

67. Richard, A.S.; Shim, B.S.; Kwon, Y.C.; Zhang, R.; Otsuka, Y.; Schmitt, K.; Berri, F.; Diamond, M.S.; Choe, H. AXL-dependent infection of human fetal endothelial cells distinguishes Zika virus from other pathogenic flaviviruses. *Proc. Natl. Acad. Sci. USA* **2017**, *114*, 2024–2029. [CrossRef] [PubMed]

68. Kumar, A.; Jovel, J.; Lopez-Orozco, J.; Limonta, D.; Airo, A.M.; Hou, S.; Stryapunina, I.; Fibke, C.; Moore, R.B.; Hobman, T.C. Human Sertoli cells support high levels of Zika virus replication and persistence. *Sci. Rep.* **2018**, *8*, 5477. [CrossRef] [PubMed]

69. Wang, H.Z.; Chen, Y.M.; Ge, Y.H.; Ma, P.P.; Ma, Q.H.; Ma, J.; Wang, H.K.; Xue, S.P.; Han, D.S. Immunoexpression of Tyro 3 family receptors—Tyro 3, Axl, and Mer—And their ligand Gas6 in postnatal developing mouse testis. *J. Histochem. Cytochem.* **2005**, *53*, 1355–1364. [CrossRef] [PubMed]

70. Shimojima, M.; Takada, A.; Ebihara, H.; Neumann, G.; Fujioka, K.; Irimura, T.; Jones, S.; Feldmann, H.; Kawaoka, Y. Tyro3 family-mediated cell entry of Ebola and Marburg viruses. *J. Virol.* **2006**, *80*, 10109–10116. [CrossRef] [PubMed]

71. Salam, A.P.; Horby, P.W. The breadth of viruses in human semen. *Emerg. Infect. Dis.* **2017**, *23*, 1922–1924. [CrossRef] [PubMed]

72. Arsuaga, M.; Bujalance, S.G.; Diaz-Menendez, M.; Vazquez, A.; Arribas, J.R. Probable sexual transmission of Zika virus from a vasectomised man. *Lancet Infect. Dis.* **2016**, *16*, 1107. [CrossRef]

73. Froeschl, G.; Huber, K.; von Sonnenburg, F.; Nothdurft, H.D.; Bretzel, G.; Hoelscher, M.; Zoeller, L.; Trottmann, M.; Pan-Montojo, F.; Dobler, G.; et al. Long-term kinetics of Zika virus RNA and antibodies in body fluids of a vasectomized traveller returning from Martinique: A case report. *BMC Infect. Dis.* **2017**, *17*, 55. [CrossRef] [PubMed]

74. Spencer, J.L.; Lahon, A.; Tran, L.L.; Arya, R.P.; Kneubehl, A.R.; Vogt, M.B.; Xavier, D.; Rowley, D.R.; Kimata, J.T.; Rico-Hesse, R.R. Replication of Zika virus in human prostate cells: A potential source of sexually transmitted virus. *J. Infect. Dis.* **2017**, *217*, 538–547. [CrossRef] [PubMed]

75. Revenig, L.; Leung, A.; Hsiao, W. Ejaculatory physiology and pathophysiology: Assessment and treatment in male infertility. *Transl. Androl. Urol.* **2014**, *3*, 41–49. [CrossRef] [PubMed]

76. Govero, J.; Esakky, P.; Scheaffer, S.M.; Fernandez, E.; Drury, A.; Platt, D.J.; Gorman, M.J.; Richner, J.M.; Caine, E.A.; Salazar, V.; et al. Zika virus infection damages the testes in mice. *Nature* **2016**, *540*, 438–442. [CrossRef] [PubMed]

77. Ma, W.Q.; Li, S.H.; Ma, S.Q.; Jia, L.N.; Zhang, F.C.; Zhang, Y.; Zhang, J.Y.; Wong, G.; Zhang, S.S.; Lu, X.C.; et al. Zika virus causes testis damage and leads to male infertility in mice. *Cell* **2016**, *167*, 1511.e10–1524.e10. [CrossRef] [PubMed]

78. Uraki, R.; Hwang, J.; Jurado, K.A.; Householder, S.; Yockey, L.J.; Hastings, A.K.; Homer, R.J.; Iwasaki, A.; Fikrig, E. Zika virus causes testicular atrophy. *Sci. Adv.* **2017**, *3*, e1602899. [CrossRef] [PubMed]

79. Sheng, Z.Y.; Gao, N.; Wang, Z.Y.; Cui, X.Y.; Zhou, D.S.; Fan, D.Y.; Chen, H.; Wang, P.G.; An, J. Sertoli cells are susceptible to ZIKV infection in mouse testis. *Front. Cell. Infect. Microbiol.* **2017**, *7*, 272. [CrossRef] [PubMed]

80. Kawiecki, A.B.; Mayton, E.H.; Dutuze, M.F.; Goupil, B.A.; Langohr, I.M.; Del Piero, F.; Christofferson, R.C. Tissue tropisms, infection kinetics, histologic lesions, and antibody response of the MR766 strain of Zika virus in a murine model. *Virol. J.* **2017**, *14*, 82. [CrossRef] [PubMed]

81. Shan, C.; Muruato, A.E.; Jagger, B.W.; Richner, J.; Nunes, B.T.D.; Medeiros, D.B.A.; Xie, X.P.; Nunes, J.G.C.; Morabito, K.M.; Kong, W.P.; et al. A single-dose live-attenuated vaccine prevents Zika virus pregnancy transmission and testis damage. *Nat. Commun.* **2017**, *8*, 676. [CrossRef] [PubMed]

82. Stein, D.R.; Golden, J.W.; Griffin, B.D.; Warner, B.M.; Ranadheera, C.; Scharikow, L.; Sloan, A.; Frost, K.L.; Kobasa, D.; Booth, S.A. Human polyclonal antibodies produced in transchromosomal cattle prevent lethal Zika virus infection and testicular atrophy in mice. *Antivir. Res.* **2017**, *146*, 164–173. [CrossRef] [PubMed]

83. Winkler, C.W.; Myers, L.M.; Woods, T.A.; Messer, R.J.; Carmody, A.B.; McNally, K.L.; Scott, D.P.; Hasenkrug, K.J.; Best, S.M.; Peterson, K.E. Adaptive immune responses to Zika virus are important for controlling virus infection and preventing infection in brain and testes. *J. Immunol.* **2017**, *198*, 3526–3535. [CrossRef] [PubMed]

84. Duggal, N.K.; Ritter, J.M.; Pestorius, S.E.; Zaki, S.R.; Davis, B.S.; Chang, G.J.J.; Bowen, R.A.; Brault, A.C. Frequent Zika virus sexual transmission and prolonged viral RNA shedding in an immunodeficient mouse model. *Cell Rep.* **2017**, *18*, 1751–1760. [CrossRef] [PubMed]

85. Lazear, H.M.; Govero, J.; Smith, A.M.; Platt, D.J.; Fernandez, E.; Miner, J.J.; Diamond, M.S. A mouse model of Zika virus pathogenesis. *Cell Host Microbe* **2016**, *19*, 720–730. [CrossRef] [PubMed]

86. Dowall, S.D.; Graham, V.A.; Rayner, E.; Hunter, L.; Atkinson, B.; Pearson, G.; Dennis, M.; Hewson, R. Lineage-dependent differences in the disease progression of Zika virus infection in type-I interferon receptor knockout (A129) mice. *PLoS Negl. Trop. Dis.* **2017**, *11*, e0005704. [CrossRef] [PubMed]

87. Griffin, B.D.; Muthumani, K.; Warner, B.M.; Majer, A.; Hagan, M.; Audet, J.; Stein, D.R.; Ranadheera, C.; Racine, T.; De La Vega, M.A.; et al. DNA vaccination protects mice against Zika virus-induced damage to the testes. *Nat. Commun.* **2017**, *8*, 15743. [CrossRef] [PubMed]

88. Chan, J.F.W.; Zhang, A.J.; Chan, C.C.S.; Yip, C.C.Y.; Mak, W.W.N.; Zhu, H.S.; Poon, V.K.M.; Tee, K.M.; Zhu, Z.; Cai, J.P.; et al. Zika virus infection in dexamethasone-immunosuppressed mice demonstrating disseminated infection with multi-organ involvement including orchitis effectively treated by recombinant type I interferons. *EBioMedicine* **2016**, *14*, 112–122. [CrossRef] [PubMed]

89. Clancy, C.S.; Van Wettere, A.J.; Siddharthan, V.; Morrey, J.D.; Julander, J.G. Comparative histopathologic lesions of the male reproductive tract during acute Infection of Zika virus in AG129 and IFNAR-/- mice. *Am. J. Pathol.* **2018**, *188*, 904–915. [CrossRef] [PubMed]

90. Prow, N.A.; Liu, L.; Nakayama, E.; Cooper, T.H.; Yan, K.X.; Eldi, P.; Hazlewood, J.E.; Tang, B.; Le, T.T.; Setoh, Y.X.; et al. A vaccinia-based single vector construct multi-pathogen vaccine protects against both Zika and chikungunya viruses. *Nat. Commun.* **2018**, *9*, 1230. [CrossRef] [PubMed]

91. Duggal, N.K.; McDonald, E.M.; Ritter, J.M.; Brault, A.C. Sexual transmission of Zika virus enhances in utero transmission in a mouse model. *Sci. Rep.* **2018**, *8*, 4510. [CrossRef] [PubMed]

92. Siddharthan, V.; Van Wettere, A.J.; Li, R.; Miao, J.X.; Wang, Z.D.; Morrey, J.D.; Julander, J.G. Zika virus infection of adult and fetal STAT2 knock-out hamsters. *Virology* **2017**, *507*, 89–95. [CrossRef] [PubMed]

93. Dudley, D.M.; Aliota, M.T.; Mohr, E.L.; Weiler, A.M.; Lehrer-Brey, G.; Weisgrau, K.L.; Mohns, M.S.; Breitbach, M.E.; Rasheed, M.N.; Newman, C.M.; et al. A rhesus macaque model of Asian-lineage Zika virus infection. *Nat. Commun.* **2016**, *7*, 12204. [CrossRef] [PubMed]

94. Li, X.F.; Dong, H.L.; Huang, X.Y.; Qiu, Y.F.; Wang, H.J.; Deng, Y.Q.; Zhang, N.N.; Ye, Q.; Zhao, H.; Liu, Z.Y.; et al. Characterization of a 2016 clinical isolate of Zika virus in non-human primates. *EBioMedicine* **2016**, *12*, 170–177. [CrossRef] [PubMed]

95. Osuna, C.E.; Lim, S.Y.; Deleage, C.; Griffin, B.D.; Stein, D.; Schroeder, L.T.; Omange, R.W.; Best, K.; Luo, M.; Hraber, P.T.; et al. Zika viral dynamics and shedding in rhesus and cynomolgus macaques. *Nat. Med.* **2016**, *22*, 1448–1455. [CrossRef] [PubMed]

96. Nguyen, S.M.; Antony, K.M.; Dudley, D.M.; Kohn, S.; Simmons, H.A.; Wolfe, B.; Salamat, M.S.; Teixeira, L.B.C.; Wiepz, G.J.; Thoong, T.H.; et al. Highly efficient maternal-fetal Zika virus transmission in pregnant rhesus macaques. *PLoS Pathog.* **2017**, *13*, e1006378. [CrossRef] [PubMed]
97. Coffey, L.L.; Pesavento, P.A.; Keesler, R.I.; Singapuri, A.; Watanabe, J.; Watanabe, R.; Yee, J.; Bliss-Moreau, E.; Cruzen, C.; Christe, K.L.; et al. Zika virus tissue and blood compartmentalization in acute infection of rhesus macaques. *PLoS ONE* **2017**, *12*, e0171148. [CrossRef] [PubMed]
98. Hirsch, A.J.; Smith, J.L.; Haese, N.N.; Broeckel, R.M.; Parkins, C.J.; Kreklywich, C.; DeFilippis, V.R.; Denton, M.; Smith, P.P.; Messer, W.B.; et al. Zika virus infection of rhesus macaques leads to viral persistence in multiple tissues. *PLoS Pathog.* **2017**, *13*, e1006219. [CrossRef] [PubMed]
99. Abbink, P.; Larocca, R.A.; De La Barrera, R.A.; Bricault, C.A.; Moseley, E.T.; Boyd, M.; Kirilova, M.; Li, Z.F.; Ng'ang'a, D.; Nanayakkara, O.; et al. Protective efficacy of multiple vaccine platforms against Zika virus challenge in rhesus monkeys. *Science* **2016**, *353*, 1129–1132. [CrossRef] [PubMed]
100. Koide, F.; Goebel, S.; Snyder, B.; Walters, K.B.; Gast, A.; Hagelin, K.; Kalkeri, R.; Rayner, J. Development of a Zika virus infection model in cynomolgus macaques. *Front. Microbiol.* **2016**, *7*, 2028. [CrossRef] [PubMed]
101. O'Meara, C.P.; Armitage, C.W.; Kollipara, A.; Andrew, D.W.; Trim, L.; Plenderleith, M.B.; Beagley, K.W. Induction of partial immunity in both males and females is sufficient to protect females against sexual transmission of Chlamydia. *Mucosal Immunol.* **2016**, *9*, 1076–1088. [CrossRef] [PubMed]
102. Aliota, M.T.; Dudley, D.M.; Newman, C.M.; Mohr, E.L.; Gellerup, D.D.; Breitbach, M.E.; Buechler, C.R.; Rasheed, M.N.; Mohns, M.S.; Weiler, A.M.; et al. Heterologous protection against Asian Zika virus challenge in rhesus macaques. *PLoS. Negl. Trop. Dis.* **2016**, *10*, e0005168. [CrossRef] [PubMed]
103. Wahid, B.; Ali, A.; Rafique, S.; Idrees, M. Current status of therapeutic and vaccine approaches against Zika virus. *Eur. J. Intern. Med.* **2017**, *44*, 12–18. [CrossRef] [PubMed]
104. Jenabian, M.A.; Costiniuk, C.T.; Mehraj, V.; Ghazawi, F.M.; Fromentin, R.; Brousseau, J.; Brassard, P.; Belanger, M.; Ancuta, P.; Bendayan, R.; et al. Immune tolerance properties of the testicular tissue as a viral sanctuary site in ART-treated HIV-infected adults. *AIDS* **2016**, *30*, 2777–2786. [CrossRef] [PubMed]
105. Kamiyama, N.; Soma, R.; Hidano, S.; Watanabe, K.; Umekita, H.; Fukuda, C.; Noguchi, K.; Gendo, Y.; Ozaki, T.; Sonoda, A.; et al. Ribavirin inhibits Zika virus (ZIKV) replication in vitro and suppresses viremia in ZIKV-infected STAT1-deficient mice. *Antivir. Res.* **2017**, *146*, 1–11. [CrossRef] [PubMed]
106. Fernandez, E.; Dejnirattisai, W.; Cao, C.; Scheaffer, S.M.; Supasa, P.; Wongwiwat, W.; Esakky, P.; Drury, A.; Mongkolsapaya, J.; Moley, K.H.; et al. Human antibodies to the dengue virus E-dimer epitope have therapeutic activity against Zika virus infection. *Nat. Immunol.* **2017**, *18*, 1261–1269. [CrossRef] [PubMed]
107. Larocca, R.A.; Abbink, P.; Peron, J.P.S.; Zanotto, P.M.D.; Iampietro, M.J.; Badamchi-Zadeh, A.; Boyd, M.; Ng'ang'a, D.; Kirilova, M.; Nityanandam, R.; et al. Vaccine protection against Zika virus from Brazil. *Nature* **2016**, *536*, 474–478. [CrossRef] [PubMed]
108. Pardi, N.; Hogan, M.J.; Pelc, R.S.; Muramatsu, H.; Andersen, H.; DeMaso, C.R.; Dowd, K.A.; Sutherland, L.L.; Scearce, R.M.; Parks, R.; et al. Zika virus protection by a single low-dose nucleoside-modified mRNA vaccination. *Nature* **2017**, *543*, 248–251. [CrossRef] [PubMed]
109. Tebas, P.; Roberts, C.C.; Muthumani, K.; Reuschel, E.L.; Kudchodkar, S.B.; Zaidi, F.I.; White, S.; Khan, A.S.; Racine, T.; Choi, H.; et al. Safety and immunogenicity of an anti-Zika virus DNA vaccine—Preliminary report. *N. Engl. J. Med.* **2017**. [CrossRef] [PubMed]
110. Vouga, M.; Baud, D. Imaging of congenital Zika virus infection: The route to identification of prognostic factors. *Prenat. Diagn.* **2016**, *36*, 799–811. [CrossRef] [PubMed]

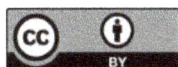

![viruses logo] *viruses*

Review

Ocular Manifestations of Emerging Flaviviruses and the Blood-Retinal Barrier

Sneha Singh [1] and Ashok Kumar [1,2,*]

[1] Department of Ophthalmology, Visual and Anatomical Sciences, Wayne State University, Detroit, MI 48201, USA; gq8860@wayne.edu
[2] Department of Biochemistry, Microbiology, and Immunology, Wayne State University, Detroit, MI 48201, USA
* Correspondence: akuma@med.wayne.edu; Tel.: +1-(313)-577-6213; Fax: +1-(313)-577-7781

Received: 12 September 2018; Accepted: 26 September 2018; Published: 28 September 2018

Abstract: Despite flaviviruses remaining the leading cause of systemic human infections worldwide, ocular manifestations of these mosquito-transmitted viruses are considered relatively uncommon in part due to under-reporting. However, recent outbreaks of Zika virus (ZIKV) implicated in causing multiple ocular abnormalities, such as conjunctivitis, retinal hemorrhages, chorioretinal atrophy, posterior uveitis, optic neuritis, and maculopathies, has rejuvenated a significant interest in understanding the pathogenesis of flaviviruses, including ZIKV, in the eye. In this review, first, we summarize the current knowledge of the major flaviviruses (Dengue, West Nile, Yellow Fever, and Japanese Encephalitis) reported to cause ocular manifestations in humans with emphasis on recent ZIKV outbreaks. Second, being an immune privilege organ, the eye is protected from systemic infections by the presence of blood-retinal barriers (BRB). Hence, we discuss how flaviviruses modulate retinal innate response and breach the protective BRB to cause ocular or retinal pathology. Finally, we describe recently identified infection signatures of ZIKV and discuss whether these system biology-predicted genes or signaling pathways (e.g., cellular metabolism) could contribute to the pathogenesis of ocular manifestations and assist in the development of ocular antiviral therapies against ZIKV and other flaviviruses.

Keywords: flavivirus; eye; zika virus; blood-retinal barrier; ocular; innate response

---

1. Introduction

Flaviviruses consist of more than 90 RNA-enveloped viruses out of which 30 can cause severe disease in humans and animals. Most members of the family are arthropod-borne and are transmitted to the host by mosquitos or ticks [1]. The genus *flavivirus* contains several members which continue to be of global concern such as mosquito-borne Dengue virus (DENV 1–4), West Nile Virus (WNV), Japanese Encephalitis virus (JEV), Yellow fever virus (YFV), Zika virus (ZIKV), Murray Valley Encephalitis Virus (MVEV), Kyasanur Forest Disease virus (KFDV), St. Louis Encephalitis Virus (SLEV) (Fenner's Veterinary Virology, 5th ed, 2017) along with Tick-borne Encephalitis Virus (TBEV). Interestingly, despite sharing a similar genomic organization and replication mechanisms, phylogenetically closely related flaviviruses can induce a spectrum of diseases. Broadly, the genus *flavivirus* is known to cause hemorrhage and vascular leakage (e.g., DENV and YFV), encephalitis (e.g., WNV and JEV) and, more recently, known to cause microcephaly and Guillain-Barre syndrome (ZIKV) [2,3].

Apart from causing systemic infections, these pathogens have been documented to cause multiple ocular complications (Figure 1) with the most common being conjunctivitis, uveitis, and diseases in the posterior segment of the eye (e.g., choroiditis, chorioretinal atrophy, retinitis) [4] (Table 1).

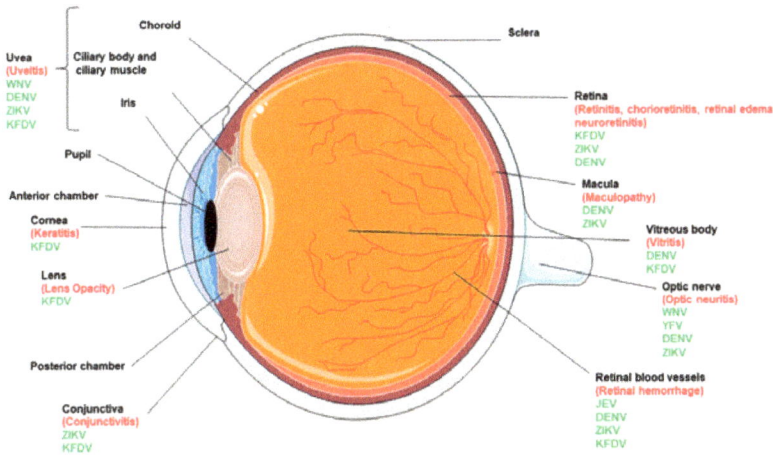

Figure 1. Eye anatomy and ocular complications caused by flaviviruses. Various components of the human eye are labelled in black. The flaviviruses responsible for causing ocular manifestations are shown in green whereas specific ocular tissue pathology is highlighted in red.

Table 1. Comparison of the major ocular findings among the different flaviviruses.

Ocular Complication	ZIKV	DENV	JEV	WNV	YFV	KFDV
Conjunctivitis/keratitis	+	+	−	−	−	+
Macular mottling	+	+	−	−	−	−
Chorioretinal atrophy	+ focal pigmentary clumping	+	−	−	−	+
Optic nerve abnormalities	+	+	−	+	+	−
Cataract	Hypoplasia, cupping, pallor	−	−	−	−	−
Microphthalmia	+	−	−	−	−	−
Iris coloboma	+	−	−	−	−	−
Uveitis	+	+	−	+	−	+
Chorioretinitis	+	+	−	−	−	+
Retinal hemorrhage	+	+	+	−	−	+

ZIKV—Zika virus; DENV—Dengue virus; JEV—Japanese Encephalitis virus; WNV—West Nile virus; YFV—Yellow Fever virus; KDFV—Kyasanur Forest Disease virus.

In the following sections, we provide an overview of ocular complications resulting from flavivirus infections in humans worldwide and elaborate on their main features, systemic complications, and ocular involvement. These viruses have evolved specific mechanisms to counteract the antiviral response from the host and exploit various metabolic pathways to cause disease. Moreover, we discuss probable interactions of viruses and their encoded proteins with ocular cells and the BRB to infect the eye and cause ophthalmic anomalies.

Molecular Pathogenesis of Flaviviruses

Flaviviruses are a family of lipid-enveloped viruses with a single-stranded ~10.5 kb positive-sense RNA genome. They encode only ten proteins which exploit host machinery to complete their infectious replication cycles. Most viral proteins have been shown to associate with host cellular functions and metabolic pathways but their biological consequence in most of these communications are not yet clearly understood [2]. The virus is introduced into the host by an infected vector (e.g., mosquito) during its blood meal. Flaviruses enter cells by receptor-mediated endocytosis [2], where they bind with host endosomes in an acidic environment triggering conformational modifications to their envelope (E) glycoprotein. Conformational changes lead to fusion of the host and viral membrane, facilitating the release of the viral genomic RNA. The polypeptide is co- and post-translationally processed by host signalases and virus encoded serine proteases to translate into the ten viral proteins: three structural proteins (Envelope (E), Capsid (C), Pre-Membrane (PrM)) and seven non-structural proteins (NS1, NS2A, NS2B, NS3, NS4A, NS4B and NS5) [1].

The non-structural proteins are involved in viral genome replication, budding, and deploying the host cell machinery. Following translation, the RNA-dependent RNA polymerase (RdRp), NS5, creates a negative-strand from genomic RNA, which then becomes a template for a new positive strand to be made. In the rough Endoplasmic Reticulum (ER), viral proteins begin to assemble, and viral RNA is packaged with structural proteins—C, E, and prM. Viral particles are then transported to the trans-Golgi network, where prM is cleaved into M, and the mature virus is then released from the host via exocytosis into the extracellular space (Figure 2).

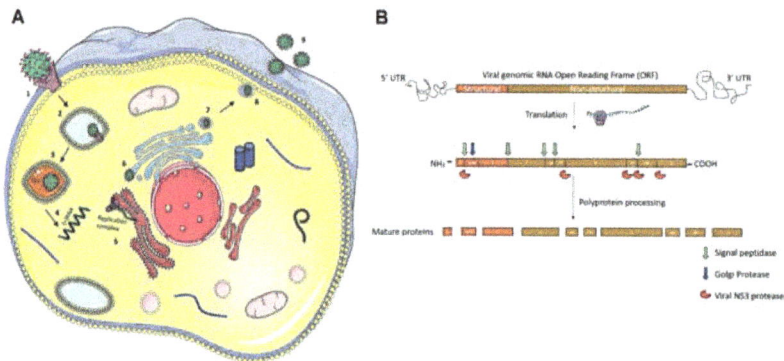

Figure 2. Flavivirus replication cycle and genome structure. (**A**) The flavivirus enters the host cell by attaching to specific receptors (1) which then leads to its endocytosis (2) followed by fusion to a lysosome into an acidic environment (3). The genome is released from the endolysosome (4) which is then translated on the Endoplasmic reticulum membrane (5) and post translational processing is done in the Golgi apparatus (6). The mature virus then buds off from the Golgi network (7) to the extracellular space via exocytosis (8, 9). (**B**) The genome consists of three structural proteins (Envelope (E), Capsid (C) and pre-membrane (prM)) and seven non-structural proteins (NS1, NS2A, NS2B, NS3, NS4A, NSB, and NS5).

2. Flaviviruses and Ocular Complications

Despite the plethora of studies on host–virus interactions to understand their pathogenesis in humans, studies of flaviviruses and their role in ocular diseases are limited. Our knowledge is incomplete regarding properties which confer an ocular tropism to particular flaviviruses and underlying molecular mechanisms which allow the breach of blood-retinal barrier (BRB) for ocular exposure. To appropriately control and treat diseases presenting with ocular complications, a more rigorous understanding of ocular symptoms is needed that can range from maculopathy to retinal hemorrhage and vision loss (Table 2).

Table 2. Flaviviruses known to cause ocular disease in humans and their symptoms.

Virus	General Symptoms	Ocular Disease in Humans	References
West Nile Virus	headache, photophobia, back pain, confusion, fever, encephalitis, meningoencephalitis, acute flaccid paralysis—poliomyelitis-like, Guillain–Barré syndrome	chorioretinitis, anterior uveitis, retinal vasculitis, optic neuritis, and congenital chorioretinal scarring	[5–8]
Yellow Fever Virus	fever, chills, malaise, headache, lower back pain, generalized myalgia, nausea, and dizziness, vomiting, epigastric pain, prostration, and dehydration, petechiae, ecchymoses, epistaxis (bleeding of the gums), and the characteristic "black vomit" (gastrointestinal bleeding)	loss of vision, optic neuritis	[9–11]
Japanese Encephalitis Virus	Fever, headache, vomiting, fits, encephalitis, and coma	Blurred vision, retinal hemorrhage, ocular fundus	[12–18]
Kyasanur Forest Disease Virus	Frontal headache, fever, hemorrhagic pneumonitis, hepatomegaly and parenchymatic degeneration, nephrosis, characteristic reticulo-endothelial cells in spleen and liver along with leucopenia, thrombocytopenia, reduced red blood cells, bradycardia, meningoencephalitis, hemorrhagic fever manifestations, coma, mental disturbance, giddiness, stiff neck, abnormality of reflexes	hemorrhages in the conjunctiva, vitreous humor, and retina, mild iritis, the opacity of lens and keratitis	[19–24]
Dengue Virus	Fever, retro-orbital pain, myalgia, thrombocytopenia, severe abdominal pain, persistent vomiting, bleeding gums, restlessness	maculopathy, blurred vision, scotoma, floaters, subconjunctival hemorrhage, uveitis, vitritis, retinal hemorrhaging, retinal venular widening, higher retinal vascular dimension, retinal vascular sheathing, RPE mottling, tortuous vessels, acute macular neuroretinopathy, intraretinal macular, retinal edema, cotton wool spots, Roth's spot, retinal detachment, retinochoroiditis, neuroretinitis, choroidal effusions, choroidal neovascularization, optic disc swelling and optic disc neuropathy, oculomotor nerve palsy, and panophthalmitis	[25–35]
Zika Virus	fever, rash, headache, joint pain, conjunctivitis, muscle pain, and may result in Guillain-Barre syndrome, microcephaly, hearing loss, seizures, impaired joint movement, facial deformities	gross macular pigment mottling, foveal reflex loss, and macular neuroretinal atrophy, chorioretinal atrophy, optic neuritis, retinal hemorrhaging, retinal mottling, iris coloboma, lens subluxation, gross macular pigment mottling, optic nerve hyperplasia, macular chorioretinal atrophy, anterior uveitis, and non-purulent conjunctivitis	[36–43]

2.1. Yellow Fever Virus (YFV)

Yellow fever (YF) has been a major threat to human health from the 18th to 20th century with repeated epidemics in North America, Europe, and the Caribbean. Described as "the original viral hemorrhagic fever (VHF)," severe YF is pan-systemic viral sepsis with viremia, fever, prostration, hepatic, renal and myocardial injury, hemorrhage, shock and lethality up to 20–50% [44]. There is an abrupt onset of severe symptoms after 3 to 6 days of fever. Patients may experience fever, chills, malaise, headache, lower back pain, generalized myalgia, nausea, and dizziness, often manifesting Faget's sign (increasing temperature with decreasing pulse rate). Infections in humans range from unapparent abortive infection to a fatal, fulminating disease with high fever, vomiting, epigastric pain, prostration, and dehydration. Hepatic-induced coagulopathy produces severe hemorrhagic manifestations including petechiae, ecchymosis, epistaxis (bleeding of the gums), and the characteristic "black vomit" (hematemesis; gastrointestinal hemorrhage) [10]. The infection rate of YFV has rapidly declined due to the successful development of two attenuated vaccines during the 1930–1940s [9]. Currently, YFV is majorly persevered in jungle environments with sporadic human outbreaks in South America and sub-Saharan Africa. The present risk of emergence and transmission of the disease is being primarily controlled by wide coverage of vulnerable populations with vaccinations [45,46].

Among reported studies in virus-induced ocular complications, there is only a single case study on a 21-year old woman traveler to Africa who suffered from irreversible loss of vision along with optic neuritis and encephalitis upon receiving vaccinations for yellow fever, hepatitis A, and B. The causal factor among the multiple vaccines could not be resolved during the investigation [11]. To our knowledge, there have been no further reports of eye infections, and therefore, the involvement of YFV in causing ocular complications is still not clear.

2.2. Japanese Encephalitis Virus (JEV)

JEV is the causal agent for Japanese Encephalitis, which can lead to severe neurological damage [47] and is known to cause 30,000 to 50,000 cases each year in the Pacific and Asia. Symptoms depend on the affected part of the nervous system and include early symptoms, such as non-specific febrile illness, diarrhea and rigor, followed by reduced levels of consciousness, seizures, headache, photophobia, and vomiting [13]. Late symptoms could include poliomyelitis-like flaccid paralysis [12] and parkinsonian syndrome. Patients exhibit the classic description of Japanese encephalitis-dull, flat, mask-like face with wide, unblinking eyes, tremor, generalized hypertonia, cogwheel rigidity, and other complications in locomotion [13]. The frequency of seizures increase with the severity of the disease [14]. In fatal cases of JEV, pathological changes are polymorphic and diffuse, involving different parts of the nervous system where the brain shows a severe degree of congestion in vasculature, microglial proliferation, and gliomesenchymal nodules formation, cystic necrosis in focal or confluent areas, cerebral edema, and trans-compartmental shift which can also lead to acute coma [15,16].

There has been a drastic reduction in the occurrence of JEV induced encephalitis cases since the use of a live attenuated vaccine (LAV) for humans [48]. There has been only a single case study published on a 53-year old woman infected with JEV leading to blurred vision with retinal hemorrhage and a clinical presentation of ocular fundus [17]. In vitro studies on JEV have shown that virus infection leads to the production of a macrophage-derived neutrophil chemotactic factor, which alters the blood-retinal barrier and thereby might have been a cause for the observed retinal hemorrhage [17,18].

2.3. Kyasanur Forest Disease Virus (KFDV)

KFDV was first reported in 1957 from Kyasanur forest in Karnataka, India and is prevalent in South Asia. It is transmitted to humans and animals by the bite of infected ticks (*Haemophysalis spinigera*) [49]. It causes biphasic illness composed of acute and convalescent phase [50]. Chief pathological features include hemorrhagic pneumonitis, hepatomegaly and parenchymatic degeneration, nephrosis, characteristic reticuloendothelial cells in spleen and liver [19] along with leucopenia, thrombocytopenia, reduced red blood cells and elevated levels of liver enzymes [20]. The second non-viremic phase may include bradycardia, meningoencephalitis, hemorrhagic fever manifestations, conjunctival inflammation, coma and neurological complications such as mental disturbance, light-headedness, stiff neck, abnormality of reflexes, confusion, and tremors [19,21]. KFDV has been classified as a risk group 4 pathogens and NIAID (National Institute of Allergy and Infectious Diseases) Category C priority pathogen due to its extreme pathogenicity and lack of US FDA approved vaccines and drugs [21].

There are around 400–500 cases reported annually during the past five decades, and the ophthalmic presentation of KFDV includes hemorrhages in the conjunctiva, vitreous humor, and retina, mild iritis, the opacity of lens and keratitis [20,22–24]. KFDV has only been reported from India, and there have been no further studies to understand the ocular anomalies and the reason behind the complications. Currently, there are no experimental models to study its pathogenesis.

2.4. West Nile Virus (WNV)

Smithburn et al. first isolated WNV, a neuro-invasive flavivirus, from the West Nile district of Uganda in 1937 [51]. The disease has gained recent global attention due to its reported multiple outbreaks in Africa, Asia, Europe, and the United States. The incubation period for the infection in humans range from 3 to 14 days along with three different systemic disease presentations: asymptomatic, fever and meningoencephalitis. Severe, potentially lethal, involvement of neurological complications (encephalitis, meningoencephalitis, acute flaccid paralysis—poliomyelitis-like, Guillain–Barré syndrome and optic neuritis) had been limited to 1%

in the past, but with time, WNV has increased its severity. WNV meningoencephalitis may be characterized by a headache, photophobia, back pain, confusion, and fever.

The ocular involvement following WNV infection was first reported during 2002–2003 with chorioretinitis, anterior uveitis, retinal vasculitis, optic neuritis, and congenital chorioretinal scarring [6]. Around 80% of the WNV infected patients with neurological complications suffered from multifocal chorioretinitis without any ocular symptoms or vaguely reduced vision. The multifocal pattern has been regarded as an early diagnostic marker for WNV infection with meningoencephalitis. Currently, there are no vaccines or antivirals against WNV infection. Clinical cases usually recover within a week and upon administration of steroids [52].

A prospective case study in India revealed that 70% of positive cases with WNV infection reported additional ocular complications apart from what was initially reported. The fundus examination revealed discrete superficial white retinitis, arteritis, phlebitis, and retinal hemorrhages with or without a macular star [5]. Moreover, areas of retinal inflammation with unclear borders, vascular and optic disc leakage, vessel wall staining, or capillary non-perfusion were also observed. One of the patients with diabetes exhibited choroidal inflammation.

Other various ocular complications reported in the past are iridocyclitis in the absence of chorioretinitis, retinitis, retinal hemorrhages, focal or diffuse vascular sheathing, vascular leakage, macular edema, occlusive vasculitis, and segmental wedge-shaped zones of atrophy and mottling of the retinal pigment epithelium [53–56]. WNV-associated optic nerve involvement may occur, including optic neuritis, neuroretinitis, optic disc swelling. WNV infection has been rarely associated with Opsoclonus-myoclonus syndrome (OMS), also known as the dancing eye syndrome in patients with rapid, involuntary, multifactorial, conjugated fast eye movements persisting during sleep [7,8]. The exact mechanisms related to optic neuropathy related to WNV are still unknown.

2.5. Dengue Virus (DENV)

DENV has been involved in causing epidemics throughout the tropics and subtropics since the 1950s, with over one-third of the world's population living at risk of infection. The transmission of DENV occurs between humans and *Aedes* mosquitoes, with incubation periods between 3 to 10 days and symptoms lasting from 3 to 7 days [57–59]. There are four serotypes of DENV reported, DENV-1, DENV-2, DENV-3, and DENV-4 [60], that can cause dengue fever (DF) as well as severe forms of dengue hemorrhagic fever (DHF) and dengue shock syndrome (DSS).

The symptoms during dengue fever usually include high fever, severe headache, retro-orbital pain, arthralgia, myalgia, nausea, vomiting, and rash. A severe form of dengue may be lethal to individuals with symptoms including bleeding gums, restlessness, fatigue, blood in vomit, and thrombocytopenia [25]. Severe forms of DENV infection mostly occur due to antibody-dependent enhancement (ADE), where pre-existing antibodies from a primary infection bind to an infecting DENV particle during secondary infection with a different DENV serotype [61]. While only 5% develop severe, life-threating infections, most dengue infections are asymptomatic. Recently, DENV NS1 protein has also been shown to be responsible for causing vascular leakage in both in vitro and in vivo models and is being used as a marker to detect DENV infection in DHF patients [62–64]. The viral NS1 protein is secreted from the cells and stays in the blood circulation of patients even after the fever and viral nucleic acid subside. At the time when severe dengue hemorrhage begins, NS1 protein levels correlate well with the degree of thrombocytopenia [65].

Traditionally, ocular pathology in dengue fever was thought to be uncommon; however, its involvement of ocular complications is now being recognized increasingly as it leads to permanent visual impairment in certain cases. Clinical studies have not seen any disease correlation with age, sex or ethnicity as risk factors [26]. Factors which have been postulated in the pathogenesis of dengue ocular diseases include viral virulence, serotypes, mutations, host susceptibility and geographic factor. Dengue eye disease can be unilateral or bilateral and the onset of ocular symptoms range from 2 to 5 days after the onset of fever and most ocular symptoms have been noted within one day after the peak of thrombocytopenia [27]. One study reported that 10% of 160 DENV seropositive hospitalized patients had maculopathy [26]. The main ocular complaints are eye pain, retro-ocular pain, blurring of vision, diplopia, foreign body sensation, photopsia, floaters, and metamorphopsia. In addition to this, other ocular symptoms include blurred vision floaters, subconjunctival hemorrhage, uveitis, and vitritis etc. (Table 2) [26–35]. Significant predictors of ocular symptoms included leukopenia and hypoalbuminemia, which could predispose patients to an opportunistic infection of ocular tissues and hyper permeability [66].

Dengue maculopathy is well recognized and studied more than other ocular manifestations, and it has been seen to be serotype and geography-related. There have been very few studies to understand the mechanism behind dengue-induced ocular implications which limit our understanding of the disease pathology. There is only one study relating maculopathy to be serotype specific with DENV-1 epidemic causing 10% incidence while there were no cases during DENV-2 epidemic [67]. Macular edema and macular hemorrhage were common findings in symptomatic patients with maculopathy.

While cellular and molecular mechanisms to understand systemic dengue has been extensively studied, there has been no studies of DENV in vitro as well as in vivo to understand the disease pathology, risk factors of eye disease and preventive measures. The serious threat to vision is dengue retinopathy, including retinal vasculopathy and macular edema. The mechanism of retinopathy is not clearly understood, but observations in patients implicate the involvement of retinal pigment epithelium (RPE) and endothelial cells. Smith et al. 2017 have recently shown that retinal epithelial and endothelial cells are susceptible to DENV infection with cytopathic effects in epithelial cells. The infection decreased the epithelial barrier integrity while the endothelial junctions were intact which correlated with the clinically observed loss of RPE in DENV infected patients [68].

Research on DENV vaccine has been a challenging path because there are four known serotypes and the associated complications of partial immunity leading to increase disease severity due to ADE. Live attenuated vaccines based on recombinant attenuated DENV serotypes (NIH) or recombinant yellow fever virus (Sanofi) or DENV-2 (Takeda) constructs expressing prM and Envelope genes from four serotypes, are currently in phase 3 or 4 clinical trials. The leading candidate, Dengvaxia, developed by Sanofi Pasteur, has been approved for use in individuals above the age of 9 years in Brazil, Mexico and the Philippines [69–71].

2.6. Zika Virus (ZIKV)

Zika virus was first isolated from a rhesus macaque from the Zika forest in Uganda, 1947 [72], with its first human detection in 1952 [72,73]. ZIKV then spread throughout parts of Africa and Asia, and in 2007 a ZIKV epidemic on Yap Island in Micronesia had 49 confirmed cases [74]. Over the last 2 years, it has raised a global alarm as it infected people in more than 70 countries causing severe deformities in newborns and neurological diseases in adults [75]. Apart from being transmitted by the vector (mosquitoes), ZIKV is capable of vertical transmission in humans during pregnancy or delivery, through sexual contact, or through contaminated blood transfusions. The incubation period for ZIKV ranges from 3 to 14 days while the symptoms last from 3 to 7 days. The risk of transmission of infection is escalated because 80% of infected adults remain asymptomatic. The usually visible signs of infection are mild and include fever, rash, headache, joint pain, conjunctivitis, muscle pain, and may result in Guillain-Barre syndrome. Congenitally contracted ZIKV causes birth defects in newborns such as microcephaly, impaired brain development, hearing loss, seizures, impaired joint movement, facial deformities, and vision problems [76].

In the eyes of adults, ZIKV presents most commonly as non-purulent conjunctivitis; however, more serious findings, such as the disruption of the RPE and iridocyclitis, have been reported in healthy and immunocompromised patients [42,77,78]. The first report on Congenital Zika Syndrome (CZS) had originated from Brazil describing ophthalmologic findings in three children with microcephaly caused by presumed ZIKV infection. There has been a steep increase in reported cases in the pathology of ocular complication in CZS, thereafter. Children present with gross macular pigment mottling, foveal reflex loss, macular neuroretinal atrophy, and fundoscopic alterations in the macular regions [79]. There have also been reports of chorioretinal atrophy, optic neuritis, retinal hemorrhaging, retinal mottling, iris coloboma, lens subluxation, gross macular pigment mottling, optic nerve hyperplasia, macular chorioretinal atrophy in other reported CZS cases [36–40]. Retinal abnormalities were also reported without microcephaly indicating the capability of ZIKV to cause ocular complications by direct infection [37]. The first study to reveal the ocular histopathologic findings of ocular tissue samples from deceased CZS fetuses by Fernandez et al., 2017 revealed pupillary membranes, immature anterior chamber angles, loss of pigment and thinning of the retinal pigment epithelium, choroidal thinning, undifferentiated nuclear layers of the retina, and a perivascular inflammatory infiltrate within the choroid. The viral antigen could be detected in iris, neural retina, choroid and the optic nerve [80].

Currently, the long-term effects of these infections are unknown, but a report in an immunocompromised patient indicates that lesions can be persistent [77]. ZIKV has been isolated from conjunctival swabs of infected patients which indicates its ability to infect the peri-ocular tissues and transmit through ocular secretions [81]. To date, there are thirteen open clinical trials at different phases, testing various concepts of ZIKV ranging from DNA vaccines, mRNA vaccines, Purified Inactivated Virus (PIV) vaccines and viral-vector-based vaccines [82,83].

3. Experimental Models of Ocular ZIKV Complications

To alleviate the disease burden associated with ocular viral infections, it is necessary to focus today's research on disease control and therapeutic strategies. An animal model for a disease would prove to be a valuable tool to shed light on the pathophysiology of infection and facilitate the assessment of therapeutics and vaccines in the offing.

3.1. In Vivo Models

There have been several animal models used to mimic the ZIKV infection. The wild-type C57BL/6, BALB/c, and CD-1 mice are resistant to flavivirus infections [84–86]. Most of the studies used immunocompromised mice, both type I and type II interferon knockout mice (AG129), for efficient infection and viral replication to mimic human symptoms [86–91]. The first model of ocular complication during ZIKV infection in mice was described by Miner et al., where subcutaneous injection of the virus in IFNAR$^{-/-}$ mice caused panuveitis and shedding of viral RNA in tears, but there was complete absence of live virus in ocular tissues and retina, as seen in humans [88]. There were no histological abnormalities evident in the eyes of congenitally infected IFNAR$^{+/-}$ fetuses from C57BL/6 IFNAR1$^{-/-}$ dams [88]. Direct inoculation of the virus in the organ/tissue of interest has been another approach used by various groups [92,93]. Singh et al. have developed a new model of ocular ZIKV infection to mimic human disease conditions by injecting the ZIKV intravitreally in the eyes of immunocompetent C57BL/6 mice or ISG15 knockout mice [94]. This model could show the observed pathological findings of retinal pigment epithelium atrophy and pigment clumping/mottling in humans. Another successful mouse model showed ocular infections mimicking humans upon subcutaneous injection of ZIKV in 1 day old pups (p1) [75]. The model showed presence of virus in the ocular tissues till 30 days pi while the inflammation subsided by 60 dpi. Therefore, these models could be used to study ocular complications in ZIKV as well as other viral infections to understand the viral pathogenesis in the ocular tissue.

In mouse models, ZIKV has been shown to infect multiple ocular cell types and that ZIKV inoculated mice developed conjunctivitis, pan-uveitis, infection of the cornea, iris, optic nerve, retina, as well as the detection of viral RNA in tears [88,94]. These studies exhibit the ability of ZIKV to infect previously unexplored cell types of the eye, and the need for research investigating these relationships is of paramount importance. The studies indicate the spread of the virus via two modes: hematogenic or axonal which is also supported by Fernandez et al. [80]. The virus could reach the fetal circulation from the placenta and infect the RPE, retinal endothelial cells, and the retina [94]. The other possible pathway would be through axonal transport into the eye along the optic nerve [95,96], leading to ganglion cell layer (GCL) loss, foveal maldevelopment, and central chorioretinal abnormalities [97]. How ZIKV and other flaviviruses enter the eye in vivo remains to be determined.

3.2. In Vitro Models

Since wild-type mice are not susceptible to ZIKV, most in vitro studies have used primary human cells or established cell lines. For example, Singh et al. have recently reported that retinal cell types lining the BRB are susceptible to ZIKV infection and cause cell death by activating Caspase 3 [94]. Zhao et al. and Aleman et al. have independently shown the Muller glia cells to be the primary target of ZIKV infection leading to decreased neurotropic functions and increased pro-inflammatory cytokines post infection with the help of murine models [96,98]. ZIKV infection in RPE was shown to disrupt its cell to cell adhesion and barrier properties [99]. Similarly, ZIKV was found to infect human fetal retinal pigment epithelial cells (FRPE), iPSC-derived retinal stem cells (iRSCs), and retinal cup (RC) organoids [100]. The underlying mechanisms and detailed sketch of the breach of BRB to cause the ocular pathology has not been addressed till now. Currently, the field of ZIKV research has been undecided on the role of the protein tyrosine kinase TAM receptors—TYRO3, AXL, and MER—in ZIKV entry into cells. The TAM receptors have been shown to be upregulated in the retinal epithelial and endothelial primary cells during ZIKV infection but their roles are still under debate [94].

4. Interaction with Blood-Retinal Barrier (BRB)

The BRB forms as an extension of the blood-brain barrier (BBB), which aids in the separation of the internal environment of the eye from the systemic vascular system. The BRB has two modules: an inner barrier, formed by retinal endothelial cells, and an outer barrier, formed by the RPE layer along with Bruch's membrane and choriocapillaries [94]. The outer BRB shields the neuroretina from blood-borne pathogens including viruses. Therefore, disruption of the RPE could create a route of entry for virus present in fenestrated choroidal capillaries to enter the tissues of the eye. The BRB is limited internally by tight junctions between the endothelial cells underlining the retinal capillaries whereas the outer barrier is formed of tight junctions between the cells of RPE, separating the choroid system from the sensory retina [101].

The development and maintenance of the BRB is needed for healthy vision and the loss of the BRB leads to the pathology of a variety of retinal diseases. A balance of the vascular endothelial and epithelial mechanisms of the BRB supports the specialized neural retina environment. The vascular endothelium and the pigment epithelium layer of the retina possess a highly developed complex of inter cellular junction complexes including the adherens and tight junctions [102,103]. These junctions impart a high degree of barrier permeability to the solute and fluid across the retina. An understanding of BRB regulation during viral infection will allow the development of therapies aimed at restoring the compromised barrier or manipulating the barrier for specific transport of therapies.

ZIKV is permissive to all cell types comprising the different layers of the eye except the photoreceptor cells and causes similar pathological findings as in human patients with chorioretinal atrophy, pigment mottling/clumping [94]. There are two models proposed for the infection and entry of ZIKV into the eye: (a) cell death caused by ZIKV infection in the outer BRB might form the portal of entry of the virus into the eye and infect the inner layers, thereby causing inflammation and vision loss in severe infected cases [94]; (b) ZIKV could possibly enter via the retinal arteries (inner BRB) which leads to infection of the retinal endothelial cells and pericytes and the virus enters the outer BRB via the choroid capillaries [104].

4.1. Modulation of Retinal Innate and Adaptive Immunity

RPE cells are multi-functional and help in transport of nutrients and waste from the retina across the choroid and impart adhesive properties to the retina (Bok, 1995, 1993). It forms the first line of defense against pathogens in the retina and has a role in innate as well as adaptive immunity [105].

These cells have been identified as an ideal target for infectious agents such as Cytomegalovirus, *Toxoplasma gondii*, Coronavirus, Zika virus [94,105]. They produce a variety of cytokines (IL6, IL8, MCP-1), chemokines, growth factors, and act as Antigen Presenting Cells (APC) in the retina upon a pathogen assault [106–108]. Few immune cells reside within the ocular tissues [41,109]. Upon infection, the peripheral immune cells can gain access to the eye leading to local inflammation [110]. Despite the upsurge of interest in the RPE cell and its critical role in retinal health and disease, the exact mechanisms of how the RPE cells participate in the regulation of the blood-retinal barrier remain largely unknown. The retina also contains specialized myeloid cells (microglia), similar to brain microglia and the central and peripheral rims of the retina contain a small population of DCIR$^+$ MHC Class II^{hi} DCs, as does the corneal periphery [111]. In addition to neurons, retina contains glial cells (microglia and Muller glia) and astrocytes which not only provide structural support but play an important role in evoking retinal innate responses to injury or infectious stimuli. How these retinal residential glial cells regulate innate immunity is an active area of investigation in our laboratory. Similarly, cells lining the BRB, also contribute to retinal immune response to microbial infections.

ZIKV infection of RPE, Muller glia and the retinal endothelial cells leads to an increase in the markers of innate immune response along with interferon and interferon stimulated gene response in a time dependent manner and causes chorioretinal atrophy, RPE mottling and cell death in in vitro as well as in vivo models [75,94,112]. ZIKV induces the expression of AXL in all the retinal cell types except the photoreceptor cells and the TAM receptor seems to be the dominant receptor used for the infection of the retinal cell types. ZIKV infection leads to an increase in innate immune response with an increase in TLR3 expression along with an increase in the expression of other viral recognition receptors—MDA5, RIG-I. There is an increase in ocular pathology due to the inflammation caused by significant production of RANTES and an increase in the expression of inflammatory genes *TNFA, IL1B, CXCL10, CCL5* leading to ocular inflammation [94,104]. The infection also leads to elevated levels of granzyme B, perforin, IFN and IFN stimulated genes—*OAS2, ISG15,* and *MX1* [75,94].

Recently, Manangeeswaran et al., 2018 reported that subcutaneous infection can also lead to symptomatic posterior uveitis that could replicate the infection in the patients by employing wild-type B6 mouse model [75]. The model demonstrated the preferential infection of cornea and retina causing chorioretinal lesions upon ZIKV infection. The infection elicits an inflammatory response characterized by increased local chemokine expression, infiltration of neutrophils, APCs, natural killer cells and CD4 and CD8 cells in the later stage. The infection subsides by 30 dpi while the cytotoxic T cells remained in the eyes along with the expression of several chemokines. The study also showed that the cornea and retina had higher levels of chemokines associated with the infiltration of CD45+ cells along with biomarkers for APCs (CD86, B2m, H2-EB1) and T-cell infiltration (CD3, CD4, GITR, CD40L, Fas-L) causing increased cytotoxicity in the infected tissues. This new model of study could prove to be very helpful in dissecting the mechanism of the breach of BRB during ZIKV infection and the various alterations occurring in the ocular tissues as it mimics vector bite followed by infection and inflammation in the eye similar to symptoms in human.

During ZIKV infection, ISG15 acts as a key player in confining viral replication in the retina/eye mostly by positive loop regulation of interferon signaling. The backfire of the antiviral immunity in the infected host leads to a huge amount of tissue inflammation and tissue damage leading to vision loss and further complications which has also been evident during the fetus development [113]. Another parallel study on primary Muller glia cells demonstrated their high susceptibility to ZIKV infection and induce a robust inflammatory response. They activate several intracellular pathways, including ERK, p38MAPK, NF-kB, STAT3 and ER stress, thereby influencing the differential expression of growth and inflammatory factors. The p38MAPK has been shown to be strongly controlling the expression of inflammatory pathways and has been proven to be highly potent during many viral infections, including ZIKV [112].

4.2. Modulation of Cellular Metabolism

As viruses are non-living entities and do not possess their individual metabolism, they alter host cellular metabolic pathways for their optimal replication. The flaviviruses are known to subvert cholesterol homeostasis using multiple mechanisms to transform lipid droplets into their replication complexes with host membranes. To identify unique molecular signature of ZIKV infection in RPE, Singh et al., performed meta-analysis of ZIKV infected RPE cells and other related flaviviruses, DENV, JEV, WNV [114]. This led to the identification of a 43 genes signature referred to as core signature genes which are dysregulated upon ZIKV infection and not by the other flaviviruses tested. The validation of some of the identified genes in the signature revealed that ZIKV modulated (upregulation) their expression at relatively higher levels than DENV. Interestingly, the pathway analysis revealed that ZIKV alters cellular metabolism involving SH3/SH2 adaptor activity, lipid metabolism and ceramide metabolism. The *SH2B3* gene may help in evading the immune system by attenuating the inflammatory response and the infiltration of innate immune cells to the site of infection [114]. The reduction in ALDH5A1 enzyme activity would lead to an increase in the endogenous levels of GHB (gamma-Hydroxybutyric acid) and GABA (gamma-aminobutyric acid) levels, leading to neurological manifestations of ZIKV infection such as microcephaly and Guillain-Barre Syndrome in adults.

ZIKV capsid protein has been recently shown to hijack host lipid metabolism for efficient viral replication and interact with nucleolar proteins to facilitate replication [115]. Among the highly altered genes, *ABCG1* and *ABCA1*, membrane transporters involved in cholesterol efflux and innate immune response, are among the top candidates. Moreover, inhibition of *ABCG1* resulted in reduced ZIKV replication in RPE cells [114]. As host cell lipids and cholesterol play an essential role in various stages of viral replication, including entry, uncoating, genome replication, assembly, and release, it is important to understand the molecules exploited by the virus and exploit the drug targets for therapeutic purposes. Recently studied global interactomics revealed the hijack of lipid metabolism machinery by the ZIKV Capsid protein and the interaction of NS2A and other ZIKV proteins with peroxisome-associated polypeptides that govern the lipid trafficking and innate immune regulation in host cells for the efficient replication of the virus [115]. The lipid metabolism machinery is centrally controlled by AMPK (5′ AMP activated protein kinase), one of the master regulators of various cellular metabolic pathways. AMPK has a prominent role during bacterial endophthalmitis with its activation by pharmacological drugs leading to a significant decrease in bacterial load in the infected eyes [116]. AMPK is known to be altered during flavivirus infection and has pro- as well as antiviral activity upon activation for different viruses [117]. Its role in ZIKV infection and ocular pathology has not been studied till now. Studies are ongoing in our laboratory to understand its role in viral replication and the breach of BRB by altering the intercellular junction machinery [118,119].

5. Conclusions

Ocular complications caused by flaviviruses and other viruses will have long-term economic, psychological and health implications. Therefore, a deeper understanding of the host–virus interaction and the viral pathogenesis in the eye will help in the discovery or re-purposing of therapeutic drugs to protect against viral-borne ocular abnormalities. As there are no known effective antiviral treatments or vaccines against emerging flaviviruses, infected patients can only be provided with palliative care upon diagnosis. The incidence of flavivirus infections can be reduced with supervised vector control and prevention of bites with vectors. A therapeutic approach to decrease viral load combined with a regulation of immune cascade response in the eye could save patients from detrimental ocular consequences in the future. Investigations in both immune-deficient and immune-competent mouse models of ZIKV infection may help to identify key host-pathogen factors and devise novel therapies to restrain the systemic and local inflammatory responses associated with ZIKV infection in the eye. The severity of ocular complications due to viral infections presents additional stress and challenges to communities that have already been devastated by the loss of life, community, and infrastructure. Flavivirus infections are seen increasingly in the endemic and non-endemic regions as the result of an increase in international travel, and therefore, ophthalmologists should have the requisite knowledge to diagnose and manage such patients and keep a track of the patient's history for exposure to viral infections for early diagnosis of viral-related ocular complications.

6. Future Directions

Viral infection epidemics pose significant challenges for healthcare and the world economy. Flavivirus infections causing ocular diseases will have significant long-term economic, psychological and health implications. Vision-related complications may be an underreported effect of flavivirus infection which has been a reason of global concern for many years. ZIKV infection and other related ocular complications in the recent epidemic in Brazil emphasizes the urgency to understand the virus pathogenesis in the eye and develop strategies to prevent potential vision loss due to viral infections. Viral infections may linger in immune privilege tissue/organs such as the central nervous system or the eye. The recent description of a patient recovering from Ebola, where the blood and urine tests were negative but ocular inflammation including anterior uveitis and vitritis continued, calls attention to the long-term effects of ocular infections and understand the role they might play in the replication cycle [120]. The precise pathogenesis of the ocular complications, development of specific antiviral therapy and vaccinations against these threatening flaviviruses are fields that require further research.

There could be various possible theories to explain the factors involved in the breach of the blood-retinal barrier and the transmission of the Zika virus to the eye. In this section, we are trying to hypothesize some of the probable ones to understand the ZIKV disease model and the increase in the severity of the disease caused and their transmission route to the ocular tissues (Figure 3).

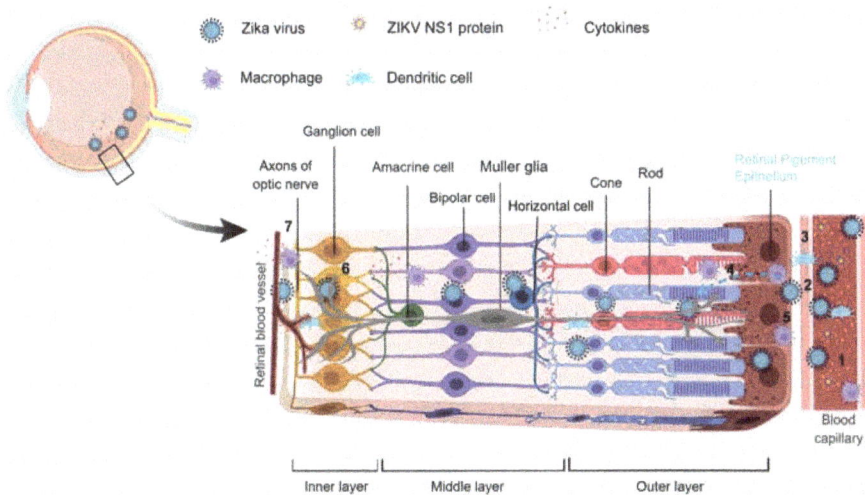

Figure 3. Probable mechanisms for the breach of blood-retinal barriers by ZIKV. Upon infection and peak viremia, there is an increased circulation of Zika virus, ZIKV NS1 protein, and immune cells in the blood (1). The virus in the retinal blood capillaries infect the endothelial lining (2) and the immune cells reach the site of infection/inflammation by diapedesis through the capillaries (3). It is followed by infection of RPE, the cell lining the outer BRB, resulting in chorioretinal atrophy. The viral infections might cause a BRB weakening by decreasing intercellular junction integrity. Being a neurotrophic virus, at later stages ZIKV can infect retinal Muller glia or neurons inside of the eye (4). The complications are worsened with the involvement of immune cells which get activated upon infection and release a "cytokine storm" as an antiviral response which damages the host cells by altering the barrier integrity (5). The virus along with the circulating immune cells can cross the inner BRB (retinal blood vessels) and infect neuronal cells such as ganglion cells (6, 7). The Image has been created with BioRender software.

6.1. Possible Involvement of ADE

Since the transmission system of flaviviruses overlap, there is a high probability that many patients who have ZIKV infection have also had a previous exposure to at least one of the DENV serotypes. Likewise, many patients now exposed to ZIKV are highly likely to be exposed to at least one of the DENV serotypes in the future. There have been reports of an increase in the severity of ZIKV infection in individuals who have been infected with DENV in the recent past via a mechanism similar to ADE [121–123]. Therefore, pre-existing immunity against one flavivirus can affect clinical outcomes and diagnosis of the disease produced by infection with a heterologous flavivirus.

6.2. Possible Role of Secreted ZIKV NS1 Protein

Secreted DENV NS1 protein, a marker for DENV infection in patients, has been shown to be a causal factor for severe dengue and hemorrhage in cell culture and in vivo studies [63,64,124]. Zika virus, being a closely related member of the same family, may also share similar antigenic roles for secreted NS1 protein and may be a potential candidate in causing retinal hemorrhage and ocular complications by being a possible mediator in breaching the blood-retinal barrier.

6.3. Involvement of Immune Response and Cytokine Storm

The ocular complications are usually the outcome of a robust immune response from the host following an infection. During DENV infection, hemorrhage caused in tissues is mostly due to the cytokine storm from invading immune cells into tissues, thereby increasing severity of the disease [125–127]. The invading immune cells in the eye could also be exacerbating the severity of the complications and damaging the retina and blood vessels due to their response to control the infection. The inflammation and infiltrating cells may play a key role in clearing the virus but may also contribute to the development of lesions. Understanding the role of the immune response in the generation and persistence of the retinal lesions may enlighten the helpfulness of using immune suppressors, such as corticoids, during the later stages in the disease.

6.4. Involvement of the Altered Host Machinery

Flaviviruses employ the host lipid metabolism machinery for its replication which makes it a potent target for therapeutic purpose [2,128,129]. Flaviviruses have been shown to impair the intercellular junction integrity via different cellular intermediates and cause a breach in the barrier via tight junction and adherens junction protein alteration and degradation. Little research has been conducted to understand the pathogenesis of ZIKV and how it breaches the blood-retinal barrier to cause ocular complications. Our recent study using a transcriptomic approach on retinal epithelial cells, a major component of the outer blood-retinal barrier, indicates the involvement of cholesterol metabolism in viral replication [114]. Targeting host cellular metabolism could alleviate ocular complications due to ZIKV infection.

Therefore, a deeper understanding of the ocular pathogenesis of viral diseases and their interaction with the various cell types involved in the blood-retinal barrier can etch a path towards the invention or re-purposing of therapeutic drugs to prevent vision loss in infected patients. The ocular complications during viral infections have been under-reported mostly due to the late or ignored investigation by ophthalmologists. Ophthalmologists have a crucial role to help in decreasing ocular complications by being aware of changing symptoms during flavivirus infections and having a complete patient history of their previous exposure to viral infections to rule out secondary infection complications.

Author Contributions: A.K. conceived the idea and both S.S. and A.K. wrote and revise the manuscript to final form. All authors read and approved the manuscript.

Funding: Research in our laboratory is supported in parts by National Institute of Health (NIH) Grants (R21AI135583, R01EY026964, and R01 EY027381 to A.K.), NIH Core Grant P30EY004068 (to Linda D. Hazlett), and an unrestricted grant from Research to Prevent Blindness Inc. (to Kresge Eye Institute, Wayne State University).

Viruses **2018**, *10*, 530

Acknowledgments: The authors would like to thank other members of the lab for their helpful discussions.

Disclaimer: The authors have made every effort to ensure that appropriate and justified references have been added to the best of their knowledge. The authors would like to apologize to the groups whose references would have been overlooked while writing the review article.

Conflicts of Interest: The authors declare no conflict of interest.

Glossary

Chorioretinitis	Inflammation of the choroid and retina of the eye. It is a form of posterior uveitis
Keratitis	Inflammation of the cornea
Iritis	Inflammation of the iris
Chorioretinal atrophy	A condition of the eye where both the choroid and retina are damaged. This causes them to wither away and stop working
Maculopathy	Any pathological condition of the macula, an area at the center of the retina that is associated with highly sensitive, accurate vision
Conjunctivitis	Inflammation of the conjunctiva of the eye
Uveitis	Inflammation of the uvea
Vitritis	Inflammation of the vitreous body
Optic neuritis	Inflammation that damages the optic nerve, a bundle of nerve fibers that transmits visual information from your eye to the brain
RPE	Retinal pigment epithelium cells
ADE	Antibody-Dependent enhancement
Scotoma	A partial loss of vision or a blind spot in an otherwise normal visual field
cotton wool spots	Fluffy white patches on the retina. They are caused by damage to nerve fibers and are a result of accumulations of axoplasmic material within the nerve fiber layer
Roth's spot	Retinal hemorrhages with white or pale centers
Panophthalmitis	Inflammation of all coats of the eye including intraocular structures
iris coloboma	A hole in the iris
BRB	Blood-retinal barrier

References

1. Ludwig, G.V.; Iacono-Connors, L.C. Insect-transmitted vertebrate viruses: Flaviviridae. *In Vitro Cell. Dev. Biol. Anim.* **1993**, *29A*, 296–309. [CrossRef] [PubMed]
2. Fernandez-Garcia, M.D.; Mazzon, M.; Jacobs, M.; Amara, A. Pathogenesis of flavivirus infections: Using and abusing the host cell. *Cell Host Microbe* **2009**, *5*, 318–328. [CrossRef] [PubMed]
3. Bharucha, T.; Breuer, J. Review: A neglected Flavivirus: An update on Zika virus in 2016 and the future direction of research. *Neuropathol. Appl. Neurobiol.* **2016**, *42*, 317–325. [CrossRef] [PubMed]
4. De Andrade, G.C.; Ventura, C.V.; Mello Filho, P.A.; Maia, M.; Vianello, S.; Rodrigues, E.B. Arboviruses and the eye. *Int. J. Retin. Vitreous* **2017**, *3*, 4. [CrossRef] [PubMed]
5. Sivakumar, R.R.; Prajna, L.; Arya, L.K.; Muraly, P.; Shukla, J.; Saxena, D.; Parida, M. Molecular diagnosis and ocular imaging of West Nile virus retinitis and neuroretinitis. *Ophthalmology* **2013**, *120*, 1820–1826. [CrossRef] [PubMed]
6. Garg, S.; Jampol, L.M. Systemic and intraocular manifestations of West Nile virus infection. *Surv. Ophthalmol.* **2005**, *50*, 3–13. [CrossRef] [PubMed]
7. Alshekhlee, A.; Sultan, B.; Chandar, K. Opsoclonus persisting during sleep in West Nile encephalitis. *Arch. Neurol.* **2006**, *63*, 1324–1326. [CrossRef] [PubMed]
8. Bîrluţiu, V.; Bîrluţiu, R.M. Opsoclonus-myoclonus syndrome attributable to West Nile encephalitis: A case report. *J. Med. Case Rep.* **2014**, *8*, 232. [CrossRef] [PubMed]
9. Monath, T.P.; Vasconcelos, P.F. Yellow fever. *J. Clin. Virol.* **2015**, *64*, 160–173. [CrossRef] [PubMed]
10. Gardner, C.L.; Ryman, K.D. Yellow fever: A reemerging threat. *Clin. Lab. Med.* **2010**, *30*, 237–260. [CrossRef] [PubMed]

11. Voigt, U.; Baum, U.; Behrendt, W.; Hegemann, S.; Terborg, C.; Strobel, J. Neuritis of the optic nerve after vaccinations against hepatitis A.; hepatitis B. and yellow fever. *Klinische Monatsblatter Augenheilkunde* **2001**, *218*, 688–690. [CrossRef] [PubMed]

12. Solomon, T.; Kneen, R.; Dung, N.M.; Khanh, V.C.; Thuy, T.T.; Ha, D.Q.; Day, N.P.; Nisalak, A.; Vaughn, D.W.; White, N.J. Poliomyelitis-like illness due to Japanese encephalitis virus. *Lancet* **1998**, *351*, 1094–1097. [CrossRef]

13. Solomon, T.; Dung, N.M.; Kneen, R.; Gainsborough, M.; Vaughn, D.W.; Khanh, V.T. Japanese encephalitis. *J. Neurol. Neurosurg. Psychiatry* **2000**, *68*, 405–415. [CrossRef] [PubMed]

14. Solomon, T. Flavivirus encephalitis. *N. Engl. J. Med.* **2004**, *351*, 370–378. [CrossRef] [PubMed]

15. Ishii, T.; Matsushita, M.; Hamada, S. Characteristic residual neuropathological features of Japanese, *B. encephalitis. Acta Neuropathol.* **1977**, *38*, 181–186. [CrossRef] [PubMed]

16. Ghosh, D.; Basu, A. Japanese encephalitis-a pathological and clinical perspective. *PLoS Negl. Trop. Dis.* **2009**, *3*, e437. [CrossRef] [PubMed]

17. Fang, S.T.; Chu, S.Y.; Lee, Y.C. Ischaemic maculopathy in Japanese encephalitis. *Eye* **2006**, *20*, 1439–1441. [CrossRef] [PubMed]

18. Mathur, A.; Khanna, N.; Chaturvedi, U.C. Breakdown of blood-brain barrier by virus-induced cytokine during Japanese encephalitis virus infection. *Int. J. Exp. Pathol* **1992**, *73*, 603–611. [PubMed]

19. Pattnaik, P. Kyasanur forest disease: An epidemiological view in India. *Rev. Med. Virol.* **2006**, *16*, 151–165. [CrossRef] [PubMed]

20. Work, T.H.; Trapido, H.; Murthy, D.P.; Rao, R.L.; Bhatt, P.N.; Kulkarni, K.G. Kyasanur forest disease. III. A preliminary report on the nature of the infection and clinical manifestations in human beings. *Indian J. Med. Sci.* **1957**, *11*, 619–645. [PubMed]

21. Shah, S.Z.; Jabbar, B.; Ahmed, N.; Rehman, A.; Nasir, H.; Nadeem, S.; Jabbar, I.; Rahman, Z.U.; Azam, S. Epidemiology, Pathogenesis, and Control of a Tick-Borne Disease- Kyasanur Forest Disease: Current Status and Future Directions. *Front. Cell. Infect. Microbiol.* **2018**, *8*, 149. [CrossRef] [PubMed]

22. Grard, G.; Moureau, G.; Charrel, R.N.; Lemasson, J.J.; Gonzalez, J.P.; Gallian, P.; Gritsun, T.S.; Holmes, E.C.; Gould, E.A.; de Lamballerie, X. Genetic characterization of tick-borne flaviviruses: New insights into evolution, pathogenetic determinants and taxonomy. *Virology* **2007**, *361*, 80–92. [CrossRef] [PubMed]

23. Rao, R.L. Clinical observations on Kyasanur Forest disease cases. *J. Indian Med. Assoc.* **1958**, *31*, 113–116. [PubMed]

24. Ocular manifestations of Kyasanur forest disease (a clinical study). *Indian J. Ophthalmol.* **1983**, *31*, 700–702.

25. Boo, Y.L.; Aris, M.A.M.; Chin, P.W.; Sulaiman, W.A.W.; Basri, H.; Hoo, F.K. Guillain-Barré syndrome complicating dengue fever: Two case reports. *Ci Ji Yi Xue Za Zhi* **2016**, *28*, 157–159. [CrossRef] [PubMed]

26. Su, D.H.; Bacsal, K.; Chee, S.P.; Flores, J.V.; Lim, W.K.; Cheng, B.C.; Jap, A.H.; Group, D.M.S. Prevalence of dengue maculopathy in patients hospitalized for dengue fever. *Ophthalmology* **2007**, *114*, 1743–1747. [CrossRef] [PubMed]

27. Chan, D.P.; Teoh, S.C.; Tan, C.S.; Nah, G.K.; Rajagopalan, R.; Prabhakaragupta, M.K.; Chee, C.K.; Lim, T.H.; Goh, K.Y.; Eye Institute Dengue-Related Ophthalmic Complications Workgroup. Ophthalmic complications of dengue. *Emerg. Infect. Dis.* **2006**, *12*, 285–289. [CrossRef] [PubMed]

28. Tabbara, K. Dengue retinochoroiditis. *Ann. Saudi Med.* **2012**, *32*, 530–533. [CrossRef] [PubMed]

29. Beral, L.; Laurence, B.; Merle, H.; Harold, M.; David, T.; Thierry, D. Ocular complications of Dengue fever. *Ophthalmology* **2008**, *115*, 1100–1101. [PubMed]

30. Lei, H.Y.; Yeh, T.M.; Liu, H.S.; Lin, Y.S.; Chen, S.H.; Liu, C.C. Immunopathogenesis of dengue virus infection. *J. Biomed. Sci.* **2001**, *8*, 377–388. [CrossRef] [PubMed]

31. Lim, W.K.; Mathur, R.; Koh, A.; Yeoh, R.; Chee, S.P. Ocular manifestations of dengue fever. *Ophthalmology* **2004**, *111*, 2057–2064. [CrossRef] [PubMed]

32. Donnio, A.; Béral, L.; Olindo, S.; Cabie, A.; Merle, H. Dengue, a new etiology in oculomotor paralysis. *Can. J. Ophthalmol.* **2010**, *45*, 183–184. [CrossRef] [PubMed]

33. Aragão, R.E.; Barreira, I.M.; Lima, L.N.; Rabelo, L.P.; Pereira, F.B. Bilateral optic neuritis after dengue viral infection: Case report. *Arq. Bras. Oftalmol.* **2010**, *73*, 175–178. [CrossRef] [PubMed]

34. Cruz-Villegas, V.; Berrocal, A.M.; Davis, J.L. Bilateral choroidal effusions associated with dengue fever. *Retina* **2003**, *23*, 576–578. [CrossRef] [PubMed]

35. Saranappa, S.B.S.; Sowbhagya, H.N. Panophthalmitis in dengue fever. *Indian Pediatr.* **2012**, *49*, 760. [CrossRef]

36. Ventura, C.V.; Maia, M.; Ventura, B.V.; Linden, V.V.; Araújo, E.B.; Ramos, R.C.; Rocha, M.A.; Carvalho, M.D.; Belfort, R.; Ventura, L.O. Ophthalmological findings in infants with microcephaly and presumable intra-uterus Zika virus infection. *Arq. Bras. Oftalmol.* **2016**, *79*, 1–3. [CrossRef] [PubMed]

37. Ventura, L.O.; Ventura, C.V.; Lawrence, L.; van der Linden, V.; van der Linden, A.; Gois, A.L.; Cavalcanti, M.M.; Barros, E.A.; Dias, N.C.; Berrocal, A.M.; et al. Visual impairment in children with congenital Zika syndrome. *J. AAPOS* **2017**, *21*, 295–299. [CrossRef] [PubMed]

38. Sarno, M.; Sacramento, G.A.; Khouri, R.; do Rosário, M.S.; Costa, F.; Archanjo, G.; Santos, L.A.; Nery, N.; Vasilakis, N.; Ko, A.I.; et al. Zika Virus Infection and Stillbirths: A Case of Hydrops Fetalis, Hydranencephaly and Fetal Demise. *PLoS Negl. Trop. Dis.* **2016**, *10*, e0004517. [CrossRef] [PubMed]

39. Miranda, H.A.; Costa, M.C.; Frazão, M.A.M.; Simão, N.; Franchischini, S.; Moshfeghi, D.M. Expanded Spectrum of Congenital Ocular Findings in Microcephaly with Presumed Zika Infection. *Ophthalmology* **2016**, *123*, 1788–1794. [CrossRef] [PubMed]

40. Miranda-Filho, D.E.B.; Martelli, C.M.; Ximenes, R.A.; Araújo, T.V.; Rocha, M.A.; Ramos, R.C.; Dhalia, R.; França, R.F.; Marques Júnior, E.T.; Rodrigues, L.C. Initial Description of the Presumed Congenital Zika Syndrome. *Am. J. Public Health* **2016**, *106*, 598–600. [CrossRef] [PubMed]

41. Furtado, J.M.; Espósito, D.L.; Klein, T.M.; Teixeira-Pinto, T.; da Fonseca, B.A. Uveitis Associated with Zika Virus Infection. *N. Engl. J. Med.* **2016**, *375*, 394–396. [CrossRef] [PubMed]

42. Kodati, S.; Palmore, T.N.; Spellman, F.A.; Cunningham, D.; Weistrop, B.; Sen, H.N. Bilateral posterior uveitis associated with Zika virus infection. *Lancet* **2017**, *389*, 125–126. [CrossRef]

43. Merle, H.; Najioullah, F.; Chassery, M.; Césaire, R.; Hage, R. Zika-Related Bilateral Hypertensive Anterior Acute Uveitis. *JAMA Ophthalmol.* **2017**, *135*, 284–285. [CrossRef] [PubMed]

44. Monath, T.P. Treatment of yellow fever. *Antivir. Res.* **2008**, *78*, 116–124. [CrossRef] [PubMed]

45. Callender, D.M. Management and control of yellow fever virus: Brazilian outbreak January–April, 2018. *Glob. Public Health* **2018**, 1–11. [CrossRef] [PubMed]

46. Sanna, A.; Andrieu, A.; Carvalho, L.; Mayence, C.; Tabard, P.; Hachouf, M.; Cazaux, C.M.; Enfissi, A.; Rousset, D.; Kallel, H. Yellow fever cases in French Guiana, evidence of an active circulation in the Guiana Shield, 2017 and 2018. *Eurosurveill* **2018**, *23*, 1800471. [CrossRef] [PubMed]

47. Erlanger, T.E.; Weiss, S.; Keiser, J.; Utzinger, J.; Wiedenmayer, K. Past, present, and future of Japanese encephalitis. *Emerg. Infect. Dis.* **2009**, *15*, 1–7. [CrossRef] [PubMed]

48. Igarashi, A. Control of Japanese encephalitis in Japan: Immunization of humans and animals, and vector control. *Curr. Top. Microbiol. Immunol.* **2002**, *267*, 139–152. [PubMed]

49. Work, T.H.; Roderiguez, F.R.; Bhatt, P.N. Virological epidemiology of the 1958 epidemic of Kyasanur Forest disease. *Am. J. Public Health Nations Health* **1959**, *49*, 869–874. [CrossRef] [PubMed]

50. Mourya, D.T.; Yadav, P.D.; Mehla, R.; Barde, P.V.; Yergolkar, P.N.; Kumar, S.R.; Thakare, J.P.; Mishra, A.C. Diagnosis of Kyasanur forest disease by nested RT-PCR, real-time RT-PCR and IgM capture ELISA. *J. Virol. Methods* **2012**, *186*, 49–54. [CrossRef] [PubMed]

51. Smithburn, K.C.; Hughes, T.P.; Burke, A.W.; Paul, J.H. A Neurotropic Virus Isolated from the Blood of a Native of Uganda1. *Am. J. Trop. Med. Hyg.* **1940**, *1*, 471–492. [CrossRef]

52. Merle, H.; Donnio, A.; Jean-Charles, A.; Guyomarch, J.; Hage, R.; Najioullah, F.; Césaire, R.; Cabié, A. Ocular manifestations of emerging arboviruses: Dengue fever, Chikungunya, Zika virus, West Nile virus, and yellow fever. *J. Fr. Ophtalmol.* **2018**, *41*, e235–e243. [CrossRef] [PubMed]

53. Abroug, F.; Ouanes-Besbes, L.; Letaief, M.; Ben Romdhane, F.; Khairallah, M.; Triki, H.; Bouzouiaia, N. A cluster study of predictors of severe West Nile virus infection. *Mayo Clin. Proc.* **2006**, *81*, 12–16. [CrossRef] [PubMed]

54. Khairallah, M.; Ben Yahia, S.; Ladjimi, A.; Zeghidi, H.; Ben Romdhane, F.; Besbes, L.; Zaouali, S.; Messaoud, R. Chorioretinal involvement in patients with West Nile virus infection. *Ophthalmology* **2004**, *111*, 2065–2070. [CrossRef] [PubMed]

55. Khairallah, M.; Ben Yahia, S.; Attia, S.; Jelliti, B.; Zaouali, S.; Ladjimi, A. Severe ischemic maculopathy in a patient with West Nile virus infection. *Ophthalmic Surg. Lasers Imaging* **2006**, *37*, 240–242. [PubMed]

56. Yahia, S.B.; Khairallah, M. Ocular manifestations of West Nile virus infection. *Int. J. Med. Sci.* **2009**, *6*, 114–115. [CrossRef] [PubMed]

57. Holmes, E.C.; Twiddy, S.S. The origin, emergence and evolutionary genetics of dengue virus. *Infect. Genet. Evol.* **2003**, *3*, 19–28. [CrossRef]

58. Bhatt, S.; Gething, P.W.; Brady, O.J.; Messina, J.P.; Farlow, A.W.; Moyes, C.L.; Drake, J.M.; Brownstein, J.S.; Hoen, A.G.; Sankoh, O.; et al. The global distribution and burden of dengue. *Nature* **2013**, *496*, 504–507. [CrossRef] [PubMed]

59. Rudolph, K.E.; Lessler, J.; Moloney, R.M.; Kmush, B.; Cummings, D.A. Incubation periods of mosquito-borne viral infections: A systematic review. *Am. J. Trop. Med. Hyg.* **2014**, *90*, 882–891. [CrossRef] [PubMed]

60. Mustafa, M.S.; Rasotgi, V.; Jain, S.; Gupta, V. Discovery of fifth serotype of dengue virus (DENV-5): A new public health dilemma in dengue control. *Med. J. Armed Forces India* **2015**, *71*, 67–70. [CrossRef] [PubMed]

61. Dejnirattisai, W.; Jumnainsong, A.; Onsirisakul, N.; Fitton, P.; Vasanawathana, S.; Limpitikul, W.; Puttikhunt, C.; Edwards, C.; Duangchinda, T.; Supasa, S.; et al. Cross-reacting antibodies enhance dengue virus infection in humans. *Science* **2010**, *328*, 745–748. [CrossRef] [PubMed]

62. Glasner, D.R.; Ratnasiri, K.; Puerta-Guardo, H.; Espinosa, D.A.; Beatty, P.R.; Harris, E. Dengue virus NS1 cytokine-independent vascular leak is dependent on endothelial glycocalyx components. *PLoS Pathog.* **2017**, *13*, e1006673. [CrossRef] [PubMed]

63. Beatty, P.R.; Puerta-Guardo, H.; Killingbeck, S.S.; Glasner, D.R.; Hopkins, K.; Harris, E. Dengue virus NS1 triggers endothelial permeability and vascular leak that is prevented by NS1 vaccination. *Sci. Transl. Med.* **2015**, *7*, 304ra141. [CrossRef] [PubMed]

64. Avirutnan, P.; Punyadee, N.; Noisakran, S.; Komoltri, C.; Thiemmeca, S.; Auethavornanan, K.; Jairungsri, A.; Kanlaya, R.; Tangthawornchaikul, N.; Puttikhunt, C.; et al. Vascular leakage in severe dengue virus infections: A potential role for the nonstructural viral protein NS1 and complement. *J. Infect. Dis.* **2006**, *193*, 1078–1088. [CrossRef] [PubMed]

65. Sirisena, N.; Noordeen, F.; Fernando, L. NS 1 lasts longer than the dengue virus nucleic acid in the clinically suspected patients with dengue fever and dengue haemorrhagic fever. *Virusdisease* **2017**, *28*, 341–344. [CrossRef] [PubMed]

66. Seet, R.C.; Quek, A.M.; Lim, E.C. Symptoms and risk factors of ocular complications following dengue infection. *J. Clin. Virol.* **2007**, *38*, 101–105. [CrossRef] [PubMed]

67. Chee, E.; Sims, J.L.; Jap, A.; Tan, B.H.; Oh, H.; Chee, S.P. Comparison of prevalence of dengue maculopathy during two epidemics with differing predominant serotypes. *Am. J. Ophthalmol.* **2009**, *148*, 910–913. [CrossRef] [PubMed]

68. Carr, J.M.; Ashander, L.M.; Calvert, J.K.; Ma, Y.; Aloia, A.; Bracho, G.G.; Chee, S.P.; Appukuttan, B.; Smith, J.R. Molecular Responses of Human Retinal Cells to Infection with Dengue Virus. *Mediat. Inflamm.* **2017**, *2017*, 3164375. [CrossRef] [PubMed]

69. Guy, B.; Jackson, N. Dengue vaccine: Hypotheses to understand CYD-TDV-induced protection. *Nat. Rev. Microbiol.* **2016**, *14*, 45–54. [CrossRef] [PubMed]

70. Murphy, B.R.; Whitehead, S.S. Immune response to dengue virus and prospects for a vaccine. *Annu. Rev. Immunol.* **2011**, *29*, 587–619. [CrossRef] [PubMed]

71. De Silva, A.M.; Harris, E. Which Dengue Vaccine Approach Is the Most Promising, and Should We Be Concerned about Enhanced Disease after Vaccination? The Path to a Dengue Vaccine: Learning from Human Natural Dengue Infection Studies and Vaccine Trials. *Cold Spring Harb. Perspect. Biol.* **2018**, *10*, a029371. [CrossRef] [PubMed]

72. Dick, G.W.; Kitchen, S.F.; Haddow, A.J. Zika virus. I. Isolations and serological specificity. *Trans. R. Soc. Trop. Med. Hyg.* **1952**, *46*, 509–520. [CrossRef]

73. Macnamara, F.N. Zika virus: A report on three cases of human infection during an epidemic of jaundice in Nigeria. *Trans. R. Soc. Trop. Med. Hyg.* **1954**, *48*, 139–145. [CrossRef]

74. Faye, O.; Freire, C.C.; Iamarino, A.; de Oliveira, J.V.; Diallo, M.; Zanotto, P.M.; Sall, A.A. Molecular evolution of Zika virus during its emergence in the 20(th) century. *PLoS Negl. Trop. Dis.* **2014**, *8*, e2636. [CrossRef] [PubMed]

75. Manangeeswaran, M.; Kielczewski, J.L.; Sen, H.N.; Xu, B.C.; Ireland, D.D.C.; McWilliams, I.L.; Chan, C.C.; Caspi, R.R.; Verthelyi, D. ZIKA virus infection causes persistent chorioretinal lesions. *Emerg. Microbes Infect.* **2018**, *7*, 96. [CrossRef] [PubMed]

76. Miner, J.J.; Diamond, M.S. Zika Virus Pathogenesis and Tissue Tropism. *Cell Host Microbe* **2017**, *21*, 134–142. [CrossRef] [PubMed]

77. Henry, C.R.; Al-Attar, L.; Cruz-Chacón, A.M.; Davis, J.L. Chorioretinal Lesions Presumed Secondary to Zika Virus Infection in an Immunocompromised Adult. *JAMA Ophthalmol.* **2017**, *135*, 386–389. [CrossRef] [PubMed]

78. Fontes, B.M. Zika virus-related hypertensive iridocyclitis. *Arq. Bras. Oftalmol.* **2016**, *79*, 63. [CrossRef] [PubMed]

79. De Paula Freitas, B.; de Oliveira Dias, J.R.; Prazeres, J.; Sacramento, G.A.; Ko, A.I.; Maia, M.; Belfort, R., Jr. Ocular Findings in Infants With Microcephaly Associated With Presumed Zika Virus Congenital Infection in Salvador, Brazil. *JAMA Ophthalmol.* **2016**, *134*, 529–535. [CrossRef] [PubMed]

80. Fernandez, M.P.; Parra Saad, E.; Ospina Martinez, M.; Corchuelo, S.; Mercado Reyes, M.; Herrera, M.J.; Parra Saavedra, M.; Rico, A.; Fernandez, A.M.; Lee, R.K.; et al. Ocular Histopathologic Features of Congenital Zika Syndrome. *JAMA Ophthalmol.* **2017**, *135*, 1163–1169. [CrossRef] [PubMed]

81. Sun, J.; Wu, D.; Zhong, H.; Guan, D.; Zhang, H.; Tan, Q.; Ke, C. Presence of Zika Virus in Conjunctival Fluid. *JAMA Ophthalmol.* **2016**, *134*, 1330–1332. [CrossRef] [PubMed]

82. Abbink, P.; Stephenson, K.E.; Barouch, D.H. Zika virus vaccines. *Nat. Rev. Microbiol.* **2018**, *16*, 594–600. [CrossRef] [PubMed]

83. Modjarrad, K.; Lin, L.; George, S.L.; Stephenson, K.E.; Eckels, K.H.; De La Barrera, R.A.; Jarman, R.G.; Sondergaard, E.; Tennant, J.; Ansel, J.L.; et al. Preliminary aggregate safety and immunogenicity results from three trials of a purified inactivated Zika virus vaccine candidate: Phase 1, randomised, double-blind, placebo-controlled clinical trials. *Lancet* **2018**, *391*, 563–571. [CrossRef]

84. Larocca, R.A.; Abbink, P.; Peron, J.P.; Zanotto, P.M.; Iampietro, M.J.; Badamchi-Zadeh, A.; Boyd, M.; Nganga, D.; Kirilova, M.; Nityanandam, R.; et al. Vaccine protection against Zika virus from Brazil. *Nature* **2016**, *536*, 474–478. [CrossRef] [PubMed]

85. Lazear, H.M.; Govero, J.; Smith, A.M.; Platt, D.J.; Fernandez, E.; Miner, J.J.; Diamond, M.S. A Mouse Model of Zika Virus Pathogenesis. *Cell Host Microbe* **2016**, *19*, 720–730. [CrossRef] [PubMed]

86. Rossi, S.L.; Tesh, R.B.; Azar, S.R.; Muruato, A.E.; Hanley, K.A.; Auguste, A.J.; Langsjoen, R.M.; Paessler, S.; Vasilakis, N.; Weaver, S.C. Characterization of a Novel Murine Model to Study Zika Virus. *Am. J. Trop. Med. Hyg.* **2016**, *94*, 1362–1369. [CrossRef] [PubMed]

87. Aliota, M.T.; Caine, E.A.; Walker, E.C.; Larkin, K.E.; Camacho, E.; Osorio, J.E. Characterization of Lethal Zika Virus Infection in AG129 Mice. *PLoS Negl. Trop. Dis.* **2016**, *10*, e0004682. [CrossRef] [PubMed]

88. Miner, J.J.; Sene, A.; Richner, J.M.; Smith, A.M.; Santeford, A.; Ban, N.; Weger-Lucarelli, J.; Manzella, F.; Rückert, C.; Govero, J.; et al. Zika Virus Infection in Mice Causes Panuveitis with Shedding of Virus in Tears. *Cell Rep.* **2016**, *16*, 3208–3218. [CrossRef] [PubMed]

89. Julander, J.G.; Siddharthan, V.; Evans, J.; Taylor, R.; Tolbert, K.; Apuli, C.; Stewart, J.; Collins, P.; Gebre, M.; Neilson, S.; et al. Efficacy of the broad-spectrum antiviral compound BCX4430 against Zika virus in cell culture and in a mouse model. *Antivir. Res.* **2017**, *137*, 14–22. [CrossRef] [PubMed]

90. Zmurko, J.; Marques, R.E.; Schols, D.; Verbeken, E.; Kaptein, S.J.; Neyts, J. The Viral Polymerase Inhibitor 7-Deaza-2′-C-Methyladenosine Is a Potent Inhibitor of In Vitro Zika Virus Replication and Delays Disease Progression in a Robust Mouse Infection Model. *PLoS Negl. Trop. Dis.* **2016**, *10*, e0004695. [CrossRef] [PubMed]

91. Weger-Lucarelli, J.; Duggal, N.K.; Bullard-Feibelman, K.; Veselinovic, M.; Romo, H.; Nguyen, C.; Rückert, C.; Brault, A.C.; Bowen, R.A.; Stenglein, M.; et al. Development and Characterization of Recombinant Virus Generated from a New World Zika Virus Infectious Clone. *J. Virol.* **2017**, *91*. [CrossRef] [PubMed]

92. Li, C.; Xu, D.; Ye, Q.; Hong, S.; Jiang, Y.; Liu, X.; Zhang, N.; Shi, L.; Qin, C.F.; Xu, Z. Zika Virus Disrupts Neural Progenitor Development and Leads to Microcephaly in Mice. *Cell Stem Cell* **2016**, *19*, 672. [CrossRef] [PubMed]

93. Wu, K.Y.; Zuo, G.L.; Li, X.F.; Ye, Q.; Deng, Y.Q.; Huang, X.Y.; Cao, W.C.; Qin, C.F.; Luo, Z.G. Vertical transmission of Zika virus targeting the radial glial cells affects cortex development of offspring mice. *Cell Res.* **2016**, *26*, 645–654. [CrossRef] [PubMed]

94. Singh, P.K.; Guest, J.M.; Kanwar, M.; Boss, J.; Gao, N.; Juzych, M.S.; Abrams, G.W.; Yu, F.S.; Kumar, A. Zika virus infects cells lining the blood-retinal barrier and causes chorioretinal atrophy in mouse eyes. *JCI Insight* **2017**, *2*, e92340. [CrossRef] [PubMed]

95. Van den Pol, A.N.; Mao, G.; Yang, Y.; Ornaghi, S.; Davis, J.N. Zika Virus Targeting in the Developing Brain. *J. Neurosci.* **2017**, *37*, 2161–2175. [CrossRef] [PubMed]

96. Aleman, T.S.; Ventura, C.V.; Cavalcanti, M.M.; Serrano, L.W.; Traband, A.; Nti, A.A.; Gois, A.L.; Bravo-Filho, V.; Martins, T.T.; Nichols, C.W.; et al. Quantitative Assessment of Microstructural Changes of the Retina in Infants With Congenital Zika Syndrome. *JAMA Ophthalmol.* **2017**, *135*, 1069–1076. [CrossRef] [PubMed]

97. De Oliveira Dias, J.R.; Ventura, C.V.; de Paula Freitas, B.; Prazeres, J.; Ventura, L.O.; Bravo-Filho, V.; Aleman, T.; Ko, A.I.; Zin, A.; Belfort, R.; et al. Zika and the Eye: Pieces of a Puzzle. *Prog. Retin. Eye Res.* **2018**. [CrossRef] [PubMed]

98. Zhao, Z.; Yang, M.; Azar, S.R.; Soong, L.; Weaver, S.C.; Sun, J.; Chen, Y.; Rossi, S.L.; Cai, J. Viral Retinopathy in Experimental Models of Zika Infection. *Investig. Ophthalmol. Vis. Sci.* **2017**, *58*, 4355–4365. [CrossRef] [PubMed]

99. Salinas, S.; Erkilic, N.; Damodar, K.; Moles, J.P.; Fournier-Wirth, C.; Van de Perre, P.; Kalatzis, V.; Simonin, Y. Zika Virus Efficiently Replicates in Human Retinal Epithelium and Disturbs Its Permeability. *J. Virol.* **2017**, *91*, e02144-16. [CrossRef] [PubMed]

100. Contreras, D.; Jones, M.; Martinez, L.E.; Gangalapudi, V.; Tang, J.; Wu, Y.; Zhao, J.J.; Chen, Z.; Wang, S.; Arumugaswami, V. Modeling Zika Virus Congenital Eye Disease: Differential Susceptibility of Fetal Retinal Progenitor Cells and iPSC-Derived Retinal Stem Cells to Zika Virus Infection. *bioRxiv* **2017**. [CrossRef]

101. Fronk, A.H.; Vargis, E. Methods for culturing retinal pigment epithelial cells: A review of current protocols and future recommendations. *J. Tissue Eng.* **2016**, *7*. [CrossRef] [PubMed]

102. Díaz-Coránguez, M.; Ramos, C.; Antonetti, D.A. The inner blood-retinal barrier: Cellular basis and development. *Vis. Res.* **2017**, *139*, 123–137. [CrossRef] [PubMed]

103. Campbell, M.; Humphries, P. The blood-retina barrier: Tight junctions and barrier modulation. *Adv. Exp. Med. Biol.* **2012**, *763*, 70–84. [PubMed]

104. Roach, T.; Alcendor, D.J. Zika virus infection of cellular components of the blood-retinal barriers: Implications for viral associated congenital ocular disease. *J. Neuroinflamm.* **2017**, *14*, 43. [CrossRef] [PubMed]

105. Kumar, M.V.; Nagineni, C.N.; Chin, M.S.; Hooks, J.J.; Detrick, B. Innate immunity in the retina: Toll-like receptor (TLR) signaling in human retinal pigment epithelial cells. *J. Neuroimmunol.* **2004**, *153*, 7–15. [CrossRef] [PubMed]

106. Chin, M.S.; Nagineni, C.N.; Hooper, L.C.; Detrick, B.; Hooks, J.J. Cyclooxygenase-2 gene expression and regulation in human retinal pigment epithelial cells. *Investig. Ophthalmol. Vis. Sci.* **2001**, *42*, 2338–2346.

107. Momma, Y.; Nagineni, C.N.; Chin, M.S.; Srinivasan, K.; Detrick, B.; Hooks, J.J. Differential expression of chemokines by human retinal pigment epithelial cells infected with cytomegalovirus. *Investig. Ophthalmol. Vis. Sci.* **2003**, *44*, 2026–2033. [CrossRef]

108. Percopo, C.M.; Hooks, J.J.; Shinohara, T.; Caspi, R.; Detrick, B. Cytokine-mediated activation of a neuronal retinal resident cell provokes antigen presentation. *J. Immunol.* **1990**, *145*, 4101–4107. [PubMed]

109. Perez, V.L.; Caspi, R.R. Immune mechanisms in inflammatory and degenerative eye disease. *Trends Immunol.* **2015**, *36*, 354–363. [CrossRef] [PubMed]

110. Taylor, A.W. Ocular Immune Privilege and Transplantation. *Front. Immunol.* **2016**, *7*, 37. [CrossRef] [PubMed]

111. Xu, H.; Dawson, R.; Forrester, J.V.; Liversidge, J. Identification of novel dendritic cell populations in normal mouse retina. *Investig. Ophthalmol. Vis. Sci.* **2007**, *48*, 1701–1710. [CrossRef] [PubMed]

112. Zhu, S.; Luo, H.; Liu, H.; Ha, Y.; Mays, E.R.; Lawrence, R.E.; Winkelmann, E.; Barrett, A.D.; Smith, S.B.; Wang, M.; et al. p38MAPK plays a critical role in induction of a pro-inflammatory phenotype of retinal Müller cells following Zika virus infection. *Antivir. Res.* **2017**, *145*, 70–81. [CrossRef] [PubMed]

113. Casazza, R.L.; Lazear, H.M. Antiviral immunity backfires: Pathogenic effects of type I interferon signaling in fetal development. *Sci. Immunol.* **2018**, *3*, eaar3446. [CrossRef] [PubMed]

114. Singh, P.K.; Khatri, I.; Jha, A.; Pretto, C.D.; Spindler, K.R.; Arumugaswami, V.; Giri, S.; Kumar, A.; Bhasin, M.K. Determination of system level alterations in host transcriptome due to Zika virus (ZIKV) Infection in retinal pigment epithelium. *Sci. Rep.* **2018**, *8*, 11209. [CrossRef] [PubMed]

115. Coyaud, E.; Ranadheera, C.; Cheng, D.T.; Goncalves, J.; Dyakov, B.; Laurent, E.; St-Germain, J.R.; Pelletier, L.; Gingras, A.C.; Brumell, J.H.; et al. Global interactomics uncovers extensive organellar targeting by Zika virus. *Mol. Cell Proteom.* **2018**. [CrossRef] [PubMed]

116. Kumar, A.; Giri, S. 5-Aminoimidazole-4-carboxamide ribonucleoside-mediated adenosine monophosphate-activated protein kinase activation induces protective innate responses in bacterial endophthalmitis. *Cell. Microbiol.* **2016**, *18*, 1815–1830. [CrossRef] [PubMed]

117. Mankouri, J.; Harris, M. Viruses and the fuel sensor: The emerging link between AMPK and virus replication. *Rev. Med. Virol.* **2011**, *21*, 205–212. [CrossRef] [PubMed]

118. Zhang, L.; Li, J.; Young, L.H.; Caplan, M.J. AMP-activated protein kinase regulates the assembly of epithelial tight junctions. *Proc. Natl. Acad. Sci. USA* **2006**, *103*, 17272–17277. [CrossRef] [PubMed]

119. Yano, T.; Matsui, T.; Tamura, A.; Uji, M.; Tsukita, S. The association of microtubules with tight junctions is promoted by cingulin phosphorylation by AMPK. *J. Cell Biol.* **2013**, *203*, 605–614. [CrossRef] [PubMed]

120. Jampol, L.M.; Ferris, F.L.; Bishop, R.J. Ebola and the eye. *JAMA Ophthalmol.* **2015**, *133*, 1105–1106. [CrossRef] [PubMed]

121. Dejnirattisai, W.; Supasa, P.; Wongwiwat, W.; Rouvinski, A.; Barba-Spaeth, G.; Duangchinda, T.; Sakuntabhai, A.; Cao-Lormeau, V.M.; Malasit, P.; Rey, F.A.; et al. Dengue virus sero-cross-reactivity drives antibody-dependent enhancement of infection with zika virus. *Nat. Immunol.* **2016**, *17*, 1102–1108. [CrossRef] [PubMed]

122. Kawiecki, A.B.; Christofferson, R.C. Zika Virus-Induced Antibody Response Enhances Dengue Virus Serotype 2 Replication In Vitro. *J. Infect. Dis.* **2016**, *214*, 1357–1360. [CrossRef] [PubMed]

123. George, J.; Valiant, W.G.; Mattapallil, M.J.; Walker, M.; Huang, Y.S.; Vanlandingham, D.L.; Misamore, J.; Greenhouse, J.; Weiss, D.E.; Verthelyi, D.; et al. Prior Exposure to Zika Virus Significantly Enhances Peak Dengue-2 Viremia in Rhesus Macaques. *Sci. Rep.* **2017**, *7*, 10498. [CrossRef] [PubMed]

124. Modhiran, N.; Watterson, D.; Muller, D.A.; Panetta, A.K.; Sester, D.P.; Liu, L.; Hume, D.A.; Stacey, K.J.; Young, P.R. Dengue virus NS1 protein activates cells via Toll-like receptor 4 and disrupts endothelial cell monolayer integrity. *Sci. Transl. Med.* **2015**, *7*, 304ra142. [CrossRef] [PubMed]

125. Guabiraba, R.; Ryffel, B. Dengue virus infection: Current concepts in immune mechanisms and lessons from murine models. *Immunology* **2014**, *141*, 143–156. [CrossRef] [PubMed]

126. Mangione, J.N.; Huy, N.T.; Lan, N.T.; Mbanefo, E.C.; Ha, T.T.; Bao, L.Q.; Nga, C.T.; Tuong, V.V.; Dat, T.V.; Thuy, T.T.; et al. The association of cytokines with severe dengue in children. *Trop. Med. Health* **2014**, *42*, 137–144. [CrossRef] [PubMed]

127. Appanna, R.; Wang, S.M.; Ponnampalavanar, S.A.; Lum, L.C.; Sekaran, S.D. Cytokine factors present in dengue patient sera induces alterations of junctional proteins in human endothelial cells. *Am. J. Trop. Med. Hyg.* **2012**, *87*, 936–942. [CrossRef] [PubMed]

128. Rothwell, C.; Lebreton, A.; Young Ng, C.; Lim, J.Y.; Liu, W.; Vasudevan, S.; Labow, M.; Gu, F.; Gaither, L.A. Cholesterol biosynthesis modulation regulates dengue viral replication. *Virology* **2009**, *389*, 8–19. [CrossRef] [PubMed]

129. Apte-Sengupta, S.; Sirohi, D.; Kuhn, R.J. Coupling of replication and assembly in flaviviruses. *Curr. Opin. Virol.* **2014**, *9*, 134–142. [CrossRef] [PubMed]

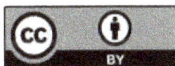

Communication

Fetal Brain Infection Is Not a Unique Characteristic of Brazilian Zika Viruses

Yin Xiang Setoh [1,†] , Nias Y. Peng [1,†] , Eri Nakayama [2,3,†], Alberto A. Amarilla [1] ,
Natalie A. Prow [2], Andreas Suhrbier [2,*] and Alexander A. Khromykh [1,*]

[1]   Australian Infectious Diseases Research Centre, School of Chemistry and Molecular Biosciences,
    The University of Queensland, St. Lucia 4072, Australia; y.setoh@uq.edu.au (Y.X.S.);
    y.g.peng@uq.net.au (N.Y.P.); a.amarillaortiz@uq.edu.au (A.A.A.)
[2]   Inflammation Biology Group, QIMR Berghofer Medical Research Institute, Brisbane 4006, Australia;
    Eri.Nakayama@qimrberghofer.edu.au (E.N.); Natalie.Prow@qimrberghofer.edu.au (N.A.P.)
[3]   Department of Virology I, National Institute of Infectious Diseases, Tokyo 162-8640, Japan
*   Correspondence: andreas.suhrbier@qimrberghofer.edu.au (A.S.); alexander.khromykh@uq.edu.au (A.A.K.)
†   These authors contributed equally to this work.

Received: 29 August 2018; Accepted: 30 September 2018; Published: 3 October 2018

Abstract: The recent emergence of Zika virus (ZIKV) in Brazil was associated with an increased number of fetal brain infections that resulted in a spectrum of congenital neurological complications known as congenital Zika syndrome (CZS). Herein, we generated *de novo* from sequence data an early Asian lineage ZIKV isolate (ZIKV-MY; Malaysia, 1966) not associated with microcephaly and compared the *in vitro* replication kinetics and fetal brain infection in interferon α/β receptor 1 knockout (IFNAR1$^{-/-}$) dams of this isolate and of a Brazilian isolate (ZIKV-Natal; Natal, 2015) unequivocally associated with microcephaly. The replication efficiencies of ZIKV-MY and ZIKV-Natal in A549 and Vero cells were similar, while ZIKV-MY replicated more efficiently in wild-type (WT) and IFNAR$^{-/-}$ mouse embryonic fibroblasts. Viremias in IFNAR1$^{-/-}$ dams were similar after infection with ZIKV-MY or ZIKV-Natal, and importantly, infection of fetal brains was also not significantly different. Thus, fetal brain infection does not appear to be a unique feature of Brazilian ZIKV isolates.

Keywords: Zika virus; pregnancy; fetal infection; congenital Zika syndrome; Asian lineage

---

1. Introduction

Zika virus (ZIKV) belongs to the genus *Flavivirus* of the Flaviviridae family [1], which includes yellow fever virus, dengue virus, West Nile virus, Japanese encephalitis virus, and tick-borne encephalitis virus. First isolated in Uganda in 1947, ZIKV has since spread across continents, emerging as a medically significant pathogen associated with Guillain–Barré syndrome in adults and, following infection of pregnant women, with a spectrum of congenital neurological complications known as congenital Zika syndrome (CZS) that manifests in the newborns [2]. ZIKV is an enveloped virus with a single-stranded positive-strand RNA genome of approximately 11 kb in length. Like all flaviviruses, the ZIKV genome encodes a single open reading frame translated into a single polyprotein that is cleaved post-translationally by cellular and viral proteases into three structural proteins, i.e., capsid (C), precursor membrane (prM), envelope (E), and seven non-structural (NS) proteins (NS1, NS2A, NS2B, NS3, NS4A, NS4B, NS5) [3].

Phylogenetically, ZIKV strains are categorized into either African or Asian lineages [4], with most epidemic-associated ZIKV strains belonging to the Asian lineage [4–8]. Several epidemiological and bioinformatics studies investigating the etiology of ZIKV emergence in the Americas have independently suggested that amino acid changes within the Asian lineage viruses were likely to have contributed to enhanced infectivity and pathogenicity, which resulted in the unprecedented increase in

CZS that was primarily associated with the Brazilian outbreak [8–12]. The ability to infect a developing fetus and cause CZS, including microcephaly [13,14], is the most distressing feature of ZIKV. In the 2015 Brazilian outbreak, microcephaly in newborns was reported to be 20 times higher than the background incidence [15], with a retrospective analysis of the 2013 outbreak in French Polynesia also showing an increased risk of microcephaly associated with ZIKV infection [16].

A central question associated with the ZIKV epidemic in Brazil (and in French Polynesia) is whether the virus strains involved had acquired mutations that enhanced their ability to cause CZS [17,18]. Several studies have supported this notion [19,20], whereas others have argued that all ZIKV strains may be similarly neurotropic [21,22].

We previously generated the contemporary Asian lineage isolate ZIKV-Natal from sequence data obtained directly from the brain tissue of an aborted ZIKV-infected human fetus during the 2015 Brazilian outbreak [14,23]. Using a pregnant IFNAR1$^{-/-}$ mouse model, we previously demonstrated that the Brazilian isolate (ZIKV-Natal) was capable of causing fetal infection and congenital malformations [23,24]. Herein, we sought to determine whether fetal infection is a newly acquired characteristic of Asian lineage strains of ZIKV by comparing ZIKV-Natal to the P6-740 Malaysian 1966 ZIKV isolate (ZIKV-MY). ZIKV-MY was chosen because it represents the earliest documented Asian lineage ZIKV strain, with no reported association with human congenital disease [25]. We show that ZIKV-MY and ZIKV-Natal produced similar viremias in pregnant interferon α/β receptor 1 knockout (IFNAR1$^{-/-}$) dams and were both capable of causing fetal brain infections.

2. Materials and Methods

2.1. Generation of ZIKV-MY and Chimeric Virus Using Circular Polymerase Extension Reaction (CPER)

The ZIKV-MY (strain P6-740) isolate whose sequence was used in this study was reported to be passaged six times in suckling mouse brains, once in baby hamster kidney (BHK) cells, once in C6/36 cells, twice in Vero cells, and five times in Vero E6 cells (GenBank accession number KX694533). Six dsDNA fragments covering the entire viral sequence (Figure 1a) were purchased from Integrated DNA Technologies (Baulkham Hills, NSW, Australia) as gBlocks, and each cloned into a pUC19 vector to produce six plasmids. The plasmids were sequenced to confirm the correct viral sequence. The fragments used for CPER (see Figure 1a) were then amplified from individual pUC19 plasmids using corresponding pairs of primers (Table 1). CPER assembly and recovery of WT ZIKV-MY virus by transfection into Vero cells were performed as previously described [23]. The WT ZIKV-Natal virus was generated previously [23]. The ZIKV-Natal/MY-prME chimeric virus was generated using CPER by replacing the ZIKV-Natal fragments 1 and part of fragment 2 encompassing E gene (Figure 1a) with those of ZIKV-MY. Chimeric primers (Table 1) were used for polymerase chain reaction (PCR) amplification of amplicons to generate chimeric virus.

Table 1. Primers used for generation of cDNA amplicons of parental P6-740 Malaysian 1966 Zika virus isolate (ZIKV-MY) and ZIKV-Natal (Brazilian isolate)/MY chimeric virus.

WT ZIKV-MY Primers	Primer Sequence (5′ to 3′)
Fragment 1 Forward	AGTTGTTGATCTGTGTGAATCAGAC
Fragment 1 Reverse	GTGAACGCCGCGGTACATAAGGAGTATG
Fragment 2 Forward	CATACTCCTTATGTACCGCGGCGTTCAC
Fragment 2 Reverse	GATGAAAGAGACCAGCAACGCGGG
Fragment 3 Forward	CCCGCGTTGCTGGTCTCTTTCATC
Fragment 3 Reverse	CAGCAGCGACAACCCTGGTTGGAG
Fragment 4 Forward	CTCCAACCAGGGTTGTCGCTGCTG
Fragment 4 Reverse	GTACATGTAGTGCGCCACGAGCAGAATG
Fragment 5 Forward	CATTCTGCTCGTGGCGCACTACATGTAC
Fragment 5 Reverse	CTCCTGGTGTGCGGCTCATTTCTTC
Fragment 6 Forward	GAAGAAATGAGCCGCACACCAGGAG
Fragment 6 Reverse	AGACCCATGGATTTCCCCACACCG

Table 1. *Cont.*

WT ZIKV-MY Primers	Primer Sequence (5′ to 3′)
Chimeric primers	Primer sequence (5′ to 3′)
Natal 5′C (MY1966) R	CTCCCACGTCTGGTGACCTCCACTGCCATAGCTGTGGTCAGCAG
MY1966prM_F	GTGGAGGTCACCAGACGTG
MY1966E_R	AGCAGAGACGGCTGTAGATAGG
Natal NS1-junc2 (MY1966) F	CTTCCTATCTACAGCCGTCTCTGCTGATGTGGGGTGCTCGGTG

2.2. Growth Kinetics

Vero (CCL-81), A549 (ATCC CCL-185), wild-type mouse embryonic fibroblasts (MEFs), and IFNAR$^{-/-}$ MEFs (44) were infected with passage 1 of C6/36-derived stock of ZIKV-MY, ZIKV-Natal, or ZIKV-Natal/MY-prME viruses at the indicated multiplicity of infection (MOI), and 200 μL of culture supernatant was collected from each sample well at the indicated times post-infection. Three independent experiments were conducted for each cell line. Viral titers were determined by standard plaque assay on Vero cells, as previously described [23].

2.3. Mice and ZIKV Infection

IFNAR1$^{-/-}$ mice on a C57BL/6J background were provided by Dr P Hertzog (Monash University, VIC, Australia) [26] and bred in-house at the Queensland Institute of Medical Research (QIMR) Berghofer Medical Research Institute. Pregnant female IFNAR1$^{-/-}$ mice (between 10–20 weeks old) were infected s.c. at the base of the tail with 100 μL of medium at a dose of 10^4 CCID$_{50}$ as described [24]. Mating was verified by the presence of a vaginal plug. Pregnancy was monitored by weight gain. In older (>10 weeks) IFNAR1$^{-/-}$ mice, infection with either ZIKA-MY or ZIKV-Natal did not result in any overt morbidity. Mice were euthanized with CO_2.

2.4. Ethics Statement

All mouse work was conducted in accordance with the "Australian code for the care and use of animals for scientific purposes", as defined by the National Health and Medical Research Council of Australia. Animal experiments and associated statistical treatments were reviewed and approved by the QIMR Berghofer Medical Research Institute animal ethics committee (P2195, A1604-611M).

2.5. ZIKV CCID$_{50}$ Assays

ZIKV cell culture infectious dose, 50% endpoint (CCID$_{50}$) assays for viremia and tissue titers were undertaken as described [27,28], with minor modifications. Briefly, serum or supernatants from tissues (bead-macerated in medium) were collected and titrated in quadruplicates in five-fold serial dilutions on low-passage C6/36 cells (ATCC CRL-1660). After five days, 25 μL of the supernatants were individually transferred onto parallel plates (i.e., A1 to A1, A2 to A2 ... H12 to H12, etc.) containing Vero E6 cells (ATCC CRL1586). After seven more days, the plates were stained with crystal violet to visualize cytopathic effects (CPE). The titers were calculated using the Reed and Münch method.

2.6. Statistics

Statistical analysis of experimental data was performed using IBM SPSS Statistics for Windows, Version 19.0. Two-sample comparison using t-test was performed when the difference in variances was <4, skewness was >−2, and kurtosis was <2. Non-parametric data with difference in variances of <4 was analyzed using Mann–Whitney U-test; if the difference of variances was >4, the Kolmogorov–Smirnov test was employed.

3. Results

3.1. De Novo Generation and Characterization of ZIKV-MY

To generate ZIKV-MY, six synthetic gBlock DNA fragments covering the full genome of ZIKV-MY (GenBank: KX694533) were purchased from Integrated DNA Technologies (Figure 1a). The first 28 nucleotides of the 5′-UTR were missing from the published sequence, and, therefore, a fully conserved sequence of this region from four complete genomes of Asian lineage ZIKV (AGTTGTTGATCTGTGTGAATCAGACTGC, GenBank: KU527068, KU501215, KU681081, KU681082) was used instead. The gBlock fragments were individually cloned into pUC19 plasmids for archival purposes and then re-amplified for assembly by CPER, with the addition of the UTR-linker fragment, as described previously [23]. The CPER DNA was transfected into Vero cells, the culture media collected at six days post-transfection, and the presence of the virus was confirmed by plaque assay method as previously described [23] (Figure 1b).

Analysis of replication efficiencies in different cell lines showed that ZIKV-MY and ZIKV-Natal replicated with similar efficiencies in Vero and A549 cells (Figure 1c,d). As reported previously [23], ZIKV-Natal was unable to replicate in wild-type (WT) mouse embryonic fibroblasts (MEFs), while, here, we show that ZIKV-MY replicated to a detectable, albeit still relatively low, level (~2.57 × 10^3 pfu/mL) (Figure 1e). Even in MEFs deficient in the type I IFN response (interferon α/β receptor-deficient MEF; IFNAR$^{-/-}$ MEF), ZIKV-MY replicated more efficiently than ZIKV-Natal (Figure 1f). To ascertain whether the structural proteins of ZIKV-MY contributed to improved replication in murine cells, a chimeric virus with ZIKV-MY prME proteins and ZIKV-Natal non-structural proteins was constructed (ZIKV-Natal/MY-prME) (Figure S1a). In both WT and IFNAR$^{-/-}$ MEFs, the chimeric virus expressing ZIKV-MY prME did not show enhanced replication compared to ZIKV-Natal (Figure S1b,c). The better replication of ZIKV-MY in MEFs is clearly unrelated to the type I IFN response and would appear to be imparted by non-structural proteins.

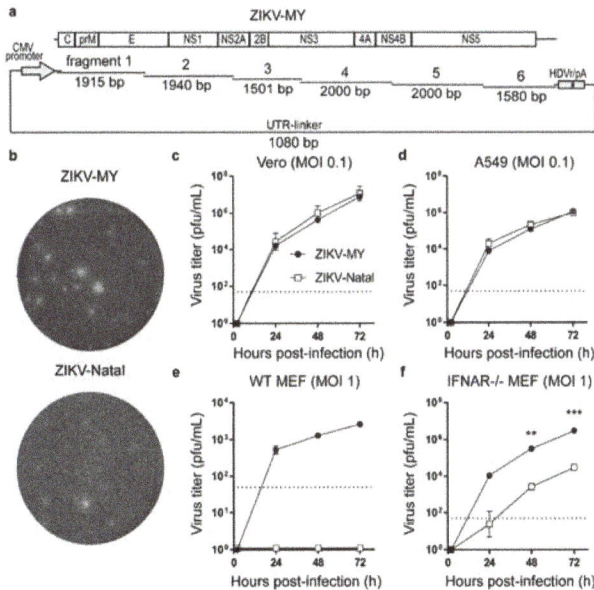

Figure 1. De novo generation and characterization of ZIKV-MY. (**a**) Schematic of Circular Polymerase Extension Reaction (CPER) fragments used for recovering ZIKV-MY. All fragments, except for the UTR-linker, are drawn to scale; (**b**) Plaque morphology on a Vero cell monolayer of ZIKV-MY recovered from the culture supernatant of CPER-transfected Vero cells, compared to ZIKV-Natal;

Growth kinetics of ZIKV-MY versus ZIKV-Natal was performed on (**c**) Vero, (**d**) A549, (**e**) WT MEF, and (**f**) IFNAR$^{-/-}$ MEF cells at their indicated multiplicity of infection (MOI), and culture supernatants were harvested at the indicated time points post-infection and titered by plaque assay. The dashed lines represent the limit of detection of the assay. Means and ± SE are shown. Statistical analyses were performed using *t*-tests (*n* = three biological replicates); statistically significant are differences shown in panel (**f**) **—*p* = 0.008, ***—*p* < 0.001.

3.2. ZIKV-MY and ZIKV-Natal Both Infect IFNAR1$^{-/-}$ Mice and Produce Similar Viraemia and Viral Titres in Different Organs

IFNAR1$^{-/-}$ mice were infected with ZIKV-MY or ZIKV-Natal at E12.5 of gestation, and viremias were determined daily for five days post-infection. No statistically significant differences in mean viremias were observed after infection with the two viruses in either pregnant or non-pregnant mice (Figure 2a). Viremia in the non-pregnant mice were measured up to day 7 post-infection and showed that the virus was cleared by 7 days post-infection (Figure 2a). The pregnant mice were euthanized on day 5 post-infection (E17.5), and a panel of organs was harvested (spleens, spinal cords, muscles, liver, kidneys, eyes, brains) to determine the viral titres. No statistically significant differences in viral titres for any organs were observed between ZIKV-MY and ZIKV-Natal infections (Figure 2b–h).

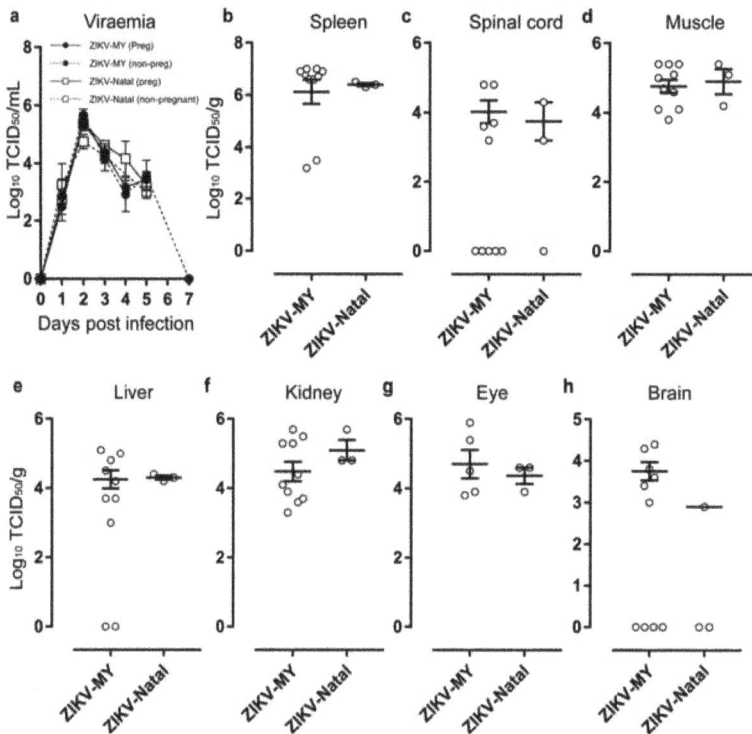

Figure 2. ZIKV-MY and ZIKV-Natal replicate to similar levels *in vivo*. (**a**) Interferon α/β receptor 1 knockout (IFNAR1$^{-/-}$) C57BL/6 female mice were infected with ZIKV-MY or ZIKV-Natal. Pregnant mice were infected at E12.5 of gestation. Viremia was determined daily for five days post-infection. Pregnant mice were euthanized at E17.5, and their (**b**) spleen, (**c**) spinal cord, (**d**) muscle, (**e**) liver, (**f**) kidney, (**g**) eye, and (**h**) brain samples were processed to determine the viral titers by the CCID$_{50}$ assay.

3.3. ZIKV-MY and ZIKV-Natal Infection of Placenta and Foetal Heads in Pregnant IFNAR1$^{-/-}$ Mice

Groups of pregnant mice were infected with ZIKV-MY or ZIKV-Natal at E12.5 of gestation and euthanized at E17.5, with fetuses and placentas collected. The viral tissue titres in fetal heads obtained from dams infected with ZIKV-MY or ZIKV-Natal were not significantly different (Figure 3a, $p = 0.077$ Kolmogorov–Smirnov test). Placental titers were about 0.8 logs higher for ZIKV-MY than for ZIKV-Natal infection ($p = 0.002$, Kolmogorov–Smirnov test). Following ZIKV infection, placenta and fetuses often form highly deformed indistinguishable masses, as described previously [23]. Viral titers in these masses were ≈2 logs higher ($p = 0.045$, Kolmogorov–Smirnov test) in ZIKV-MY- than in ZIKV-Natal-infected dams (Figure 3c). These data provide no support for the notion that ZIKV-Natal (unequivocally associated with microcephaly) has acquired elevated capacity to infect fetal brains.

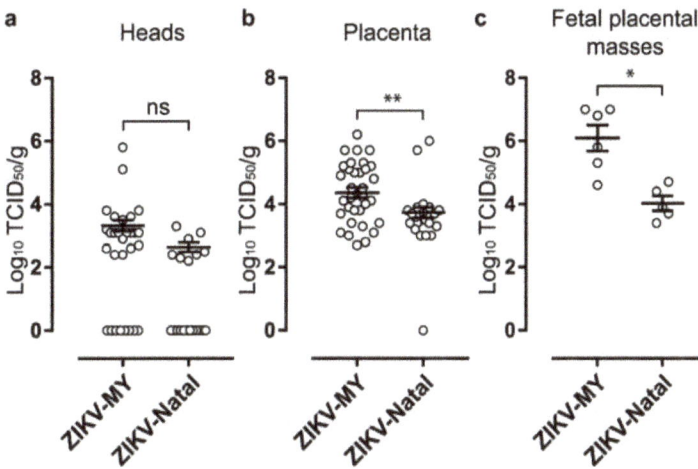

Figure 3. Fetal and placental virus titers after infection with ZIKV-MY or ZIKV-Natal. IFNAR1$^{-/-}$ C57BL/6 pregnant mice were infected with ZIKV-MY or ZIKV-Natal at E12.5 and were euthanized at E17.5 of gestation. (**a**) Fetal heads, (**b**) placenta, and (**c**) deformed fetal–placental masses were collected, and tissue viral titers determined by the CCID$_{50}$ assay. *—$p = 0.002$; **—$p = 0.045$.

4. Discussion

Herein, a 1966 Malaysian isolate of ZIKV was generated de novo directly from a published sequence and was shown to cause fetal brain infection in pregnant IFNAR1$^{-/-}$ mice, with similar efficiency to the 2015 Natal isolate from Brazil. Both ZIKV-MY and ZIKV-Natal also generated indistinguishable viremia and viral loads in a panel of organs tested. Thus, the propensity for congenital infection does not appear to be a unique feature of contemporary Brazilian ZIKV strains.

The use of mice as a ZIKV animal model remains the main practical approach for *in vivo* characterization of ZIKV virulence. Because of the inability of ZIKV to degrade murine STAT2 [29], IFN response-deficient mice are required, and previously we have validated the use of IFNAR1$^{-/-}$ C57BL/6 as a congenital infection model [23]. In other studies that investigated fetal infection by ZIKV in a mouse model [18,30–34], direct comparisons between pre-outbreak versus outbreak ZIKV strains were not performed. Although one study [35] did compare the pre-outbreak 1966 Malaysian strain to an outbreak Puerto Rico 2015 strain of Asian lineage, viral pathogenesis was examined only in the context of an infection in non-pregnant adult mice, rather than investigating fetal infection in pregnant dams. Here, we have directly compared the infection of pregnant dams and their fetuses after subcutaneous infection with Malaysian and Brazilian isolates and show that both strains are capable of infecting fetal brains.

A potential limitation of our study is that the Malaysian isolate generated herein was derived from the sequence of an isolate that had undergone six passages in suckling mouse brain (Table 2). Potentially, such passaging may have resulted in the selection of a virus with increased ability to mediate congenital infections in mouse models. However, on the basis of the amino acid alignment, only two amino acids in ZIKV-MY (NS4B I180 and NS5 Y720) are found in one of two other mouse-adapted isolates (Table 2), and the rest of the amino acid changes are either found in non-mouse-adapted isolates or not found in any other isolates (Table 2). NS4B I180 and NS5 Y720 are also unlikely to be associated with congenital ZIKV syndrome [9].

Table 2. Amino acid differences between ZIKV-MY and ZIKV-Natal.

Protein	Amino Acid Position (Within Protein)	African, MR766 1947 (146× SM, 1× C6/36, 1× Vero)	African, Nigeria 1968 (21× SM, 1× Vero)	Malaysian ZIKV-MY 1966 (6× SM, 1× BHK, 1× C6/36, 8× Vero)	African, DakAr41525 1985 (5× Vero, 1× C6/36, 2× Vero)	Brazilian ZIKV-Natal 2015 (No Passaging)	Brazilian, Suriname 2015 (4× Vero)
prM	1	A	A	V	A	A	A
	17	S	S	S	S	N	N
	21	K	K	K	K	E	E
	31	V	V	V	V	M	M
E	154–156	NDT	Deleted	NDI	NDT	NDT	NDT
	393	D	D	D	D	E	E
	473	V	V	V	V	M	M
	487	T	T	T	T	M	M
NS1	146	E	K	K	K	E	K
	188	V	V	A	V	V	V
	233	T	T	T	T	A	T
	264	V	V	V	V	M	M
	349	M	M	M	M	V	M
NS2A	117	A	A	V	A	A	A
	143	A	A	A	A	V	V
NS3	400	N	N	N	N	H	H
	472	M	M	M	M	L	L
	584	Y	Y	Y	Y	H	H
NS4B	14	A	A	G	A	S	S
	26	M	V	M	M	I	I
	49	L	L	L	L	F	F
	98	M	M	M	M	I	I
	180	I	A	I	V	V	V
	184	V	V	V	V	I	I
	186	L	L	L	L	S	S
	240	T	T	T	T	I	T
NS5	115	M	M	T	M	V	V
	140	P	P	S	P	P	P
	230	I	I	I	I	T	T
	268	A	A	A	A	V	V
	276	M	M	L	M	M	M
	283	I	I	V	I	I	I
	377	N	N	N	N	S	S
	527	A	A	T	A	I	I
	531	K	K	K	K	R	R
	588	G	G	R	G	K	K
	643	P	P	P	P	S	S
	648	R	R	S	R	N	N
	704	S	S	S	S	D	D
	714	H	H	Y	H	H	H
	720	Y	H	Y	H	H	H
	868	D	D	D	D	N	N

Accession numbers: ZIKV-MY (KX694533), ZIKV-Natal (KU527068), MR766 (HQ234498), Nigeria (HQ234500) DakAr41525 (KU955591), Suriname (KU312312). SM—suckling mouse brain.

In conclusion, our results argue that ZIKV has an intrinsic ability to cause congenital infection, irrespective of the sequence evolution that has been documented in recent years.

Supplementary Materials: The following are available online at http://www.mdpi.com/1999-4915/10/10/541/s1, Figure S1: Chimeric ZIKV encoding prM-E genes from ZIKV-MY and the remaining genome of ZIKV-Natal.

Author Contributions: Conceptualization, A.A.K., A.S., Y.X.S.; methodology, A.A.K., A.S., Y.X.S., N.A.P., A.A.A.; investigation: Y.X.S., N.Y.P., E.N., A.A.A.; formal analysis, Y.X.S., E.N., A.A.K., A.S.; writing—original draft preparation, Y.X.S., N.Y.P., A.A.K., A.S.; writing—review and editing, Y.X.S., A.A.K., A.S.; supervision, Y.X.S., A.A.K., A.S.; project administration, Y.X.S., A.A.K., A.S.; funding acquisition, A.A.K., A.S., Y.X.S.

Funding: This research was funded by the National Health and Medical Research Council (NHMRC) of Australia, grant number APP1144950. A.A.K. and A.S. are Research Fellows with the NHMRC. N.A.P. was supported by an Advance Queensland Research Fellowship from the Queensland Government, Australia. E.N. was supported in part by the Daiichi Sankyo Foundation of Life Science, Japan.

Acknowledgments: The authors would like to thank the animal house staff of QIMR B for their assistance with the animal work.

Conflicts of Interest: The authors declare no conflict of interest. The funders had no role in the design of the study; in the collection, analyses, or interpretation of data; in the writing of the manuscript, or in the decision to publish the results.

References

1. Kuno, G.; Chang, G.J. Full-length sequencing and genomic characterization of Bagaza, Kedougou, and Zika viruses. *Arch. Virol.* **2007**, *152*, 687–696. [CrossRef] [PubMed]
2. Wikan, N.; Smith, D.R. Zika virus: History of a newly emerging arbovirus. *Lancet Infect. Dis.* **2016**, *16*, e119–e126. [CrossRef]
3. Roby, J.A.; Setoh, Y.X.; Hall, R.A.; Khromykh, A.A. Post-translational regulation and modifications of flavivirus structural proteins. *J. Gen. Virol.* **2015**, *96*, 1551–1569. [CrossRef] [PubMed]
4. Lanciotti, R.S.; Kosoy, O.L.; Laven, J.J.; Velez, J.O.; Lambert, A.J.; Johnson, A.J.; Stanfield, S.M.; Duffy, M.R. Genetic and serologic properties of Zika virus associated with an epidemic, yap state, Micronesia, 2007. *Emerg. Infect. Dis.* **2008**, *14*, 1232–1239. [CrossRef] [PubMed]
5. Faye, O.; Freire, C.C.; Iamarino, A.; Faye, O.; de Oliveira, J.V.; Diallo, M.; Zanotto, P.M.; Sall, A.A. Molecular evolution of Zika virus during its emergence in the 20(th) century. *PLoS Negl. Trop. Dis.* **2014**, *8*, e2636. [CrossRef] [PubMed]
6. Gatherer, D.; Kohl, A. Zika virus: A previously slow pandemic spreads rapidly through the Americas. *J. Gen. Virol.* **2016**, *97*, 269–273. [CrossRef] [PubMed]
7. Faria, N.R.; Azevedo Rdo, S.; Kraemer, M.U.; Souza, R.; Cunha, M.S.; Hill, S.C.; Theze, J.; Bonsall, M.B.; Bowden, T.A.; Rissanen, I.; et al. Zika virus in the Americas: Early epidemiological and genetic findings. *Science* **2016**, *352*, 345–349. [CrossRef] [PubMed]
8. Wang, L.; Valderramos, S.G.; Wu, A.; Ouyang, S.; Li, C.; Brasil, P.; Bonaldo, M.; Coates, T.; Nielsen-Saines, K.; Jiang, T.; et al. From mosquitos to humans: Genetic evolution of Zika virus. *Cell Host Microbe* **2016**, *19*, 561–565. [CrossRef] [PubMed]
9. Pettersson, J.H.; Eldholm, V.; Seligman, S.J.; Lundkvist, A.; Falconar, A.K.; Gaunt, M.W.; Musso, D.; Nougairede, A.; Charrel, R.; Gould, E.A.; et al. How did Zika virus emerge in the pacific islands and Latin America? *MBio* **2016**, *7*, e01239-16. [CrossRef] [PubMed]
10. Weaver, S.C. Emergence of epidemic Zika virus transmission and congenital Zika syndrome: Are recently evolved traits to blame? *MBio* **2017**, *8*, e02063–16. [CrossRef] [PubMed]
11. Yokoyama, S.; Starmer, W.T. Possible roles of new mutations shared by Asian and American Zika viruses. *Mol. Biol. Evol.* **2017**, *34*, 525–534. [CrossRef] [PubMed]
12. Liu, Y.; Liu, J.; Du, S.; Shan, C.; Nie, K.; Zhang, R.; Li, X.F.; Zhang, R.; Wang, T.; Qin, C.F.; et al. Evolutionary enhancement of Zika virus infectivity in *Aedes aegypti* mosquitoes. *Nature* **2017**, *545*, 482–486. [CrossRef] [PubMed]
13. Seferovic, M.; Martin, C.S.; Tardif, S.D.; Rutherford, J.; Castro, E.C.C.; Li, T.; Hodara, V.L.; Parodi, L.M.; Giavedoni, L.; Layne-Colon, D.; et al. Experimental Zika virus infection in the pregnant common marmoset induces spontaneous fetal loss and neurodevelopmental abnormalities. *Sci. Rep.* **2018**, *8*, 6851. [CrossRef] [PubMed]
14. Mlakar, J.; Korva, M.; Tul, N.; Popovic, M.; Poljsak-Prijatelj, M.; Mraz, J.; Kolenc, M.; Resman Rus, K.; Vesnaver Vipotnik, T.; Fabjan Vodusek, V.; et al. Zika virus associated with microcephaly. *N. Engl. J. Med.* **2016**, *374*, 951–958. [CrossRef] [PubMed]
15. Ventura, C.V.; Maia, M.; Bravo-Filho, V.; Gois, A.L.; Belfort, R., Jr. Zika virus in Brazil and macular atrophy in a child with microcephaly. *Lancet* **2016**, *387*, 228. [CrossRef]
16. Cauchemez, S.; Besnard, M.; Bompard, P.; Dub, T.; Guillemette-Artur, P.; Eyrolle-Guignot, D.; Salje, H.; Van Kerkhove, M.D.; Abadie, V.; Garel, C.; et al. Association between zika virus and microcephaly in French polynesia, 2013–15: A retrospective study. *Lancet* **2016**, *387*, 2125–2132. [CrossRef]

17. Simonin, Y.; van Riel, D.; Van de Perre, P.; Rockx, B.; Salinas, S. Differential virulence between Asian and African lineages of Zika virus. *PLoS Negl. Trop. Dis.* **2017**, *11*, e0005821. [CrossRef] [PubMed]

18. Cugola, F.R.; Fernandes, I.R.; Russo, F.B.; Freitas, B.C.; Dias, J.L.; Guimaraes, K.P.; Benazzato, C.; Almeida, N.; Pignatari, G.C.; Romero, S.; et al. The Brazilian Zika virus strain causes birth defects in experimental models. *Nature* **2016**, *534*, 267–271. [CrossRef] [PubMed]

19. Xia, H.; Luo, H.; Shan, C.; Muruato, A.E.; Nunes, B.T.D.; Medeiros, D.B.A.; Zou, J.; Xie, X.; Giraldo, M.I.; Vasconcelos, P.F.C.; et al. An evolutionary ns1 mutation enhances Zika virus evasion of host interferon induction. *Nat. Commun.* **2018**, *9*, 414. [CrossRef] [PubMed]

20. Smith, D.R.; Sprague, T.R.; Hollidge, B.S.; Valdez, S.M.; Padilla, S.L.; Bellanca, S.A.; Golden, J.W.; Coyne, S.R.; Kulesh, D.A.; Miller, L.J.; et al. African and Asian Zika virus isolates display phenotypic differences both in vitro and in vivo. *Am. J. Trop. Med. Hyg.* **2018**, *98*, 432–444. [CrossRef] [PubMed]

21. Rosenfeld, A.B.; Doobin, D.J.; Warren, A.L.; Racaniello, V.R.; Vallee, R.B. Replication of early and recent Zika virus isolates throughout mouse brain development. *Proc. Natl. Acad. Sci. USA* **2017**, *114*, 12273–12278. [CrossRef] [PubMed]

22. Nutt, C.; Adams, P. Zika in Africa-the invisible epidemic? *Lancet* **2017**, *389*, 1595–1596. [CrossRef]

23. Setoh, Y.X.; Prow, N.A.; Peng, N.; Hugo, L.E.; Devine, G.; Hazlewood, J.E.; Suhrbier, A.; Khromykh, A.A. De novo generation and characterization of new Zika virus isolate using sequence data from a microcephaly case. *mSphere* **2017**, *2*, e00190-17. [CrossRef] [PubMed]

24. Prow, N.A.; Liu, L.; Nakayama, E.; Cooper, T.H.; Yan, K.; Eldi, P.; Hazlewood, J.E.; Tang, B.; Le, T.T.; Setoh, Y.X.; et al. A vaccinia-based single vector construct multi-pathogen vaccine protects against both Zika and Chikungunya viruses. *Nat. Commun.* **2018**, *9*, 1230. [CrossRef] [PubMed]

25. Marchette, N.J.; Garcia, R.; Rudnick, A. Isolation of Zika virus from *Aedes aegypti* mosquitoes in Malaysia. *Am. J. Trop. Med. Hyg.* **1969**, *18*, 411–415. [CrossRef] [PubMed]

26. Swann, J.B.; Hayakawa, Y.; Zerafa, N.; Sheehan, K.C.; Scott, B.; Schreiber, R.D.; Hertzog, P.; Smyth, M.J. Type I IFN contributes to NK cell homeostasis, activation, and antitumor function. *J. Immunol.* **2007**, *178*, 7540–7549. [CrossRef] [PubMed]

27. Gardner, J.; Anraku, I.; Le, T.T.; Larcher, T.; Major, L.; Roques, P.; Schroder, W.A.; Higgs, S.; Suhrbier, A. Chikungunya virus arthritis in adult wild-type mice. *J. Virol.* **2010**, *84*, 8021–8032. [CrossRef] [PubMed]

28. Hugo, L.E.; Prow, N.A.; Tang, B.; Devine, G.; Suhrbier, A. Chikungunya virus transmission between *Aedes albopictus* and laboratory mice. *Parasit. Vectors* **2016**, *9*, 555. [CrossRef] [PubMed]

29. Grant, A.; Ponia, S.S.; Tripathi, S.; Balasubramaniam, V.; Miorin, L.; Sourisseau, M.; Schwarz, M.C.; Sanchez-Seco, M.P.; Evans, M.J.; Best, S.M.; et al. Zika virus targets human stat2 to inhibit type I interferon signaling. *Cell Host Microbe* **2016**, *19*, 882–890. [CrossRef] [PubMed]

30. Cui, L.; Zou, P.; Chen, E.; Yao, H.; Zheng, H.; Wang, Q.; Zhu, J.N.; Jiang, S.; Lu, L.; Zhang, J. Visual and motor deficits in grown-up mice with congenital Zika virus infection. *EBioMedicine* **2017**, *20*, 193–201. [CrossRef] [PubMed]

31. Vermillion, M.S.; Lei, J.; Shabi, Y.; Baxter, V.K.; Crilly, N.P.; McLane, M.; Griffin, D.E.; Pekosz, A.; Klein, S.L.; Burd, I. Intrauterine Zika virus infection of pregnant immunocompetent mice models transplacental transmission and adverse perinatal outcomes. *Nat. Commun.* **2017**, *8*, 14575. [CrossRef] [PubMed]

32. Yockey, L.J.; Varela, L.; Rakib, T.; Khoury-Hanold, W.; Fink, S.L.; Stutz, B.; Szigeti-Buck, K.; Van den Pol, A.; Lindenbach, B.D.; Horvath, T.L.; et al. Vaginal exposure to Zika virus during pregnancy leads to fetal brain infection. *Cell* **2016**, *166*, 1247–1256. [CrossRef] [PubMed]

33. Tang, W.W.; Young, M.P.; Mamidi, A.; Regla-Nava, J.A.; Kim, K.; Shresta, S. A mouse model of Zika virus sexual transmission and vaginal viral replication. *Cell Rep.* **2016**, *17*, 3091–3098. [CrossRef] [PubMed]

34. Miner, J.J.; Cao, B.; Govero, J.; Smith, A.M.; Fernandez, E.; Cabrera, O.H.; Garber, C.; Noll, M.; Klein, R.S.; Noguchi, K.K.; et al. Zika virus infection during pregnancy in mice causes placental damage and fetal demise. *Cell* **2016**, *165*, 1081–1091. [CrossRef] [PubMed]

35. Tripathi, S.; Balasubramaniam, V.R.; Brown, J.A.; Mena, I.; Grant, A.; Bardina, S.V.; Maringer, K.; Schwarz, M.C.; Maestre, A.M.; Sourisseau, M.; et al. A novel Zika virus mouse model reveals strain specific differences in virus pathogenesis and host inflammatory immune responses. *PLoS Pathog.* **2017**, *13*, e1006258. [CrossRef] [PubMed]

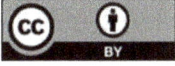

Article

Comparative Pathogenesis of Asian and African-Lineage Zika Virus in Indian Rhesus Macaque's and Development of a Non-Human Primate Model Suitable for the Evaluation of New Drugs and Vaccines

Jonathan O. Rayner [1,2,†] [iD], Raj Kalkeri [3,†], Scott Goebel [3], Zhaohui Cai [3], Brian Green [3], Shuling Lin [3], Beth Snyder [3], Kimberly Hagelin [3], Kevin B. Walters [3] and Fusataka Koide [3,*]

[1]   Department of Infectious Disease Research, Southern Research Institute, Birmingham, AL 35205, USA; jrayner@southalabama.edu
[2]   Department of Microbiology and Immunology, University of South Alabama, Mobile, AL 36688, USA
[3]   Department of Infectious Disease Research, Southern Research Institute, Frederick, MD 21701, USA; rkalkeri@southernresearch.org (R.K.); sgoebel@southernresearch.org (S.G.); zcai@southernresearch.org (Z.C.); bgreen@southernresearch.org (B.G.); slin@southernresearch.org (S.L.); bsnyder@southernresearch.org (B.S.); khagelin@southernresearch.org (K.H.); kwalters@southernresearch.org (K.B.W.)
*   Correspondence: fkoide@southernresearch.org
†   These authors contributed equally to this work.

Received: 6 April 2018; Accepted: 27 April 2018; Published: 1 May 2018

Abstract: The establishment of a well characterized non-human primate model of Zika virus (ZIKV) infection is critical for the development of medical interventions. In this study, challenging Indian rhesus macaques (IRMs) with ZIKV strains of the Asian lineage resulted in dose-dependent peak viral loads between days 2 and 5 post infection and a robust immune response which protected the animals from homologous and heterologous re-challenge. In contrast, viremia in IRMs challenged with an African lineage strain was below the assay's lower limit of quantitation, and the immune response was insufficient to protect from re-challenge. These results corroborate previous observations but are contrary to reports using other African strains, obviating the need for additional studies to elucidate the variables contributing to the disparities. Nonetheless, the utility of an Asian lineage ZIKV IRM model for countermeasure development was verified by vaccinating animals with a formalin inactivated reference vaccine and demonstrating sterilizing immunity against a subsequent subcutaneous challenge.

Keywords: Zika virus; ZIKV; rhesus macaques; Non-human primates; NHP; infection; natural history; Asian-lineage; African-lineage

1. Introduction

Since its introduction into the Americas, Zika virus (ZIKV) has been the subject of a widespread outbreak linked to a number of different fetal abnormalities including congenital microcephaly [1–6] and neurological disorders such as Guillain-Barre syndrome (GBS) [7]. Previously, human infections with ZIKV were infrequent or underreported and associated with only mild symptoms including headache, myalgia, rash and a self-limiting fever; thus, no vaccines or therapeutics have been developed against ZIKV despite the fact that the virus has been known since 1947 [8]. Given the magnitude of the recent outbreak and association with significant clinical manifestations, there is a heightened need for medical interventions to prevent or treat ZIKV infections in humans. Concomitant with the need for new vaccines and therapeutics is the need for appropriate animal models which can be used to support pre-clinical efficacy studies.

ZIKV is a mosquito-borne virus belonging to the *Flavivirus* genus of the *Flaviviridae* family and was first isolated in the Zika forest region of Uganda from the blood of a sentinel rhesus macaque [9]. Since that time, the virus has spread from Africa into Asia with little incidence until 2007 when it was associated with an outbreak characterized by rash, conjunctivitis, and arthralgia on the Island of Yap in the Federal States of Micronesia [10]. This outbreak was followed by an epidemic of ZIKV infection in French Polynesia in 2013 and 2014 that was correlated retrospectively with a 20-fold higher incidence rate of GBS [11,12]. A retrospective case-control study confirmed the association of ZIKV with increased incidence of GBS [13], and a second study identified an increased incidence of congenital cerebral malformations in fetuses and newborns associated with ZIKV infection during this time [14]. Subsequent ZIKV outbreaks were reported from numerous islands in the Pacific prior to its emergence in Brazil in March of 2015 [15,16]. As of March 2017, the World Health Organization Situation Report identified 84 countries, territories and subnational areas with evidence of vector-borne ZIKV transmission; 31 countries or territories who have reported microcephaly and other central nervous system malformations possibly associated with ZIKV infection; and 33 countries or territories who have reported and increased incidence of GBS potentially associated with ZIKV infection [17].

Prior to 2015, animal models of ZIKV infection were limited. However, with the increased magnitude of the recent ZIKV outbreaks and severity of clinical disease in both adults and in the developing fetus, there has been a heightened interest in developing animal models to better understand the pathogenesis of different geographic and temporal ZIKV isolates [18]. Recent research efforts with mice have focused predominantly on the use of immunocompromised strains which lack receptors for type I interferon (IFN α/β), type II interferon (IFN γ) or which lack other components of the innate antiviral response [19–23]. Infection of immunocompromised mice with ZIKV is frequently lethal depending on the specific immune deficiency; however, most of these studies used different ZIKV strains, doses, and routes of administration, making it difficult to draw conclusions. While a lethal challenge model provides a definite endpoint for efficacy studies, a central tenant to animal model development under the animal rule (21 CFR Parts 314.600–314.650 and 21 CFR Parts 601.90–601.95) is that disease progression in the model recapitulates that observed in humans. The immunocompromised nature of these models also limits their utility for vaccine efficacy studies. Although no overt disease is observed in wild-type immunocompetent mice challenged with ZIKV, viral RNA in addition to infectious viruses can be detected in serum and tissues depending on the ZIKV isolate and the route of inoculation, and these models have been used for vaccine efficacy studies [19,23–25].

Non-human primates (NHP's) have also been studied extensively following the emergence of ZIKV in the America's, and rhesus macaques are an obvious first choice given the fact that the virus was originally isolated from this species in 1947 [9]. Consequently, several different groups have evaluated ZIKV pathogenesis in rhesus macaques and the resultant model has been used for vaccine efficacy studies [26–31]. Cynomolgus macaques and pigtail macaques have also been evaluated [28,32,33] and all species have been found to be similarly susceptible and affectively recapitulate the human condition; however, each of these studies utilized different ZIKV isolates of either African or Asian lineages, different routes of inoculation, and different challenge doses, again making it difficult to make comparisons. The objective of this study is to provide a definitive evaluation of ZIKV natural history utilizing highly characterized virus stocks of African and Asian lineages to establish an Indian rhesus macaque (IRM) model for product evaluation under the animal rule. In the process, significant differences in the infectivity of IRMs to ZIKV strains of Asian and African lineages were noted and are contrary to previous reports with other strains of the African lineage [34]. The implications of these differences are discussed below.

2. Materials and Methods

2.1. Care and Use of Animals

This study was designed to use the fewest number of animals possible, consistent with the objective of the study, the scientific needs, contemporary scientific standards, and in consideration of applicable regulatory requirements. The study design was reviewed by the Institutional Animal Care and Use Committee (IACUC) at Southern Research (ACUP#16-08-037F, approved 13 October 2016). Animals were socially housed during the quarantine and pre-study phases, then single housed following challenge phases of the study. Animals were housed in stainless steel cages that meet requirements as set forth in the Animal Welfare Act (Public Law 99–198) and the *Guide for the Care and Use of Laboratory Animals* (8th Edition, Institute of Animal Resources, Commission on Life Sciences, National Research Council; National Academy Press; Washington, DC, USA; 2011). Animals were housed in an environmentally monitored and ventilated room. Fluorescent lighting provided illumination approximately 12 h per day to simulate the natural diurnal lighting and minimize housing-associated stress.

2.2. Viruses, Cell Culture

Vero cells were grown in Dulbecco's Minimal Essential Medium (DMEM, Lonza, Walkersville, MD, USA), supplemented with 10% Fetal Bovine Serum (FBS), NEAA and L-Glutamine according to standard culture conditions. ZIKV strain PRVABC59 was isolated in 2015 from human serum collected in Puerto Rico and obtained from the Centers for Disease Control and Prevention (Division of Vector-borne Infectious Diseases, CDC, Fort Collins, CO, USA). The PLCal_ZV strain (NR-50234) was isolated from a human who had traveled to Thailand in 2013 and was obtained through the Biodefense and Emerging Infections Research Resources Repository (BEI Resources, Manassas, VA, USA), National Institute of Allergy and Infectious Diseases (NIAD), of the National Institute of Health (NIH). ZIKV, IbH_30656, NR-50066 was obtained through BEI Resources, NIAID, NIH, as part of the WRCEVA program and was isolated from human blood collected in Nigeria in 1968. Master and working stocks of each virus strain were amplified in Vero cells (with minimal passages after receiving them in house from the primary source) and quantified using standard plaque assay on Vero cells to determine the plaque forming unit (PFU) titer. All stocks were determined to be free of mycoplasma using a MycoAlert Mycoplasma Detection Kit (Lonza, LT07-118). Endotoxin levels for stocks were determined by a QCL-1000 kit (Lonza, 50-647U) and found to be <0.1 EU/mL. Sterility was also verified by both blood agar and potato dextrose slant cultures for at least 14 days.

2.3. Natural History Study

A total of 36 IRM's seronegative by ELISA for Dengue, West Nile and ZIKV were subdivided into nine groups, each group containing 2 males and 2 females assigned randomly based on body weight. Animals weighed between 3.0 to 7.5 kg and 2–5 years age at the study start.

For the initial challenge, animals were inoculated subcutaneously (SC) with a ZIKV isolate from either the Asian-lineage (PRVABC59 or PLCal_ZV) or the African-lineage (IbH_30656) at the indicated doses (Table 1). Biological fluid samples (blood, urine, and saliva) were collected between days 0–30 post initial challenge (Figure 1). Following a 2-week resting period, the 12 animals originally challenged with each isolate in Phase 1 were distributed into two groups composed of one male and one female from each low, medium and high dosing group and re-challenged at a dose of 1×10^6 PFU/animal using either the identical strain they were previously exposed to or a different strain as indicated in Table 2. Serum collection during the re-challenge phase paralleled the periodicity of the collection time points of the initial challenge phase, between days 45–75 as per Figure 1.

Table 1. Animal groupings of (36) Indian Rhesus Macaques subdivided into 9 groups for initial challenge with the ZKV isolate at the dose indicated.

Group Number	Animal Number	Isolate	Target Dose (PFU/Animal)	Delivered Dose (PFU/Animal)
1	4 (2M/2F)	PRVABC59	1×10^4	5.5×10^3
2	4 (2M/2F)	PRVABC59	1×10^5	9.1×10^4
3	4 (2M/2F)	PRVABC59	1×10^6	7.6×10^5
4	4 (2M/2F)	PLCal_ZV	1×10^4	3.0×10^3
5	4 (2M/2F)	PLCal_ZV	1×10^5	9.0×10^4
6	4 (2M/2F)	PLCal_ZV	1×10^6	6.5×10^5
7	4 (2M/2F)	IbH_30656	1×10^4	2.8×10^3
8	4 (2M/2F)	IbH_30656	1×10^5	3.4×10^4
9	4 (2M/2F)	IbH_30656	1×10^6	3.9×10^5

Table 2. Animal groupings of (36) Indian Rhesus Macaques for the re-challenge phase resulting in some animals being re-challenged with the identical geographical isolate or cross challenged with a ZKV isolate from a different geographical location at the dose indicated.

Group Number	Animal Number	Initial Challenge	Secondary Challenge	Target Dose (PFU/Animal)	Delivered Dose (PFU/Animal)
1	6 (3M/3F)	PRVABC59	PRVABC59	1×10^6	5.9×10^5
2	6 (3M/3F)	PRVABC59	PLCal_ZV	1×10^6	1.4×10^6
3	6 (3M/3F)	PLCal_ZV	PLCal_ZV	1×10^6	1.4×10^6
4	6 (3M/3F)	PLCal_ZV	PRVABC59	1×10^6	5.9×10^5
5	6 (3M/3F)	IbH_30656	IbH_30656	1×10^6	1.0×10^6
6	6 (3M/3F)	IbH_30656	PRVABC59	1×10^6	5.9×10^5

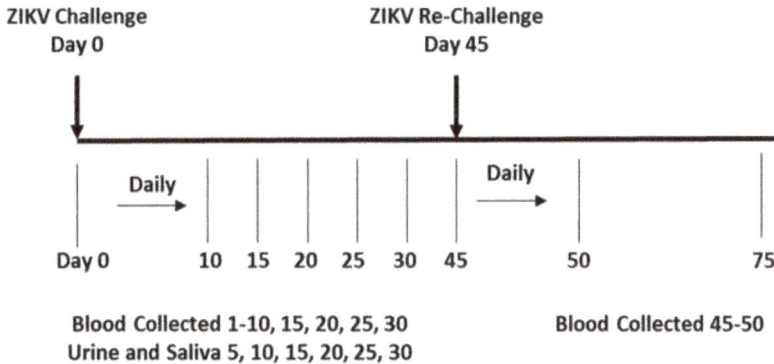

Figure 1. Key Study Challenge and Sample Collection Time Points. Challenge Phase I animals were subdivided into cohorts and inoculated on day 0 with a primary challenge ZIKV isolate. After the primary challenge and a resting period, animals were regrouped and challenged on day 45 with either the same isolate or cross-challenged with an isolate of different geographic origin. Blood, saliva and urine samples were collected as indicated for viral load analysis by qRT-PCR or plaque assay.

2.4. Primers and Probes

PCR primers and probes were designed to the viral Envelope region of each ZIKV genome, proximal to those described in [35] utilizing modified sequences optimizing primer/probe binding for strains PRVABC59 (Genbank Accession KU501215.1), PLCal_ZV (Genbank Accession KX694532.1) and IbH_30656 (Genbank Accession HQ234500.1). All genomic ZIKV strain analysis used for primer and probe design for PRVABC59 and IbH_30656 were as previously described [36]. For the PLCal_ZV strain, we used the previously described primers Zika Dual-For and Zika Dual-Rev [36] and a sequence optimized probe (5′6FAM-TGC-CCA-ACA/ZEN/CAA-GGC-GAA-GCC-TAC-CT-3′IABkFQ). The probe contains a 5′-6FAM reporter, an internal ZEN quencher and a 3′ IBFQ Iowa Black quencher. All primers and probes were synthesized by Integrated DNA Technologies (IDT, Coralville, IA, USA). Primer and probe combinations were fully characterized for compatible melting temperatures (Tm), self-dimer and hairpin potential as previously described [32]. Primers and protocols used for the generation of the RNA template used for the standard curve for absolute quantitation were as described in [36].

2.5. Biological Sample Collection

Biological fluid samples (serum, urine and saliva) were collected from anesthetized IRM at multiple times after the initial challenge on days 0–30 and re-challenge on days 45–79 (Figure 1). Briefly, for the initial challenge (day 0), blood was collected daily (day 0–10) and then on days 15, 20, 25 and 30. After the re-challenge on day 45, blood was collected daily from days 45–55 and thereafter on days 60, 65, 70 and 75. Collected blood samples were immediately processed to serum using serum separator tubes (SST) with brief centrifugation and stored at or below −70 °C. Urine was collected by either cystocentesis (needle) or catheter. Saliva (or drool) was collected directly; if saliva could not be collected, oral cavity swabs were taken and immersed in 1 mL DPBS without Calcium and Magnesium (Cat. # 17-512F, Lonza Walkersville, MD, USA). Both urine and saliva collections occurred on the same schedule, post initial challenge on days 5, 10, 15, 20, 25, and 30 and post re-challenge on days 50, 55, 60, 65, 70 and 75. Upon collection and the preparation of small aliquots, urine and saliva were frozen at or below −70 °C.

2.6. Viral Load by qRT-PCR

Viral RNA was extracted from collected biological fluids to quantify viral load. Briefly, using the QIAmp Viral RNA Mini kit, (Qiagen, 52906, Germantown, MD, USA) total RNA was extracted and purified from a biological sample volume of 140 μL (as per the manufacturer) and eluted into 60 μL of nuclease-free water (Ambion, AM9939). Five μL of purified RNA from each test article was used in a 20 μL qRT-PCR reaction consisting of Fast Virus 4× Master Mix (Applied Biosystems, 4444436, Foster City, CA, USA) containing 500 nM forward and reverse primers with a 200 nM probe. Cycling parameters for the QuantStudio Flex 6 instrument include: an initial reverse transcription (RT) step for 5 min at 53 °C, followed by 1 min at 95 °C and 45 cycles of 2-step cycling at 95 °C for 5 s and 60 °C for 50 s. A standard curve for absolute quantitation using a positive control RNA template was established over the dynamic range of 6-logs (1×10^6–1×10^1) with each dilution in triplicate of test samples. As reported in [32] the Ct values obtained for each of the 6-log dilutions for each strain specific primer/probe combination performed consistently (within 1 Ct) with each other. NCBI Sequence alignment was used for the development of primers and probes that would work specifically with IbH_30656 and other strains used in this study. Additionally, the lower limit of quantitative detection (LLOQ) is approximately 10 copies/20 μL PCR reaction. Depending on the volume/weight of the extracted test sample and the elution volumes, the resulting dilution factor is typically between 80 and 100 fold, thus the LLOQ for this assay is recorded as 500 copies/mL.

2.7. Viral Load by Plaque Assay

The 3 serum samples from each primary and secondary challenge containing the highest viral load as determined by qRT-PCR were further assessed by plaque assay on Vero cells. Briefly, Vero cells were cultured in 6-well plates to approximately 90–100% confluent monolayers and cells were exposed to 200 μL of 4-fold serially diluted samples. Three dilutions of each sample were tested in duplicate. Plates were incubated at 37 °C and 5% CO_2 for 1 h before the addition of an overlay media consisting of EMEM and 0.5% agarose. Plates were incubated for 3 to 5 days until discernable plaques were formed then fixed and stained with crystal violet.

2.8. Indirect ELISA

Purified African lineage ZIKV lysate (The Native Antigen Company, Oxfordshire, UK) was diluted to 0.5 µg/mL in carbonate-bicarbonate buffer (Thermo Fisher Scientific, Waltham, MA, USA). Lysate was generated by culturing virus in Vero cells, clarified, concentrated via sucrose gradient ultracentrifugation, then lysed in Triton X-100, and heat-inactivated. Use of a whole virus lysate provides magnitudes of additional linear epitopes, when compared to use of a single viral protein (Env or NS1 only). This allows for increased epitope presentation, presumably including targets present on both African and Asian lineages.

High binding MAXISORP™ 96-well plates (Thermo Fisher Scientific) were coated with 100 µL of diluted antigen and refrigerated at 2–8 °C overnight. Plates were washed five times with 0.05% Tween 20 in PBS, then blocked for 30 min at 37 °C using 5% dry milk (Quality Biological, Gathersburg, MD, USA). Plates were washed five times then incubated for 1 h at 37 °C with serially diluted sera samples. Signal was detected using goat anti-human HRP conjugated IgG (SeraCare, Milford, MA, USA) diluted 1:2000 in 5% milk. Following washing, 100 µL of ABTS 1-component peroxidase substrate (SeraCare, Milford, MA, USA) was added to each well under low light. Plates were covered and incubated at room temperature for fifteen to twenty minutes, then 100 µL of 1% sodium dodecyl sulfate (Fisher Scientific) was added to stop the reaction. Absorbance optical density (OD) was read at 405 nm on a SpectraMax i3 using Softmax Pro software (Version 6.3 GxP, Sunnyvale, CA, USA). Averaged OD values were plotted against the log of the reciprocal of their dilution (ex. $Log_{10}100$, $Log_{10}12800$). A four-parameter non-linear regression method (GraphPad Prism 5 software, La Jolla, CA, USA) was used for data analysis. Using the formula from curve fitting, data points between each dilution step were extrapolated, expanding the data from eight to one thousand OD values. The log of the reciprocal dilution that corresponded to the extrapolated OD value at a cut-point was identified. The antilog of each identified value at the cut-point was calculated. This value is the reciprocal of the lowest serum dilution capable of producing a positive result for anti-ZIKV IgG antibodies.

An endpoint cut-off was defined as follows: more than twenty IRM serum samples were tested using commercially available kits for ZIKV (XpressBio, Frederick, MD, USA) and Dengue Virus (Calbiotech, El Cajon, CA, USA and Abcam, Cambridge, MA, USA). Sera testing negative for both viruses on all kits were run on the above ELISA, with the exception that samples were diluted 1:100 only. Naive sera averaged an OD value of 0.064. The cut point OD value (0.148) was calculated by adding two times the standard deviation of the OD values to the average OD value.

2.9. Focus Reduction Neutralization Test (FRNT)

The FRNT assay for ZIKV was performed on serum samples collected at the time points indicated. Briefly, Vero cells seeded at a concentration of approximately 1×10^5 to 2×10^5 cells/mL in a 96-well plate were incubated for approximately 24 h. On the day of the assay, input virus and serially diluted serum samples were mixed and incubated for 1 h at 37 °C $\pm$ 1 °C in the dilution plate. The supernatant was decanted from cell-seeded 96-well plates and then 100 µL of virus/serum mixture was transferred from the dilution plate and added to the cells. After adsorption for 1 h, overlay medium was added to the plate and incubated at 5% CO_2 overnight. The following day, the plates were stained using broad spectrum pan-flavivirus antibody (MAB10216, Millipore, Burlington, MA, USA) and Goat anti-mouse IgG (H + L) HRP-conjugated secondary antibody (5220-0341, SeraCare Life Sciences, Milford, MA, USA). TrueBlue Peroxidase Substrate (5510-0030, SeraCare Life Sciences, Milford, MA, USA) was added to the plates and spots were analyzed by BioSpot scanner. Each dilution of sera was tested in triplicate. Neutralizing antibody titers were reported as the inverse of the serum dilution estimated to reduce the number of input virus by 50% ($FRNT_{50}$). The percent neutralization at each dilution was calculated by the ratio of average foci counts of the replicates to the average foci of the input virus wells. $FRNT_{50}$ titers were estimated by point-to-point linear regression between the two dilutions that spanned 50% neutralization.

2.10. Efficacy and Immunogenicity Testing of Inactivated Vaccine

Formalin Inactivated PRVABC59 Vaccine (lot number 2016) [37], with a concentration of 5 µg/0.5 mL, obtained from Walter Reed Army Institute of Research (WRAIR, Springfield, MD, USA) was used for the study. Prior to Study day 0, four (4) IRMs were randomized into two groups (2 animals/group) according to gender/weight using Provantis Software. On days 0 and 28, all animals were anesthetized and inoculated intramuscularly (IM) with inactivated-PRVABC59 vaccine (Group 1) or SC with Minimal Essential Medium supplemented with 1% FBS as a vehicle control (Group 2). On day 56, all macaques were anesthetized and challenged SC with 0.5 mL of ZIKV strain PRVABC59 with a target challenge dose of 1×10^5 PFU per animal. Blood samples were collected on day 0 (prior to immunization), day 14, day 28 (prior to boost) and day 56 (prior to challenge) to determine anti-ZIKV neutralizing antibody (Nab) titer's by FRNT. Viral load was assessed by qRT-PCR on serum samples collected daily between days 56 and 66 and again on day 85.

3. Results

3.1. Clinical Observations

All of the animals were monitored twice daily during the challenge and re-challenge phases. With the exception of some mild erythema, described below, none of the animals showed overt signs of clinical manifestations associated with ZIKV infection throughout the study. On day 1, ZIKV challenge-associated mild erythema at the injection site was observed in 5 animals; however, there was no correlation with challenge dose or strain, and lesions resolved by day 2. Mild erythema at the inguinal region was also observed in one animal challenged with PLCal_ZV at 1×10^6 PFU on day 6 and another challenged with the PRVABC59 strain at 1×10^5 PFU on day 21. Mild erythema was detectable for only one day and lesions were barely perceptible in these monkeys. ZIKV re-challenge-associated mild erythema at the injection site was observed in a total of 13 animals distributed throughout the study groups on day 46 and one animal on day 47, but resolved afterwards without progressing further. Overall, mild erythema detected post primary and secondary challenge was mostly limited to the local injection site and completely resolved without desquamation.

3.2. Virus Detection Following Primary Infection

Following the challenge, the dose preparations were back titered via plaque assay, and targeted doses were confirmed for all but the high, medium and low dose groups for IbH_30656 and the low dose group for PLCal_ZV, which were slightly more than 0.5 logs below the targeted dose (Table 1). Serum, saliva and urine samples collected at the time points indicated in Figure 1 were tested by qRT-PCR to estimate the relative level of virus replication in each animal. Analysis of the serum viral RNA load (Figure 2) showed that animals challenged with PRVABC59 developed peak concentrations on day 2 in the mid and high dose groups as compared to day 3 in the low dose group (Figure 2A). Regardless of the dose concentration, viral RNA fell below the LLOQ after day 4 in serum from animals challenged with PRVABC59. Animals challenged with PLCal_ZV demonstrated similar serum viral RNA kinetics to PRVABC59 at the mid and high dose levels, but peak RNA concentration was delayed until day 4 and persisted until after day 6 in the low dose group (Figure 2B). Animals challenged with the IbH_30656 (African) strain demonstrated only low levels of viral RNA in serum samples collected throughout the study that were generally at or below the LLOQ (Figure 2C). Only the highest dose group produced an average viral RNA concentration above the LLOQ on day 2 that was transient.

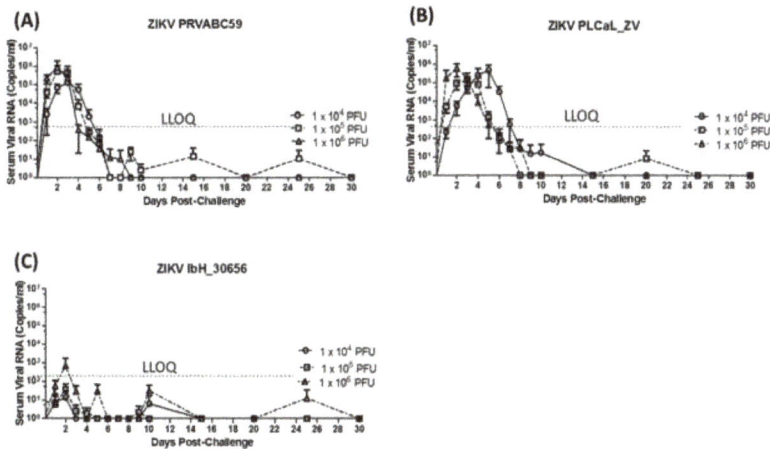

Figure 2. Serum viral RNA copies in IRMs infected with different ZIKV isolates: Serum viral RNA copies in the IRM's (*N* = 4 per dose group) infected with different doses of ZIKV isolates as indicated in the figures. (**A**) PRVABC59 (**B**) PLCal_ZV (**C**) IbH_30656. Viral RNA is reported as copies/mL from serum purified from blood collected at multiple time points post challenge between days 0–30. Lower Limit of Quantitation (LLOQ) is shown by the dotted line.

Serum samples with high viral RNA concentrations in the qRT-PCR assay (above the LLOQ) were selected for testing by standard plaque assay to quantify infectious virus particles present in serum, and the comparative results are presented in Tables S1 and S2. Based on these criteria, the viral plaque assay was only performed on samples from IRMs challenged with PRVABC59 and PLCal_ZV. Infectious virus particles were detected in most samples confirming viremia; however, viral PFU titers were generally 2 to 3 logs lower as compared to viral genome levels. In some cases, no plaque titers were detected despite RNA copy numbers as high as 1.12×10^5/mL; thus, there was no consistent correlation between RNA copy number and plaque titer, and qRT-PCR analysis was confirmed to be a more reliable method for the detection of the virus in serum.

Detectable levels of viral RNA were also observed in urine and saliva samples collected throughout the study from animals challenged with the PRVABC59 and PLCal_ZV strains. However, RNA detection from individual animals was sporadic and independent of dose concentration as demonstrated in Figure 3 for animals challenged with PRVABC59. In this case, low levels of viral RNA (5.3 to 69 copies/mL on average) were detected in urine samples up to day 30 (Figure 3A), yet only one animal challenged with the lowest dose had RNA levels above the LLOQ on day 10 post infection. Viral RNA ranging from 3.9 to 970 copies/mL on average was also observed in saliva samples up to day 25, but again only two samples from animals in the medium dose group had detectable RNA above the LLOQ on days 5 and 10 post-infection (Figure 3B). Results were similar for samples collected from animals challenged with PLCal_ZV; however, viral RNA was only detected in 4 urine samples from animals challenged with IbH_30656 collected over the course of this study while none of the saliva samples had detectable RNA levels [38]. The most notable observation from the analysis of urine and saliva samples from animals challenged with Asian lineage viruses is that viral RNA is most reliably detected (though below the LLOQ) in saliva samples collected 5 days post infection as demonstrated for PRVABC59 in Figure 3.

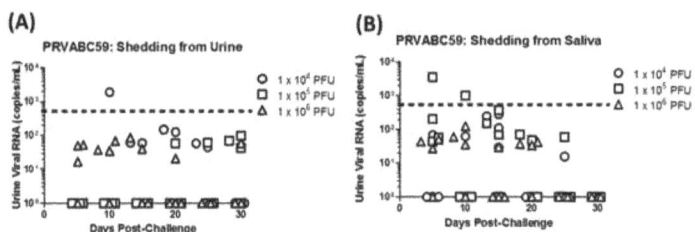

Figure 3. Viral RNA shedding in PRVABC59 infected IRM: Urine and saliva were collected at multiple time points post challenge between days 0–30 from IRM infected with ZIKV PRVABC59 and subjected to qRT-PCR assay. ZIKV RNA concentrations (copies/mL) in the urine (**A**) and saliva (**B**). Circles represent data from single animals in the 1×10^4 dose group, squares represent the 1×10^5 dose group, and triangles represent the 1×10^6 dose group. Urine could not be collected from one IRM on day 5 (dose 1×10^4) and day 25 (dose 1×10^5). Lower Limit of Quantitation (LLOQ) is shown by the dotted line.

3.3. Immune Response Following Primary Infection

Anti-ZIKV antibodies induced following challenge with varying doses of ZIKV are illustrated in Figure 4 and Table S3. IgG antibodies were measured using an in-house quantitative ZIKV ELISA against a purified African lineage ZIKV lysate and enumerated using four-point non-linear regression analysis. Following the challenge, a dose-dependent anti-ZIKV immune response was detected by day 10 in all groups though higher levels of IgG were observed in IRMs challenged with Asian lineage strains (PRVABC59 and PLCal_ZV) as compared to the African lineage strain (IbH_30656). Antibody titers were weak for IbH_30656-infected animals presumably due to very low infection of the animals. The highest average IgG titers on day 10 were observed in the high dose groups challenged with PLCal_ZV, followed by PRVABC59 and IbH_30656. By day 15, antibody titers in the high dose groups of each isolate increased; however, by day 30, average IgG antibody titers from IRMs challenged with PLCal_ZV and IbH_30656 began to decrease while PRVABC59 continued to increase. IRMs challenged with PLCal_ZV and PRVABC59 at the median dose level had averaged titers of 732 and 1026, respectively, on day 10 as compared to an average titer of 226 in those challenged with IbH_30656. Titers peaked at this dose level in all groups on day 15. By day 30, PLCal_ZV titers in the median dose group were retained, while PRVABC59 and IbH_30656 titers decreased. In the lowest dose groups, only one of four animals challenged with IbH_30656 and three of four animals challenged with PLCal_ZV had an IgG Antibody titer above the LLOQ, whereas all animals challenged with PRVABC59 at this dose on this day had a detectable titer. By day 15, the average IgG titers increased in IRMs challenged with PRVABC59 and PLCal_ZV and titers continued to increase on day 30. IgG antibody titers in IRMs challenged with the low dose of IbH_30656 also increased on day 15 but fell on day 30.

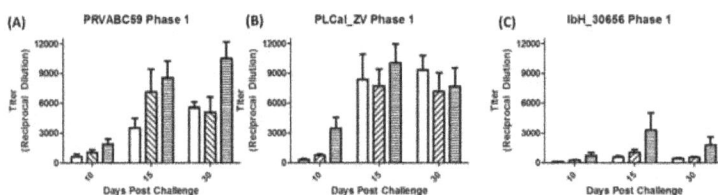

Figure 4. Anti-ZIKV IgG production after initial challenge with ZIKV. Animals were challenged with 1×10^4 PFU, 1×10^5 PFU, or 1×10^6 PFU with either ZIKV (**A**) PRVABC59, (**B**) PLCal_ZV or (**C**) IbH_30656 and anti-ZIKV IgG was detected in serum by ELISA. Bars with no fill 1×10^4 PFU, hatched lines 1×10^5 PFU, or horizontal lines 1×10^6 PFU.

3.4. Virus Detection Following Secondary Challenge

After primary challenge and the conclusion of the natural history study, animals were regrouped as described in the materials and methods section and were challenged on day 45 either with the same isolate they were previously exposed to or cross-challenged with an isolate of different geographic origin (Table 2). The targeted dose of 2×10^6 PFU/mL was confirmed by plaque assay (Table 2), and serum was collected to assess viral load and immunological responses as before (Figure 1). In animals previously challenged with PRVABC59, viral RNA that was below the LLOQ was detected in only 4 samples following re-challenge with PRVABC59 and two samples from animals challenged with PCal_ZV (Figure 5). Following homologous challenge, no viral RNA was detected in serum samples from IRMs previously challenged with PLCal_ZV; however, RNA that was below the LLOQ was detected in at least one animal at various times when challenged with the heterologous PRVABC59. Re-challenging IRMs with IbH_30656 resulted in detectable levels of RNA in multiple samples that were similar to the levels seen following primary challenge but again below the LLOQ. In contrast, challenging IRMs with PRVABC59 following a primary challenge with IbH_30656 resulted in detectable levels of viral RNA that were attenuated by only two logs as compared to naïve animals challenged with PRVABC59 (Figure 5 vs. Figure 2A). In this case, peak concentrations of viral RNA were achieved between days 2 and 3 post challenge and persisted to day 5 before falling below the LLOQ (Figure 4).

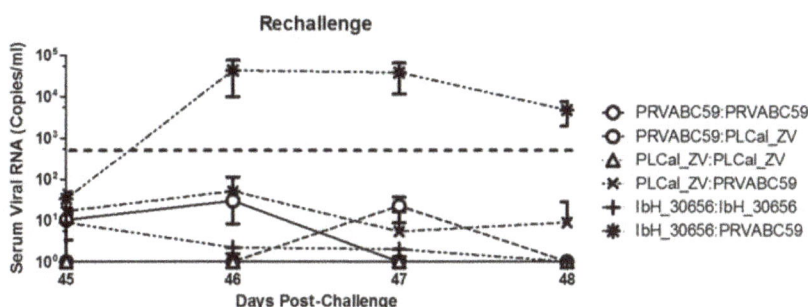

Figure 5. Serum viral RNA copies post rechallenge in IRMs: Serum viral RNA copies were determined by qRT-PCR in IRMs (*N* = 6 per group) previously infected and re-challenged with either PRVABC59, PLCal_ZV, or IbH_30656 at a dose of 1×10^6 PFU/IRM. Viral RNA is reported as copies/mL of serum purified from blood collected at multiple time points post re-challenge between days 45–50. Note, for the IbH_30656:IbH_30656 group day (50) viral RNA copies were determined from *N* = 3. Lower Limit of Quantitation (LLOQ) is shown by the dotted line.

3.5. Immune Response Following Secondary Challenge

Figure 6 and Table S4 illustrate the anti-ZIKV immune response at 5 and 30 days post-secondary challenge (Study days 50 and 75, respectively) with homologous and heterologous ZIKV challenge. Average IgG antibody titers ranged between 10,141 and 12,099 on day 50 when IRMs received homologous or heterologous secondary challenges with high doses of PRVABC59 or PLCal_ZV. IgG concentrations remained high on day 75 for IRMs that received a secondary challenge with PLCal_ZV (Figure 6A,B), while titers of animals re-challenged with PRVABC59 decreased. Re-challenging IRMs with IbH_30656 did not increase the average IgG immune response on days 50 or 75; however, challenging IRMs with PRVABC59 following an initial exposure to IbH_30656 resulted in increased IgG concentrations on day 75 of 10,456 on average as shown in Figure 6C.

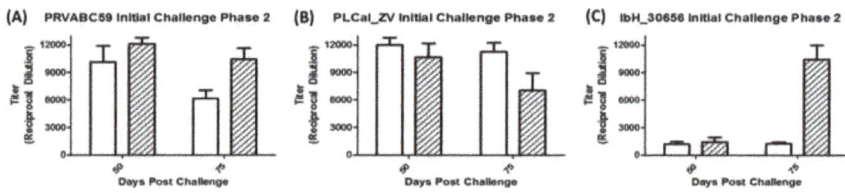

Figure 6. Anti-ZIKV IgG production after secondary challenge with ZIKV. Antibody titers on Study days 50 and 75 during Phase II. Animals from each group in Phase I were reassigned based on previous challenge strain and titer, then re-challenged with 1×10^6 PFU of PRVABC59, PLCal_ZV, or IbH_30656. (**A**) Primary challenge with PRVABC59 followed by secondary challenge with PRVABC59 (No fill) or PLCal_ZV (Hatched lines); (**B**) Primary challenge with PLCal_ZV followed by secondary challenge with PLCal_ZV (No fill) or PRVABC59 (Hatched lines); and (**C**) Primary challenge with IbH_30656 followed by secondary challenge with IbH_30656 (No fill) or PRVABC59 (Hatched lines).

3.6. Immunogenicity and Efficacy of Inactivated ZIKV Vaccine

To demonstrate the utility of the resultant model, groups of 2 IRMs were immunized twice (day 0 and 28) with inactivated PRVABC59 vaccine (Group 1) or vehicle alone (Group 2) followed by SC challenge with PRVABC59 virus on day 56. Immunogenicity of the inactivated vaccine was evaluated by measuring Nab's as shown in Figure 7A. FRNTs in sera collected on day 14 demonstrated seroconversion in both animals in the vaccinated group with an average FRNT$_{50}$ titer of 294. By day 28, prior to boost, FRNT$_{50}$ titers had decreased to 127 on average; however, following the boost and prior to challenge on day 56, FRNT$_{50}$ titers averaged 3270 in the two vaccinated animals. In contrast, ZIKV neutralizing antibodies were not observed in the vehicle control animals.

Efficacy of the vaccine was evaluated by assessing serum viral loads in the vaccinated and control animals via qRT-PCR as shown in Figure 7B. Viremia was below the LLOQ in vaccinated animals throughout the study, whereas control animals showed significant viremia starting on day 57 and peaking on day 58. Individual peak viral titers in the unvaccinated animals ranged from 6.2×10^4 to 2.8×10^5 GE/mL and viral titers fell below the LLOQ by day 62, 6 days post challenge, similar to what was observed in preliminary studies.

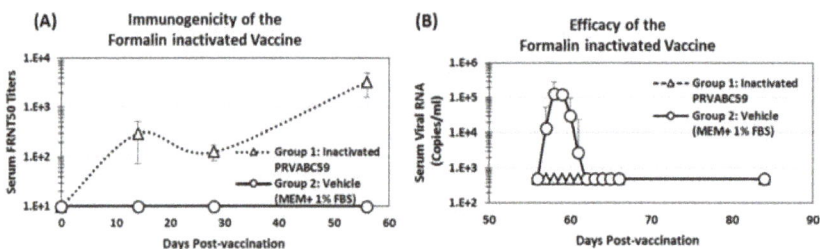

Figure 7. Immunogenicity (**A**) and Efficacy (**B**) of Formalin-inactivated ZIKV vaccine in the IRM model: IRMs were vaccinated with formalin-inactivated ZIKV vaccine or the sham control on day 0, followed by challenge with 1×10^5 PFU of PRVABC59 per IRM on day 54. Serum viral RNA copies after the challenge and FRNT50 titers after vaccination were measured by using qRT-PCR assay and ZIKV neutralization assay as described in the method section. Triangles—Vaccinated animals, Circles—Vehicle control.

4. Discussion

In 2016, more than 40,000 symptomatic Zika disease cases, not including congenital disease cases, were reported in the United States and its territories alone (https://www.cdc.gov/zika/reporting).

In 2017, the number decreased to less than 1000; however, the global incidence remained high with as many as 84 countries, territories or subnational areas reporting evidence of vector-borne ZIKV transmission [17]. In the same report, at least 13 countries have also reported evidence of person-to-person transmission, underscoring the need to better understand the factors contributing to the epidemiology and pathogenesis of ZIKV and to develop new vaccines and therapies to prevent or treat disease in humans. Paramount to addressing these needs are animal models which recapitulate the human condition, and NHPs have arguably proven to be the most appropriate model to fulfill these requirements. The rhesus macaque in particular has been the most extensively utilized to study the pathogenesis of multiple different ZIKV isolates from the Asian-lineage following SC exposure; however, only one isolate of the African-lineage, MR766, has been evaluated via this route to this point [34]. MR766 represents the prototype ZIKV strain originally isolated from rhesus macaques in Uganda in 1947 and was passaged at least 149 times in suckling mouse brains [9]. IRMs challenged with ZIKV strain MR766 via the SC route resulted in plasma viral loads that were similar to those seen in IRMs challenged with a French Polynesian strain (H/FP/2013) isolated in 2013 [34]. Primary infection of IRMs with the MR766 strain also resulted in a robust immune response, which protected the animals from subsequent challenge with H/FP/2013. In a separate study, cynomolgus macaques were demonstrated to be refractory to infection with the IbH_30656 strain of ZIKV which was isolated in Nigeria in 1968 [32]. The IbH_30656 strain falls under the West African subclade of the African-lineage ZIKV isolates as compared to MR766 which falls under the East African subclade [39,40]; thus, it is unclear if the disparity in these results is related to the phylogenetic differences, the extensive passage history of MR766 in mouse brains, or the genetic background of the NHPs. In yet another study, both rhesus macaques and cynomolgus macaques developed detectable viremia following intravaginal (IVAG) and intrarectal (IR) challenge with a ZIKV strain isolated from mosquitoes collected in Senegal in 1984 [29]. This strain (ArD 41525) is also of the West African subclade and closely related to IbH_30656 [39,40], further complicating the interpretation of these results. The IbH_30656 strain was chosen for this comparative study because it is a historical African isolate but unlike MR766 was not passaged in animals with the intent of increasing virulence. The objective of this study was not to provide an exhaustive comparison of Asian and African lineage viruses but to verify previous data with the IbH_30656 strain in cynomolgus macaques and to challenge the dogma from a single study with MR766 that African lineage isolates are equally pathogenic to Asian lineage isolates in rhesus and that an immune response generated to the African-lineage isolates is protective against Asian-lineage viruses. The ultimate goal of these studies was to perform a definitive analysis of ZIKV isolates from Asian and African-lineage using qualified virus stocks and to establish an NHP model of ZIKV suitable for vaccine and antiviral evaluation.

To this end, master and working stocks of ZIKV isolates PRVABC59, PLCal_ZV, and IbH_30656 were prepared in a qualified bank of Vero cells and were confirmed for purity, quantity, mycoplasma contamination, and endotoxin levels. All stocks met the acceptance criteria prior to use in the study. Comparison of the genome copies (as measured by qRT-PCR) and PFU data suggested that generally the genome copies were about 2–3 log higher than the PFU levels. These differences are most likely due to the sensitivities of the assays which are much greater for qRT-PCR that will detect all viral RNA as compared to the plaque assays, which will only detect viable virus able to infect cells in culture. IRMs determined to be naïve to flavivirus exposure were challenged with ZIKV via the SC route and at doses between 1×10^4 and 1×10^6 PFU as has been done previously [27] to most closely mimic the natural route of vector-borne transmission and at theoretical concentrations reported for West Nile Virus in mosquito saliva [41]. More recent studies suggest that the maximum concentration of ZIKV in mosquito saliva is closer to 1×10^3 PFU and that replication kinetics are delayed when ZIKV is delivered via mosquito bite as compared to the SC route at a dose of 1×10^4 PFU [42]. However, the number of mosquitoes feeding on any given animal was not controlled in that study, adding variability to the actual challenge dose, and other aspects of ZIKV infection including tissue distribution were not significantly altered, justifying the dose and route used in these studies. Following the challenge, a transient rash was observed in some IRMs similar to previous reports [34,43]. Previous reports have also reported mild weight loss after infection of IRMs with the French Polynesian strain H/FP/2013 [27] and elevations in body temperatures [26,28]. In contrast, no significant changes in body weight or temperatures were observed in these experiments.

Similar to previously published IRM studies with Asian lineage ZIKV strains and MR766 [27,28,34,44,45], serum RNA levels in PRVABC59 and PLCal_ZV infected NHPs peaked at day 2 to 3 depending on the dose and persisted until day 6). Virus shedding in urine and saliva that persisted to day 30 and day 25, respectively, was also observed similar to previous reports [26,27,43] but at significantly reduced concentrations (1×10^2–1×10^3 genome copies/mL here versus 1×10^4–1×10^6 genome copies/mL in other reports). Differences in virus shedding in urine and saliva might be due to the ZIKV strain used, the method by which the sample was collected, or differences in the sensitivities and detection limits of the qRT-PCR assays, and highlight the need to standardize these methods between laboratories so that accurate comparisons can be made. Regardless, the sporadic nature of virus shedding in urine and saliva reported here and elsewhere limits the utility of these specimens for assessing clinical progression of ZIKV and efficacy of medical interventions as compared to viremia. The immune response to ZIKV PRVABC59 and PLCal_ZV as measured by IgG response was also similar to previous reports [43,44]. All animals challenged with these strains had detectable IgG titers by day 10 that peaked at day 15 or day 30 depending on the challenge dose. Higher IgG titers were generally observed in IRMs challenged with PLCal_ZV as compared with PRVABC59; however, the immune response following exposure to either PLCal_ZV or PRVABC59 was sufficient to protect IRMs from homologous and heterologous re-challenge as demonstrated by serum viral RNA titers that were below the LLOQ.

In contrast to IRMs challenged with PRVABC59 and PLCal_ZV, viremia following primary challenge with ZIKV strain IbH_30656 was below the LLOQ consistent with what was observed previously in cynomolgus macaques [32]. Consistent with the low level infectivity, the immune response to challenge with the IbH_30656 isolate was also low, and although detectable serum IgG responses were observed in all animals by day 15, they were insufficient to protect IRMs from heterologous challenge with the PRVABC59 strain. While these results appear contrary to what was reported previously in IRMs challenged with the MR766 strain, it is most likely that this failure to protect is due to the low level immune response as opposed to the failure of the antibodies to cross protect [34].

These results serve to rule out the genetic background of the NHP model as a factor contributing to the differential infectivity of African-lineage ZIKV strains; however, it is yet to be determined what viral genetic factors contribute to the disparity. Both the IbH_30656 and MR766 isolates have been subject to multiple laboratory passages since their initial isolation more than 50 years ago. Sequence comparisons performed in 2012 demonstrated that MR766 and IbH_30656 differ by 7% at the nucleotide level and 2.2% at the amino acid level, whereas the ArD 41519 strain which was isolated more recently and also productively infected IRMs via the IVAG and IR routes differs from MR766 by 1.7% at the amino acid level despite a 7% nucleotide divergence [40]. These results serve to narrow the amino acid changes to be assessed in future studies aimed at discerning the viral genetic factors that contribute to differential pathologies of ZIKV strains from the African-lineage and should aid in determining the changes that have contributed to recently emerging pathologies associated with Asian-lineage strains.

Until then, the results presented here and elsewhere support the use of IRMs and the ZIKV PRVABC59 strain as a model of Asian-lineage ZIKV infection for the evaluation of new vaccines and therapeutics. The PRVABC59 strain represents a human clinical isolate of low passage which is a prerequisite for animal model development under the animal rule. Additionally, infection of IRMs with as little as 1×10^4 PFU of virus results in detectable viremia that can be assessed by qRT-PCR. Vaccinating IRMs with an inactivated PRVABC59 vaccine resulted in Nab's of similar titers and kinetics to those reported previously [31], and vaccinated animals were protected from challenge with 1×10^5 PFU of live ZIKV PRVABC59 as determined by the absence of viremia as compared to sham vaccinated animals. This model utilizing qualified master and working virus banks will serve as a valuable resource suitable for submission of preclinical efficacy data on new ZIKV vaccines and therapeutics to the FDA.

Supplementary Materials: The following are available online at http://www.mdpi.com/1999-4915/10/5/229/s1.

Author Contributions: Jonathan O. Rayner was the original Principal Investigator for the research, responsible for overseeing design and implementation of the model development studies. Raj Kalkeri is a scientist who developed the in vitro protocols for this project, provided technical guidance to Brian Green and Beth Snyder. Jonathan O. Rayner and Raj Kalkeri equally contributed to the manuscript preparation. Scott Goebel and Brian Green developed the qRT-PCR assay and ELISA respectively, analyzed the results and contributed to manuscript preparation. Beth Snyder is a scientist who propagated Zika virus and performed Zika virus plaque assays. Kevin B. Walters is a scientist who directed virus propagation and characterization as an in vitro Study Director, contributed to the protocols and manuscript preparation. Zhaohui Cai and Shuling Lin are scientists who performed RNA extractions and contributed to qRT-PCR. Kimberly Hagelin conducted NHP handling, virus dosing of NHPs, sample collections and necropsy of animals. Fusataka Koide was the Study Director of in-life studies and led protocol development and technical report writing for NIH/NIAID. Fusataka Koide is the current Principal Investigator for the research.

Acknowledgments: The research reported in this publication was supported by the National Institutes of Health (NIH)/National Institute of Allergy and Infectious Diseases (NIAID) contract HHSN272201000022I; C33 Task Order No. HHSN2720006 (Development of a Non-Human Primate Model of Zika Virus Infection for Product Evaluation).

Conflicts of Interest: The authors declare no conflict of interest.

References

1. Schuler-Faccini, L.; Ribeiro, E.M.; Feitosa, I.M.; Horovitz, D.D.; Cavalcanti, D.P.; Pessoa, A.; Doriqui, M.J.; Neri, J.I.; Neto, J.M.; Wanderley, H.Y.; et al. Possible association between zika virus infection and microcephaly—Brazil, 2015. *MMWR Morb. Mortal. Wkly. Rep.* **2016**, *65*, 59–62. [CrossRef] [PubMed]

2. Brasil, P.; Pereira, J.P., Jr.; Moreira, M.E.; Ribeiro Nogueira, R.M.; Damasceno, L.; Wakimoto, M.; Rabello, R.S.; Valderramos, S.G.; Halai, U.A.; Salles, T.S.; et al. Zika virus infection in pregnant women in Rio de Janeiro. *N. Engl. J. Med.* **2016**, *375*, 2321–2334. [CrossRef] [PubMed]

3. Sarno, M.; Sacramento, G.A.; Khouri, R.; do Rosario, M.S.; Costa, F.; Archanjo, G.; Santos, L.A.; Nery, N., Jr.; Vasilakis, N.; Ko, A.I.; et al. Zika virus infection and stillbirths: A case of hydrops fetalis, hydranencephaly and fetal demise. *PLoS Negl. Trop. Dis.* **2016**, *10*, e0004517. [CrossRef] [PubMed]

4. Franca, G.V.; Schuler-Faccini, L.; Oliveira, W.K.; Henriques, C.M.; Carmo, E.H.; Pedi, V.D.; Nunes, M.L.; Castro, M.C.; Serruya, S.; Silveira, M.F.; et al. Congenital zika virus syndrome in brazil: A case series of the first 1501 livebirths with complete investigation. *Lancet* **2016**, *388*, 891–897. [CrossRef]

5. Melo, A.S.; Aguiar, R.S.; Amorim, M.M.; Arruda, M.B.; Melo, F.O.; Ribeiro, S.T.; Batista, A.G.; Ferreira, T.; Dos Santos, M.P.; Sampaio, V.V.; et al. Congenital zika virus infection: Beyond neonatal microcephaly. *JAMA Neurol.* **2016**, *73*, 1407–1416. [CrossRef] [PubMed]

6. De Oliveira, W.K.; Carmo, E.H.; Henriques, C.M.; Coelho, G.; Vazquez, E.; Cortez-Escalante, J.; Molina, J.; Aldighieri, S.; Espinal, M.A.; Dye, C. Zika virus infection and associated neurologic disorders in Brazil. *N. Engl. J. Med.* **2017**, *376*, 1591–1593. [CrossRef] [PubMed]

7. Brasil, P.; Sequeira, P.C.; Freitas, A.D.; Zogbi, H.E.; Calvet, G.A.; de Souza, R.V.; Siqueira, A.M.; de Mendonca, M.C.; Nogueira, R.M.; de Filippis, A.M.; et al. Guillain-barre syndrome associated with zika virus infection. *Lancet* **2016**, *387*, 1482. [CrossRef]

8. Musso, D.; Gubler, D.J. Zika virus. *Clin. Microbiol. Rev.* **2016**, *29*, 487–524. [CrossRef] [PubMed]

9. Dick, G.W.; Kitchen, S.F.; Haddow, A.J. Zika virus. I. Isolations and serological specificity. *Trans. R. Soc. Trop. Med. Hyg.* **1952**, *46*, 509–520. [CrossRef]

10. Duffy, M.R.; Chen, T.-H.; Hancock, W.T.; Powers, A.M.; Kool, J.L.; Lanciotti, R.S.; Pretrick, M.; Marfel, M.; Holzbauer, S.; Dubray, C.; et al. Zika virus outbreak on yap island, federated states of micronesia. *N. Engl. J. Med.* **2009**, *360*, 2536–2543. [CrossRef] [PubMed]

11. Musso, D.; Nilles, E.J.; Cao-Lormeau, V.M. Rapid spread of emerging zika virus in the Pacific area. *Clin. Microbiol. Infect.* **2014**, *20*, O595–O596. [CrossRef] [PubMed]

12. Cao-Lormeau, V.M.; Roche, C.; Teissier, A.; Robin, E.; Berry, A.L.; Mallet, H.P.; Sall, A.A.; Musso, D. Zika virus, French Polynesia, South Pacific, 2013. *Emerg. Infect. Dis.* **2014**, *20*, 1085–1086. [CrossRef] [PubMed]

13. Cao-Lormeau, V.M.; Blake, A.; Mons, S.; Lastere, S.; Roche, C.; Vanhomwegen, J.; Dub, T.; Baudouin, L.; Teissier, A.; Larre, P.; et al. Guillain-barre syndrome outbreak associated with zika virus infection in French Polynesia: A case-control study. *Lancet* **2016**, *387*, 1531–1539. [CrossRef]

14. Besnard, M.; Eyrolle-Guignot, D.; Guillemette-Artur, P.; Lastere, S.; Bost-Bezeaud, F.; Marcelis, L.; Abadie, V.; Garel, C.; Moutard, M.L.; Jouannic, J.M.; et al. Congenital cerebral malformations and dysfunction in fetuses and newborns following the 2013 to 2014 zika virus epidemic in French Polynesia. *Eur. Surveill.* **2016**, *21*. [CrossRef] [PubMed]

15. Campos, G.S.; Bandeira, A.C.; Sardi, S.I. Zika virus outbreak, bahia, brazil. *Emerg. Infect. Dis.* **2015**, *21*, 1885–1886. [CrossRef] [PubMed]

16. Zanluca, C.; Melo, V.C.; Mosimann, A.L.; Santos, G.I.; Santos, C.N.; Luz, K. First report of autochthonous transmission of zika virus in Brazil. *Mem. Inst. Oswaldo. Cruz.* **2015**, *110*, 569–572. [CrossRef] [PubMed]

17. World Health Organization. *Zika Virus, Microcephaly and Guillain-Barre Syndrome*; WHO: Geneva, Switzerland, 2017.

18. Morrison, T.E.; Diamond, M.S. Animal models of zika virus infection, pathogenesis, and immunity. *J. Virol.* **2017**, *91*, e00009-17. [CrossRef] [PubMed]

19. Lazear, H.M.; Govero, J.; Smith, A.M.; Platt, D.J.; Fernandez, E.; Miner, J.J.; Diamond, M.S. A mouse model of zika virus pathogenesis. *Cell Host Microbe.* **2016**, *19*, 720–730. [CrossRef] [PubMed]

20. Dowall, S.D.; Graham, V.A.; Rayner, E.; Atkinson, B.; Hall, G.; Watson, R.J.; Bosworth, A.; Bonney, L.C.; Kitchen, S.; Hewson, R. A susceptible mouse model for zika virus infection. *PLoS Negl. Trop. Dis.* **2016**, *10*, e0004658. [CrossRef] [PubMed]

21. Tripathi, S.; Balasubramaniam, V.R.M.T.; Brown, J.A.; Mena, I.; Grant, A.; Bardina, S.V.; Maringer, K.; Schwarz, M.C.; Maestre, A.M.; Sourisseau, M.; et al. A novel zika virus mouse model reveals strain specific differences in virus pathogenesis and host inflammatory immune responses. *PLOS Pathog.* **2017**, *13*, e1006258. [CrossRef] [PubMed]

22. Aliota, M.T.; Caine, E.A.; Walker, E.C.; Larkin, K.E.; Camacho, E.; Osorio, J.E. Characterization of lethal zika virus infection in ag129 mice. *PLoS Negl. Trop. Dis.* **2016**, *10*, e0004682. [CrossRef] [PubMed]

23. Rossi, S.L.; Tesh, R.B.; Azar, S.R.; Muruato, A.E.; Hanley, K.A.; Auguste, A.J.; Langsjoen, R.M.; Paessler, S.; Vasilakis, N.; Weaver, S.C. Characterization of a novel murine model to study zika virus. *Am. J. Trop. Med. Hyg.* **2016**, *94*, 1362–1369. [CrossRef] [PubMed]

24. Larocca, R.A.; Abbink, P.; Peron, J.P.; Zanotto, P.M.; Iampietro, M.J.; Badamchi-Zadeh, A.; Boyd, M.; Nganga, D.; Kirilova, M.; Nityanandam, R.; et al. Vaccine protection against zika virus from brazil. *Nature* **2016**, *536*, 474–478. [CrossRef] [PubMed]

25. Duggal, N.K.; Ritter, J.M.; McDonald, E.M.; Romo, H.; Guirakhoo, F.; Davis, B.S.; Chang, G.-J.J.; Brault, A.C. Differential neurovirulence of african and asian genotype zika virus isolates in outbred immunocompetent mice. *Am. J. Trop. Med. Hyg.* **2017**, *97*, 1410–1417. [CrossRef] [PubMed]

26. Li, X.F.; Dong, H.L.; Huang, X.Y.; Qiu, Y.F.; Wang, H.J.; Deng, Y.Q.; Zhang, N.N.; Ye, Q.; Zhao, H.; Liu, Z.Y.; et al. Characterization of a 2016 clinical isolate of zika virus in non-human primates. *EBioMedicine* **2016**, *12*, 170–177. [CrossRef] [PubMed]

27. Dudley, D.M.; Aliota, M.T.; Mohr, E.L.; Weiler, A.M.; Lehrer-Brey, G.; Weisgrau, K.L.; Mohns, M.S.; Breitbach, M.E.; Rasheed, M.N.; Newman, C.M.; et al. A rhesus macaque model of asian-lineage zika virus infection. *Nat. Commun.* **2016**, *7*, 12204. [CrossRef] [PubMed]

28. Osuna, C.E.; Lim, S.Y.; Deleage, C.; Griffin, B.D.; Stein, D.; Schroeder, L.T.; Omange, R.; Best, K.; Luo, M.; Hraber, P.T.; et al. Zika viral dynamics and shedding in rhesus and cynomolgus macaques. *Nat. Med.* **2016**, *22*, 1448–1455. [CrossRef] [PubMed]

29. Haddow, A.D.; Nalca, A.; Rossi, F.D.; Miller, L.J.; Wiley, M.R.; Perez-Sautu, U.; Washington, S.C.; Norris, S.L.; Wollen-Roberts, S.E.; Shamblin, J.D.; et al. High infection rates for adult macaques after intravaginal or intrarectal inoculation with zika virus. *Emerg. Infect. Dis.* **2017**, *23*, 1274–1281. [CrossRef] [PubMed]

30. Dowd, K.A.; Ko, S.-Y.; Morabito, K.M.; Yang, E.S.; Pelc, R.S.; DeMaso, C.R.; Castilho, L.R.; Abbink, P.; Boyd, M.; Nityanandam, R.; et al. Rapid development of a DNA vaccine for zika virus. *Science* **2016**, *354*, 237–240. [CrossRef] [PubMed]

31. Abbink, P.; Larocca, R.A.; De La Barrera, R.A.; Bricault, C.A.; Moseley, E.T.; Boyd, M.; Kirilova, M.; Li, Z.; Ng'ang'a, D.; Nanayakkara, O.; et al. Protective efficacy of multiple vaccine platforms against zika virus challenge in rhesus monkeys. *Science* **2016**, *353*, 1129–1132. [CrossRef] [PubMed]
32. Koide, F.; Goebel, S.; Snyder, B.; Walters, K.B.; Gast, A.; Hagelin, K.; Kalkeri, R.; Rayner, J. Development of a zika virus infection model in cynomolgus macaques. *Front. Microbiol.* **2016**, *7*, 2028. [CrossRef] [PubMed]
33. Adams Waldorf, K.M.; Stencel-Baerenwald, J.E.; Kapur, R.P.; Studholme, C.; Boldenow, E.; Vornhagen, J.; Baldessari, A.; Dighe, M.K.; Thiel, J.; Merillat, S.; et al. Fetal brain lesions after subcutaneous inoculation of zika virus in a pregnant nonhuman primate. *Nat. Med.* **2016**, *22*, 1256. [CrossRef] [PubMed]
34. Aliota, M.T.; Dudley, D.M.; Newman, C.M.; Mohr, E.L.; Gellerup, D.D.; Breitbach, M.E.; Buechler, C.R.; Rasheed, M.N.; Mohns, M.S.; Weiler, A.M.; et al. Heterologous protection against asian zika virus challenge in *Rhesus macaques*. *PLoS Negl. Trop. Dis.* **2016**, *10*, e0005168. [CrossRef] [PubMed]
35. Lanciotti, R.S.; Kosoy, O.L.; Laven, J.J.; Velez, J.O.; Lambert, A.J.; Johnson, A.J.; Stanfield, S.M.; Duffy, M.R. Genetic and serologic properties of zika virus associated with an epidemic, yap state, Micronesia, 2007. *Emerg. Infect. Dis.* **2008**, *14*, 1232–1239. [CrossRef] [PubMed]
36. Goebel, S.; Snyder, B.; Sellati, T.; Saeed, M.; Ptak, R.; Murray, M.; Bostwick, R.; Rayner, J.; Koide, F.; Kalkeri, R. A sensitive virus yield assay for evaluation of antivirals against zika virus. *J. Virol. Methods* **2016**, *238*, 13–20. [CrossRef] [PubMed]
37. Modjarrad, K.; Lin, L.; George, S.L.; Stephenson, K.E.; Eckels, K.H.; de la Barrera, R.A.; Jarman, R.G.; Sondergaard, E.; Tennant, J.; Ansel, J.L.; et al. Preliminary aggregate safety and immunogenicity results from three trials of a purified inactivated zika virus vaccine candidate: Phase 1, randomised, double-blind, placebo-controlled clinical trials. *Lancet* **2017**, *391*, 563–571. [CrossRef]
38. Rayner, J.O.; Kalkeri, R.; Goebel, S.; Cai, Z.; Green, B.; Lin, S.; Snyder, B.; Hagelin, K.; Walters, K.B.; Koide, F. *Viral RNA Was Only Detected in 4 Urine Samples from Animals Challenged with IbH_30656 While None of the Saliva Samples Had Detectable RNA Levels*; Southern Research: Frederick, MD, USA, 2016.
39. Gong, Z.; Xu, X.; Han, G.Z. The diversification of zika virus: Are there two distinct lineages? *Genome Biol. Evol.* **2017**, *9*, 2940–2945. [CrossRef] [PubMed]
40. Haddow, A.D.; Schuh, A.J.; Yasuda, C.Y.; Kasper, M.R.; Heang, V.; Huy, R.; Guzman, H.; Tesh, R.B.; Weaver, S.C. Genetic characterization of zika virus strains: Geographic expansion of the asian lineage. *PLoS Negl. Trop. Dis.* **2012**, *6*, e1477. [CrossRef] [PubMed]
41. Styer, L.M.; Kent, K.A.; Albright, R.G.; Bennett, C.J.; Kramer, L.D.; Bernard, K.A. Mosquitoes inoculate high doses of west nile virus as they probe and feed on live hosts. *PLoS Pathog.* **2007**, *3*, 1262–1270. [CrossRef] [PubMed]
42. Dudley, D.M.; Newman, C.M.; Lalli, J.; Stewart, L.M.; Koenig, M.R.; Weiler, A.M.; Semler, M.R.; Barry, G.L.; Zarbock, K.R.; Mohns, M.S.; et al. Infection via mosquito bite alters zika virus tissue tropism and replication kinetics in *Rhesus macaques*. *Nat. Commun.* **2017**, *8*, 2096. [CrossRef] [PubMed]
43. Hirsch, A.J.; Smith, J.L.; Haese, N.N.; Broeckel, R.M.; Parkins, C.J.; Kreklywich, C.; DeFilippis, V.R.; Denton, M.; Smith, P.P.; Messer, W.B.; et al. Zika virus infection of rhesus macaques leads to viral persistence in multiple tissues. *PLoS Pathog.* **2017**, *13*, e1006219. [CrossRef] [PubMed]
44. Aid, M.; Abbink, P.; Larocca, R.A.; Boyd, M.; Nityanandam, R.; Nanayakkara, O.; Martinot, A.J.; Moseley, E.T.; Blass, E.; Borducchi, E.N.; et al. Zika virus persistence in the central nervous system and lymph nodes of rhesus monkeys. *Cell* **2017**, *169*, 610–620. [CrossRef] [PubMed]
45. Magnani, D.M.; Rogers, T.F.; Beutler, N.; Ricciardi, M.J.; Bailey, V.K.; Gonzalez-Nieto, L.; Briney, B.; Sok, D.; Le, K.; Strubel, A.; et al. Neutralizing human monoclonal antibodies prevent zika virus infection in macaques. *Sci. Transl. Med.* **2017**, *9*, eaan8184. [CrossRef] [PubMed]

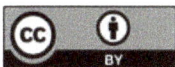

Article

Strain-Dependent Consequences of Zika Virus Infection and Differential Impact on Neural Development

Forrest T. Goodfellow [1], Katherine A. Willard [2] (ID), Xian Wu [1], Shelley Scoville [3], Steven L. Stice [1,*] and Melinda A. Brindley [4,*] (ID)

[1] Department of Animal and Dairy Science, Regenerative Bioscience Center, College of Agriculture and Environmental Science, University of Georgia, Athens, GA 30602, USA; forrestgoodfellow@gmail.com (F.T.G.); xian.wu@nih.gov (X.W.)

[2] Department of Infectious Diseases, College of Veterinary Medicine, University of Georgia, Athens, GA 30602, USA; katherine.willard@duke.edu

[3] ArunA Biomedical, Athens, GA 30602, USA; sscoville@arunabio.com

[4] Department of Infectious Diseases, Department of Population Health, Center for Vaccines and Immunology, College of Veterinary Medicine, University of Georgia, Athens, GA 30602, USA

* Correspondence: sstice@uga.edu (S.L.S.); mbrindle@uga.edu (M.A.B.); Tel.: +1-706-542-5796 (M.A.B.)

Received: 22 August 2018; Accepted: 4 October 2018; Published: 9 October 2018

Abstract: Maternal infection with Zika virus (ZIKV) during pregnancy can result in neonatal abnormalities, including neurological dysfunction and microcephaly. Experimental models of congenital Zika syndrome identified neural progenitor cells as a target of viral infection. Neural progenitor cells are responsible for populating the developing central nervous system with neurons and glia. Neural progenitor dysfunction can lead to severe birth defects, namely, lissencephaly, microcephaly, and cognitive deficits. For this study, the consequences of ZIKV infection in human pluripotent stem cell-derived neural progenitor (hNP) cells and neurons were evaluated. ZIKV isolates from Asian and African lineages displayed lineage-specific replication kinetics, cytopathic effects, and impacts on hNP function and neuronal differentiation. The currently circulating ZIKV isolates exhibit a unique profile of virulence, cytopathic effect, and impaired cellular functions that likely contribute to the pathological mechanism of congenital Zika syndrome. The authors found that infection with Asian-lineage ZIKV isolates impaired the proliferation and migration of hNP cells, and neuron maturation. In contrast, the African-lineage infections resulted in abrupt and extensive cell death. This work furthers the understanding of ZIKV-induced brain pathology.

Keywords: Zika virus; neural progenitor cells; neurons

1. Introduction

Zika virus (ZIKV) was recognized in the 1950s as an arbovirus that could infect humans, though it garnered little attention until the substantial outbreaks in French Polynesia and other South Pacific islands were reported in 2013–2014 [1,2]. ZIKV causes mild febrile illness, joint pain, and conjunctivitis when symptomatic, yet remains asymptomatic in 80% of infected individuals [3]. Beginning in 2016, an epidemic of ZIKV in Brazil established an evidentiary link between congenital infection and placental insufficiency, spontaneous abortion, ocular defects, and microcephaly [4–7]. However, these severe clinical manifestations of congenital ZIKV infection had not been previously reported in areas where ZIKV was endemic. A phylogenetic comparison of ZIKV isolates demonstrated a distinction between older African-lineage isolates of the virus and contemporary Asian-lineage isolates [8]. Further characterization of ZIKV isolates that are directly associated with congenital abnormalities suggests that genetic mutations distinguishing African-lineage and Asian-lineage ZIKV isolates may be responsible for the unique pathologies observed in Latin America.

Efforts to understand the pathological mechanism of congenital ZIKV infection were initiated using in vitro and in vivo model systems. Murine models of vector-borne, vertical, and sexual transmission were established [9–13]. Both vertically transmitted infections and direct infection of the developing mouse brain highlighted the susceptibility of human neural progenitor (hNP) cells and immature neurons to ZIKV infection [13–15]. This neurotropism was confirmed using in vitro organoid and 2D-cultures of hNP cells derived from pluripotent stem cells [16–21]. Experimental models of congenital ZIKV syndrome prompted the current hypothesis that ZIKV infects and damages the developing central nervous system (CNS) and, to a lesser extent, the peripheral nervous system (PNS) [20,22–24]. Initial studies suggest that African-lineage ZIKV isolates cause more profound cell death in hNP cells and neurons than Asian-lineage ZIKV [25].

To further address the lineage-specific effects of ZIKV infection, the authors employed a representative in vitro model of CNS development to directly evaluate the effects of ZIKV infection using both African-lineage and Asian-lineage isolates of ZIKV. Previously, the authors demonstrated that hNP cells could yield mature neurons in a predictable and well-defined manner representative of in vivo human development [26–28]. In vitro culture of hNP cells and hNP-derived neurons enabled the evaluation of viral replication and cytopathic effect of both Asian and African lineages of ZIKV. Although African isolates displayed more rapid viral replication and detriment to cell viability, the Asian isolates disrupted key functional aspects of hNP cells and hNP-derived neurons including proliferation, migration, and neurite outgrowth. The authors surmised that the less dramatic cell death allowed for a population of functionally damaged neurons to remain. Deficient neural maturation caused by the Asian lineages correlates to pronounced effects on in vivo human neural development. The defects in hNP maturation due to Asian-lineage infections increase the understanding of the underlying mechanisms of CNS malformation resulting from congenital ZIKV infection.

2. Materials and Methods

2.1. Culture and In Vitro Differentiation of hNP Cells

hPSC line WA09 (WiCell 0062, Madison, WI, USA) was used to derive hNP cells (hNP1^{TM} 00001) as previously described and was obtained from ArunA Biomedical, Inc. (Athens, GA, USA) [29]. hNP cells were thawed in proliferation medium containing AB2^{TM} basal medium supplemented with ANS^{TM} neural supplement (both from ArunA Biomedical Inc.), 2 mM L-glutamine (Gibco, Waltham, MA, USA), 2 U/mL penicillin (Gibco), 2 µg/mL streptomycin (Gibco), 20 ng/mL fibroblast growth factor 2 (FGF2) (R&D Systems Inc. Inc., Minneapolis, MN, USA), and 10 ng/mL leukemia inhibitory factor (LIF) (Millipore, Billerica, MA, USA) and subsequently plated on cell culture dishes coated with Matrigel 1:100 (B&D Biosciences, Bedford, MA, USA). Differentiation of hNP cultures was induced by substituting the proliferation medium with differentiation medium (the proliferation medium lacking FGF2). Cultures were maintained for up to 28 days in vitro (DIV) with the fresh differentiation medium applied every two or three days. All cell cultures were maintained at 37 °C in a humidified incubator with a 5% CO_2 atmosphere.

2.2. ZIKV Stock Production

ZIKV stocks were grown in Vero cells. Cell supernatant was collected when cells showed >80% cytopathic effect. Supernatants were cleared of cell debris (5000× *g*, 5 min, 4 °C), aliquoted into cryovials, and frozen at −80 °C for one week before titers were determined. The amount of infectious virus was quantified by either TCID$_{50}$ or plaque assays. African isolate MR766 was derived from the original ZIKV isolation and underwent extensive passaging in both mice and tissue culture cells. African isolate IbH 30656 (VR-1829™, ATCC) was also extensively passaged in cell culture before it was obtained. The IbH stock was obtained from ATCC. Asian isolate MEX1-44 was isolated from a mosquito in Chiapas, Mexico, and the virus was obtained after being passaged four times. The lab passaged the virus three additional times in Vero cells before completing these studies. Asian isolate SPH was isolated from a male ZIKV patient in Brazil. The virus was passaged two times in Vero cells before the stock was received, and the virus was passaged three times in Vero cells before performing the experiments. Prior to experimentation, all ZIKV isolates tested negative for Mycoplasma contamination (MycoSensor PCR Assay Kit, Agilent, West Cedar Creek, TX, USA).

2.3. ZIKV Infection of hNP Cells and Neurons

hNP cells, 14 DIV nascent neurons, or 28 DIV mature neurons were seeded into 12-well tissue culture treated dishes for viral replication assays at a density of 400,000 cells/well or Costar® 96-well cell culture plates for viability and proliferation assays at a density of 30,000 cells/well. In all cases, wells were treated with Matrigel 1:200 (B&D) for one hour and rinsed with phosphate buffered saline (PBS) prior to plating. Cells adhered to the plate prior to ZIKV infection (12 h). Cells were infected by multiplicity of infection (MOI) ranging from 0.1 to 10. Viral inoculum was removed 12 h following infection. The cells were washed once with PBS and restored with the respective culture medium.

2.4. Virus Quantification

ZIKV isolates MR766, IbH, and MEX1-44 produced easily discernable plaques on Vero cells and therefore titers were determined using plaque assays. The differential plaque morphologies may be a result of the variation of amino acid deletions in the E protein glycosylation sites, which have been previously noted [30]. For plaque assays, Vero cells were infected with 10-fold serial dilutions of sample for 1–2 h. The inoculum was then removed, replaced with 1.5% semi-solid agar overlay, and the cells were incubated for 4–5 days at 37 °C, 5% CO_2. The cells were fixed in 4% formalin in PBS and stained with crystal violet, and the number of viral plaques was enumerated. ZIKV-SPH stocks titers were determined by 50% tissue culture infectious dose ($TCID_{50}$) titration on Vero cells according to the Spearmann–Karber method and scored 6–7 days later.

2.5. Cell Viability Assay

Cell viability was measured either two or six days following infection with CellTiter-Glo® Luminescent Cell Viability Assay (Promega, Fitchburg, WA, USA) according to manufacturer specifications. Briefly, cells were lysed in CellTiter-Glo® Reagent. After a 15-min incubation, luminescence was measured with a GloMax-96 Microplate Luminometer (Promega).

2.6. Immunocytochemistry to Assess Viral Infection or Proliferation

hNP, neurons, or Vero cells were fixed with 4% paraformaldehyde 48 h following infection by applying 100 µL of warm (37 °C) 8% paraformaldehyde solution to wells containing 100 µL of medium and incubated at room temperature for 20 min [31]. Following fixation, cells were washed three times with PBS. The following steps were performed with the epMotion® 5073l liquid handling station (Eppendorf, Hauppauge, NY, USA). Cells were permeabilized with 0.5% saponin in PBS and blocked for 1 h in 0.1% saponin in PBS containing 2% bovine serum albumin (BSA). Anti-Ki67 antibody (ab15580) (ABCAM, Cambridge, MA, USA) or mouse anti-flavivirus group antigen monoclonal antibody (MAB10216) (Millipore, Temecula, CA, USA) were diluted 1:1000 or 1:400 respectively, in 0.1% saponin containing 2% BSA and incubated with cells for 2 h. Following incubation with these primary antibodies, cells were washed three times with 0.1% saponin containing 2% BSA and incubated with a 1:1000 dilution DyLight® 488-conjugated donkey anti-rabbit IgG secondary antibody in 0.1% saponin containing 2% BSA for 1 h at room temperature while protected from light. Cells were then incubated in 0.1% Hoechst 33342 dye in 0.1% saponin containing 2% BSA for 20 min, then washed three times with PBS, and stored at 4 °C. Images and quantifications were done with the Thermo Scientific ArrayScanVTI HCS Reader (Thermo Fisher Scientific/Cellomics, Waltham, MA, USA). A minimum of eight wells per treatment group and three biological replicates were analyzed.

2.7. ORIS^{TM} Cell Migration Assay

60,000 hNP cells were seeded onto Oris Cell Migration Assay plates with seeding stoppers. After 12 h, wells were infected with ZIKV at an MOI of 10, 1, or 0.1. At 12 h post-infection, the seeding stoppers were removed, cells were washed once with PBS, and fresh differentiation medium was applied to all wells. Cells were allowed to migrate into the exclusion zone for 48 h and were then fixed and stained following the method previously stated to assess cellular proliferation. The migration assay was quantified with the attachment of the Oris^{TM} detection mask and the Thermo Scientific ArrayScanVTI HCS Reader (Thermo Fisher Scientific/Cellomics).

2.8. Neurite Outgrowth Assay

The neurite outgrowth assay was conducted as previously described [32]. Briefly, 28 DIV neurons were seeded onto Costar® 96-well cell culture plates at a density of 15,000 cells per well. Cells were infected with ZIKV 12 h after plating, then the culture medium was washed and refreshed after an additional 12 h. At 48 h following infection, cells were fixed and stained with Anti-MAP2 antibody (5622) (Millipore, Temecula, CA, USA) at a dilution of 1:200. Following incubation in primary antibodies, DyLight® 488-conjugated donkey anti-rabbit IgG secondary antibody and 0.1% Hoechst 33,342 dye were used following an identical method as the one used for the hNP immunocytochemistry assays reported in this study.

2.9. Statistics

All analyses were conducted in *R* [33]. All measurements were compared by ANOVA and Tukey honest significant difference (HSD) test. A *p*-value of <0.05 indicated statistically significant differences between groups.

3. Results

3.1. Isolate-Specific ZIKV Growth and Cytotoxicity in Human Neural Progenitor Cells

Proliferating naïve hNP and differentiating hNP cells were infected with multiple isolates of ZIKV. As previously demonstrated, hNP cells self-renew when the culture medium contains FGF2 and LIF (Figure 1A) and neuronal differentiation is induced by the removal of FGF2 [34]. Two prototypical isolates of African-lineage ZIKV, MR766 and IbH [35], were juxtaposed against two contemporary ZIKV isolates of the Asian lineage, MEX1-44 and SPH [30]. Infection with African and Asian isolates resulted in differential temporal dynamics and peak titers. African isolates (MR766 and IbH) produced high viral titers within four days of initial infection and subsequently diminished (Figures 1B and S1A). Asian isolates (MEX1-44 and SPH) demonstrated delayed growth, but ultimately achieved equal or greater peak titers compared to African isolates (Figures 1B and S1A). In addition to robust virion production, both African and Asian isolates significantly reduced hNP and differentiating hNP viability six days post-infection compared to uninfected control cells (Figures 1C,E and S1B,D). African stains were significantly more cytopathic than Asian isolates at comparable MOIs (Supplementary Tables S1 and S2). This result complemented the observed decrease in viral titers over time in the African-lineage infections. Cumulatively, ZIKV infection has an isolate-specific impact on viral replication and viability in both hNP and differentiating hNP cells.

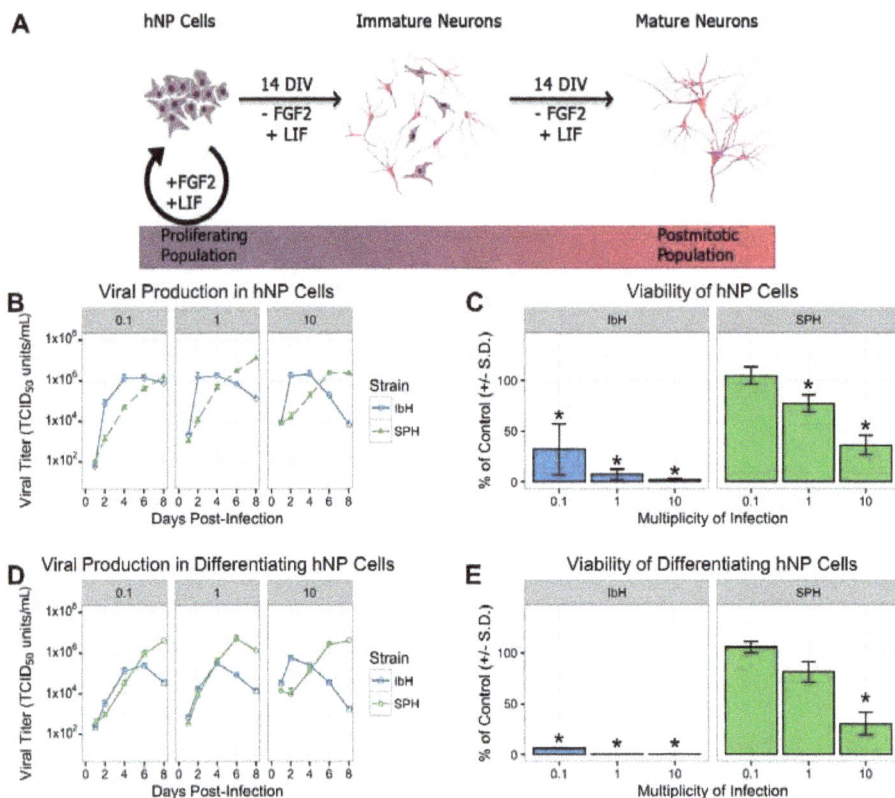

Figure 1. Zika virus (ZIKV) isolate-specific growth and cytotoxicity in human pluripotent stem cell-derived neural progenitor (hNP) cells at six days post-infection. (**A**) hNP cells are maintained as a proliferating population in media with fibroblast growth factor (FGF) and leukemia inhibitory factor (LIF). Withdrawal of FGF and LIF from the media leads to differentiation and a population of immature neurons after 14 DIV, then post-mitotic neurons exclusively emerge after 28 DIV. (**B–E**) African-lineage ZIKV isolate (IbH) grew robustly and induced cell death in undifferentiated hNP cells and differentiating hNP cells, while Asian isolate (SPH) replicated more slowly with less extensive cell death. * demonstrates *p* < 0.05.

3.2. Isolate-Specific Cell Death and Growth in hNP-Derived Neurons

The differentiation process from hNP to highly enriched mature neurons requires 28 days (28 DIV), whereas nascent neurons are evident halfway through the process (14 DIV). The authors, using their well-characterized hNP to neuron differentiation process, could characterize the pathogenic effects of ZIKV infection on populations of both immature and mature neurons. After 14 DIV in the absence of FGF2, hNP cell cultures presented a neuronal phenotype with reduced SOX1 expression and a portion of HuC/HuD+ and βIII-tubulin+ cells, indicative of maturing neurons (Figure 1A) [28]. The full 28 DIV of differentiation in vitro resulted in a highly homogeneous population of post-mitotic and mature neurons characterized by microtubule-associated protein 2 (MAP2) expression (Figure 1A) [34,36]. One African Zika isolate, IbH, and one Asian isolate, SPH, were selected to evaluate the isolate-specific effects of ZIKV on 14 DIV and 28 DIV neurons. The phenotypic differences between ZIKV lineages were again apparent when immature neurons were infected with African and Asian ZIKV. The African isolate, IbH, quickly reached peak viral production four days following infection. Peak IbH titers were followed by a marked reduction in viral production caused by virus-induced death of the cell population (Figure 2A,B). In contrast, cells infected with SPH continued to produce virions, resulting in higher viral titers peaking six or eight days post-infection. SPH-induced cell death was less apparent than with IbH, resulting in more viable immature neurons six days post-infection (Figure 2A,B). Mature neurons infected with SPH produced similar phenotypes to the nascent 14 DIV neurons (Figure 2C,D). Altogether, both isolates of the ZIKV effectively replicated in immature and mature neurons, although the Asian lineage produced higher viral titers while inducing less cell death.

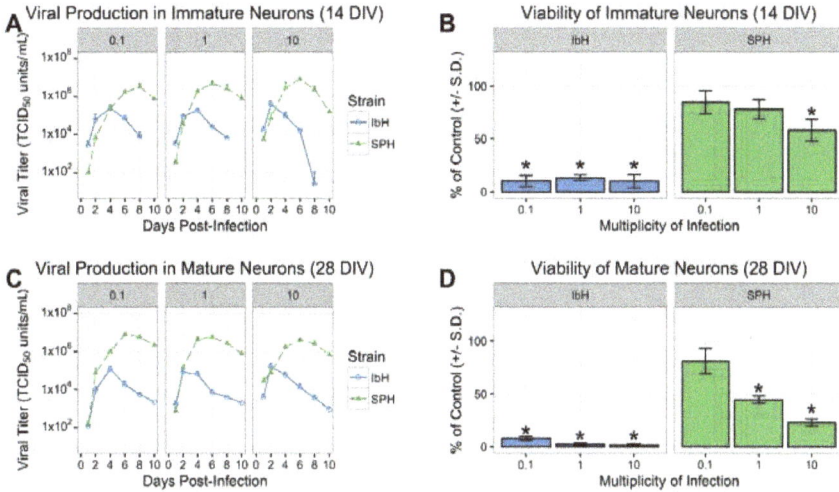

Figure 2. ZIKV isolate-specific growth and cytotoxicity in human neurons. (**A,B**) Viral replication and viability of hNP-derived nascent neurons (14 DIV) and (**C,D**) mature neurons (28 DIV) six days post-infection. * demonstrates $p < 0.05$.

3.3. ZIKV Infects Neural Progenitor Cells and Mature Neurons

The differences observed in cell viability between the ZIKV lineages may be influenced by the isolates' abilities to initially infect the cells. A previous study found that African isolates were able to infect significantly more hNP cells than an Asian isolate [37,38]. To evaluate the ability of two prototypical Asian and African ZIKV isolates to infect hNP cells and mature neurons, the number of hNP cell or neurons containing ZIKV E protein was compared to infected Vero cells 12 h after infection. Vero cells readily produced viral proteins, and pervasive infection was observed independent of the ZIKV isolate (Figure 3A,D). hNP cells and 28 DIV mature neurons displayed lower susceptibility/permissivity relative to Vero cells. Only a fraction of the hNP cells and 28 DIV neurons expressed ZIKV E protein, and lineage-specific susceptibility was observed in these cell lines. The high MOI infection (MOI 10) of hNP cells resulted in 13% of the IbH-infected cells expressing ZIKV E protein after 48 h, whereas only 7% of hNPs and 28 DIV neurons were infected by Asian isolate SPH (Figure 3B–D).

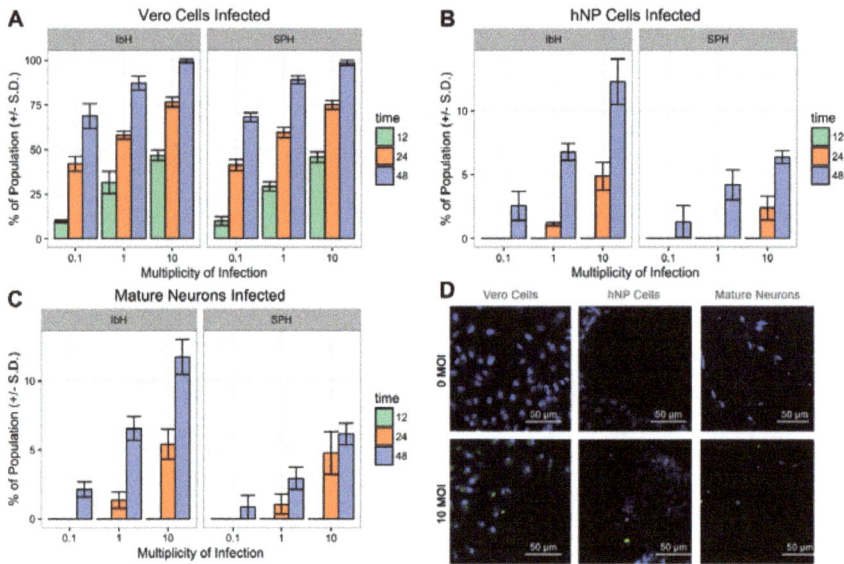

Figure 3. Isolate-dependent ability of ZIKV to infect hNP cells and mature neurons. (**A**) ZIKV isolates IbH and SPH readily infect Vero cells within 48 h. (**B**) hNP cells are more susceptible to IbH infection than SPH infection, however neither isolate infected more than 13% of the population. (**C**) Mature neurons (28 DIV) were similarly more susceptible to ZIKV IbH infection than SPH infection. (**D**) Non-infected (0 MOI) did not demonstrate ZIKV E protein's presence, but infected (SPH 10 MOI) cells after 48 h did contain ZIKV E protein in all three cell types.

3.4. Neural Progenitor Cell Proliferation and Migration Decreases after ZIKV Infection

Proper hNP cell proliferation and migration are two fundamental cellular activities needed to construct the human cerebral cortex [26]. The impact of ZIKV infection on hNP cell function was evaluated 48 h after infection. At this time point, hNP cells infected with both IbH and SPH exhibited significant viral replication, yet minimal impact on cell viability (Figures 1B and 4A). Proliferation of hNP cells diminished when infected with African and Asian ZIKV isolates, indicated by a decrease in the number of Ki67 positive cells (Figure 4B). However, infection with SPH decreased hNP cell proliferation without impacting cell viability (Figure 4A,B). hNP cell motility was evaluated by enumerating the cells migrating into the exclusion zone. hNP cells infected with either IbH or SPH exhibited a reduced ability to migrate compared to non-infected hNP cells (Figure 4C). IbH-infected populations had significantly fewer mobile hNP cells at all MOIs. In contrast, SPH-infected hNP cells only significantly impaired migration when infected at a high MOI (Figure 4C). Overall, ZIKV infection impacted the proliferation and migration of hNP cells, and these impacts occurred prior to reduced cell viability resulting from ZIKV infection.

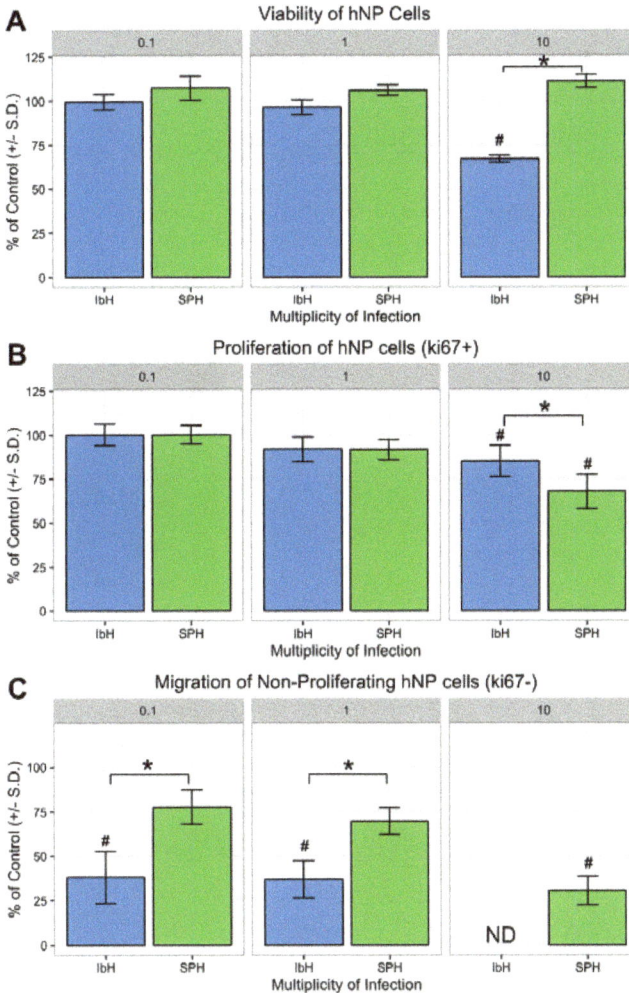

Figure 4. ZIKV infection decreased hNP cell proliferation and migration. (**A**) Only infection with MOI 10 of African-lineage ZIKV demonstrated a significant impact on cell viability after 48 h, whereas infection with SPH did not decrease viability. (**B**) The proliferation of hNP cells after ZIKV infection was significantly decreased following infection with SPH as determined by quantification of Ki67 expression. (**C**) The migration of hNP cells was disrupted by both IbH and SPH infections. IbH infection severely inhibited migration at MOI 10 to such an extent that no acceptable data were collected (shown as ND). * demonstrates $p < 0.05$ significance between IbH and SPH and # demonstrates $p < 0.05$ significance difference from non-infected control.

3.5. Neuronal Maturation is Hindered by ZIKV Infection

Neurite outgrowth of cortical neurons is a critical step near the conclusion of neural maturation, and pathological perturbation of neurite outgrowth contributes to defects in cognitive function [39]. The impact of ZIKV infection on neurite outgrowth was assessed prior to significant viral-induced cell death. Both IbH and SPH Zika isolates actively produced virus in mature 28 DIV neurons 48 h after initial infection despite a relatively small proportion of the cell population exhibiting an active infection (Figures 3C and 2C). The acute infection with IbH, but not SPH, induced significant cell death at high MOI (Figure 5A,C). Infection of 28 DIV neurons with SPH significantly diminished the number of neurites, attenuated the neurite length, and decreased the number of branch points (Figure 5B–F). The total number of neurites extending from neurons infected with IbH was unaltered, but the length and number of branch points were decreased. Infection with Asian isolate SPH did not impact cell viability but altered the neurite outgrowth. Collectively, Asian isolate ZIKV infection impacted neurite outgrowth prior to decreased viability of the infected 28 DIV neurons. This result suggested an exceptional ability of the Asian isolates to functionally damage populations of neurons differently than African isolates.

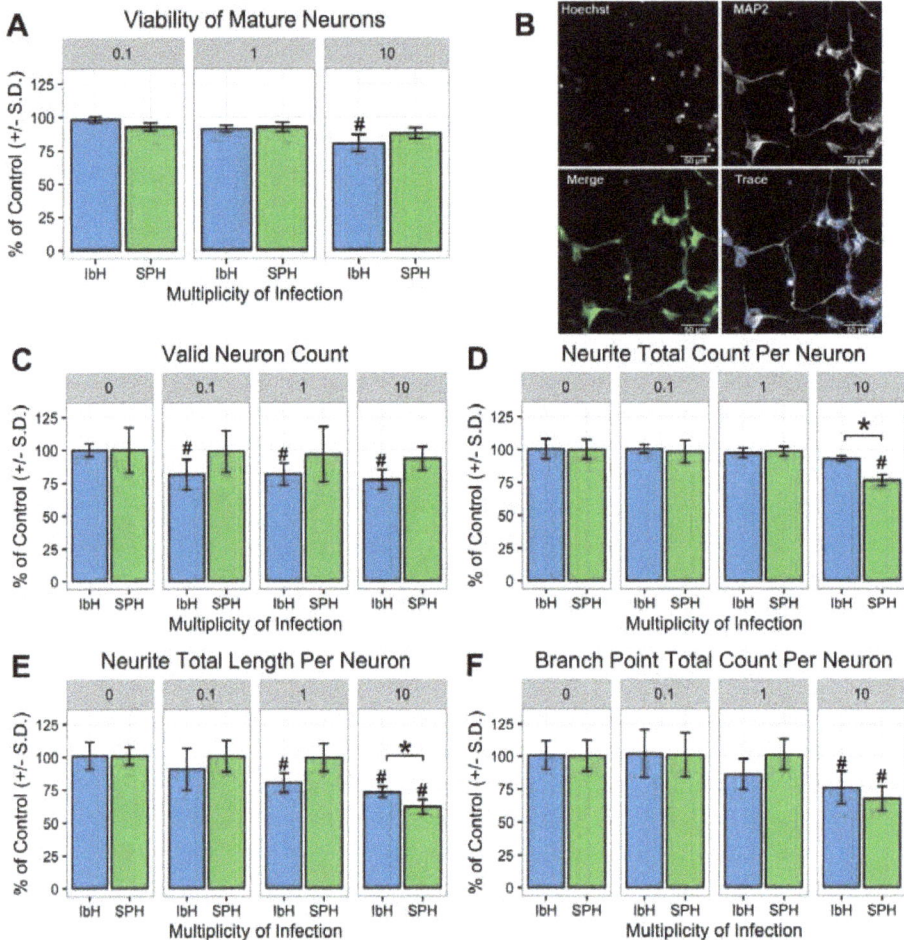

Figure 5. ZIKV infection perturbs neurite outgrowth in human neural progenitor cell-derived neurons. (**A**) At 48 h post-infection, both African (IbH) and Asian (SPH) isolates had minimal impact on neuron viability. (**B**) Representative images of neurite outgrowth quantification. Hoechst stain labels nuclei of neurons and MAP2 identifies neurites. Both images contribute to the enumeration and quantification of neurite outgrowth characteristics. Scale bar = 50 micrometers (**C–F**). Infection with Asian-lineage ZIKV (SPH) did not reduce the number of valid neurons observed, yet infection with SPH (MOI 10) proved detrimental to neurite outgrowth by decreasing the quantity, length, and number of branch points per neuron. * demonstrates $p < 0.05$ significance between IbH and SPH and # demonstrates $p < 0.05$ significance difference from non-infected control.

4. Discussion

hNP cells and hNP-derived neurons are advantageous when assessing developmental malformations and provide a platform to examine the effects toxins and pathogens exert in a controlled, homogenous, and reproducible setting [39]. In vitro assays designed to evaluate critical functions of hNP and hNP-derived neurons provide critical insight into how environmental stresses and pathogens can alter normal functions including cell migration and neurite outgrowth [28,39,40]. In order to evaluate the impact of Asian and African isolates of ZIKV on human neural cell development, both undifferentiated hNP cells and hNP-derived neurons were infected to observe ZIKV-induced changes in differentiation, proliferation, migration, and neurite outgrowth.

Initially, the authors compared African and Asian isolates' abilities to infect, replicate, and induce cell death in hNP cells and neurons. Genetic divergence between African and Asian isolates of ZIKV has been implicated in differential infection phenotypes [8,35,38]. Embryonic mice infected with African ZIKV isolates exhibited more pronounced apoptosis and a larger decrease in progenitor cell proliferation than mice infected with an Asian isolate [25]. African isolates of ZIKV induced higher chicken embryo mortality than Asian isolates [30]. These observations were confirmed with in vitro model systems using hNP cells and other cell types within the developing brain derived from pluripotent stem cells. However, the possibility remains that pluripotent stem cell-derived hNP cells and neurons could respond differently than cells of primary origins [16–20,41]. The observation of viral replication in hNP cells and hNP-derived neurons in this study provides further evidence that African and Asian isolates generate distinct differences in neural developmental processes.

Both isolates displayed infection in the hNP cells and neurons compared to the Vero cells. Adding equivalent volumes of ZIKV resulted in nearly 100% of the Vero cells infected with ZIKV, whereas only a fraction of hNP cells and neurons produced viral protein E (Figure 3). The relatively poor rates of infection in hNPs and neurons compared to Vero cells may be due to a functional interferon response in the CNS lines compared to the interferon deficient Vero cells [42,43]. The African-lineage virus was able to infect twice as many hNPs and mature neurons compared to Asian isolates (Figure 3). The African isolates used in this study were extensively cultured in fetal mouse brains for several decades, which may have created viral isolates more adept at infecting the primordial mammalian CNS [44]. Conversely, Asian isolates infected fewer neural cells initially, yet were able to remain in the population longer by inducing only modest cell death (Figures 1–3). Perhaps this trait is an indication of the Asian ZIKV isolate's ability to more effectively evade host anti-viral defenses [45].

The authors suspect that the African-lineage isolates produced lower viral titers because of virus-induced cell death. Only a small percentage of the hNP or neuron populations contained the ZIKV E protein, but the viability of the neural populations dramatically decreased. This result suggested that some of the cell death could be due to bystander killing rather than primary ZIKV infection (Figure 3) [46]. This hypothesis of bystander effects of ZIKV infection altering the proliferation of infected cells and the paracrine stimulation of hNP cells could trigger apoptotic pathways independent of infection [41,47]. Mutations could enable the Asian-lineage isolates to prevent cell death pathways or decrease bystander cell death. Such changes may allow Asian-lineage ZIKV to persist in the prenatal or neonatal CNS without fatal consequences [48].

Beyond evaluating ZIKV growth and viral-induced cell death, the authors tested how ZIKV infection disturbed the functional attributes of hNP cells and hNP-derived neurons. Neural progenitor cell function is critical for CNS growth and maturation [26]. Previous in vitro models reported that ZIKV caused perturbation of the cell cycle and transcription of neurodevelopmental pathways in hNP cells [17,49]. Murine experimental models and autopsies of newborns with congenital Zika syndrome exhibited altered neural cell proliferation and migration after ZIKV infection [14,15,50]. This study's data demonstrated that SPH uniquely inhibited proliferation prior to any detrimental effect on cell viability (Figure 4A,B), suggesting the in vitro infection model could be used in further examining the mechanisms of ZIKV-induced microcephaly.

hNP cell migration is the culmination of intracellular processes and interactions with the extracellular matrix [51]. Monitoring hNP cell migration after ZIKV infection indicated that both IbH and SPH could subvert normal cell mobility prior to the cytotoxic effects of ZIKV. Deficiencies in the cell motility likely contributed to the observation of CNS malformation in mouse models when exposed to either African- or Asian-lineage viruses [11,52]. This study's results suggested that Asian ZIKV isolates caused diminished proliferation and migration of hNP cells while avoiding significant cell death. In combination, these events likely contribute to how ZIKV infection leads to congenital brain malformations.

The architecture of the cortex is established by the proliferation and migration of hNP cells [53]. Later, neurons mature within the cortex by extending neurites and synaptogenesis [54]. The integrity of neurite structure is critical for CNS function, and the precise organization of the cytoskeleton, microtubule dynamics, and neurite outgrowth can be pathologically disrupted [55]. The impact of ZIKV infection in neurons was evaluated by measuring the degree of neurite outgrowth and branching. High MOI infections with Asian isolate SPH caused significant loss in the number of neurites, the length of the neurites, and the number of branch points. Clinical reports from congenital ZIKV infection included ocular defects and seizures [56]. The attenuated proliferation, migration, and neurite outgrowth reported in this study appears to resemble other pathologies leading to seizures and cognitive defects [53,57].

5. Conclusions

In conclusion, the authors' use of well-defined cell types and assays allowed them to evaluate the functional consequences of ZIKV infection in cells of the developing brain. The direct comparison of African and Asian isolates of the ZIKV revealed the ability of the Asian ZIKV isolate, SPH, to disturb hNP and neuronal cell function. The diminished hNP cell proliferation, migration, and altered neurite outgrowth in neurons suggested that Asian-lineage ZIKV infection altered cellular function in the developing CNS while slowly inducing cytopathic effects, which could result in congenital Zika syndrome. The evidence indicates that ZIKV isolates of Asian origin may have a unique ability to alter critical cellular processes. Further work comparing viral evolutionary changes should provide evidence of how Asian isolates of the ZIKV are capable of altering cells of the developing brain without inducing extensive cell death and will help elucidate the mechanism behind ZIKV congenital syndrome.

Supplementary Materials: The following are available online at http://www.mdpi.com/1999-4915/10/10/550/s1. Figure S1. ZIKV isolate-specific growth and cytotoxicity in hNP cells at six days post-infection. Table S1. Comparison of ZIKV isolates at unique MOI (* indicates $p < 0.05$). Table S2. Comparison of MOI within each ZIKV isolate.

Author Contributions: Conceptualization, F.T.G., S.L.S. and M.A.B.; Methodology, F.T.G., S.S. and X.W.; Software, F.T.G. and X.W.; Validation, F.T.G., S.S. and X.W.; Formal Analysis, F.T.G. and K.A.W.; Investigation, F.T.G. and K.A.W.; Resources, S.L.S. and M.A.B.; Data Curation, F.T.G. and K.A.W.; Writing—Original Draft Preparation, F.T.G.; Writing—Review and Editing, K.A.W., M.A.B. and S.L.S.; Visualization, F.T.G.; Supervision, S.L.S. and M.A.B.; Funding Acquisition, S.L.S. and M.A.B.

Funding: This research received no external funding; the project was supported by funds from the University of Georgia.

Acknowledgments: The authors would like to thank all remaining members of the Stice, Brindley, and Tripp laboratories at the University of Georgia.

Conflicts of Interest: The authors declare no conflict of interest. The funders had no role in the design of the study; in the collection, analyses, or interpretation of data; in the writing of the manuscript; and in the decision to publish the results.

References

1. Dick, G.W.; Kitchen, S.F.; Haddow, A.J. Zika virus. I. Isolations and serological specificity. *Trans. R. Soc. Trop. Med. Hyg.* **1952**, *46*, 509–520. [CrossRef]

2. Ioos, S.; Mallet, H.P.; Leparc Goffart, I.; Gauthier, V.; Cardoso, T.; Herida, M. Current Zika virus epidemiology and recent epidemics. *Med. Mal. Infect.* **2014**, *44*, 302–307. [CrossRef] [PubMed]

3. Petersen, E.; Wilson, M.E.; Touch, S.; McCloskey, B.; Mwaba, P.; Bates, M.; Dar, O.; Mattes, F.; Kidd, M.; Ippolito, G.; et al. Rapid Spread of Zika Virus in The Americas–Implications for Public Health Preparedness for Mass Gatherings at the 2016 Brazil Olympic Games. *Int J. Infect. Dis.* **2016**, *44*, 11–15. [CrossRef] [PubMed]

4. Driggers, R.W.; Ho, C.Y.; Korhonen, E.M.; Kuivanen, S.; Jaaskelainen, A.J.; Smura, T.; Rosenberg, A.; Hill, D.A.; DeBiasi, R.L.; Vezina, G.; et al. Zika Virus Infection with Prolonged Maternal Viremia and Fetal Brain Abnormalities. *N. Engl. J. Med.* **2016**, *374*, 2142–2151. [CrossRef] [PubMed]

5. Mlakar, J.; Korva, M.; Tul, N.; Popovic, M.; Poljsak-Prijatelj, M.; Mraz, J.; Kolenc, M.; Resman Rus, K.; Vesnaver Vipotnik, T.; Fabjan Vodusek, V.; et al. Zika Virus Associated with Microcephaly. *N. Engl. J. Med.* **2016**, *374*, 951–958. [CrossRef] [PubMed]

6. Sarno, M.; Sacramento, G.A.; Khouri, R.; do Rosario, M.S.; Costa, F.; Archanjo, G.; Santos, L.A.; Nery, N., Jr.; Ko, A.I.; et al. Zika Virus Infection and Stillbirths: A Case of Hydrops Fetalis, Hydranencephaly and Fetal Demise. *PLoS Negl. Trop. Dis.* **2016**, *10*, e0004517. [CrossRef] [PubMed]

7. Ventura, C.V.; Maia, M.; Dias, N.; Ventura, L.O.; Belfort, R., Jr. Zika: Neurological and ocular findings in infant without microcephaly. *Lancet* **2016**, *387*, 2502. [CrossRef]

8. Yun, S.I.; Song, B.H.; Frank, J.C.; Julander, J.G.; Polejaeva, I.A.; Davies, C.J.; White, K.L.; Lee, Y.M. Complete Genome Sequences of Three Historically Important, Spatiotemporally Distinct, and Genetically Divergent Strains of Zika Virus: MR-766, P6-740, and PRVABC-59. *Genome Announc.* **2016**, *4*. [CrossRef] [PubMed]

9. Miner, J.J.; Sene, A.; Richner, J.M.; Smith, A.M.; Santeford, A.; Ban, N.; Weger-Lucarelli, J.; Manzella, F.; Ruckert, C.; Govero, J. Zika Virus Infection in Mice Causes Panuveitis with Shedding of Virus in Tears. *Cell Rep.* **2016**, *16*, 3208–3218. [CrossRef] [PubMed]

10. Govero, J.; Esakky, P.; Scheaffer, S.M.; Fernandez, E.; Drury, A.; Platt, D.J.; Gorman, M.J.; Richner, J.M.; Caine, E.A.; Salazar, V.; et al. Zika virus infection damages the testes in mice. *Nature* **2016**, *540*, 438–442. [CrossRef] [PubMed]

11. Cugola, F.R.; Fernandes, I.R.; Russo, F.B.; Freitas, B.C.; Dias, J.L.; Guimaraes, K.P.; Benazzato, C.; Almeida, N.; Pignatari, G.C.; Romero, S.; et al. The Brazilian Zika virus strain causes birth defects in experimental models. *Nature* **2016**, *534*, 267–271. [CrossRef] [PubMed]

12. Yockey, L.J.; Varela, L.; Rakib, T.; Khoury-Hanold, W.; Fink, S.L.; Stutz, B.; Szigeti-Buck, K.; van den Pol, A.; Lindenbach, B.D.; Horvath, T.L.; et al. Vaginal Exposure to Zika Virus during Pregnancy Leads to Fetal Brain Infection. *Cell* **2016**, *166*, 1247–1256. [CrossRef] [PubMed]

13. Miner, J.J.; Cao, B.; Govero, J.; Smith, A.M.; Fernandez, E.; Cabrera, O.H.; Garber, C.; Noll, M.; Klein, R.S.; Noguchi, K.K.; et al. Zika Virus Infection during Pregnancy in Mice Causes Placental Damage and Fetal Demise. *Cell* **2016**, *165*, 1081–1091. [CrossRef] [PubMed]

14. Wu, K.Y.; Zuo, G.L.; Li, X.F.; Ye, Q.; Deng, Y.Q.; Huang, X.Y.; Cao, W.C.; Qin, C.F.; Luo, Z.G. Vertical transmission of Zika virus targeting the radial glial cells affects cortex development of offspring mice. *Cell Res.* **2016**, *26*, 645–654. [CrossRef] [PubMed]

15. Li, H.; Saucedo-Cuevas, L.; Regla-Nava, J.A.; Chai, G.; Sheets, N.; Tang, W.; Terskikh, A.V.; Shresta, S.; Gleeson, J.G. Zika Virus Infects Neural Progenitors in the Adult Mouse Brain and Alters Proliferation. *Cell Stem Cell* **2016**, *19*, 593–598. [CrossRef] [PubMed]

16. Hanners, N.W.; Eitson, J.L.; Usui, N.; Richardson, R.B.; Wexler, E.M.; Konopka, G.; Schoggins, J.W. Western Zika Virus in Human Fetal Neural Progenitors Persists Long Term with Partial Cytopathic and Limited Immunogenic Effects. *Cell Rep.* **2016**, *15*, 2315–2322. [CrossRef] [PubMed]

17. Tang, H.; Hammack, C.; Ogden, S.C.; Wen, Z.; Qian, X.; Li, Y.; Yao, B.; Shin, J.; Zhang, F.; Lee, E.M.; et al. Zika Virus Infects Human Cortical Neural Progenitors and Attenuates Their Growth. *Cell Stem Cell* **2016**, *18*, 587–590. [CrossRef] [PubMed]

18. Dang, J.; Tiwari, S.K.; Lichinchi, G.; Qin, Y.; Patil, V.S.; Eroshkin, A.M.; Rana, T.M. Zika Virus Depletes Neural Progenitors in Human Cerebral Organoids through Activation of the Innate Immune Receptor TLR3. *Cell Stem Cell* **2016**, *19*, 258–265. [CrossRef] [PubMed]

19. Onorati, M.; Li, Z.; Liu, F.; Sousa, A.M.; Nakagawa, N.; Li, M.; Dell'Anno, M.T.; Gulden, F.O.; Pochareddy, S.; Tebbenkamp, A.T.; et al. Zika Virus Disrupts Phospho-TBK1 Localization and Mitosis in Human Neuroepithelial Stem Cells and Radial Glia. *Cell Rep.* **2016**, *16*, 2576–2592. [CrossRef] [PubMed]

20. Ghouzzi, V.E.; Bianchi, F.T.; Molineris, I.; Mounce, B.C.; Berto, G.E.; Rak, M.; Lebon, S.; Aubry, L.; Tocco, C.; Gai, M.; et al. ZIKA virus elicits P53 activation and genotoxic stress in human neural progenitors similar to mutations involved in severe forms of genetic microcephaly and p53. *Cell Death Dis.* **2016**, *7*, e2440. [CrossRef] [PubMed]

21. Rosenfeld, A.B.; Doobin, D.J.; Warren, A.L.; Racaniello, V.R.; Vallee, R.B. Replication of early and recent Zika virus isolates throughout mouse brain development. *Proc. Natl. Acad. Sci. USA* **2017**, *114*, 12273–12278. [CrossRef] [PubMed]

22. Barkovich, A.J.; Guerrini, R.; Kuzniecky, R.I.; Jackson, G.D.; Dobyns, W.B. A developmental and genetic classification for malformations of cortical development: Update 2012. *Brain* **2012**, *135*, 1348–1369. [CrossRef] [PubMed]

23. Oh, Y.; Zhang, F.; Wang, Y.; Lee, E.M.; Choi, I.Y.; Lim, H.; Mirakhori, F.; Li, R.; Huang, L.; Xu, T.; et al. Zika virus directly infects peripheral neurons and induces cell death. *Nat. Neurosci.* **2017**, *20*, 1209–1212. [CrossRef] [PubMed]

24. Cumberworth, S.L.; Barrie, J.A.; Cunningham, M.E.; de Figueiredo, D.P.G.; Schultz, V.; Wilder-Smith, A.J.; Brennan, B.; Pena, L.J.; Freitas de Oliveira Franca, R.; Linington, C.; et al. Zika virus tropism and interactions in myelinating neural cell cultures: CNS cells and myelin are preferentially affected. *Acta Neuropathol. Commun.* **2017**, *5*, 50. [CrossRef] [PubMed]

25. Shao, Q.; Herrlinger, S.; Zhu, Y.N.; Yang, M.; Goodfellow, F.; Stice, S.L.; Qi, X.P.; Brindley, M.A.; Chen, J.F. The African Zika virus MR-766 is more virulent and causes more severe brain damage than current Asian lineage and dengue virus. *Development* **2017**, *144*, 4114–4124. [CrossRef] [PubMed]

26. Gokoffski, K.K.; Wu, H.H.; Beites, C.L.; Kim, J.; Kim, E.J.; Matzuk, M.M.; Johnson, J.E.; Lander, A.D.; Calof, A.L. Activin and GDF11 collaborate in feedback control of neuroepithelial stem cell proliferation and fate. *Development* **2011**, *138*, 4131–4142. [CrossRef] [PubMed]

27. Dhara, S.K.; Stice, S.L. Neural differentiation of human embryonic stem cells. *J. Cell Biochem.* **2008**, *105*, 633–640. [CrossRef] [PubMed]

28. Wu, X.; Majumder, A.; Webb, R.; Stice, S.L. High content imaging quantification of multiple in vitro human neurogenesis events after neurotoxin exposure. *BMC Pharmacol. Toxicol.* **2016**, *17*, 62. [CrossRef] [PubMed]

29. Shin, S.; Mitalipova, M.; Noggle, S.; Tibbitts, D.; Venable, A.; Rao, R.; Stice, S.L. Long-term proliferation of human embryonic stem cell-derived neuroepithelial cells using defined adherent culture conditions. *Stem Cells* **2006**, *24*, 125–138. [CrossRef] [PubMed]

30. Willard, K.A.; Demakovsky, L.; Tesla, B.; Goodfellow, F.T.; Stice, S.L.; Murdock, C.C.; Brindley, M.A. Zika Virus Exhibits Lineage-Specific Phenotypes in Cell Culture, in Aedes aegypti Mosquitoes, and in an Embryo Model. *Viruses* **2017**, *9*. [CrossRef] [PubMed]

31. Doherty, P.; Williams, G.; Williams, E.J. CAMs and axonal growth: A critical evaluation of the role of calcium and the MAPK cascade. *Mol. Cell Neurosci.* **2000**, *16*, 283–295. [CrossRef] [PubMed]

32. Goodfellow, F.T.; Simchick, G.A.; Mortensen, L.J.; Stice, S.L.; Zhao, Q. Tracking and Quantification of Magnetically Labeled Stem Cells Using Magnetic Resonance Imaging. *Adv. Funct. Mater.* **2016**, *26*, 3899–3915. [CrossRef] [PubMed]

33. R Stats Program. Available online: https://www.R-project.org/ (accessed on 7 November 2015).

34. Young, A.; Machacek, D.W.; Dhara, S.K.; Macleish, P.R.; Benveniste, M.; Dodla, M.C.; Sturkie, C.D.; Stice, S.L. Ion channels and ionotropic receptors in human embryonic stem cell derived neural progenitors. *Neuroscience* **2011**, *192*, 793–805. [CrossRef] [PubMed]

35. Haddow, A.D.; Schuh, A.J.; Yasuda, C.Y.; Kasper, M.R.; Heang, V.; Huy, R.; Guzman, H.; Tesh, R.B.; Weaver, S.C. Genetic characterization of Zika virus strains: geographic expansion of the Asian lineage. *PLoS Negl. Trop. Dis.* **2012**, *6*, e1477. [CrossRef] [PubMed]

36. Young, A.; Assey, K.S.; Sturkie, C.D.; West, F.D.; Machacek, D.W.; Stice, S.L. Glial cell line-derived neurotrophic factor enhances in vitro differentiation of mid-/hindbrain neural progenitor cells to dopaminergic-like neurons. *J. Neurosci. Res.* **2010**, *88*, 3222–3232. [CrossRef] [PubMed]

37. Gabriel, E.; Ramani, A.; Karow, U.; Gottardo, M.; Natarajan, K.; Gooi, L.M.; Goranci-Buzhala, G.; Krut, O.; Peters, F.; Nikolic, M.; et al. Recent Zika Virus Isolates Induce Premature Differentiation of Neural Progenitors in Human Brain Organoids. *Cell Stem Cell* **2017**, *20*, 397–406. [CrossRef] [PubMed]

38. Simonin, Y.; Loustalot, F.; Desmetz, C.; Foulongne, V.; Constant, O.; Fournier-Wirth, C.; Leon, F.; Moles, J.P.; Goubaud, A.; Lemaitre, J.M.; et al. Zika Virus Strains Potentially Display Different Infectious Profiles in Human Neural Cells. *EBioMedicine* **2016**, *12*, 161–169. [CrossRef] [PubMed]
39. Harrill, J.A.; Freudenrich, T.M.; Machacek, D.W.; Stice, S.L.; Mundy, W.R. Quantitative assessment of neurite outgrowth in human embryonic stem cell-derived hN2 cells using automated high-content image analysis. *Neurotoxicology* **2010**, *31*, 277–290. [CrossRef] [PubMed]
40. Wu, X.; Yang, X.; Majumder, A.; Swetenburg, R.; Goodfellow, F.; Bartlett, M.G.; Stice, S.L. Astrocytes are protective against chlorpyrifos developmental neurotoxicity in human pluripotent stem cell derived astrocyte-neuron co-cultures. *Toxicol. Sci.* **2017**. [CrossRef] [PubMed]
41. McGrath, E.L.; Rossi, S.L.; Gao, J.; Widen, S.G.; Grant, A.C.; Dunn, T.J.; Azar, S.R.; Roundy, C.M.; Xiong, Y.; Prusak, D.J.; et al. Differential Responses of Human Fetal Brain Neural Stem Cells to Zika Virus Infection. *Stem Cell Rep.* **2017**, *8*, 715–727. [CrossRef] [PubMed]
42. Emeny, J.M.; Morgan, M.J. Regulation of the interferon system: Evidence that Vero cells have a genetic defect in interferon production. *J. Gen. Virol.* **1979**, *43*, 247–252. [CrossRef] [PubMed]
43. Osada, N.; Kohara, A.; Yamaji, T.; Hirayama, N.; Kasai, F.; Sekizuka, T.; Kuroda, M.; Hanada, K. The genome landscape of the african green monkey kidney-derived vero cell line. *DNA Res.* **2014**, *21*, 673–683. [CrossRef] [PubMed]
44. Ming, G.L.; Tang, H.; Song, H. Advances in Zika Virus Research: Stem Cell Models, Challenges, and Opportunities. *Cell Stem Cell* **2016**, *19*, 690–702. [CrossRef] [PubMed]
45. Grant, A.; Ponia, S.S.; Tripathi, S.; Balasubramaniam, V.; Miorin, L.; Sourisseau, M.; Schwarz, M.C.; Sanchez-Seco, M.P.; Evans, M.J.; Best, S.M.; et al. Zika Virus Targets Human STAT2 to Inhibit Type I Interferon Signaling. *Cell Host Microbe* **2016**, *19*, 882–890. [CrossRef] [PubMed]
46. Ho, C.Y.; Ames, H.M.; Tipton, A.; Vezina, G.; Liu, J.S.; Scafidi, J.; Torii, M.; Rodriguez, F.J.; du Plessis, A.; DeBiasi, R.L. Differential neuronal susceptibility and apoptosis in congenital Zika virus infection. *Ann. Neurol.* **2017**, *82*, 121–127. [CrossRef] [PubMed]
47. Ivanov, V.N.; Hei, T.K. A role for TRAIL/TRAIL-R2 in radiation-induced apoptosis and radiation-induced bystander response of human neural stem cells. *Apoptosis* **2014**, *19*, 399–413. [CrossRef] [PubMed]
48. Bhatnagar, J.; Rabeneck, D.B.; Martines, R.B.; Reagan-Steiner, S.; Ermias, Y.; Estetter, L.B.; Suzuki, T.; Ritter, J.; Keating, M.K.; Hale, G.; et al. Zika Virus RNA Replication and Persistence in Brain and Placental Tissue. *Emerg. Infect. Dis.* **2017**, *23*. [CrossRef] [PubMed]
49. Yi, L.; Pimentel, H.; Pachter, L. Zika infection of neural progenitor cells perturbs transcription in neurodevelopmental pathways. *PLoS ONE* **2017**, *12*, e0175744. [CrossRef] [PubMed]
50. Chimelli, L.; Melo, A.S.O.; Avvad-Portari, E.; Wiley, C.A.; Camacho, A.H.S.; Lopes, V.S.; Machado, H.N.; Andrade, C.V.; Dock, D.C.A.; Moreira, M.E.; et al. The spectrum of neuropathological changes associated with congenital Zika virus infection. *Acta Neuropathol.* **2017**, *133*, 983–999. [CrossRef] [PubMed]
51. Bertipaglia, C.; Goncalves, J.C.; Vallee, R.B. Nuclear migration in mammalian brain development. *Semin. Cell Dev. Biol.* **2017**. [CrossRef] [PubMed]
52. Huang, W.C.; Abraham, R.; Shim, B.S.; Choe, H.; Page, D.T. Zika virus infection during the period of maximal brain growth causes microcephaly and corticospinal neuron apoptosis in wild type mice. *Sci. Rep.* **2016**, *6*, 34793. [CrossRef] [PubMed]
53. Bizzotto, S.; Francis, F. Morphological and functional aspects of progenitors perturbed in cortical malformations. *Front. Cell Neurosci.* **2015**, *9*, 30. [CrossRef] [PubMed]
54. Harrill, J.A.; Chen, H.; Streifel, K.M.; Yang, D.; Mundy, W.R.; Lein, P.J. Ontogeny of biochemical, morphological and functional parameters of synaptogenesis in primary cultures of rat hippocampal and cortical neurons. *Mol. Brain.* **2015**, *8*, 10. [CrossRef] [PubMed]
55. Gomme, E.A.; Wirblich, C.; Addya, S.; Rall, G.F.; Schnell, M.J. Immune clearance of attenuated rabies virus results in neuronal survival with altered gene expression. *PLoS Pathog.* **2012**, *8*, e1002971. [CrossRef] [PubMed]

56. Panchaud, A.; Stojanov, M.; Ammerdorffer, A.; Vouga, M.; Baud, D. Emerging Role of Zika Virus in Adverse Fetal and Neonatal Outcomes. *Clin. Microbiol. Rev.* **2016**, *29*, 659–694. [CrossRef] [PubMed]
57. Liu, J.S.; Schubert, C.R.; Walsh, C.A. Rare genetic causes of lissencephaly may implicate microtubule-based transport in the pathogenesis of cortical dysplasias. In *Jasper's Basic Mechanisms of the Epilepsies*, 4th ed.; Noebels, J.L., Avoli, M., Eds.; National Center for Biotechnology Information (US): Bethesda, MD, USA, 2012.

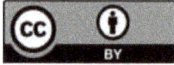

![viruses logo] *viruses*

MDPI

Article

An Alanine-to-Valine Substitution in the Residue 175 of Zika Virus NS2A Protein Affects Viral RNA Synthesis and Attenuates the Virus In Vivo

Silvia Márquez-Jurado [1],[†] , Aitor Nogales [2],[†], Ginés Ávila-Pérez [2], Francisco J. Iborra [1], Luis Martínez-Sobrido [2],* and Fernando Almazán [1],*

1   Department of Molecular and Cell Biology, Centro Nacional de Biotecnología (CNB-CSIC), Campus Universidad Autónoma de Madrid, 3 Darwin street, 28049 Madrid, Spain; smarquez@cnb.csic.es (S.M.-J.); fjiborra@cnb.csic.es (F.J.I.)
2   Department of Microbiology and Immunology, University of Rochester Medical Center, 601 Elmwood Avenue, Rochester, NY 14642, USA; aitor_nogales@urmc.rochester.edu (A.N.); Gines_Perez@urmc.rochester.edu (G.Á.P.)
*   Correspondence: luis_martinez@urmc.rochester.edu (L.M.-S.); falmazan@cnb.csic.es (F.A.); Tel.: +1-585-276-4733 (L.M.-S.); +34-91-585-4561 (F.A.)
†   These authors contributed equally to this work.

Received: 12 September 2018; Accepted: 4 October 2018; Published: 7 October 2018

Abstract: The recent outbreaks of Zika virus (ZIKV), its association with Guillain–Barré syndrome and fetal abnormalities, and the lack of approved vaccines and antivirals, highlight the importance of developing countermeasures to combat ZIKV disease. In this respect, infectious clones constitute excellent tools to accomplish these goals. However, flavivirus infectious clones are often difficult to work with due to the toxicity of some flavivirus sequences in bacteria. To bypass this problem, several alternative approaches have been applied for the generation of ZIKV clones including, among others, in vitro ligation, insertions of introns and using infectious subgenomic amplicons. Here, we report a simple and novel DNA-launched approach based on the use of a bacterial artificial chromosome (BAC) to generate a cDNA clone of Rio Grande do Norte Natal ZIKV strain. The sequence was identified from the brain tissue of an aborted fetus with microcephaly. The BAC clone was fully stable in bacteria and the infectious virus was efficiently recovered in Vero cells through direct delivery of the cDNA clone. The rescued virus yielded high titers in Vero cells and was pathogenic in a validated mouse model (A129 mice) of ZIKV infection. Furthermore, using this infectious clone we have generated a mutant ZIKV containing a single amino acid substitution (A175V) in the NS2A protein that presented reduced viral RNA synthesis in cell cultures, was highly attenuated in vivo and induced fully protection against a lethal challenge with ZIKV wild-type. This BAC approach provides a stable and reliable reverse genetic system for ZIKV that will help to identify viral determinants of virulence and facilitate the development of vaccine and therapeutic strategies.

Keywords: Zika virus; Full-length cDNA infectious clones; Bacterial artificial chromosome; NS2A protein

---

1. Introduction

Zika virus (ZIKV) is a recently emerged mosquito-borne member of the family *Flaviviridae*, which was declared by the Word Health Organization (WHO) as a global public health emergency on February 2016 [1,2]. Like other flaviviruses, the viral particle is constituted by an inner nucleocapsid composed of the capsid (C) protein associated with the viral genomic RNA (gRNA), surrounded by a lipid bilayer that contains the structural membrane (M) and envelope (E) proteins, which are arranged with icosahedral symmetry on the surface [3]. The viral genome consists in a positive single-stranded RNA molecule of about 10.8 kb that, similarly to cellular mRNAs, contains a cap structure at the 5′ end and a single open reading frame (ORF) flanked by 5′ and 3′ untranslated regions (UTRs). The ORF encodes a large polyprotein of approximately 3423 amino acids, which is co- and post-translationally processed by viral and cellular proteases into three structural proteins (C, pre-membrane (prM) and E) and seven non-structural (NS) proteins (NS1, NS2A, NS2B, NS3, NS4A, NS4B and NS5). The structural proteins are essential components of the virion and are involved in viral entry, fusion, and assembly. The NS proteins are required for viral RNA synthesis, virion assembly and evasion of the host antiviral responses [4,5].

Human illness caused by ZIKV infection was first recognized in Nigeria in 1953 [6] and only a few cases of ZIKV infections across Africa and Asia were reported over 50 years. Historically, ZIKV was considered as a modest public health concern, causing a mild febrile illness with similar symptoms to those of dengue (DENV) and chikungunya (CHIKV) viruses, hampering differential diagnosis [7]. In general, over 80% of ZIKV cases are asymptomatic, while the remaining cases typically exhibit mild fever, maculopapular rash, and joint pain for a period of several days to a week [8]. However, the recent large outbreaks in the Island of Yap in 2007 [9], French Polynesia in 2013 [10], and the massive epidemic that emerge from Brazil in 2015 to rapidly spread throughout South and Central America, the Caribbean, and more recently the United States [1,11–13], have changed the historic perspective of ZIKV infection due its association with Guillain–Barré syndrome (a debilitating neuronal disease in adults) and severe congenital abnormalities such us stillbirth, hydrocephaly and microcephaly, which are collectively known as congenital ZIKV syndrome (CZVS) [14–19]. Human health concerns posed by ZIKV are further aggravated due to the non-vector-borne transmission of ZIKV. The virus is spread to people primarily through the bite of infected mosquitoes of the genus *Aedes* [20,21], however, at difference to most other flaviviruses, ZIKV can also be transmitted from mother to child during pregnancy or spread through sexual contact, breastfeeding, blood transfusion, and non-human primate bites [1,22,23]. Due to the recent emergence of ZIKV as an important human pathogen, there are not currently approved vaccines or antivirals available to combat ZIKV infection. The only available disease prevention measures consist in protection from mosquito bites, excluding pregnant females from travelling to ZIKV-endemic areas, and practicing safe sex.

The significance of ZIKV in human health, together with the lack of prophylactic and therapeutic interventions to combat ZIKV infection, highlight the importance of developing safe and effective countermeasures to control or prevent ZIKV disease in humans. In this sense, the development of ZIKV reverse genetic systems constitute an essential tool for basic research and development of vaccine and antiviral strategies. Likewise other flaviviruses, construction of ZIKV infectious clones has been hampered due to the toxicity of some flavivirus sequences during its propagation in bacteria using standard high copy number plasmids, which can be attributed to the leaky expression of toxic viral proteins from cryptic bacterial promoters (CBPs) encoded in the viral genome [24–26]. Recently, this toxicity problem was overcome using non-traditional approaches based on in vitro ligation of cDNA fragments [27,28], low-copy plasmids [29,30], intron insertion in the toxic region [31–33], Gibson assembly method [34], infectious subgenomic amplicons (ISA) [35,36], in silico prediction and mutational silencing of CBPs present in the viral genome [37], and the use of circular polymerase extension reaction (CPER) [38]. All these systems are valuable tools to study viral pathogenesis, vector transmission and for the development of attenuated forms of ZIKV for their implementation as safe vaccines or for the identification of therapeutics.

In the present study, we report a different and efficient ZIKV reverse genetic approach, based on the use of a bacterial artificial chromosome (BAC), that overcomes the toxicity problems and allows the generation of ZIKV cDNA clones on single bacterial plasmid. Following a similar strategy to that used for DENV [39], the full-length cDNA copy of the viral genome of ZIKV Rio Grande do Norte Natal (RGN) was assembled in a BAC under the control of the cytomegalovirus (CMV) immediate-early promoter. This DNA-launched system couples expression of the viral RNA in the

Viruses 2018, 10, 547

nucleus from the CMV promoter with a second amplification step in the cytoplasm driven by the viral polymerase. The recombinant virus rescued from the BAC clone was fully infectious in vitro and in vivo. The ZIKV-RGN infectious clone was further used to evaluate the effect of a single amino acid change (alanine to valine) at residue 175 of the NS2A protein on viral RNA synthesis and pathogenesis in vivo. We found that this unique single amino acid substitution impairs viral RNA synthesis in cell culture and results in viral attenuation in A129 mice. Remarkably, a single dose of the mutant virus was sufficient to induce protection against challenge with the parental wild-type (WT) ZIKV. These results demonstrate the reliability and potential of our BAC approach to study ZIKV biology and to facilitate the development of vaccine and antiviral strategies.

2. Materials and Methods

2.1. Cell Culture and Virus Infection

Vero (a kidney epithelial cell line from an African green monkey) and A549 (an human adenocarcinomic alveolar epithelial cell line) cells were purchased from the American Type Culture Collection (ATCC, CCL-81) and were grown and maintained at 37 °C and 5% CO_2 in growth medium, consisting in Dulbecco's modified Eagle's medium (DMEM) supplemented with 5% fetal bovine serum (FBS) (HyClone, ThermoFisher Scientific, Madrid, Spain), 2 mM L-glutamine (Sigma-Aldrich, Madrid, Spain), 1% nonessential amino acids (Sigma-Aldrich), 100 U/mL penicillin (Sigma-Aldrich) and 100 µg/mL streptomycin (Sigma-Aldrich).

The recombinant ZIKV-RGN WT (rZIKV-RGN) or NS2A mutant (rZIKV-RGN-mNS2A) viruses were propagated in Vero cells with virus growth medium (DMEM supplemented with 2% FBS, 2 mM L-glutamine, 1% nonessential amino acids, 100 U/mL penicillin and 100 µg/mL streptomycin) at 37 °C and 5% CO_2. For virus stocks preparation, 80 to 90% confluent monolayers of Vero cells were infected with a multiplicity of infection (MOI) of 0.1 plaque forming units (PFU) per cell in virus growth medium and incubated at 37 °C under 5% CO_2. After 3–4 days of infection, the tissue culture supernatants were collected, clarified by centrifugation at 6000× g for 5 min, and stored in small aliquots at −80 °C.

2.2. Plasmids and Bacteria Strains

The BAC plasmid pBeloBAC11 [40], kindly provided by H. Shizuya (California Institute of Technology, Pasadena, CA, USA), was used to assemble the ZIKV-RGN infectious cDNA clone. This plasmid is a synthetic low-copy-number plasmid (one copy per cell) based on the Escherichia coli (E. coli) F-factor [41] that minimize the toxicity problems in the bacteria of exogenous sequences. E. coli DH10B cells (Invitrogen, ThermoFisher Scientific) were used to amplify the BAC plasmids. Electrocompetent DH10B cells (Invitrogen, ThermoFisher Scientific) were transformed by electroporation using a MicroPulser unit (Bio-Rad, Madrid, Spain), according to the manufacturer's instructions. BAC-based plasmids were isolated and purified using the Large-Construct kit (Qiagen, Hilden, Germany), following the manufacturer's specifications.

2.3. Construction of ZIKV-RGN Infectious cDNA Clone

We have assembled a ZIKV infectious cDNA clone in the BAC plasmid pBeloBAC11, based on the data of the full-length sequence of the ZIKV clinical strain RGN [19] deposited in the GenBanK (accession number KU527068). This strain was selected because the full-length sequence was obtained directly from the virus-infected brain tissue of an aborted fetus with microcephaly in Brazil in 2015 and therefore represents a good candidate to study ZIKV pathogenesis. The first step for the assembly of the full-length cDNA clone was the selection of the restriction sites PmlI, AfeI, and BstBI (genomic positions 3347, 5969 and 9127, respectively), which are unique in the viral genome (Figure 1A). After that, four overlapping DNA fragments covering the entire viral genome (ZIKV 1 to ZIKV 4) and flanked by the appropriate restriction sites, were generated by chemical synthesis (Bio Basic,

321

Inc., Toronto, Canada) (Figure 1B). ZIKV 1 fragment contained the CMV promoter precisely fused to the first 3350 nucleotides of the viral genome flanked at the 5′-end by ApaLI and AscI (absent in the viral genome) sites and at the 3′-end by a multiple-cloning site containing the selected restriction sites (PmlI, AfeI and BstBI) followed by MluI (absent in the viral genome) and BamHI. Fragments ZIKV 2 (flanked by PmlI and AfeI) and ZIKV 3 (flanked by AfeI and BstBI) covered the genomic regions 3346–5972 and 5967–9131, respectively. ZIKV 4 fragment contained the restriction site BstBI, the last 1683 nucleotides of the viral genome, the hepatitis delta virus (HDV) ribozyme, the bovine growth hormone (BGH) termination and polyadenylation sequences, and the MluI restriction site. The infectious clone was assembled into pBeloBAC11 by sequential cloning of these four overlapping DNA fragments. Briefly, fragment ZIKV 1 was digested with ApaLI and BamHI and cloned into pBeloBAC11^{-AfeI} (a pBeloBAC11 without the AfeI restriction site) digested with the same enzymes, to generate the intermediate plasmid pBAC-ZIKV1. Then, this plasmid was used as the backbone for the sequential cloning of the remaining overlapping DNA fragments (ZIKV 2 to ZIKV 4) into the multicloning site of the intermediate plasmid (contains the restriction sites selected, PmlI, AfeI, BstBI and MluI) to generate the full-length cDNA clone pBAC-ZIKV-RGN (Figure 1B). The genetic integrity of the cDNA clone was verified throughout the assembly process by extensive restriction analysis and sequencing. In all cases, the bacterial strain DH10B (Invitrogen, ThermoFisher Scientific) was used as the *E. coli* host for all the cloning steps and the propagation of the BAC cDNA clone.

2.4. Recovery of Infectious Virus from the BAC cDNA Clones

To recover the infectious virus, Vero cells on 6-well plates were grown to 90% confluence in growth medium without antibiotics, and transfected with 4 µg of the BAC cDNA clone using 12 µL of Lipofectamine 2000 (Invitrogen, ThermoFisher Scientific), following the manufacturer's specifications. After 6 h of incubation at 37 °C, the transfection medium was replaced with fresh growth medium and the cells incubated at 37 °C. Aliquots of the culture supernatants were collected at 24 h intervals for virus titer determination by plaque assay on Vero cells. After five to seven days of transfection, when the cytopathic effect (CPE) was clear, cell culture supernatants were harvested and the recovered virus was cloned by three rounds of plaque purification.

2.5. Sequencing of Viral RNA

To determine the complete genome sequence of the rescued viruses, virions from supernatant of infected Vero cells (MOI of 0.01 PFU/cell) were purified through a 20% (w/v) sucrose cushion. Viral RNA was isolate from the purified virus with the QIAamp viral RNA minikit (Qiagen) following the manufacturer's instructions and deep-sequenced at the University of Rochester Genomics Research Center using Illumina MiSeq (Illumina, San Diego, CA, USA). Briefly, 0.5 µg of total viral RNA was fragmented by controlled sonication and a DNA library was generated using the NEBNext mRNA library prep master mix set for Illumina (New England Biolabs, Ipswich, MA, USA), according to the manufacturer's instructions. After analyzing the library for size and quality (Bio-Analyzer; Agilent Technologies, Inc., Santa Clara, CA, USA), deep-sequencing was performed using MiSeq (Illumina) and the raw sequencing reads analyzed using SWARM custom software. The genomic 5′- and 3′-terminal sequences were determined by the rapid amplification of cDNA ends (RACE) using the 5′/3′ RACE second generation kit (Roche, Basilea, Switzerland) with a polyA-tail added to the cDNA prior to the 3′ RACE reaction using polyA polymerase (New England Biolabs), following the manufacturer's instructions.

To analyze the genetic stability of the recombinant ZIKV harboring the point mutation A175V in the coding region of the NS2A protein (rZIKV-RGN-mNS2A), total RNA was purified from Vero cells infected with viruses from passage 1 (P1) to passage 5 (P5) using the RNeasy minikit (Qiagen), according to the manufacturer's specifications. Purified RNA (600 ng) was reverse transcribed (RT) with random hexamer primers using the High-Capacity cDNA Transcription kit (Life Technologies, ThermoFisher Scientific), and the cDNA was amplified by PCR with the forward primer ZIKV-3414VS

(5′-GAGGAATGGTGCTGCAGG-3′), spanning nucleotides 3414 to 3431 of the viral genome, and the reverse primer ZIKV-4817RS (5′-GCTTGACATCTCCCCAG-3′), complementary to nucleotides 4817 to 4833 of the viral genome. Finally, the amplicons generated covering the region encoding NS2A and NS2B proteins (genomic region 3414–4833) were sequenced by Sanger sequencing (Macrogen Europe, Amsterdam, Netherlands) using specific oligonucleotides.

2.6. Virus Titrations

Vero cells seeded into 12-well plates at 80–90% of confluence were infected with 150 µL of serial 10-fold dilutions of the virus in virus growth medium without FBS for 1 h at 37 °C. After viral absorption, the viral inoculum was removed and the cells overlaid with 2 mL of virus growth medium containing 1% DEAE-Dextran (Sigma-Aldrich) and 0.6% Agar Noble (Difco, ThermoFisher Scientific). After 3–4 days of incubation at 37 °C under 5% CO_2, the cells were fixed with 4% formaldehyde for 1 h at room temperature, the overlaid removed, and the viral plaques visualized by staining with 0.1% crystal violet in 20% methanol or by immunostaining with 1 µg/mL of the pan-flavivirus E protein monoclonal antibody (mAb) 4G2 (BEI Resources; NR-50327) using the Vectastain ABC kit (Vector Laboratories Inc., Burlingame, CA, USA). Visible plaques were counted and virus titers were calculated as PFU/mL.

2.7. Virus Growth Kinetics

Vero and A549 cells seeded into 24-well plates at 90% of confluence were infected with the indicated viruses diluted in virus growth medium without FBS at the specified MOIs. After 1 h of absorption at 37 °C in 5% CO_2, the virus inoculum was removed, the cell monolayers washed twice with PBS, and 0.5 mL of fresh virus growth medium was added to each well. Cells were incubated at 37 °C under 5% CO_2 and at selected time points, aliquots of tissue culture supernatants were collected and virus titers determined by plaque assay in Vero cells as described above.

2.8. Analysis of Viral RNA Synthesis

Viral RNA synthesis was evaluated by quantitative RT-PCR (RT-qPCR). Total intracellular RNA from uninfected or infected Vero cells was purified using the RNeasy minikit (Qiagen) and total cDNA was synthetized from 100 ng of purified RNA using random hexamer primers and the High-Capacity cDNA Transcription kit (Life Technologies, ThermoFisher Scientific), following the manufacturer's specifications. Using this cDNA, the level of viral RNA was further quantified by qPCR using a custom TaqMan assay specific for ZIKV-RGN RNA. This TaqMan assay is constituted by the forward primer 5′-GAAGAGCATCCAGCCAGAGAA-3′ (spanning nucleotides 1358 to 1378 of the viral genome), the reverse primer 5′-CTGGGAGCCATGAACTGACA-3′ (complementary to nucleotides 1399 to 1418 of the viral genome), and the probe 5′-FAM-TGGAGTACCGGATAATG-3IABKFQ-3′ (covering nucleotides 1381 to 1397 of the viral genome). To normalize for differences in RNA sampling, the expression of the histone H2B (reference housekeeping gene) was analyzed using a specific TaqMan gene expression assay (Rh04253068_s1; Life Technologies, ThermoFisher Scientific). Data were acquired with a 7500 real-time PCR system (Life Technologies, ThermoFisher Scientific) and analyzed with ABI PRISM 7500 software v2.0.6. The relative quantifications were performed using the cycle threshold ($2^{-\Delta\Delta CT}$) method [42]. All experiments and data analysis were MIQE (Minimum Information for Publication of Quantitative Real-Time PCR Experiments) compliant [43].

2.9. Indirect Immunofluorescence Assay

The expression of ZIKV E protein was analyzed by indirect immunofluorescence assay (IFA). Vero cells grown on coverslips in 24-well plates at 80–90% of confluence were infected with the rescued rZIKVs at the indicated MOIs. At selected time points post-infection, cells were fixed with 4% paraformaldehyde in 250 mM Hepes pH 7.4 during 20 min at room temperature and then permeabilized with 0.5% Triton X-100 in PBS for 10 min. After that, cells were treated for 1 h at room temperature with blocking solution (10% FBS in PBS) and incubated with 1 µg/mL of the pan-flavivirus E protein mAb 4G2 (BEI Resources; NR-50327) in blocking solution for 2 h at room temperature. After three washed with PBS, cells were incubated at room temperature for 1 h with donkey anti-mouse antibody conjugated to Alexa Fluor 488 (Invitrogen, ThermoFisher Scientific) diluted 1:500 in blocking solution, extensively washed with PBS, and incubated for 10 min with DAPI (4′,6′-diamidino-2-phenylindole) (Sigma-Aldrich) diluted 1:200 in PBS for nuclear staining. Finally, coverslips were mounted in ProLong Gold antifade reagent (Invitrogen, ThermoFisher Scientific) and analyzed on a Leica SP5 confocal microscope. Immunofluorescence acquired images were processed and analyzed with ImageJ 1.52b software [44].

2.10. Enzyme-Linked Immunosorbent Assay

For the evaluation of the virus-specific antibodies levels present in the sera of vaccinated mice, enzyme-linked immunosorbent assays (ELISAs) were performed as previously described [45]. Briefly, 96-well plates were coated with cell lysates from mock- or ZIKV-infected Vero cells and incubated overnight at 4 °C. The coated wells were washed with PBS, blocked with 1% BSA in PBS, and then incubated with two-fold dilutions (starting dilution of 1:50) of mice sera for 1 h at 37 °C. After that, plates were washed with water and incubated with HRP-conjugated goat anti-mouse IgG (1:2000; Southern Biotech, Birmingham, AL, USA) for 1 h at 37 °C. Reactions were developed with tetramethylbenzidine (TMB) substrate (BioLegend, San Diego, CA, USA) for 10 min at room temperature, quenched with 2 N H_2SO_4, and read at 450 nm in a Vmax Kinetic microplate reader (Molecular devices, San Jose, CA, USA).

2.11. Mice Experiments

The in vivo studies were performed in type-I interferon (IFN) receptor deficient (IFNR-/-) A129 mice (The Jackson Laboratory, Bar Harbor, ME, USA) maintained in the animal care facility at the University of Rochester under specific pathogen-free conditions. In this animal model, subcutaneous (s.c.) or intraperitoneal (i.p.) infection with ZIKV induces neurological disease and the animals succumb to viral infection, with high viral load in blood, brain, spin cord, and testes, consistent with manifestations of ZIKV infection in humans. Although deficient in innate IFN responses, A129 mice retain their adaptive immunity and have been successfully used as a suitable model for testing antivirals and vaccines [46–48].

To evaluate virus pathogenicity, female 4-to-6-week-old A129 mice ($n = 5$) were first anesthetized i.p. with a mixture of ketamine (100 µg per gram of body weight) and xylazine (20 µg per gram of body weight), and then mock-infected (PBS) or infected s.c. in the footpad with the indicated doses of rZIKV-RGN or rZIKV-RGN-mNS2A diluted in PBS in a final volume of 50 µL. After viral infection, animals were monitored daily for morbidity (body weight loss and disease signs, including hunching, ruffling and hind limb paralysis) and mortality (survival) over 14 days. Mice showing more than 20% of body weight loss or severe paralysis were considered to have reached the experimental endpoint and were humanely euthanized. To correlate development of clinical symptoms and death with virus replication, 4-to-6-week-old mice ($n = 6$) were infected as described above and the viral titers in serum were determined at days 2 ($n = 3$) and 4 ($n = 3$) by plaque assay and immunostaining using the pan-flavivirus E protein mAb 4G2 as indicated before.

To evaluate the protection efficacy of the rZIKV-RGN-mNS2A, female 4-to-6-week-old A129 mice ($n = 5$) were first anesthetized i.p. as indicated above, and then mock-immunized (PBS) or immunized s.c. in the footpad with 10^5 PFU of rZIKV-RGN-mNS2A diluted in PBS in a final volume of 50 µL. At 20 days post-immunization, mouse sera were collected by submandibular bleeding and the presence of total antibodies against ZIKV-RGN was evaluated by ELISA. Twenty-four hours after bleeding, mice were challenged s.c. in the footpad with 10^5 PFU of rZIKV-RGN and their morbidity and mortality monitored over 14 days as previously described. To determine viral replication, challenged 4-to-6-week-old A129 mice ($n = 6$) were bleeding at days 2 ($n = 3$) and 4 ($n = 3$) post-challenge and

ZIKV viremia was determined by plaque assay and immunostaining using the pan-flavivirus E protein mAb 4G2 as previously described.

2.12. Statistical Analysis

For quantitative analyses, a two-tailed, unpaired Student *t* test was used to analyze differences in mean values between groups. All results were expressed as mean ± standard deviations of the means. *P* values of <0.05 were considered significant. For mice experiments, the Meier Log-Rank test was used to compare survival data and the Reed and Muench method to determine the mouse lethal dose 50 (MLD_{50}). GraphPad Prism v7.0 software was used for all statistical analysis.

2.13. Ethics Statement

All animal protocols were approved by the University of Rochester Committee of Animal Resources (Protocol number: UCAR-2017-005/101851; approval date: 05/05/2017) and complied with the recommendations in the Guide for the Care and Use of Laboratory animals of the National Research Council [49].

3. Results

3.1. Development of a ZIKV-RGN Reverse Genetic System Using a BAC

To overcome the toxicity problems associated to several flavivirus sequences during its propagation in bacteria, we used the BAC plasmid pBeloBAC11 (a single-copy plasmid derived from the *E. coli* F-factor) [40] to assemble a ZIKV infectious cDNA clone, based on the genome sequence of the RGN strain of ZIKV (GenBank accession number KU527068) [19] (Figure 1). This ZIKV-RGN strain was selected because it has no laboratory passage history and the full-length genome sequence was obtained from a ZIKV-infected fetus with microcephaly in 2015 [19], constituting a good candidate to further study ZIKV pathogenesis.

After appropriate selection of unique restriction sites in the ZIKV-RGN genome (Figure 1A), four overlapping DNA fragments (ZIKV 1 to ZIKV 4), spanning the full-length viral genome and flanked for the selected restriction sites, were chemically synthesized, and sequentially cloned into pBeloBAC11 to generate the infectious cDNA clone pBAC-ZIKV-RGN (Figure 1B). Fragment ZIKV 1 contained the CMV immediate-early promoter to allow the expression of the viral RNA in the nucleus by the cellular RNA polymerase II [50] and fragment ZIKV 4 was flanked at the 3'-end by the HDV ribozyme followed by the BGH termination and polyadenylation sequences to produce synthetic RNAs bearing authentic 3'-ends of the viral genome. This DNA-lunched system ensures capping of the viral RNA and allows the recovery of infectious virus from the transfected cDNA clone without the need of an in vitro transcription step. Once assembled, the full-length sequence of the ZIKV-RGN BAC clone was determined and no changes were detected to that reported for the ZIKV-RGN strain (GenBank accession number KU527068). Finally, to confirm the stability of this synthetic infectious cDNA clone in bacteria, the BAC clone was passaged in *E. coli* DH10B cells for more than two hundred generations and the genetic integrity of the passaged infectious clone analyzed by restriction endonuclease analysis and sequencing. No differences were detected, demonstrating that the ZIKV-RGN BAC clone was fully stable in bacteria and that the BAC approach is a reliable and simple method to generate ZIKV infectious cDNA clones.

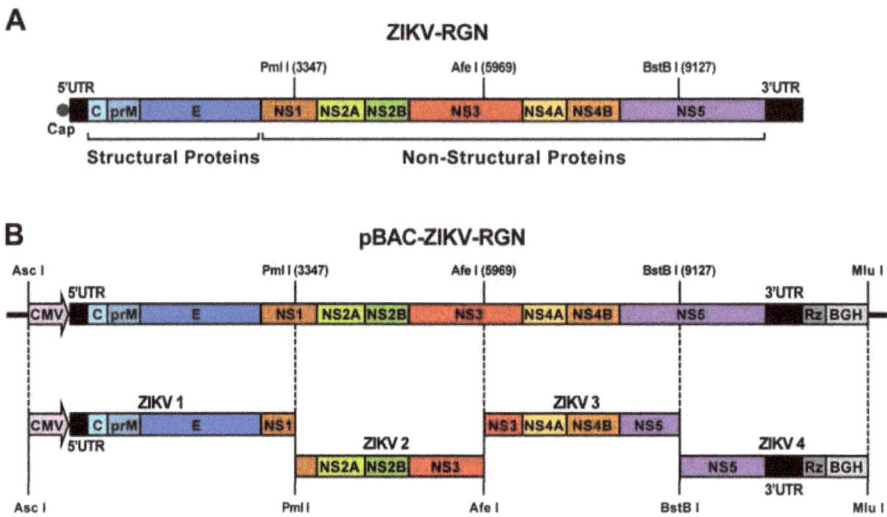

Figure 1. Assembly of a Zika Virus-Rio Grande do Norte Natal (ZIKV-RGN) infectious cDNA clone as a bacterial artificial chromosome (BAC). (**A**) Genetic structure of the ZIKV-RGN strain genome. The coding region from the structural (C, prM and E) and NS (NS1, NS2A, NS2B, NS3, NS4A, NS4B and NS5) proteins are illustrated by colored boxes. Relevant unique restriction sites in the viral genome used for the assembly of the infectious clone and their genomic positions (in brackets) are indicated. 5′ and 3′ UTR: 5′ and 3′ untranslated regions; cap: cap structure. (**B**) Strategy to assemble the ZIKV-RGN infectious cDNA clone. Four overlapping DNA fragments (ZIKV 1 to ZIKV 4, left to right), covering the entire viral genome and flanked by the indicated restriction sites, were generated by chemical synthesis and sequentially cloned into the BAC plasmid pBeloBAC11 to generate the infectious BAC clone pBAC-ZIKV-RGN. The full-length cDNA was assembled under the control of the cytomegalovirus (CMV) immediate-early promoter and flanked at the 3′-end by the hepatitis delta virus (HDV) ribozyme (Rz) followed by the bovine growth hormone (BGH) termination and polyadenylation sequences. Acronyms for coding regions and regulatory elements are as described in panel A.

3.2. Rescue and In Vitro Characterization of rZIKV-RGN

To recover the infectious virus (Figure 2), Vero cells were transiently transfected with the BAC cDNA clone using Lipofectamine 2000 and virus production analyzed during seven days. In contrast to mock-transfected cells, increasing amounts of infectious virus were detected in the tissue culture supernatant of cells transfected with the infectious clone, with peak titers around 10^7 PFU/mL on day five (Figure 2A). To further confirm the identity of the rescued virus, Vero cells were infected with an MOI of 0.5 PFU/cell of the rescue virus and monitored for CPE induction and viral E protein expression by IFA using the pan-flavivirus E protein mAb 4G2 (Figure 2B). The rescued virus induced a clear CPE, characterized by the presence of rounded and birefringent cells, and high levels of E protein expression were detected in the perinuclear region of infected cells. These results demonstrated that the ZIKV-RGN infectious BAC cDNA clone produces high titers of rZIKV-RGN directly after transfection of susceptible Vero cells.

Once the identity of the rescued virus was confirmed, it was cloned by three round of plaque purification, and its phenotypic and genotypic properties were determined. Analysis of the growth kinetics revealed that the rZIKV-RGN replicated efficiently in both Vero and A549 cells, reaching peak titers of approximately 10^7 and 10^6 PFU/mL at 48 hpi, respectively (Figure 3A). In addition, the rescued virus generated homogeneous plaques of about 2 mm in size after four days of infection in Vero cells (Figure 3B). Finally, the genetic identity of the virus was analyzed by deep-sequencing of two independent clones. Full-genome sequencing of both viral clones revealed that both clones presented the same sequence that the cDNA clone. Overall, these results demonstrate the feasibility of generating infectious rZIKVs using a BAC-based approach.

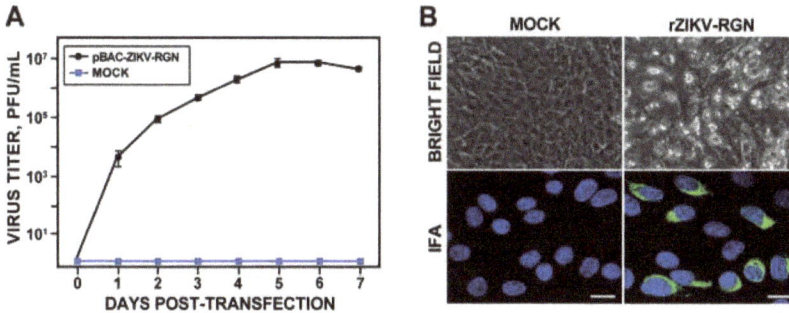

Figure 2. Recovery of infectious rZIKV-RGN from the BAC cDNA clone. (**A**) Virus rescue. Vero cells at 90% of confluence (6-well plate format; triplicates) were mock-transfected (Mock) or transfected with 4 μg/well of the ZIKV BAC cDNA clone (pBAC-ZIKV-RGN) and at the indicated times post-transfection, virus titers in the tissue culture supernatant of transfected cells were determined by plaque assay. Error bars represent standard deviations of the means from three experiments. (**B**) Analysis of the cytopathic effect (CPE) induction and ZIKV E protein expression. Vero cells were mock-infected (left) or infected (right) with 0.5 PFU/cell of the rescued virus (rZIKV-RGN) and at 48 h post-infection (hpi) analyzed for the induction of CPE by light microscopy (top) and for viral E protein expression by immunofluorescence assay (IFA) using the pan-flavivirus E protein mAb 4G2 (bottom). Bars, 20 μm.

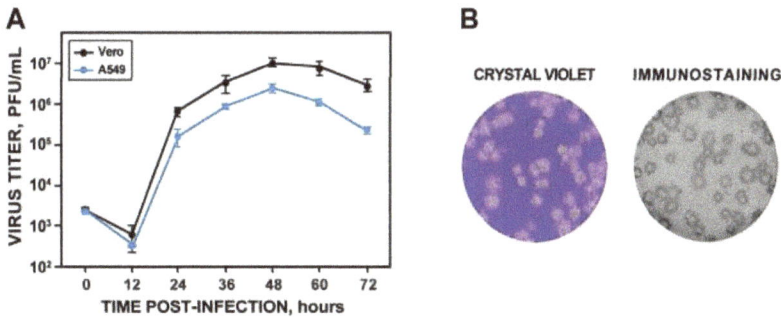

Figure 3. Viral growth kinetics and plaque phenotype of rZIKV-RGN. (**A**) Growth kinetics. Vero and A549 cells at 90% confluence (24-well plate format; triplicates) were infected at a multiplicity of infection (MOI) of 1 PFU/cell and at the indicated hpi, virus titers in the tissue culture supernatants were determined by plaque assay on Vero cells. Error bars represent standard deviations of the mean from three experiments. (**B**) Plaque morphology. Vero cells at 90% confluence (6-well plate format) were infected with 50 PFU of rZIKV-RGN and at four days post-infection viral plaques were visualized by staining with crystal violet (left) or immunostaining (right) using the pan-flavivirus E protein mAb 4G2.

3.3. Pathogenesis of rZIKV-RGN in Mice

To determine whether the rescued rZIKV-RGN was pathogenic in vivo (Figure 4), groups of five female 4-to-6-week-old A129 mice (IFNR-/-) were inoculated s.c. in the footpad with PBS (as negative control) or with different doses of rZIKV-RGN (10^3, 10^4 and 10^5 PFU per animal) and the morbidity (body weight loss and disease signs) and survival were monitored daily over 14 days (Figure 4A). As expected, weight loss and survival correlated with the inoculated dose. Mice infected with 10^3 PFU did not show disease symptoms, only a slight reduction in body weight was detected on days 8 to 12, and all of them survived. In the case of mice infected with 10^4 PFU, they presented some symptoms of disease (hunching and reduced mobility) and weight loss from days seven to nine (with a maximum of 10% on day nine), but all of them recovered the initial body weight and survived. In contrast, animals infected with 10^5 PFU showed hind limb paralysis, rapidly lost weight, and all of them succumbed to viral infection between days seven and eight post-infection (Figure 4A). Using the Reed & Muench method we determined that the MLD_{50} of rZIKV-RGN was approximately 5×10^4 PFU. To further analyze whether the virulence observed correlated with viral replication, viral titers in mouse sera were analyzed at days two and four post-infection (Figure 4B). As expected, the viremia in the infected animals was dose dependent, reaching the highest titers at day two after inoculation. At day four post-inoculation a significant reduction of the viral titers was observed. In the case of animals infected with 10^3 or 10^4 PFU, viremia was not detected or only detected in one of the three infected mice, respectively (Figure 4B). Overall, these results indicated that the rZIKV-RGN recovered from the infectious clone is virulent in mice but only at high (10^5 PFU) dose.

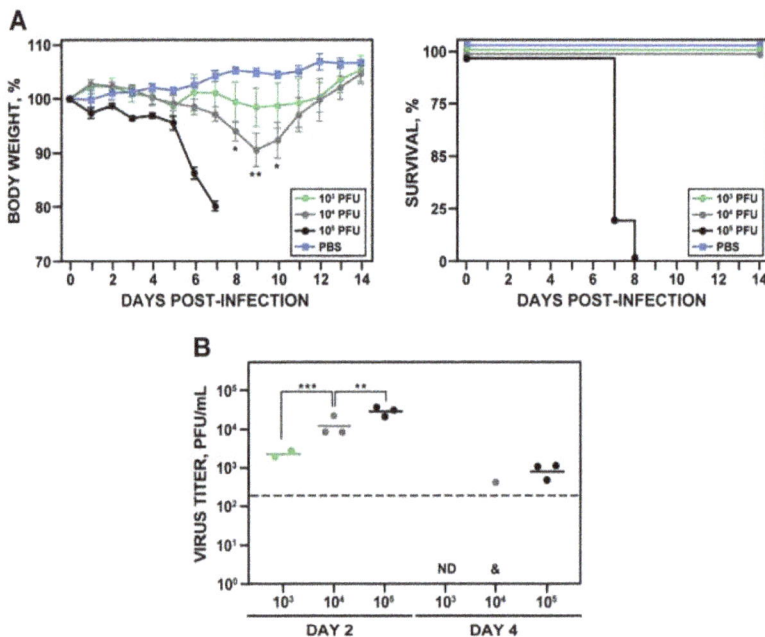

Figure 4. Pathogenesis of rZIKV-RGN in A129 mice. (**A**) Weight loss and mortality. Female 4-to-6-week-old A129 mice (five mice per group) were mock-infected (PBS) or infected s.c. in the footpad with the indicated PFU of rZIKV-RGN, and body weight loss (expressed as the percentage of starting weight, left panel) and survival (right panel) were monitored daily during 14 days. Mice that lost more than 20% of their initial body weight or presented hind limb paralysis were humanely euthanized. Error bars represent standard deviations of the mean for each group of mice. Asterisks indicate that the differences between viral doses of 10^3 and 10^4 are statistically significant when data are compared using the unpaired *t* test (*, $P < 0.05$; **, $P < 0.01$). (**B**) Viral titers in mice sera. Female 4-to-6-week-old A129 mice (six mice per group) were infected with the indicated PFU of rZIKV-RGN as described above, and viral titers in sera were determined at days two and four after infection (three animals per time point) by plaque assay and immunostaining using the pan-flavivirus E protein mAb 4G2. Symbols represent data from individual mice and bars the geometric means of viral titers. Asterisks indicate that the differences in viral titers between experimental samples are statistically significant when data are compared using the unpaired *t* test (**, $P < 0.01$; ***, $P < 0.001$). &: virus not detected in two mice; ND: virus not detected. The detection limit of the assay (200 PFU/mL) is indicate as a dashed line.

3.4. Rescue and In Vitro Charazterization of a rZIKV-RGN Harboring a Point Mutation in the NS2A Protein

During the assembly of the pBAC-ZIKV-RGN infectious clone, we detected the presence of a point mutation in the NS2A protein, which was introduced during the chemical synthesis of fragment ZIKV 2. This mutation consists in a cytosine-to-thymidine substitution at genomic position 4069, resulting in an alanine-to-valine change in the residue 175 of the NS2A protein (A175V). Because this mutation consists of a conservative amino acid change, we decided to explore the possibility of using this mutation as a genetic marker. To this end, the infectious clone pBAC-ZIKV-RGN-mNS2A was generated by replacing the ZIKV 2 WT fragment for that containing the NS2A A175V mutation. This infectious clone was fully stable in bacteria and no additional mutations were observed after sequencing the full-length clone. After that, Vero cells were transfected with the mutant infectious clone and the recovery efficiency of the rZIKV-RGN-mNS2A mutant virus was compared to that of the parental rZIKV-RGN virus (Figure 5). Although the infectious virus was recovered in both cases, virus production was one logarithm lower in the case of the mutant rZIKV-RGN-mNS2A, reaching maximum titers of 10^6 PFU/mL at seven days post-transfection (Figure 5A). When the plaque phenotype was analyzed, we found that the plaque size of the mutant rZIKV-RGN-mNS2A was smaller (more than a 5-fold reduction) than that of the parental rZIKV-RGN (Figure 5B), indicating that the A175V mutation, despite of being a conservative substitution, caused reduction in plaque size and virus production. In addition, an in silico analysis was performed to evaluate the frequency of amino acid residues 175 of the NS2A protein in more than 700 ZIKV strains sequences deposited in the database [51] (https://www.viprbrc.org/brc/home.spg?decorator=flavi). This analysis indicated that amino acid A175 is highly conserved, since the 100% of the analyzed ZIKV sequences contained an alanine residue at this position.

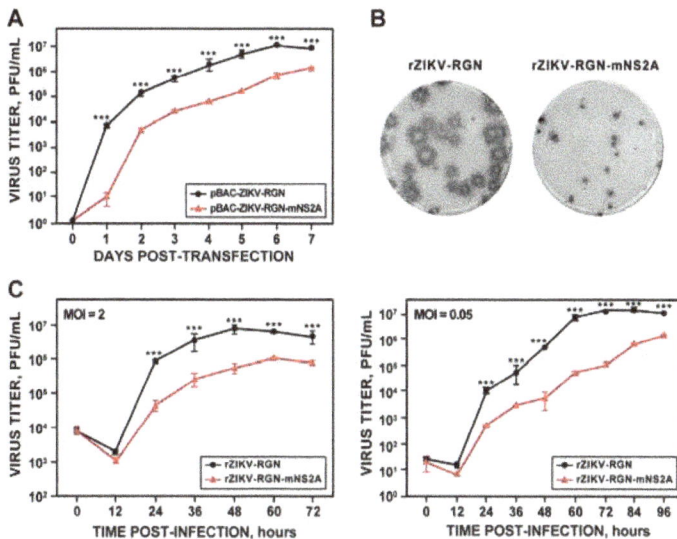

Figure 5. *Cont.*

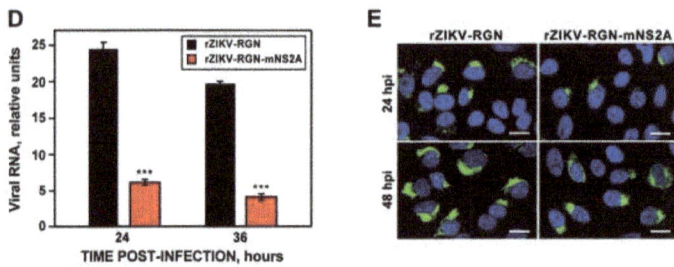

Figure 5. Rescue and growth properties of rZIKV-RGN-mNS2A in Vero cells. (**A**) Virus rescue. Vero cells at 90% of confluence (6-well plate format; triplicates) were transiently transfected with 4 μg/well of the infectious clones pBAC-ZIKV-RGN or pBAC-ZIKV-RGN-mNS2A, and at the indicated times post-transfection, virus titers in tissue culture supernatants were determined by plaque assay. Error bars represent standard deviations of the means from three experiments. (**B**) Plaque morphology. Vero cells at 90% confluence (6-well plate format) were infected with 25 PFU of rZIKV-RGN or rZIKV-RGN-mNS2A and at four days post-infection the viral plaques were visualized by immunostaining using the pan-flavivirus E protein mAb 4G2. (**C**) Growth kinetics. Vero cells at 90% confluence (24-well plate format; triplicates) were infected with rZIKV-RGN or rZIKV-RGN-mNS2A at high (2 PFU/cell, left) or low (0.05 PFU/cell, right) MOI, and at the indicated hpi virus titers were determined by plaque assay. Error bars represent standard deviations of the mean from three experiments. (**D**) Analysis of viral RNA synthesis. Vero cells at 90% confluence (12-well plate format; triplicates) were infected (MOI of 0.5 PFU/cell) with rZIKV-RGN or rZIKV-RGN-mNS2A and at the indicated hpi, viral RNA levels were quantified by RT-qPCR. Error bars represent standard deviations of the mean from three experiments. (**E**) Analysis of viral E protein expression. Vero cells were infected (MOI of 0.5 PFU/cell) with rZIKV-RGN or rZIKV-RGN-mNS2A and at the indicated hpi, viral E protein expression was analyzed by IFA using the pan-flavivirus E protein mAb 4G2. Bars, 20 μm. Asterisks in panels A, C, and D indicate that the differences between rZIKV-RGN and rZIKV-RGN-mNS2A are statistically significant when data are compared using the unpaired *t* test (***, $P < 0.001$).

To further confirm the effect of the NS2A A175V mutation on virus production, the growth kinetics at high (2 PFU/cell) and low (0.05 PFU/cell) MOI of the mutant virus were compared to those of the parental virus (Figure 5C). Again, a reduction of about one logarithmic unit in virus production was detected in Vero cells infected with the mutant virus both at high and low MOI (Figure 5C). Taken into consideration that flavivirus NS2A protein is involved in regulation of RNA replication and virus assembly [5], we further analyzed whether the reduction in plaque size and virus production of the mutant virus was associated with reduced viral RNA synthesis. To this end, the production of viral RNA in Vero cells infected with either the parental or mutant viruses at an MOI of 0.5 PFU/cell was analyzed at 24 and 36 hpi by RT-qPCR using a custom TaqMan assay specific for ZIKV-RGN genome (Figure 5D). At both times, a 5-fold reduction in the levels of viral RNA was observed in cells infected with the mutant virus (Figure 5D), confirming that NS2A A175V mutation at least impairs viral RNA synthesis. In agreement with these data, a reduction in the expression levels of ZIKV E protein was observed by IFA in Vero cells infected with the mutant virus in comparison to cells infected with the parental virus (Figure 5E). Finally, to discard the presence of other undesired mutations, the full-length sequence of the mutant virus was determined by deep-sequencing, and no mutations other than NS2A A175V were detected. Collectively, these results indicated that NS2A A175V mutation alone affected ZIKV growth in Vero cells at least by impairing viral RNA synthesis.

3.5. Pathogenesis of rZIKV-RGN-mNS2A in Mice

To investigate whether the reduced RNA synthesis of rZIKV-RGN-mNS2A in Vero cells could result in viral attenuation in vivo, the ability of the mutant virus to induce pathogenesis was analyzed in A129 mice and compared with that of the parental rZIKV-RGN (Figure 6). To that end, groups of five female 4-to-6-week-old A129 mice were inoculated s.c. in the footpad with 10^5 PFU of either rZIKV-RGN or rZIKV-RGN-mNS2A, or with PBS as a negative control, and the body weight loss and survival were monitored daily over 14 days. In contrast to mice infected with rZIKV-RGN that quickly lost weight and all of them died at day eight after infection, mice infected with the mutant rZIKV-RGN-mNS2A did not presented any clinical signs of infection or weight loss and all of them survived to viral infection (Figure 6A). To further analyze the correlation of the attenuation of the mutant virus with viral replication, presence of the virus in mice sera was analyzed at days two and four post-infection. In agreement with the pathogenicity data, mice infected with the mutant virus presented lower viremia than mice infected with the parental virus (Figure 6B). The mutant virus was only detected at day two after infection and at lower titers (approximately 1.5 logarithms lower) than the parental virus. As an internal control of the experiment, the plaque phenotype of the viruses recovered from the blood of infected mice were analyzed. As expected, rZIKV-RGN formed big plaques while the mutant rZIKV-RGN-mNS2A formed small plaques (Figure 6C). These results indicated that rZIKV-RGN-mNS2A was highly attenuated in mice, as compared to rZIKV-RGN, and that this attenuation may be due to a lower replication of the rZIKV-RGN-mNS2A mutant virus.

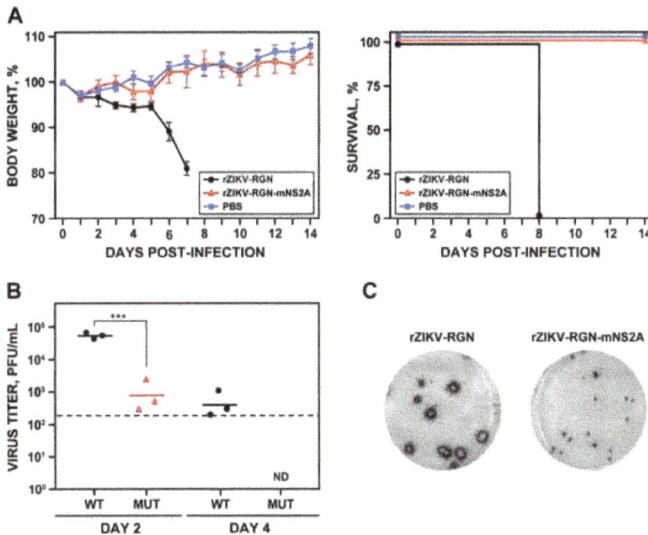

Figure 6. Pathogenesis of rZIKV-RGN-mNS2A in A129 mice. (**A**) Weight loss and mortality. Female 4-to-6-week-old A129 mice (five mice per group) were mock-infected (PBS) or infected s.c. in the footpad with 10^5 PFU of rZIKV-RGN or rZIKV-RGN-mNS2A, and body weight loss (expressed as the percentage of starting weight, left panel) and survival (right panel) were monitored daily during 14 days. Mice that lost more than 20% of their initial body weight or presented hind limb paralysis were humanely euthanized. Error bars represent standard deviations of the mean for each group of mice. (**B**) Viral titers in mice sera. Female 4-to-6-week-old A129 mice (six mice per group) were infected with 10^5 PFU of rZIKV-RGN (WT) or rZIKV-RGN-mNS2A (MUT) as described above, and viral titers in sera were determined at days two and four after infection (three animals per time point) by plaque assay and immunostaining using the pan-flavivirus E protein mAb 4G2. Symbols represent data from individual mice and bars the geometric means of viral titers. Asterisks indicate that the differences between rZIKV-RGN and rZIKV-RGN-mNS2A are statistically significant when data are compared using the unpaired *t* test (***, $P < 0.001$). ND: virus not detected. The detection limit of the assay (200 PFU/mL) is indicate as a dashed line. (**C**) Plaque phenotype. Vero cells at 90% confluence (6-well plate format) were infected with 25 PFU of rZIKV-RGN (left) or rZIKV-RGN-mNS2A (right) recovered from infected mice at day two post-infection and the plaque size evaluated by plaque assay and immunostaining using the pan-flavivirus E protein mAb 4G2.

3.6. Analysis of the Protection Efficacy in Mice of rZIKV-RGN-mNS2A

After elucidating that rZIKV-RGN-mNS2A was attenuated in vivo, its ability to induce protection against a challenge with the parental rZIKV-RGN was analyzed (Figure 7). To that end, groups of five female 4-to-6-week-old A129 mice were vaccinated s.c. in the footpad with 10^5 PFU of rZIKV-RGN-mNS2A or mock-vaccinated with PBS. Twenty days after vaccination, blood samples were collected to evaluate the humoral response. One day later, mice were challenged with a lethal dose (10^5 PFU) of rZIKV-RGN and the body weight loss and survival were analyzed daily over 14 days. As expected, mice vaccinated with PBS lost weight rapidly, showed clear symptoms of disease, and all of them succumbed to challenge with rZIKV-RGN. In contrast, mice vaccinated with rZIKV-RGN-mNS2A did not lose weight and all of them survived the challenge with rZIKV-RGN (Figure 7A), indicating that a single immunization dose with rZIKV-RGN-mNS2A is enough to induce full protection against ZIKV-RGN. In agreement with these data, a strong humoral response against ZIKV-RGN was observed in mice vaccinated with rZIKV-RGN-mNS2A (Figure 7B) and no viremia was detected in sera samples of vaccinated mice at days two and four after challenge (Figure 7C).

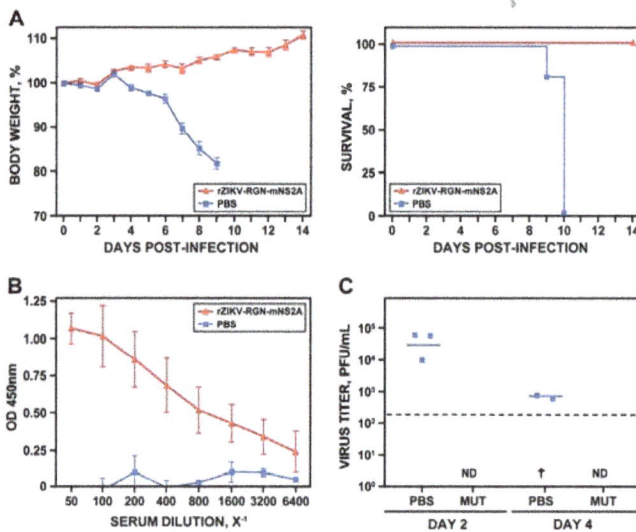

Figure 7. Protection efficacy of rZIKV-RGN-mNS2A. (**A**) Weight loss and mortality. Female 4-to-6-week-old A129 mice (five mice per group) were mock-vaccinated (PBS) or vaccinated s.c. in the footpad with 10^5 PFU of rZIKV-RGN-mNS2A. At 21 days after vaccination, mice were challenged with 10^5 PFU of rZIKV-RGN and the body weight loss (expressed as the percentage of starting weight, left panel) and survival (right panel) were monitored daily during 14 days. Mice that lost more than 20% of their initial body weight or presented hind limb paralysis were humanely euthanized. Error bars represent standard deviations of the mean for each group of mice. (**B**) Induction of humoral response. One day before challenge with rZIKV-RGN, sera samples were collected from mock-vaccinated (PBS) and rZIKV-RGN-mNS2A vaccinated mice, and total IgG antibodies against ZIKV-RGN were evaluated by ELISA. OD, optical density. Error bars represent standard deviations of the mean for each group of mice. (**C**) Viral titers in mice sera. Female 4-to-6-week-old A129 mice (six mice per group) mock-vaccinated (PBS) or vaccinated with 10^5 PFU of rZIKV-RGN-mNS2A (MUT) were challenged with 10^5 PFU of rZIKV-RGN as described above, and viral titers in sera were determined at days two and four after challenge (three animals per time point) by plaque assay and immunostaining using the pan-flavivirus E protein mAb 4G2. Symbols represent data from individual mice and bars the geometric means of viral titers. †: virus not detected in one mouse; ND: virus not detected. The limit of detection of the assay (200 PFU/mL) is indicate as a dashed line.

3.7. Genetic Stability of rZIKV-RGN-mNS2A In Vero Cells

Once confirmed that rZIKV-RGN-mNS2A was attenuated in vivo and induces protection against ZIKV-RGN in mice, the genetic stability of the mutant virus was analyzed in Vero cells, in order to test the possible use of this mutant virus as a base for the development of a live-attenuated ZIKV vaccine (Figure 8). To this end, both mutant (rZIKV-RGN-mNS2A) and parental (rZIKV-RGN) viruses were passaged five times in Vero cells (P1 to P5) and the virus plaque phenotype, growth kinetics and the sequence of NS2A were analyzed for each passage.

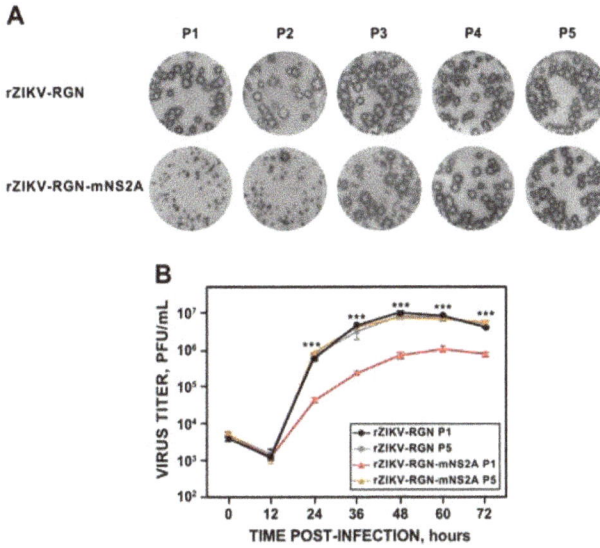

Figure 8. Stability of rZIKV-RGN-mNS2A in cultured cells. Vero cells growth in 6-well plates at 90% of confluence were infected with 0.1 PFU/cell of rZIKV-RGN or rZIKV-RGN-mNS2A. At 72 hpi, cell culture supernatants were collected and used to infect fresh Vero cells. This process was repeated four more times and virus stocks of passages 1 to 5 (P1 to P5) were generated. (**A**) Plaque size. Vero cells were infected with the different passages (P1 to P5) of rZIKV-RGN or rZIKV-RGN-mNS2A, and at four days post-infection the viral plaques were visualized by immunostaining using the pan-flavivirus E protein mAb 4G2. (**B**) Growth kinetics. Vero cells at 90% confluence (24-well plate format; triplicates) were infected (MOI of 1 PFU/cell) with P1 and P5 of rZIKV-RGN or rZIKV-RGN-mNS2A and at the indicated hpi, virus titers were determined by plaque assay. Error bars represent standard deviations of the mean from three experiments. Asterisks indicate that the differences between rZIKV-RGN-mNS2A P1 and the experimental samples, rZIKV-RGN P1, rZIKV-RGN P5 and rZIKV-RGN-mNS2A P5, are statistically significant when data are compared using the unpaired t test (***, $P < 0.001$).

Analysis of the plaque phenotype showed that the parental virus presented the expected plaque size throughout all passaging. In contrast, for the mutant virus a reversion to parental plaque phenotype was observed. This reversion started at P2 (2% of big plaques), clearly increased at P3 (45% of big plaques) and was complete at P4 (Figure 8A). After that, we analyzed whether this plaque size reversion of the mutant rZIKV-RGN-mNS2A correlated with an increase in virus replication to levels of that of the parental virus. To that end, the growth kinetics (MOI of 1 PFU/cell) of the mutant virus from P1 and P5 were compared to those of the parental virus. Growth curve analysis showed that in contrast to the mutant virus from P1, the virus from P5 replicated to the same levels as the parental virus (Figure 8B), suggesting that the mutant virus reverted to the WT sequence during its propagation in Vero cells. To confirm these observations, the NS2A coding region of mutant viruses from P1 to P5 was amplified by RT-PCR and sequenced. Sequence analysis confirmed the reversion of the A175V mutation to the WT sequence. Although the instability and reversion of the mutant virus to the WT sequence during its propagation in Vero cells limits the use of this mutant for vaccine development, these data further support the importance of this NS2A residue for virus replication. Moreover, these data also suggest that ZIKV NS2A protein represents a good target for the development of antivirals against ZIKV infection.

4. Discussion

The significance of ZIKV to public health due its association with Guillain–Barré syndrome and fetal abnormalities [14–19], together with the lack of approved antiviral agents or vaccines, have triggered a global effort to study this flavivirus in order to develop effective strategies to prevent and control ZIKV infection in humans. In this respect, the development and implementation of reverse genetic approaches for ZIKV provide investigators with a novel and powerful experimental tool to study both the biology and pathogenesis of ZIKV as well as the development of attenuated forms of ZIKV for their implementation as live-attenuated vaccines. However, as described for other flaviviruses, the generation of ZIKV infectious clones using traditional approaches are very difficult due to the toxicity and instability of some viral sequences when they were propagated as cloned cDNA in bacteria [24–26]. In the past two years, several approaches that overcomes this toxicity problem have been applied for the successfully generation of ZIKV infectious clones. These include the use of low-copy plasmids [29,30], insertion of introns to disrupt toxic sequences [31–33], mutational silencing of CBPs present in the viral genome [37], in vitro ligation of cDNA fragments [27,28,34], the ISA method [35,36], and the CPER approach [38]. Although very useful, some of these approaches are laborious, time consuming and present several disadvantages. For instance, most of them need in vitro ligation and transcription steps that complicate the assembly and reduce the recovery efficiency. Moreover, these low recovery efficiencies increase the presence of undesired mutations that could result in in vitro and/or in vivo attenuation, limiting the use of these infectious clones for certain studies. Others, such as the mutational silencing of CBPs, in which a high number of silent mutations have to be introduced, could affect viral fitness. Finally, the use of low-copy plasmids has been shown to be effective for several ZIKV strains but not for others, probably due the different degrees of toxicity of RNA sequences of different strains [28,32,34,36].

Here, we describe a powerful approach for the generation of an infectious cDNA clone of the ZIKV-RGN strain in a single plasmid, based on the use of a combination of synthetic biology and BACs. The full-length cDNA copy of the ZIKV-RGN strain was generated from four synthetic DNA fragments and cloned in the BAC plasmid pBeloBAC11 [40] under the control of the CMV promoter, which allows the expression of the viral RNA in the nucleus [50], and flanked at the 3'-end by the HDV ribozyme and the BGH polyadenylation and termination sequences to produce synthetic RNAs bearing authentic 3'-ends of the viral genome. The BAC cDNA clone was fully stable during its propagation in bacteria and the functional infectious virus was rescued after direct transfection of susceptible Vero cells that was pathogenic in A129 mice. A ZIKV-RGN infectious clone generated using the CPER approach has been recently reported [38]. However, in contrast to our results, the rescued virus was asymptomatic and nonlethal in female 8-to-12-week-old A129 mice infected with doses of 10^3 to 10^6 CCID$_{50}$ (50% cell culture infective doses) via the s.c. route. Whether the differences in pathogenicity among this rZIKV-RGN and ours are related to the experimental approach (CPER versus BAC), the age of the mice (8-to-12-week-old versus 4-to-6-week-old) or the MOI used to infect the mice (10^3–10^6 CCID$_{50}$ versus 10^5 PFU) remain to be evaluated.

Although other ZIKV reverse genetic systems have been reported (discussed above), the BAC approach constitutes an useful alternative that presents important advantages: (i) The BAC plasmids present a strictly controlled replication leading to only one plasmid per cell and therefore minimize the toxicity associated with several flavivirus sequences when amplified in bacteria [41]. This allows the easy and direct manipulation of the viral genome for molecular studies; (ii) Similarly to other approaches using polII-driven promoters, the BAC approach results in intracellular expression of the viral RNA [32,33,35,36,38], allowing the capping of the viral RNA and the recovery of infectious virus without the need of an in vitro transcription step. Although some splicing events could occur during the nuclear expression of the viral genome, mainly due to the presence of donor and acceptor putative sequences in the viral genome, the efficiency of this phenomenon is very low and does not affect the recovery of infectious viruses [52]; (iii) Like other systems based on transfection of DNA constructs [32,33,35,36,38], BAC cDNA clones present a higher efficiency of transfection than RNA transcripts in mammalian cells. This allows higher efficiencies of virus recovery, reducing the passages in cell culture to get a viral stock and therefore, the possibility of introducing undesired mutations by cell culture adaptation; (iv) The manipulation of BAC cDNA clones is relatively easy and similar to that of conventional plasmids with slight modifications due to the presence of only one plasmid copy per cell. In addition to standard protocols, the BAC cDNA clones could also be efficiently modified into *E. coli* by homologous recombination using a two-step approach that combine the Red recombination system and counterselection with the homing endonuclease I-SceI [53–56]; and (v) The BAC approach has been successfully used to engineer infectious clones of other flaviviruses, including DENV [39], and several coronaviruses that contain the largest viral RNA genome known and similar toxicity problems to those described for flaviviruses [52,57–60]. These data highlight the potential of the BAC approach for the rapid and reliable construction of stable infectious clones of emerging flavivirus and other similar RNA viruses with unstable viral genomes when amplified as cDNAs in bacteria.

The ZIKV reverse genetic system described in this article was further used to study the effect of a single amino acid substitution (A175V) in the viral NS2A protein on virus growth in cultured cells and pathogenesis in vivo. Our results suggested that this single amino acid change impaired viral RNA synthesis and virus production in cell culture and highly attenuated the virus in mice. However, we cannot discard that this mutation in the NS2A protein could affect other steps in the replication cycle of the virus. Flavivirus NS2A protein is a 22-kDa hydrophobic protein associated with the endoplasmic reticulum that contains eight transmembrane domains. It is a multifunctional protein that has been involved in viral RNA synthesis [61,62], virus assembly [63,64], membrane rearrangement [64], and immunomodulation of innate immune response [65–67]. By homology with the DENV NS2A topology, the ZIKV NS2A A175V mutation maps in the last transmembrane domain, for which no specific function has been reported. Therefore, our data constitute the first evidence of a role of this NS2A domain in viral RNA synthesis. On the other hand, it is important to note that the NS2A A175V mutation promoted a 5-fold reduction in viral RNA synthesis and more than 10-fold reduction in virus production. This reduced virus production could be a consequence of the RNA synthesis impairment. However, since the reduction in virus production is higher than that observed in RNA synthesis and that flavivirus NS2A protein is also involved in virus assembly, we cannot discard an additional effect of A175V mutation in ZIKV assembly. In addition, we have found that the mutant virus was attenuated in A129 mice. This attenuation could be explained as a consequence of the lower RNA synthesis of the mutant virus. However, an additional effect of the A175V mutation on the putative immunomodulatory role of NS2A protein [65–67], leading to virulence attenuation, cannot be discarded. Future studies will be required to determine whether this mutation affects only viral RNA synthesis or also virus assembly and immunomodulation of the host defenses.

Importantly, we have shown that immunization with a single dose of 10^5 PFU of the mutant rZIKV-RGN-mNS2A induced protection against a lethal challenge with the parental rZIKV-RGN, suggesting the potential implementation of this NS2A mutant as the base of a live-attenuated vaccine. Unfortunately, the mutant rZIKV-RGN-mNS2A was instable and reverted to the WT sequence during its propagation in Vero cells, limiting the use of this mutation alone for vaccine development. However, this instability and the high conservation of the amino acid A175 of the NS2A protein among ZIKV strains highlights the importance of this NS2A residue for virus replication, and therefore the potential use of NS2A protein as a good target for antiviral development against ZIKV infection.

In summary, we have developed a powerful ZIKV reverse genetic system based on the use of BACs that has allowed us to identify a single point mutation in the NS2A protein that attenuates

Viruses **2018**, *10*, 547

the virus in vitro and in vivo. This infectious clone system provides a valuable tool to the research community to explore ZIKV molecular biology, viral determinants of ZIKV pathogenesis, virus-host interactions, and vaccine and antivirals developments.

Author Contributions: Conceived, designed and supervised the research: F.A. and L.M.-S.; Conducted in vitro experiments: S.M.-J. and F.A.; Conducted in vivo experiments: A.N. and G.A.-P.; Analyzed and interpreted the data: S.M.-J., A.N., G.A.-P., L.M.-S., and F.A.; Contributed to discussion and provide important advice: F.J.I.; Wrote original draft of the manuscript: F.A.; Reviewed and edited the manuscript: F.A., L.M.-S., A.N., S.M.-J., G.A.-P., and F.J.I. All authors read and approved the final version of the manuscript.

Funding: This research was funded by the Spanish Ministry of Economy and Competitiveness (MINECO) (grant number BFU2016-79127-R) to F.A. and F.J.I. and the National Institute of Health (NIH) (grant number 1R21AI120500) to L.M.-S. and F.A.

Acknowledgments: We are grateful to Carla Gómez and Snezhana Dimitrova for technical assistance in the BAC clone generation and mice experiments, respectively. We also thank Sylvia Gutiérrez and Ana Oña at the CNB Advanced Microscopy Facility for their valuable support in immunofluorescence microscopy analysis.

Conflicts of Interest: The authors declare no conflict of interest. The funders had no role in the design of the study, in the collection, analyses, or interpretation of data, in the writing of the manuscript, and in the decision to publish the results.

References

1. Baud, D.; Gubler, D.J.; Schaub, B.; Lanteri, M.C.; Musso, D. An update on zika virus infection. *Lancet* **2017**, *390*, 2099–2109. [CrossRef]
2. Friedrich, M.J. Who calls off global zika emergency. *J. Am. Med. Assoc.* **2017**, *317*, 246. [CrossRef] [PubMed]
3. Sirohi, D.; Chen, Z.; Sun, L.; Klose, T.; Pierson, T.C.; Rossmann, M.G.; Kuhn, R.J. The 3.8 å resolution cryo-em structure of zika virus. *Science* **2016**, *352*, 467–470. [CrossRef] [PubMed]
4. Lee, I.; Bos, S.; Li, G.; Wang, S.; Gadea, G.; Despres, P.; Zhao, R.Y. Probing molecular insights into zika virus(-)host interactions. *Viruses* **2018**, *10*, 233. [CrossRef] [PubMed]
5. Lindenbach, B.D.; Murray, C.J.; Thiel, H.J.; Rice, C.M. Flaviviridae. In *Fields virology*, 6th ed.; Knipe, D.M., Howley, P.M., Eds.; Wolters Kluwer, Lippincott Williams & Wilkins: Philadelphia, PA, USA, 2013; Volume 1, pp. 712–748.
6. Macnamara, F.N. Zika virus: A report on three cases of human infection during an epidemic of jaundice in nigeria. *Trans. R. Soc. Trop. Med. Hyg.* **1954**, *48*, 139–145. [CrossRef]
7. Moulin, E.; Selby, K.; Cherpillod, P.; Kaiser, L.; Boillat-Blanco, N. Simultaneous outbreaks of dengue, chikungunya and zika virus infections: Diagnosis challenge in a returning traveller with nonspecific febrile illness. *New Microbes New Infect.* **2016**, *11*, 6–7. [CrossRef] [PubMed]
8. Boeuf, P.; Drummer, H.E.; Richards, J.S.; Scoullar, M.J.; Beeson, J.G. The global threat of zika virus to pregnancy: Epidemiology, clinical perspectives, mechanisms, and impact. *BMC Med.* **2016**, *14*, 112. [CrossRef] [PubMed]
9. Duffy, M.R.; Chen, T.H.; Hancock, W.T.; Powers, A.M.; Kool, J.L.; Lanciotti, R.S.; Pretrick, M.; Marfel, M.; Holzbauer, S.; Dubray, C.; et al. Zika virus outbreak on yap island, federated states of micronesia. *N. Engl. J. Med.* **2009**, *360*, 2536–2543. [CrossRef] [PubMed]
10. Cao-Lormeau, V.M.; Roche, C.; Teissier, A.; Robin, E.; Berry, A.L.; Mallet, H.P.; Sall, A.A.; Musso, D. Zika virus, french polynesia, south pacific, 2013. *Emerg. Infect. Dis.* **2014**, *20*, 1085–1086. [CrossRef] [PubMed]
11. Faria, N.R.; Azevedo Rdo, S.; Kraemer, M.U.; Souza, R.; Cunha, M.S.; Hill, S.C.; Theze, J.; Bonsall, M.B.; Bowden, T.A.; Rissanen, I.; et al. Zika virus in the americas: Early epidemiological and genetic findings. *Science* **2016**, *352*, 345–349. [CrossRef] [PubMed]
12. McCarthy, M. Four in florida are infected with zika from local mosquitoes. *Br. Med. J.* **2016**, *354*, i4235. [CrossRef] [PubMed]
13. McCarthy, M. Zika virus was transmitted by sexual contact in texas, health officials report. *Br. Med. J.* **2016**, *352*, i720. [CrossRef] [PubMed]
14. Costello, A.; Dua, T.; Duran, P.; Gulmezoglu, M.; Oladapo, O.T.; Perea, W.; Pires, J.; Ramon-Pardo, P.; Rollins, N.; Saxena, S. Defining the syndrome associated with congenital zika virus infection. *Bull. World Health Organ.* **2016**, *94*, 406–406a. [CrossRef] [PubMed]

15. Cugola, F.R.; Fernandes, I.R.; Russo, F.B.; Freitas, B.C.; Dias, J.L.; Guimaraes, K.P.; Benazzato, C.; Almeida, N.; Pignatari, G.C.; Romero, S.; et al. The brazilian zika virus strain causes birth defects in experimental models. *Nature* **2016**, *534*, 267–271. [CrossRef] [PubMed]

16. Do Rosario, M.S.; de Jesus, P.A.; Vasilakis, N.; Farias, D.S.; Novaes, M.A.; Rodrigues, S.G.; Martins, L.C.; Vasconcelos, P.F.; Ko, A.I.; Alcantara, L.C.; et al. Guillain-barre syndrome after zika virus infection in brazil. *Am. J. Trop. Med. Hyg.* **2016**, *95*, 1157–1160. [CrossRef] [PubMed]

17. Li, C.; Xu, D.; Ye, Q.; Hong, S.; Jiang, Y.; Liu, X.; Zhang, N.; Shi, L.; Qin, C.F.; Xu, Z. Zika virus disrupts neural progenitor development and leads to microcephaly in mice. *Cell. Stem Cell* **2016**, *19*, 672. [CrossRef] [PubMed]

18. Miner, J.J.; Cao, B.; Govero, J.; Smith, A.M.; Fernandez, E.; Cabrera, O.H.; Garber, C.; Noll, M.; Klein, R.S.; Noguchi, K.K.; et al. Zika virus infection during pregnancy in mice causes placental damage and fetal demise. *Cell* **2016**, *165*, 1081–1091. [CrossRef] [PubMed]

19. Mlakar, J.; Korva, M.; Tul, N.; Popovic, M.; Poljsak-Prijatelj, M.; Mraz, J.; Kolenc, M.; Resman Rus, K.; Vesnaver Vipotnik, T.; Fabjan Vodusek, V.; et al. Zika virus associated with microcephaly. *N. Engl. J. Med.* **2016**, *374*, 951–958. [CrossRef] [PubMed]

20. Diagne, C.T.; Diallo, D.; Faye, O.; Ba, Y.; Faye, O.; Gaye, A.; Dia, I.; Faye, O.; Weaver, S.C.; Sall, A.A.; et al. Potential of selected senegalese aedes spp. Mosquitoes (diptera: Culicidae) to transmit zika virus. *BMC Infect. Dis.* **2015**, *15*, 492. [CrossRef] [PubMed]

21. Tham, H.W.; Balasubramaniam, V.; Ooi, M.K.; Chew, M.F. Viral determinants and vector competence of zika virus transmission. *Front. Microbiol.* **2018**, *9*, 1040. [CrossRef] [PubMed]

22. Colt, S.; Garcia-Casal, M.N.; Pena-Rosas, J.P.; Finkelstein, J.L.; Rayco-Solon, P.; Weise Prinzo, Z.C.; Mehta, S. Transmission of zika virus through breast milk and other breastfeeding-related bodily-fluids: A systematic review. *PLoS Negl. Trop. Dis.* **2017**, *11*, e0005528. [CrossRef] [PubMed]

23. Rodriguez-Morales, A.J.; Bandeira, A.C.; Franco-Paredes, C. The expanding spectrum of modes of transmission of zika virus: A global concern. *Ann. Clin. Microbiol. Antimicrob.* **2016**, *15*, 13. [CrossRef] [PubMed]

24. Aubry, F.; Nougairede, A.; Gould, E.A.; de Lamballerie, X. Flavivirus reverse genetic systems, construction techniques and applications: A historical perspective. *Antivir. Res.* **2015**, *114*, 67–85. [CrossRef] [PubMed]

25. Pu, S.Y.; Wu, R.H.; Yang, C.C.; Jao, T.M.; Tsai, M.H.; Wang, J.C.; Lin, H.M.; Chao, Y.S.; Yueh, A. Successful propagation of flavivirus infectious cDNAs by a novel method to reduce the cryptic bacterial promoter activity of virus genomes. *J. Virol.* **2011**, *85*, 2927–2941. [CrossRef] [PubMed]

26. Ruggli, N.; Rice, C.M. Functional cDNA clones of the flaviviridae: Strategies and applications. *Adv. Virus Res.* **1999**, *53*, 183–207. [PubMed]

27. Deng, C.-L.; Zhang, Q.-Y.; Chen, D.-D.; Liu, S.-Q.; Qin, C.-F.; Zhang, B.; Ye, H.-Q. Recovery of the zika virus through an in vitro ligation approach. *J. Gen. Virol.* **2017**, *98*, 1739–1743. [CrossRef] [PubMed]

28. Widman, D.G.; Young, E.; Yount, B.L.; Plante, K.S.; Gallichotte, E.N.; Carbaugh, D.L.; Peck, K.M.; Plante, J.; Swanstrom, J.; Heise, M.T.; et al. A reverse genetics platform that spans the zika virus family tree. *mBio* **2017**, *8*. [CrossRef] [PubMed]

29. Annamalai, A.S.; Pattnaik, A.; Sahoo, B.R.; Muthukrishnan, E.; Natarajan, S.K.; Steffen, D.; Vu, H.L.X.; Delhon, G.; Osorio, F.A.; Petro, T.M.; et al. Zika virus encoding nonglycosylated envelope protein is attenuated and defective in neuroinvasion. *J. Virol.* **2017**, *91*. [CrossRef] [PubMed]

30. Shan, C.; Xie, X.; Muruato, A.E.; Rossi, S.L.; Roundy, C.M.; Azar, S.R.; Yang, Y.; Tesh, R.B.; Bourne, N.; Barrett, A.D.; et al. An infectious cDNA clone of zika virus to study viral virulence, mosquito transmission, and antiviral inhibitors. *Cell. Host Microbe.* **2016**, *19*, 891–900. [CrossRef] [PubMed]

31. Liu, Z.-Y.; Yu, J.-Y.; Huang, X.-Y.; Fan, H.; Li, X.-F.; Deng, Y.-Q.; Ji, X.; Cheng, M.-L.; Ye, Q.; Zhao, H.; et al. Characterization of cis-acting rna elements of zika virus by using a self-splicing ribozyme-dependent infectious clone. *J. Virol.* **2017**, *91*. [CrossRef] [PubMed]

32. Schwarz, M.C.; Sourisseau, M.; Espino, M.M.; Gray, E.S.; Chambers, M.T.; Tortorella, D.; Evans, M.J. Rescue of the 1947 zika virus prototype strain with a cytomegalovirus promoter-driven cDNA clone. *mSphere* **2016**, *1*. [CrossRef] [PubMed]

33. Tsetsarkin, K.A.; Kenney, H.; Chen, R.; Liu, G.; Manukyan, H.; Whitehead, S.S.; Laassri, M.; Chumakov, K.; Pletnev, A.G. A full-length infectious cDNA clone of zika virus from the 2015 epidemic in brazil as a genetic platform for studies of virus-host interactions and vaccine development. *mBio* **2016**, *7*. [CrossRef] [PubMed]

34. Weger-Lucarelli, J.; Duggal, N.K.; Bullard-Feibelman, K.; Veselinovic, M.; Romo, H.; Nguyen, C.; Ruckert, C.; Brault, A.C.; Bowen, R.A.; Stenglein, M.; et al. Development and characterization of recombinant virus generated from a new world zika virus infectious clone. *J. Virol.* **2017**, *91*. [CrossRef] [PubMed]

35. Atieh, T.; Baronti, C.; de Lamballerie, X.; Nougairede, A. Simple reverse genetics systems for asian and african zika viruses. *Sci. Rep.* **2016**, *6*, 39384. [CrossRef] [PubMed]

36. Gadea, G.; Bos, S.; Krejbich-Trotot, P.; Clain, E.; Viranaicken, W.; El-Kalamouni, C.; Mavingui, P.; Desprès, P. A robust method for the rapid generation of recombinant zika virus expressing the *gfp* reporter gene. *Virology* **2016**, *497*, 157–162. [CrossRef] [PubMed]

37. Munster, M.; Plaszczyca, A.; Cortese, M.; Neufeldt, C.J.; Goellner, S.; Long, G.; Bartenschlager, R. A reverse genetics system for zika virus based on a simple molecular cloning strategy. *Viruses* **2018**, *10*, 368. [CrossRef] [PubMed]

38. Setoh, Y.X.; Prow, N.A.; Peng, N.; Hugo, L.E.; Devine, G.; Hazlewood, J.E.; Suhrbier, A.; Khromykh, A.A. De novo generation and characterization of new zika virus isolate using sequence data from a microcephaly case. *mSphere* **2017**, *2*. [CrossRef] [PubMed]

39. Usme-Ciro, J.A.; Lopera, J.A.; Enjuanes, L.; Almazan, F.; Gallego-Gomez, J.C. Development of a novel DNA-launched dengue virus type 2 infectious clone assembled in a bacterial artificial chromosome. *Virus Res.* **2014**, *180*, 12–22. [CrossRef] [PubMed]

40. Wang, K.; Boysen, C.; Shizuya, H.; Simon, M.I.; Hood, L. Complete nucleotide sequence of two generations of a bacterial artificial chromosome cloning vector. *BioTechniques* **1997**, *23*, 992–994. [CrossRef] [PubMed]

41. Shizuya, H.; Birren, B.; Kim, U.J.; Mancino, V.; Slepak, T.; Tachiiri, Y.; Simon, M. Cloning and stable maintenance of 300-kilobase-pair fragments of human DNA in *Escherichia coli* using an f-factor-based vector. *Proc. Natl. Acad. Sci. USA* **1992**, *89*, 8794–8797. [CrossRef] [PubMed]

42. Livak, K.J.; Schmittgen, T.D. Analysis of relative gene expression data using real-time quantitative PCR and the 2(−ΔΔ c(t)) method. *Methods* **2001**, *25*, 402–408. [CrossRef] [PubMed]

43. Bustin, S.A.; Benes, V.; Garson, J.A.; Hellemans, J.; Huggett, J.; Kubista, M.; Mueller, R.; Nolan, T.; Pfaffl, M.W.; Shipley, G.L.; et al. The miqe guidelines: Minimum information for publication of quantitative real-time PCR experiments. *Clin. Chem.* **2009**, *55*, 611–622. [CrossRef] [PubMed]

44. Schindelin, J.; Arganda-Carreras, I.; Frise, E.; Kaynig, V.; Longair, M.; Pietzsch, T.; Preibisch, S.; Rueden, C.; Saalfeld, S.; Schmid, B.; et al. Fiji: An open-source platform for biological-image analysis. *Nat. Methods* **2012**, *9*, 676–682. [CrossRef] [PubMed]

45. Nogales, A.; Huang, K.; Chauche, C.; DeDiego, M.L.; Murcia, P.R.; Parrish, C.R.; Martinez-Sobrido, L. Canine influenza viruses with modified ns1 proteins for the development of live-attenuated vaccines. *Virology* **2017**, *500*, 1–10. [CrossRef] [PubMed]

46. Dowall, S.D.; Graham, V.A.; Rayner, E.; Atkinson, B.; Hall, G.; Watson, R.J.; Bosworth, A.; Bonney, L.C.; Kitchen, S.; Hewson, R. A susceptible mouse model for zika virus infection. *PLoS Negl. Trop. Dis.* **2016**, *10*, e0004658. [CrossRef] [PubMed]

47. Lazear, H.M.; Govero, J.; Smith, A.M.; Platt, D.J.; Fernandez, E.; Miner, J.J.; Diamond, M.S. A mouse model of zika virus pathogenesis. *Cell. Host Microbe* **2016**, *19*, 720–730. [CrossRef] [PubMed]

48. Rossi, S.L.; Tesh, R.B.; Azar, S.R.; Muruato, A.E.; Hanley, K.A.; Auguste, A.J.; Langsjoen, R.M.; Paessler, S.; Vasilakis, N.; Weaver, S.C. Characterization of a novel murine model to study zika virus. *Am. J. Trop. Med. Hyg.* **2016**, *94*, 1362–1369. [CrossRef] [PubMed]

49. National Research Council (U.S.). Committee for the Update of the Guide for the Care and Use of Laboratory Animals. In *Guide for the Care and Use of Laboratory Animals*, 8th ed.; Institute for Laboratory Animal Research (U.S.) & National Academies Press (U.S.): Washington, DC, USA, 2011.

50. Dubensky, T.W., Jr.; Driver, D.A.; Polo, J.M.; Belli, B.A.; Latham, E.M.; Ibanez, C.E.; Chada, S.; Brumm, D.; Banks, T.A.; Mento, S.J.; et al. Sindbis virus DNA-based expression vectors: Utility for in vitro and in vivo gene transfer. *J. Virol.* **1996**, *70*, 508–519. [PubMed]

51. Virus Pathogen Resource (ViPR), *Faviviridae*. Available online: https://www.viprbrc.org/brc/home.spg?decorator=flavi (accessed on 24 May 2018).

52. Almazan, F.; Gonzalez, J.M.; Penzes, Z.; Izeta, A.; Calvo, E.; Plana-Duran, J.; Enjuanes, L. Engineering the largest RNA virus genome as an infectious bacterial artificial chromosome. *Proc. Natl. Acad. Sci. USA* **2000**, *97*, 5516–5521. [CrossRef] [PubMed]

53. Jamsai, D.; Orford, M.; Nefedov, M.; Fucharoen, S.; Williamson, R.; Ioannou, P.A. Targeted modification of a human β-globin locus bac clone using get recombination and an i-scei counterselection cassette. *Genomics* **2003**, *82*, 68–77. [CrossRef]
54. Lee, E.C.; Yu, D.; Martinez de Velasco, J.; Tessarollo, L.; Swing, D.A.; Court, D.L.; Jenkins, N.A.; Copeland, N.G. A highly efficient *Escherichia coli*-based chromosome engineering system adapted for recombinogenic targeting and subcloning of bac DNA. *Genomics* **2001**, *73*, 56–65. [CrossRef] [PubMed]
55. Tischer, B.K.; von Einem, J.; Kaufer, B.; Osterrieder, N. Two-step red-mediated recombination for versatile high-efficiency markerless DNA manipulation in *Escherichia coli*. *BioTechniques* **2006**, *40*, 191–197. [PubMed]
56. Zhang, Y.; Buchholz, F.; Muyrers, J.P.; Stewart, A.F. A new logic for DNA engineering using recombination in *Escherichia coli*. *Nat. Genet.* **1998**, *20*, 123–128. [CrossRef] [PubMed]
57. Almazan, F.; Dediego, M.L.; Galan, C.; Escors, D.; Alvarez, E.; Ortego, J.; Sola, I.; Zuniga, S.; Alonso, S.; Moreno, J.L.; et al. Construction of a severe acute respiratory syndrome coronavirus infectious cDNA clone and a replicon to study coronavirus RNA synthesis. *J. Virol.* **2006**, *80*, 10900–10906. [CrossRef] [PubMed]
58. Almazan, F.; DeDiego, M.L.; Sola, I.; Zuniga, S.; Nieto-Torres, J.L.; Marquez-Jurado, S.; Andres, G.; Enjuanes, L. Engineering a replication-competent, propagation-defective middle east respiratory syndrome coronavirus as a vaccine candidate. *mBio* **2013**, *4*, e00650-13. [CrossRef] [PubMed]
59. Balint, A.; Farsang, A.; Zadori, Z.; Hornyak, A.; Dencso, L.; Almazan, F.; Enjuanes, L.; Belak, S. Molecular characterization of feline infectious peritonitis virus strain df-2 and studies of the role of orf3abc in viral cell tropism. *J. Virol.* **2012**, *86*, 6258–6267. [CrossRef] [PubMed]
60. St-Jean, J.R.; Desforges, M.; Almazan, F.; Jacomy, H.; Enjuanes, L.; Talbot, P.J. Recovery of a neurovirulent human coronavirus oc43 from an infectious cDNA clone. *J. Virol.* **2006**, *80*, 3670–3674. [CrossRef] [PubMed]
61. Mackenzie, J.M.; Khromykh, A.A.; Jones, M.K.; Westaway, E.G. Subcellular localization and some biochemical properties of the flavivirus kunjin nonstructural proteins ns2a and ns4a. *Virology* **1998**, *245*, 203–215. [CrossRef] [PubMed]
62. Rossi, S.L.; Fayzulin, R.; Dewsbury, N.; Bourne, N.; Mason, P.W. Mutations in west nile virus nonstructural proteins that facilitate replicon persistence in vitro attenuate virus replication in vitro and in vivo. *Virology* **2007**, *364*, 184–195. [CrossRef] [PubMed]
63. Kummerer, B.M.; Rice, C.M. Mutations in the yellow fever virus nonstructural protein ns2a selectively block production of infectious particles. *J. Virol.* **2002**, *76*, 4773–4784. [CrossRef] [PubMed]
64. Leung, J.Y.; Pijlman, G.P.; Kondratieva, N.; Hyde, J.; Mackenzie, J.M.; Khromykh, A.A. Role of nonstructural protein ns2a in flavivirus assembly. *J. Virol.* **2008**, *82*, 4731–4741. [CrossRef] [PubMed]
65. Liu, W.J.; Chen, H.B.; Wang, X.J.; Huang, H.; Khromykh, A.A. Analysis of adaptive mutations in kunjin virus replicon RNA reveals a novel role for the flavivirus nonstructural protein ns2a in inhibition of β interferon promoter-driven transcription. *J. Virol.* **2004**, *78*, 12225–12235. [CrossRef] [PubMed]
66. Liu, W.J.; Wang, X.J.; Clark, D.C.; Lobigs, M.; Hall, R.A.; Khromykh, A.A. A single amino acid substitution in the west nile virus nonstructural protein ns2a disables its ability to inhibit α/β interferon induction and attenuates virus virulence in mice. *J. Virol.* **2006**, *80*, 2396–2404. [CrossRef] [PubMed]
67. Munoz-Jordan, J.L. Subversion of interferon by dengue virus. *Curr. Top. Microbiol. Immunol.* **2010**, *338*, 35–44. [PubMed]

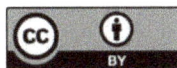

viruses

MDPI

Article

The Roles of prM-E Proteins in Historical and Epidemic Zika Virus-Mediated Infection and Neurocytotoxicity

Ge Li [1,†], Sandra Bos [2,†], Konstantin A. Tsetsarkin [3], Alexander G. Pletnev [3], Philippe Desprès [2], Gilles Gadea [2,*] and Richard Y. Zhao [1,4,5,6,*]

[1] Department of Pathology, University of Maryland School of Medicine, Baltimore, MD 21201, USA; lige_cn@hotmail.com
[2] Unité Mixte Processus Infectieux en Milieu Insulaire Tropical, Plateforme Technologique CYROI, Université de La Réunion, INSERM U1187, CNRS UMR 9192, IRD UMR 249, Sainte-Clotilde, 97400 La Réunion, France; SandraBos.Lab@gmail.com (S.B.); philippe.despres@univ-reunion.fr (P.D.)
[3] Laboratory of Infectious Diseases, NIAID, NIH, Bethesda, MD 20892, USA; konstantin.tsetsarkin@nih.gov (K.A.T.); apletnev@niaid.nih.gov (A.G.P.)
[4] Department of Microbiology-Immunology, University of Maryland School of Medicine, Baltimore, MD 21201, USA
[5] Institute of Global Health, University of Maryland School of Medicine, Baltimore, MD 21201, USA
[6] Institute of Human Virology, University of Maryland School of Medicine, Baltimore, MD 21201, USA
* Correspondence: gilles.gadea@inserm.fr (G.G.); rzhao@som.umaryland.edu (R.Y.Z.); Tel.: +410-706-6301 (R.Y.Z.)
† These authors contributed equally to this work.

Received: 18 December 2018; Accepted: 9 February 2019; Published: 14 February 2019

Abstract: The Zika virus (ZIKV) was first isolated in Africa in 1947. It was shown to be a mild virus that had limited threat to humans. However, the resurgence of the ZIKV in the most recent Brazil outbreak surprised us because it causes severe human congenital and neurologic disorders including microcephaly in newborns and Guillain-Barré syndrome in adults. Studies showed that the epidemic ZIKV strains are phenotypically different from the historic strains, suggesting that the epidemic ZIKV has acquired mutations associated with the altered viral pathogenicity. However, what genetic changes are responsible for the changed viral pathogenicity remains largely unknown. One of our early studies suggested that the ZIKV structural proteins contribute in part to the observed virologic differences. The objectives of this study were to compare the historic African MR766 ZIKV strain with two epidemic Brazilian strains (BR15 and ICD) for their abilities to initiate viral infection and to confer neurocytopathic effects in the human brain's SNB-19 glial cells, and further to determine which part of the ZIKV structural proteins are responsible for the observed differences. Our results show that the historic African (MR766) and epidemic Brazilian (BR15 and ICD) ZIKV strains are different in viral attachment to host neuronal cells, viral permissiveness and replication, as well as in the induction of cytopathic effects. The analysis of chimeric viruses, generated between the MR766 and BR15 molecular clones, suggests that the ZIKV E protein correlates with the viral attachment, and the C-prM region contributes to the permissiveness and ZIKV-induced cytopathic effects. The expression of adenoviruses, expressing prM and its processed protein products, shows that the prM protein and its cleaved Pr product, but not the mature M protein, induces apoptotic cell death in the SNB-19 cells. We found that the Pr region, which resides on the N-terminal side of prM protein, is responsible for prM-induced apoptotic cell death. Mutational analysis further identified four amino-acid residues that have an impact on the ability of prM to induce apoptosis. Together, the results of this study show that the difference of ZIKV-mediated viral pathogenicity, between the historic and epidemic strains, contributed in part the functions of the structural prM-E proteins.

Keywords: Zika virus; prM-E proteins; viral pathogenicity; virus attachment; viral replication; viral permissiveness; viral survival; apoptosis; cytopathic effects; mutagenesis; chimeric viruses; human brain glial cells

---

1. Introduction

The 2015 Zika virus (ZIKV) outbreak in South America has a tremendous impact on public health. It was estimated that it left more than three thousand babies who were born with microcephaly, due to ZIKV infection in Brazil alone [1]. Monitoring those babies after birth continue to show various developmental and neurologic disorders that are now known as the congenital ZIKV syndrome [2,3]. Even though the causal relationship between ZIKV infection and ZIKV-induced microcephaly and other neurologic disorders have been firmly established [4–6], the reason for the sudden ZIKV virulence, and resulting neurologic disorders in humans, remain largely unknown.

ZIKV was originally isolated in 1947 from caged monkeys in the Zika forest of Uganda, Africa [7]. It was thought to be a mild virus that causes mild flu-like symptoms [7,8] and having a limited threat to humans [9,10]. A number of small-scale ZIKV outbreaks, with increasing number of individuals affected, took place in Asia and in Pacific Islands in past years [11,12] until it reached the Americas in a large-scale outbreak in 2015 [1]. In the most recent ZIKV outbreak, the virus spread to eighty-four countries, territories, or sub-national areas, with an estimate of over 1.5 million affected individuals [13]. Brazil was the most affected country, with an estimated 440,000 to 1.3 million cases reported [14]. The fact that the epidemic ZIKV causes severe human congenital and neurologic disorders, suggests that the epidemic ZIKV must have acquired enhanced viral pathogenicity through adaptive viral gene mutations.

ZIKV is a member of the flaviviruses (the family of *Flaviviridae*), which include a number of well-known human pathogens such as Dengue Virus (DENV), West Nile Virus (WNV), and Japanese Encephalitis Virus (JEV). It is a single-stranded, positive-sense RNA virus with a viral genome of approximately 10.7 kilobases (kb). The ZIKV genome encodes a single large open reading frame that produces a polyprotein, which is subsequently processed by viral and host proteases to produce a total of fourteen immature proteins, mature proteins, and small peptides [10,15]. A total of ten mature viral proteins, i.e., three structural proteins and seven non-structural proteins are produced after viral processing [16,17]. The structural proteins consist of an anchor capsid (anaC) protein, a precursor membrane (prM) protein, and an envelope (E) protein. In non-infectious and immature viral particles, the prM protein forms a heterodimer with the E protein [18,19]. The E protein, composed of the majority of the virion surface, is involved in binding to the host cell surface and triggering subsequent membrane fusion and endocytosis [10,20,21]. For virus maturation, the mature capsid (C) protein is produced by the proteolytic cleavage of the anaC protein in a post-Golgi compartment, which in turn triggers the cleavage of the prM protein by a host protease furin to produce a mature membrane (M) protein (75 a.a) and a Pr protein product (93 a.a) [15,22,23]. The transition of prM to M by furin cleavage results in mature and infectious particles [19,24]. Thus, one of our research interests here was to examine the effect of prM and its processed proteins, the mature M protein and a cleaved Pr protein product, on ZIKV-mediated cytopathic effect.

Based on phylogenetic analysis, ZIKV can be classified into two viral lineages, i.e., the African lineage, that includes ZIKV strains from Africa; and the Asian lineage that includes both Asian strains and those ZIKV strains that were isolated from the Americas, such as the Brazilian strains [25,26]. Comparative studies of the African and Asian ZIKV strains in vivo, ex vivo, and in animal models suggest that these two ZIKV lineages are intrinsically different in their pathogenicity and virulence [10,25,27,28]. Those virologic differences could potentially explain why the Brazilian ZIKV, which belongs to the Asian lineage, has acquired the epidemic potential and become highly virulent in humans. Conceivably, those epidemic and virologic potentials to cause the observed congenital ZIKV syndromes could be acquired through evolution by adaptive viral gene mutations [10,28,29]. Nevertheless, which viral gene(s) is responsible for the observed phenotypic transition, and what type of viral gene mutations were adapted for this transition remain elusive.

Potential virologic differences between the African and Asian ZIKV lineages could be elucidated by exchanging different components of the ZIKV genome between the two viral lineages by generating chimeric viruses. Through such analysis of chimeric viral infection, any virologic changes, due to the swapping alteration would allow us to correlate a virologic change with a specific domain or gene of the ZIKV genome. By using this strategy and comparative analysis of a historic African ZIKV MR766 strain and an epidemic Brazilian BR15 strain in human host cells, we discovered in our earlier study that the structural proteins of the BR15 and MR766 ZIKV strains differ in their ability to initiate viral infection [30]. In line with our findings, an earlier comparative study of the ZIKV protein evolution from the pre-epidemic to the epidemic ZIKV, suggested that some of the amino acid (a.a.) sites in the E protein were negatively selected during ZIKV evolution, indicating possible functional alterations might have occurred during evolution [29]. In addition, another evolutionary study suggested that the S139N substitution in the prM protein was positively selected for in the pre-epidemic to the epidemic transition, and this single mutation alone led to more severe microcephaly than the pre-epidemic ZIKV strain [31]. The objectives of this study were (1) to further compare the historic African MR766 ZIKV strain with two epidemic Brazilian strains (molecular clones of BR15 and ICD) for their abilities to initiate viral infection and to confer neurocytopathic effects in human brain SNB-19 glial cells, and (2) to evaluate the contribution of prM-E proteins in the susceptibility of human brain glial cells to ZIKV infection.

2. Materials and Methods

2.1. Cell Culture

The SNB-19 (RRID:CVCL_0535), provided by Dr. HL Tang [32], is a human astrocytoma cell line, which was maintained in Corning RPMI 1640 medium (Product number: 10-040-CV, Mediatech, Inc., Manassas, VA, USA) supplemented with 10% fetal bovine serum (FBS) and 100 units/mL penicillin plus 100 μg/mL streptomycin. Vero76 cell is a derivative of the original Vero cells, which were originally isolated from the kidney of a normal adult African green monkey. Vero76 cells (ATCC-CRL-1587, Manassas, VA) were grown in Dulbecco's Modified Eagle Medium (DMEM) medium (Product number: 10-017-CV, Mediatech, Inc., Manassas, VA, USA), supplemented with 10% FBS and 100 units/mL penicillin, plus 100 μg/mL streptomycin.

2.2. Zika Virus Molecular Clones and Infection

The MR766 ZIKV strain was the first documented Zika strain that was isolated from caged monkey in the Zika forest in Uganda in 1947 [9]. Hence, it is called the historical strain. This viral strain has been passaged countless times in new-born mouse brains. The molecular clone of ZIKV-ZIKV-MR766-NIID was generated, based on the sequence of ZIKV strain MR766 Uganda 47-NIID (Genbank access # LC002520), using the infectious sub-genomic amplicon (ISA) method as described previously [33]. The BR15 ZIKV strain (BeH819015) was isolated from a blood sample of a patient and sequenced after one passage in mosquito C6/36 cells. It was one of the earliest Zika viral sequences that was isolated from one of the Northern states of Brazil (Pará) in July 2015 from a large clade [34,35]. The molecular clone of BR15 was generated, based on the BeH819015 sequence (Genbank Accession number: KU365778), using the same strategy as that of the ZIKV-MR766-NIID [30,33]. BR15 is available to BEI resources (Manssas, VA, USA) under the catalog number NR-51129. The ZIKV Paraíba_01/2015 strain (Genbank Accession number: KX280026) was originally isolated from the northeast state of Paraíba (Brazil) in 2015 from a serum sample of a febrile female. The virus was passed twice in Vero cells, and a molecular clone (ZIKV-ICD *aka* 674v4) was generated as described [36].

For viral infection, the cells were seeded in culture plates and incubated at 37 °C/5% CO_2 overnight to allow the cells to attach to the wells. The second day, ZIKV was added to the cells with the multiplicity of infection (MOI) of 1.0, unless specifically indicated. The cells were incubated for 2 h at 37 °C, with gentle agitation every 30 min. Next, the inoculum was removed, and the cells were washed twice with PBS. The culture medium was added to each well, and the cells were incubated at 37 °C/5% CO_2 for the duration of the experiment.

2.3. Generation and Production of the Chimeric Viruses

Two chimeric ZIKV molecular clones were generated. The M/B chimeric virus consisted of the C-prM viral sequence of MR766, with the rest of the viral genome replaced with the counterpart sequence of BR15 ZIKV molecular clone. Conversely, the B/M chimeric virus consists of the C-prM viral sequence of BR15 with the rest of the viral genome replaced with the counterpart sequence of MR766 ZIKV molecular clone. The general approach used for the construction of chimeric molecular clones was previously described [30,33]. To generate the M/B or B/M chimeric molecular clones, the respective C-prM regions from the MR766 or from the BR15 were extracted from the Z1 fragment. It was then introduced into the BR15 or the MR766 backbone respectively, by using the following shared primers: 5′-GCCAAAAAGTCATATACTTGGTCATGATACTGCTGATTGCCCCGGC-3′ and 5′-GCCGGGGCAATCAGCAGTATCATGACCAAGTATATGACTTTTTGGC-3′.

The procedure to generate and produce chimeric ZIKV viruses was essentially the same as described [30,33]. Briefly, the purified PCR fragments were electroporated into Vero76 cells. After 5 days, cell supernatants were recovered, usually in absence of cytopathic effects and were used to infect fresh Vero76 cells (DMEM with 2% FBS) in a first round of amplification (P1). Viral clones M/B or B/M were recovered 3–7 days later until cytopathic effect was observed under microscope and amplified for another 2 days on Vero76 cells to produce working P2 stocks of the viruses that were used for all studies. The viral titers were determined using the standard plaque-forming assay, as described previously, and expressed as plaque-forming units per mL (PFU/mL) [30]. The sequences of all the viruses and plasmid used in the study are available from the authors upon request.

2.4. Adenoviral Constructs and Cell Transduction

All of the Adenoviral (Adv) constructs, that were used in this study, were custom-made by ViGene (Rockville, MD, USA). The viral titers were determined using an ELISA Adeno-X rapid titer kit (Cat#: 631028, Clontech, Mountain View, CA, USA), which detects the Adenoviral Hexon surface antigen. For Adv transduction, SNB-19 cells in the concentration of 1×10^4/well in 96 well plate were seeded and incubated at 37 °C/5% CO_2 overnight to allow the cells to attach to the wells. The second day, the SNB-19 cells were transduced with Adv with the MOI of 1000. The Adv transduced cells were incubated at 37 °C/5% CO_2 and the cells were collected at indicated times for analyses.

2.5. Viral Binding Assay

SNB-19 cells were cultured at sub-confluent density in 60 mm dishes. Cell monolayers were washed in cold PBS and cooled at 4 °C for at least 20 min in the presence of RPMI 1640, supplemented with 2% FBS. Pre-chilled cells were then incubated at 4 °C with ZIKV at MOI of 1.0 in 1.5 mL of RPMI 1640 medium supplemented with 2% FBS. After 1 h of incubation, the virus inputs were removed, and the cells were washed with RPMI 1640 medium, supplemented with 2% FBS. Total cellular RNA was extracted using TRIzol reagent (Life technologies, Carlsbad, CA, USA). The RT-qPCR analysis on viral RNA was performed using the primers amplifying a conserved ZIKV region between the NS5 and 3′UTR. The nucleotide sequences of these primer pairs are ZIKV-F: 5′-AGGATCATAGGTGATGAAGAAAAGT-3′ and ZIKV-R: 5′-CCTGACAACACTAAGATTG-GTGC-3′. For viral binding assay in A549 cells, the RT-qPCR analysis on viral RNA was performed using the primers amplifying a region of the E protein, as described [30]. ZIKV E primers were designed to match both MR766-NIID and BeH819015 sequences. A house-keeping gene glyceraldehyde 3-phosphate dehydrogenase (GAPDH) was used as an endogenous control for the measurement of viral bindings.

2.6. Immunofluorescence Staining

The immunostaining method was used to determine ZIKV infectivity and induction of apoptosis, as described in [32]. Briefly, SNB-19 cells were infected with ZIKV, as described above. ZIKV-infected cells were fixed at 48 h post-infection (p.i.) with 3.7% paraformaldehyde in PBS for 1 h at room temperature on Labtek II slides. After washing three times for 5 min in PBS, the cells were blocked and permeabilized for 30 min in blocking buffer (10% FBS, 0.25% Triton X-100 in PBS). To determine viral infectivity, i.e., the percent of cells infected with ZIKV with MOI of 1.0, cells were first incubated with mouse anti-Flaviviridae group antigen (clone name: D1-4G2-15, Cat# MAB10216, MilliporeSigma, Burlington, MA) primary antibody with proper dilutions in the incubation buffer (1% BSA in PBS) for 2 h at 37 °C. After washing, cells were incubated with Texas Red-conjugated goat anti-mouse IgG secondary antibody (Cat# T-862, ThermoFisher, Waltham, MA, USA) at suggested concentration in the incubation buffer for 1 h at room temperature. After washing, cells were stained with DAPI for 5 min and washed again. Cells were then mounted with mounting medium and visualized on a Leica DM4500B microscope (Leica Microsystems, Buffalo Grove, IL) with Openlab software (Improvision, Lexington, MA, USA). ZIKV-induced caspase-3 cleavage, a hallmark of cellular apoptosis, was measured, by using the same immunostaining method, as described except cells was tested at 72 h p.i., and the primary antibody used was Cleaved Caspase-3 (Asp175) (5A1E) Rabbit mAb (Cat#9664, Cell Signaling, Danvers, MA, USA). The secondary antibody used was the FITC-conjugated goat anti-rabbit IgG secondary antibody (Cat# 31635, ThermoFisher, Waltham, MA, USA).

2.7. Measurement of ZIKV Viral Replication

ZIKV viral replication was measured over time, by using real-time reverse transcription polymerase chain reaction (RT-PCR) analysis, essentially as described previously [37]. Briefly, the total RNA was extracted from SNB-19 cells using TRIzol reagent (Life technologies, Carlsbad, CA, USA) according to the manufacturer's protocol. The RNA pellet was re-suspended in RNase-free distilled water and stored at −80 °C. Five hundred nanograms of RNA was used for real-time RT-PCR analysis, using iTaq universal SYBR Green one-step kit (BioRad, Hercules, CA, USA), according to the manufacturer's instruction. The primer sequences used here are the same conserved ZIKV region between the NS5 and 3'UTR as that described in the Section 2.5. The amplification in BioRad CFX96 real-time PCR system involved a reverse transcription reaction at 50 °C for 10 min, activation and DNA denaturation at 95 °C for 1 min, followed by 40 amplification cycles of 95 °C for 15 s and 60 °C for 30 s. The mRNA expression (fold-induction) was quantified by calculating the $2^{-\Delta CT}$ value, with GAPDH mRNA as an endogenous control.

Besides the RT-PCR, the conventional plaque forming assay was also used to measure viral replication. Viral titers were determined by a standard plaque-forming assay, as previously described, with minor modifications [38]. Briefly, Vero76 cells, grown in 48-well culture plate, were infected with tenfold dilutions of virus samples for 2 h at 37 °C and then incubated with 0.8% carboxymethylcellulose (CMC) for 4 days. CMC was removed from plate. The cells were washed two times with PBS and fixed by 3.7% FA in PBS and stained with 0.5% crystal violet in 20% ethanol. Viral titers were expressed as PFU/mL.

2.8. MTT Assay

The MTT assay was used to measure cell proliferation and viability as described previously [39]. SNB-19 cells were plated in 100 µL media in 96-well plate, with 10,000 cells per well, and incubated at 37 °C/5% CO_2 overnight to allow the cells to attach to the wells. At the indicated time intervals post-treatment, 10 µL of MTT solution (Thiazolyl Blue Tetrazolium Bromide, 5mg/mL in PBS) was added to each well, thoroughly mixed and incubated at 37 °C for 4 h to allow the MTT to be metabolized. Then the media was removed and resuspended in 100 μL DMSO to solubilize formazan (the MTT metabolized product). After shaking at 150 rpm for 5 min, the plate was subjected to optical density measurement at 562 nm by a SYNERGY-H1 microplate reader (BioTek Instruments, Winooski, VT, USA).

2.9. Measurement of Cellular Necrosis and Apoptosis

Cellular necrosis and apoptosis were measured by a RealTime-Glo™ Annexin V Apoptosis and Necrosis Assay kit (Promega, Madison, WI, USA) according to manufacturer's instruction. Briefly, 1×10^4 SNB-19 cells/well were seeded into a 96-well plate (Costar 3610, Corning, NY, USA) and cultured at 37 °C/5% CO_2 overnight. The cells were transduced with adenovirus, and 2x detection reagent (which included Annexin V NanoBiT®substrate, $CaCl_2$, Necrosis Detection Reagent, Annexin V-SmBiT and Annexin V-LgBiT) was added into each tested well of 96-well plate. The plates were incubated at 37 °C/5%, followed by measurements of luminance (RLU) for apoptosis, and fluorescence (RFU, 485 nm_{Ex}/520–30 nm_{Em}) for necrosis at the indicated time intervals post infection using a SYNERGY-H1 microplate reader.

2.10. Statistical Analysis

Unless indicated, two-tailed and paired student *t*-test was used for a pair-wise comparison of data, using Microsoft Excel software. Two-way ANOVA analysis was used to analyze results generated for Figure 1B, Figure 2A, Figure 3C, Figure 4A, Figure 5B,C and Figure 6C,D, respectively using Prism 7 (GraphPad Software, San Diego, CA, USA). A difference is considered statistically significant if $p \leq 0.1$ (*), $p \leq 0.05$ (**) or $p \leq 0.01$ (***) according to conventional definitions.

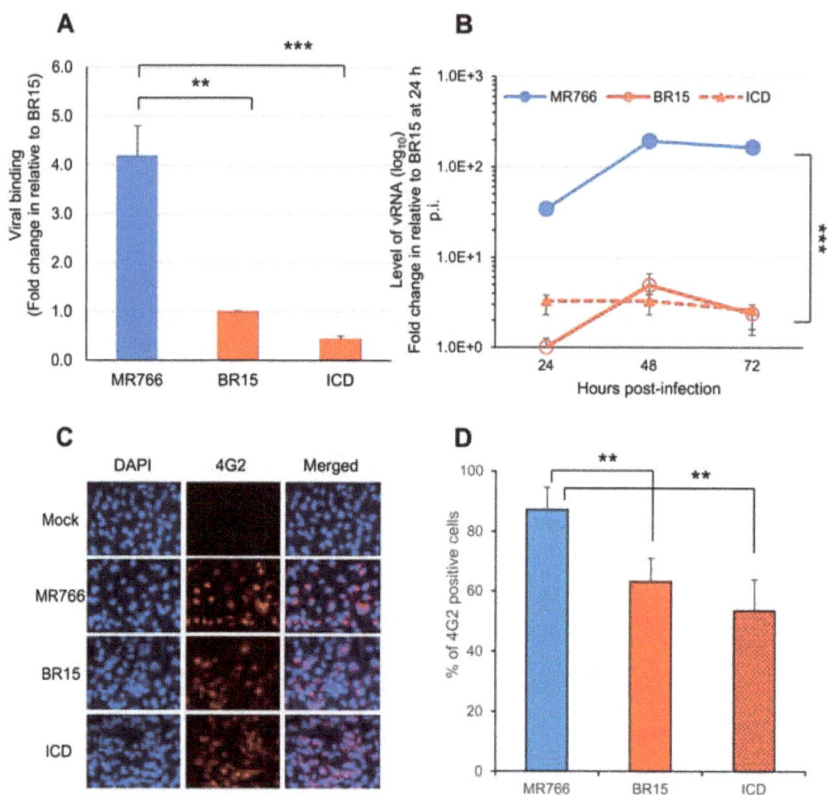

Figure 1. Different infectivity between the epidemic Brazilian Zika virus (BR15 and ICD) molecular clones and the historical African MR766 molecular clone in human brain glial SNB-19 cells. (**A**) Viral binding to SNB-19 cells was measured by presence of cell-associated vRNA one-hour post-infection (p.i.). A housekeeping gene GAPDH was used as an endogenous control for the measurement of viral bindings. (**B**) Zika virus (ZIKV) replication was measured by quantitative RT-PCR with timeframe as indicated. SNB-19 cells were infected by Zika viruses with multiplicity of infection (MOI) 1.0. Results represent average and standard deviation ($X \pm SD$) of four independent experiments. (**C**) Viral infectivity measured by anti-E mAb 4G2 at 48 h p.i. (**D**) Viral infectivity is shown as an average of three different experiments, each carried out in triplicates. Average cell number counted was about 100–200. Results represent average and standard deviation ($X \pm SD$). Levels of statistical significance were calculated by two-tailed and paired t-test for (**A**), and Two-way ANOVA was used for (**B**). **, $p < 0.05$; ***, $p < 0.01$.

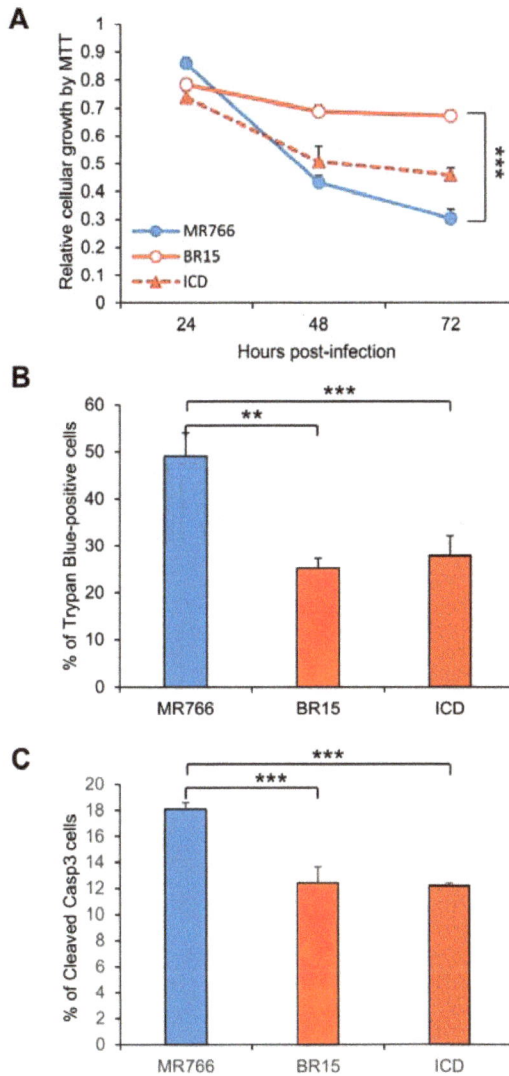

Figure 2. Different neuro-cytopathic effects of epidemic and historical molecular clones of Zika viruses on human brain glial SNB-19 cells. (**A**) Cellular survival was measured by the MTT assay. The graph is plotted as the relative growth in relevance to mock infected SNB19 cells. Statistic t-test shows that the differences among three viruses are not statistically significant. (**B**) ZIKV-induced cell death as measured by the Trypan blue assay. ******, $p < 0.05$ for BR15 and *******, $p < 0.01$ for ICD. Three different experiments were carried out. Average cell number counted was about 100–200. (**C**) ZIKV-induced apoptosis was measured by caspase-3 cleavages using immunostaining as reported previously [32]. Cells were collected at 72 h p.i. Two experiments were conducted and cells showing caspase-3 cleavages were counted at 10 different areas with an average number of cells counted at 25–75. All results represent average and standard deviation (X + SD). Levels of statistical significance were calculated by Two-way ANOVA for (**A**). The difference between MR766 and BR15 is highly significant with $p < 0.01$ (*******).

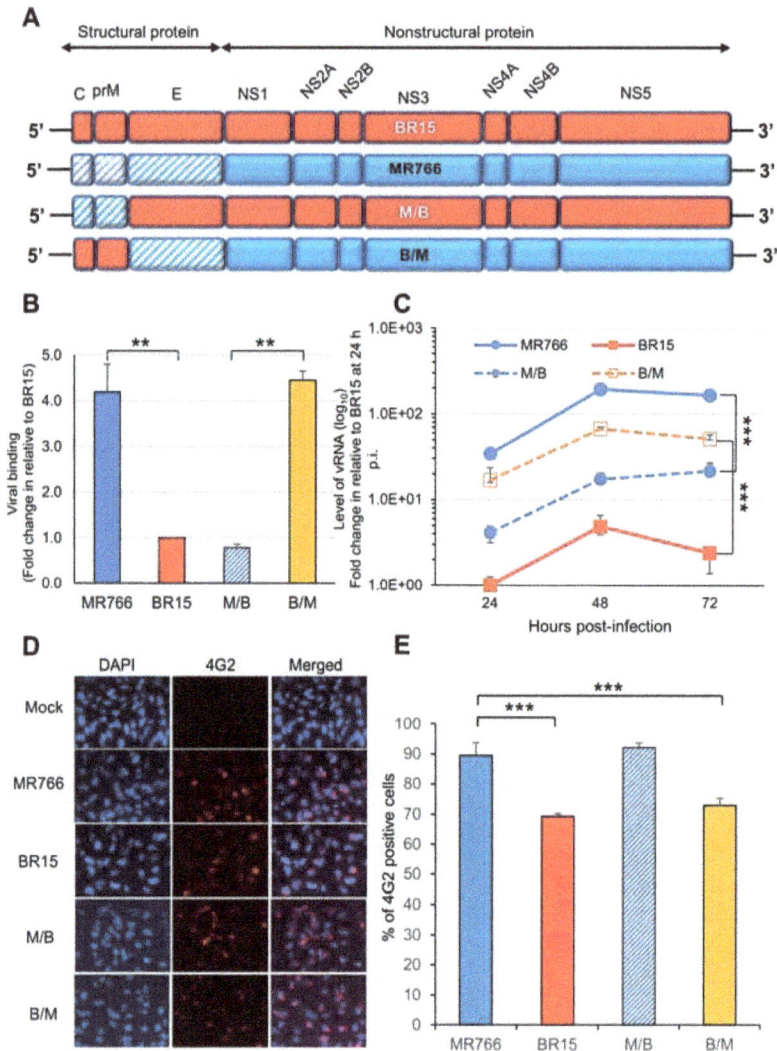

Figure 3. Correlation of the ZIKV C-prM with viral attachment and viral infection. (**A**) Generation of chimeric ZIKV molecular clones are shown along with their parental clones. The chimeric viruses were made between the MR766 and the BR15 ZIKV molecular clones. The viral genome exchange is at the junction of prM and E protein. (**B**) Viral binding was measured by presence of cell-associated vRNA 1 h p.i. A housekeeping gene GAPDH was used as an endogenous control for the measurement of viral bindings. Results represent average and standard deviation (X ± SD) of four independent experiments. (**C**) ZIKV viral replication was measured by RT-qPCR with timeframe as indicated. (**D**) Viral infection was measured by anti-E mAb 4G2 at 48 h p.i. (**E**) Quantification of the results shown in (**D**). SNB-19 cells were infected with Zika viruses with MOI of 1.0. Three different experiments were carried out in triplicates. Average cell number counted was about 100–200. All quantitative results represent average and standard deviation (X ± SD). Levels of statistical significance were calculated by two-tailed and paired t-test for (**B**), and Two-way ANOVA was used for (**C**). **, $p < 0.05$; ***, $p < 0.01$.

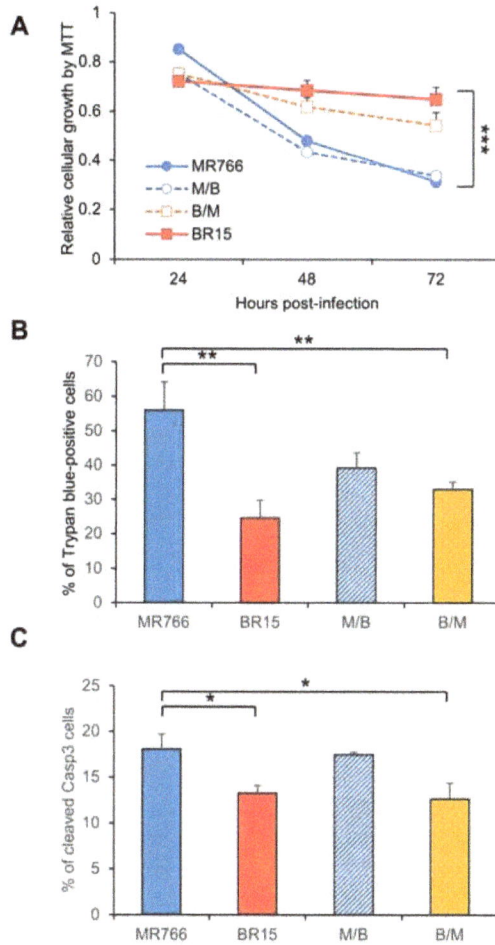

Figure 4. Correlation of the C-prM with ZIKV-induced growth restriction and apoptotic cell death. (**A**) Cell proliferation was measured by the MTT assay. Statistic t-test shows the differences shown among three viruses are not significant. (**B**) ZIKV-induced cell death was measured by the Trypan blue assay 72 h p.i. Two different experiments were carried out. Average number of cells counted was about 100-200. Differences between MR766 vs. BR15, and MR766 vs. B/M were both high significant with $p \leq 0.05$ (**) for both comparisons. The difference between MR766 and M/B was not significant with $p = 0.11$. (**C**) ZIKV-induced apoptosis was measured by cleavage of caspase-3. Cells were collected at 72 h p.i. All results represent average and standard deviation (X ± SD). Levels of statistical significance were calculated by Two-way ANOVA for (**A**). The difference between MR766 and BR15 is highly significant with $p < 0.01$ (***).

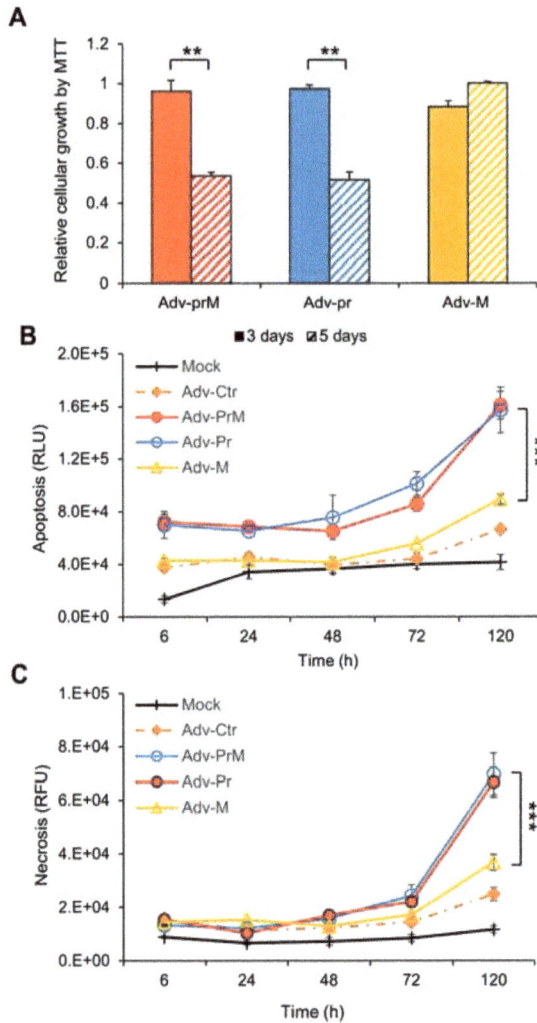

Figure 5. Effect of prM protein processing on ZIKV-induced neurocytotoxicity. (**A**) Cell proliferation and viability was measured overtime by the MTT assay. The graph is plotted as the relative growth in relevance to mock infected SNB-19 cells. The differences shown were highly significant with $p < 0.05$ (**). (**B**) Measurement of apoptosis by Annexin V over time. The difference between Adv-prM and Adv-M was highly significant with $p < 0.01$ (***), but the difference between Adv-prM and Adv-Pr was not significant with $p = 0.84$. (**C**) Measurement of cellular necrosis over time. Two-way ANOVA was used to calculate the difference between Adv-prM and Adv-M for (**B**) and (**C**). The differences between Adv-prM and Adv-M were highly significant with $p < 0.01$ (***). More than two different experiments were conducted to evaluate apoptosis and necrosis. All results represent average and standard deviation (X ± SD).

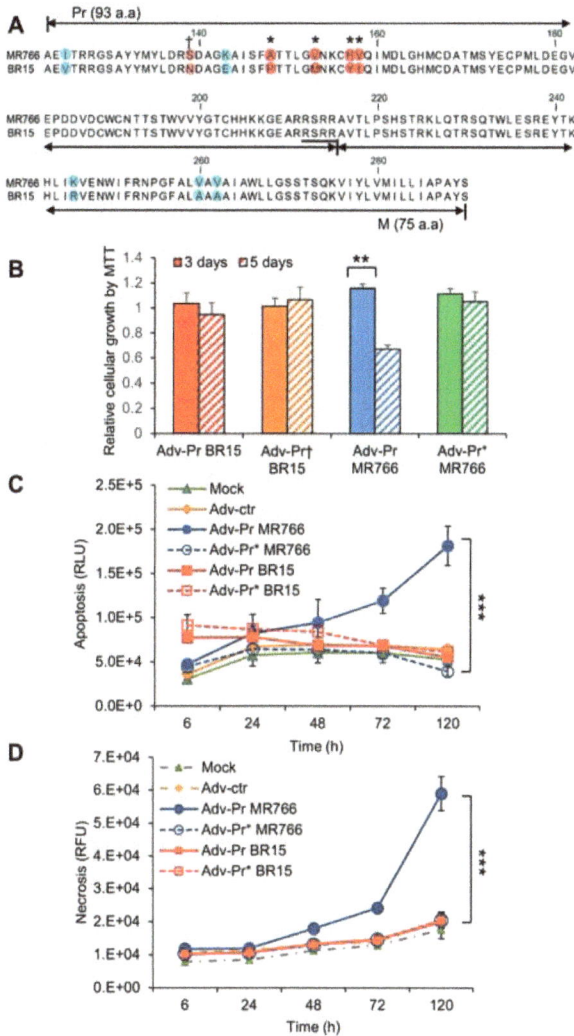

Figure 6. Mutational analysis of the Pr region of the prM protein. (**A**) Mutagenesis of the Pr protein. Four amino acids mutations (A148P, V153M, H157Y and V158I) were generated as shown by "*" on the top of the prM sequence alignments between MR766 (top) and BR15 (bottom). The resulting mutant adenoviral construct is labeled as Adv-Pr*$_{MR766}$. The site of the reverse N139S mutation is shown by "+" on the top of the prM sequence. The corresponding mutant adenoviral construct is labeled as Adv-Pr+$_{BR15}$. (**B**) Cell proliferation and viability by the MTT assay. Only Adv-prM showed significant differences overtime with $p < 0.05$ (**). Adv-Pr-induced cell death was measured by (**C**) apoptosis, and (**D**) necrosis over time. The underlined RSRR sequence indicates the putative furin cleavage site on the prM protein, based on its consensus target site Arg-X-Lys/Arg-Arg↓, where the arrow indicates the location of furin cleavage site. Two-way ANOVA was used to calculate the differences between Adv-prM and Adv-M for (**C**) and (**D**). The differences between Adv-Pr MR766 and Adv-Pr* MR766 were highly significant with $p < 0.01$ (***). However, the difference between Adv-Pr BR15 and Adv-Pr+ BR15 was not significant with $p > 0.99$ for both apoptosis and necrosis. All quantitative results represent average and standard deviation (X ± SD).

3. Results

3.1. Comparison of Viral Infectivity Between the Historical African Zika Virus and the Epidemic Brazilian Zika Viruses in Human Brain Glial SNB-19 Cells

Viral infectivity is defined as the ability of the ZIKV to bind, enter, and to replicate in host cells over time [40]. The goal of this experiment was to compare the viral infectivity between the epidemic Brazilian ZIKV molecular clones (BR15 and ICD) and the historical African ZIKV molecular clone (MR766). We first compared the viral attachment between molecular clones derived from epidemic Brazilian ZIKV strains (BR15 and ICD) and from the historical African ZIKV strain (MR766). All three ZIKV molecular clones have been reported previously [30,36]. The historical MR766 ZIKV strain is the first documented Zika strain that was isolated from caged monkey in the Zika forest in Uganda in 1947 [9]. Two epidemic ZIKV strains, BR15 (BeH819015) and ICD (Paraiba_01/2015) were isolated from Brazil in 2015 during the ZIKV epidemic [34,36]. A human brain glial cell line SNB-19 was used in this study because it is highly permissive to ZIKV infection [32].

The SNB-19 cells were infected with these three ZIKV molecular clones at the MOI of 1.0. After 1 h of incubation on ice, the free viruses were removed by washing the infected cells with cold RPMI 1640 medium supplemented with 2% FBS. Cell-associated viral RNA (vRNA), which represents the viruses attached to the cell surface, was isolated and quantified by real-time RT-PCR. A housekeeping gene, GAPDH, was used as an endogenous control for the measurement of viral bindings. As shown in Figure 1A, statistically significant differences in the virus binding to the SNB-19 cells were observed. Specifically, the numbers of ZIKV ICD or BR15 viral particles, that bound to the cells were about 4.2- to 9.5-fold lower, compared to the MR766 molecular clone.

We next monitored ZIKV viral replication over a time period of 3 days by real-time RT-PCR analysis (Figure 1B). The infection of the MR766 results, in consistently high viral RNA levels, were about 30-fold higher than that of BR15 or ICD over time. Both MR766 and BR15 displayed comparable replication kinetics, with a replication rate of 5.9 ± 0.71 fold-increase, and 4.4 ± 0.47 fold-increase, from 24 h, to 48 h p.i., respectively. The rate of vRNA decreased thereafter, presumably due to cytotoxicity. Notably, the vRNA in the ICD-infected cells was relatively stable over time, with an average replication rate of 1.3 ± 0.27 fold-increase, from 24 h to 48 h p.i.

Since there were clearly differences in the levels of viral bindings and the rates of vRNA production between the two types of molecular clones, we tested whether they were due to the viral permissiveness to SNB-19 cells, which typically represents the result of viral circumvention to host antiviral responses. The percentage of cells producing ZIKV particles was measured at 48 h p.i. Cells were immune-stained using the monoclonal antibody 4G2, which is directed against the flavivirus E protein [32]. The results of the immunostaining are shown in (Figure 1C), and the percentages of infected cells with each molecular clone are shown in (Figure 1D). Infection with the MR766 molecular clone resulted in statistically higher percentages of infected cells, with an average of 81.9% than the two Brazilian molecular clones, that displayed 57.8% for BR15 and 46.1% for ICD.

Together, these data indicate that the historical African strain MR766 showed a higher rate vRNA production and better infectivity in SNB-19 cells than that of the epidemic Brazilian ZIKV molecular clones (BR15 and ICD) presumably due to, at least in part, higher level of virus binding.

3.2. Comparison of the Historical Zika Virus with the Brazilian Epidemic Zika Viruses in Their Abilities to Induce Cytotoxicity

We next tested ZIKV-mediated cytotoxicity of the three ZIKV molecular clones. The SNB-19 cells were infected with the three molecular clones separately, as described in the Materials and Methods section. The MTT assay, which measures cell proliferation and viability [39], was used to measure the impacts of ZIKV infection on cellular metabolic activities. As shown in Figure 2A, cell proliferation and viability decreased rather rapidly in the MR766-infected cells between 24 h to 72 h p.i., whereas BR15- and ICD-infected cells were less affected. Even though the trend was clear, the differences are not statistically significant. ZIKV-mediated cell death was then measured over the same period of time by Trypan blue staining that specifically detects dead cells. Time-dependent cell death was observed in cells infected with all three molecular clones. ZIKV-induced cell death was the most pronounced at 72 h p.i., in which the rate of MR766-induced cell death was significantly increased with 49.0 ± 5.0% of Trypan blue-positive cells than that of BR15 or ICD both with 25.3 ± 2.1%, and 27.9 ± 4.4% of dead cells, respectively (Figure 2B; two-tailed t-test). To further assess whether ZIKV-induced cell death in the SNB-19 cells was caused by apoptosis, we carried out an immunostaining assay to measure in situ Caspase-3 (Casp-3) cleavages, a hallmark of apoptosis [30,32]. In mock-infected cells, little or no cells showed background staining (Supplemental Figure S1A); whereas ZIKV-infected cells showed Casp-3 cleavages, and MR766-infected cells showed significantly higher percentage of apoptotic cells (Figure 2C; two-tailed *t*-test, $p \leq 0.001$). These data show that the historical MR766 molecular clone is more apoptotic than the two Brazilian molecular clones (BR15 and ICD), suggesting that mutations within the epidemic strains might contribute to the reduced cytotoxicity.

3.3. Effects of the C-prM Region on Viral Infectivity

Since there were clear differences in viral infectivity between the historic and epidemic ZIKV strains in SNB-19 cells (Figure 1), we were interested in identifying which part of the ZIKV genome is responsible for the observed differences. Hereafter, we only focused on MR766 and BR15 molecular clones, as BR15 and ICD were very similar. Our previous study showed that the structural protein region (C-prM-E) of the ZIKV genome contributed to initiation of viral infection [30]. In this study, we decided to generate chimeric viruses, by separating the C-prM region from the E region of the structural proteins, using the ISA method [33]. In this way, we were able to differentiate the possible contribution of the C-prM region to viral infectivity or cytotoxicity from that of the E region. Specifically, the C-prM region of the MR766 was exchanged with that of the BR15 molecular clone, or vice versa. The two resulting new chimeric viruses were designated as M/B or B/M, in which the chimeric M/B virus carries the C-prM region of the MR766 with the rest of viral genome from the BR15; conversely, the chimeric B/M virus carries the BR15 C-prM region and the rest of the genomic structure is from MR766 (Figure 3A). These two chimeric viral genomes were assembled separately in Vero 76 cells, as previously described [30]. The viruses were recovered from cell supernatants, and were then amplified twice in Vero76 cells. The final viral titers were determined using the plaque-forming assay [38].

The ability of the two chimeric viruses to bind SNB-19 cells was firstly evaluated (Figure 3B). As the E protein is responsible for viral attachment to cells [10,21], the levels of cell attachment indeed corresponded to which ZIKV strain the E region originated from. For example, as we previously demonstrated [30], significantly high levels of cell-attached vRNA were observed with ZIKV clones harboring the MR766 structural proteins. Similar levels of cell-associated vRNA were detected with the B/M virus, in which the MR766-derived E protein is presented. In contrast, both the BR15 and the M/B viruses were less efficient in attaching to SNB-19 cells. The same viral binding test was also conducted in a different cell line A549, and similar results were observed (Supplemental Figure S2A). These results confirm the link between the E protein and cell attachment, and demonstrate that C-prM region is not directly involved in viral attachment to the host-cells. In addition, the initial levels of ZIKV viral replication as measured by RT-PCR correlated with the levels of virus attachment to SNB-19 cells (Figure 3C). MR766 and B/M showed significantly higher levels of vRNA over time than BR15 and M/B, with similar kinetics. Consistently, the conventional plaque-forming assay was also used to test viral infectivity of newly generated chimeric viruses in A549 cells. The test results showed a strong correlation between 4G2-positive cell percentages and viral progeny productions (Supplemental Figure S2B).

We next analyzed the percentages of SNB-19 cells infected with these two chimeric viruses and their parental controls. As shown in (Figure 3D,E), both chimeric viruses were able to infect the SNB-19 cells. Interestingly, an opposite correlation was observed between the chimeric viruses and the parental viruses in the percentages of viral infection to the SNB-19 cells. Statistical two-tailed and paired *t*-test analyses showed that the differences between MR766 vs. BR15, and MR766 vs. B/M were highly significant with $p \leq 0.01$ (***) for both comparisons; whereas the difference between MR766 and M/B was not significant with $p = 0.64$. Thus, the levels of infected cells, with a given chimeric virus, correlated with the C-prM region of its parental virus, not the E region. Indeed, in the cells infected by the M/B chimeric virus, the percentage of infected cells was significantly higher than that of BR15, but it was comparable with that of MR766 ($p = 0.64$, two-tailed and paired t-test). A similar correlative relationship was also observed between the B/M chimeric virus and the BR15 virus (Figure 3E).

These results confirm that ZIKV E region correlates with viral attachment to the host cells, and suggest that ZIKV C-prM region contributes to the permissiveness of viral infection.

3.4. Contribution of the ZIKV C-prM Region to ZIKV-Induced Growth Restriction and Apoptotic Cell Death

The data shown in Figure 3D,E were unexpected. It is believed that if the virus has high binding efficiency to the host cells, it should result in higher percentage of viral infected cells. Since ZIKV induces cytotoxicity, we reasoned that the C-prM region could contribute to ZIKV-induced cytotoxicity, which affects the outcome of the measured levels of viral infection. To test this possibility, we measured the effects of chimeric viruses on cell proliferation and viability. As shown in Figure 4A, genetic determinant(s) of cell viability was associated with of the C-prM region of the viral genome. For instance, both MR766 and M/B showed similar cell growth pattern, which was clearly distinguishable from that of BR15 and B/M. Nevertheless, a statistical t-test showed those differences were not statistically significant. However and consistent with the trend shown in Figure 4A, a similar but statistically significant correlation was detected in ZIKV-induced cell death (Figure 4B), and in apoptosis, as shown by the casp-3 cleavages (Figure 4C). Together, these data supported the idea that the C-prM domain of African ZIKV molecular clone contributes to ZIKV-induced growth restriction and apoptotic cell death.

3.5. Effect of prM Protein and Its Processed Protein Products (M and Pr) on ZIKV-Induced Cytotoxicity

Considering the association of the C-prM region of ZIKV genome with virus-induced cytotoxicity, it was interesting to evaluate whether the proteolytic processing of the C-prM protein precursor relates to cytotoxicity. Here, we focused on testing prM protein and its processed protein products (M and Pr). The C protein was studied separately. The proteolytic cleavage of prM by furin protease generates two proteins: a virion-associated M protein of 75 a.a. and an extracellularly released Pr polypeptide of 99 a.a. The M protein is only found in mature and fully infectious virus particles [10,41].

The SNB-19 cells were transduced with MOI of 1000 by Adv-prM, Adv-Pr or Adv-M, that were derived from MR766. They represent the precursor prM and a processed mature M protein and a Pr protein product, respectively. Mock-transduced cells were used as a background control. Cell viability was first measured at day 3 and day 5 p.i. as shown in Figure 5A. Both the prM and the Pr caused approximately 50% reduction of the cell viability while no clear change in cell viability was observed in the Adv-M-transduced cells. The prM effect on cell viability was further confirmed in different cell lines including human brain microvascular endothelial cells (HBMEC) and a neuronal cell line SH-SY5Y (Supplemental Figure S3A). Time-dependent measurements of cellular necrosis (Figure 5B) and apoptosis (Figure 5C), by real-time Annexin V Apoptosis and Necrosis assays, showed comparable results, in total agreement with the MTT assay at end of the time course. Note that the differences among the three Adv constructs were relatively small at early time points and only became significant at 120 h p.i.

Overall, our data indicated that ZIKV prM protein and its cleaved Pr protein product, but not the matured M protein, induced apoptotic cell death in SNB-19 cells.

3.6. Mutational Analysis of the Pr Region of the prM Protein and Their Effects on ZIKV-Induced Cytotoxicity

In Figure 2, we showed that the MR766 was more cytotoxic than the BR15. Our data further showed that the MR766 prM, and its cleaved product, Pr protein contributed to ZIKV-induced cytotoxicity, suggesting that the Pr region of the prM protein might be the source of prM-mediated cytotoxicity (Figure 5). However, we did not know whether Pr-induced apoptosis is ZIKV strain-specific. There is a total of 10 known divergent a.a. mutations of prM protein between MR766 and BR15 (Figure 6A) [31]. Seven of those mutations are within the Pr region. Thus, we tested whether the Pr-induced cell death is only restricted to MR766, or whether we could alter the Pr-induced cell death by introducing divergent genetic mutations, that are present in the Pr protein of the BR15 molecular clone into the MR766 Pr protein. The residue 139 was first selected for reverse genetic analysis because the pre-epidemic to epidemic mutational transition from S to N at the residue 139 (S139N) of the Pr region was reported to be a crucial site for ZIKV-induced microcephaly [31]. Here, we reversed this mutational transition by generating the N139S mutation on the backbone of the BR15 Pr nucleotide sequence (Adv-Pr$_{BR15}$) to generate the Pr mutant (Adv-Pr$^{\dagger}_{BR15}$). Another four additional a.a. mutational sites (A148P, V153M, H157Y and V158I) were selected for the forward genetic mutagenesis. This region was of particular interest because the A148P mutation could have a major impact on protein folding. We decided to replace the entire cluster 148→158 as adjacent mutations could support putative structure changes associated with A148P mutation. The wildtype MR766 Pr nucleotide sequence (Adv-Pr$_{MR766}$) was used to generate the MR766 Pr mutant clone (Adv-Pr$^{*}_{MR766}$), that carries the four selected mutants to represent forward genetic mutations.

The effect of Adv-Pr$^{\dagger}_{BR15}$ or Adv-Pr$^{*}_{MR766}$ on the SNB-19 cell viability was measured by the MTT assay and compared to the wild type Adv-Pr$_{BR15}$ or the Adv-Pr$_{MR766}$. The expression of Adv-Pr$_{BR15}$ showed comparable proliferation and viability at day 3 and day 5 p.i., suggesting that the BR15 Pr is not as cytotoxic as the MR766 (Figure 6B). Next, we analyzed the effect of the N139S reverse mutation in the BR15 Pr protein. The introduction of the N139S substitution into the BR15 Pr protein showed little or no significant changes of BR15 Pr-induced growth restriction and cell death. In contrast and similar to what we showed in Figure 5A, about 50% decrease of cellular growth was observed in cells transduced with the wildtype Adv-Pr$_{MR766}$ at 5 days *p.i.* (Figure 6B). However, cells infected with the mutant Adv-Pr$^{*}_{MR766}$ displayed no viability decrease in cellular growth, in marked contrast with cells transduced with the wildtype Adv-Pr$_{MR766}$ at 5 days p.i. (Figure 6B). Similarly, the induction of necrosis (Figure 6C) and apoptosis (Figure 6D) by Adv-Pr$_{MR766}$ was completely blocked by the four a.a. mutations generated in the Pr region.

These data suggest that the Pr region of the MR766 prM protein is indeed responsible for prM-induced cytotoxicity. By introducing the four epidemic and divergent a.a. variants (A148, V153, H157 and V158) to the MR766 Pr region of the prM protein, by forward mutagenesis, alleviated MR766 Pr-induced apoptotic cell killing. This suggests that the acquisition of these four a.a. in BR15 could be responsible for its attenuated cytotoxic phenotype. However, reverse genetic mutation at the residue 139 (N139S) did not improve Adv-Pr$_{BR15}$-induced cytotoxicity, indicating the N139S mutation does not seem to play a role in prM-induced cytotoxicity.

4. Discussion

In this study, we showed that the historic African MR766 ZIKV strain displays different characteristics from that of the epidemic Brazilian strains BR15 and ICD. Those differences include the levels of virus attachment to the human brain glial SNB-19 cells, viral infection and replication overtime (Figure 1), as well as cytotoxicity, as measured by cell proliferation and apoptotic cell death (Figure 2). Since our early study showed that the structural protein region is responsible for the initiation of viral infection, in this study, we further examined the contribution of ZIKV structural prM-E proteins to viral infectivity and cytopathic effects. This was accomplished by generating chimeric viruses (M/B and B/M) that swap the C-prM and E regions of the structural proteins between the MR766 and the BR15 viral genomes. We showed that the E protein is associated with viral attachment to host cells (Figure 3B,C) and the C-prM region is correlated with viral permissiveness and ZIKV-induced cytotoxicity (Figure 3D,E; Figure 4). Further analysis of the prM and its processed protein product, the mature M protein and the Pr protein, indicated that the Pr region of the prM is responsible for the prM-induced cytopathic effects (Figure 5). To further pinpoint where exactly the specific changes occurred in the Pr region of the prM protein, which contributes to the differences observed between MR766 and BR15, we carried out genetic mutagenesis (Figure 6A) to test whether we could reverse or mimic the respective effects observed in MR766 or BR15. As a result, we showed that the forward genetic mutation at four a.a. changes (A148P, V153M, H157Y and V158I) reversed MR766 Pr-induced cytopathic effects (Figure 6B–D). However, the reverse genetic mutation at the residue of 139 (S139N) did not show any clear effect (Figure 6B–D).

Differences between the historic African MR766 strain and the epidemic Brazilian ZIKV strains have been reported previously [for reviews, see [27,28]]. Although the specific causes of those differences are currently unknown, it is possible that the neurological defects caused by the epidemic Brazilian ZIKV in humans were attributed by subtle but important changes. Those newly adapted changes could include the alteration of viral infection patterns to human brain cells, the ability to establish replication in host cells, and the induction of neuropathic damages that lead to those observed ZIKV-associated neurological disorders [27]. Overall, the historic African MR766 strain has been shown to be more virulent and to cause more severe brain damage than that of the epidemic Asian lineages, including the Brazilian strains [25,42–44]. Indeed, the results of our comparative studies, described here between the historic African MR766 and the epidemic Brazilian BR15 and ICD molecular clones, supported this general notion that MR766 strain is more pathogenic than Brazilian strains.

One of our earlier studies suggested that the structural proteins contribute in part to the differences we observed between historical MR766 and epidemic BR15 strains of Zika viruses [30]. Following that lead, we further dissected the structural proteins of those two ZIKV molecular clones and evaluated the effect of separating the C-prM proteins from the E protein in viral infectivity and induction of cytotoxicity. This objective was achieved by swapping the C-prM region of the viral genome between the two viruses (Figure 3A). Our results suggested that the E protein is likely associated with viral attachment to host cells (Figure 3B,C) whilst the C-prM region is responsible for ZIKV permissiveness and ZIKV-induced cytopathic effects (Figure 3D,E; Figure 4). The finding that, E protein is linked to viral attachment to host cells, is expected because E protein is a major viral surface protein that is responsible for the viral entry. It is a crucial that the viral determinant for initiating the ZIKV-host interaction and for determining viral pathogenesis, and further investigations are needed [10,21]. Our study also suggests a possible relationship between ZIKV permissiveness and ZIKV-induced apoptosis, which would be based on the Pr, a processed protein product by furin cleavage of the prM protein. It would be interesting to clarify the exact contribution of the Pr protein in this relationship.

Here, we provide evidences showing that the function of the prM protein is linked to ZIKV-induced cytotoxicity that could affect the outcome of viral infection (Figure 3D,E; Figure 4). This finding is consistent with our previous reporting showing that the prM protein induces cytopathic effects in fission yeast cells [15]. The dissection analysis of the prM processing further indicated that the functional domain of the prM-mediated cytotoxicity resides within the Pr region of the protein (Figure 5). Most interestingly, reverse genetic analysis by converting asparagine (N) at residue 139 of the BR15 molecular clone to serine (S) of the MR766 molecular clone (N139S) did not significantly alter the cytopathic effects of BR15 Pr (Figure 6B–D). In contrast, forward genetic mutation analysis completely reversed the MR766 Pr-induced cell growth restriction and apoptotic cell death (Figure 6B–D), by replacing four divergent a.a. at residues 148, 153, 157 and 158 presented in MR766, with that of BR15 (A148P, V153M, H157Y and V158I). Note that, ideally, a reciprocal mutant construct should also be generated using BR15 backbone to test whether the opposite effect can be observed. However, the presence of additional divergent amino acids in the Pr protein (Fig. 6A) could contribute to the observed phenotypes that will complicate the interpretation of the experimental results using reciprocal constructs. Similarly, to confirm the mutant effect of Pr during viral infection, it would be desirable to generate a MR766 mutant molecular clone that contains the four described a.a. and test their mutant effect in the context of viral infection. This is not possible because, besides the prM, the ZIKV-induced apoptotic phenotype is also contributed by other viral proteins, such as

Viruses **2019**, *11*, 157

non-structural proteins during viral infection. For these reasons, we decided not to generate this reciprocal adenoviral mutant construct or the mutant viral molecular clones.

It should be mentioned that an early study indicates that the pre-epidemic to epidemic mutational transition (S139N) of the prM protein is a crucial site for ZIKV-induced microcephaly [31]. This forward genetic substitution in the viral polyprotein of a presumably less neurovirulent Cambodian ZIKVFSS13025 strain [45], substantially increased ZIKV infectivity in both human and mouse neuronal cells, that led to more severe microcephaly in the mouse fetus, as well as higher mortality rates in neonatal mice [31]. The results of this study suggested an important contribution of prM to fetal microcephaly. However, the molecular mechanism in which prM contributes to microcephaly, and the functional impact of S139N mutation on the prM function in human host cells, are presently unknown. It is intriguing to note that residue 139 is located in the Pr region of the prM protein. Since neither prM nor Pr are present in the mature and infectious viral particles [24,46], it would be interesting to test whether the N139S substitution in the MR766 strain or the four divergent mutations in the BR15 strain will have any effects on their abilities to infect human brain cells.

Supplementary Materials: The following are available online at http://www.mdpi.com/1999-4915/11/2/157/s1, Figure S1: Representative pictures of the immunostaining assay to measure caspase 3 cleavages (A) as shown in Figure 2C; Figure S2: Correlation of viral attachment and viral infection between chimeric viruses and their parental viruses in A549 cells; Figure S3: Effect of Adv-prM expression on ZIKV-induced cell viability in different cell lines.

Author Contributions: Conceptualization, P.D., G.G. and R.Z.; Formal analysis, R.Z.; Investigation, G.L. and S.B.; Methodology, K.T. and A.P.; Writing—original draft, R.Z.; Writing—review and editing, P.D. and G.G.

Funding: This study was funded in part by National Institute of Health (NIH R21 AI129369) and the University of Maryland Medical Center (to R.Y.Z.). A.P. and K.T. were supported by National Institute of Allergy and Infectious Diseases (NIAID) Intramural Program. This work was also supported by the ZIKAlert project (European Union-Région Réunion program under grant agreement n SYNERGY: RE0001902). S.B. is the recipient of a PhD degree scholarship from La Réunion Island University (Ecole Doctorale STS), funded by the French ministry MEESR (Ministère de l'Education, de l'Enseignement Supérieur et de la Recherche).

Acknowledgments: The authors would like to thank: Hengli Tang from Florida State University for providing the SNB-19 cell line, Kim Kwang Sik from Johns Hopkins University for the human brain microvascular endothelial cells (HBMEC) cell line, and Mohammed Rahman from University of Maryland School of Medicine for the Vero76 cells.

Conflicts of Interest: The authors declare no conflict of interest.

References

1. Victora, C.G.; Schuler-Faccini, L.; Matijasevich, A.; Ribeiro, E.; Pessoa, A.; Barros, F.C. Microcephaly in Brazil: How to interpret reported numbers? *Lancet* **2016**, *387*, 621–624. [CrossRef]
2. Melo, A.S.; Aguiar, R.S.; Amorim, M.M.; Arruda, M.B.; Melo, F.O.; Ribeiro, S.T.; Batista, A.G.; Ferreira, T.; Dos Santos, M.P.; Sampaio, V.V.; et al. Congenital Zika Virus Infection: Beyond Neonatal Microcephaly. *JAMA Neurol.* **2016**, *73*, 1407–1416. [CrossRef] [PubMed]
3. Del Campo, M.; Feitosa, I.M.; Ribeiro, E.M.; Horovitz, D.D.; Pessoa, A.L.; Franca, G.V.; Garcia-Alix, A.; Doriqui, M.J.; Wanderley, H.Y.; Sanseverino, M.V.; et al. The phenotypic spectrum of congenital Zika syndrome. *Am. J. Med. Genet. A* **2017**, *173*, 841–857. [CrossRef] [PubMed]
4. Mlakar, J.; Korva, M.; Tul, N.; Popovic, M.; Poljsak-Prijatelj, M.; Mraz, J.; Kolenc, M.; Resman Rus, K.; Vesnaver Vipotnik, T.; Fabjan Vodusek, V.; et al. Zika Virus Associated with Microcephaly. *N. Engl. J. Med.* **2016**. [CrossRef] [PubMed]
5. Driggers, R.W.; Ho, C.Y.; Korhonen, E.M.; Kuivanen, S.; Jaaskelainen, A.J.; Smura, T.; Rosenberg, A.; Hill, D.A.; DeBiasi, R.L.; Vezina, G.; et al. Zika Virus Infection with Prolonged Maternal Viremia and Fetal Brain Abnormalities. *N. Engl. J. Med.* **2016**. [CrossRef] [PubMed]
6. Qian, X.; Nguyen, H.N.; Song, M.M.; Hadiono, C.; Ogden, S.C.; Hammack, C.; Yao, B.; Hamersky, G.R.; Jacob, F.; Zhong, C.; et al. Brain-Region-Specific Organoids Using Mini-bioreactors for Modeling ZIKV Exposure. *Cell* **2016**, *165*, 1238–1254. [CrossRef] [PubMed]
7. Dick, G.W. Zika virus. II. Pathogenicity and physical properties. *Trans. R Soc. Trop. Med. Hyg.* **1952**, *46*, 521–534. [CrossRef]

8. Bell, T.M.; Field, E.J.; Narang, H.K. Zika virus infection of the central nervous system of mice. *Arch. Gesamte Virusforsch.* **1971**, *35*, 183–193. [CrossRef]
9. Dick, G.W.; Kitchen, S.F.; Haddow, A.J. Zika virus. I. Isolations and serological specificity. *Trans. R Soc. Trop Med. Hyg.* **1952**, *46*, 509–520. [CrossRef]
10. Lee, I.; Bos, S.; Li, G.; Wang, S.; Gadea, G.; Despres, P.; Zhao, R.Y. Probing Molecular Insights into Zika Virus(-)Host Interactions. *Viruses* **2018**, *10*. [CrossRef]
11. Musso, D.; Nhan, T.; Robin, E.; Roche, C.; Bierlaire, D.; Zisou, K.; Shan Yan, A.; Cao-Lormeau, V.M.; Broult, J. Potential for Zika virus transmission through blood transfusion demonstrated during an outbreak in French Polynesia, November 2013 to February 2014. *Eurosurveillance* **2014**, *19*. [CrossRef]
12. Duffy, M.R.; Chen, T.H.; Hancock, W.T.; Powers, A.M.; Kool, J.L.; Lanciotti, R.S.; Pretrick, M.; Marfel, M.; Holzbauer, S.; Dubray, C.; et al. Zika virus outbreak on Yap Island, Federated States of Micronesia. *N. Engl. J. Med.* **2009**, *360*, 2536–2543. [CrossRef] [PubMed]
13. Hennessey, M.; Fischer, M.; Staples, J.E. Zika Virus Spreads to New Areas-Region of the Americas, May 2015-January 2016. *Morb. Mortal. Wkly. Rep.* **2016**, *65*, 55–58. [CrossRef] [PubMed]
14. Talero-Gutierrez, C.; Rivera-Molina, A.; Perez-Pavajeau, C.; Ossa-Ospina, I.; Santos-Garcia, C.; Rojas-Anaya, M.C.; de-la-Torre, A. Zika virus epidemiology: From Uganda to world pandemic, an update. *Epidemiol. Infect.* **2018**, *146*, 673–679. [CrossRef] [PubMed]
15. Li, G.; Poulsen, M.; Fenyvuesvolgyi, C.; Yashiroda, Y.; Yoshida, M.; Simard, J.M.; Gallo, R.C.; Zhao, R.Y. Characterization of cytopathic factors through genome-wide analysis of the Zika viral proteins in fission yeast. *Proc. Natl. Acad. Sci. USA* **2017**, *114*, E376–E385. [CrossRef] [PubMed]
16. Chambers, T.J.; Hahn, C.S.; Galler, R.; Rice, C.M. Flavivirus genome organization, expression, and replication. *Annu. Rev. Microbiol.* **1990**, *44*, 649–688. [CrossRef]
17. Harris, E.; Holden, K.L.; Edgil, D.; Polacek, C.; Clyde, K. Molecular biology of flaviviruses. *Novartis. Found. Symp.* **2006**, *277*, 23–39, discussion 40, 71–23, 251–253.
18. Yu, I.M.; Zhang, W.; Holdaway, H.A.; Li, L.; Kostyuchenko, V.A.; Chipman, P.R.; Kuhn, R.J.; Rossmann, M.G.; Chen, J. Structure of the immature dengue virus at low pH primes proteolytic maturation. *Science* **2008**, *319*, 1834–1837. [CrossRef]
19. Mecharles, S.; Herrmann, C.; Poullain, P.; Tran, T.H.; Deschamps, N.; Mathon, G.; Landais, A.; Breurec, S.; Lannuzel, A. Acute myelitis due to Zika virus infection. *Lancet* **2016**. [CrossRef]
20. Faye, O.; Freire, C.C.; Iamarino, A.; Faye, O.; de Oliveira, J.V.; Diallo, M.; Zanotto, P.M.; Sall, A.A. Molecular evolution of Zika virus during its emergence in the 20(th) century. *PLoS Negl. Trop Dis.* **2014**, *8*, e2636. [CrossRef]
21. Fontes-Garfias, C.R.; Shan, C.; Luo, H.; Muruato, A.E.; Medeiros, D.B.A.; Mays, E.; Xie, X.; Zou, J.; Roundy, C.M.; Wakamiya, M.; et al. Functional Analysis of Glycosylation of Zika Virus Envelope Protein. *Cell Rep.* **2017**, *21*, 1180–1190. [CrossRef] [PubMed]
22. Lobigs, M.; Lee, E.; Ng, M.L.; Pavy, M.; Lobigs, P. A flavivirus signal peptide balances the catalytic activity of two proteases and thereby facilitates virus morphogenesis. *Virology* **2010**, *401*, 80–89. [CrossRef] [PubMed]
23. Amberg, S.M.; Nestorowicz, A.; McCourt, D.W.; Rice, C.M. NS2B-3 proteinase-mediated processing in the yellow fever virus structural region: In vitro and in vivo studies. *J. Virol.* **1994**, *68*, 3794–3802. [PubMed]
24. Elshuber, S.; Allison, S.L.; Heinz, F.X.; Mandl, C.W. Cleavage of protein prM is necessary for infection of BHK-21 cells by tick-borne encephalitis virus. *J. Gen. Virol.* **2003**, *84*, 183–191. [CrossRef] [PubMed]
25. Anfasa, F.; Siegers, J.Y.; van der Kroeg, M.; Mumtaz, N.; Stalin Raj, V.; de Vrij, F.M.S.; Widagdo, W.; Gabriel, G.; Salinas, S.; Simonin, Y.; et al. Phenotypic Differences between Asian and African Lineage Zika Viruses in Human Neural Progenitor Cells. *mSphere* **2017**, *2*. [CrossRef] [PubMed]
26. Abushouk, A.I.; Negida, A.; Ahmed, H. An updated review of Zika virus. *J. Clin. Virol.* **2016**, *84*, 53–58. [CrossRef] [PubMed]
27. Simonin, Y.; van Riel, D.; Van de Perre, P.; Rockx, B.; Salinas, S. Differential virulence between Asian and African lineages of Zika virus. *PLoS Negl. Trop Dis.* **2017**, *11*, e0005821. [CrossRef] [PubMed]
28. Beaver, J.T.; Lelutiu, N.; Habib, R.; Skountzou, I. Evolution of Two Major Zika Virus Lineages: Implications for Pathology, Immune Response, and Vaccine Development. *Front. Immunol.* **2018**, *9*, 1640. [CrossRef] [PubMed]

29. Ramaiah, A.; Dai, L.; Contreras, D.; Sinha, S.; Sun, R.; Arumugaswami, V. Comparative analysis of protein evolution in the genome of pre-epidemic and epidemic Zika virus. *Infect. Genet. Evol.* **2017**, *51*, 74–85. [CrossRef] [PubMed]

30. Bos, S.; Viranaicken, W.; Turpin, J.; El-Kalamouni, C.; Roche, M.; Krejbich-Trotot, P.; Despres, P.; Gadea, G. The structural proteins of epidemic and historical strains of Zika virus differ in their ability to initiate viral infection in human host cells. *Virology* **2018**, *516*, 265–273. [CrossRef] [PubMed]

31. Yuan, L.; Huang, X.Y.; Liu, Z.Y.; Zhang, F.; Zhu, X.L.; Yu, J.Y.; Ji, X.; Xu, Y.P.; Li, G.; Li, C.; et al. A single mutation in the prM protein of Zika virus contributes to fetal microcephaly. *Science* **2017**, *358*, 933–936. [CrossRef] [PubMed]

32. Tang, H.; Hammack, C.; Ogden, S.C.; Wen, Z.; Qian, X.; Li, Y.; Yao, B.; Shin, J.; Zhang, F.; Lee, E.M.; et al. Zika Virus Infects Human Cortical Neural Progenitors and Attenuates Their Growth. *Cell Stem. Cell* **2016**, *18*, 587–590. [CrossRef] [PubMed]

33. Gadea, G.; Bos, S.; Krejbich-Trotot, P.; Clain, E.; Viranaicken, W.; El-Kalamouni, C.; Mavingui, P.; Despres, P. A robust method for the rapid generation of recombinant Zika virus expressing the GFP reporter gene. *Virology* **2016**, *497*, 157–162. [CrossRef] [PubMed]

34. Faria, N.R.; Azevedo Rdo, S.; Kraemer, M.U.; Souza, R.; Cunha, M.S.; Hill, S.C.; Theze, J.; Bonsall, M.B.; Bowden, T.A.; Rissanen, I.; et al. Zika virus in the Americas: Early epidemiological and genetic findings. *Science* **2016**, *352*, 345–349. [CrossRef]

35. Widman, D.G.; Young, E.; Yount, B.L.; Plante, K.S.; Gallichotte, E.N.; Carbaugh, D.L.; Peck, K.M.; Plante, J.; Swanstrom, J.; Heise, M.T.; et al. A Reverse Genetics Platform That Spans the Zika Virus Family Tree. *MBio* **2017**, *8*. [CrossRef]

36. Tsetsarkin, K.A.; Kenney, H.; Chen, R.; Liu, G.; Manukyan, H.; Whitehead, S.S.; Laassri, M.; Chumakov, K.; Pletnev, A.G. A Full-Length Infectious cDNA Clone of Zika Virus from the 2015 Epidemic in Brazil as a Genetic Platform for Studies of Virus-Host Interactions and Vaccine Development. *MBio* **2016**, *7*. [CrossRef] [PubMed]

37. Xu, M.Y.; Liu, S.Q.; Deng, C.L.; Zhang, Q.Y.; Zhang, B. Detection of Zika virus by SYBR green one-step real-time RT-PCR. *J. Virol. Methods* **2016**, *236*, 93–97. [CrossRef] [PubMed]

38. Frumence, E.; Roche, M.; Krejbich-Trotot, P.; El-Kalamouni, C.; Nativel, B.; Rondeau, P.; Misse, D.; Gadea, G.; Viranaicken, W.; Despres, P. The South Pacific epidemic strain of Zika virus replicates efficiently in human epithelial A549 cells leading to IFN-beta production and apoptosis induction. *Virology* **2016**, *493*, 217–226. [CrossRef]

39. Mosmann, T. Rapid colorimetric assay for cellular growth and survival: Application to proliferation and cytotoxicity assays. *J. Immunol. Methods* **1983**, *65*, 55–63. [CrossRef]

40. Rodriguez, R.A.; Pepper, I.L.; Gerba, C.P. Application of PCR-based methods to assess the infectivity of enteric viruses in environmental samples. *Appl. Environ. Microbiol.* **2009**, *75*, 297–307. [CrossRef]

41. Zheng, A.; Umashankar, M.; Kielian, M. In vitro and in vivo studies identify important features of dengue virus pr-E protein interactions. *PLoS Pathog.* **2010**, *6*, e1001157. [CrossRef]

42. Shao, Q.; Herrlinger, S.; Zhu, Y.N.; Yang, M.; Goodfellow, F.; Stice, S.L.; Qi, X.P.; Brindley, M.A.; Chen, J.F. The African Zika virus MR-766 is more virulent and causes more severe brain damage than current Asian lineage and dengue virus. *Development* **2017**, *144*, 4114–4124. [CrossRef] [PubMed]

43. Simonin, Y.; Loustalot, F.; Desmetz, C.; Foulongne, V.; Constant, O.; Fournier-Wirth, C.; Leon, F.; Moles, J.P.; Goubaud, A.; Lemaitre, J.M.; et al. Zika Virus Strains Potentially Display Different Infectious Profiles in Human Neural Cells. *EBioMedicine* **2016**, *12*, 161–169. [CrossRef] [PubMed]

44. McGrath, E.L.; Rossi, S.L.; Gao, J.; Widen, S.G.; Grant, A.C.; Dunn, T.J.; Azar, S.R.; Roundy, C.M.; Xiong, Y.; Prusak, D.J.; et al. Differential Responses of Human Fetal Brain Neural Stem Cells to Zika Virus Infection. *Stem Cell Rep.* **2017**, *8*, 715–727. [CrossRef] [PubMed]

45.   Shan, C.; Xie, X.; Muruato, A.E.; Rossi, S.L.; Roundy, C.M.; Azar, S.R.; Yang, Y.; Tesh, R.B.; Bourne, N.; Barrett, A.D.; et al. An Infectious cDNA Clone of Zika Virus to Study Viral Virulence, Mosquito Transmission, and Antiviral Inhibitors. *Cell Host Microbe* **2016**, *19*, 891–900. [CrossRef]
46.   Stadler, K.; Allison, S.L.; Schalich, J.; Heinz, F.X. Proteolytic activation of tick-borne encephalitis virus by furin. *J. Virol.* **1997**, *71*, 8475–8481.

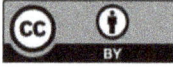

viruses

MDPI

Article

An Evolutionary Insight into Zika Virus Strains Isolated in the Latin American Region

Diego Simón [1,2] , Alvaro Fajardo [1] , Pilar Moreno [1] , Gonzalo Moratorio [1,3,*] and Juan Cristina [1,*]

[1] Laboratorio de Virología Molecular, Centro de Investigaciones Nucleares, Facultad de Ciencias, Universidad de la República, Iguá 4225, Montevideo 11400, Uruguay; dsimon@fcien.edu.uy (D.S.); afajardo32@gmail.com (A.F.); pmoreno@cin.edu.uy (P.M.)
[2] Laboratorio de Organización y Evolución del Genoma, Unidad de Genómica Evolutiva, Facultad de Ciencias, Universidad de la República, Iguá 4225, Montevideo 11400, Uruguay
[3] Laboratorio de Inmunovirología, Institut Pasteur de Montevideo, Mataojo 2020, Montevideo 11400, Uruguay
* Correspondence: gonzalo.moratorio@pasteur.fr (G.M.); cristina@cin.edu.uy (J.C.); Tel.: +598-25250901 (J.C.)

Received: 30 September 2018; Accepted: 20 November 2018; Published: 8 December 2018

Abstract: Zika virus (ZIKV) is an emerging pathogen member of the *Flaviviridae* family. ZIKV has spread rapidly in the Latin American region, causing hundreds of thousands of cases of ZIKV disease, as well as microcephaly in congenital infections. Detailed studies on the pattern of evolution of ZIKV strains have been extremely important to our understanding of viral survival, fitness, and evasion of the host's immune system. For these reasons, we performed a comprehensive phylogenetic analysis of ZIKV strains recently isolated in the Americas. The results of these studies revealed evidence of diversification of ZIKV strains circulating in the Latin American region into at least five different genetic clusters. This diversification was also reflected in the different trends in dinucleotide bias and codon usage variation. Amino acid substitutions were found in E and prM proteins of the ZIKV strains isolated in this region, revealing the presence of novel genetic variants circulating in Latin America.

Keywords: Zika; viral evolution; genetic variability; Bayesian analyses

1. Introduction

Zika virus (ZIKV) is an emerging pathogen member of the *Flaviviridae* family, naturally transmitted between *Aedes* spp. mosquito vectors and human/non-human primates, which serve as amplifying hosts in urban and sylvatic cycles, respectively [1]. The ZIKV genome consists of a single-stranded positive sense RNA molecule of about 10.7 kb with two flanking non-coding regions (5' and 3'NCR), and a single long open reading frame encoding a polyprotein: 5'-C-prM-E-NS1-NS2A-NS2B-NS3-NS4A-NS4B-NS5-3'. This polyprotein is cleaved into capsid (C), precursor of membrane (prM), envelope (E), and seven non-structural proteins (NS) [2]. ZIKV was isolated for the first time in 1947, from the blood of a sentinel Rhesus monkey stationed in the Zika forest, Uganda [3]. Although ZIKV enzootic activity was reported in diverse countries within Africa and Asia, only a few human cases were reported until 2007, when an epidemic occurred in Micronesia [4]. A large ZIKV outbreak took place in French Polynesia during 2013–2014, and then spread to other Pacific Islands [5]. In early 2015, a ZIKV epidemic outbreak took place in Brazil, estimated at 440,000–1,300,000 cases [6]. By January 2016, locally transmitted ZIKV cases were reported by most countries and territories of the American region to the Pan American Health Organization [7].

ZIKV has spread rapidly across the Americas, causing hundreds of thousands of cases of ZIKV disease in this region, as well as microcephaly associated with congenital infection and other neurological disorders [8]. To date, ZIKV has been classified into two major genetic lineages, namely African and Asian. The African lineage is comprised of two groups: The West African (Nigerian cluster) and East African (MR766 prototype cluster) [9,10]. Previous studies have shown that the Asian genetic lineage is responsible for the Pacific Islands and American outbreaks [11,12].

The two viral envelope proteins, prM/M and E, have been used as major targets for vaccine development against ZIKV infections [13], since they are the main determinants for the high stability of ZIKV, and where epitopes for CD4[+] and CD8[+] T-cell adaptive immune responses and neutralizing antibodies are located [13,14]. The most promising vaccines currently in trials are the ones that use a combination of both prM and E proteins [13]. A detailed characterization of prM and E proteins of ZIKV strains circulating in all regions of the world are very important for our understanding of the antigenicity and pathogenesis of ZIKV, as well as for the development of suitable ZIKV vaccines.

For all these reasons, a detailed analysis on the molecular evolution of ZIKV populations is of extreme importance to understand the relation among viruses and hosts, viral survival, fitness, and evasion from the host's immune system [15,16]. In order to gain insight into these matters, we performed a comprehensive phylogenetic analysis of recently isolated ZIKV strains in the Latin American region. Five different genetic clades were observed revealing a process of diversification among the ZIKV strains circulating in this region. Besides, these genetic clades displayed distinct compositional properties. Amino acid substitutions were found in E and prM proteins of the ZIKV strains isolated, revealing the presence of novel genetic variants circulating in the American region.

2. Materials and Methods

2.1. Sequences

Complete coding sequences of 61 available and comparable ZIKV strains, isolated from humans in the Latin American region, from December 2014 through to August 2017, as well as comparable 10 ZIKV strains isolated in the south region of the USA were obtained from GenBank (available at http://www.ncbi.nlm.nih.gov). For strains, accession numbers, geographic location, and date of isolation, see Supplementary Material Table S1. Only strains for which the day, month, and year of isolation was known were included. Sequences were aligned using MUSCLE [17].

2.2. Recombination Analysis

GARD program was used to detect any possible recombination event [18]. There was no evidence of recombination in the dataset.

2.3. Bayesian Coalescent Markov Chain Monte Carlo (MCMC) Analysis

To investigate the evolutionary rate and patterns of ZIKV strains circulating in the Latin American region, we used a Bayesian Markov Chain Monte Carlo (MCMC) approach as implemented in the BEAST package v.1.8.0 [19]. We started by identifying the evolutionary model that best fit our sequence dataset by using the FindModel software (available at http://hiv.lanl.gov/content/sequence/findmodel/findmodel.html). Bayesian Information Criterion (BIC), Akaike Information Criterion (AIC), and the log of the likelihood (LnL), indicated that the Tamura-Nei (TN93) + Γ model was the most suitable model (BIC = 41,048.518; AIC = 39,356.515; and LnL = $-19,531.228$). Importantly, the strict and the relaxed molecular clock models were implemented to test different models (constant population size, exponential population growth, expansion population growth, logistic population growth, and Bayesian Skyline). Statistical uncertainty in the data was reflected by the 95% highest posterior density (HPD) values. By using the TRACER program v1.6 (available at http://beast.bio.ed.ac.uk/Tracer) we assessed the results. Fourty-million generations were needed to obtain convergence, after a burn-in of 4 million steps, which were enough to acquire a suitable sample for the posterior, assessed by effective sample sizes (ESS) with values over 200. The comparison of models was done by measuring AIC in a Bayesian Monte Carlo (AICM) from the posterior output of each of the models using TRACER v1.6 program. Lower AICM values indicated better model fit. The Bayesian Skyline model was the best model to analyze the data (see Appendix A). Through the Tree Annotator program, maximum clade credibility trees were generated, and then visualized in the FigTree program v1.4.2 (available at http://tree.bio.ed.ac.uk).

2.4. Compositional Analyses

For each ZIKV, we determined for the whole polyprotein: Dinucleotide observed/expected ratios (dinucleotide bias), relative synonymous codon usage (RSCU) values for each degenerate codon (all triplets excluding AUG, UGG, and stop codons), and amino acid frequencies; as was described in previous work on the genus *Flavivirus* [20]. These compositional analyses were performed using the R package seqinr [21], with count, rho, and AAstat functions. The relationship between compositional variables and samples was obtained using multivariate statistical analyses; principal component analysis (PCA) is a type of multivariate analysis that allows a dimensionality reduction. Compositional properties of each strain included in this study were obtained, and the distribution of these strains in the plane defined by the first two principal axes of a PCA (PC1 and PC2) examined. Major trends within a dataset were determined using measures of relative inertia and sequences ordered according to their position along the different axes, and correlation between the axes and original variables. For the values obtained from the compositional analyses, see Table S2.

2.5. Prediction of Exposed Residues and Structural Regions of E and prM Proteins

To identify exposed residues and coiled regions of E and prM ZIKV proteins, we used the BepiPred approach [22]. BepiPred uses hidden Markov algorithms in combination with propensity scale methods to predict epitopes in protein sequences. From a FASTA file as input, the method outputs a GFF file with prediction scores and classifications, given a threshold. We used the BepiPred online server (available at http://www.cbs.dtu.dk/services/BepiPred) with 0.5 as threshold.

3. Results

3.1. Bayesian Coalescent Analysis of ZIKV Strains Recently Isolated in the Latin American Region

To address the degree of genetic variability and mode of evolution of the ZIKV strains recently isolated in the Latin American region, a Bayesian MCMC approach was employed [17]. The results shown in Table A1 were the outcome of 40 million steps of the MCMC, using the Tamura-Ney (TN93) + Γ model, a relaxed molecular clock, and the Bayesian Skyline model. The date of the most common ancestor to all ZIKV strains isolated in Latin America was estimated to be in early 2014 (95% HPD October 2013 to December 2014), in agreement with recent results [23–25]. A mean rate of evolution of 1.21×10^{-3} substitutions per site per year (s/s/y) was found for the ZIKV sequences included in these studies (95% HPD 7.55×10^{-4} to 1.66×10^{-3}). This was also in agreement with recent estimations of 1.15×10^{-3} s/s/y [23].

The phylogenetic relationships among ZIKV strains recently isolated in the Latin American region were explored and summarized in a maximum clade credibility tree shown in Figure 1. ZIKV strains isolated in the Latin American region from 2014 to 2017 clustered in at least five different genetic groups, revealing a significant local genetic diversification of the ZIKV strains isolated in this region. Co-circulation of different genetic lineages was observed in several countries in the region (see for instance the ZIKV strains recently isolated in Cuba in 2017).

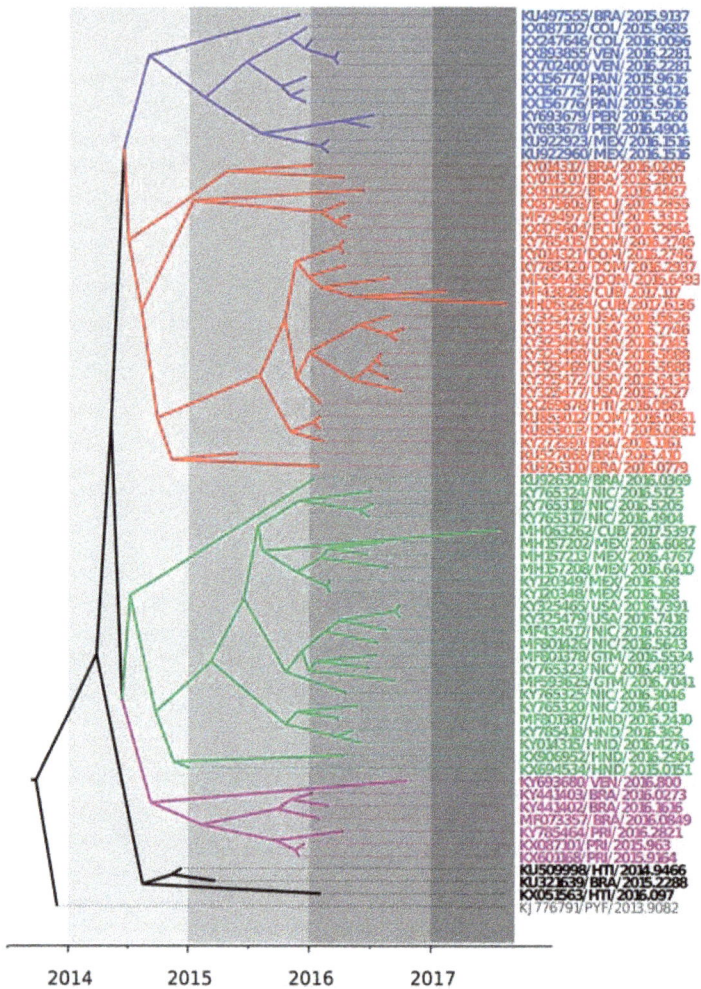

Figure 1. Bayesian maximum clade credibility tree representing the time-scale of ZIKV, obtained by the analysis of 61 complete coding sequences using the Tamura-Ney (TN93) + Γ model, the Bayesian Skyline model, and a relaxed exponential clock. The tree is rooted to the Most Recent Common Ancestor (MRCA) of strains included. The scale at the bottom is in units of evolutionary time and represents the years before the last sampling date. Strains in the tree are shown by their accession number, geographical location, and year of isolation expressed in decimal format. Clades are indicated in blue, red, green, violet, and black.

3.2. Trends in Compositional Properties Across ZIKV Strains Isolated in the Latin American Region

Principal component analysis (PCA) has shown different patterns among the genetic clusters examined (Figure 2; also see Supplementary Material Figure S1 for the loadings of the compositional variables). The phylogenetic clusters of the Zika strains presented in Figure 1 displayed a similar behavior for each compositional property analyzed (i.e., dinucleotide bias, RSCU, and amino acid frequencies).

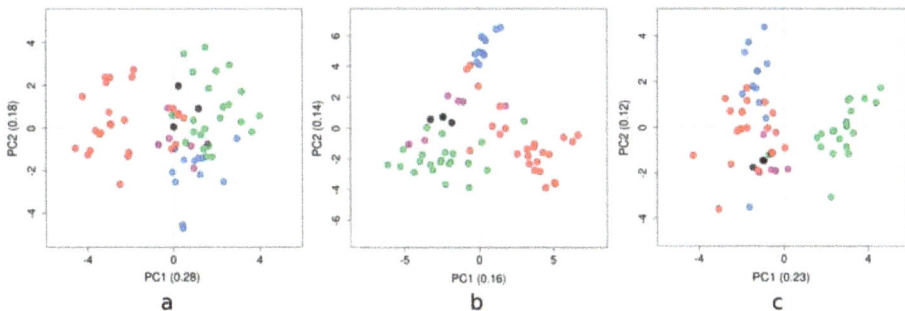

Figure 2. Positions of the ZIKV strains for the first two major axes of principal component analysis of the (**a**) dinucleotide observed/expected ratios, (**b**) relative synonymous codon usage, and (**c**) amino acid frequencies. The proportion of variance explained by each axis is displayed, placed between parentheses. Strains in the plot are colored according to their clade assignment depicted in Figure 1 (i.e., in blue, red, green, violet, and black).

Dinucleotide biases account for the dinucleotides over- and/or under-represented in a genome. For these Zika strains, the first axis (PC1) generated by the PCA accounted for 28% of the total variation, while the second axis (PC2) accounted for 18%. The results of this study are shown in Figure 2a. PC1 tended to separate the majority of clade red sequences from the rest; this axis had strong positive correlations with dinucleotides ApC and GpG, and correlated negatively with UpC and ApG. The other axis tended to distinguish blue and green clades; PC2 correlated positively with UpA and negatively with both UpG and GpU.

The redundancy of the genetic code confers the possibility to tune the efficiency and accuracy of protein production to various levels, while maintaining the same amino acid sequences [26]. The relation of codon usage among viruses and their host's is expected to affect viral survival, fitness, evasion from the host's immune system, and evolution [27]. PC1 accounted for 16% of the total variation, while the PC2 accounted for 14% (Figure 2b). PC1 discriminated the red clade from the green clade; this axis was explained by relatively high usage of CUC, AAU, UAC, and AUC codons, and relatively low usage of GUC, AAC, CUU, and UAU (towards the positive values of the PC1; the opposite towards the negative ones).

Amino acid frequencies vary as a result of non-synonymous mutations across a coding sequence. PC1 and PC2 accounted for 23% and 12% of the total variation, respectively (Figure 2c). PC1 separated the green clade from the other clades, due to a relative enrichment in cysteine and leucine, based on the highest correlations of this axis with the amino acid frequencies. Finally, PC2 was associated with glutamic acid and tryptophan.

3.3. Mapping of Amino Acid Substitutions in the ZIKV E Protein

ZIKV enters the host cell by receptor-mediated endocytosis. Importantly, the E protein has been associated with attachment and endosomal membrane fusion. Thus, the action of E-binding antibodies can impair receptor interaction and/or membrane fusion, making this protein the main target for virus-neutralizing antibodies [28]. Three domains constitute the ZIKV E protein: A central β-barrel domain (DI), an extended dimerization domain (DII), and an immunoglobulin-like segment (DIII) [29]. A fusion loop (FL) is located at the distal end of DII. This loop is inserted directly into the endosomal membrane of the host cell and then triggers fusion thanks to pH-dependent conformational changes. Furthermore, antiparallel dimers are packed in the E protein in a herringbone pattern that lies against the lipid envelope [30].

To investigate if the genetic variability observed among America´s ZIKV strains was associated with antigenic changes displayed by their E protein sequences, we explored their inferred amino acid substitutions. From the 61 strains isolated in this region, amino acid substitutions were found in only eight ZIKV strains with respect to the H/PF/2013 strain of the Asian genotype (accession number KJ776791; Table A2). Intriguingly, three substitutions were found at the DIII domain (V330L, T335A, and T369I) of E proteins from strains isolated in Latin America with respect to the H/PF/2013 strain (Figure 3).

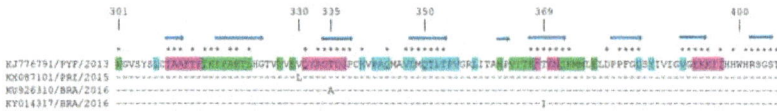

Figure 3. An amino acid sequence alignment of the DIII domain of ZIKV E proteins. Strains are shown by accession number, geographic location, and year of isolation. Identity of the strain H/PF/2013 from the Asian genotype (accession number KJ776791) is shown by a dash. Sequence position relative to the E protein of that strain is shown on the top of the figure. Predicted coiled regions of the protein are indicated by a blue arrow on top of the alignment. Predicted exposed residues are indicated by an asterisk on the upper part of the alignment. Previously described conformational epitopes ABDE, C-C', and LR [30] are shown in green, blue, and magenta.

3.4. Mapping Amino Acid Substitutions in the ZIKV prM Protein

ZIKV virion assembly involves the interaction among prM and E proteins in the endoplasmic reticulum, the encapsulation of the RNA genome with C protein, and the coverage of a lipid bilayer containing a prM-E protein complex to form immature virions. Then, the cleavage of prM to M protein by furin or furin-like proteases in the trans-Golgi network will permit the release of mature virions [31]. Therefore, due to the important function of prM in the ZIKV life cycle, we studied the amino acid substitutions found in the ZIKV strains isolated in the American region. From the 61 strains isolated in this region, only four strains had amino acid substitutions in the prM protein, by comparison with the H/PF/2013 strain of the Asian genotype (Figure 4). All Latin American strains revealed an asparagine (N) at position 139; previous studies revealed that a serine to asparagine amino acid substitution at this position (S139N) of the ZIKV prM protein exhibited the greatest neurovirulence in neonatal mice [32]. Moreover, recent studies revealed that when pre-epidemic strains were compared with epidemic strains, several amino acid substitutions were found among pre-epidemic and epidemic ZIKV prM proteins [11,33]. Interestingly, two new substitutions were found in strains isolated in 2017 in Cuba, in positions where differences among pre-epidemic and epidemic strains were previously reported [11,33]: MF438286 had a lysine at position 143 only observed in pre-epidemic strains (substitution E143K), and MH063264 had a threonine at position 266 (substitution A266T).

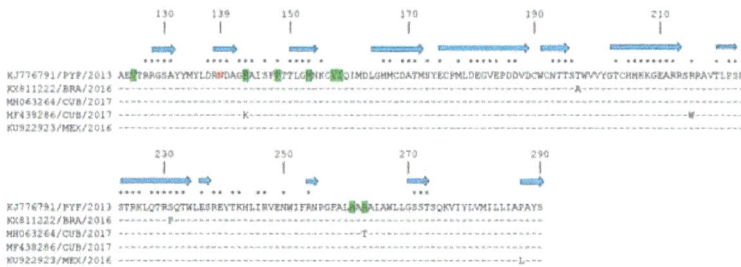

Figure 4. An amino acid sequence alignment of ZIKV prM proteins. Strains are shown by accession number, geographic location, and year of isolation. Identity of the strain H/PF/2013 from the Asian genotype (accession number KJ776791) is shown by a dash. Sequence position relative to the prM protein of that strain is shown on the top of the figure. Predicted coiled regions of the protein are indicated by a blue arrow on top of the alignment. Predicted exposed residues are indicated by an asterisk on the upper part of the alignment. Positions where amino acid substitutions were found between pre-epidemic and epidemic strains are highlighted in green. Position 139 is shown in red.

4. Discussion

Studying the degree of genetic variability and evolution of ZIKV strains would be crucial for diagnostics, vaccine development, and disease management [9]. Previous studies have shown that ZIKV strains from the Asian genotype have evolved and spread to geographically distinct continents since approximately 1960 [34]. These studies also suggest that the strain H/PF/2013 (KJ776791) is likely the ancestor of ZIKV strains of the Asian genotype currently circulating in the American region [12,34,35]. The shape of the tree, near the root, suggested rapid early spread of the outbreak, consistent with the introduction of a new virus to an immunologically naive population. This is also in agreement with recent results [23]. ZIKV genomes from strains isolated in the Latin American region and included in these studies fell into five different genetic lineages (Figure 1). This result highlighted an important degree of diversification in the ZIKV strains in this region, in agreement with previous studies done in America [23,25].

ZIKV strains belonging to distinct genetic clades were placed at different sides in the plane formed by axes 1 and 2 of each PCA (Figure 2). The patterns shown in these figures revealed that the emergence and diversification of ZIKV in this region of the world were also reflected by their dinucleotide biases and codon usage, because the clustering in these PCA plots was comparable to the topology presented in the phylogenetic tree. Previous studies have suggested that ZIKV has evolved host- and vector-specific codon usage patterns to maintain successful replication and transmission chains within multiple hosts and vectors [36], and ZIKV strains are in the process of evolutionary fine-tuning their codon usage [37]. Moreover, selection pressure from *Homo sapiens* on the ZIKV RSCU patterns was found to be dominant compared to *Ae. aegypti* and *Ae. albopictus* vectors [38]. Recent reports identified RNA-editing by the double-stranded RNA-specific adenosine deaminase ADAR as a mechanism that may have contributed to the mutational pressure on the ZIKV genome [39], suggesting that the lower amount of areas associated with ADAR-editing in the RNA minus strand of the Asian ZIKV lineage could be the major cause behind the rise in the number of outbreaks in past decade.

Furthermore, the pattern shown by the use of amino acids (Figure 2c) reflected poorly their phylogeny. The green clade, interestingly, presented a singular behavior in their protein composition that couldn't be explained solely by the divergence assessed in Figure 1. More studies are needed to take into account the extent of selective pressures on the ZIKV polyprotein, or in some subproducts.

Importantly, E protein is a primary antigenic target for neutralizing antibodies, which bind epitopes in all three structural domains, with many type-specific protective antibodies recognizing determinants in the DIII domain [30]. Recent studies identified the ZIKV DIII domain as a potential target for neutralizing antibodies and thus a possible immunogen for vaccines [30]. DIII has been used previously in the context of different flavivirus vaccines [40,41]. In order to discern if the diversification observed among the ZIKV strains isolated in the Latin American region may affect the antigenic structure of E proteins, we mapped the substitutions found in the E protein of ZIKV strains isolated in this region by comparison with the ZIKV strain H/PF/2013 E protein, representative of the Asian genotype [31]. Interestingly, substitutions were observed in the DIII domain of E proteins from strains isolated in this region (Figure 3). Substitution T335A mapped to a previously described DIII LR conformational epitope [30], and two of the three substitutions found mapped to exposed amino acid residues (Figure 3). More studies will be needed to address the biological relevance of these substitutions in ZIKV biology.

ZIKV has a similar structure to other known flaviviruses [42], and prM protein studies revealed that this protein is critical for viral assembly [43]. Therefore, studying the degree of genetic variability and evolution of the prM may contribute to our understanding of ZIKV infectivity and pathogenicity [13]. ZIKV prM, together with E proteins, are being used in most ZIKV vaccines currently undergoing clinical trials [44].

Among several amino acid substitutions found in ZIKV proteins, a serine to asparagine amino acid substitution (S139N) in the ZIKV prM protein, which is observed in most human epidemic strains, exhibited the greatest neurovirulence in neonatal mice [32]. These findings suggested that this serine to asparagine amino acid substitution in prM proteins of epidemic strains may have contributed to the recently observed congenital birth defects associated with ZIKV outbreaks in the American region [8]. Nevertheless, the contributions of other prM substitutions to ZIKV neurovirulence remain to be established.

When pre-epidemic and epidemic strains were compared, amino acid substitutions were identified in ZIKV prM proteins [11,33]. This genomic variability may have been driven by the adaptation of ZIKV to an urban-based transmission cycle targeting humans as hosts instead of the original sylvatic mode of transmission, as recently suggested [36]. Whether the two amino acid substitutions found in these studies at positions 21 and 140 of the prM protein may be related to these facts remains to be studied.

The relative contributions of prM amino acid substitutions to E protein structural biology are not yet well understood. However, amino acid changes may affect prM protein structure and induce structural changes in the E protein since its assembly is dependent on prM protein expression [45].

5. Conclusions

Altogether, these studies showed patterns of diversification of ZIKV strains circulating in the Latin American region in five different genetic groups. Moreover, different trends in dinucleotide bias and in codon usage variation among distinct genetic linages were observed, probably as a result of this diversification. Amino acid substitutions were found in E and prM proteins of ZIKV strains isolated in this region, revealing the presence of novel genetic variants circulating in the American region.

Supplementary Materials: The following are available online at http://www.mdpi.com/1999-4915/10/12/698/s1; Table S1: Origins of the ZIKV strains; Tables S2: Compositional analyses; Figure S1: Loadings of each original variable for the first two major axes of principal component analysis.

Author Contributions: Conceptualization, P.M., G.M. and J.C.; methodology and formal analysis, D.S., A.F.; writing and original draft preparation, G.M. and J.C.; writing, reviewing, and editing, D.S., A.F., P.M. and G.M.

Funding: This research was funded by Agencia Nacional de Investigación e Innovación and PEDECIBA, Uruguay. We acknowledge the Comisión Sectorial de Investigaciones Científica, Universidad de la República, Uruguay, for support through Grupos I + D grant. This work was also funded by the DARPA PREEMPT program managed by Jim Gimlett and administered though DARPA Cooperative Agreement #HR001118S0017-PREEMPT-FP001 (the content of the information does not necessarily reflect the position or the policy of the U.S. government, and no official endorsement should be inferred).

Acknowledgments: We acknowledge Sistema Nacional de Becas, Agencia Nacional de Investigación e Innovación, Uruguay (POS_NAC_2016_1_130463).

Conflicts of Interest: The authors declare no conflict of interest.

Appendix A

Table A1. Bayesian coalescent inference of ZIKV strains.

Parameter	Value [a]	HPD [b]	ESS [c]
Log likelihood	−21,802.85	−21,852.01 to −21,744.02	3179.90
Clock rate [d]	1.21×10^{-3}	7.55×10^{-4} to 1.66×10^{-3}	4823.21
tMRCA [e] All	4.20	3.70 to 5.03	291.75
	29/6/2013	**3/10/2012 to 2/13/2014**	
tMRCA [e] Latin American clade	3.37	2.87 to 6.33	
	3/27/2014	**10/24/2013 to 11/13/2014**	

[a] In all cases, the mean values are shown; [b] HPD, highest posterior density values; [c] ESS, effective sample size; [d] clock rate was calculated in substitutions/site/year; [e] tMRCA, time of the most common recent ancestor is shown in years. The date estimated is indicated in bold.

Appendix B

Table A2. Mapping of amino acid substitutions in E proteins of ZIKV strains isolated in Latin America.

Strain [a]	Amino Acid Position [b]							
	23	51	68	260	330	335	369	443
KU321639/BRA/2015	I							
MH157202/MEX/2016		T						
MF801378/GMT/2016			T					
KU497555/BRA/2015				T				
KX087101/PRI/2015					L			
KU926310/BRA/2016						A		
KY014317/BRA/2016							S	
KX694534/HND/2015								R

[a] Strains are shown by accession number, geographic location, and date of isolation; [b] amino acid positions are relative to strain H/PF/2013 (KJ776791) of the Asian genotype.

References

1. Fajardo, A.; Cristina, J.; Moreno, P. Emergence and Spreading Potential of Zika Virus. *Front. Microbiol.* **2016**, *7*, 1667. [CrossRef] [PubMed]
2. Kuno, G.; Chang, G. Full-length sequencing and genomic characterization of Bagaza, Kedougou, and Zika viruses. *Arch. Virol.* **2007**, *152*, 687–696. [CrossRef] [PubMed]
3. Dick, G.W.; Kitchen, S.F.; Haddow, A.J. Zika virus. I. Isolations and serological specificity. *Trans. R. Soc. Trop. Med. Hyg.* **1952**, *46*, 509–520. [CrossRef]
4. Duffy, M.R.; Chen, T.H.; Hancock, W.T.; Powers, A.M.; Kool, J.L.; Lanciotti, R.S.; Pretrick, M.; Marfel, M.; Holzbauer, S.; Dubray, C.; et al. Zika Virus Outbreak on Yap Island, Federated States of Micronesia. *N. Engl. J. Med.* **2009**, *360*, 2536–2543. [CrossRef] [PubMed]
5. Musso, D. Zika virus transmission from French Polynesia to Brazil. *Emerg. Infect. Dis.* **2015**, *21*, 1887. [CrossRef] [PubMed]
6. Campos, G.S.; Bandeira, A.C.; Sardi, S.I. Zika virus outbreak, Bahia, Brazil. *Emerg. Infect. Dis.* **2015**, *21*, 1885–1886. [CrossRef] [PubMed]
7. Hennessey, M.; Fischer, M.; Staples, E. Zika Virus Spreads to New Areas—Region of the Americas, May 2015–January 2016. *Morb. Mortal. Wkly. Rep.* **2016**, *65*, 55–58. [CrossRef]
8. Krauer, F.; Riesen, M.; Reveiz, L.; Oladapo, O.T.; Martínez-Vega, R.; Porgo, T.V.; Haefliger, A.; Broutet, N.J.; Low, N.; WHO Zika Causality Working Group. Zika Virus Infection as a Cause of Congenital Brain Abnormalities and Guillain-Barré Syndrome: Systematic Review. *PLoS Med.* **2017**, *14*, e1002203. [CrossRef]
9. Faye, O.; Freire, C.C.; Iamarino, A.; Faye, O.; de Oliveira, J.V.; Diallo, M. Molecular evolution of Zika virus during its emergence in the 20(th) century. *PLoS Negl. Trop. Dis.* **2014**, *8*, 2636. [CrossRef]
10. Lanciotti, R.S.; Kosoy, O.L.; Laven, J.J.; Velez, J.O.; Lambert, A.J.; Johnson, A.J.; Stanfield, S.M.; Duffy, M.R. Genetic and serologic properties of Zika virus associated with an epidemic, Yap State, Micronesia, 2007. *Emerg. Infect. Dis.* **2008**, *14*, 1232–1239. [CrossRef]
11. Zhu, Z.; Chan, J.F.; Tee, K.M.; Choi, G.K.; Lau, S.K.; Woo, P.C.; Tse, H.; Yuen, K.Y. Comparative genomic analysis of pre-epidemic and epidemic Zika virus strains for virological factors potentially associated with the rapidly expanding epidemic. *Emerg. Microbes Infect.* **2016**, *5*, e22. [CrossRef] [PubMed]
12. Fajardo, A.; Soñora, M.; Moreno, P.; Moratorio, G.; Cristina, J. Bayesian coalescent inference reveals high evolutionary rates and diversification of Zika virus populations. *J. Med. Virol.* **2016**, *88*, 1672–1676. [CrossRef] [PubMed]
13. Nambala, P.; Su, W.C. Role of Zika Virus prM Protein in Viral Pathogenicity and Use in Vaccine Development. *Front. Microbiol.* **2018**, *9*, 1797. [CrossRef]
14. Goo, L.; DeMaso, C.R.; Pelc, R.S.; Ledgerwood, J.E.; Graham, B.S.; Kuhn, R.J.; Pierson, T.C. The Zika virus envelope protein glycan loop regulates virion antigenicity. *Virology* **2018**, *515*, 191–202. [CrossRef]
15. Holmes, E.C. *The Evolution and Emergence of RNA Viruses*, 1st ed.; Oxford University Press: Oxford, UK, 2009; pp. 113–155. ISBN 978-0-19-921112-8.
16. Domingo, E.; Perales, C. Quasispecies and viruses. *Eur. Biophys. J.* **2018**, *47*, 443–457. [CrossRef] [PubMed]

17. Edgar, R.C. MUSCLE: A multiple sequence alignment method with reduced time and space complexity. *BMC Bioinform.* **2004**, *5*, 113. [CrossRef] [PubMed]
18. Kosakovski-Pond, S.L.; Posada, D.; Gravenor, M.B.; Woelk, C.H.; Frost, S.D. Automated phylogenetic detection of recombination using a genetic algorithm. *Mol. Biol. Evol.* **2006**, *23*, 1891–1901. [CrossRef]
19. Drummond, A.J.; Rambaut, A. BEAST: Bayesian evolutionary analysis by sampling trees. *BMC Evol. Biol.* **2007**, *7*, 214. [CrossRef]
20. Simón, D.; Fajardo, A.; Sóñora, M.; Delfraro, A.; Musto, H. Host influence in the genomic composition of flaviviruses: A multivariate approach. *Biochem. Biophys. Res. Commun.* **2017**, *492*, 572–578. [CrossRef]
21. Charif, D.; Lobry, J.R. SeqinR 1.0-2: A Contributed Package to the R Project for Statistical Computing Devoted to Biological Sequences Retrieval and Analysis. In *Structural Approaches to Sequence Evolution: Molecules, Networks, Populations*, 1st ed.; Bastolla, U., Porto, M., Roman, H.E., Vendruscolo, M., Eds.; Springer: New York, NY, USA, 2007; pp. 207–232. ISBN 978-3-540-35306-5.
22. Larsen, J.E.P.; Lund, O.; Nielsen, M. Improved method for predicting linear B-cell epitopes. *Immunome Res.* **2006**, *2*, e2. [CrossRef]
23. Metsky, H.C.; Matranga, C.B.; Wohl, S.; Schaffner, S.F.; Freije, C.A.; Winnicki, S.M.; West, K.; Qu, J.; Baniecki, M.L.; Gladden-Young, A.; et al. Zika virus evolution and spread in the Americas. *Nature* **2017**, *546*, 411–415. [CrossRef] [PubMed]
24. Massad, E.; Burattini, M.N.; Khan, K.; Struchiner, C.J.; Coutinho, F.A.B.; Wilder-Smith, A. On the origin and timing of Zika virus introduction in Brazil. *Epidemiol. Infect.* **2017**, *15*, 1–10. [CrossRef]
25. Aldunate, F.; Gámbaro, F.; Fajardo, A.; Soñora, M.; Cristina, J. Evidence of increasing diversification of Zika virus strains isolated in the American continent. *J. Med. Virol.* **2017**, *89*, 2059–2063. [CrossRef] [PubMed]
26. Stoletzki, N.; Eyre-Walker, A. Synonymous codon usage in *Escherichia coli*: Selection for translational accuracy. *Mol. Biol. Evol.* **2007**, *24*, 374–381. [CrossRef] [PubMed]
27. Costafreda, M.I.; Pérez-Rodriguez, F.J.; D'Andrea, L.; Guix, S.; Ribes, E.; Bosch, A.; Pintó, R.M. Hepatitis A virus adaptation to cellular shutoff is driven by dynamic adjustments of codon usage and results in the selection of populations with altered capsids. *J. Virol.* **2014**, *88*, 5029–5041. [CrossRef] [PubMed]
28. Heinz, F.X.; Stiasny, K. The Antigenic Structure of Zika Virus and Its Relation to Other Flaviviruses: Implications for Infection and Immunoprophylaxis. Microbiol. *Mol. Biol. Rev.* **2017**, *81*, e00055-16. [CrossRef] [PubMed]
29. Dai, L.; Song, J.; Lu, X.; Deng, Y.Q.; Musyoki, A.M.; Cheng, H.; Zhang, Y.; Yuan, Y.; Song, H.; Haywood, J.; et al. Structures of the Zika Virus Envelope Protein and Its Complex with a Flavivirus Broadly Protective Antibody. *Cell Host Microbe* **2016**, *19*, 696–704. [CrossRef]
30. Zhao, H.; Fernandez, E.; Dowd, K.A.; Speer, S.D.; Platt, D.J.; Gorman, M.J.; Govero, J.; Nelson, C.A.; Pierson, T.C.; Diamond, M.S.; et al. Structural Basis of Zika Virus-Specific Antibody Protection. *Cell* **2016**, *166*, 1016–1027. [CrossRef]
31. Lin, H.H.; Yip, B.S.; Huang, L.M.; Wu, S.C. Zika virus structural biology and progress in vaccine development. *Biotechnol. Adv.* **2018**, *36*, 47–53. [CrossRef]
32. Yuan, L.; Huang, X.Y.; Liu, Z.Y.; Zhang, F.; Zhu, X.L.; Yu, J.Y.; Ji, X.; Xu, Y.P.; Li, G.; Li, C.; et al. A single mutation in the prM protein of Zika virus contributes to fetal microcephaly. *Science* **2017**, *358*, 933–936. [CrossRef]
33. Bos, S.; Viranaicken, W.; Turpin, J.; El-Kalamouni, C.; Roche, M.; Krejbich-Trotot, P.; Desprès, P.; Gadea, G. The structural proteins of epidemic and historical strains of Zika virus differ in their ability to initiate viral infection in human host cells. *Virology* **2018**, *516*, 265–273. [CrossRef] [PubMed]
34. Kostyuchenko, V.A.; Lim, E.X.; Zhang, S.; Fibriansah, G.; Ng, T.S.; Ooi, J.S.; Shi, J.; Lok, S.M. Structure of the thermally stable Zika virus. *Nature* **2016**, *533*, 425–428. [CrossRef] [PubMed]
35. Lanciotti, R.S.; Lambert, A.J.; Holodniy, M.; Saavedra, S.; Signor, L. Phylogeny of Zika virus in Western Hemisphere, 2015. *Emerg. Infect. Dis.* **2016**, *22*, 933–935. [CrossRef] [PubMed]
36. Ramaiah, A.; Dai, L.; Contreras, D.; Sinha, S.; Sun, R.; Arumugaswami, V. Comparative analysis of protein evolution in the genome of pre-epidemic and epidemic Zika virus. *Infect. Genet. Evol.* **2017**, *51*, 74–85. [CrossRef] [PubMed]
37. Wang, H.; Liu, S.; Zhang, B.; Wei, W. Analysis of Synonymous Codon Usage Bias of Zika Virus and Its Adaption to the Hosts. *PLoS ONE* **2016**, *11*, e0166260. [CrossRef] [PubMed]

38. Butt, A.M.; Nasrullah, I.; Qamar, R.; Tong, Y. Evolution of codon usage in Zika virus genomes is host and vector specific. *Emerg. Microbes Infect.* **2016**, *5*, e107. [CrossRef] [PubMed]
39. Khrustalev, V.V.; Khrustaleva, T.A.; Sharma, N.; Giri, R. Mutational pressure in Zika virus: Local ADAR-editing areas associated with pauses in translation and replication. *Front. Cell Infect. Microbiol.* **2017**, *7*, 1–17. [CrossRef] [PubMed]
40. Piontkivska, H.; Frederick, M.; Miyamoto, M.M.; Wayne, M.L. RNA editing by the host ADAR system affects the molecular evolution of the Zika virus. *Ecol. Evol.* **2017**, *7*, 4475–4485. [CrossRef]
41. Martina, B.E.; Koraka, P.; van den Doel, P.; van Amerongen, G.; Rimmelzwaan, G.F.; Osterhaus, A.D. Immunization with West Nile virus envelope domain III protects mice against lethal infection with homologous and heterologous virus. *Vaccine* **2008**, *26*, 153–157. [CrossRef]
42. Sirohi, D.; Chen, Z.; Sun, L.; Klose, T.; Pierson, T.C.; Rossmann, M.G.; Kuhn, R.J. The 3.8 Å resolution cryo-EM structure of Zika virus. *Science* **2016**, *352*, 467–470. [CrossRef]
43. Yoshii, K.; Igarashi, M.; Ichii, O.; Yokozawa, K.; Ito, K.; Kariwa, H.; Takashima, I. A conserved region in the prM protein is a critical determinant in the assembly of flavivirus particles. *J. Gen. Virol.* **2012**, *93*, 27–38. [CrossRef] [PubMed]
44. WHO. WHO Vaccine Pipeline Tracker. 2018. Available online: http://www.who.int/immunization/research/vaccine_pipeline_tracker_spreadsheet/en/ (accessed on 18 November 2018).
45. Oliveira, E.R.A.; de Alencastro, R.B.; Horta, B.A.C. New insights into flavivirus biology: The influence of pH over interactions between prM and E. proteins. *J. Comput. Aided Mol. Des.* **2017**, *31*, 1009–1019. [CrossRef] [PubMed]

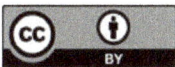

viruses

MDPI

Review

Recent Advances in Zika Virus Vaccines

Himanshu Garg *, Tugba Mehmetoglu-Gurbuz and Anjali Joshi *

Center of Emphasis in Infectious Diseases, Department of Biomedical Science,
Texas Tech University Health Sciences Center, El Paso, TX 79905, USA; tugba.gurbuz@ttuhsc.edu
* Correspondence: himanshu.garg@ttuhsc.edu (H.G.); anjali.joshi@ttuhsc.edu (A.J.); Tel.: +1-915-215-4263 (A.J.)

Received: 16 October 2018; Accepted: 11 November 2018; Published: 14 November 2018

Abstract: The recent outbreaks of Zika virus (ZIKV) infections and associated microcephaly in newborns has resulted in an unprecedented effort by researchers to target this virus. Significant advances have been made in developing vaccine candidates, treatment strategies and diagnostic assays in a relatively short period of time. Being a preventable disease, the first line of defense against ZIKV would be to vaccinate the highly susceptible target population, especially pregnant women. Along those lines, several vaccine candidates including purified inactivated virus (PIV), live attenuated virus (LAV), virus like particles (VLP), DNA, modified RNA, viral vectors and subunit vaccines have been in the pipeline with several advancing to clinical trials. As the primary objective of Zika vaccination is the prevention of vertical transmission of the virus to the unborn fetus, the safety and efficacy requirements for this vaccine remain unique when compared to other diseases. This review will discuss these recent advances in the field of Zika vaccine development.

Keywords: Zika virus; flaviviruses; vaccines; virus like particles; clinical trials; ZIKV

1. Introduction

Zika virus (ZIKV) is a flavivirus that was first isolated in 1947 form a sentinel rhesus monkey in Uganda [1]. Since the identification of this new member of the *Flaviviridae* family, the virus has been implicated in several localized outbreaks. Currently, this mosquito borne flavivirus has been reported to be circulating in 26 countries and territories in Latin America and the Caribbean [2,3]. The natural transmission cycle of the virus involves vectors mainly from the *Aedes* genus, with monkeys as intermediate hosts and humans as occasional hosts [2]. Clinical symptoms of ZIKV infection include asymptomatic cases to an influenza like syndrome with fever, headache, malaise and cutaneous rash [4,5]. However recently, more cases of ZIKV in pregnant women with fetal microcephaly, a range of disorders referred to as congenital Zika syndrome (CZS), and other neurological disorders such as the Guillain–Barre syndrome have been described [6]. The sudden appearance of fetal defects associated with the current outbreaks has drawn international attention, with the primary objective of developing effective vaccines and therapeutics to combat the virus.

2. ZIKV Genomic Organization

The ZIKV genome consists of a single stranded positive sense RNA of 10.749 Kb. The genome consists of a single open reading frame encoding a polyprotein 5′-C-PrM-E-NS1-NS2A-NS2B-NS3-NS4A-NS4B-NS5-3′ [7,8] (Figure 1). This polyprotein is then cleaved into capsid (C), precursor of membrane (prM), envelope (E) and seven non-structural proteins. The E protein (~53 Kd) is the major surface protein involved in the virus binding to the cell surface and membrane fusion [8,9]. As the E protein is the primary target for neutralizing antibodies, it is the preferred antigen in most vaccine platforms. Expression of the structural proteins (prME) of most flaviviruses is sufficient for the formation of sub-viral particles (SVPs) which makes these proteins prime candidates for vaccine development [10–13]. SVPs share several properties with wild-type viruses, such as fusogenic activity [14] and the induction of a neutralizing antibody response [12,13]. The flaviviral capsid protein is important for encapsidation of the viral genome along with interactions with lipids for particle formation [15]. While presence of the capsid protein is not required for the generation of sub-viral particles, inclusion of the protein has proven to be beneficial for vaccine purposes, for a better cell mediated immune response [16]. The flaviviral nonstructural proteins are important for several key aspects of virus replication. With regards to virus assembly, NS3 is the key protein that cleaves the terminal capsid and prME via its N terminal region in conjunction with NS2B, known as NS2B3 [10]. The non-structural proteins also help in evasion of the host's innate immune response by inhibiting production of anti-viral molecules, like the interferons [17].

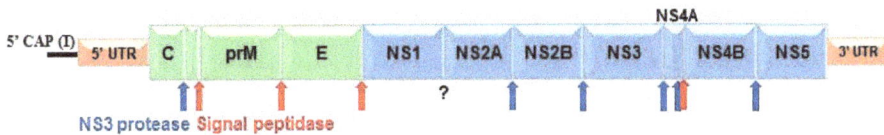

Figure 1. Zika virus genome. The viral genome comprises of a positive sense RNA that encodes a polyprotein that is processed by viral and host cell proteases. The amino terminus of the genome encodes the structural proteins (C-prM-E) essential for virion morphogenesis. The non-structural proteins NS1–NS5 are important for virus replication, polyprotein processing and invoking a cell mediated immune response, along with immune evasion.

3. Zika Disease Outbreak and Pathogenesis

The recent outbreaks of ZIKV were highly concerning due to the devastating outcome of microcephaly and other birth defects in the unborn fetus. Although identified in 1947, ZIKV remained obscure, circulating in certain African and Asian countries with limited number of reported cases. The 2007 outbreak in the Yap island, Micronesia, was the first outbreak beyond Africa and Asia followed by the 2013 outbreak in the French Polynesia with 11% of the population seeking medical attention. Soon thereafter, Brazil saw one of the worst outbreaks of ZIKV in 2015 with some areas reporting sero-positivity as high as 60% [18]. While the recent virus outbreaks have clearly been associated with marked fetal defects and congenital Zika syndrome, the reason for the sudden appearance of these defects, particularly with the current outbreak, remains unknown. Several theories have been proposed for the phenomenon including infection of neuronal progenitor stem cells during pregnancy [19], enhancement of infection due to pre-existing antibodies to Dengue virus (DENV) and/or West Nile virus (WNV) [20], presence of mutations in the envelope glycoprotein of the Asian lineage [21], environmental factors, etc. The incidence of microcephaly during the 2015 ZIKV outbreak was ~100 fold higher than the baseline microcephaly cases in the US, providing the first evidence of a link between Zika infection and birth defects. [22]. Furthermore, the isolation of ZIKV from placental tissue and infected fetuses directly linked the virus to the birth defects, although it remains uncertain if the virus alone is sufficient to induce congenital brain defects [23]. A recent study by Reynolds et al., found that in the United States, 15% of pregnant women with confirmed ZIKV infection in the first trimester had babies with Zika-associated birth defects [22].

4. Need for a Vaccine

Currently there are no ZIKV specific antivirals approved for clinical use, making prophylactic vaccination the best approach to combat the disease. As of now, control of mosquito vectors, prophylaxis against mosquito bites and prevention of pregnancy in endemic areas are the only feasible prophylaxis measures available to reduce the risk of fetal transmission. Although the mortality rate for ZIKV infections is low, the incidence of Guillain Barré syndrome following ZIKV infection warrants vaccination in endemic areas. More importantly, the high incidence of ZIKV induced fetal development disorders like microcephaly in pregnant women suggests an urgent need for an effective vaccine. Although the WHO has declared that the ZIKV outbreak is no longer a Public Health Emergency of

International Concern (PHEIC), due to a decline in the number of cases seen in 2018, the risk of a new outbreak in the near or distant future cannot be ignored. As per the WHO Target Product Profile (TPP) for ZIKV vaccines, the immunization of women of reproductive age, including pregnant women, is the highest priority. Various models have suggested that prioritizing ZIKV vaccination in women of child bearing age is likely to control ZIKV mediated prenatal infections and Congenital Zika Syndrome (CZS) [24]. A ZIKV vaccine that is safe for use in pregnant women is needed not only to combat an outbreak like the recent one in Brazil, but also for routine vaccination in endemic areas [25] that propagate/sustain the mosquito vectors imperative for virus transmission.

5. Characteristics of a Zika Vaccine

Experience from vaccines against other flaviviruses like Japanese Encephalitis Virus (JEV) and Yellow Fever Virus (YFV), suggest that a vaccine against ZIKV will need to fulfill unique criteria. As per Centers for Disease Control (CDC) guidelines, the Purified Inactivated Virus (PIV) vaccine against JEV and the live attenuated vaccine against YFV are largely contraindicated, in pregnant women unless the benefits outweigh the risk. As the target population of the ZIKV vaccine is largely women who are or may become pregnant, the vaccine will need to meet high safety standards. While safety remains a top priority, the efficacy of the ZIKV vaccine also needs to be high as vertical transmission of virus during pregnancy is associated with CZS. Although sterilizing immunity is unlikely to be achieved by a flaviviral vaccine, candidates that elicit a strong enough immune response to prevent trans-placental transfer of the virus to the fetus would be desirable. However, it is unclear what titer of neutralizing antibodies will achieve this, although results from vaccine studies in mouse model show promising results [26]. As ZIKV infections are spreading largely in developing and under developed countries, the cost of vaccination will also be a key consideration point for mass vaccination campaigns. Thus, it would be safe to say that any platform for a ZIKV vaccine must overcome the safety, efficacy and economical barriers to be successful.

6. Zika Vaccine Development

The response by the research community to the recent Zika outbreak has been unprecedented. In less than three years, multiple vaccine candidates have gone through preclinical testing and several have made it to clinical trials (Table 1). The vaccine candidates currently being pursued are discussed below.

Table 1. Zika vaccine platforms in clinical trials.

Clinical Trial No	Platform	Phase	Sponsor	Vaccine Name	Antigen	Dosage	Application	Intervals	N	Planned End Date
NCT02840487	DNA Vaccine	I	NIAID	VRC 319	prME	4 mg	Needle and syringe (Deltoid, IM)	0–8; 0–12; 0–4–8; 0–4–20 week	80–120	Dec 2018
NCT02996461	DNA Vaccine	I	NIAID	VRC 320	prME	4 mg	Single or Split-dose needle or PharmaJet (Deltoid, IM)	0–4–8 week	45	Dec 2018
NCT03110770	DNA Vaccine	II	NIAID	VRC 705	prME	4 or 8 mg	PharmaJet (Deltoid, IM)	0–4–8 week	2400	Jan 2020
NCT02887482	DNA Vaccine	I	Inovio Pharmaceuticals and GeneOne Life Sciences	GLS 5700	prME	2mg	CELLECTRA-3P electroporation (ID)	0–4–12 weeks	160	Jun 2018
NCT02809443	DNA Vaccine	I	Inovio Pharmaceuticals and GeneOne Life Sciences	GLS 5700	prME	1 or 2 mg	CELLECTRA-3P electroporation (ID)	0–4–12 weeks	40	Nov 2017
NCT02963909	Purified Inactivated Virus	I	Walter Reed Army Institute of Research and NIAID	ZPIV	Whole Virus	5 mcg	IXIARO(JEV) prime ZPIV+Alum or YF-VAX (YFV) prime ZPIV+Alum (IM)	0–4–ZPIV; 0–4 JEV-16–20 ZPIV; 0-YFV-12–16–ZPIV week	75	Feb 2019
NCT02952833	Purified Inactivated Virus	I	Walter Reed Army Institute of Research and NIAID	ZPIV	Whole Virus	2.5, 5.0 and 10 mcg	Injection of vaccine with Alum (IM)	0–4–12 weeks	91	Jun 2019
NCT02937233	Purified Inactivated Virus	I	Walter Reed Army Institute of Research and NIAID	ZPIV	Whole Virus	5 mcg	Injection of vaccine with Alum (IM)	0; 0–2; 0–4 week	36	Jun 2018
NCT03008122	Purified Inactivated Virus	I	Walter Reed Army Institute of Research and NIAID	ZPIV	Whole Virus	2.5 or 5 mcg	Injection of vaccine with Alum (IM)	0–4 week	90	Jan 2020
NCT03425149	Purified Inactivated Virus	I	Valneva	VLA1601	Whole Virus	3 or 6 AU (Antigen Units) of ZIKV	Injection of vaccine with Alum (IM)	0–1; 0–4 week	67	Nov 2018
NCT02996890	Live attenuated recombinant vaccine	I	Themis Bioscience	MV-ZIKA	prME in measles vector	High and Low dose	IM Injection	0; 0–4 week	48	Apr 2018
NCT03014089	mRNA vaccine	I/II	Moderna Therapeutics	mRNA-1325	prME	NA	NA	NA	90	Sep 2018
NCT03343626	Purified Inactivated Virus	I	Takeda	TAK-426	Whole Virus	2, 5, 10 mcg	Injection of vaccine with Alum (IM)	0, 4 week	240	Sep 2020
NCT03611946	Live Attenuated Virus	I	NIAID	rZIKV/D4Δ30-713	Whole genome	10^3 plaque-forming units (PFU)	SC	0 week only	28	Sep 2019
NA	Purified Inactivated Virus	I	Bharat BioTech	MR 766	Whole Virus	5, 10 mcg	IM	0–4 week	48	Not Known

NIAID = National Institute of Allergy and Infectious Diseases; mcg = micrograms; mg = milligrams; NA = Not available; IM = Intramuscular; ID = Intradermal; SC = Subcutaneous.

6.1. DNA Vaccines

DNA vaccines against ZIKV were amongst the first platform to be developed concurrently by several groups [26]. All of these approaches utilize the expression of prME proteins from ZIKV, as expression of these proteins in mammalian cells leads to assembly of sub-viral particles that are non-infectious, but retain structure and antigenicity similar to native virions. Larocca et al. were the first to demonstrate that a DNA vaccine expressing codon optimized prME from Brazil (BeH815744 strain, Accession # KU365780) was immunogenic and protected mice against a virus challenge [27]. Similarly, Dowd et al. developed a DNA vaccine incorporating the prME proteins (French Polynesian strain H/PF/2013, Accession # KJ776791) which was immunogenic and provided protection against viremia in mice, as well as non-human primates [28]. Similar studies were conducted by Muthumani et al. who also showed that a DNA vaccine generated via a synthetic prME construct was protective in mice and non-human primates [29]. Additionally, in this study IFNAR$-/-$ mice that were highly susceptible to Zika infection, were protected after DNA vaccination. These vaccine platforms have now progressed to clinical trials (Table 1) and preliminary safety data shows that the DNA vaccines are safe and effective. Gaudinski et al. [30] tested the safety and efficacy of two DNA vaccines; VRC 5288 that expresses a chimeric E protein containing Zika and Japanese encephalitis sequences, and VRC 5283 that expresses the wild type Zika E protein. In both vaccines, the prM signal sequence comprised of the JEV signal to improve particle secretion. In phase 1 clinical trials, the neutralizing response to VRC 5283 was superior to VRC 5288 with 100% of the participants showing neutralizing antibodies in the split needle-free dose group, making it a better candidate to progress to phase 2 clinical trials. Similarly, Tebas et al. [31] tested the efficacy of a Zika DNA vaccine (GLS5700) expressing prME regions of ZIKV from a synthetic construct derived from a consensus sequence. The vaccine showed development of neutralizing antibodies in 63% of the participants. Other DNA platforms have also progressed to clinical trials and are listed in Table 1. Although DNA vaccines provide many advantages like ease of production and rapid adaptation to new and emerging infectious agents, a head to head comparison of DNA vaccine with Purified Inactivated Virus (PIV) vaccine showed that PIV vaccines fare better in terms of immunogenicity, at least in the rhesus monkeys [32].

6.2. Purified Inactivated Virus (PIV) Vaccines

Larocca et al. described the use of a PIV ZIKV vaccine in June 2016, immediately after the 2015 outbreaks [27]. They used the Puerto Rican strain (PRVABC59) for the vaccine candidate that was passaged in Vero cells followed by inactivation with formalin. The alum adjuvanated vaccine provided complete protection in mice after a single immunization followed by challenge with ZIKV-BR (Brazil ZKV2015). Interestingly, higher antibody titers were achieved in the intramuscular versus subcutaneous immunized mice that also correlated with better protection after challenge. In the same study, the authors also compared a DNA based prME vaccine which protected mice completely against ZIKV challenge, after a single immunization. Simultaneously, in September 2016, the same group [32] evaluated the efficacy of the PIV vaccine platform against ZIKV in rhesus monkeys which provided complete protection against virus challenge. The PRVABC59 isolate was used in two doses (weeks 0 and 4) in conjunction with alum and protected monkeys against challenge with the Brazilian and Puerto Rico ZIKV isolate. Moreover, passive transfer of antibodies from immunized monkeys protected both mice and monkeys from ZIKV challenge, in a dose dependent manner. Two doses of the formalin inactivated PRVABC59 vaccine provided protection in monkeys even when challenged a year after immunization [33]. This was superior to two immunizations with a DNA counterpart that conferred protection early at the peak of antibody titers, but efficacy against challenge declined after a year.

The Walter Reed Army Institute conducted three phase 1 trials [34] of the above PIV vaccine using alum adjuvant ($N = 55$) and placebo controls ($N = 12$). The objective was to test the safety and efficacy of the PIV candidate in humans. Healthy participants were administered two doses of the PIV vaccine 29 days apart which was well tolerated with minimal side effects like pain, tenderness at the injection site or generalized fatigue. The neutralizing antibody titers obtained were ≥1:10 at day 43 and adoptive transfer of purified IgG from immunized recipients into Balb/c mice offered protection after challenge evident by reduced viral loads. Sumathy et al. developed a PIV vaccine using the African ZIKV isolate (MR766) and formalin inactivation [35]. Two doses of the vaccine provided 100% protection against the homotypic and heterotypic (FSS 13025, Accession #KU955593) ZIKV strains in AG129 mice. Moreover, passive transfer of immune sera generated in rabbits protected Balb/c mice against live virus challenge. On a related note, Yang et al. [36] described a cDNA clone of PRVABC59 with mutations in the NS1 (K265E) prME (H83R) and NS3 (S356F) proteins that increased virus yield by more than 25 fold when compared to the WT clone. This would not only facilitate high titer virus yield for PIV production in less time, but also minimize the introduction of unwanted mutations upon continuous virus passage.

6.3. Live Attenuated Virus (LAV) Vaccines

Experience from vaccination studies with other flaviviruses like YFV and JEV suggest that live attenuated vaccines (LAV) for ZIKV are likely to be effective. The most widely used LAV for YFV is derived from the 17D strain that has been in use since 1937, and shows significant protection [37]. Similarly, the JEV vaccine based on the attenuated SA14-14-2 strain has been extensively used in endemic areas [38]. With regards to ZIKV, Shan et al. [39] developed a LAV vaccine by deleting 10 nucleotides in the 3′ untranslated region (UTR) of a Cambodian strain of ZIKV (FSS 13025, Accession #KU955593). This attenuated virus provided sterilizing immunity with saturating neutralizing antibody titers in WT adult mice, and did not induce pathology after intracranial injection in 1 day old immunocompetent mice. A single dose of the vaccine also protected rhesus macaques against viremia upon challenge. Further analysis of this LAV vaccine showed that a single dose significantly reduced vertical transmission of Zika in pregnant mice, and prevented testicular damage in male mice [40]. Zou et al. [41] developed a DNA launched version of the LAV vaccine with a 20 bp deletion in the 3′-UTR, and demonstrated the efficacy of the vaccine at extremely low doses (0.5 μg), compared to other DNA vaccines. Besides the direct attenuation of ZIKV, other approaches like chimeric viruses have been used for making attenuated vaccines. Xie et al. [42] showed that a chimeric virus containing Zika prME in a DENV-2 backbone was highly attenuated in A129 mice and provided protective immunity against Zika challenge. Similarly Li et al. [43] used the attenuated JEV strain SA14-14-2 as the backbone to introduce the Zika prME region of an Asian ZIKV strain FSS 13025. When administered as a single dose, this vaccine provided protection against placental and fetal damage in pregnant mice and protected the offspring against intracranial virus challenge. A single vaccine dose was also protective in rhesus monkeys that were challenged with the virus.

6.4. Virus like Particles (VLP) Vaccines

In case of flaviviruses, expression of the structural proteins (prME or CprME) gives rise to non-infectious virus like particles that resemble infectious virions. This provides a method for presentation of viral antigens in a highly native conformation. Thus, VLP vaccines often surpass the elicited immune response when compared to subunit vaccines that are comprised of single proteins [44]. Moreover, VLPs present antigens in their native conformation in a repetitive manner that is recognized effectively by B cells leading to their activation and production of high titers of specific antibodies. Another advantage of VLP vaccines is their ease of production and scalability providing an economic platform, especially by generation of stable cell lines. Due to their non-infectious nature, VLPs are safe for administration in immunocompromised adults, children and pregnant women.

Surprisingly, with regards to ZIKV, the description of VLP platforms came much later than the PIV, DNA and mRNA counterparts. Garg et al. [45] reported the development of prME and CprME VLPs (Suriname 2015, Accession # KU312312.1) and compared them to their DNA counterparts in efficacy studies in mice. Immunization with CprME VLPs generated higher neutralizing antibody titers than prME VLPs. DNA vaccination with prME was less effective than VLPs with CprME

DNA, failing to generate neutralizing antibodies in mice. An advantage of the approach by Garg et al. was the generation of stable cell line secreting the prME VLPs, thereby eliminating the need for routine transfections and DNA amplification for large scale VLP production. This study also brought forth the advantage of incorporating the capsid protein in the VLPs for an enhanced immune response. In a similar study, Boigard et al. [46] compared CprME VLPs (Strain H/PF/2013, Accession # KJ776791.1) with formalin inactivated ZIKV (PIV) and found superior antibody generation with CprME VLPs, versus inactivated virus. While using a transient transfection protocol for VLP generation, their study emphasized the deleterious effects of chemical inactivation on neutralizing epitopes for vaccine production.

Thereafter, a number of studies described the use of different VLP platforms for ZIKV. Yang et al [47] developed a VLP displaying the EIII domain of ZIKV (PRVABC59 (amino acids 1–403, Accession # AMC13911)) on the Hepatitis B core antigen. The advantage of this system was the easy production and purification from Nicotiana plants. The vaccine elicited a strong neutralizing and cellular immune response against different ZIKV strains, and the elicited antibodies did not cause enhancement of Dengue virus infection in cells expressing the Fcγ receptor. Espinoza et al. [48] also developed a prME VLP vaccine ((prM sequence from the African MR766 strain (Accession # KU955594); the E ectodomain from the Brazilian SPH2015 strain (Accession # KU321639) and the stem-anchor from the African MR766 strain (Accession # KU955594)) containing a heterologous IL-2 signal sequence and found that the immune sera generated in WT CB6F1 mice was protective of ZIKV infection in AG129 mice. Basu et al. [49] displayed highly immunogenic potential B cell epitopes from the E protein of ZIKV (strain MR-766) on bacteriophage particles, and saw moderate protection in challenge studies in Balb/c mice. Baculovirus expressed Zika VLPs [50] displaying the prME proteins (strain SZ-WIV01) elicited a potent neutralizing and T cell response in immunized mice. Salvo et al. [51] used the Zika CPrME (strain H/PF/2013, Accession # KJ776791) VLPs to immunize Balb/c and AG129 mice followed by challenge studies and observed decreased viremia or increased survival in respective models.

6.5. Modified mRNA Vaccines

mRNA technology has recently gained popularity in the field of vaccination as mRNA's pose minimal risk of integration into the host genome making them safer than DNA vaccines. mRNA vaccines make use of the host cell processes to translate viral proteins and generally encode the protein of interest, untranslated regions at the 5′ and 3′ end give stability in cells and replacement of uridine residues in the sequence with other natural modifications, prevent indiscriminate innate immune activation [52,53]. Moreover, encapsulation of naked mRNA into lipids not only increases stability, but also helps in high protein expression by aiding in intramuscular delivery. After the 2015 ZIKV outbreaks, one of the first vaccine strategies to be described was the use of modified mRNA to protect against ZIKV infection in two simultaneous reports published in March 2017 [54,55]. Richner et al. developed a modified RNA with a type-1 cap, a signal sequence from human IgE or JEV, and the prME genes of ZIKV Asian strain (Micronesia 2007, Accession # EU545988). The modified RNA was encapsulated in lipid nanoparticles to aid in intramuscular delivery and showed excellent protection in WT C57BL/6 and AG129 mice upon virus challenge leading to sterilizing immunity. The authors also tested the role of Antibody dependent enhancement (ADE) inducing epitopes in the DII region of the flavivirus E protein by generating modified mRNA vaccines containing mutations in the E-DII-FL region. Interestingly, they showed that mutations of the DII-Fusion loop epitope diminished generation of antibodies that would enhance Dengue virus infection. The same group [56] also showed protection against "ZIKV induced congenital disease", after vaccination of pregnant dams with the lipid nanoparticle vaccine, containing the modified mRNA followed by virus challenge. Similarly, Pardi et al. [54] simultaneously demonstrated that immunization with a modified mRNA encoding the prME of ZIKV (H/PF/2013, Accession # KJ776791) encapsulated into lipid nanoparticles was able to confer potent B and T cell responses in mice and strong ZIKV specific neutralizing antibody titers in non-human primates, after a single immunization. Moreover, low doses of the vaccine (30 µg in mice and 50 μg in non-human primates) was sufficient to protect the animals against live virus challenge. Thereafter Chahal et al. [57] developed a modified dendrimer nanoparticle (MDNP)-RNA vaccine that expressed the prME proteins of ZIKV (Accession # KU312312, Asian lineage virus isolated from a patient in Suriname in 2015) cloned into an RNA replicon vector. Their approach identified a 9 amino acid long highly conserved MHC-1 restricted epitope in the E protein capable of inducing a CD8 specific T cell response in mice.

Soon after the reports of ZIKV mRNA vaccines, Moderna therapeutics in collaboration with Biomedical Advanced Research and Development Authority (BARDA) initiated clinical trials of the vaccine in 2016. The objective was to "evaluate the safety and immunogenicity of mRNA 1325 Zika vaccine in healthy adults in a non-endemic Zika region", via a phase 1, randomized, and placebo controlled trial. The study is set to complete in February 2019, enrolling 90 participants to assess any adverse events and seroconversion when compared to placebo controls. The Phase 1 study was funded by BARDA with $8 million, which will pave way for Phase 2 and 3 clinical studies with $117 million, along with supporting large scale manufacturing of the vaccine for worldwide dissemination.

6.6. Subunit Vaccines

As the E protein of flaviviruses is the major antigen for generation of neutralizing response, this protein has been used in various forms as a subunit vaccine candidate for DENV [58] and WNV [59]. Building on the same premise, To et al. [60] expressed and purified soluble ZIKV E protein produced in Drosophila melanogaster cells. The expression vector contained an insect cell optimized synthetic gene, expressing the entire prM and amino acids 1–408 of the E protein from the French Polynesian strain (Accession # KJ776791). Immunization of mice with purified recombinant E protein in combination with adjuvant resulted in neutralizing antibody titers that were protective against viremia in immunocompetent mice. Tai et al. [61] fused the ZIKV E domain III region to the C terminal Fc region of human IgG, to generate a recombinant immunogen. This recombinant E protein contained amino acids 298–409 of ZIKV E (ZIKV SPH2015 Accession # KU321639.1) and was found to be highly immunogenic, resulting in neutralizing antibody generation and protection of mice in various models. Yang et al. [62] developed a subunit vaccine derived from the EIII domain of strain PRVABC59 produced as *E. coli* inclusion bodies. The vaccine evoked a high titer neutralizing antibody response that did not enhance DENV infection in vitro, along with production of Th1 and Th2 cytokines by splenocytes. The same group [63] also described a plant produced subunit E vaccine that was found to be highly immunogenic, as seen via neutralizing antibody and T cell responses. Qu et al [64] described ZIKV subunit vaccines produced in insect cells and comprised of the domain III or the 80% N terminal region of the E protein (Accession # KU312312). Both vaccines generated antibody and T cell specific responses with the domain III vaccine being superior. Recently, Zhu et al [65] described a subunit vaccine comprising of the N terminus (450 amino acids) of the E glycoprotein that was capable of inducing long term protection in mice. Immunization of pregnant dams with the subunit vaccine also protected the fetal brains in utero and neonates against microcephaly.

6.7. Viral Vectors

Using viral vectors to deliver antigens for the purpose of developing immunity is a new and emerging field. Adenoviruses and vaccinia virus are perhaps the most well studied and widely used platforms for vaccine development. Replication deficient versions of these viruses are safe and potent inducers of immunity against antigens of choice. Abbink et al. [32] used rhesus Adenovirus 52 (RhAd52) as vector expressing ZIKV prME in rhesus monkeys. In the same study they compared multiple vaccine platforms and found that a RhAd52-prME vaccine generated neutralizing antibodies, and complete protection from challenge in rhesus monkeys after a single immunization. Xu et al. [66] developed a recombinant chimpanzee adenovirus type 7 (AdC7) expressing ZIKV M and E proteins from the Asian linage of ZIKV FSS13025 (Accession # MH158236), isolated in Cambodia. In mouse models of ZIKV, a single immunization protected the mice against ZIKV viremia and testicular damage after challenge.

Similarly, Cox et al [67] developed an Adenovirus serotype 26 (Ad26) based vaccine containing the ME region of ZIKV strain BeH815744 (Accession # KU365780.1). Single immunization with this adenoviral vaccine provided protection against challenge in both mice and Non-human primates (NHP) models. To improve upon the antigenicity of ZIKV adenoviral vaccines, Lopez-Camacho et al. [68] modified the prME region (consensus sequence) by deleting the transmembrane (TM) region of Envelope (Env). This prMEΔTM region in a chimpanzee adenoviral vector (ChAdOx1) provided better neutralizing response than the full length prME, suggesting that modification of antigen membrane anchor can enhance immunogenicity. Liu et al. [69] recently included the NS1 gene of ZIKV along with prME (isolate 1_0080_PF, Accession # KX447521) in an Adenovirus serotype 2 vector system to generate Ad2-prME-NS1 vector. The Ad2-prME-NS1 vector resulted in both Env as well as NS1 specific antibodies, and protected pups born to immunized dams against Zika induced pathology.

Recently, Prow et al. [70] incorporated ZIKV prME (Brazilian isolate SPH2015, Accession # KU321639) as well as a Chikungunya virus (CHIKV) structural protein cassette into a vaccinia derived Sementis Copenhagen Vector (SCV) system. This multi pathogen vaccine provided protection against both ZIKV and CHIKV in wild type and IFNAR−/− mice. Development of a similar multivalent vaccine against arboviruses that circulate in the same geographical region may have added advantages. Betancourt et al [71] were the first group to use the recombinant Vesicular stomatitis virus (VSV) platform to express either Zika Env or Zika prME proteins from a SPH2015 isolate (Accession # KU321639). Two immunizations with these vectors resulted in an anti Zika antibody response that protected newborn mice born to vaccinated mothers against lethal Zika challenge. Emanuel et al. [72] recently used a recombinant VSV that expressed the codon optimized prME (Accession # KU681081.3) region of Zika along with an Ebola GP protein. This vector was built upon the previous Ebola vaccine vector, VSV-EBOV vaccine [73,74]. The vector was tested in IFNAR−/− mice and provided protection from lethal challenge after a single immunization as late as 3 days prior to ZIKV challenge. However, the replicating nature of the recombinant VSV vectors make them less likely to be used in vulnerable populations like pregnant mothers. The rapid nature of protection makes them ideal for controlling outbreaks in certain geographical regions.

7. Conclusions

There is no doubt that the response from the research community with respect to a Zika vaccine has been unprecedented. With the tremendous progress made in this field, a viable vaccine for ZIKV is both possible and closer than expected. However, the lack of new Zika cases in 2018 has dampened the enthusiasm as well as urgency for the vaccine. Moreover, lack of uniformity in the assays being used to determine vaccine efficacies makes comparison of different candidates difficult. The reduction in Zika cases also makes it difficult to study the efficacy of the vaccine in clinical trials. Moreover, conducting placebo control trials in pregnant women in Zika endemic areas has serious ethical issues. Nevertheless, a safe effective and economical vaccine for Zika should be developed in order to prepare for a subsequent outbreak which remains a real possibility. This lesson has already been learned from the overwhelming 2015 outbreaks, more than 50 years after the identification of the virus.

Author Contributions: H.G., T.G. and A.J. reviewed the literature and wrote the manuscript.

Funding: This research received no external funding.

Conflicts of Interest: The authors declare no conflicts of interest.

References

1. Weaver, S.C.; Costa, F.; Garcia-Blanco, M.A.; Ko, A.I.; Ribeiro, G.S.; Saade, G.; Shi, P.Y.; Vasilakis, N. Zika virus: History, emergence, biology, and prospects for control. *Antivir. Res.* **2016**, *130*, 69–80. [CrossRef] [PubMed]
2. Hayes, E.B. Zika virus outside Africa. *Emerg. Infect. Dis.* **2009**, *15*, 1347–1350. [CrossRef] [PubMed]

3. Duffy, M.R.; Chen, T.H.; Hancock, W.T.; Powers, A.M.; Kool, J.L.; Lanciotti, R.S.; Pretrick, M.; Marfel, M.; Holzbauer, S.; Dubray, C.; et al. Zika virus outbreak on Yap Island, Federated States of Micronesia. *N. Engl. J. Med.* **2009**, *360*, 2536–2543. [CrossRef] [PubMed]
4. Bearcroft, W.G. Zika virus infection experimentally induced in a human volunteer. *Trans. R. Soc. Trop. Med. Hyg.* **1956**, *50*, 442–448. [CrossRef]
5. Simpson, D.I. Zika Virus Infection in Man. *Trans. R. Soc. Trop. Med. Hyg.* **1964**, *58*, 335–338. [CrossRef]
6. Enfissi, A.; Codrington, J.; Roosblad, J.; Kazanji, M.; Rousset, D. Zika virus genome from the Americas. *Lancet* **2016**, *387*, 227–228. [CrossRef]
7. Chambers, T.J.; Hahn, C.S.; Galler, R.; Rice, C.M. Flavivirus genome organization, expression, and replication. *Annu. Rev. Microbiol.* **1990**, *44*, 649–688. [CrossRef] [PubMed]
8. Kuno, G.; Chang, G.J. Full-length sequencing and genomic characterization of Bagaza, Kedougou, and Zika viruses. *Arch. Virol.* **2007**, *152*, 687–696. [CrossRef] [PubMed]
9. Lindenbach, B.D.; Rice, C.M. Molecular biology of flaviviruses. *Adv. Virus Res.* **2003**, *59*, 23–61. [PubMed]
10. Lobigs, M. Flavivirus premembrane protein cleavage and spike heterodimer secretion require the function of the viral proteinase NS3. *Proc. Natl. Acad. Sci. USA* **1993**, *90*, 6218–6222. [CrossRef] [PubMed]
11. Lorenz, I.C.; Kartenbeck, J.; Mezzacasa, A.; Allison, S.L.; Heinz, F.X.; Helenius, A. Intracellular assembly and secretion of recombinant subviral particles from tick-borne encephalitis virus. *J. Virol.* **2003**, *77*, 4370–4382. [CrossRef] [PubMed]
12. Pincus, S.; Mason, P.W.; Konishi, E.; Fonseca, B.A.; Shope, R.E.; Rice, C.M.; Paoletti, E. Recombinant vaccinia virus producing the prM and E proteins of yellow fever virus protects mice from lethal yellow fever encephalitis. *Virology* **1992**, *187*, 290–297. [CrossRef]
13. Pugachev, K.V.; Mason, P.W.; Shope, R.E.; Frey, T.K. Double-subgenomic Sindbis virus recombinants expressing immunogenic proteins of Japanese encephalitis virus induce significant protection in mice against lethal JEV infection. *Virology* **1995**, *212*, 587–594. [CrossRef] [PubMed]
14. Schalich, J.; Allison, S.L.; Stiasny, K.; Mandl, C.W.; Kunz, C.; Heinz, F.X. Recombinant subviral particles from tick-borne encephalitis virus are fusogenic and provide a model system for studying flavivirus envelope glycoprotein functions. *J. Virol.* **1996**, *70*, 4549–4557. [PubMed]
15. Oliveira, E.R.A.; Mohana-Borges, R.; de Alencastro, R.B.; Horta, B.A.C. The flavivirus capsid protein: Structure, function and perspectives towards drug design. *Virus Res.* **2017**, *227*, 115–123. [CrossRef] [PubMed]
16. Duenas-Carrera, S.; Alvarez-Lajonchere, L.; Alvarez-Obregon, J.C.; Herrera, A.; Lorenzo, L.J.; Pichardo, D.; Morales, J. A truncated variant of the hepatitis C virus core induces a slow but potent immune response in mice following DNA immunization. *Vaccine* **2000**, *19*, 992–997. [CrossRef]
17. Chen, S.; Wu, Z.; Wang, M.; Cheng, A. Innate Immune Evasion Mediated by Flaviviridae Non-Structural Proteins. *Viruses* **2017**, *9*, 291. [CrossRef] [PubMed]
18. Netto, E.M.; Moreira-Soto, A.; Pedroso, C.; Hoser, C.; Funk, S.; Kucharski, A.J.; Rockstroh, A.; Kummerer, B.M.; Sampaio, G.S.; Luz, E.; et al. High Zika Virus Seroprevalence in Salvador, Northeastern Brazil Limits the Potential for Further Outbreaks. *mBio* **2017**, *8*, e01390-17. [CrossRef] [PubMed]
19. Tang, H.; Hammack, C.; Ogden, S.C.; Wen, Z.; Qian, X.; Li, Y.; Yao, B.; Shin, J.; Zhang, F.; Lee, E.M.; et al. Zika Virus Infects Human Cortical Neural Progenitors and Attenuates Their Growth. *Cell Stem Cell* **2016**, *18*, 587–590. [CrossRef] [PubMed]
20. Bardina, S.V.; Bunduc, P.; Tripathi, S.; Duehr, J.; Frere, J.J.; Brown, J.A.; Nachbagauer, R.; Foster, G.A.; Krysztof, D.; Tortorella, D.; et al. Enhancement of Zika virus pathogenesis by preexisting antiflavivirus immunity. *Science* **2017**, *356*, 175–180. [CrossRef] [PubMed]
21. Fontes-Garfias, C.R.; Shan, C.; Luo, H.; Muruato, A.E.; Medeiros, D.B.A.; Mays, E.; Xie, X.; Zou, J.; Roundy, C.M.; Wakamiya, M.; et al. Functional Analysis of Glycosylation of Zika Virus Envelope Protein. *Cell Rep.* **2017**, *21*, 1180–1190. [CrossRef] [PubMed]
22. Reynolds, M.R.; Jones, A.M.; Petersen, E.E.; Lee, E.H.; Rice, M.E.; Bingham, A.; Ellington, S.R.; Evert, N.; Reagan-Steiner, S.; Oduyebo, T.; et al. Vital Signs: Update on Zika Virus-Associated Birth Defects and Evaluation of All U.S. Infants with Congenital Zika Virus Exposure—U.S. Zika Pregnancy Registry, 2016. *MMWR Morb. Mortal. Wkly. Rep.* **2017**, *66*, 366–373. [CrossRef] [PubMed]

23. Krauer, F.; Riesen, M.; Reveiz, L.; Oladapo, O.T.; Martinez-Vega, R.; Porgo, T.V.; Haefliger, A.; Broutet, N.J.; Low, N.; WHO Zika Causality Working Group. Zika Virus Infection as a Cause of Congenital Brain Abnormalities and Guillain-Barre Syndrome: Systematic Review. *PLoS Med.* **2017**, *14*, e1002203. [CrossRef] [PubMed]
24. Durham, D.P.; Fitzpatrick, M.C.; Ndeffo-Mbah, M.L.; Parpia, A.S.; Michael, N.L.; Galvani, A.P. Evaluating Vaccination Strategies for Zika Virus in the Americas. *Ann. Intern. Med.* **2018**, *168*, 621–630. [CrossRef] [PubMed]
25. Durbin, A.; Wilder-Smith, A. An update on Zika vaccine developments. *Expert Rev. Vaccines* **2017**, *16*, 781–787. [CrossRef] [PubMed]
26. Kudchodkar, S.B.; Choi, H.; Reuschel, E.L.; Esquivel, R.; Jin-Ah Kwon, J.; Jeong, M.; Maslow, J.N.; Reed, C.C.; White, S.; Kim, J.J.; et al. Rapid response to an emerging infectious disease—Lessons learned from development of a synthetic DNA vaccine targeting Zika virus. *Microbes Infect.* **2018**. [CrossRef] [PubMed]
27. Larocca, R.A.; Abbink, P.; Peron, J.P.; Zanotto, P.M.; Iampietro, M.J.; Badamchi-Zadeh, A.; Boyd, M.; Ng'ang'a, D.; Kirilova, M.; Nityanandam, R.; et al. Vaccine protection against Zika virus from Brazil. *Nature* **2016**, *536*, 474–478. [CrossRef] [PubMed]
28. Dowd, K.A.; Ko, S.Y.; Morabito, K.M.; Yang, E.S.; Pelc, R.S.; DeMaso, C.R.; Castilho, L.R.; Abbink, P.; Boyd, M.; Nityanandam, R.; et al. Rapid development of a DNA vaccine for Zika virus. *Science* **2016**, *354*, 237–240. [CrossRef] [PubMed]
29. Muthumani, K.; Griffin, B.D.; Agarwal, S.; Kudchodkar, S.B.; Reuschel, E.L.; Choi, H.; Kraynyak, K.A.; Duperret, E.K.; Keaton, A.A.; Chung, C.; et al. In vivo protection against ZIKV infection and pathogenesis through passive antibody transfer and active immunisation with a prMEnv DNA vaccine. *NPJ Vaccines* **2016**, *1*, 16021. [CrossRef] [PubMed]
30. Gaudinski, M.R.; Houser, K.V.; Morabito, K.M.; Hu, Z.; Yamshchikov, G.; Rothwell, R.S.; Berkowitz, N.; Mendoza, F.; Saunders, J.G.; Novik, L.; et al. Safety, tolerability, and immunogenicity of two Zika virus DNA vaccine candidates in healthy adults: Randomised, open-label, phase 1 clinical trials. *Lancet* **2018**, *391*, 552–562. [CrossRef]
31. Tebas, P.; Roberts, C.C.; Muthumani, K.; Reuschel, E.L.; Kudchodkar, S.B.; Zaidi, F.I.; White, S.; Khan, A.S.; Racine, T.; Choi, H.; et al. Safety and Immunogenicity of an Anti-Zika Virus DNA Vaccine—Preliminary Report. *N. Engl. J. Med.* **2017**. [CrossRef] [PubMed]
32. Abbink, P.; Larocca, R.A.; De La Barrera, R.A.; Bricault, C.A.; Moseley, E.T.; Boyd, M.; Kirilova, M.; Li, Z.; Ng'ang'a, D.; Nanayakkara, O.; et al. Protective efficacy of multiple vaccine platforms against Zika virus challenge in rhesus monkeys. *Science* **2016**, *353*, 1129–1132. [CrossRef] [PubMed]
33. Abbink, P.; Larocca, R.A.; Visitsunthorn, K.; Boyd, M.; De La Barrera, R.A.; Gromowski, G.D.; Kirilova, M.; Peterson, R.; Li, Z.; Nanayakkara, O.; et al. Durability and correlates of vaccine protection against Zika virus in rhesus monkeys. *Sci. Transl. Med.* **2017**, *9*, eaao4163. [CrossRef] [PubMed]
34. Modjarrad, K.; Lin, L.; George, S.L.; Stephenson, K.E.; Eckels, K.H.; De La Barrera, R.A.; Jarman, R.G.; Sondergaard, E.; Tennant, J.; Ansel, J.L.; et al. Preliminary aggregate safety and immunogenicity results from three trials of a purified inactivated Zika virus vaccine candidate: Phase 1, randomised, double-blind, placebo-controlled clinical trials. *Lancet* **2018**, *391*, 563–571. [CrossRef]
35. Sumathy, K.; Kulkarni, B.; Gondu, R.K.; Ponnuru, S.K.; Bonguram, N.; Eligeti, R.; Gadiyaram, S.; Praturi, U.; Chougule, B.; Karunakaran, L.; et al. Protective efficacy of Zika vaccine in AG129 mouse model. *Sci. Rep.* **2017**, *7*, 46375. [CrossRef] [PubMed]
36. Yang, Y.; Shan, C.; Zou, J.; Muruato, A.E.; Bruno, D.N.; de Almeida Medeiros Daniele, B.; Vasconcelos, P.F.C.; Rossi, S.L.; Weaver, S.C.; Xie, X.; et al. A cDNA Clone-Launched Platform for High-Yield Production of Inactivated Zika Vaccine. *EBioMedicine* **2017**, *17*, 145–156. [CrossRef] [PubMed]
37. Collins, N.D.; Barrett, A.D. Live Attenuated Yellow Fever 17D Vaccine: A Legacy Vaccine Still Controlling Outbreaks in Modern Day. *Curr. Infect. Dis. Rep.* **2017**, *19*, 14. [CrossRef] [PubMed]
38. Monath, T.P. Japanese encephalitis vaccines: Current vaccines and future prospects. *Curr. Top. Microbiol. Immunol.* **2002**, *267*, 105–138. [PubMed]
39. Shan, C.; Muruato, A.E.; Nunes, B.T.D.; Luo, H.; Xie, X.; Medeiros, D.B.A.; Wakamiya, M.; Tesh, R.B.; Barrett, A.D.; Wang, T.; et al. A live-attenuated Zika virus vaccine candidate induces sterilizing immunity in mouse models. *Nat. Med.* **2017**, *23*, 763–767. [CrossRef] [PubMed]

40. Shan, C.; Muruato, A.E.; Jagger, B.W.; Richner, J.; Nunes, B.T.D.; Medeiros, D.B.A.; Xie, X.; Nunes, J.G.C.; Morabito, K.M.; Kong, W.P.; et al. A single-dose live-attenuated vaccine prevents Zika virus pregnancy transmission and testis damage. *Nat. Commun.* **2017**, *8*, 676. [CrossRef] [PubMed]

41. Zou, J.; Xie, X.; Luo, H.; Shan, C.; Muruato, A.E.; Weaver, S.C.; Wang, T.; Shi, P.Y. A single-dose plasmid-launched live-attenuated Zika vaccine induces protective immunity. *EBioMedicine* **2018**, *36*, 92–102. [CrossRef] [PubMed]

42. Xie, X.; Yang, Y.; Muruato, A.E.; Zou, J.; Shan, C.; Nunes, B.T.; Medeiros, D.B.; Vasconcelos, P.F.; Weaver, S.C.; Rossi, S.L.; et al. Understanding Zika Virus Stability and Developing a Chimeric Vaccine through Functional Analysis. *mBio* **2017**, *8*, e02134-16. [CrossRef] [PubMed]

43. Li, X.F.; Dong, H.L.; Wang, H.J.; Huang, X.Y.; Qiu, Y.F.; Ji, X.; Ye, Q.; Li, C.; Liu, Y.; Deng, Y.Q.; et al. Development of a chimeric Zika vaccine using a licensed live-attenuated flavivirus vaccine as backbone. *Nat. Commun.* **2018**, *9*, 673. [CrossRef] [PubMed]

44. Wang, L.; Wang, Y.C.; Feng, H.; Ahmed, T.; Compans, R.W.; Wang, B.Z. Virus-like particles containing the tetrameric ectodomain of influenza matrix protein 2 and flagellin induce heterosubtypic protection in mice. *BioMed Res. Int.* **2013**, *2013*, 686549. [CrossRef] [PubMed]

45. Garg, H.; Sedano, M.; Plata, G.; Punke, E.B.; Joshi, A. Development of Virus-Like-Particle Vaccine and Reporter Assay for Zika Virus. *J. Virol.* **2017**, *91*, e00834-17. [CrossRef] [PubMed]

46. Boigard, H.; Alimova, A.; Martin, G.R.; Katz, A.; Gottlieb, P.; Galarza, J.M. Zika virus-like particle (VLP) based vaccine. *PLoS Negl. Trop. Dis.* **2017**, *11*, e0005608. [CrossRef] [PubMed]

47. Yang, M.; Lai, H.; Sun, H.; Chen, Q. Virus-like particles that display Zika virus envelope protein domain III induce potent neutralizing immune responses in mice. *Sci. Rep.* **2017**, *7*, 7679. [CrossRef] [PubMed]

48. Espinosa, D.; Mendy, J.; Manayani, D.; Vang, L.; Wang, C.; Richard, T.; Guenther, B.; Aruri, J.; Avanzini, J.; Garduno, F.; et al. Passive Transfer of Immune Sera Induced by a Zika Virus-Like Particle Vaccine Protects AG129 Mice Against Lethal Zika Virus Challenge. *EBioMedicine* **2018**, *27*, 61–70. [CrossRef] [PubMed]

49. Basu, R.; Zhai, L.; Contreras, A.; Tumban, E. Immunization with phage virus-like particles displaying Zika virus potential B-cell epitopes neutralizes Zika virus infection of monkey kidney cells. *Vaccine* **2018**, *36*, 1256–1264. [CrossRef] [PubMed]

50. Dai, S.; Zhang, T.; Zhang, Y.; Wang, H.; Deng, F. Zika Virus Baculovirus-Expressed Virus-Like Particles Induce Neutralizing Antibodies in Mice. *Virol. Sin.* **2018**, *33*, 213–226. [CrossRef] [PubMed]

51. Salvo, M.A.; Kingstad-Bakke, B.; Salas-Quinchucua, C.; Camacho, E.; Osorio, J.E. Zika virus like particles elicit protective antibodies in mice. *PLoS Negl. Trop. Dis.* **2018**, *12*, e0006210. [CrossRef] [PubMed]

52. Anderson, B.R.; Muramatsu, H.; Jha, B.K.; Silverman, R.H.; Weissman, D.; Kariko, K. Nucleoside modifications in RNA limit activation of $2'$-$5'$-oligoadenylate synthetase and increase resistance to cleavage by RNase L. *Nucleic Acids Res.* **2011**, *39*, 9329–9338. [CrossRef] [PubMed]

53. Kariko, K.; Ni, H.; Capodici, J.; Lamphier, M.; Weissman, D. mRNA is an endogenous ligand for Toll-like receptor 3. *J. Biol. Chem.* **2004**, *279*, 12542–12550. [CrossRef] [PubMed]

54. Pardi, N.; Hogan, M.J.; Pelc, R.S.; Muramatsu, H.; Andersen, H.; DeMaso, C.R.; Dowd, K.A.; Sutherland, L.L.; Scearce, R.M.; Parks, R.; et al. Zika virus protection by a single low-dose nucleoside-modified mRNA vaccination. *Nature* **2017**, *543*, 248–251. [CrossRef] [PubMed]

55. Richner, J.M.; Himansu, S.; Dowd, K.A.; Butler, S.L.; Salazar, V.; Fox, J.M.; Julander, J.G.; Tang, W.W.; Shresta, S.; Pierson, T.C.; et al. Modified mRNA Vaccines Protect against Zika Virus Infection. *Cell* **2017**, *169*, 176. [CrossRef] [PubMed]

56. Richner, J.M.; Jagger, B.W.; Shan, C.; Fontes, C.R.; Dowd, K.A.; Cao, B.; Himansu, S.; Caine, E.A.; Nunes, B.T.D.; Medeiros, D.B.A.; et al. Vaccine Mediated Protection Against Zika Virus-Induced Congenital Disease. *Cell* **2017**, *170*, 273–283. [CrossRef] [PubMed]

57. Chahal, J.S.; Fang, T.; Woodham, A.W.; Khan, O.F.; Ling, J.; Anderson, D.G.; Ploegh, H.L. An RNA nanoparticle vaccine against Zika virus elicits antibody and CD8+ T cell responses in a mouse model. *Sci. Rep.* **2017**, *7*, 252. [CrossRef] [PubMed]

58. Clements, D.E.; Coller, B.A.; Lieberman, M.M.; Ogata, S.; Wang, G.; Harada, K.E.; Putnak, J.R.; Ivy, J.M.; McDonell, M.; Bignami, G.S.; et al. Development of a recombinant tetravalent dengue virus vaccine: Immunogenicity and efficacy studies in mice and monkeys. *Vaccine* **2010**, *28*, 2705–2715. [CrossRef] [PubMed]

59. Jarvi, S.I.; Lieberman, M.M.; Hofmeister, E.; Nerurkar, V.R.; Wong, T.; Weeks-Levy, C. Protective efficacy of a recombinant subunit West Nile virus vaccine in domestic geese (Anser anser). *Vaccine* **2008**, *26*, 5338–5344. [CrossRef] [PubMed]

60. To, A.; Medina, L.O.; Mfuh, K.O.; Lieberman, M.M.; Wong, T.A.S.; Namekar, M.; Nakano, E.; Lai, C.Y.; Kumar, M.; Nerurkar, V.R.; et al. Recombinant Zika Virus Subunits Are Immunogenic and Efficacious in Mice. *mSphere* **2018**, *3*, e00576-17. [CrossRef] [PubMed]

61. Tai, W.; He, L.; Wang, Y.; Sun, S.; Zhao, G.; Luo, C.; Li, P.; Zhao, H.; Fremont, D.H.; Li, F.; et al. Critical neutralizing fragment of Zika virus EDIII elicits cross-neutralization and protection against divergent Zika viruses. *Emerg. Microbes Infect.* **2018**, *7*, 7. [CrossRef] [PubMed]

62. Yang, M.; Dent, M.; Lai, H.; Sun, H.; Chen, Q. Immunization of Zika virus envelope protein domain III induces specific and neutralizing immune responses against Zika virus. *Vaccine* **2017**, *35*, 4287–4294. [CrossRef] [PubMed]

63. Yang, M.; Sun, H.; Lai, H.; Hurtado, J.; Chen, Q. Plant-produced Zika virus envelope protein elicits neutralizing immune responses that correlate with protective immunity against Zika virus in mice. *Plant Biotechnol. J.* **2018**, *16*, 572–580. [CrossRef] [PubMed]

64. Qu, P.; Zhang, W.; Li, D.; Zhang, C.; Liu, Q.; Zhang, X.; Wang, X.; Dai, W.; Xu, Y.; Leng, Q.; et al. Insect cell-produced recombinant protein subunit vaccines protect against Zika virus infection. *Antivir. Res.* **2018**, *154*, 97–103. [CrossRef] [PubMed]

65. Zhu, X.; Li, C.; Afridi, S.K.; Zu, S.; Xu, J.W.; Quanquin, N.; Yang, H.; Cheng, G.; Xu, Z. E90 subunit vaccine protects mice from Zika virus infection and microcephaly. *Acta Neuropathol. Commun.* **2018**, *6*, 77. [CrossRef] [PubMed]

66. Xu, K.; Song, Y.; Dai, L.; Zhang, Y.; Lu, X.; Xie, Y.; Zhang, H.; Cheng, T.; Wang, Q.; Huang, Q.; et al. Recombinant Chimpanzee Adenovirus Vaccine AdC7-M/E Protects against Zika Virus Infection and Testis Damage. *J. Virol.* **2018**, *92*, e01722-17. [CrossRef] [PubMed]

67. Cox, F.; van der Fits, L.; Abbink, P.; Larocca, R.A.; van Huizen, E.; Saeland, E.; Verhagen, J.; Peterson, R.; Tolboom, J.; Kaufmann, B.; et al. Adenoviral vector type 26 encoding Zika virus (ZIKV) M-Env antigen induces humoral and cellular immune responses and protects mice and nonhuman primates against ZIKV challenge. *PLoS ONE* **2018**, *13*, e0202820. [CrossRef] [PubMed]

68. Lopez-Camacho, C.; Abbink, P.; Larocca, R.A.; Dejnirattisai, W.; Boyd, M.; Badamchi-Zadeh, A.; Wallace, Z.R.; Doig, J.; Velazquez, R.S.; Neto, R.D.L.; et al. Rational Zika vaccine design via the modulation of antigen membrane anchors in chimpanzee adenoviral vectors. *Nat. Commun.* **2018**, *9*, 2441. [CrossRef] [PubMed]

69. Liu, X.; Qu, L.; Ye, X.; Yi, C.; Zheng, X.; Hao, M.; Su, W.; Yao, Z.; Chen, P.; Zhang, S.; et al. Incorporation of NS1 and prM/M are important to confer effective protection of adenovirus-vectored Zika virus vaccine carrying E protein. *NPJ Vaccines* **2018**, *3*, 29. [CrossRef] [PubMed]

70. Prow, N.A.; Liu, L.; Nakayama, E.; Cooper, T.H.; Yan, K.; Eldi, P.; Hazlewood, J.E.; Tang, B.; Le, T.T.; Setoh, Y.X.; et al. A vaccinia-based single vector construct multi-pathogen vaccine protects against both Zika and chikungunya viruses. *Nat. Commun.* **2018**, *9*, 1230. [CrossRef] [PubMed]

71. Betancourt, D.; de Queiroz, N.M.; Xia, T.; Ahn, J.; Barber, G.N. Cutting Edge: Innate Immune Augmenting Vesicular Stomatitis Virus Expressing Zika Virus Proteins Confers Protective Immunity. *J. Immunol.* **2017**, *198*, 3023–3028. [CrossRef] [PubMed]

72. Emanuel, J.; Callison, J.; Dowd, K.A.; Pierson, T.C.; Feldmann, H.; Marzi, A. A VSV-based Zika virus vaccine protects mice from lethal challenge. *Sci. Rep.* **2018**, *8*, 11043. [CrossRef] [PubMed]

73. Garbutt, M.; Liebscher, R.; Wahl-Jensen, V.; Jones, S.; Moller, P.; Wagner, R.; Volchkov, V.; Klenk, H.D.; Feldmann, H.; Stroher, U. Properties of replication-competent vesicular stomatitis virus vectors expressing glycoproteins of filoviruses and arenaviruses. *J. Virol.* **2004**, *78*, 5458–5465. [CrossRef] [PubMed]

74. Suder, E.; Furuyama, W.; Feldmann, H.; Marzi, A.; de Wit, E. The vesicular stomatitis virus-based Ebola virus vaccine: From concept to clinical trials. *Hum. Vaccines Immunother.* **2018**, *14*, 2107–2113. [CrossRef] [PubMed]

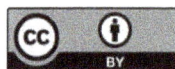

viruses

MDPI

Review

Research Models and Tools for the Identification of Antivirals and Therapeutics against Zika Virus Infection

Marco P. Alves [1,2,*], **Nathalie J. Vielle** [1,2,3], **Volker Thiel** [1,2,*] and **Stephanie Pfaender** [1,2,*]

[1] Institute of Virology and Immunology, 3012 Bern, Switzerland; nathalie.vielle@vetsuisse.unibe.ch
[2] Department of Infectious Diseases and Pathobiology, Vetsuisse Faculty, University of Bern, 3012 Bern, Switzerland
[3] Graduate School for Cellular and Biomedical Sciences, University of Bern, 3012 Bern, Switzerland
* Correspondence: marco.alves@vetsuisse.unibe.ch (M.P.A.); volker.thiel@vetsuisse.unibe.ch (V.T.); stephanie.pfaender@vetsuisse.unibe.ch (S.P.); Tel.: +41-31-631-24-83 (M.P.A.); +41-31-631-24-13 (V.T.); +41-31-631-25-02 (S.P.)

Received: 2 October 2018; Accepted: 26 October 2018; Published: 30 October 2018

Abstract: Zika virus recently re-emerged and caused global outbreaks mainly in Central Africa, Southeast Asia, the Pacific Islands and in Central and South America. Even though there is a declining trend, the virus continues to spread throughout different geographical regions of the world. Since its re-emergence in 2015, massive advances have been made regarding our understanding of clinical manifestations, epidemiology, genetic diversity, genomic structure and potential therapeutic intervention strategies. Nevertheless, treatment remains a challenge as there is no licensed effective therapy available. This review focuses on the recent advances regarding research models, as well as available experimental tools that can be used for the identification and characterization of potential antiviral targets and therapeutic intervention strategies.

Keywords: Zika virus; antivirals; therapeutics; research models and tools

1. Introduction

Zika virus (ZIKV) was first isolated in 1947 in the Zika forest in Uganda from an infected rhesus macaque monkey [1]. Since its discovery, the virus has been detected in different species of *Aedes* mosquitos followed by the identification of the first infected human case in Uganda in 1962 [2–5]. Since then, human infections had only been sporadically reported in Africa and Asia [6] before the first major outbreak occurred in 2007 in Micronesia [6,7]. After this, the virus continued to spread and caused another major outbreak in 2013–2014 in French Polynesia [8], which was retrospectively associated with an unusual high frequency of newborns with microcephaly, a cerebral congenital anomaly, and an increase in the number of cases of Guillain-Barré syndrome (GBS) in adults [9]. ZIKV received global attention in 2015, following its emergence in Brazil due to its association with several thousand cases of microcephaly in newborn children [10–12]. Since then, the virus has spread further, with a total of 86 countries reporting evidence of Zika infection (WHO 2018). Mosquito bites present the major route of transmission of ZIKV, after which viral replication is believed to occur in skin fibroblasts/keratinocytes and skin-associated dendritic cells (DCs) with subsequent dissemination to lymph nodes and the bloodstream [13]. In addition, sporadic non-vector borne human-to-human transmissions have been described. ZIKV has been reported to be transmitted perinatally (reviewed in [14]), sexually [15] and via blood transfusion products [16,17]. Recently, the virus was suspected to transmit through breastfeeding [18]. Furthermore, viral RNA, as well as in some cases infectious virus, has been isolated from various body fluids (reviewed in [14]) including saliva, urine, vaginal secretions, breast milk, semen and conjunctival fluid [19].

ZIKV infection is in most cases asymptomatic or can lead to mild, self-limiting symptoms including rash, fever, joint pain, as well as conjunctivitis [20]. Infrequently, severe neurological conditions such as GBS [21], meningoencephalitis [22] and acute myelitis [23] have been reported in association with ZIKV infection. However, exposure to ZIKV during pregnancy can have severe consequences for the fetus including several fetal malformations such as microcephaly and hydrocephaly, as well as spontaneous abortion, stillbirth and placental insufficiency [20,24]. In addition, it is becoming clear that the long-term neurological defects in affected children are not yet fully elucidated. Up to date, there is still no protective vaccine available. Mosquito control practices are the primary measures to impede further spread and transmission of the virus. Even though much progress was made regarding potential treatment options, no specific antiviral has been licensed against ZIKV, emphasizing the need for the development of effective therapeutics.

2. Replication Cycle and Potential Intervention Strategies

2.1. Genomic Organization

ZIKV belongs to the genus flavivirus within the Flaviviridae family. It has a positive-sense single-stranded RNA genome of 10.8 kb, containing a single open reading frame, flanked by a 5′ and 3′ untranslated region (UTR), encoding for three structural and seven nonstructural proteins, which are co- and post-translationally processed by viral and host proteases [25]. The three structural proteins, the envelope protein (E), the membrane protein (M), which is expressed in the immature virion as precursor preM, as well as the capsid (C) form the mature virion. The nonstructural (NS) proteins NS1, NS2A, NS2B, NS3, NS4A, NS4B and NS5 are involved in viral replication and assembly and participate in the evasion of the host immune system [26].

2.2. Replication Cycle

After binding to specific receptors on the host cell, the virus is internalized by clathrin-mediated endocytosis. The low pH within the endosomes triggers viral uncoating and release of the viral genome into the cytosol [27]. The genomic RNA is translated, resulting in the synthesis of a polyprotein that is co- and post-translationally processed; the RNA-dependent RNA polymerase (RdRp) NS5 replicates viral RNA in close association with cell-derived membranes [28]. Immature virions containing newly synthesized RNA assemble through budding within the endoplasmatic reticulum (ER), followed by transition from the ER through the trans-Golgi network (TGN) to the cell surface, upon which protease- and pH-dependent maturation occurs, and subsequent budding and release of mature virus particles through the secretory pathway [29].

2.3. Intervention Strategies

Several therapeutic approaches that target the different steps of the viral replication cycle (Figure 1) have been developed (reviewed in [30–32]). In general, drug candidates can be classified according to their mode of action, either directed against viral targets (direct-acting antivirals) or acting against cellular targets (host-targeting antivirals). To inhibit the binding of a virus particle to a target cell, strategies include, among others, blocking of the receptor-virus interactions via various compounds [33, 34], direct interaction with the viral lipid envelop [35], targeting of the viral surface by structurally mimicking cellular receptors, binding to carbohydrates that interact directly with the glycosylated viral envelope proteins or binding to other peptide regions of the viral envelope (reviewed in [32]). Another antiviral strategy is to target endocytosis and subsequent pH-dependent endosomal fusion and uncoating of the viral particle. This includes, e.g., drugs that alter host-cell membrane properties [36] or blocking of endosomal pH acidification [37–41]. Interference with translation of the viral polyprotein and polyprotein processing via host and viral proteases also represents an attractive target for antiviral drugs. Especially, interference with the viral NS2B-NS3 protease, which post-translationally cleaves the polyprotein, has been extensively evaluated (reviewed in [30–32]). Next to its protease activity,

NS3 displays a nucleoside-tri-phosphatase (NTPase) and RNA helicase activity that is crucial for viral replication. However, there are only a few studies investigating NS3 helicase inhibitors so far [42]. This might be due to some difficulties, e.g., limited access to the active site of the NS3 helicase-RNA complex as described for Dengue virus (DENV) [43]. NS5offers a very attractive target for intervention with the viral replication complex, which is one of the most conserved among the NS proteins. NS5 contains the RdRp at the C-terminus, which is required for RNA synthesis, and there are several drugs described to interfere with its function (reviewed in [30–32]). Next to its polymerase function, NS5 encodes an N-terminal methyltransferase (MTase) domain, which is required for mRNA capping and stabilization to facilitate the translation process, to escape detection of the viral mRNA by the host innate immune sensors, as well as for cap-independent methylation [44]. Interference with the MTase domain offers an additional therapeutic target [42,45–48]. Furthermore, interference with other viral proteins that are crucial for viral RNA replication, e.g., NS4B, which has been shown to be a therapeutic target for other flaviviruses [49–52] or NS1 [53], could be attractive for the development of new antivirals. In addition, host proteins could be targeted to inhibit viral replication. These include host cell nucleoside biosynthesis inhibitors, host cell lipid biosynthesis inhibitors and host kinase inhibitors (reviewed in [53]). To inhibit viral assembly, maturation and budding, interference with the host metabolism by targeting proteins involved in protein synthesis, folding and degradation can be employed (reviewed in [30]). Furthermore, targeting of intracellular membrane trafficking can inhibit several steps of the viral replication cycle, including entry, assembly and release of infectious particles [54]. Compounds that presumably directly interfere with glycosylation and maturation of ZIKV during its trafficking through the secretory pathway can also inhibit the release of infectious particles [55]. Finally, the capsid protein could be targeted by antivirals. The protein has multiple functions during the viral replication cycle, and studies with other flaviviruses have shown an effect of specific capsid inhibitors on viral assembly and/or release and entry of infectious particles [56–58]. In conclusion, several strategies have been employed for interfering with the viral replication cycle (Figure 1). However, to avoid the surge of resistance mutation, several strategies could and should be used in combination to treat an acute ZIKV infection.

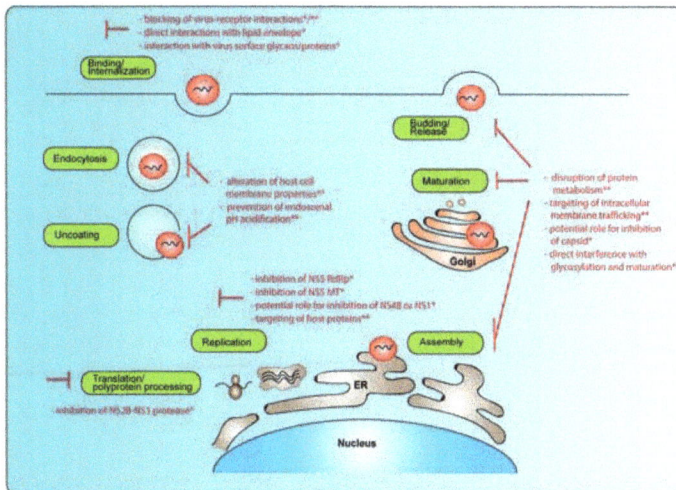

Figure 1. Intervention strategies to interfere with the different stages of the viral replication cycle. (*) direct-acting antivirals; (**) host-targeting antiviral intervention strategies. RdRp: RNA-dependent RNA polymerase, MT: methyltransferase.

3. In Vitro Models and Screening Approaches

The first prerequisite with respect to the development of antiviral compounds is the availability of in vitro systems including virus isolates and/or recombinant constructs and robust in vitro cellular models (Figure 2).

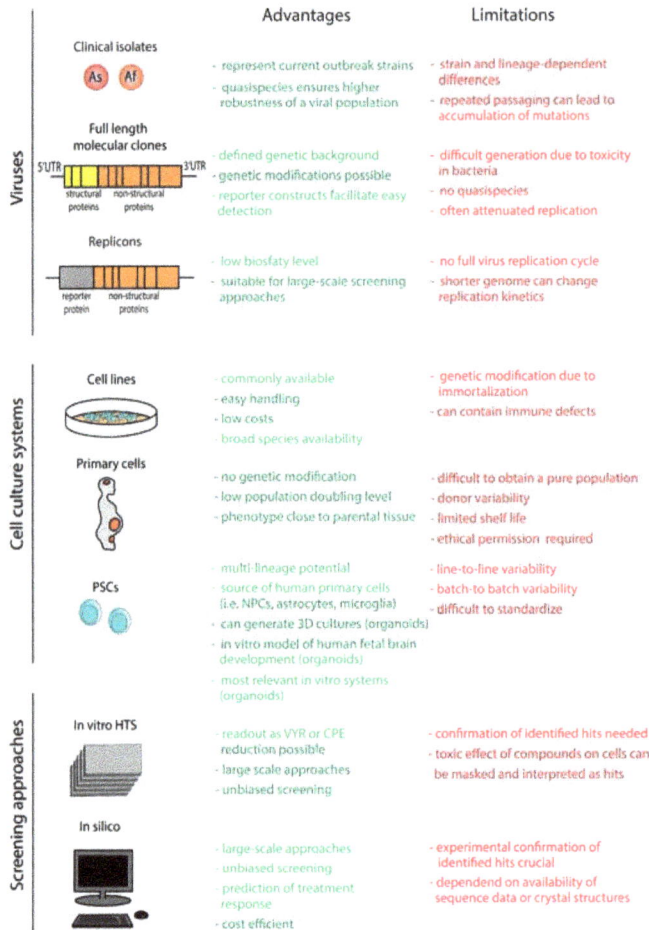

Figure 2. In vitro systems and screening approaches used for antiviral compound development against ZIKV. The text highlighted in green and red indicates advantages and limitations, respectively. PSCs: pluripotent stem cells, HTS: high-throughput screening, VYR: virus yield reduction, CPE: cytopathic effect.

3.1. Viruses

3.1.1. Clinical Viral Isolates

Clinical viral isolates are the best representatives of the currently circulating ZIKV strains. Among ZIKV strains, there are two distinct lineages described, the African and the Asian lineages [59]. Phylogenetic analysis revealed that the currently circulating and pathogenic ZIKV strains most likely descended from the Asian lineage [60]. The "historical" ZIKV strain from Uganda (MR766) has been most consistently used in several in vitro and in vivo studies. Even though it has been passaged over

147 times in different culture models, there seems to be only a low number of nucleotide changes compared to some primary ancient African lineage isolates [61]. Interestingly, of all the ZIKV genomes isolated so far, all African strains have been recovered from mosquitos or non-human primates (NHPs), whereas the Asian strains have been isolated from mosquitos or humans [62]. Phylogenetic analysis revealed that the virus has changed significantly since its initial isolation, with regard to both the nucleotide sequences and amino acid composition with several lineage-specific differences between the African and Asian isolates [59,63,64]. These changes can have a substantial impact on pathogenesis, viral fitness, transmissibility and replication kinetics. Indeed, there are several studies that have analyzed the lineage-dependent properties in animal and cell culture models and found differences between the African and the Asian lineages with respect to plaque phenotype, infectivity, replication kinetics and virulence, with most studies showing that the African lineages display faster replication kinetics, high viral titers, as well as higher virulence in mice [64–68]. On the other hand, there is a significant number of studies with primary human cells and mouse models suggesting that the strains from the African lineage are also neurovirulent and sometimes even more than the contemporary Asian strains [64,69–73]. Thus, there is currently no definitive evidence that the rise in microcephaly cases is exclusively caused by the Asian lineage viruses [74,75]. Of note, all these results have to be interpreted with care as variations including viral strain passage number, cell culture system used and utilization of different mouse background strains can have an impact on the observed phenotypes. For instance, it has been speculated that a high passage number of some ZIKV isolates has resulted in a distinct loss of glycosylation sites, which could have an impact on ZIKV-associated pathogenesis [61]. Nevertheless, for the development and characterization of antivirals, it is important to take into account potential differences between viral isolates, as well as culture systems, since variations in infectivity and replication kinetics can have a significant influence on drug efficacy.

3.1.2. Full-Length Infectious Clones

Next to clinical isolates, reverse genetic systems for the generation of recombinant ZIKV are of great advantage to study virus properties, including virulence/attenuation, replication, host range and tropism. Especially with respect to the identification and development of antivirals, molecular infectious clones are crucial for the understanding of the molecular mechanisms of viral replication and consequently development of potential intervention strategies. To generate an infectious clone, a complementary DNA (cDNA) copy of an RNA virus is usually stably incorporated into a plasmid vector and amplified in *Escherichia coli*. This cDNA can be modified and manipulated as required before genomic RNA is obtained via in vitro transcription and subsequent virus recovery upon transfection of suitable cells [76]. Generation of a ZIKV infectious clone has not been that simple to establish as flavivirus sequences are often not compatible with growth in *E. coli* and may contain viral proteins with bacterial toxicity expressed through cryptic bacterial promoters, which hamper the propagation of the viral cDNA via bacterial plasmids (reviewed in [76,77]). Nevertheless, several strategies have been reported to generate ZIKV molecular clones (Table 1). These include the insertion of a synthetic intron into the molecular construct, which is later removed upon splicing in mammalian cells [78,79], or the separation of the viral genome and generation of subgenomic fragments. Several approaches have been used to circumvent toxicity in bacteria including usage of low copy plasmids [80], usage of bacterial artificial chromosomes [81] and separation of the genome to disrupt toxic regions [82,83]. Furthermore, a more elaborated approach using a bacterium-free reverse genetic method called ISA (infectious subgenomic-amplicons) [84] based on the in vitro generation of overlapping subgenomic amplicons covering the ZIKV genome, subsequent transfection into susceptible host cells and recovery of recombinant virus by "in cellulo" recombination was applied [85–87]. Furthermore, a circular polymerase extension cloning (CPEC) protocol [88] based on the polymerase extension mechanism to join overlapping DNA fragments into a double-stranded circular form has been used [89,90]. Another recent approach used mutational inactivation of several cryptic *E. coli* promoters [91]. All these efforts have resulted in the construction of several molecular clones encompassing various viral strains, with or without the presence of reporter proteins for easier detection. These proteins can easily be manipulated to study molecular functions and to identify potential targets for therapeutic intervention (Table 1). Furthermore, the appearance of possible resistance mutations can be studied upon repeated passaging of the virus in the presence of a compound of interest, thereby anticipating possible viral counter mechanisms. Nevertheless, it is important to keep in mind that, due to a high mutation rate of viral RNA polymerases, it is believed that RNA viruses exist not as a homogeneous entity, but rather as quasispecies of genomes that are centered around a consensus sequence, which facilitates a higher robustness of a viral population [92,93], features that are not recapitulated in molecular clones. This leads, for most ZIKV clones described so far, to an attenuation in cell lines in comparison to the parental strains. Furthermore, reporter-protein expression can additionally attenuate viral replication and/or can show low genomic stability limited to few passage numbers.

3.1.3. Replicons

Compared to full-length infectious clones, ZIKV replicons offer an alternative for the identification and characterization of antiviral compounds. Subgenomic replicons contain the genetic elements crucial for viral replication, but lacking the structural genes required for assembly and release of infectious progeny virus [94]. This renders the replicon system non-infectious, thereby reducing possible biosafety concerns, an issue to consider when used for large screening approaches of compound libraries. In general, flavivirus replicons encompass an in-frame deletion in the structural genes; however, the first 20 codons of the C protein, as well as the 3′ end of the E gene need to be retained as they contain important elements for replication, as well as the signal peptide for the downstream NS1 protein, respectively [94]. Incorporation of a reporter protein, either luminescence- or fluorescence-based, allows for easy detection of viral replication. Stable replicon cell lines can be generated by introducing resistance genes and thus facilitate large-scale antiviral screenings [94]. Several approaches have been described to generate and use ZIKV replicons for the characterization of antivirals [95,96]. Future studies using this molecular tool might facilitate the characterization and development of new therapeutic strategies to inhibit ZIKV replication.

3.2. Cell Culture Systems

Cell culture models are crucial tools to study the molecular mechanisms of ZIKV life cycle and to develop and identify therapeutics. ZIKV has been shown to display a broad tissue tropism with several cell surface receptors facilitating ZIKV entry. These include receptor tyrosine kinase family members like AXL and Tyro-3, as well as the innate immune receptor DC-SIGN and the receptor TIM-1, also known as hepatitis A virus cellular receptor 1 (HAVcr-1) (reviewed in [97]). However, none of these receptors seems to be unique for ZIKV. Genetic ablations of, e.g., the AXL receptor, which has been discussed as a crucial attachment factor for ZIKV, could not confer resistance to ZIKV infection in vitro and in vivo [98]. This might indicate that ZIKV either concordantly uses several receptors as attachment factors or that receptor usage differs between different cell types and tissues. In accordance with its clinical manifestation, the virus infects several brain cells including cortical neurons, neuronal progenitor cells (NPCs), as well as glial cells, astrocytes and microglia. Furthermore, given its classical route of transmission, skin cells with dermal fibroblasts and epidermal keratinocytes, as well as skin-associated immune cells, including DCs, have also been described to be susceptible. Other susceptible tissues include testis, with Sertoli cells suspected to act as a ZIKV reservoir, and placenta with Hofbauer cells, trophoblasts and placental endothelial cells being susceptible to ZIKV infection (reviewed in [97]). A comprehensive list of the currently identified susceptible human primary cells to ZIKV infection is presented in Table 2.

Table 1. Reverse genetic systems for ZIKV, full-length infectious clones.

ZIKV Isolate	Lineage	Isolation	Cloning Strategy	Plasmid Name	Reporter	Tested	Reference
Paraiba_01/2015	Asian	Brazil, 2015	Synthetic intron insertion	ZIKV-1 ZIKV-ICD ZIKV-NS3m	-	Cell culture	[78]
MR766	African	Uganda, 1947	Synthetic intron insertion		-	Cell culture	[79]
FSS13025	Asian	Cambodia, 2010	Subgenomic fragments	pFLZIKV	RLuc	Cell culture mosquito-mouse model	[80]
MR766 H/PF/2013 SPH2015 BeH819015	African Asian Asian Asian	Uganda, 1947 French Polynesia, 2013 Brazil, 2015 Brazil, 2015	Subgenomic fragments		-	Cell culture mouse model	[82]
BeH819015	Asian	Brazil, 2015	Subgenomic fragments	icDNA BeH819015	nLuc GFP mCherry	Cell culture	[83]
MR766^{NIID}	African	Uganda 1947	Subgenomic fragments	ZIKV-MR766$^{NIID-MC}$ ZIKV$_{GFP}$	GFP	Cell culture	[85]
PF DAK (MART)	Asian African Asian	French Polynesia, 2013 Dakar, 1984 Martinique, 2015	Subgenomic fragments	PF DAK PF/DAK DAK/PF PF/MART	-	Cell culture	[86]
MR766^M BeH819015	African Asian	Uganda, 1947 Brazil, 2015	Subgenomic fragments	MR766^{MC} BR15^{MC} CHIM	-	Cell culture	[87]
ZIKV$_{Natal}$	Asian	Natal, 2015	Subgenomic fragments			Cell culture	[89]
PRVABC59	Asian	Puerto Rico, 2015	Subgenomic fragments			Cell culture mosquito-mouse model	[90]
MR-766 P6-740 PRVABC-59	African Asian Asian	Uganda, 1947 Malaysia, 1966 Puerto Rico, 2015	Subgenomic fragments	pBac/MR-766, pBac/P6-740 pBac/PRVABC-59	-	Cell culture	[81]
MR766 H/PF/2013	African Asian	Uganda 1947 French Polynesia, 2013	Mutational inactivation CEPs	synZIKV-MR766 synZIKV-H/PF/2013	*RLuc* FP635	Cell culture	[91]

nLuc, nano-luciferase; RLuc, Renilla luciferase; FP635, turbo far-red fluorescent protein; icDNA, infectious cDNA clone; CEPs, cryptic *E. coli* promoters.

Table 2. Susceptible human primary cells to ZIKV infection.

Primary Cell Type	Tissue/Source	Reference
Dermal fibroblasts	Skin	[99,100]
Epidermal keratinocytes	Skin	[99]
Blood dendritic cells	Peripheral blood	[101]
Monocyte-derived dendritic cells	Peripheral blood	[73,99,102,103]
Monocyte-derived macrophages	Peripheral blood	[104,105]
Monocytes	Peripheral blood	[104,106,107]
NPCs	Brain/PSCs	[108,109]
Astrocytes	Brain	[66,110–112]
Microglia	Brain	[110]
Endothelial cells	Brain	[113]
Hofbauer cells	Placenta	[114–117]
Trophoblasts	Placenta	[114,116,118–120]
Fibroblasts	Placenta	[116]
Endothelial cells	Placenta	[116]
Fibroblasts	Uterus	[34,114]
Mesenchymal stem cells	Umbilical cord	[114]
Epithelial cells	Vagina and cervix	[121]
Sertoli cells	Testis	[122–124]
Spermatozoa	Testis	[125]
Germ cells	Testis	[126,127]
Retinal endothelial cells	Eye	[128]
Retinal pericytes	Eye	[128]
Retinal pigmented cells	Eye	[128]

3.2.1. Human and Animal Cell Lines

Cell lines can be used as a platform to produce high-titer ZIKV stocks, but also to study various aspects of virus replication, including replication kinetics, susceptibility and, to a certain extent, immune response. Especially for the identification and initial characterization of antivirals, they offer a solid basis and have been used to test several approaches. One of the most commonly-used cell lines in ZIKV research is the Vero cell line derived from epithelial kidney cells from African green monkeys. These cells are deficient in type I interferon (IFN) production, making them suitable to yield high virus titers [129]. Other cell lines that have been shown to be susceptible and support ZIKV replication include human kidney, skin, liver, muscle, retina, placental and lung epithelial cell lines, as well as human and murine neuronal cell lines. Interestingly, even though ZIKV was able to replicate efficiently in various cell lines, the amount of intracellular infectious particles, as well as virus release and extent of cytopathic effect varied among the cell lines tested [87,113,130–132]. Furthermore, it was shown that next to human, NHPs and murine cells, ZIKV is able to replicate within a wide range of animal cell lines, expanding the variety of cell lines that can be used to study ZIKV infections [81,130,133]. Given their usefulness regarding availability, cost and handling, cell lines offer a powerful tool for the identification and characterization of antivirals. However, cell line-specific differences with respect to viral kinetics, observed phenotypes, genetic manipulation, as well as innate immune defects should be considered when interpreting results.

3.2.2. Human Primary Cell Cultures

In contrast to cell lines which often differ genetically and phenotypically from their parental tissue, primary cells have a low population doubling level and therefore more closely recapitulate the physiological conditions observed in vivo (Table 2). Primary cells are characterized by their high degree of specialization, are often fully differentiated and thus require optimal defined culture conditions in order to preserve their original phenotype. This means that the use of serum-free specific formulated media is required in order to prevent undesired differentiation or promote the growth of contaminating cells, typically fibroblasts. A large majority of the studies for searching/screening potential therapeutics against ZIKV infection focused on a specific in vitro system often based on cell lines. Considering the wide tissue and cellular tropism of ZIKV and the different possible routes of transmission, broader approaches are mandatory. Thus, when evaluating a potential antiviral approach against ZIKV infection, the selection of the appropriate in vitro system is of central importance, particularly when evaluating compounds targeting cellular host factors involved in viral life cycle. For instance, when the experimental paradigm is to pharmacologically modulate host factors to interfere with vector-borne transmission, the primary cellular targets of ZIKV infection should be selected for therapeutics screening, including skin fibroblasts, epidermal keratinocytes or skin-associated immune cells such as DCs. On the other hand, when screening for therapeutics in the context of vertical transmission, placental, amniotic and/or fetal primary cultures are a more appropriate in vitro system and have already been used by some investigators for the screening of antivirals [34,116,134]. Furthermore, the ability of ZIKV to be transmitted sexually and to persist in the genital tract led to the use of human primary vaginal/cervical epithelial and male germ cells to test the efficacy of anti-ZIKV compounds [121,127]. Although primary cell cultures are relevant biological systems for the identification of potential anti-ZIKV therapeutics, there are technical difficulties limiting their use. Depending on the tissue of interest, obtaining a pure population of primary cells can be laborious, and phenotypic variability is commonly observed between donors. Furthermore, the vast majority of isolated primary cells have a limited shelf life and eventually undergo cellular senescence after a short number of passages. Finally, yet importantly, work with human-derived primary cells from native tissue requires patient-approved consent and the evaluation by an institutional ethical review board.

3.2.3. Human Pluripotent Stem Cell-Derived Cultures

When screening for anti-ZIKV therapeutics targeting host factors with a protective effect on the human neuronal tissue, the use of primary human cell-based systems is challenging for ethical and technical reasons. In addition, in the context of congenital neurotropic ZIKV infection, there is currently no robust in vivo system modelling early human brain development. These obstacles can be bypassed using elaborated in vitro systems exploiting the possibilities offered by human embryonic stem cells (ESCs) and/or human induced pluripotent stem cells (iPSCs) (collectively PSCs) (Table 2). PSCs proliferate extensively and retain multi-lineage activity allowing one to generate virtually any cell type of the body, making them a precious source of primary cells. While ESCs are isolated from surplus human embryos for in vitro fertilization, iPSCs are obtained by reprogramming somatic cells and can be used as a replacement of ESCs to generate distinct brain cells, including cortical neurons, NPCs, glial cells and complex cerebral three-dimensional (3D) cultures termed organoids [135,136]. In the fetal brain, ZIKV targets NPCs, and several investigators used PSC-derived NPCs to investigate the efficacy of antivirals and their ability to prevent microcephaly in vitro [137,138]. Furthermore, there are now established methods to generate primary glial cultures, astrocytes and microglia from PSCs ([139–141]. Additionally, a more advanced in vitro system generated from PSCs, namely 3D cerebral organoids, is to date the only available in vitro system modelling early human brain development [142]. Contrary to NPCs and glial cultures, the cerebral organoid approach allows the screening for therapeutics using an in vitro system mimicking the cellular and architectural complexity of the brain tissue and is thus more predictive of how a potential treatment responds in vivo. This advanced in vitro model helped to unravel the link between microcephaly and ZIKV infection during pregnancy [143,144]. Given the neurotropism of ZIKV, brain organoids have already been used to validate anti-ZIKV compounds [38,138,145]. Although the cerebral organoid technology is currently the most relevant model of the developing human brain, this system has some limitations such as PSCs' line-to-line and organoid batch-to-batch variability, leading to some level of variability and in general to a limited degree of standardization.

3.3. Screening Approaches

In addition to testing specific compounds that have been described to inhibit related viruses or have been shown to possess a known antiviral activity, unbiased screening approaches offer an alternative to identify new antiviral compounds based on libraries containing hundreds of bioactive molecules. Several of these libraries contain FDA-approved drugs and clinical investigational agents, which have shown good safety and pharmacokinetics in vivo, thereby facilitating drug-repurposing strategies. Drug repurposing plays a very important role, given that a considerable risk of an infection exists during pregnancy, which can complicate medical intervention. Identification of antiviral drugs that are already approved during pregnancy could greatly accelerate the availability of therapeutic interventions.

3.3.1. In Vitro Screening Approaches

Different in vitro screening approaches exist, which are usually based on an automated readout, mostly microscopy- or luminescence-based. This readout can be either based on virus yield reduction (VYR) or on cytopathic effect (CPE) reduction [30]. VYR assays include luciferase reporter activity assays, where the reduction in reporter signal correlates to VYR, which in the case of ZIKV has been described either upon usage of replicon cell lines [95,96], pseudo-viruses [146], full-length infectious clones [80,83,91], assays based on immuno-labeling of viral proteins and/or cell proliferation markers and fluorescent or histochemical microscopic analysis [34,134,138,147] and assays based on quantification of viral RNA via quantitative PCR [148]. CPE reduction assays generally monitor the ability of the compound to reduce or inhibit virus-mediated CPE, thereby monitoring cell viability [30]. In the case of ZIKV, several assays have been utilized including colorimetric or luminometric cell death assays [149–151], bright-field microscopy-based phenotypic assays analyzing the percentage of cells undergoing ZIKV-induced morphology changes detected by automated image analysis software [152], viral plaque forming assays [153] and assays measuring caspase-3 activity, which precedes cell death in ZIKV-infected human NPCs [38]. However, CPE reduction assays lack some specificity as alterations in the cellular morphology or viability based on the compound treatment can sometimes not be distinguished from the effects mediated by a reduced CPE due to reduced virus replication and should therefore be interpreted carefully. An alternative approach is to utilize purified recombinant ZIKV proteins, e.g., the NS2-NS3 protease or the NS5 RdRp, and to monitor their enzymatic activity upon compound treatment [154,155] or utilization of a split luciferase complementation assay for the identification of orthosteric inhibitors, which block specific viral protein interactions (e.g., NS2B-NS3) [156].

3.3.2. In Silico Screening Approaches

Computational in silico approaches have proven to be powerful tools in predicting drug targets and the evaluation of treatment strategies. In general, these in silico systems use computational models to describe macromolecule–ligand interactions. Structure-based approaches mimic the binding of the putatively active ligand within the relevant binding site and are therefore frequently able to facilitate further chemical optimization of the compound [157]. Structure-based drug discovery approaches include in silico homology modeling, which predicts the tertiary structure of an amino acid sequence based on a homologous experimentally-determined structure [158]. Homology modeling techniques and molecular docking analyses, which essentially reflect the ligand-receptor binding process of a virtual library of compounds, can be utilized to identify compounds that can target directly viral proteins and have been applied to ZIKV protease [42,159], methyltransferase [42] and RdRp [42,160]. Furthermore, homology models have been designed to predict the ability of potential compounds to inhibit allosterically the binding of viral envelope proteins to cellular glycoproteins [161]. As an alternative to homology modeling, consensus scoring can be used if the target 3D structure is known. This method involves the comparison of two or more methods of docking process, thereby enhancing the performance of virtual screening by improving the rates at which potential hit compounds are reached, which improves the prediction of bound conformations and poses [162]. As ZIKV proteins have been crystalized and ZIKV virions have been studied by electron microscopy [163–165], this method could be used to identify potential hit compounds that have good binding affinities for a real matured ZIKV protein structure obtained with cryo-electron microscopy [166]. A complementary approach to that of molecular docking analysis is to use pharmacophore searching algorithms to find ligands similar to one of known activity and chemical features (such as hydrogen bonds, charges, lipophilic areas) [167,168], which has recently been utilized to identify potent inhibitors of ZIKV NS2B-NS3 [169]. Next to structure-based drug discovery approaches, mathematical analysis of viral replication dynamics and antiviral treatment strategies have been performed for several viruses, including human immunodeficiency virus, hepatitis C virus, influenza A virus, Ebola virus, DENV and ZIKV [170]. A recent study predicted ZIKV replication dynamics in an NHP model including the potential effects of antiviral treatments, data that can be used to optimize and evaluate in silico the impact of antiviral strategies [171]. In conclusion, in silico screening approaches accelerate the drug development process combined with low costs.

4. In Vivo Models

In vitro models greatly facilitate the initial screening and identification of new antivirals. However, they do not fully reflect the complexity and physiology of living organisms. To this end, several in vivo models have been developed to study virus pathogenesis and to test new drugs and vaccines (Figure 3).

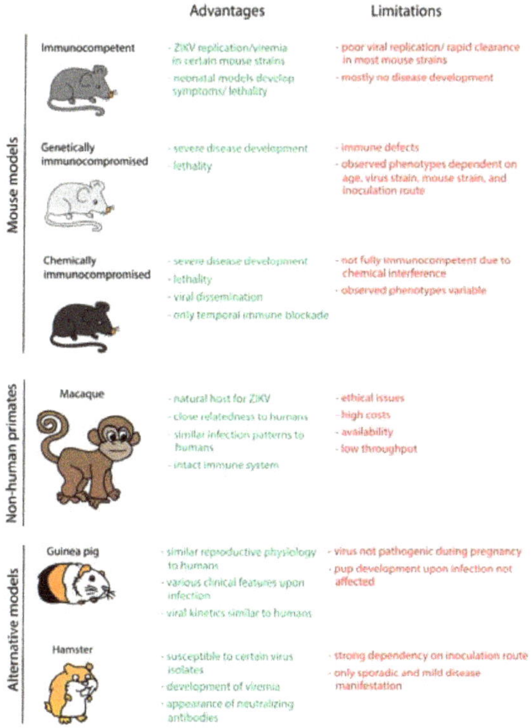

Figure 3. Overview of the currently available in vivo models for the study of ZIKV pathogenesis and for possible antiviral approaches. The text highlighted in green and red indicates advantages and limitations, respectively.

4.1. Mouse Models

Mouse models are widely used to study various aspects of virus infection in vivo, such as pathogenesis and transmission. Several mouse models have been developed to study ZIKV infection (Table 3). Very early studies have shown that mice are susceptible to ZIKV infection, with intracranial inoculation causing neurological symptoms in suckling mice, whereas consistent disease in adult white mice was not clearly manifested ([172–174]. It has been shown that peripheral inoculation of most wildtype (WT) mice results in poor replication, as well as a rapid clearance of infection with no disease development [70,175,176]. One major obstacle appears to be innate immune responses, namely the murine IFN system [177,178]. Similarly to other WT mouse strains, ZIKV infection of the Balb/c mouse model does not result in a fatal outcome; however, it seems to support ZIKV replication more efficiently compared to C57BL/6 WT mice and leads to viremia that is comparable to human in its magnitude and duration [179]. Furthermore, neonatal mouse models have been shown to be susceptible to ZIKV and to develop symptoms and even lead to fetal death depending on the age and virus dose [180–183]. Another exception seems to be the WT SJL mouse model, which supports ZIKV replication and results after intravenous ZIKV inoculation of pregnant mice in growth restriction of developing fetuses, cortical malformations and ocular defects [144,179]. However, SJL mice have been described to have impaired IFN signaling and several immunological defects, rendering them not fully immunocompetent, which might explain the observed susceptibility and fetal pathogenesis [178, 184,185]. To overcome these limitations, immunocompromised mouse systems have been developed. Especially, interference with the type I IFN signaling pathway has been proven to be useful to facilitate viral replication [186]. Genetically modified mice lacking either the type I IFN receptor ifnar1 gene (Ifnar1$^{-/-}$) or the transcription factors Irf3, Irf5 and Irf7 (Irf3$^{-/-}$, Irf5$^{-/-}$, Irf7$^{-/-}$ triple knockout) in 129 (A129) or C57BL/6 background have been shown to be highly susceptible to ZIKV infection and to develop severe diseases following peripheral inoculation, including development of neurological disease and death [70,175,176,180,187–190]. Severity of ZIKV infection in these immunocompromised mice seems to be age dependent, with older mice (>11 weeks-old) being less susceptible to infection than younger mice (3–5 weeks-old) [175,176]. Double knockout mice, lacking both the type I IFN receptor and type II IFN receptor (AG129), displayed even greater susceptibility and more severe disease following ZIKV infection compared to Ifnar1$^{-/-}$-deficient A129 mice [175,191]. Furthermore, in an attempt to better model vertical ZIKV transmission, it could be shown that crossing of female immunocompromised mice with WT males produced heterozygous, IFN competent (Ifnar$^{+/-}$) fetuses, which better resembled the immune status of human fetuses, with ZIKV maternal inoculation resulting in fetal demise that was associated with ZIKV infection of the placenta and fetal brain [192]. Besides directly targeting the IFN receptors, blockage of type I and type III IFN signaling via interference with STAT signaling in Stat1$^{-/-}$- or Stat2$^{-/-}$-deficient mice has also been shown to facilitate ZIKV infection and spreading [70,193]. Furthermore, blockage of type I IFN signaling upon administration of a monoclonal antibody (Mab) targeting the Ifnar1 receptor has been tested as a means to only temporally block IFN signaling in an otherwise immunocompetent mouse and has been shown to increase susceptibility to ZIKV infections [176,194–196]. Increased susceptibility to ZIKV infection has also been demonstrated by pretreatment of mice with dexamethasone, resulting in temporal immunocompromised animals, rendering them susceptible to ZIKV infections [197]. Recently, a transgenic immunocompetent mouse model has been described in which murine Stat2 was replaced with human STAT2, thereby allowing evasion of IFN signaling cascades in infected cells. This model was combined with the generation of a mouse-adapted strain of ZIKV containing a key mutation in the viral NS4B gene and resulted in reduced induction of IFN-β and greater replication in the brain. This approach of establishing an immunocompetent mouse model of ZIKV infection allowed analyses on virus replication, trans-placental transmission, as well as fetal infection [196]. Mouse models can be very well suited to analyze pharmacokinetics of drug candidates, including stability and in vivo retention, as well as the protective efficacy of antivirals and new therapeutics in vivo. There are several studies showing that infection of immunocompromised AG129 (IFN type I and

II receptors deficiency), A129 (IFN type I receptor deficiency) or Stat1$^{-/-}$ mice with ZIKV and subsequent treatment with potential antiviral compounds can lead to decreased viral burden in various tissues, reduced pathology, as well as reduced or delayed morbidity and mortality [156,193, 198–203]. Furthermore, dexamethasone-immunosuppressed mice have been used to evaluate the therapeutic potential of antivirals [159], and in addition, immunocompetent or neonatal mouse models have been shown to be useful to evaluate the efficacy of potential antiviral candidates to reduce viremia [40,204–207]. Even though mouse models can give important insights into viral transmission and pathogenesis and can be used for the initial characterization of therapeutics, it is important to keep in mind that they differ significantly from humans, with respect to several features including placental anatomy and gestation period, as well as disease manifestation, rendering more complex animal models necessary to study specific aspects of ZIKV infection.

Table 3. Mouse models of ZIKV infection.

Model	Strain	Deficiency	ZIKV Inoculation	Pathogenesis	Reference
Immunocompetent	Balb/c		ZIKV2015 (Brazil, 2015) PRVABC59 (Puerto Rico, 2015)	ZIKV replication Viremia Lethality: No	[179]
	SJL	Immunological defects	ZIKV2015 (Brazil, 2015)	ZIKV replication Viremia Lethality: No	[179]
			ZIKV^BR (Brazil, 2015)	Whole-body growth delay or intra-uterine growth restriction (IUGR) in pups	[144]
	C57BL/6		PRVABC59 (Puerto Rico, 2015)	Neurological symptoms	[180]
	C57BL/6 Kunming ICR		MR766 (Uganda, 1947) PRVABC59 (Puerto Rico, 2015) SZ-WIV01 (China, 2016)	Neurological symptoms Lethality: Yes (age and dose-dependent)	[183]
Neonatal	Balb/c C57BL/6 Kunming		Z16006 (China, 2016)	Neurological symptoms Lethality: Yes/No (mouse strain-specific differences)	[181]
	Balb/c		MRS_OPY_Martinique_PaRi_2015 (Martinique, 2015) GZ01 (Venezuela, 2016) SZ01 (Samoa, 2016) FSS13025 (Cambodia, 2010)	Neurological symptoms Lethality: Yes (viral strain-specific differences)	[182]
	C57Bl/6		Dakar 41519 (Senegal, 1984)	Lethality: Yes (partly)	[176]
Partially immunocompetent	hSTAT2 KI Mice (C57BL/6)	hSTAT2 under control mStat2 promotor	Mouse adapted ZIKV-Dak-41525 (=ZIKV-Dak-MA) (Senegal, 1984)	Placental transmission Lethality: Yes (partially)	[196]

Table 3. *Cont.*

Model	Strain	Deficiency	ZIKV Inoculation	Pathogenesis	Reference
Genetically Immunocompromised	A192 (129sV)	Ifnar1$^{-/-}$	MP1751 (Uganda, 1962)	Sever disease Lethality: Yes	[187]
			FSS13025 (Cambodia, 2010)	Signs of illness Severe disease (age dependent) Lethality: Yes (age dependent)	[175]
	IFNAR$^{-/-}$ (C57BL/6)	Ifnar$^{-/-}$	MR 766 (Uganda, 1947) Dakar 41519, 41667, 4167 (Senegal, 1984) H/PF/2013 (FP, 2013)	Severe disease Neurological symptoms Lethality: Yes (age dependent)	[176]
			PRVABC59 (Puerto Rico, 2015)	Severe disease Lethality: Yes	[180]
			FSS13025 (Cambodia, 2010)	Severe disease Lethality: Yes	[188]
			MR 766 (Uganda, 1947 DAKAR 41519 (Senegal, 1984) P6-740 (Malaysia, 1966) FSS13025 (Cambodia, 2010) PRVABC59 (Puerto Rico, 2015)	Severe disease Neurological symptoms Lethality: Yes (virus strain-specific differences in morbidity and lethality)	[70]
	Irf3$^{-/-}$, Irf5$^{-/-}$, Irf7$^{-/-}$ TKO (C57BL/6)	Irf3$^{-/-}$, Irf5$^{-/-}$, Irf7$^{-/-}$	MR 766 (Uganda, 1947), H/PF/2013 (French Polynesia, 2013)	Severe Disease Neurological symptoms Lethality: Yes	[176]
			FSS13025 (Cambodia, 2010)	Signs of disease Neurological symptoms	[189]
	Irf3$^{-/-}$, Irf7$^{-/-}$ DKO (C57BL/6)	Irf3$^{-/-}$, Irf7$^{-/-}$	MR766 (Uganda, 1947)	Viremia Lethality: Infrequent	[190]
	AG129 (129/Sv)	Ifnar$^{-/-}$, Ifngr1$^{-/-}$	FSS13025 (Cambodia, 2010)	Severe disease Neurological symptoms Lethality: Yes	[175]
			H/PF/2013 (French Polynesia, 2013)	Severe disease Lethality: Yes	[191]
	Stat2$^{-/-}$ (C57BL/6)	Stat2$^{-/-}$	MR 766 (Uganda, 1947) DAKAR 41519 (Senegal, 1984) P6-740 (Malaysia, 1966) FSS13025 (Cambodia, 2010) PRVABC59 (Puerto Rico, 2015)	Severe disease Neurological symptoms Lethality: Yes (virus strain-specific differences in morbidity and lethality)	[70]

Table 3. *Cont.*

Model	Strain	Deficiency	ZIKV Inoculation	Pathogenesis	Reference
	Stat1−/−	Stat1−/−	MR 766 (Uganda, 1947)	Viremia Disease development Lethality: Yes	[193]
	C57Bl/6	IFNAR1-blocking monoclonal antibody (MAb-5A3	H/PF/2013 (French Polynesia, 2013)	Viremia / Increased replication Lethality: No	[176]
			DAK AR D 41525 (Senegal, 1984)	Viremia Severe disease Lethality: Yes (differences depending on inoculation route)	[195]
Chemically immunocompromised			Mouse adapted ZIKV-Dak-41525 (=ZIKV-Dak-MA) (Senegal, 1984)	Viremia Severe Disease Lethality: Yes	[194]
			ZIKV-DAK-41525 (Senegal, 1984) ZIKV-DAK-MA (mouse adapted)	Lethality: Yes	[196]
	C57BL/6		H/PF/2013 (French Polynesia, 2013) Mouse adapted ZIKV-Dak-41525 (=ZIKV-Dak-MA) (Senegal, 1984)	Viremia in testis and epididymis	[208]
	Balb/c	Dexamethasone	PRVABC59 (Puerto Rico, 2015)	Viral dissemination Severe disease (after withdrawal) Lethality: Yes (after withdrawal)	[197]

4.2. Non-Human Primate Models

NHPs seem to be natural hosts for ZIKV and are believed to represent the major animal reservoir [209]. ZIKV was first isolated from a rhesus macaque [2], and several monkey species in forests were found to be seropositive for ZIKV [210]. Given their close relatedness to humans, they offer great potential as surrogate models to study specific aspects of ZIKV infection and pathogenesis. It has been shown that macaques are susceptible to infection by both African and Asian ZIKV lineages and that infection results in similar patterns comparable to human infections regarding transmission, cellular tropism, immune responses and viral replication. Infection with ZIKV resulted in viremia that peaked around 2–6 days post-infection, followed by viral clearance. Importantly, viral RNA could be detected in various body fluids including urine, saliva, seminal fluid, vaginal secretions and cerebrospinal fluid, indicating similar dissemination patterns compared to humans [211–217]. Furthermore, mucosal viral inoculation (vaginal or rectal) was shown to lead to productive infection in macaques, mimicking the anogenital transmission route in humans [218]. Importantly, in contrast to mice, NHPs display similarities in gestation, placental barrier and fetal development to humans, rendering them suitable to model ZIKV infections physiologically during pregnancy in humans [219,220]. Indeed, subcutaneous ZIKV inoculation of pregnant macaques with an Asian lineage ZIKV resulted in vertical maternal-fetal ZIKV transmission and reduced growth of the fetal brain, as well as substantial pathology to the central nervous system [216,221]. Even though NHPs offer a more physiological animal model for the study of ZIKV, there are several limitations including ethical issues, high costs, availability and low throughput. These limitations have so far hampered the usage of NHPs for the development and characterization of vaccines and antiviral approaches [214,222–225].

4.3. Alternative Animal Models

Several other animal models have been investigated for the study of ZIKV infections, including guinea pigs, cotton-rats and rabbits, all of which failed to show clinical signs of infection after intracerebral inoculation with the prototype African ZIKV strain MR766 [172]. However, recent studies described the susceptibility of guinea pigs to infection with Asian strains of ZIKV and the development of various clinical features, immune activation and viral kinetics, similar to what has been observed in humans [226]. In addition to subcutaneous infection, other infection routes including intranasal infection and contact transmission of Zika virus could be demonstrated using the guinea pig model, highlighting its suitability to study transmission pathways [227]. However, not all clinical aspects can be reproduced, as circulating ZIKV strains seemed not to be pathogenic during the pregnancy of immunocompetent guinea pigs and did not interfere with offspring development [228]. Nevertheless, in contrast to other small animal models, the guinea pig model is physiologically and immunologically more similar to humans [229]. Especially in the context of ZIKV infection, the similarity of the guinea pig's reproductive physiology, placentation and estrous cycle to humans, as well as the fact that pups are born with a mature central nervous system can be of great advantage for the study of ZIKV pathogenesis and transmission [229–231]. Next to guinea pigs, Syrian golden hamsters have recently also been shown to be to some extent susceptible to certain ZIKV isolates and dependent on the route of inoculation, development of viremia and appearance of virus neutralizing antibodies, and in some cases, mild disease manifestations were observed, rendering them an interesting model to study phenotypic variations between ZIKV strains [232].

These studies show that the host range of ZIKV might be broader than originally anticipated, and different animal models might be useful for the study of different aspects of ZIKV infections. However, the value of these alternative animal models for the characterization and development of antivirals and therapeutics still needs to be fully explored.

5. Concluding Remarks

In recent years, significant advances were made regarding our understanding of ZIKV-associated morbidity in human. Consequently, significant progress was achieved regarding the availability of research models and new experimental tools for the identification of therapeutic and antiviral strategies against ZIKV. However, treatment remains a challenge. Given that treatment needs to be safe and efficient especially in the context of pregnancy further complicates drug development. In addition, a declining trend in ZIKV infections could limit clinical trials. As there is no licensed effective therapy available yet, further efforts are required in order to find potential drug candidates with ideally a wide spectrum of action against flaviviruses found in similar geographical regions with often overlapping symptoms. Furthermore, assuming the broad cellular tropism and the different routes of ZIKV transmission of ZIKV, a variety of models should be applied in order to validate a promising drug. Ultimately, beyond the potential clinical benefits, the knowledge derived from the screening of anti-ZIKV drugs using relevant models will reveal new insights into the understanding of the molecular mechanisms of ZIKV-associated morbidity and greatly contribute to increase our knowledge on flavivirus biology.

Author Contributions: Conceptualization, S.P. Writing, original draft, S.P., M.P.A. Writing, review and editing, all authors.

Funding: S.P. was supported by the European Union's Horizon 2020 research and innovation program under the Marie Skłodowska-Curie Grant Agreement No. 748627. V.T. was supported by the Marie Skłodowska-Curie Innovative Training Network "Honours" (Grant Agreement No. 721367). M.P.A and N.J.V. were supported by the European Union's Horizon 2020 research and innovation program under Grant Agreement No. 735548 ZIKAlliance.

Conflicts of Interest: The authors declare no conflict of interest.

References

1. Dick, G.W. Epidemiological notes on some viruses isolated in Uganda; Yellow fever, Rift Valley fever, Bwamba fever, West Nile, Mengo, Semliki forest, Bunyamwera, Ntaya, Uganda S and Zika viruses. *Trans. R. Soc. Trop. Med. Hyg.* **1953**, *47*, 13–48. [CrossRef]
2. Dick, G.W.; Kitchen, S.F.; Haddow, A.J. Zika virus. I. Isolations and serological specificity. *Trans. R. Soc. Trop. Med. Hyg.* **1952**, *46*, 509–520. [CrossRef]
3. Weinbren, M.P.; Williams, M.C. Zika virus: Further isolations in the Zika area, and some studies on the strains isolated. *Trans. R. Soc. Trop. Med. Hyg.* **1958**, *52*, 263–268. [CrossRef]
4. Haddow, A.J.; Williams, M.C.; Woodall, J.P.; Simpson, D.I.; Goma, L.K. Twelve Isolations of Zika Virus from Aedes (Stegomyia) Africanus (Theobald) Taken in and above a Uganda Forest. *Bull. World Health Organ.* **1964**, *31*, 57–69. [PubMed]
5. Simpson, D.I. Zika Virus Infection in Man. *Trans. R. Soc. Trop. Med. Hyg.* **1964**, *58*, 335–338. [CrossRef]
6. Faye, O.; Freire, C.C.; Iamarino, A.; Faye, O.; de Oliveira, J.V.; Diallo, M.; Zanotto, P.M.; Sall, A.A. Molecular evolution of Zika virus during its emergence in the 20(th) century. *PLoS Negl. Trop. Dis.* **2014**, *8*, e2636. [CrossRef] [PubMed]
7. Duffy, M.R.; Chen, T.H.; Hancock, W.T.; Powers, A.M.; Kool, J.L.; Lanciotti, R.S.; Pretrick, M.; Marfel, M.; Holzbauer, S.; Dubray, C.; et al. Zika virus outbreak on Yap Island, Federated States of Micronesia. *N. Engl. J. Med.* **2009**, *360*, 2536–2543. [CrossRef] [PubMed]
8. Cao-Lormeau, V.M.; Roche, C.; Teissier, A.; Robin, E.; Berry, A.L.; Mallet, H.P.; Sall, A.A.; Musso, D. Zika virus, French polynesia, South pacific, 2013. *Emerg. Infect. Dis.* **2014**, *20*, 1085–1086. [CrossRef] [PubMed]
9. Jouannic, J.M.; Friszer, S.; Leparc-Goffart, I.; Garel, C.; Eyrolle-Guignot, D. Zika virus infection in French Polynesia. *Lancet* **2016**, *387*, 1051–1052. [CrossRef]
10. Campos, G.S.; Bandeira, A.C.; Sardi, S.I. Zika Virus Outbreak, Bahia, Brazil. *Emerg. Infect. Dis.* **2015**, *21*, 1885–1886. [CrossRef] [PubMed]
11. Schuler-Faccini, L.; Ribeiro, E.M.; Feitosa, I.M.; Horovitz, D.D.; Cavalcanti, D.P.; Pessoa, A.; Doriqui, M.J.; Neri, J.I.; Neto, J.M.; Wanderley, H.Y.; et al. Possible Association Between Zika Virus Infection and Microcephaly—Brazil, 2015. *MMWR Morb. Mortal. Wkly. Rep.* **2016**, *65*, 59–62. [CrossRef] [PubMed]

12. Martines, R.B.; Bhatnagar, J.; Keating, M.K.; Silva-Flannery, L.; Muehlenbachs, A.; Gary, J.; Goldsmith, C.; Hale, G.; Ritter, J.; Rollin, D.; et al. Notes from the Field: Evidence of Zika Virus Infection in Brain and Placental Tissues from Two Congenitally Infected Newborns and Two Fetal Losses—Brazil, 2015. *MMWR Morb. Mortal. Wkly. Rep.* **2016**, *65*, 159–160. [CrossRef] [PubMed]

13. Boyer, S.; Calvez, E.; Chouin-Carneiro, T.; Diallo, D.; Failloux, A.B. An overview of mosquito vectors of Zika virus. *Microbes Infect.* **2018**. [CrossRef] [PubMed]

14. Grischott, F.; Puhan, M.; Hatz, C.; Schlagenhauf, P. Non-vector-borne transmission of Zika virus: A systematic review. *Travel Med. Infect. Dis.* **2016**, *14*, 313–330. [CrossRef] [PubMed]

15. Hills, S.L.; Russell, K.; Hennessey, M.; Williams, C.; Oster, A.M.; Fischer, M.; Mead, P. Transmission of Zika Virus Through Sexual Contact with Travelers to Areas of Ongoing Transmission—Continental United States, 2016. *MMWR Morb. Mortal. Wkly. Rep.* **2016**, *65*, 215–216. [CrossRef] [PubMed]

16. Musso, D.; Nhan, T.; Robin, E.; Roche, C.; Bierlaire, D.; Zisou, K.; Shan Yan, A.; Cao-Lormeau, V.M.; Broult, J. Potential for Zika virus transmission through blood transfusion demonstrated during an outbreak in French Polynesia, November 2013 to February 2014. *Euro Surveill* **2014**, *19*, 20761. [CrossRef] [PubMed]

17. Gallian, P.; Cabie, A.; Richard, P.; Paturel, L.; Charrel, R.N.; Pastorino, B.; Leparc-Goffart, I.; Tiberghien, P.; de Lamballerie, X. Zika virus in asymptomatic blood donors in Martinique. *Blood* **2017**, *129*, 263–266. [CrossRef] [PubMed]

18. Blohm, G.M.; Lednicky, J.A.; Marquez, M.; White, S.K.; Loeb, J.C.; Pacheco, C.A.; Nolan, D.J.; Paisie, T.; Salemi, M.; Rodriguez-Morales, A.J.; et al. Evidence for Mother-to-Child Transmission of Zika Virus Through Breast Milk. *Clin. Infect. Dis.* **2018**, *66*, 1120–1121. [CrossRef] [PubMed]

19. Tan, J.J.L.; Balne, P.K.; Leo, Y.S.; Tong, L.; Ng, L.F.P.; Agrawal, R. Persistence of Zika virus in conjunctival fluid of convalescence patients. *Sci. Rep.* **2017**, *7*, 11194. [CrossRef] [PubMed]

20. Petersen, L.R.; Jamieson, D.J.; Powers, A.M.; Honein, M.A. Zika Virus. *N. Engl. J. Med.* **2016**, *374*, 1552–1563. [CrossRef] [PubMed]

21. Cao-Lormeau, V.M.; Blake, A.; Mons, S.; Lastere, S.; Roche, C.; Vanhomwegen, J.; Dub, T.; Baudouin, L.; Teissier, A.; Larre, P.; et al. Guillain-Barre Syndrome outbreak associated with Zika virus infection in French Polynesia: A case-control study. *Lancet* **2016**, *387*, 1531–1539. [CrossRef]

22. Carteaux, G.; Maquart, M.; Bedet, A.; Contou, D.; Brugieres, P.; Fourati, S.; Cleret de Langavant, L.; de Broucker, T.; Brun-Buisson, C.; Leparc-Goffart, I.; et al. Zika Virus Associated with Meningoencephalitis. *N. Engl. J. Med.* **2016**, *374*, 1595–1596. [CrossRef] [PubMed]

23. Mecharles, S.; Herrmann, C.; Poullain, P.; Tran, T.H.; Deschamps, N.; Mathon, G.; Landais, A.; Breurec, S.; Lannuzel, A. Acute myelitis due to Zika virus infection. *Lancet* **2016**, *387*, 1481. [CrossRef]

24. Costello, A.; Dua, T.; Duran, P.; Gulmezoglu, M.; Oladapo, O.T.; Perea, W.; Pires, J.; Ramon-Pardo, P.; Rollins, N.; Saxena, S. Defining the syndrome associated with congenital Zika virus infection. *Bull. World Health Organ.* **2016**, *94*, 406–406A. [CrossRef] [PubMed]

25. Kuno, G.; Chang, G.J. Full-length sequencing and genomic characterization of Bagaza, Kedougou, and Zika viruses. *Arch. Virol.* **2007**, *152*, 687–696. [CrossRef] [PubMed]

26. Chambers, T.J.; Hahn, C.S.; Galler, R.; Rice, C.M. Flavivirus genome organization, expression, and replication. *Annu. Rev. Microbiol.* **1990**, *44*, 649–688. [CrossRef] [PubMed]

27. Bressanelli, S.; Stiasny, K.; Allison, S.L.; Stura, E.A.; Duquerroy, S.; Lescar, J.; Heinz, F.X.; Rey, F.A. Structure of a flavivirus envelope glycoprotein in its low-pH-induced membrane fusion conformation. *EMBO J.* **2004**, *23*, 728–738. [CrossRef] [PubMed]

28. Cortese, M.; Goellner, S.; Acosta, E.G.; Neufeldt, C.J.; Oleksiuk, O.; Lampe, M.; Haselmann, U.; Funaya, C.; Schieber, N.; Ronchi, P.; et al. Ultrastructural Characterization of Zika Virus Replication Factories. *Cell Rep.* **2017**, *18*, 2113–2123. [CrossRef] [PubMed]

29. Hasan, S.S.; Sevvana, M.; Kuhn, R.J.; Rossmann, M.G. Structural biology of Zika virus and other flaviviruses. *Nat. Struct. Mol. Biol.* **2018**, *25*, 13–20. [CrossRef] [PubMed]

30. Mottin, M.; Borba, J.; Braga, R.C.; Torres, P.H.M.; Martini, M.C.; Proenca-Modena, J.L.; Judice, C.C.; Costa, F.T.M.; Ekins, S.; Perryman, A.L.; et al. The A-Z of Zika drug discovery. *Drug Discov. Today* **2018**. [CrossRef] [PubMed]

31. da Silva, S.; Oliveira Silva Martins, D.; Jardim, A.C.G. A Review of the Ongoing Research on Zika Virus Treatment. *Viruses* **2018**, *10*, 255. [CrossRef] [PubMed]

32. Qadir, A.; Riaz, M.; Saeed, M.; Shahzad-Ul-Hussan, S. Potential targets for therapeutic intervention and structure based vaccine design against Zika virus. *Eur. J. Med. Chem.* **2018**, *156*, 444–460. [CrossRef] [PubMed]

33. Carvalho, C.A.M.; Casseb, S.M.M.; Goncalves, R.B.; Silva, E.V.P.; Gomes, A.M.O.; Vasconcelos, P.F.C. Bovine lactoferrin activity against Chikungunya and Zika viruses. *J. Gen. Virol.* **2017**, *98*, 1749–1754. [CrossRef] [PubMed]

34. Rausch, K.; Hackett, B.A.; Weinbren, N.L.; Reeder, S.M.; Sadovsky, Y.; Hunter, C.A.; Schultz, D.C.; Coyne, C.B.; Cherry, S. Screening Bioactives Reveals Nanchangmycin as a Broad Spectrum Antiviral Active against Zika Virus. *Cell Rep.* **2017**, *18*, 804–815. [CrossRef] [PubMed]

35. Carneiro, B.M.; Batista, M.N.; Braga, A.C.S.; Nogueira, M.L.; Rahal, P. The green tea molecule EGCG inhibits Zika virus entry. *Virology* **2016**, *496*, 215–218. [CrossRef] [PubMed]

36. Tricarico, P.M.; Caracciolo, I.; Gratton, R.; D'Agaro, P.; Crovella, S. 25-hydroxycholesterol reduces inflammation, viral load and cell death in ZIKV-infected U-87 MG glial cell line. *Inflammopharmacology* **2018**. [CrossRef] [PubMed]

37. Delvecchio, R.; Higa, L.M.; Pezzuto, P.; Valadao, A.L.; Garcez, P.P.; Monteiro, F.L.; Loiola, E.C.; Dias, A.A.; Silva, F.J.; Aliota, M.T.; et al. Chloroquine, an Endocytosis Blocking Agent, Inhibits Zika Virus Infection in Different Cell Models. *Viruses* **2016**, *8*, 322. [CrossRef] [PubMed]

38. Xu, M.; Lee, E.M.; Wen, Z.; Cheng, Y.; Huang, W.K.; Qian, X.; Tcw, J.; Kouznetsova, J.; Ogden, S.C.; Hammack, C.; et al. Identification of small-molecule inhibitors of Zika virus infection and induced neural cell death via a drug repurposing screen. *Nat. Med.* **2016**, *22*, 1101–1107. [CrossRef] [PubMed]

39. Shiryaev, S.A.; Mesci, P.; Pinto, A.; Fernandes, I.; Sheets, N.; Shresta, S.; Farhy, C.; Huang, C.T.; Strongin, A.Y.; Muotri, A.R.; et al. Repurposing of the anti-malaria drug chloroquine for Zika Virus treatment and prophylaxis. *Sci. Rep.* **2017**, *7*, 15771. [CrossRef] [PubMed]

40. Li, C.; Zhu, X.; Ji, X.; Quanquin, N.; Deng, Y.Q.; Tian, M.; Aliyari, R.; Zuo, X.; Yuan, L.; Afridi, S.K.; et al. Chloroquine, a FDA-approved Drug, Prevents Zika Virus Infection and its Associated Congenital Microcephaly in Mice. *EBioMedicine* **2017**, *24*, 189–194. [CrossRef] [PubMed]

41. Kuivanen, S.; Bespalov, M.M.; Nandania, J.; Ianevski, A.; Velagapudi, V.; De Brabander, J.K.; Kainov, D.E.; Vapalahti, O. Obatoclax, saliphenylhalamide and gemcitabine inhibit Zika virus infection in vitro and differentially affect cellular signaling, transcription and metabolism. *Antiviral Res.* **2017**, *139*, 117–128. [CrossRef] [PubMed]

42. Byler, K.G.; Ogungbe, I.V.; Setzer, W.N. In-silico screening for anti-Zika virus phytochemicals. *J. Mol. Graph. Model.* **2016**, *69*, 78–91. [CrossRef] [PubMed]

43. Lim, S.P.; Wang, Q.Y.; Noble, C.G.; Chen, Y.L.; Dong, H.; Zou, B.; Yokokawa, F.; Nilar, S.; Smith, P.; Beer, D.; et al. Ten years of dengue drug discovery: Progress and prospects. *Antiviral Res.* **2013**, *100*, 500–519. [CrossRef] [PubMed]

44. Coutard, B.; Barral, K.; Lichiere, J.; Selisko, B.; Martin, B.; Aouadi, W.; Lombardia, M.O.; Debart, F.; Vasseur, J.J.; Guillemot, J.C.; et al. Zika Virus Methyltransferase: Structure and Functions for Drug Design Perspectives. *J. Virol.* **2017**, *91*, e02202-16. [CrossRef] [PubMed]

45. Stephen, P.; Baz, M.; Boivin, G.; Lin, S.X. Structural Insight into NS5 of Zika Virus Leading to the Discovery of MTase Inhibitors. *J. Am. Chem. Soc.* **2016**, *138*, 16212–16215. [CrossRef] [PubMed]

46. Zhang, C.; Feng, T.; Cheng, J.; Li, Y.; Yin, X.; Zeng, W.; Jin, X.; Li, Y.; Guo, F.; Jin, T. Structure of the NS5 methyltransferase from Zika virus and implications in inhibitor design. *Biochem. Biophys. Res. Commun.* **2017**, *492*, 624–630. [CrossRef] [PubMed]

47. Duan, W.; Song, H.; Wang, H.; Chai, Y.; Su, C.; Qi, J.; Shi, Y.; Gao, G.F. The crystal structure of Zika virus NS5 reveals conserved drug targets. *EMBO J.* **2017**, *36*, 919–933. [CrossRef] [PubMed]

48. Hercik, K.; Brynda, J.; Nencka, R.; Boura, E. Structural basis of Zika virus methyltransferase inhibition by sinefungin. *Arch. Virol.* **2017**, *162*, 2091–2096. [CrossRef] [PubMed]

49. Xie, X.; Wang, Q.Y.; Xu, H.Y.; Qing, M.; Kramer, L.; Yuan, Z.; Shi, P.Y. Inhibition of dengue virus by targeting viral NS4B protein. *J. Virol.* **2011**, *85*, 11183–11195. [CrossRef] [PubMed]

50. van Cleef, K.W.; Overheul, G.J.; Thomassen, M.C.; Kaptein, S.J.; Davidson, A.D.; Jacobs, M.; Neyts, J.; van Kuppeveld, F.J.; van Rij, R.P. Identification of a new dengue virus inhibitor that targets the viral NS4B protein and restricts genomic RNA replication. *Antiviral Res.* **2013**, *99*, 165–171. [CrossRef] [PubMed]

51. Hernandez-Morales, I.; Geluykens, P.; Clynhens, M.; Strijbos, R.; Goethals, O.; Megens, S.; Verheyen, N.; Last, S.; McGowan, D.; Coesemans, E.; et al. Characterization of a dengue NS4B inhibitor originating from an HCV small molecule library. *Antiviral Res.* **2017**, *147*, 149–158. [CrossRef] [PubMed]

52. Wang, S.; Liu, Y.; Guo, J.; Wang, P.; Zhang, L.; Xiao, G.; Wang, W. Screening of FDA-Approved Drugs for Inhibitors of Japanese Encephalitis Virus Infection. *J. Virol.* **2017**, *91*. [CrossRef] [PubMed]

53. Watterson, D.; Modhiran, N.; Young, P.R. The many faces of the flavivirus NS1 protein offer a multitude of options for inhibitor design. *Antiviral Res.* **2016**, *130*, 7–18. [CrossRef] [PubMed]

54. Bekerman, E.; Neveu, G.; Shulla, A.; Brannan, J.; Pu, S.Y.; Wang, S.; Xiao, F.; Barouch-Bentov, R.; Bakken, R.R.; Mateo, R.; et al. Anticancer kinase inhibitors impair intracellular viral trafficking and exert broad-spectrum antiviral effects. *J. Clin. Investig.* **2017**, *127*, 1338–1352. [CrossRef] [PubMed]

55. Albulescu, I.C.; Kovacikova, K.; Tas, A.; Snijder, E.J.; van Hemert, M.J. Suramin inhibits Zika virus replication by interfering with virus attachment and release of infectious particles. *Antiviral Res.* **2017**, *143*, 230–236. [CrossRef] [PubMed]

56. Kota, S.; Takahashi, V.; Ni, F.; Snyder, J.K.; Strosberg, A.D. Direct binding of a hepatitis C virus inhibitor to the viral capsid protein. *PLoS ONE* **2012**, *7*, e32207. [CrossRef] [PubMed]

57. Scaturro, P.; Trist, I.M.; Paul, D.; Kumar, A.; Acosta, E.G.; Byrd, C.M.; Jordan, R.; Brancale, A.; Bartenschlager, R. Characterization of the mode of action of a potent dengue virus capsid inhibitor. *J. Virol.* **2014**, *88*, 11540–11555. [CrossRef] [PubMed]

58. Oliveira, E.R.A.; Mohana-Borges, R.; de Alencastro, R.B.; Horta, B.A.C. The flavivirus capsid protein: Structure, function and perspectives towards drug design. *Virus Res.* **2017**, *227*, 115–123. [CrossRef] [PubMed]

59. Wang, L.; Valderramos, S.G.; Wu, A.; Ouyang, S.; Li, C.; Brasil, P.; Bonaldo, M.; Coates, T.; Nielsen-Saines, K.; Jiang, T.; et al. From Mosquitos to Humans: Genetic Evolution of Zika Virus. *Cell Host Microbe* **2016**, *19*, 561–565. [CrossRef] [PubMed]

60. Wang, L.; Zhao, H.; Oliva, S.M.; Zhu, H. Modeling the transmission and control of Zika in Brazil. *Sci. Rep.* **2017**, *7*, 7721. [CrossRef] [PubMed]

61. Haddow, A.D.; Schuh, A.J.; Yasuda, C.Y.; Kasper, M.R.; Heang, V.; Huy, R.; Guzman, H.; Tesh, R.B.; Weaver, S.C. Genetic characterization of Zika virus strains: Geographic expansion of the Asian lineage. *PLoS Negl. Trop. Dis.* **2012**, *6*, e1477. [CrossRef] [PubMed]

62. Beaver, J.T.; Lelutiu, N.; Habib, R.; Skountzou, I. Evolution of Two Major Zika Virus Lineages: Implications for Pathology, Immune Response, and Vaccine Development. *Front. Immunol.* **2018**, *9*, 1640. [CrossRef] [PubMed]

63. Pettersson, J.H.; Eldholm, V.; Seligman, S.J.; Lundkvist, A.; Falconar, A.K.; Gaunt, M.W.; Musso, D.; Nougairede, A.; Charrel, R.; Gould, E.A.; et al. How Did Zika Virus Emerge in the Pacific Islands and Latin America? *MBio* **2016**, *7*, e01239-16. [CrossRef] [PubMed]

64. Anfasa, F.; Siegers, J.Y.; van der Kroeg, M.; Mumtaz, N.; Stalin Raj, V.; de Vrij, F.M.S.; Widagdo, W.; Gabriel, G.; Salinas, S.; Simonin, Y.; et al. Phenotypic Differences between Asian and African Lineage Zika Viruses in Human Neural Progenitor Cells. *mSphere* **2017**, *2*, e00292-17. [CrossRef] [PubMed]

65. Simonin, Y.; van Riel, D.; Van de Perre, P.; Rockx, B.; Salinas, S. Differential virulence between Asian and African lineages of Zika virus. *PLoS Negl. Trop. Dis.* **2017**, *11*, e0005821. [CrossRef] [PubMed]

66. Hamel, R.; Ferraris, P.; Wichit, S.; Diop, F.; Talignani, L.; Pompon, J.; Garcia, D.; Liegeois, F.; Sall, A.A.; Yssel, H.; et al. African and Asian Zika virus strains differentially induce early antiviral responses in primary human astrocytes. *Infect. Genet. Evol.* **2017**, *49*, 134–137. [CrossRef] [PubMed]

67. Zhang, F.; Wang, H.J.; Wang, Q.; Liu, Z.Y.; Yuan, L.; Huang, X.Y.; Li, G.; Ye, Q.; Yang, H.; Shi, L.; et al. American Strain of Zika Virus Causes More Severe Microcephaly Than an Old Asian Strain in Neonatal Mice. *EBioMedicine* **2017**, *25*, 95–105. [CrossRef] [PubMed]

68. Smith, D.R.; Sprague, T.R.; Hollidge, B.S.; Valdez, S.M.; Padilla, S.L.; Bellanca, S.A.; Golden, J.W.; Coyne, S.R.; Kulesh, D.A.; Miller, L.J.; et al. African and Asian Zika Virus Isolates Display Phenotypic Differences Both In Vitro and In Vivo. *Am. J. Trop. Med. Hyg.* **2018**, *98*, 432–444. [CrossRef] [PubMed]

69. Simonin, Y.; Loustalot, F.; Desmetz, C.; Foulongne, V.; Constant, O.; Fournier-Wirth, C.; Leon, F.; Moles, J.P.; Goubaud, A.; Lemaitre, J.M.; et al. Zika Virus Strains Potentially Display Different Infectious Profiles in Human Neural Cells. *EBioMedicine* **2016**, *12*, 161–169. [CrossRef] [PubMed]

70. Tripathi, S.; Balasubramaniam, V.R.; Brown, J.A.; Mena, I.; Grant, A.; Bardina, S.V.; Maringer, K.; Schwarz, M.C.; Maestre, A.M.; Sourisseau, M.; et al. A novel Zika virus mouse model reveals strain specific differences in virus pathogenesis and host inflammatory immune responses. *PLoS Pathog.* **2017**, *13*, e1006258. [CrossRef] [PubMed]

71. Dowall, S.D.; Graham, V.A.; Rayner, E.; Hunter, L.; Atkinson, B.; Pearson, G.; Dennis, M.; Hewson, R. Lineage-dependent differences in the disease progression of Zika virus infection in type-I interferon receptor knockout (A129) mice. *PLoS Negl. Trop. Dis.* **2017**, *11*, e0005704. [CrossRef] [PubMed]

72. Shao, Q.; Herrlinger, S.; Zhu, Y.N.; Yang, M.; Goodfellow, F.; Stice, S.L.; Qi, X.P.; Brindley, M.A.; Chen, J.F. The African Zika virus MR-766 is more virulent and causes more severe brain damage than current Asian lineage and dengue virus. *Development* **2017**, *144*, 4114–4124. [CrossRef] [PubMed]

73. Vielle, N.J.; Zumkehr, B.; Garcia-Nicolas, O.; Blank, F.; Stojanov, M.; Musso, D.; Baud, D.; Summerfield, A.; Alves, M.P. Silent infection of human dendritic cells by African and Asian strains of Zika virus. *Sci. Rep.* **2018**, *8*, 5440. [CrossRef] [PubMed]

74. Meda, N.; Salinas, S.; Kagone, T.; Simonin, Y.; Van de Perre, P. Zika virus epidemic: Africa should not be neglected. *Lancet* **2016**, *388*, 337–338. [CrossRef]

75. Wetsman, N. The missing pieces: Lack of Zika data from Africa complicates search for answers. *Nat. Med.* **2017**, *23*, 904–906. [CrossRef] [PubMed]

76. Aubry, F.; Nougairede, A.; Gould, E.A.; de Lamballerie, X. Flavivirus reverse genetic systems, construction techniques and applications: A historical perspective. *Antiviral Res.* **2015**, *114*, 67–85. [CrossRef] [PubMed]

77. Ruggli, N.; Rice, C.M. Functional cDNA clones of the Flaviviridae: Strategies and applications. *Adv. Virus Res.* **1999**, *53*, 183–207. [PubMed]

78. Tsetsarkin, K.A.; Kenney, H.; Chen, R.; Liu, G.; Manukyan, H.; Whitehead, S.S.; Laassri, M.; Chumakov, K.; Pletnev, A.G. A Full-Length Infectious cDNA Clone of Zika Virus from the 2015 Epidemic in Brazil as a Genetic Platform for Studies of Virus-Host Interactions and Vaccine Development. *MBio* **2016**, *7*, e01114-16. [CrossRef] [PubMed]

79. Schwarz, M.C.; Sourisseau, M.; Espino, M.M.; Gray, E.S.; Chambers, M.T.; Tortorella, D.; Evans, M.J. Rescue of the 1947 Zika Virus Prototype Strain with a Cytomegalovirus Promoter-Driven cDNA Clone. *mSphere* **2016**, *1*, e00246-16. [CrossRef] [PubMed]

80. Shan, C.; Xie, X.; Muruato, A.E.; Rossi, S.L.; Roundy, C.M.; Azar, S.R.; Yang, Y.; Tesh, R.B.; Bourne, N.; Barrett, A.D.; et al. An Infectious cDNA Clone of Zika Virus to Study Viral Virulence, Mosquito Transmission, and Antiviral Inhibitors. *Cell Host Microbe* **2016**, *19*, 891–900. [CrossRef] [PubMed]

81. Yun, S.I.; Song, B.H.; Frank, J.C.; Julander, J.G.; Olsen, A.L.; Polejaeva, I.A.; Davies, C.J.; White, K.L.; Lee, Y.M. Functional Genomics and Immunologic Tools: The Impact of Viral and Host Genetic Variations on the Outcome of Zika Virus Infection. *Viruses* **2018**, *10*, 422. [CrossRef] [PubMed]

82. Widman, D.G.; Young, E.; Yount, B.L.; Plante, K.S.; Gallichotte, E.N.; Carbaugh, D.L.; Peck, K.M.; Plante, J.; Swanstrom, J.; Heise, M.T.; et al. A Reverse Genetics Platform That Spans the Zika Virus Family Tree. *MBio* **2017**, *8*, e02014-16. [CrossRef] [PubMed]

83. Mutso, M.; Saul, S.; Rausalu, K.; Susova, O.; Zusinaite, E.; Mahalingam, S.; Merits, A. Reverse genetic system, genetically stable reporter viruses and packaged subgenomic replicon based on a Brazilian Zika virus isolate. *J. Gen. Virol.* **2017**, *98*, 2712–2724. [CrossRef] [PubMed]

84. Aubry, F.; Nougairede, A.; de Fabritus, L.; Querat, G.; Gould, E.A.; de Lamballerie, X. Single-stranded positive-sense RNA viruses generated in days using infectious subgenomic amplicons. *J. Gen. Virol.* **2014**, *95*, 2462–2467. [CrossRef] [PubMed]

85. Gadea, G.; Bos, S.; Krejbich-Trotot, P.; Clain, E.; Viranaicken, W.; El-Kalamouni, C.; Mavingui, P.; Despres, P. A robust method for the rapid generation of recombinant Zika virus expressing the GFP reporter gene. *Virology* **2016**, *497*, 157–162. [CrossRef] [PubMed]

86. Atieh, T.; Baronti, C.; de Lamballerie, X.; Nougairede, A. Simple reverse genetics systems for Asian and African Zika viruses. *Sci. Rep.* **2016**, *6*, 39384. [CrossRef] [PubMed]

87. Bos, S.; Viranaicken, W.; Turpin, J.; El-Kalamouni, C.; Roche, M.; Krejbich-Trotot, P.; Despres, P.; Gadea, G. The structural proteins of epidemic and historical strains of Zika virus differ in their ability to initiate viral infection in human host cells. *Virology* **2018**, *516*, 265–273. [CrossRef] [PubMed]

88. Quan, J.; Tian, J. Circular polymerase extension cloning. *Methods Mol. Biol.* **2014**, *1116*, 103–117. [CrossRef] [PubMed]

89. Setoh, Y.X.; Prow, N.A.; Peng, N.; Hugo, L.E.; Devine, G.; Hazlewood, J.E.; Suhrbier, A.; Khromykh, A.A. De Novo Generation and Characterization of New Zika Virus Isolate Using Sequence Data from a Microcephaly Case. *mSphere* **2017**, *2*, e00190-17. [CrossRef] [PubMed]

90. Weger-Lucarelli, J.; Duggal, N.K.; Bullard-Feibelman, K.; Veselinovic, M.; Romo, H.; Nguyen, C.; Ruckert, C.; Brault, A.C.; Bowen, R.A.; Stenglein, M.; et al. Development and Characterization of Recombinant Virus Generated from a New World Zika Virus Infectious Clone. *J. Virol.* **2017**, *91*, e01765-16. [CrossRef] [PubMed]

91. Munster, M.; Plaszczyca, A.; Cortese, M.; Neufeldt, C.J.; Goellner, S.; Long, G.; Bartenschlager, R. A Reverse Genetics System for Zika Virus Based on a Simple Molecular Cloning Strategy. *Viruses* **2018**, *10*, 368. [CrossRef] [PubMed]

92. de Visser, J.A.; Hermisson, J.; Wagner, G.P.; Ancel Meyers, L.; Bagheri-Chaichian, H.; Blanchard, J.L.; Chao, L.; Cheverud, J.M.; Elena, S.F.; Fontana, W.; et al. Perspective: Evolution and detection of genetic robustness. *Evolution* **2003**, *57*, 1959–1972. [CrossRef] [PubMed]

93. Elena, S.F.; Carrasco, P.; Daros, J.A.; Sanjuan, R. Mechanisms of genetic robustness in RNA viruses. *EMBO Rep.* **2006**, *7*, 168–173. [CrossRef] [PubMed]

94. Kummerer, B.M. Establishment and Application of Flavivirus Replicons. *Adv. Exp. Med. Biol.* **2018**, *1062*, 165–173. [CrossRef] [PubMed]

95. Xie, X.; Zou, J.; Shan, C.; Yang, Y.; Kum, D.B.; Dallmeier, K.; Neyts, J.; Shi, P.Y. Zika Virus Replicons for Drug Discovery. *EBioMedicine* **2016**, *12*, 156–160. [CrossRef] [PubMed]

96. Li, J.Q.; Deng, C.L.; Gu, D.; Li, X.; Shi, L.; He, J.; Zhang, Q.Y.; Zhang, B.; Ye, H.Q. Development of a replicon cell line-based high throughput antiviral assay for screening inhibitors of Zika virus. *Antiviral Res.* **2018**, *150*, 148–154. [CrossRef] [PubMed]

97. Lee, I.; Bos, S.; Li, G.; Wang, S.; Gadea, G.; Despres, P.; Zhao, R.Y. Probing Molecular Insights into Zika Virus−Host Interactions. *Viruses* **2018**, *10*, 233. [CrossRef] [PubMed]

98. Wells, M.F.; Salick, M.R.; Wiskow, O.; Ho, D.J.; Worringer, K.A.; Ihry, R.J.; Kommineni, S.; Bilican, B.; Klim, J.R.; Hill, E.J.; et al. Genetic Ablation of AXL Does Not Protect Human Neural Progenitor Cells and Cerebral Organoids from Zika Virus Infection. *Cell Stem Cell* **2016**, *19*, 703–708. [CrossRef] [PubMed]

99. Hamel, R.; Dejarnac, O.; Wichit, S.; Ekchariyawat, P.; Neyret, A.; Luplertlop, N.; Perera-Lecoin, M.; Surasombatpattana, P.; Talignani, L.; Thomas, F.; et al. Biology of Zika Virus Infection in Human Skin Cells. *J. Virol.* **2015**, *89*, 8880–8896. [CrossRef] [PubMed]

100. Kim, J.A.; Seong, R.K.; Son, S.W.; Shin, O.S. Insights into ZIKV-Mediated Innate Immune Responses in Human Dermal Fibroblasts and Epidermal Keratinocytes. *J. Investig. Dermatol.* **2018**. [CrossRef] [PubMed]

101. Sun, X.; Hua, S.; Chen, H.R.; Ouyang, Z.; Einkauf, K.; Tse, S.; Ard, K.; Ciaranello, A.; Yawetz, S.; Sax, P.; et al. Transcriptional Changes during Naturally Acquired Zika Virus Infection Render Dendritic Cells Highly Conducive to Viral Replication. *Cell Rep.* **2017**, *21*, 3471–3482. [CrossRef] [PubMed]

102. Bowen, J.R.; Zimmerman, M.G.; Suthar, M.S. Taking the defensive: Immune control of Zika virus infection. *Virus Res.* **2018**, *254*, 21–26. [CrossRef] [PubMed]

103. Bowen, J.R.; Quicke, K.M.; Maddur, M.S.; O'Neal, J.T.; McDonald, C.E.; Fedorova, N.B.; Puri, V.; Shabman, R.S.; Pulendran, B.; Suthar, M.S. Zika Virus Antagonizes Type I Interferon Responses during Infection of Human Dendritic Cells. *PLoS Pathog.* **2017**, *13*, e1006164. [CrossRef] [PubMed]

104. Lum, F.M.; Lee, D.; Chua, T.K.; Tan, J.J.L.; Lee, C.Y.P.; Liu, X.; Fang, Y.; Lee, B.; Yee, W.X.; Rickett, N.Y.; et al. Zika Virus Infection Preferentially Counterbalances Human Peripheral Monocyte and/or NK Cell Activity. *mSphere* **2018**, *3*, e00120-18. [CrossRef] [PubMed]

105. Carlin, A.F.; Vizcarra, E.A.; Branche, E.; Viramontes, K.M.; Suarez-Amaran, L.; Ley, K.; Heinz, S.; Benner, C.; Shresta, S.; Glass, C.K. Deconvolution of pro- and antiviral genomic responses in Zika virus-infected and bystander macrophages. *Proc. Natl. Acad. Sci. USA* **2018**, *115*, E9172–E9181. [CrossRef] [PubMed]

106. Michlmayr, D.; Andrade, P.; Gonzalez, K.; Balmaseda, A.; Harris, E. CD14+CD16+ monocytes are the main target of Zika virus infection in peripheral blood mononuclear cells in a paediatric study in Nicaragua. *Nat. Microbiol.* **2017**, *2*, 1462–1470. [CrossRef] [PubMed]

107. Foo, S.S.; Chen, W.; Chan, Y.; Bowman, J.W.; Chang, L.C.; Choi, Y.; Yoo, J.S.; Ge, J.; Cheng, G.; Bonnin, A.; et al. Asian Zika virus strains target CD14+ blood monocytes and induce M2-skewed immunosuppression during pregnancy. *Nat. Microbiol.* **2017**, *2*, 1558–1570. [CrossRef] [PubMed]

108. Tang, H.; Hammack, C.; Ogden, S.C.; Wen, Z.; Qian, X.; Li, Y.; Yao, B.; Shin, J.; Zhang, F.; Lee, E.M.; et al. Zika Virus Infects Human Cortical Neural Progenitors and Attenuates Their Growth. *Cell Stem Cell* **2016**, *18*, 587–590. [CrossRef] [PubMed]

109. Qian, X.; Nguyen, H.N.; Song, M.M.; Hadiono, C.; Ogden, S.C.; Hammack, C.; Yao, B.; Hamersky, G.R.; Jacob, F.; Zhong, C.; et al. Brain-Region-Specific Organoids Using Mini-bioreactors for Modeling ZIKV Exposure. *Cell* **2016**, *165*, 1238–1254. [CrossRef] [PubMed]

110. Meertens, L.; Labeau, A.; Dejarnac, O.; Cipriani, S.; Sinigaglia, L.; Bonnet-Madin, L.; Le Charpentier, T.; Hafirassou, M.L.; Zamborlini, A.; Cao-Lormeau, V.M.; et al. Axl Mediates ZIKA Virus Entry in Human Glial Cells and Modulates Innate Immune Responses. *Cell Rep.* **2017**, *18*, 324–333. [CrossRef] [PubMed]

111. Stefanik, M.; Formanova, P.; Bily, T.; Vancova, M.; Eyer, L.; Palus, M.; Salat, J.; Braconi, C.T.; Zanotto, P.M.A.; Gould, E.A.; et al. Characterisation of Zika virus infection in primary human astrocytes. *BMC Neurosci.* **2018**, *19*, 5. [CrossRef] [PubMed]

112. Chen, J.; Yang, Y.F.; Yang, Y.; Zou, P.; Chen, J.; He, Y.; Shui, S.L.; Cui, Y.R.; Bai, R.; Liang, Y.J.; et al. AXL promotes Zika virus infection in astrocytes by antagonizing type I interferon signalling. *Nat. Microbiol.* **2018**, *3*, 302–309. [CrossRef] [PubMed]

113. Mladinich, M.C.; Schwedes, J.; Mackow, E.R. Zika Virus Persistently Infects and Is Basolaterally Released from Primary Human Brain Microvascular Endothelial Cells. *MBio* **2017**, *8*, e00952-17. [CrossRef] [PubMed]

114. El Costa, H.; Gouilly, J.; Mansuy, J.M.; Chen, Q.; Levy, C.; Cartron, G.; Veas, F.; Al-Daccak, R.; Izopet, J.; Jabrane-Ferrat, N. ZIKA virus reveals broad tissue and cell tropism during the first trimester of pregnancy. *Sci. Rep.* **2016**, *6*, 35296. [CrossRef] [PubMed]

115. Jurado, K.A.; Simoni, M.K.; Tang, Z.; Uraki, R.; Hwang, J.; Householder, S.; Wu, M.; Lindenbach, B.D.; Abrahams, V.M.; Guller, S.; et al. Zika virus productively infects primary human placenta-specific macrophages. *JCI Insight* **2016**, *1*. [CrossRef] [PubMed]

116. Tabata, T.; Petitt, M.; Puerta-Guardo, H.; Michlmayr, D.; Wang, C.; Fang-Hoover, J.; Harris, E.; Pereira, L. Zika Virus Targets Different Primary Human Placental Cells, Suggesting Two Routes for Vertical Transmission. *Cell Host Microbe* **2016**, *20*, 155–166. [CrossRef] [PubMed]

117. Quicke, K.M.; Bowen, J.R.; Johnson, E.L.; McDonald, C.E.; Ma, H.; O'Neal, J.T.; Rajakumar, A.; Wrammert, J.; Rimawi, B.H.; Pulendran, B.; et al. Zika Virus Infects Human Placental Macrophages. *Cell Host Microbe* **2016**, *20*, 83–90. [CrossRef] [PubMed]

118. Bayer, A.; Lennemann, N.J.; Ouyang, Y.; Bramley, J.C.; Morosky, S.; Marques, E.T., Jr.; Cherry, S.; Sadovsky, Y.; Coyne, C.B. Type III Interferons Produced by Human Placental Trophoblasts Confer Protection against Zika Virus Infection. *Cell Host Microbe* **2016**, *19*, 705–712. [CrossRef] [PubMed]

119. Sheridan, M.A.; Yunusov, D.; Balaraman, V.; Alexenko, A.P.; Yabe, S.; Verjovski-Almeida, S.; Schust, D.J.; Franz, A.W.; Sadovsky, Y.; Ezashi, T.; et al. Vulnerability of primitive human placental trophoblast to Zika virus. *Proc. Natl. Acad. Sci. USA* **2017**, *114*, e1587–e1596. [CrossRef] [PubMed]

120. Aagaard, K.M.; Lahon, A.; Suter, M.A.; Arya, R.P.; Seferovic, M.D.; Vogt, M.B.; Hu, M.; Stossi, F.; Mancini, M.A.; Harris, R.A.; et al. Primary Human Placental Trophoblasts are Permissive for Zika Virus (ZIKV) Replication. *Sci. Rep.* **2017**, *7*, 41389. [CrossRef] [PubMed]

121. Fink, S.L.; Vojtech, L.; Wagoner, J.; Slivinski, N.S.J.; Jackson, K.J.; Wang, R.; Khadka, S.; Luthra, P.; Basler, C.F.; Polyak, S.J. The Antiviral Drug Arbidol Inhibits Zika Virus. *Sci. Rep.* **2018**, *8*, 8989. [CrossRef] [PubMed]

122. Siemann, D.N.; Strange, D.P.; Maharaj, P.N.; Shi, P.Y.; Verma, S. Zika Virus Infects Human Sertoli Cells and Modulates the Integrity of the In Vitro Blood-Testis Barrier Model. *J. Virol.* **2017**, *91*, e00623-17. [CrossRef] [PubMed]

123. Strange, D.P.; Green, R.; Siemann, D.N.; Gale, M., Jr.; Verma, S. Immunoprofiles of human Sertoli cells infected with Zika virus reveals unique insights into host-pathogen crosstalk. *Sci. Rep.* **2018**, *8*, 8702. [CrossRef] [PubMed]

124. Kumar, A.; Jovel, J.; Lopez-Orozco, J.; Limonta, D.; Airo, A.M.; Hou, S.; Stryapunina, I.; Fibke, C.; Moore, R.B.; Hobman, T.C. Human Sertoli cells support high levels of Zika virus replication and persistence. *Sci. Rep.* **2018**, *8*, 5477. [CrossRef] [PubMed]

125. Joguet, G.; Mansuy, J.M.; Matusali, G.; Hamdi, S.; Walschaerts, M.; Pavili, L.; Guyomard, S.; Prisant, N.; Lamarre, P.; Dejucq-Rainsford, N.; et al. Effect of acute Zika virus infection on sperm and virus clearance in body fluids: A prospective observational study. *Lancet Infect. Dis.* **2017**, *17*, 1200–1208. [CrossRef]

126. Matusali, G.; Houzet, L.; Satie, A.P.; Mahe, D.; Aubry, F.; Couderc, T.; Frouard, J.; Bourgeau, S.; Bensalah, K.; Lavoue, S.; et al. Zika virus infects human testicular tissue and germ cells. *J. Clin. Investig.* **2018**. [CrossRef] [PubMed]

127. Robinson, C.L.; Chong, A.C.N.; Ashbrook, A.W.; Jeng, G.; Jin, J.; Chen, H.; Tang, E.I.; Martin, L.A.; Kim, R.S.; Kenyon, R.M.; et al. Male germ cells support long-term propagation of Zika virus. *Nat. Commun.* **2018**, *9*, 2090. [CrossRef] [PubMed]

128. Roach, T.; Alcendor, D.J. Zika virus infection of cellular components of the blood-retinal barriers: Implications for viral associated congenital ocular disease. *J. Neuroinflamm.* **2017**, *14*, 43. [CrossRef] [PubMed]

129. Mosca, J.D.; Pitha, P.M. Transcriptional and posttranscriptional regulation of exogenous human beta interferon gene in simian cells defective in interferon synthesis. *Mol. Cell. Biol.* **1986**, *6*, 2279–2283. [CrossRef] [PubMed]

130. Chan, J.F.; Yip, C.C.; Tsang, J.O.; Tee, K.M.; Cai, J.P.; Chik, K.K.; Zhu, Z.; Chan, C.C.; Choi, G.K.; Sridhar, S.; et al. Differential cell line susceptibility to the emerging Zika virus: Implications for disease pathogenesis, non-vector-borne human transmission and animal reservoirs. *Emerg. Microbes Infect.* **2016**, *5*, e93. [CrossRef] [PubMed]

131. Offerdahl, D.K.; Dorward, D.W.; Hansen, B.T.; Bloom, M.E. Cytoarchitecture of Zika virus infection in human neuroblastoma and Aedes albopictus cell lines. *Virology* **2017**, *501*, 54–62. [CrossRef] [PubMed]

132. Himmelsbach, K.; Hildt, E. Identification of various cell culture models for the study of Zika virus. *World J. Virol.* **2018**, *7*, 10–20. [CrossRef] [PubMed]

133. Barr, K.L.; Anderson, B.D.; Prakoso, D.; Long, M.T. Working with Zika and Usutu Viruses In Vitro. *PLoS Negl. Trop. Dis.* **2016**, *10*, e0004931. [CrossRef] [PubMed]

134. Barrows, N.J.; Campos, R.K.; Powell, S.T.; Prasanth, K.R.; Schott-Lerner, G.; Soto-Acosta, R.; Galarza-Munoz, G.; McGrath, E.L.; Urrabaz-Garza, R.; Gao, J.; et al. A Screen of FDA-Approved Drugs for Inhibitors of Zika Virus Infection. *Cell Host Microbe* **2016**, *20*, 259–270. [CrossRef] [PubMed]

135. Takahashi, K.; Yamanaka, S. Induction of pluripotent stem cells from mouse embryonic and adult fibroblast cultures by defined factors. *Cell* **2006**, *126*, 663–676. [CrossRef] [PubMed]

136. Papapetrou, E.P. Induced pluripotent stem cells, past and future. *Science* **2016**, *353*, 991–992. [CrossRef] [PubMed]

137. Lanko, K.; Eggermont, K.; Patel, A.; Kaptein, S.; Delang, L.; Verfaillie, C.M.; Neyts, J. Replication of the Zika virus in different iPSC-derived neuronal cells and implications to assess efficacy of antivirals. *Antiviral Res.* **2017**, *145*, 82–86. [CrossRef] [PubMed]

138. Zhou, T.; Tan, L.; Cederquist, G.Y.; Fan, Y.; Hartley, B.J.; Mukherjee, S.; Tomishima, M.; Brennand, K.J.; Zhang, Q.; Schwartz, R.E.; et al. High-Content Screening in hPSC-Neural Progenitors Identifies Drug Candidates that Inhibit Zika Virus Infection in Fetal-like Organoids and Adult Brain. *Cell Stem Cell* **2017**, *21*, 274–283.e5. [CrossRef] [PubMed]

139. Krencik, R.; Weick, J.P.; Liu, Y.; Zhang, Z.J.; Zhang, S.C. Specification of transplantable astroglial subtypes from human pluripotent stem cells. *Nat. Biotechnol.* **2011**, *29*, 528–534. [CrossRef] [PubMed]

140. Shaltouki, A.; Peng, J.; Liu, Q.; Rao, M.S.; Zeng, X. Efficient generation of astrocytes from human pluripotent stem cells in defined conditions. *Stem Cells* **2013**, *31*, 941–952. [CrossRef] [PubMed]

141. Muffat, J.; Li, Y.; Yuan, B.; Mitalipova, M.; Omer, A.; Corcoran, S.; Bakiasi, G.; Tsai, L.H.; Aubourg, P.; Ransohoff, R.M.; et al. Efficient derivation of microglia-like cells from human pluripotent stem cells. *Nat. Med.* **2016**, *22*, 1358–1367. [CrossRef] [PubMed]

142. Lancaster, M.A.; Renner, M.; Martin, C.A.; Wenzel, D.; Bicknell, L.S.; Hurles, M.E.; Homfray, T.; Penninger, J.M.; Jackson, A.P.; Knoblich, J.A. Cerebral organoids model human brain development and microcephaly. *Nature* **2013**, *501*, 373–379. [CrossRef] [PubMed]

143. Garcez, P.P.; Loiola, E.C.; Madeiro da Costa, R.; Higa, L.M.; Trindade, P.; Delvecchio, R.; Nascimento, J.M.; Brindeiro, R.; Tanuri, A.; Rehen, S.K. Zika virus impairs growth in human neurospheres and brain organoids. *Science* **2016**, *352*, 816–818. [CrossRef] [PubMed]

144. Cugola, F.R.; Fernandes, I.R.; Russo, F.B.; Freitas, B.C.; Dias, J.L.; Guimaraes, K.P.; Benazzato, C.; Almeida, N.; Pignatari, G.C.; Romero, S.; et al. The Brazilian Zika virus strain causes birth defects in experimental models. *Nature* **2016**, *534*, 267–271. [CrossRef] [PubMed]

145. Watanabe, M.; Buth, J.E.; Vishlaghi, N.; de la Torre-Ubieta, L.; Taxidis, J.; Khakh, B.S.; Coppola, G.; Pearson, C.A.; Yamauchi, K.; Gong, D.; et al. Self-Organized Cerebral Organoids with Human-Specific Features Predict Effective Drugs to Combat Zika Virus Infection. *Cell Rep.* **2017**, *21*, 517–532. [CrossRef] [PubMed]

146. Pan, T.; Peng, Z.; Tan, L.; Zou, F.; Zhou, N.; Liu, B.; Liang, L.; Chen, C.; Liu, J.; Wu, L.; et al. Non-Steroidal Anti-Inflammatory Drugs (NSAIDs) Potently Inhibit the Replication of Zika Viruses by Inducing the Degradation of AXL. *J. Virol.* **2018**, *92*, e01018-18. [CrossRef] [PubMed]

147. Pascoalino, B.S.; Courtemanche, G.; Cordeiro, M.T.; Gil, L.H.; Freitas-Junior, L. Zika antiviral chemotherapy: Identification of drugs and promising starting points for drug discovery from an FDA-approved library. *F1000Research* **2016**, *5*, 2523. [CrossRef] [PubMed]

148. Goebel, S.; Snyder, B.; Sellati, T.; Saeed, M.; Ptak, R.; Murray, M.; Bostwick, R.; Rayner, J.; Koide, F.; Kalkeri, R. A sensitive virus yield assay for evaluation of Antivirals against Zika Virus. *J. Virol. Methods* **2016**, *238*, 13–20. [CrossRef] [PubMed]

149. Eyer, L.; Nencka, R.; Huvarova, I.; Palus, M.; Joao Alves, M.; Gould, E.A.; De Clercq, E.; Ruzek, D. Nucleoside Inhibitors of Zika Virus. *J. Infect. Dis.* **2016**, *214*, 707–711. [CrossRef] [PubMed]

150. Muller, J.A.; Harms, M.; Schubert, A.; Mayer, B.; Jansen, S.; Herbeuval, J.P.; Michel, D.; Mertens, T.; Vapalahti, O.; Schmidt-Chanasit, J.; et al. Development of a high-throughput colorimetric Zika virus infection assay. *Med. Microbiol. Immunol.* **2017**, *206*, 175–185. [CrossRef] [PubMed]

151. Adcock, R.S.; Chu, Y.K.; Golden, J.E.; Chung, D.H. Evaluation of anti-Zika virus activities of broad-spectrum antivirals and NIH clinical collection compounds using a cell-based, high-throughput screen assay. *Antiviral Res.* **2017**, *138*, 47–56. [CrossRef] [PubMed]

152. Bernatchez, J.A.; Yang, Z.; Coste, M.; Li, J.; Beck, S.; Liu, Y.; Clark, A.E.; Zhu, Z.; Luna, L.A.; Sohl, C.D.; et al. Development and Validation of a Phenotypic High-Content Imaging Assay for Assessing the Antiviral Activity of Small-Molecule Inhibitors Targeting Zika Virus. *Antimicrob. Agents Chemother.* **2018**, *62*. [CrossRef] [PubMed]

153. Micewicz, E.D.; Khachatoorian, R.; French, S.W.; Ruchala, P. Identification of novel small-molecule inhibitors of Zika virus infection. *Bioorg. Med. Chem. Lett.* **2017**. [CrossRef] [PubMed]

154. Roy, A.; Lim, L.; Srivastava, S.; Lu, Y.; Song, J. Solution conformations of Zika NS2B-NS3pro and its inhibition by natural products from edible plants. *PLoS ONE* **2017**, *12*, e0180632. [CrossRef] [PubMed]

155. Xu, H.T.; Hassounah, S.A.; Colby-Germinario, S.P.; Oliveira, M.; Fogarty, C.; Quan, Y.; Han, Y.; Golubkov, O.; Ibanescu, I.; Brenner, B.; et al. Purification of Zika virus RNA-dependent RNA polymerase and its use to identify small-molecule Zika inhibitors. *J. Antimicrob. Chemother.* **2017**, *72*, 727–734. [CrossRef] [PubMed]

156. Li, Z.; Brecher, M.; Deng, Y.Q.; Zhang, J.; Sakamuru, S.; Liu, B.; Huang, R.; Koetzner, C.A.; Allen, C.A.; Jones, S.A.; et al. Existing drugs as broad-spectrum and potent inhibitors for Zika virus by targeting NS2B-NS3 interaction. *Cell Res.* **2017**, *27*, 1046–1064. [CrossRef] [PubMed]

157. Murgueitio, M.S.; Bermudez, M.; Mortier, J.; Wolber, G. In silico virtual screening approaches for anti-viral drug discovery. *Drug Discov. Today Technol.* **2012**, *9*, e219–e225. [CrossRef] [PubMed]

158. Franca, T.C. Homology modeling: An important tool for the drug discovery. *J. Biomol. Struct. Dyn.* **2015**, *33*, 1780–1793. [CrossRef] [PubMed]

159. Yuan, S.; Chan, J.F.; den-Haan, H.; Chik, K.K.; Zhang, A.J.; Chan, C.C.; Poon, V.K.; Yip, C.C.; Mak, W.W.; Zhu, Z.; et al. Structure-based discovery of clinically approved drugs as Zika virus NS2B-NS3 protease inhibitors that potently inhibit Zika virus infection in vitro and in vivo. *Antiviral Res.* **2017**, *145*, 33–43. [CrossRef] [PubMed]

160. Singh, A.; Jana, N.K. Discovery of potential Zika virus RNA polymerase inhibitors by docking-based virtual screening. *Comput. Biol. Chem.* **2017**, *71*, 144–151. [CrossRef] [PubMed]

161. Airapetian, K.V.; Nikitin, S.S.; Pavlov, E.V. [Electroneuromyography in patients with severe diphtheric polyneuropathy under conditions of artificial ventilation of the lungs]. *Anesteziol. Reanimatol.* **1996**, 21–23.

162. Feher, M. Consensus scoring for protein-ligand interactions. *Drug Discov. Today* **2006**, *11*, 421–428. [CrossRef] [PubMed]

163. Sirohi, D.; Chen, Z.; Sun, L.; Klose, T.; Pierson, T.C.; Rossmann, M.G.; Kuhn, R.J. The 3.8 A resolution cryo-EM structure of Zika virus. *Science* **2016**, *352*, 467–470. [CrossRef] [PubMed]

164. Lei, J.; Hansen, G.; Nitsche, C.; Klein, C.D.; Zhang, L.; Hilgenfeld, R. Crystal structure of Zika virus NS2B-NS3 protease in complex with a boronate inhibitor. *Science* **2016**, *353*, 503–505. [CrossRef] [PubMed]

165. Chen, X.; Yang, K.; Wu, C.; Chen, C.; Hu, C.; Buzovetsky, O.; Wang, Z.; Ji, X.; Xiong, Y.; Yang, H. Mechanisms of activation and inhibition of Zika virus NS2B-NS3 protease. *Cell Res.* **2016**, *26*, 1260–1263. [CrossRef] [PubMed]

166. Onawole, A.T.; Sulaiman, K.O.; Adegoke, R.O.; Kolapo, T.U. Identification of potential inhibitors against the Zika virus using consensus scoring. *J. Mol. Graph. Model.* **2017**, *73*, 54–61. [CrossRef] [PubMed]

167. Jayanthi, C.J.; Tosatti, E.; Fasolino, A. Erratum: Self-consistent phonons, thermal properties, and vibrational instability of the copper crystal. *Phys. Rev. B Condens. Matter* **1985**, *31*, 7465. [CrossRef] [PubMed]

168. McInnes, C. Virtual screening strategies in drug discovery. *Curr. Opin. Chem. Biol.* **2007**, *11*, 494–502. [CrossRef] [PubMed]

169. Rohini, K.; Agarwal, P.; Preethi, B.; Shanthi, V.; Ramanathan, K. Exploring the Lead Compounds for Zika Virus NS2B-NS3 Protein: An e-Pharmacophore-Based Approach. *Appl. Biochem. Biotechnol.* **2018**. [CrossRef] [PubMed]

170. Zitzmann, C.; Kaderali, L. Mathematical Analysis of Viral Replication Dynamics and Antiviral Treatment Strategies: From Basic Models to Age-Based Multi-Scale Modeling. *Front. Microbiol.* **2018**, *9*, 1546. [CrossRef] [PubMed]

171. Best, K.; Guedj, J.; Madelain, V.; de Lamballerie, X.; Lim, S.Y.; Osuna, C.E.; Whitney, J.B.; Perelson, A.S. Zika plasma viral dynamics in nonhuman primates provides insights into early infection and antiviral strategies. *Proc. Natl. Acad. Sci. USA* **2017**, *114*, 8847–8852. [CrossRef] [PubMed]

172. Dick, G.W. Zika virus. II. Pathogenicity and physical properties. *Trans. R. Soc. Trop. Med. Hyg.* **1952**, *46*, 521–534. [CrossRef]

173. Bell, T.M.; Field, E.J.; Narang, H.K. Zika virus infection of the central nervous system of mice. *Arch. Gesamte Virusforsch.* **1971**, *35*, 183–193. [CrossRef] [PubMed]

174. Way, J.H.; Bowen, E.T.; Platt, G.S. Comparative studies of some African arboviruses in cell culture and in mice. *J. Gen. Virol.* **1976**, *30*, 123–130. [CrossRef] [PubMed]

175. Rossi, S.L.; Tesh, R.B.; Azar, S.R.; Muruato, A.E.; Hanley, K.A.; Auguste, A.J.; Langsjoen, R.M.; Paessler, S.; Vasilakis, N.; Weaver, S.C. Characterization of a Novel Murine Model to Study Zika Virus. *Am. J. Trop. Med. Hyg.* **2016**, *94*, 1362–1369. [CrossRef] [PubMed]

176. Lazear, H.M.; Govero, J.; Smith, A.M.; Platt, D.J.; Fernandez, E.; Miner, J.J.; Diamond, M.S. A Mouse Model of Zika Virus Pathogenesis. *Cell Host Microbe* **2016**, *19*, 720–730. [CrossRef] [PubMed]

177. Grant, A.; Ponia, S.S.; Tripathi, S.; Balasubramaniam, V.; Miorin, L.; Sourisseau, M.; Schwarz, M.C.; Sanchez-Seco, M.P.; Evans, M.J.; Best, S.M.; et al. Zika Virus Targets Human STAT2 to Inhibit Type I Interferon Signaling. *Cell Host Microbe* **2016**, *19*, 882–890. [CrossRef] [PubMed]

178. Morrison, T.E.; Diamond, M.S. Animal Models of Zika Virus Infection, Pathogenesis, and Immunity. *J. Virol.* **2017**, *91*. [CrossRef] [PubMed]

179. Larocca, R.A.; Abbink, P.; Peron, J.P.; Zanotto, P.M.; Iampietro, M.J.; Badamchi-Zadeh, A.; Boyd, M.; Ng'ang'a, D.; Kirilova, M.; Nityanandam, R.; et al. Vaccine protection against Zika virus from Brazil. *Nature* **2016**, *536*, 474–478. [CrossRef] [PubMed]

180. Manangeeswaran, M.; Ireland, D.D.; Verthelyi, D. Zika (PRVABC59) Infection Is Associated with T cell Infiltration and Neurodegeneration in CNS of Immunocompetent Neonatal C57Bl/6 Mice. *PLoS Pathog.* **2016**, *12*, e1006004. [CrossRef] [PubMed]

181. Yu, J.; Liu, X.; Ke, C.; Wu, Q.; Lu, W.; Qin, Z.; He, X.; Liu, Y.; Deng, J.; Xu, S.; et al. Effective Suckling C57BL/6, Kunming, and BALB/c Mouse Models with Remarkable Neurological Manifestation for Zika Virus Infection. *Viruses* **2017**, *9*, 165. [CrossRef] [PubMed]

182. Yuan, L.; Huang, X.Y.; Liu, Z.Y.; Zhang, F.; Zhu, X.L.; Yu, J.Y.; Ji, X.; Xu, Y.P.; Li, G.; Li, C.; et al. A single mutation in the prM protein of Zika virus contributes to fetal microcephaly. *Science* **2017**, *358*, 933–936. [CrossRef] [PubMed]

183. Li, S.; Armstrong, N.; Zhao, H.; Hou, W.; Liu, J.; Chen, C.; Wan, J.; Wang, W.; Zhong, C.; Liu, C.; et al. Zika Virus Fatally Infects Wild Type Neonatal Mice and Replicates in Central Nervous System. *Viruses* **2018**, *10*, 49. [CrossRef] [PubMed]

184. Hutchings, P.R.; Varey, A.M.; Cooke, A. Immunological defects in SJL mice. *Immunology* **1986**, *59*, 445–450. [PubMed]

185. Izumi, K.; Mine, K.; Inoue, Y.; Teshima, M.; Ogawa, S.; Kai, Y.; Kurafuji, T.; Hirakawa, K.; Miyakawa, D.; Ikeda, H.; et al. Reduced Tyk2 gene expression in beta-cells due to natural mutation determines susceptibility to virus-induced diabetes. *Nat. Commun.* **2015**, *6*, 6748. [CrossRef] [PubMed]

186. Haller, O.; Kochs, G.; Weber, F. The interferon response circuit: Induction and suppression by pathogenic viruses. *Virology* **2006**, *344*, 119–130. [CrossRef] [PubMed]

187. Dowall, S.D.; Graham, V.A.; Rayner, E.; Atkinson, B.; Hall, G.; Watson, R.J.; Bosworth, A.; Bonney, L.C.; Kitchen, S.; Hewson, R. A Susceptible Mouse Model for Zika Virus Infection. *PLoS Negl. Trop. Dis.* **2016**, *10*, e0004658. [CrossRef] [PubMed]

188. Yockey, L.J.; Varela, L.; Rakib, T.; Khoury-Hanold, W.; Fink, S.L.; Stutz, B.; Szigeti-Buck, K.; Van den Pol, A.; Lindenbach, B.D.; Horvath, T.L.; et al. Vaginal Exposure to Zika Virus during Pregnancy Leads to Fetal Brain Infection. *Cell* **2016**, *166*, 1247–1256.e4. [CrossRef] [PubMed]

189. Li, H.; Saucedo-Cuevas, L.; Regla-Nava, J.A.; Chai, G.; Sheets, N.; Tang, W.; Terskikh, A.V.; Shresta, S.; Gleeson, J.G. Zika Virus Infects Neural Progenitors in the Adult Mouse Brain and Alters Proliferation. *Cell Stem Cell* **2016**, *19*, 593–598. [CrossRef] [PubMed]

190. Kawiecki, A.B.; Mayton, E.H.; Dutuze, M.F.; Goupil, B.A.; Langohr, I.M.; Del Piero, F.; Christofferson, R.C. Tissue tropisms, infection kinetics, histologic lesions, and antibody response of the MR766 strain of Zika virus in a murine model. *Virol. J.* **2017**, *14*, 82. [CrossRef] [PubMed]

191. Aliota, M.T.; Caine, E.A.; Walker, E.C.; Larkin, K.E.; Camacho, E.; Osorio, J.E. Characterization of Lethal Zika Virus Infection in AG129 Mice. *PLoS Negl. Trop. Dis.* **2016**, *10*, e0004682. [CrossRef] [PubMed]

192. Miner, J.J.; Cao, B.; Govero, J.; Smith, A.M.; Fernandez, E.; Cabrera, O.H.; Garber, C.; Noll, M.; Klein, R.S.; Noguchi, K.K.; et al. Zika Virus Infection during Pregnancy in Mice Causes Placental Damage and Fetal Demise. *Cell* **2016**, *165*, 1081–1091. [CrossRef] [PubMed]

193. Kamiyama, N.; Soma, R.; Hidano, S.; Watanabe, K.; Umekita, H.; Fukuda, C.; Noguchi, K.; Gendo, Y.; Ozaki, T.; Sonoda, A.; et al. Ribavirin inhibits Zika virus (ZIKV) replication in vitro and suppresses viremia in ZIKV-infected STAT1-deficient mice. *Antiviral Res.* **2017**, *146*, 1–11. [CrossRef] [PubMed]

194. Zhao, H.; Fernandez, E.; Dowd, K.A.; Speer, S.D.; Platt, D.J.; Gorman, M.J.; Govero, J.; Nelson, C.A.; Pierson, T.C.; Diamond, M.S.; et al. Structural Basis of Zika Virus-Specific Antibody Protection. *Cell* **2016**, *166*, 1016–1027. [CrossRef] [PubMed]

195. Smith, D.R.; Hollidge, B.; Daye, S.; Zeng, X.; Blancett, C.; Kuszpit, K.; Bocan, T.; Koehler, J.W.; Coyne, S.; Minogue, T.; et al. Neuropathogenesis of Zika Virus in a Highly Susceptible Immunocompetent Mouse Model after Antibody Blockade of Type I Interferon. *PLoS Negl. Trop. Dis.* **2017**, *11*, e0005296. [CrossRef] [PubMed]

196. Gorman, M.J.; Caine, E.A.; Zaitsev, K.; Begley, M.C.; Weger-Lucarelli, J.; Uccellini, M.B.; Tripathi, S.; Morrison, J.; Yount, B.L.; Dinnon, K.H., 3rd; et al. An Immunocompetent Mouse Model of Zika Virus Infection. *Cell Host Microbe* **2018**, *23*, 672–685.e6. [CrossRef] [PubMed]

197. Chan, J.F.; Zhang, A.J.; Chan, C.C.; Yip, C.C.; Mak, W.W.; Zhu, H.; Poon, V.K.; Tee, K.M.; Zhu, Z.; Cai, J.P.; et al. Zika Virus Infection in Dexamethasone-immunosuppressed Mice Demonstrating Disseminated Infection with Multi-organ Involvement Including Orchitis Effectively Treated by Recombinant Type I Interferons. *EBioMedicine* **2016**, *14*, 112–122. [CrossRef] [PubMed]

198. Zmurko, J.; Marques, R.E.; Schols, D.; Verbeken, E.; Kaptein, S.J.; Neyts, J. The Viral Polymerase Inhibitor 7-Deaza-2'-C-Methyladenosine Is a Potent Inhibitor of In Vitro Zika Virus Replication and Delays Disease Progression in a Robust Mouse Infection Model. *PLoS Negl. Trop. Dis.* **2016**, *10*, e0004695. [CrossRef] [PubMed]

199. Deng, Y.Q.; Zhang, N.N.; Li, C.F.; Tian, M.; Hao, J.N.; Xie, X.P.; Shi, P.Y.; Qin, C.F. Adenosine Analog NITD008 Is a Potent Inhibitor of Zika Virus. *Open Forum Infect. Dis.* **2016**, *3*, ofw175. [CrossRef] [PubMed]

200. Bullard-Feibelman, K.M.; Govero, J.; Zhu, Z.; Salazar, V.; Veselinovic, M.; Diamond, M.S.; Geiss, B.J. The FDA-approved drug sofosbuvir inhibits Zika virus infection. *Antiviral Res.* **2017**, *137*, 134–140. [CrossRef] [PubMed]

201. Julander, J.G.; Siddharthan, V.; Evans, J.; Taylor, R.; Tolbert, K.; Apuli, C.; Stewart, J.; Collins, P.; Gebre, M.; Neilson, S.; et al. Efficacy of the broad-spectrum antiviral compound BCX4430 against Zika virus in cell culture and in a mouse model. *Antiviral Res.* **2017**, *137*, 14–22. [CrossRef] [PubMed]

202. Chen, L.; Liu, Y.; Wang, S.; Sun, J.; Wang, P.; Xin, Q.; Zhang, L.; Xiao, G.; Wang, W. Antiviral activity of peptide inhibitors derived from the protein E stem against Japanese encephalitis and Zika viruses. *Antiviral Res.* **2017**, *141*, 140–149. [CrossRef] [PubMed]

203. Costa, V.V.; Del Sarto, J.L.; Rocha, R.F.; Silva, F.R.; Doria, J.G.; Olmo, I.G.; Marques, R.E.; Queiroz-Junior, C.M.; Foureaux, G.; Araujo, J.M.S.; et al. N-Methyl-d-Aspartate (NMDA) Receptor Blockade Prevents Neuronal Death Induced by Zika Virus Infection. *MBio* **2017**, *8*, e00350-17. [CrossRef] [PubMed]

204. Li, C.; Deng, Y.Q.; Wang, S.; Ma, F.; Aliyari, R.; Huang, X.Y.; Zhang, N.N.; Watanabe, M.; Dong, H.L.; Liu, P.; et al. 25-Hydroxycholesterol Protects Host against Zika Virus Infection and Its Associated Microcephaly in a Mouse Model. *Immunity* **2017**, *46*, 446–456. [CrossRef] [PubMed]

205. Ferreira, A.C.; Zaverucha-do-Valle, C.; Reis, P.A.; Barbosa-Lima, G.; Vieira, Y.R.; Mattos, M.; Silva, P.P.; Sacramento, C.; de Castro Faria Neto, H.C.; Campanati, L.; et al. Sofosbuvir protects Zika virus-infected mice from mortality, preventing short- and long-term sequelae. *Sci. Rep.* **2017**, *7*, 9409. [CrossRef] [PubMed]

206. Shiryaev, S.A.; Farhy, C.; Pinto, A.; Huang, C.T.; Simonetti, N.; Elong Ngono, A.; Dewing, A.; Shresta, S.; Pinkerton, A.B.; Cieplak, P.; et al. Characterization of the Zika virus two-component NS2B-NS3 protease and structure-assisted identification of allosteric small-molecule antagonists. *Antiviral Res.* **2017**, *143*, 218–229. [CrossRef] [PubMed]

207. Pattnaik, A.; Palermo, N.; Sahoo, B.R.; Yuan, Z.; Hu, D.; Annamalai, A.S.; Vu, H.L.X.; Correas, I.; Prathipati, P.K.; Destache, C.J.; et al. Discovery of a non-nucleoside RNA polymerase inhibitor for blocking Zika virus replication through in silico screening. *Antiviral Res.* **2018**, *151*, 78–86. [CrossRef] [PubMed]

208. Govero, J.; Esakky, P.; Scheaffer, S.M.; Fernandez, E.; Drury, A.; Platt, D.J.; Gorman, M.J.; Richner, J.M.; Caine, E.A.; Salazar, V.; et al. Zika virus infection damages the testes in mice. *Nature* **2016**, *540*, 438–442. [CrossRef] [PubMed]

209. Bueno, M.G.; Martinez, N.; Abdalla, L.; Duarte Dos Santos, C.N.; Chame, M. Animals in the Zika Virus Life Cycle: What to Expect from Megadiverse Latin American Countries. *PLoS Negl. Trop. Dis.* **2016**, *10*, e0005073. [CrossRef] [PubMed]

210. McCrae, A.W.; Kirya, B.G. Yellow fever and Zika virus epizootics and enzootics in Uganda. *Trans. R. Soc. Trop. Med. Hyg.* **1982**, *76*, 552–562. [CrossRef]

211. Osuna, C.E.; Lim, S.Y.; Deleage, C.; Griffin, B.D.; Stein, D.; Schroeder, L.T.; Omange, R.W.; Best, K.; Luo, M.; Hraber, P.T.; et al. Zika viral dynamics and shedding in rhesus and cynomolgus macaques. *Nat. Med.* **2016**, *22*, 1448–1455. [CrossRef] [PubMed]

212. Li, X.F.; Dong, H.L.; Huang, X.Y.; Qiu, Y.F.; Wang, H.J.; Deng, Y.Q.; Zhang, N.N.; Ye, Q.; Zhao, H.; Liu, Z.Y.; et al. Characterization of a 2016 Clinical Isolate of Zika Virus in Non-human Primates. *EBioMedicine* **2016**, *12*, 170–177. [CrossRef] [PubMed]

213. Dudley, D.M.; Aliota, M.T.; Mohr, E.L.; Weiler, A.M.; Lehrer-Brey, G.; Weisgrau, K.L.; Mohns, M.S.; Breitbach, M.E.; Rasheed, M.N.; Newman, C.M.; et al. A rhesus macaque model of Asian-lineage Zika virus infection. *Nat. Commun.* **2016**, *7*, 12204. [CrossRef] [PubMed]

214. Aliota, M.T.; Dudley, D.M.; Newman, C.M.; Mohr, E.L.; Gellerup, D.D.; Breitbach, M.E.; Buechler, C.R.; Rasheed, M.N.; Mohns, M.S.; Weiler, A.M.; et al. Heterologous Protection against Asian Zika Virus Challenge in Rhesus Macaques. *PLoS Negl. Trop. Dis.* **2016**, *10*, e0005168. [CrossRef] [PubMed]

215. Koide, F.; Goebel, S.; Snyder, B.; Walters, K.B.; Gast, A.; Hagelin, K.; Kalkeri, R.; Rayner, J. Development of a Zika Virus Infection Model in Cynomolgus Macaques. *Front. Microbiol.* **2016**, *7*, 2028. [CrossRef] [PubMed]

216. Nguyen, S.M.; Antony, K.M.; Dudley, D.M.; Kohn, S.; Simmons, H.A.; Wolfe, B.; Salamat, M.S.; Teixeira, L.B.C.; Wiepz, G.J.; Thoong, T.H.; et al. Highly efficient maternal-fetal Zika virus transmission in pregnant rhesus macaques. *PLoS Pathog.* **2017**, *13*, e1006378. [CrossRef] [PubMed]

217. Rayner, J.O.; Kalkeri, R.; Goebel, S.; Cai, Z.; Green, B.; Lin, S.; Snyder, B.; Hagelin, K.; Walters, K.B.; Koide, F. Comparative Pathogenesis of Asian and African-Lineage Zika Virus in Indian Rhesus Macaque's and Development of a Non-Human Primate Model Suitable for the Evaluation of New Drugs and Vaccines. *Viruses* **2018**, *10*, 229. [CrossRef] [PubMed]

218. Haddow, A.D.; Nalca, A.; Rossi, F.D.; Miller, L.J.; Wiley, M.R.; Perez-Sautu, U.; Washington, S.C.; Norris, S.L.; Wollen-Roberts, S.E.; Shamblin, J.D.; et al. High Infection Rates for Adult Macaques after Intravaginal or Intrarectal Inoculation with Zika Virus. *Emerg. Infect. Dis.* **2017**, *23*, 1274–1281. [CrossRef] [PubMed]

219. Grigsby, P.L. Animal Models to Study Placental Development and Function throughout Normal and Dysfunctional Human Pregnancy. *Semin. Reprod. Med.* **2016**, *34*, 11–16. [CrossRef] [PubMed]

220. Mysorekar, I.U.; Diamond, M.S. Modeling Zika Virus Infection in Pregnancy. *N. Engl. J. Med.* **2016**, *375*, 481–484. [CrossRef] [PubMed]

221. Adams Waldorf, K.M.; Stencel-Baerenwald, J.E.; Kapur, R.P.; Studholme, C.; Boldenow, E.; Vornhagen, J.; Baldessari, A.; Dighe, M.K.; Thiel, J.; Merillat, S.; et al. Fetal brain lesions after subcutaneous inoculation of Zika virus in a pregnant nonhuman primate. *Nat. Med.* **2016**, *22*, 1256–1259. [CrossRef] [PubMed]

222. Abbink, P.; Larocca, R.A.; De La Barrera, R.A.; Bricault, C.A.; Moseley, E.T.; Boyd, M.; Kirilova, M.; Li, Z.; Ng'ang'a, D.; Nanayakkara, O.; et al. Protective efficacy of multiple vaccine platforms against Zika virus challenge in rhesus monkeys. *Science* **2016**, *353*, 1129–1132. [CrossRef] [PubMed]

223. Dowd, K.A.; Ko, S.Y.; Morabito, K.M.; Yang, E.S.; Pelc, R.S.; DeMaso, C.R.; Castilho, L.R.; Abbink, P.; Boyd, M.; Nityanandam, R.; et al. Rapid development of a DNA vaccine for Zika virus. *Science* **2016**, *354*, 237–240. [CrossRef] [PubMed]

224. Muthumani, K.; Griffin, B.D.; Agarwal, S.; Kudchodkar, S.B.; Reuschel, E.L.; Choi, H.; Kraynyak, K.A.; Duperret, E.K.; Keaton, A.A.; Chung, C.; et al. In vivo protection against ZIKV infection and pathogenesis through passive antibody transfer and active immunisation with a prMEnv DNA vaccine. *NPJ Vaccines* **2016**, *1*, 16021. [CrossRef] [PubMed]

225. Pardi, N.; Hogan, M.J.; Pelc, R.S.; Muramatsu, H.; Andersen, H.; DeMaso, C.R.; Dowd, K.A.; Sutherland, L.L.; Scearce, R.M.; Parks, R.; et al. Zika virus protection by a single low-dose nucleoside-modified mRNA vaccination. *Nature* **2017**, *543*, 248–251. [CrossRef] [PubMed]

226. Kumar, M.; Krause, K.K.; Azouz, F.; Nakano, E.; Nerurkar, V.R. A guinea pig model of Zika virus infection. *Virol. J.* **2017**, *14*, 75. [CrossRef] [PubMed]

227. Deng, Y.Q.; Zhang, N.N.; Li, X.F.; Wang, Y.Q.; Tian, M.; Qiu, Y.F.; Fan, J.W.; Hao, J.N.; Huang, X.Y.; Dong, H.L.; et al. Intranasal infection and contact transmission of Zika virus in guinea pigs. *Nat. Commun.* **2017**, *8*, 1648. [CrossRef] [PubMed]

228. Bierle, C.J.; Fernandez-Alarcon, C.; Hernandez-Alvarado, N.; Zabeli, J.C.; Janus, B.C.; Putri, D.S.; Schleiss, M.R. Assessing Zika virus replication and the development of Zika-specific antibodies after a mid-gestation viral challenge in guinea pigs. *PLoS ONE* **2017**, *12*, e0187720. [CrossRef] [PubMed]

229. Padilla-Carlin, D.J.; McMurray, D.N.; Hickey, A.J. The guinea pig as a model of infectious diseases. *Comp. Med.* **2008**, *58*, 324–340. [PubMed]

230. Griffith, B.P.; McCormick, S.R.; Fong, C.K.; Lavallee, J.T.; Lucia, H.L.; Goff, E. The placenta as a site of cytomegalovirus infection in guinea pigs. *J. Virol.* **1985**, *55*, 402–409. [PubMed]

231. Mess, A. The Guinea pig placenta: Model of placental growth dynamics. *Placenta* **2007**, *28*, 812–815. [CrossRef] [PubMed]

232. Miller, L.J.; Nasar, F.; Schellhase, C.W.; Norris, S.L.; Kimmel, A.E.; Valdez, S.M.; Wollen-Roberts, S.E.; Shamblin, J.D.; Sprague, T.R.; Lugo-Roman, L.A.; et al. Zika Virus Infection in Syrian Golden Hamsters and Strain 13 Guinea Pigs. *Am. J. Trop. Med. Hyg.* **2018**, *98*, 864–867. [CrossRef] [PubMed]

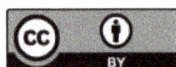

![viruses logo] *viruses*

MDPI

Review

Host-Directed Antivirals: A Realistic Alternative to Fight Zika Virus

Juan-Carlos Saiz *, Nereida Jiménez de Oya ⓘ, Ana-Belén Blázquez ⓘ,
Estela Escribano-Romero ⓘ and Miguel A. Martín-Acebes * ⓘ

Department of Biotechnology, Instituto Nacional de Investigación y Tecnología Agraria y Alimentaria (INIA), 28040 Madrid, Spain; jdeoya@inia.es (N.J.d.O.); blazquez@inia.es (A.-B.B.); eescribano@inia.es (E.E.-R.)
* Correspondence: jcsaiz@inia.es (J.-C.S.); martin.mangel@inia.es (M.A.M.-A.); Tel.: +34-91-347-1497 (J.-C.S.); +34-91-347-8770 (M.A.M.-A.)

Received: 19 July 2018; Accepted: 22 August 2018; Published: 24 August 2018

Abstract: Zika virus (ZIKV), a mosquito-borne flavivirus, was an almost neglected pathogen until its introduction in the Americas in 2015, where it has been responsible for a threat to global health, causing a great social and sanitary alarm due to its increased virulence, rapid spread, and an association with severe neurological and ophthalmological complications. Currently, no specific antiviral therapy against ZIKV is available, and treatments are palliative and mainly directed toward the relief of symptoms, such as fever and rash, by administering antipyretics, anti-histamines, and fluids for dehydration. Nevertheless, lately, search for antivirals has been a major aim in ZIKV investigations. To do so, screening of libraries from different sources, testing of natural compounds, and repurposing of drugs with known antiviral activity have allowed the identification of several antiviral candidates directed to both viral (structural proteins and enzymes) and cellular elements. Here, we present an updated review of current knowledge about anti-ZIKV strategies, focusing on host-directed antivirals as a realistic alternative to combat ZIKV infection.

Keywords: flavivirus; Zika virus; therapy; host-directed antivirals

---

1. Introduction

Since the beginning of the 21st century, a number of infectious disease threats have emerged that demand a global response. Among them, severe acute respiratory syndrome virus, avian influenza in humans, pandemic influenza A (H1N1), Middle East respiratory syndrome coronavirus, chikungunya virus, and Ebola virus have been the most threatening ones. Nonetheless, the emergency of a vector-borne virus, Zika virus (ZIKV), which is responsible for congenital malformations and other neurological and ophthalmological disorders, was hard to predict.

ZIKV is a mosquito-borne virus belonging to the Spondweni serocomplex in the genus *Flavivirus* of the family *Flaviviridae* [1]. The virus has been isolated from various mosquito species, although it seems that the natural transmission vectors are mosquitoes of the genus *Aedes* [2,3]. Besides mosquito bites, viral direct human-to-human transmission can occur perinatally, sexually, and through breastfeeding and blood transfusion [4]. The ZIKV genome is a single-stranded RNA molecule ($\approx$10.7 kb) of positive polarity encoding a single open reading frame (ORF) flanked by two untranslated regions at the 5$'$ and 3$'$ ends [5].

ZIKV was first isolated from the serum of a monkey in 1947, and one year later from *Aedes africanus* mosquitoes caught in the same area, the Zika forest [6]. Until it was detected in Asia in the 1980s, the virus had been confined to Africa. Later on, human outbreaks were reported in the Pacific islands, Micronesia in 2007 and, then, in French Polynesia in 2013 [4]. The natural course of ZIKV infection was usually asymptomatic or produce a relatively mild illness and an uneventful recovery [7], hence, the virus was considered an almost neglected pathogen until its recent introduction into the Americas in 2015, when it became a threat to global health, showing increased virulence, rapid spread, and an association with severe neurological complications such as an unexpected rise of microcephaly cases in fetuses and newborns and a remarkable increase in Guillain-Barré syndrome (GBS) cases [8]. This drove the World Health Organization (WHO) to declare a public health emergency of international concern (PHEIC) in 2016 [9].

ZIKV is a neurotropic virus with a wide tissue tropism [10–12], including reproductive tissues and organs. In males, ZIKV can infect testes, the prostate, and seminal vesicles [12,13], and in females it can infect the vagina, uterus, vaginal epithelium, uterine fibroblasts, Hofbauer cells, trophoblasts, and endothelial cells from the placenta [12,14]. ZIKV has also been detected in the cornea, neurosensory retina, optic nerve, aqueous humor, and tears [15]. Because of this, ZIKV infection can lead to severe neurological and ophthalmological disorders.

Lack of effective prophylactics, vaccines, or therapeutics hampers the fight against ZIKV. Consequently, inactivated viruses, live vector-based, and nucleic acid (DNA or RNA)-based candidates, subunit elements, virus-like particles, and recombinant viruses are been rehearsed, some of them already in clinical trials [16]. Likewise, many different compounds are being tested as possible therapeutic agents against ZIKV that target either viral or cellular components.

The present review discusses recent advances in the design and development of antivirals and therapeutics for ZIKV infection, focusing in those directed against host factors needed for the viral life cycle as a realistic alternative for the treatment of ZIKV infection.

2. Therapeutic Approaches

Since the recent outbreak in 2015 in the Americas, a quite high number of possible antiviral candidates are being tested *in vitro* and *in vivo*. However, until now, no specific therapy has been approved against any flavivirus [17], including ZIKV [18], and, thus, current treatments are mainly directed toward the relief of symptoms, such as fever and rash, by administering antipyretics, anti-histamines, and fluids for dehydration [15]. Nevertheless, it should be noted that some commonly used drugs, such as acetylsalicylic acid, are contraindicated in ZIKV-infected patients, since they increase the risk of internal bleeding, and other arboviruses (dengue or chikungunya viruses) that can co-infect the patients may produce hemorrhages [3].

Due to the natural course of ZIKV infection, which is usually asymptomatic or produce a relatively mild illness and an uneventful recovery, when facing anti-ZIKV strategies, a very important point to take into account is the main target population that would benefit from it, namely immunocompromised patients and pregnant women and their fetuses [4]. In this sense, only for some of the tested drugs their safety profiles are known [19]. However, in cases of Food and Drug Administration (FDA) (https://www.drugs.com/) category B compounds (*animal reproduction studies have failed to demonstrate a risk to the fetus and there are no adequate and well-controlled studies in pregnant women*), or even in those of category C (*animal reproduction studies have shown an adverse effect on the fetus and there are no adequate and well-controlled studies in humans, but potential benefits may warrant use of the drug in pregnant women despite potential risks*), or D (*there is positive evidence of human fetal risk based on adverse reaction data from investigational or marketing experience or studies in humans, but potential benefits may warrant use of the drug in pregnant women despite potential risks*), their use in pregnancy can be contemplated if the potential benefit outweighs the risks. Even more, some of the assayed compounds cross the placenta and, thus, can also benefit the fetus. Nonetheless, if used, this should be done in an individualized way, conditioning dosage and timings, and always under a clinician's control where the patient is informed of the pros and cons.

Current search for ZIKV antivirals is being conducted with different approaches: by screening of compounds libraries; by the repurposing of drugs of known active efficacy against other diseases now in use in clinical practice, many of which display broad-spectrum activity; and by testing natural products. Two different strategies can be applied when pursuing for antivirals, those searching for compounds directed to viral targets (direct-acting antivirals) and those aimed to target cellular components needed for the viral life cycle (host-directed antivirals).

3. Direct-Acting Antivirals

Among the virus-directed drugs tested [18,20] are those acting against the viral RNA-dependent RNA polymerase (non-structural protein 5 (NS5)) catalytic domain, including nucleoside analogs and polymerase inhibitors; the methyltransferase catalytic domain of the NS5 responsible for transferring the mRNA cap; the NS2B-NS3 trypsin-like serine protease needed for proper processing of the viral polyprotein; and the NS3 helicase. The crystal structures of all these proteins have already been resolved and will certainly help to find new antivirals [21–32]. In the same way, structures from other viral proteins are also available that could help to design ZIKV therapeutic alternatives, such as those of the capsid C protein [33], whose destabilization may impair ZIKV multiplication, the NS1 [34,35], an immuno-modulator, or the envelope glycoprotein [36–38], which mediates cell binding and endosomal fusion, constitutes a major target for neutralizing antibodies, and could be also the target for virucidal compounds [39].

On the other hand, it has also been reported that passive transfer of neutralizing antibodies to pregnant mice suppresses ZIKV multiplication, inhibits cell death, reduces the number of progenitor neuronal cells, and prevents microcephaly [40,41]. Likewise, administration of monoclonal antibodies (MAbs) recognizing the domain III of the ZIKV-E protein protect mice of lethal ZIKV challenge [42,43] and other MAbs are able to bind and neutralize ZIKV, including those directed against the E dimer epitope [44]. Human polyclonal antibodies produced in transchromosomal bovines also protect mice from ZIKV lethal infection, eliminated ZIKV induced tissue damage in the brain and testes, and protected against testicular atrophy [45]. Thus, administration of therapeutic antibodies seems to also be a potential strategy against ZIKV. Nevertheless, it should be noted that, although still controvertial in the case of ZIKV infection [46], the well-known antibody dependent enhancement effect (ADE) [47], of which dengue virus (DENV) is the prototypic model, may potentiate the risk of disease exacerbation.

4. Host-Acting Antivirals

Flaviviruses have small RNA genomes (around 10.7 kb in length) and thus require many host factors and co-option of cellular metabolic pathways to successfully infect host cells and propagate efficiently [48]. This offers an opportunity to search for host targets as therapeutic tools that, in many instances, as they are shared by different members of the *Flaviviridae* family, can be envisaged as pan-flaviviral antivirals [48–50]. This strategy can be directed to host factors implicated in infection, pathogenesis, and in the immune response, as it has been shown for DENV and the West Nile virus (WNV) [51]. In addition, their effect would be less prone to the emergence of mutants that will escape their action, as often occurs with drugs targeting viral components. Consequently, this kind of approach could ideally lead to the discovery of broad spectrum antivirals that could provide low cost but effective tools for the control of flaviviral threats.

Different approaches are being used to identify potential host factors as therapeutic targets against flaviviruses including the analyses of transcript levels (e.g., next generation RNA sequencing) for altered expression patterns during infection, proteome changes, kinases activities variations, and protein-RNA interactions (e.g., two-hybrid screenings and affinity chromatography). Likewise, functional analysis can be applied by overexpressing cDNAs or by RNAi-mediated loss of function screens using dsRNA, siRNA, or shRNA libraries, although it should be noted that in some cases downregulation is inefficient and some genes have redundant functions [51]. Replicons may also be used to specifically assay replication activity [52,53].

Theoretically, host-acting antivirals can be directed to any molecule or pathway implicated in the different steps of the viral life cycle, from early events (binding, entry, and fusion), to the formation of the replication complex, and the viral maturation and egress.

4.1. Early Steps: Binding, Entry, and Endosomal Fusion

The first step of ZIKV infection is its binding to the cellular receptor (Figure 1). Several molecules have been proposed as a ZIKV receptor (members of the Tyro3/Axl/Mer (TAM) family of receptor tyrosine kinases, T-cell immunoglobulin and mucin domain (TIM) and dendritic cell-specific intercellular adhesion molecule 3-grabbing nonintegrin (DC-SIGN)) that are expressed in different neuronal and non-neuronal permissive cell types. These molecules are also receptors for other viruses, including flaviviruses such as DENV and WNV, regulate several cellular activities (adhesion, migration, proliferation, and survival, release of inflammatory cytokines, antigen uptake, and signaling), and play important roles in the host's response to infection [54]. However, elimination of a known receptor does not necessarily result in complete protection from viral infection, since flaviviruses use different receptors and, thus, there is always redundancy and alternatives. For instances, inhibiting, downregulating, knocking-down, or ablating AXL, although in some cases they reduce ZIKV infection, they do not completely abolish it, pointing to the use of different cell surface receptors on different cell types [55–58].

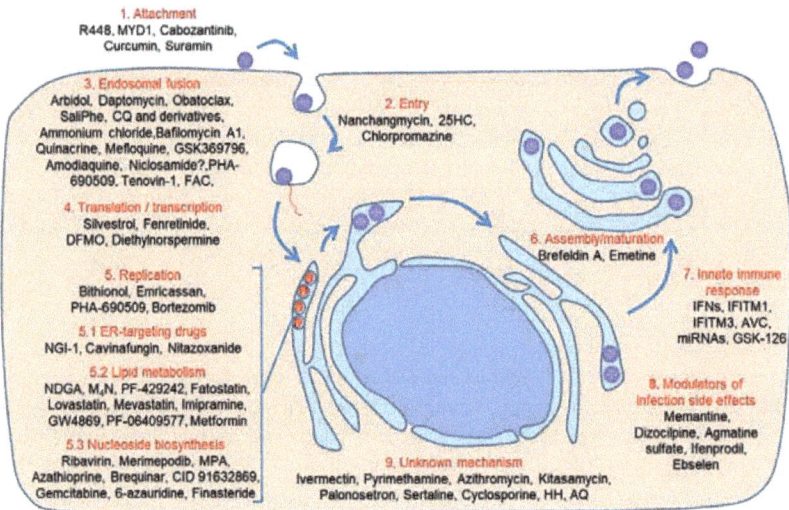

Figure 1. Life cycle of Zika virus (ZIKV) and drugs targeting cellular components. Drugs targeting: attachment (1); entry (2); endosomal fusion (3); translation/transcription (4); replication (5) by affecting the endoplasmic reticulum (ER) (5.1), the lipid metabolism (5.2), the pyrimidine and the purine biosynthesis (5.3); assembly or maturation of the virions (6); or innate immune response (7). Drugs effective for ZIKV infection side effects (8). Drugs with unknown mechanism (9). MYD1: AXL decoy receptor; 25HC: 25-hydroxycholesterol; CQ: chloroquine; FAC: iron salt ferric ammonium citrate; DFMO: difluoromethylornithine; NGI-1: N-linked Glycosylation Inhibitor-1; NDGA: nordihydroguaiaretic acid; M_4N: teramceprocol; MPA: mycophenolic acid; IFNs: interferons; IFITM: interferon-induced transmembrane proteins; AVC: (1-(2-fluorophenyl)-2-(5-isopropyl-1,3,4-thiadiazol-2-yl)-1,2-ihydrochromeno[2,3-c]pyrrole-3,9-dione; HH: hippeastrine hydrobromide; AQ: amodiaquine dihydrochloride dehydrate.

4.1.1. Binding/Entry

Different molecules have been shown to inhibit ZIKV infection at the entry step (Figure 1). R448 (an AXL kinase inhibitor) and MYD1 (an AXL decoy receptor) compromises, but do not completely abolish, ZIKV infection of glial cells [57]. R448, as well as cabozantinib, an inhibitor of AXL phosphorylation, that are currently in clinical trials for anticancer activities, significantly impairs ZIKV infection of human endothelial cells in a dose-dependent manner by affecting a post-binding step [59]. Likewise, curcumin, a widely used food additive and herbal supplement, reduces ZIKV infection in cell culture inhibiting cell binding while maintaining viral RNA integrity [60], as does suramin, an anti-parasitic that interferes with attachment to host cells and with virion biogenesis by affecting glycosylation and maturation [61,62].

4.1.2. Endosomal Fusion

Once ZIKV binds to the cell receptor, like other flaviviruses, it is internalized through clathrin-mediated endocytosis and transported to the endosomes with the involvement of cellular actin and microtubules to establish a productive infection (Figure 1) [57]. After internalization, to start translation and replication, the viral genome is released inside the cytoplasm by fusing the viral envelope with the membranes of the cellular endosomes, a process triggered by acidic pH inside them [63,64]. Nanchangmycin, an insecticide and antibacterial polyether, inhibits ZIKV multiplication and, although the exact mechanism of action has not been completely elucidated, it probably targets AXL and blocks clathrin-mediated endocytosis [65]. Acid endosomal pH triggers rapid conformational changes on viral envelope protein that result in its fusion with endosomal membrane in a pH-dependent manner, thus allowing nucleocapsid release to the cytoplasm for genome uncoating (Figure 1). The optimal pH for conformational rearrangements and viral fusion is 6.3–6.4, and these processes are likely dependent on the presence of cholesterol and specific lipids in the target membrane [66]. These processes can be potentially druggable, and in fact, arbidol, a broad-spectrum antiviral and immunomodulatory use for human influenza A and B infections, inhibits ZIKV multiplication in cell culture probably because it intercalates into membrane lipids leading to the inhibition of membrane fusion between virus particles and plasma membranes, and between virus particles and the membranes of endosomes [67]. Chlorpromazine, an antipsychotic drug that also inhibits clathrin-mediated endocytosis, reduced ZIKV infection, confirming the requirement for clathrin-mediated endocytosis of ZIKV [68]. In addition, 25-hydroxycholesterol (25HC) is increased in ZIKV-infected human embryonic cells and brain organoids, and reduces viremia and viral loads without affecting viral binding, but blocking internalization and suppressing viral and cell membranes fusion [69]. Even more, 25HC reduces mortality and prevents microcephaly in ZIKV-infected mice, and also decreases viral loads in the urine and serum of treated non-human infected primates [69]. Daptomycin, a lipopeptide antibiotic that inserts into cell membranes rich in phosphatidylglycerol, which suggests an effect on late endosomal membranes enriched in this lipid, has also been described as a ZIKV inhibitor [70].

The dependence on endosomal acidification for ZIKV infection also provides a host target suitable for antiviral intervention. For instance, Obatoclax (or GX15-070), an anti-neoplastic and pro-apoptotic inhibitor of the Bcl-2 that targets cellular Mcl-1, impairs ZIKV endocytic uptake by reducing the pH of the endosomal vesicles in cell culture, and thereby most likely inhibits viral fusion [71,72]. However, Obatoclax, which presents a low solubility, has not produced satisfactory results in clinical trials for hematological and myeloid diseases. Saliphenylhalamide (SaliPhe), which targets vacuolar adenosine triphosphatase enzyme (ATPase) and blocks the acidification of endosomes, inhibits ZIKV multiplication in human retinal pigment epithelial cells [71] that are natural targets for ZIKV infection [12]. Similar results were found by Adcock et al. (2017) with SaliPhe using a different screening [73]; however, they reported that, contrary to that described by others [65], other compounds that interfere with the endocytic pathway, such as dynasore, that blocks clathrin-mediated endocytosis, or monensin, a cation transporter, were either toxic for the cells used or did not show any anti-ZIKV activity, as neither did chloroquine (CQ). These contradictory results are probably explained by the different methodologies, cell types, and, to a lower extent, viral strains used to analyze the antiviral activities of the compounds and suggest that compounds showing different activities should be carefully evaluated before going further with investigations. In this line, and contrary to above mentioned report [73], CQ, an FDA-approved anti-inflammatory 4-aminoquinoline and an autophagy inhibitor widely used as an anti-malaria drug that is administered to pregnant women at risk of exposure to Plasmodium parasites, was shown to have anti-ZIKV activity in different cell types (Vero cells, human brain microvascular endothelial cells (hBMECs), and human neural stem cells (NSCs)), affecting early stages of the viral life cycle, possibly by raising the endosomal pH and inhibiting the fusion of the envelope protein to the endosomal membrane [74,75]. CQ has been shown to reduce placental and fetal ZIKV infection [76], and also attenuate ZIKV-associated morbidity and mortality in mice and protect the fetus from microcephaly [77]. Even more, CQ attenuated vertical transmission in ZIKV-infected pregnant interferon signaling-competent Swiss Jim Lambert (SJL) mice, significantly reducing fetal brain viral loads [78]. Similarly, CQ, and other lysosomotropic agents (ammonium chloride, bafilomycin A1, quinacrine, mefloquine, and *N*-tert-Butyl Isoquine (GSK369796)) that neutralize the acidic pH of endosomal compartments, block infection of a human fibroblast cell line and Vero cells [68,75].

Additionally, by medicinal chemistry-driven approaches, a series of new 2,8-bis(trifluoromethyl)quinoline and *N*-(2-(arylmethylimino)ethyl)-7-chloroquinolin-4-amine derivatives have been proved to inhibit ZIKV replication *in vitro* with a higher potency than chloroquine or mefloquine [79,80]. More recently, by screening FDA-approved drugs using a cell-based assay, it has been shown that amodiaquine, another antimalarial drug, also has anti-ZIKV activity in cell culture by targeting early events of the viral replication cycle [81]. Niclosamide, a category B antihelmintic drug approved by FDA, was capable of inhibiting ZIKV infection, and although its antiflaviviral effect has been associated to its ability to neutralize endolysosomal pH and interfere with pH-dependent membrane fusion, in the case of ZIKV, it seems that it was affecting other post-entry steps [82]. In addition, recently, it has been reported that niclosamide decreases ZIKV production, partially restores differentiation, and prevents apoptosis in human induced NSCs; even more, it can partially rescue ZIKV-induced microcephaly and attenuate infection in a developed humanized ZIKV-infected embryo model *in vivo* [83]. Likewise, tenovin-1, which represses cell growth and induces apoptosis in cells expressing p53 by inhibiting the protein-deacetylating activities of SirT1 and SirT2 and, thus, affects endosome functions, potently inhibits ZIKV infection in primary placental fibroblast cells [65]. Iron salt ferric ammonium citrate (FAC) also inhibits ZIKV infection through inducing viral fusion and blocking endosomal viral release by promoting liposome aggregation and intracellular vesicle fusion [84]. Overall, these studies evidence the potential of targeting viral entry to combat ZIKV.

4.2. Translation/Transcription

Once ZIKV-RNA is released from the endosomes in the cytoplasm, it acts as mRNA to synthesize the negative-strand viral RNA that directs positive-strand RNA synthesis (Figure 1) [4]. Silvestrol, a natural compound isolated from the plant *Aglaia foveolata* that it is known to inhibit the Asp-Glu-Ala-Asp (DEAD)-box RNA helicase eukaryotic initiation factor-4A (eIF4A) required to unwind structured 5′-untranslated regions and thus impairing RNA translation, exerts a significant inhibition of ZIKV replication in A549 cells and primary human hepatocytes [85]. *N*-(4-hydroxyphenyl) retinamide (fenretinide or 4-HPR), an activator of retinoid receptors that inhibits the proliferation of cancer cells and can induce apoptosis, inhibits ZIKV in cell culture and significantly reduces both serum viremia and brain viral burden in mice by decreasing the rate of viral RNA synthesis, though not via direct inhibition of the activity of the viral replicase [86]. ZIKV relies on polyamines for both translation and transcription [87], so that, drugs targeting the polyamine biosynthetic pathway, such as difluoromethylornithine (DFMO or eflornithine), an FDA-approved drug that is used to treat trypanosomiasis, hirsutism, and some cancers, as well as diethylnorspermine (DENSpm) limit viral replication in BHK-21 cells [88].

4.3. Replication, Assembly, and Maturation

ZIKV replication and particle morphogenesis take place associated with a virus-induced organelle-like structure derived from the membrane of the endoplasmic reticulum (ER) (Figure 1) [4]. *De novo* synthesized positive strand-RNA, once packaged, form enveloped immature virions in the ER, enter the secretory pathway and, then, in the trans-Golgi network, the prM is cleaved before the virus is released from the infected cell (Figure 1) [89,90].

ER-membrane multiprotein complexes, such as the oligosaccharyltransferase (OST) complex, have been reported to be critical host factors for flavivirus multiplication. In this regard, it has been shown that the N-linked Glycosylation Inhibitor-1 (NGI-1) chemical modulator of the OST complex blocks ZIKV-RNA replication in different cell types [91]. Similarly, the host ER-associated signal peptidase (SPase) is an essential, membrane-bound serine protease complex involved in cleavage of the signal peptides of newly synthesized secretory and membrane proteins at the ER and also for processing of the flavivirus prM and E structural proteins [92]. It has also been reported that cavinafungin, an alaninal-containing lipopeptide of fungal origin, potently inhibits growth of ZIKV-infected cells [93]. Nitazoxanide, a broad-spectrum antiviral agent approved by the FDA as an antiprotozoan and with potential activity against several viruses in clinical trials (rotavirus and norovirus gastroenteritis, chronic hepatitis B, chronic hepatitis C, and influenza), also inhibits virus infection targeting a post-attachment step, most likely virus genome replication [94]. Likewise, Brefeldin A, a *Penicillium* sp. product that inhibits protein transport from the ER to the Golgi apparatus, inhibits ZIKV multiplication [95], as does Emetine, an anti-protozoal agent that inhibits both ZIKV NS5 polymerase activity and disrupts lysosomal function [96].

ZIKV infection leads to cell-death by inducing host caspase-3 and neuronal apoptosis during its propagation [97]. Thereby, bithionol, a caspase inhibitor, inhibits ZIKV strains of different geographical origin in Vero cells and human astrocytes [98]. Similarly, by using a drug repurposing screening of over 6000 molecules, it was found that emricasan, a pan-caspase inhibitor that restrains ZIKV-induced increases in caspase-3 activity and is currently in phase 2 clinical trials in chronic hepatitis C virus (HCV)-infected patients, protected human cortical neural progenitor cells (NPC) in both monolayer and three-dimensional organoid cultures, showing neuroprotective activity without suppression of viral replication [82]. Additionally, bortezomib, a dipeptide boronate proteasome inhibitor approved for treatment of multiple myeloma and mantle cell non-Hodgkin's lymphoma that regulates the Bcl-2 family of proteins, has also been described as a ZIKV inhibitor [70]. Similarly, different cyclin-dependent kinase (CDK) inhibitors, such as (alphaS)-4-(Acetylamino)-alpha-methyl-*N*-(5-(1-methylethyl)-2-thiazolyl)benzeneacetamide (PHA-690509), reduced ZIKV-infection and propagation [82]. However, CDK inhibitors should not be suitable for the treatment of pregnant women but could be useful for the treatment of other non-pregnant patients, preventing the complications associated with ZIKV infection.

4.3.1. Lipid Metabolism Modulators

The need for specific host lipids for flavivirus replication and particle envelopment make lipid metabolism a potential target for an antiviral search [66,99], and, even though manipulating a major metabolic pathway such as lipid biosynthesis can be envisaged as a dangerous antiviral approach due to the undesirable effects that could be detrimental for the host, current use of drugs such as ibuprofen and aspirin (cyclooxygenase-2 (COX-2) inhibitors) or statins (3-hidroxi-3-metil-glutaril-CoA (HMG-CoA) reductase inhibitors) highlights the feasibility of lipid-based therapeutics [100,101]. Accordingly, inhibition of key enzymes involved in fatty acid synthesis, such as acetyl-CoA carboxylase (ACC) [102], and fatty acid synthase (FASN) [103–105], are potential targets for anti-ZIKV therapy. In this line, we have reported that nordihydroguaiaretic acid (NDGA) and its derivative tetra-O-methyl nordihydroguaiaretic (M4N or terameprocol), two compounds that disturb the lipid metabolism probably by interfering with the sterol regulatory element-binding proteins (SREBP) pathway, inhibit the infection of ZIKV and WNV, likely by impairing viral replication, as did other structurally unrelated inhibitors of the SREBP pathway, such as 4-[(Diethylamino)methyl]-*N*-[2-(2-methoxyphenyl)ethyl]-*N*-(3R)-3-pyrrolidinyl-benzamide dihydrochloride (PF-429242) and fatostatin [106]. In the same way, the dependence on cholesterol for different processes during flavivirus infection also provides a suitable target for antiviral strategies. As mentioned above, 25HC reduces viremia and viral loads *in vitro*, and also reduces mortality and prevent microcephaly in mice, and decreases viral loads in the urine and serum in non-human infected primates [69]. Lovastatin and mevastatin are hypolipidemic agents (HMG-CoA inhibitors) belonging to the family of statins that are widely used for lowering cholesterol in patients with hypercholesterolemia and have been previously shown to present antiviral activity against dengue and hepatitis C viruses. Both agents have been proposed as therapeutic candidates against ZIKV [107]. In fact, lovastatin attenuates nervous injury in animal models of GBS [108]. Likewise, imipramine, an FDA-approved antidepressant, inhibits ZIKV-RNA replication and virion production in human skin fibroblasts, probably by interfering with intracellular cholesterol transport [109]. Regarding sphingolipid metabolism, which has been involved in flavivirus infection [66], treatment with the neutral sphingomyelinase inhibitor GW4869 reduced ZIKV production by affecting viral morphogenesis [110] as described for other flaviviruses [111]. Finally, since adenosine monophosphate-activated protein kinase (AMPK) is a master regulator of lipid metabolism, its activation by PF-06409577 or metformin reduced ZIKV infection by impairing viral replication [112,113]. Thus, targeting lipid metabolism could provide therapeutic alternatives for the discovery of host-directed antivirals against ZIKV.

4.3.2. Nucleosides Biosynthesis Inhibitors

The NS5 protein is the viral RNA-dependent RNA polymerase responsible for the RNA synthesis that also inhibits interferon (IFN) signaling by acting over the signal transducer and activator of transcription 2 (STAT2) protein [114], being, thus, a major target for antiviral design. Besides the proven antiviral activities of different nucleosides analogs and inhibitors of the ZIKV-NS5 [18], several inhibitors of the biosynthesis of nucleosides (purines and pyrimidines) also impair ZIKV replication (Figure 1). Ribavirin is an inhibitor of the inosine monophosphate dehydrogenase (IMPDH) with antiviral activity to several RNA viruses [115], but its mechanism of action is not entirely clear. It may act as a guanosine synthesis inhibitor, a viral cap synthesis inhibitor, a viral RNA mutagen, and as an inducer of lethal mutagenesis [116–118]. By using a cell-based assay, no antiviral activity of the drug was initially observed [73] but, later on, it was reported that although no activity against ZIKV was detected in Vero cells, the drug did inhibit virus multiplication in human cell lines, including liver Huh-7 and rhabdomyosarcoma (RD) cells [119]. Further studies have confirmed an inhibitory activity of ribavirin against ZIKV strains of different geographical origin in various types of cells, such as human neural progenitor cells (hNPCs), human dermal fibroblasts (HDFs), human lung adenocarcinoma cells (A549), and even in Vero cells [120–122]. Still more, the drug was shown to abrogate viremia in ZIKV-infected STAT-1-deficient mice [121], which lack type I IFN signaling, are highly sensitive to ZIKV infection, and exhibit a lethal outcome. Two other inhibitors of IMPDH, merimepodib (MMPD or VX-497) [123] and mycophenolic acid (MPA) [65,70,124] also inhibit ZIKV-RNA replication in different cell types, including Huh-7 cells, human cervical placental cells, and neural stem and primary amnion cells. However, other authors [73] have described that MPA have little effect on ZIKV replication and showed significant cell toxicity. Likewise, azathioprine, another inhibitor of purine synthesis and immunosuppressant, impaired ZIKV replication in HeLa and JEG3 cells [70]; nonetheless, its use in pregnant women is not recommended. The above described contradictory results stress again the differences that drug treatments may have as a consequence of the different viral strains, cell types, and methodologies used to assess them.

As with the inhibitors of purine biosynthesis, compounds inhibiting the synthesis of pyrimidines have also effect on ZIKV replication (Figure 1). So that, the virus was highly susceptible to brequinar and CID 91632869 treatments in cell culture [73]. However, it should be noted that it has been reported that brequinar, as well as DD264, antiviral activity may not be due to pyrimidine deprivation, but rather to the induction of the cellular immune response [125,126]. Similarly, other inhibitors of the pyrimidine synthesis, such as gemcitabine, an activator of cellular caspases [65,71], and, although with a lower efficiency probably due to its lower solubility, 6-azauridine and finasteride, a 4-azasteroid analog of testosterone that inhibit type II and type III 5α-reductase and is being tested for benign prostatic hyperplasia and male pattern baldness, reduce ZIKV replication [73,107].

4.3.3. Unknown Mechanisms

Several other compounds have been shown to have anti-ZIKV activity by inhibiting viral entry and/or RNA synthesis, although their mechanisms of action have not yet been fully elucidated. Among them are antiparasitics such as ivermectin (used mainly against worms infections) and pyrimethamine (a folic acid antagonist that inhibits the dihydrofolate reductase and, thus, DNA and RNA synthesis, is classified as a pregnancy category C, and was initially used to treat malaria and now toxoplasmosis and cystoisosporiasis) [70]; antibiotics such as azithromycin that prevents infection, replication, and virus-mediated cell dead [55], and kitasamycin (a natural product from Streptomyces narbonensis that inhibits protein biosynthesis) [107]; drugs used to prevent chemotherapy-induced nausea and vomiting as palonosetron (a FDA-approved 5-HT3 antagonist) [107]; antidepressants like sertraline (a selective serotonin reuptake inhibitor) [107] and cyclosporine (that is also use for rheumatoid arthritis, psoriasis, Crohn's disease, nephrotic syndrome, and in organ transplants, is believed to lower the activity of T-cells, and is currently in clinical trials for tis possible use in ameliorate neuronal cellular damage) [70]. Similarly, after chemical screening, it was found that hippeastrine hydrobromide (HH), an active component of traditional Chinese medicine, and amodiaquine dihydrochloride dihydrate (AQ), an FDA-approved drug for treatment of malaria, inhibit ZIKV infection of human pluripotent stem cell-derived cortical NPCs and in adult mouse brain *in vivo* even when the infection was already ongoing but, again, their mechanisms of action are not known [127].

5. Drugs Preventing ZIKV Infection Side Effects

Besides drugs that act against host targets directly implicated in the viral cycle, there are compounds that can prevent undesirable effects of ZIKV infection. In this regard, ZIKV infection leads to massive neuronal damage, especially of neural progenitor cells, and neurodegeneration [128–130], via both direct replication in neuronal cells and possibly through increased excitotoxicity via over activation of N-methyl-D-aspartate receptor (NMDAR)-dependent neuronal excitotoxicity in nearby cells. Memantine, a pregnancy category B FDA-approved drug widely used to treat patients with Alzheimer's disease, as well as other NMDAR blockers (dizocilpine, agmatine sulfate, or ifenprodil), prevents neuronal damage and death and intraocular pressure increase induced by ZIKV infection in infected mice, but it does not affect virus replication, pointing to its possible use to prevent or minimize ZIKV-related microcephaly during pregnancy [131]. Ebselen (EBS), an antioxidant that reduces oxidative stress and improves histopathological features in a testicular injury study model and is currently in clinical trials for various diseases, showed minor effects in reducing ZIKV progeny production and viral E protein expression and on overall survival and viremia level of challenged AG129 mice; however, it should be noted that EBS reduced some ZIKV-induced effects, such as testicular oxidative stress, leucocyte infiltration, and production of pro-inflammatory response, whereas, in a model of male-to-female mouse sperm transfer, the drug improved testicular pathology and prevented the sexual transmission of ZIKV [132].

6. Innate Immunity Modulation

IFNs play a key role in the elimination of pathogens and they are release upon the activation of the innate immune response by infecting viruses. In this way, ZIKV infection induces IFN signaling pathways and further activates cytoplasmic retinoic acid inducible gene 1 protein (RIG1)-like receptors (RLRs) and several type I and III IFN-stimulated genes, driving to the subsequent activation of the Janus kinase (JAK)/STAT innate immune pathway that confer resistance to ZIKV infection [54]. Different studies showed that IFN-α, IFN-β, and IFN-γ inhibit ZIKV replication in cell culture [124,133,134], and that treatment of pregnant mice with IFN-λ reduced ZIKV infection [135]. In addition, IFITM1 and IFITM3, which are interferon-induced transmembrane proteins, impair early stages of ZIKV infection. Even more, IFITM3 prevents ZIKV-induced cell death [136]. Likewise, it has been reported that an interferon-activating small molecule

(1-(2-fluorophenyl)-2-(5-isopropyl-1,3,4-thiadiazol-2-yl)-1,2-ihydrochromeno[2,3-c]pyrrole-3,9-dione (AVC) strongly inhibits replication of ZIKV in cell culture [137]. However, it is also known that the virus is capable of evading type I IFN responses by acting over the JAK/STAT signaling pathway [114,138–140], and that type I IFNs might be mediators of pregnancy complications, including spontaneous abortions and growth restriction [141]. In any case, use of IFN against ZIKV, alone or in combination with other antivirals, deserve further studies.

By screening a library of known human microRNAs (miRNAs), small, noncoding RNAs (sncRNAs) that modulate gene expression post-transcriptionally and regulate a broad range of cellular processes, several miRNAs were found to inhibit ZIKV by increasing the capability of infected cells to respond to infection through the interferon-based innate immune pathway [142]. Another alternative is intervening over epigenetic regulation by using epigenetics modulators. For instance, histone H3K27 methyltransferases (EZH1 and EZH2) suppress gene transcription and it has been shown that inhibitors such as 1-[(2S)-butan-2-yl]-N-[(4,6-dimethyl-2-oxo-1H-pyridin-3-yl)methyl]-3-methyl-6-(6-piperazin-1-ylpyridin-3-yl)indole-4-carboxamide (GSK-126) reduce ZIKV multiplication in cell culture through the activation of cellular antiviral and immune responses [143]. In any case, further studies are needed to evaluate the potential therapeutic capability of these immunomodulators against ZIKV infection.

7. Conclusions

A great effort is being lately made to find compounds to fight ZIKV infection by applying different approaches, from repurposing of drugs with known antiviral activity to the screening of bioactive molecules from different libraries, as well as natural products. However, most of the already tested drugs have been found to inhibit viral replication *in vitro*, and only a few have been tested *in vivo*. Hence, since, in many instances, the results will be difficult to extrapolate to humans, it would be hard for most of the tested antivirals to complete the entire drug development pipeline. In addition, it should be remarked that many drugs could have untoward effects and, thus, careful evaluation should be conducted before using them in clinical practice, as the main target populations for anti-ZIKV therapy will be pregnant women and patients with other medical complications.

Many of the already tested drugs are directed against viral structural and enzymatic proteins, including, for instance, anticancer and anti-inflammatory molecules, antibiotics, and antiparasitics; however, it is well known that this approach can easily lead to the appearance of resistance. Since flaviviruses require many host factors and co-option of cellular metabolic pathways to successfully infect host cells and propagate efficiently, this offers an opportunity to search for host targets as therapeutic tools that, in many instances, can be broad spectrum agents, and which effect would be less prone to the emergence of mutants that will escape their action. Because of that, and even though manipulating host metabolic pathways can be seen as dangerous due to the undesirable effects that could be detrimental for the host, its success for other diseases make of them a realistic option for the treatment of ZIKV infection.

Funding: This study was funded by The Spanish Ministry of Economy and Competitiveness (MINECO) grant numbers RTA2015-00009 and E-RTA2017-00003-C02 (to J.-C.S.) and AGL2014-56518-JIN (to M.A.M.-A.).

Conflicts of Interest: The authors declare no conflict of interest. The funders had no role in in the writing of the manuscript or in the decision to publish.

References

1. Kuno, G.; Chang, G.J.; Tsuchiya, K.R.; Karabatsos, N.; Cropp, C.B. Phylogeny of the genus flavivirus. *J. Virol.* **1998**, *72*, 73–83. [PubMed]
2. Diagne, C.T.; Diallo, D.; Faye, O.; Ba, Y.; Gaye, A.; Dia, I.; Weaver, S.C.; Sall, A.A.; Diallo, M. Potential of selected senegalese *Aedes* spp. Mosquitoes (*Diptera*: *Culicidae*) to transmit Zika virus. *BMC Infect. Dis.* **2015**, *15*, 492. [CrossRef] [PubMed]
3. Musso, D.; Gubler, D.J. Zika virus. *Clin. Microbiol. Rev.* **2016**, *29*, 487–524. [CrossRef] [PubMed]

4. Saiz, J.C.; Vazquez-Calvo, A.; Blazquez, A.B.; Merino-Ramos, T.; Escribano-Romero, E.; Martin-Acebes, M.A. Zika virus: The latest newcomer. *Front. Microbiol.* **2016**, *7*, 496. [CrossRef] [PubMed]

5. Kuno, G.; Chang, G.J. Full-length sequencing and genomic characterization of bagaza, kedougou, and Zika viruses. *Arch. Virol.* **2007**, *152*, 687–696. [CrossRef] [PubMed]

6. Dick, G.W.; Kitchen, S.F.; Haddow, A.J. Zika virus. I. Isolations and serological specificity. *Trans. R. Soc. Trop. Med. Hyg.* **1952**, *46*, 509–520. [CrossRef]

7. Duffy, M.R.; Chen, T.H.; Hancock, W.T.; Powers, A.M.; Kool, J.L.; Lanciotti, R.S.; Pretrick, M.; Marfel, M.; Holzbauer, S.; Dubray, C.; et al. Zika virus outbreak on yap island, federated states of micronesia. *N. Engl. J. Med.* **2009**, *360*, 2536–2543. [CrossRef] [PubMed]

8. Blazquez, A.B.; Saiz, J.C. Neurological manifestations of Zika virus infection. *World J. Virol.* **2016**, *5*, 135–143. [CrossRef] [PubMed]

9. WHO. The History of Zika Virus. Available online: http://www.who.int/emergencies/zika-virus/history/en/ (accessed on 17 July 2018).

10. Gourinat, A.C.; O'Connor, O.; Calvez, E.; Goarant, C.; Dupont-Rouzeyrol, M. Detection of Zika virus in urine. *Emerg. Infect. Dis.* **2015**, *21*, 84–86. [CrossRef] [PubMed]

11. Coffey, L.L.; Pesavento, P.A.; Keesler, R.I.; Singapuri, A.; Watanabe, J.; Watanabe, R.; Yee, J.; Bliss-Moreau, E.; Cruzen, C.; Christe, K.L.; et al. Zika virus tissue and blood compartmentalization in acute infection of rhesus macaques. *PLoS ONE* **2017**, *12*, e0171148. [CrossRef] [PubMed]

12. Miner, J.J.; Diamond, M.S. Zika virus pathogenesis and tissue tropism. *Cell Host Microbe* **2017**, *21*, 134–142. [CrossRef] [PubMed]

13. Govero, J.; Esakky, P.; Scheaffer, S.M.; Fernandez, E.; Drury, A.; Platt, D.J.; Gorman, M.J.; Richner, J.M.; Caine, E.A.; Salazar, V.; et al. Zika virus infection damages the testes in mice. *Nature* **2016**, *540*, 438–442. [CrossRef] [PubMed]

14. Hirsch, A.J.; Smith, J.L.; Haese, N.N.; Broeckel, R.M.; Parkins, C.J.; Kreklywich, C.; DeFilippis, V.R.; Denton, M.; Smith, P.P.; Messer, W.B.; et al. Zika virus infection of rhesus macaques leads to viral persistence in multiple tissues. *PLoS Pathog.* **2017**, *13*, e1006219. [CrossRef] [PubMed]

15. Saiz, J.C.; Martin-Acebes, M.A.; Bueno-Mari, R.; Salomon, O.D.; Villamil-Jimenez, L.C.; Heukelbach, J.; Alencar, C.H.; Armstrong, P.K.; Ortiga-Carvalho, T.M.; Mendez-Otero, R.; et al. Zika virus: What have we learnt since the start of the recent epidemic? *Front. Microbiol.* **2017**, *8*, 1554. [CrossRef] [PubMed]

16. WHO. Who Vaccine Pipeline Tracker. Available online: http://www.who.int/immunization/research/vaccine_pipeline_tracker_spreadsheet/en/ (accessed on 17 July 2018).

17. Menendez-Arias, L.; Richman, D.D. Editorial overview: Antivirals and resistance: Advances and challenges ahead. *Curr. Opin. Virol.* **2014**, *8*, iv–vii. [CrossRef] [PubMed]

18. Saiz, J.C.; Martin-Acebes, M.A. The race to find antivirals for Zika virus. *Antimicrob. Agents Chemother.* **2017**, *61*. [CrossRef] [PubMed]

19. Khandia, R.; Munjal, A.; Dhama, K. Consequences of Zika virus infection during fetal stage and pregnancy safe drugs: An update. *Int. J. Pharmacol.* **2017**, *13*, 370–377.

20. Munjal, A.; Khandia, R.; Dhama, K.; Sachan, S.; Karthik, K.; Tiwari, R.; Malik, Y.S.; Kumar, D.; Singh, R.K.; Iqbal, H.M.N.; et al. Advances in developing therapies to combat Zika virus: Current knowledge and future perspectives. *Front. Microbiol.* **2017**, *8*, 1469. [CrossRef] [PubMed]

21. Lei, J.; Hansen, G.; Nitsche, C.; Klein, C.D.; Zhang, L.; Hilgenfeld, R. Crystal structure of Zika virus NS2B-NS3 protease in complex with a boronate inhibitor. *Science* **2016**, *353*, 503–505. [CrossRef] [PubMed]

22. Jain, R.; Coloma, J.; Garcia-Sastre, A.; Aggarwal, A.K. Structure of the NS3 helicase from Zika virus. *Nat. Struct. Mol. Biol.* **2016**, *23*, 752–754. [CrossRef] [PubMed]

23. Zhang, Z.; Li, Y.; Loh, Y.R.; Phoo, W.W.; Hung, A.W.; Kang, C.; Luo, D. Crystal structure of unlinked NS2B-NS3 protease from Zika virus. *Science* **2016**, *354*, 1597–1600. [CrossRef] [PubMed]

24. Godoy, A.S.; Lima, G.M.; Oliveira, K.I.; Torres, N.U.; Maluf, F.V.; Guido, R.V.; Oliva, G. Crystal structure of Zika virus NS5 RNA-dependent RNA polymerase. *Nat. Commun.* **2017**, *8*, 14764. [CrossRef] [PubMed]

25. Coloma, J.; Jain, R.; Rajashankar, K.R.; Garcia-Sastre, A.; Aggarwal, A.K. Structures of NS5 methyltransferase from Zika virus. *Cell. Rep.* **2016**, *16*, 3097–3102. [CrossRef] [PubMed]

26. Duan, W.; Song, H.; Wang, H.; Chai, Y.; Su, C.; Qi, J.; Shi, Y.; Gao, G.F. The crystal structure of Zika virus NS5 reveals conserved drug targets. *EMBO J.* **2017**, *36*, 919–933. [CrossRef] [PubMed]

27. Wang, B.; Tan, X.F.; Thurmond, S.; Zhang, Z.M.; Lin, A.; Hai, R.; Song, J. The structure of Zika virus NS5 reveals a conserved domain conformation. *Nat. Commun.* **2017**, *8*, 14763. [CrossRef] [PubMed]

28. Zhao, B.; Yi, G.; Du, F.; Chuang, Y.C.; Vaughan, R.C.; Sankaran, B.; Kao, C.C.; Li, P. Structure and function of the Zika virus full-length NS5 protein. *Nat. Commun.* **2017**, *8*, 14762. [CrossRef] [PubMed]

29. Phoo, W.W.; Li, Y.; Zhang, Z.; Lee, M.Y.; Loh, Y.R.; Tan, Y.B.; Ng, E.Y.; Lescar, J.; Kang, C.; Luo, D. Structure of the NS2B-NS3 protease from Zika virus after self-cleavage. *Nat. Commun.* **2016**, *7*, 13410. [CrossRef] [PubMed]

30. Li, Y.; Zhang, Z.; Phoo, W.W.; Loh, Y.R.; Wang, W.; Liu, S.; Chen, M.W.; Hung, A.W.; Keller, T.H.; Luo, D.; et al. Structural dynamics of Zika virus NS2b-NS3 protease binding to dipeptide inhibitors. *Structure* **2017**, *25*, 1242–1250.e3. [CrossRef] [PubMed]

31. Li, Y.; Phoo, W.W.; Loh, Y.R.; Zhang, Z.; Ng, E.Y.; Wang, W.; Keller, T.H.; Luo, D.; Kang, C. Structural characterization of the linked NS2b-NS3 protease of Zika virus. *FEBS Lett.* **2017**, *591*, 2338–2347. [CrossRef] [PubMed]

32. Li, Y.; Zhang, Z.; Phoo, W.W.; Loh, Y.R.; Li, R.; Yang, H.Y.; Jansson, A.E.; Hill, J.; Keller, T.H.; Nacro, K.; et al. Structural insights into the inhibition of Zika virus NS2B-NS3 protease by a small-molecule inhibitor. *Structure* **2018**, *26*, 555–564.e3. [CrossRef] [PubMed]

33. Shang, Z.; Song, H.; Shi, Y.; Qi, J.; Gao, G.F. Crystal structure of the capsid protein from Zika virus. *J. Mol. Biol.* **2018**, *430*, 948–962. [CrossRef] [PubMed]

34. Song, H.; Qi, J.; Haywood, J.; Shi, Y.; Gao, G.F. Zika virus NS1 structure reveals diversity of electrostatic surfaces among flaviviruses. *Nat. Struct. Mol. Biol.* **2016**, *23*, 456–458. [CrossRef] [PubMed]

35. Xu, X.; Song, H.; Qi, J.; Liu, Y.; Wang, H.; Su, C.; Shi, Y.; Gao, G.F. Contribution of intertwined loop to membrane association revealed by Zika virus full-length NS1 structure. *EMBO J.* **2016**, *35*, 2170–2178. [CrossRef] [PubMed]

36. Kostyuchenko, V.A.; Lim, E.X.; Zhang, S.; Fibriansah, G.; Ng, T.S.; Ooi, J.S.; Shi, J.; Lok, S.M. Structure of the thermally stable Zika virus. *Nature* **2016**, *533*, 425–428. [CrossRef] [PubMed]

37. Dai, L.; Song, J.; Lu, X.; Deng, Y.Q.; Musyoki, A.M.; Cheng, H.; Zhang, Y.; Yuan, Y.; Song, H.; Haywood, J.; et al. Structures of the Zika virus envelope protein and its complex with a flavivirus broadly protective antibody. *Cell Host Microbe* **2016**, *19*, 696–704. [CrossRef] [PubMed]

38. Prasad, V.M.; Miller, A.S.; Klose, T.; Sirohi, D.; Buda, G.; Jiang, W.; Kuhn, R.J.; Rossmann, M.G. Structure of the immature Zika virus at 9 A resolution. *Nat. Struct. Mol. Biol.* **2017**, *24*, 184–186. [CrossRef] [PubMed]

39. Vazquez-Calvo, A.; Jimenez de Oya, N.; Martin-Acebes, M.A.; Garcia-Moruno, E.; Saiz, J.C. Antiviral properties of the natural polyphenols delphinidin and epigallocatechin gallate against the flaviviruses West Nile virus, Zika virus, and dengue virus. *Front. Microbiol.* **2017**, *8*, 1314. [CrossRef] [PubMed]

40. Wang, S.; Hong, S.; Deng, Y.Q.; Ye, Q.; Zhao, L.Z.; Zhang, F.C.; Qin, C.F.; Xu, Z. Transfer of convalescent serum to pregnant mice prevents Zika virus infection and microcephaly in offspring. *Cell Res.* **2016**, *27*, 158–160. [CrossRef] [PubMed]

41. Sapparapu, G.; Fernandez, E.; Kose, N.; Bin, C.; Fox, J.M.; Bombardi, R.G.; Zhao, H.; Nelson, C.A.; Bryan, A.L.; Barnes, T.; et al. Neutralizing human antibodies prevent Zika virus replication and fetal disease in mice. *Nature* **2016**, *540*, 443–447. [CrossRef] [PubMed]

42. Stettler, K.; Beltramello, M.; Espinosa, D.A.; Graham, V.; Cassotta, A.; Bianchi, S.; Vanzetta, F.; Minola, A.; Jaconi, S.; Mele, F.; et al. Specificity, cross-reactivity, and function of antibodies elicited by Zika virus infection. *Science* **2016**, *353*, 823–826. [CrossRef] [PubMed]

43. Wang, J.; Bardelli, M.; Espinosa, D.A.; Pedotti, M.; Ng, T.S.; Bianchi, S.; Simonelli, L.; Lim, E.X.Y.; Foglierini, M.; Zatta, F.; et al. A human bi-specific antibody against Zika virus with high therapeutic potential. *Cell* **2017**, *171*, 229–241.e15. [CrossRef] [PubMed]

44. Abbink, P.; Larocca, R.A.; Dejnirattisai, W.; Peterson, R.; Nkolola, J.P.; Borducchi, E.N.; Supasa, P.; Mongkolsapaya, J.; Screaton, G.R.; Barouch, D.H. Therapeutic and protective efficacy of a dengue antibody against zika infection in rhesus monkeys. *Nat. Med.* **2018**, *24*, 721–723. [CrossRef] [PubMed]

45. Stein, D.R.; Golden, J.W.; Griffin, B.D.; Warner, B.M.; Ranadheera, C.; Scharikow, L.; Sloan, A.; Frost, K.L.; Kobasa, D.; Booth, S.A.; et al. Human polyclonal antibodies produced in transchromosomal cattle prevent lethal Zika virus infection and testicular atrophy in mice. *Antivir. Res.* **2017**, *146*, 164–173. [CrossRef] [PubMed]

46. Martin-Acebes, M.A.; Saiz, J.C.; Jimenez de Oya, N. Antibody-dependent enhancement and zika: Real threat or phantom menace? *Front. Cell. Infect. Microbiol.* **2018**, *8*, 44. [CrossRef] [PubMed]
47. Halstead, S.B. Pathogenic exploitation of Fc activity. In *Antibody Fc Linking Adaptive and Innate Immunity*; Ackerman, M., Ed.; Academic Press: Cambridge, MA, USA, 2014; pp. 333–350.
48. Fernandez-Garcia, M.D.; Mazzon, M.; Jacobs, M.; Amara, A. Pathogenesis of flavivirus infections: Using and abusing the host cell. *Cell Host Microbe* **2009**, *5*, 318–328. [CrossRef] [PubMed]
49. Pastorino, B.; Nougairede, A.; Wurtz, N.; Gould, E.; de Lamballerie, X. Role of host cell factors in flavivirus infection: Implications for pathogenesis and development of antiviral drugs. *Antivir. Res.* **2010**, *87*, 281–294. [CrossRef] [PubMed]
50. Boldescu, V.; Behnam, M.A.M.; Vasilakis, N.; Klein, C.D. Broad-spectrum agents for flaviviral infections: Dengue, zika and beyond. *Nat. Rev. Drug Discov.* **2017**, *16*, 565–586. [CrossRef] [PubMed]
51. Krishnan, M.N.; Garcia-Blanco, M.A. Targeting host factors to treat West Nile and dengue viral infections. *Viruses* **2014**, *6*, 683–708. [CrossRef] [PubMed]
52. Xie, X.; Zou, J.; Shan, C.; Yang, Y.; Kum, D.B.; Dallmeier, K.; Neyts, J.; Shi, P.Y. Zika virus replicons for drug discovery. *EBioMedicine* **2016**, *12*, 156–160. [CrossRef] [PubMed]
53. Kummerer, B.M. Establishment and application of flavivirus replicons. *Adv. Exp. Med. Biol.* **2018**, *1062*, 165–173. [PubMed]
54. Lee, I.; Bos, S.; Li, G.; Wang, S.; Gadea, G.; Despres, P.; Zhao, R.Y. Probing molecular insights into Zika virus (-)host interactions. *Viruses* **2018**, *10*, 233. [CrossRef] [PubMed]
55. Retallack, H.; Di Lullo, E.; Arias, C.; Knopp, K.A.; Laurie, M.T.; Sandoval-Espinosa, C.; Mancia Leon, W.R.; Krencik, R.; Ullian, E.M.; Spatazza, J.; et al. Zika virus cell tropism in the developing human brain and inhibition by azithromycin. *Proc. Natl. Acad. Sci. USA* **2016**, *113*, 14408–14413. [CrossRef] [PubMed]
56. Wells, M.F.; Salick, M.R.; Wiskow, O.; Ho, D.J.; Worringer, K.A.; Ihry, R.J.; Kommineni, S.; Bilican, B.; Klim, J.R.; Hill, E.J.; et al. Genetic ablation of axl does not protect human neural progenitor cells and cerebral organoids from Zika virus infection. *Cell Stem Cell* **2016**, *19*, 703–708. [CrossRef] [PubMed]
57. Meertens, L.; Labeau, A.; Dejarnac, O.; Cipriani, S.; Sinigaglia, L.; Bonnet-Madin, L.; Le Charpentier, T.; Hafirassou, M.L.; Zamborlini, A.; Cao-Lormeau, V.M.; et al. Axl mediates Zika virus entry in human glial cells and modulates innate immune responses. *Cell Rep.* **2017**, *18*, 324–333. [CrossRef] [PubMed]
58. Wang, Z.Y.; Wang, Z.; Zhen, Z.D.; Feng, K.H.; Guo, J.; Gao, N.; Fan, D.Y.; Han, D.S.; Wang, P.G.; An, J. Axl is not an indispensable factor for Zika virus infection in mice. *J. Gen. Virol.* **2017**, *98*, 2061–2068. [CrossRef] [PubMed]
59. Liu, S.; DeLalio, L.J.; Isakson, B.E.; Wang, T.T. Axl-mediated productive infection of human endothelial cells by Zika virus. *Circ. Res.* **2016**, *119*, 1183–1189. [CrossRef] [PubMed]
60. Mounce, B.C.; Cesaro, T.; Carrau, L.; Vallet, T.; Vignuzzi, M. Curcumin inhibits zika and chikungunya virus infection by inhibiting cell binding. *Antivir. Res.* **2017**, *142*, 148–157. [CrossRef] [PubMed]
61. Tan, C.W.; Sam, I.C.; Chong, W.L.; Lee, V.S.; Chan, Y.F. Polysulfonate suramin inhibits Zika virus infection. *Antivir. Res.* **2017**, *143*, 186–194. [CrossRef] [PubMed]
62. Albulescu, I.C.; Kovacikova, K.; Tas, A.; Snijder, E.J.; van Hemert, M.J. Suramin inhibits Zika virus replication by interfering with virus attachment and release of infectious particles. *Antivir. Res.* **2017**, *143*, 230–236. [CrossRef] [PubMed]
63. Stiasny, K.; Fritz, R.; Pangerl, K.; Heinz, F.X. Molecular mechanisms of flavivirus membrane fusion. *Amino Acids* **2011**, *41*, 1159–1163. [CrossRef] [PubMed]
64. Vazquez-Calvo, A.; Saiz, J.C.; McCullough, K.C.; Sobrino, F.; Martin-Acebes, M.A. Acid-dependent viral entry. *Virus Res.* **2012**, *167*, 125–137. [CrossRef] [PubMed]
65. Rausch, K.; Hackett, B.A.; Weinbren, N.L.; Reeder, S.M.; Sadovsky, Y.; Hunter, C.A.; Schultz, D.C.; Coyne, C.B.; Cherry, S. Screening bioactives reveals nanchangmycin as a broad spectrum antiviral active against Zika virus. *Cell Rep.* **2017**, *18*, 804–815. [CrossRef] [PubMed]
66. Martin-Acebes, M.A.; Vazquez-Calvo, A.; Saiz, J.C. Lipids and flaviviruses, present and future perspectives for the control of dengue, zika, and West Nile viruses. *Prog. Lipid Res.* **2016**, *64*, 123–137. [CrossRef] [PubMed]
67. Haviernik, J.; Stefanik, M.; Fojtikova, M.; Kali, S.; Tordo, N.; Rudolf, I.; Hubalek, Z.; Eyer, L.; Ruzek, D. Arbidol (umifenovir): A broad-spectrum antiviral drug that inhibits medically important arthropod-borne flaviviruses. *Viruses* **2018**, *10*, 184. [CrossRef] [PubMed]

68. Persaud, M.; Martinez-Lopez, A.; Buffone, C.; Porcelli, S.A.; Diaz-Griffero, F. Infection by Zika viruses requires the transmembrane protein AXL, endocytosis and low pH. *Virology* **2018**, *518*, 301–312. [CrossRef] [PubMed]

69. Li, C.; Deng, Y.Q.; Wang, S.; Ma, F.; Aliyari, R.; Huang, X.Y.; Zhang, N.N.; Watanabe, M.; Dong, H.L.; Liu, P.; et al. 25-hydroxycholesterol protects host against Zika virus infection and its associated microcephaly in a mouse model. *Immunity* **2017**, *46*, 446–456. [CrossRef] [PubMed]

70. Barrows, N.J.; Campos, R.K.; Powell, S.T.; Prasanth, K.R.; Schott-Lerner, G.; Soto-Acosta, R.; Galarza-Munoz, G.; McGrath, E.L.; Urrabaz-Garza, R.; Gao, J.; et al. A screen of FDA-approved drugs for inhibitors of Zika virus infection. *Cell Host Microbe* **2016**, *20*, 259–270. [CrossRef] [PubMed]

71. Kuivanen, S.; Bespalov, M.M.; Nandania, J.; Ianevski, A.; Velagapudi, V.; De Brabander, J.K.; Kainov, D.E.; Vapalahti, O. Obatoclax, saliphenylhalamide and gemcitabine inhibit Zika virus infection in vitro and differentially affect cellular signaling, transcription and metabolism. *Antivir. Res.* **2017**, *139*, 117–128. [CrossRef] [PubMed]

72. Varghese, F.S.; Rausalu, K.; Hakanen, M.; Saul, S.; Kummerer, B.M.; Susi, P.; Merits, A.; Ahola, T. Obatoclax inhibits alphavirus membrane fusion by neutralizing the acidic environment of endocytic compartments. *Antimicrob. Agents Chemother.* **2017**, *61*. [CrossRef] [PubMed]

73. Adcock, R.S.; Chu, Y.K.; Golden, J.E.; Chung, D.H. Evaluation of anti-Zika virus activities of broad-spectrum antivirals and NIH clinical collection compounds using a cell-based, high-throughput screen assay. *Antivir. Res.* **2017**, *138*, 47–56. [CrossRef] [PubMed]

74. Delvecchio, R.; Higa, L.M.; Pezzuto, P.; Valadao, A.L.; Garcez, P.P.; Monteiro, F.L.; Loiola, E.C.; Dias, A.A.; Silva, F.J.; Aliota, M.T.; et al. Chloroquine, an endocytosis blocking agent, inhibits Zika virus infection in different cell models. *Viruses* **2016**, *8*, 322. [CrossRef] [PubMed]

75. Balasubramanian, A.; Teramoto, T.; Kulkarni, A.A.; Bhattacharjee, A.K.; Padmanabhan, R. Antiviral activities of selected antimalarials against dengue virus type 2 and Zika virus. *Antivir. Res.* **2017**, *137*, 141–150. [CrossRef] [PubMed]

76. Cao, B.; Parnell, L.A.; Diamond, M.S.; Mysorekar, I.U. Inhibition of autophagy limits vertical transmission of Zika virus in pregnant mice. *J. Exp. Med.* **2017**, *214*, 2303–2313. [CrossRef] [PubMed]

77. Li, C.; Zhu, X.; Ji, X.; Quanquin, N.; Deng, Y.Q.; Tian, M.; Aliyari, R.; Zuo, X.; Yuan, L.; Afridi, S.K.; et al. Chloroquine, a FDA-approved drug, prevents Zika virus infection and its associated congenital microcephaly in mice. *EBioMedicine* **2017**, *24*, 189–194. [CrossRef] [PubMed]

78. Shiryaev, S.A.; Mesci, P.; Pinto, A.; Fernandes, I.; Sheets, N.; Shresta, S.; Farhy, C.; Huang, C.T.; Strongin, A.Y.; Muotri, A.R.; et al. Repurposing of the anti-malaria drug chloroquine for Zika virus treatment and prophylaxis. *Sci. Rep.* **2017**, *7*, 15771. [CrossRef] [PubMed]

79. Barbosa-Lima, G.; da Silveira Pinto, L.S.; Kaiser, C.R.; Wardell, J.L.; De Freitas, C.S.; Vieira, Y.R.; Marttorelli, A.; Cerbino Neto, J.; Bozza, P.T.; Wardell, S.; et al. *N*-(2-(arylmethylimino)ethyl)-7-chloroquinolin-4-amine derivatives, synthesized by thermal and ultrasonic means, are endowed with anti-Zika virus activity. *Eur. J. Med. Chem.* **2017**, *127*, 434–441. [CrossRef] [PubMed]

80. Barbosa-Lima, G.; Moraes, A.M.; Araujo, A.D.S.; da Silva, E.T.; de Freitas, C.S.; Vieira, Y.R.; Marttorelli, A.; Neto, J.C.; Bozza, P.T.; de Souza, M.V.N.; et al. 2,8-*bis*(trifluoromethyl)quinoline analogs show improved anti-Zika virus activity, compared to mefloquine. *Eur. J. Med. Chem.* **2017**, *127*, 334–340. [CrossRef] [PubMed]

81. Han, Y.; Mesplede, T.; Xu, H.; Quan, Y.; Wainberg, M.A. The antimalarial drug amodiaquine possesses anti-Zika virus activities. *J. Med. Virol.* **2018**, *90*, 796–802. [CrossRef] [PubMed]

82. Xu, M.; Lee, E.M.; Wen, Z.; Cheng, Y.; Huang, W.K.; Qian, X.; Tcw, J.; Kouznetsova, J.; Ogden, S.C.; Hammack, C.; et al. Identification of small-molecule inhibitors of Zika virus infection and induced neural cell death via a drug repurposing screen. *Nat. Med.* **2016**, *22*, 1101–1107. [CrossRef] [PubMed]

83. Cairns, D.M.; Boorgu, D.; Levin, M.; Kaplan, D.L. Niclosamide rescues microcephaly in a humanized in vivo model of zika infection using human induced neural stem cells. *Biol. Open* **2018**, *7*. [CrossRef] [PubMed]

84. Wang, H.; Li, Z.; Niu, J.; Xu, Y.; Ma, L.; Lu, A.; Wang, X.; Qian, Z.; Huang, Z.; Jin, X.; et al. Antiviral effects of ferric ammonium citrate. *Cell Discov.* **2018**, *4*, 14. [CrossRef] [PubMed]

85. Elgner, F.; Sabino, C.; Basic, M.; Ploen, D.; Grunweller, A.; Hildt, E. Inhibition of Zika virus replication by silvestrol. *Viruses* **2018**, *10*, 149. [CrossRef] [PubMed]

86. Pitts, J.D.; Li, P.C.; de Wispelaere, M.; Yang, P.L. Antiviral activity of *N*-(4-hydroxyphenyl) retinamide (4-HPR) against Zika virus. *Antivir. Res.* **2017**, *147*, 124–130. [CrossRef] [PubMed]

87. Mounce, B.C.; Poirier, E.Z.; Passoni, G.; Simon-Loriere, E.; Cesaro, T.; Prot, M.; Stapleford, K.A.; Moratorio, G.; Sakuntabhai, A.; Levraud, J.P.; et al. Interferon-induced spermidine-spermine acetyltransferase and polyamine depletion restrict zika and chikungunya viruses. *Cell Host Microbe* **2016**, *20*, 167–177. [CrossRef] [PubMed]

88. Mounce, B.C.; Cesaro, T.; Moratorio, G.; Hooikaas, P.J.; Yakovleva, A.; Werneke, S.W.; Smith, E.C.; Poirier, E.Z.; Simon-Loriere, E.; Prot, M.; et al. Inhibition of polyamine biosynthesis is a broad-spectrum strategy against rna viruses. *J. Virol.* **2016**, *90*, 9683–9692. [CrossRef] [PubMed]

89. Mukhopadhyay, S.; Kuhn, R.J.; Rossmann, M.G. A structural perspective of the flavivirus life cycle. *Nat. Rev. Microbiol.* **2005**, *3*, 13–22. [CrossRef] [PubMed]

90. Roby, J.A.; Setoh, Y.X.; Hall, R.A.; Khromykh, A.A. Post-translational regulation and modifications of flavivirus structural proteins. *J. Gen. Virol.* **2015**, *96*, 1551–1569. [CrossRef] [PubMed]

91. Puschnik, A.S.; Marceau, C.D.; Ooi, Y.S.; Majzoub, K.; Rinis, N.; Contessa, J.N.; Carette, J.E. A small-molecule oligosaccharyltransferase inhibitor with pan-flaviviral activity. *Cell Rep.* **2017**, *21*, 3032–3039. [CrossRef] [PubMed]

92. Zhang, R.; Miner, J.J.; Gorman, M.J.; Rausch, K.; Ramage, H.; White, J.P.; Zuiani, A.; Zhang, P.; Fernandez, E.; Zhang, Q.; et al. A CRISPR screen defines a signal peptide processing pathway required by flaviviruses. *Nature* **2016**, *535*, 164–168. [CrossRef] [PubMed]

93. Estoppey, D.; Lee, C.M.; Janoschke, M.; Lee, B.H.; Wan, K.F.; Dong, H.; Mathys, P.; Filipuzzi, I.; Schuhmann, T.; Riedl, R.; et al. The natural product cavinafungin selectively interferes with zika and dengue virus replication by inhibition of the host signal peptidase. *Cell Rep.* **2017**, *19*, 451–460. [CrossRef] [PubMed]

94. Cao, R.Y.; Xu, Y.F.; Zhang, T.H.; Yang, J.J.; Yuan, Y.; Hao, P.; Shi, Y.; Zhong, J.; Zhong, W. Pediatric drug nitazoxanide: A potential choice for control of zika. *Open Forum Infect. Dis.* **2017**, *4*, ofx009. [CrossRef] [PubMed]

95. Raekiansyah, M.; Mori, M.; Nonaka, K.; Agoh, M.; Shiomi, K.; Matsumoto, A.; Morita, K. Identification of novel antiviral of fungus-derived brefeldin A against dengue viruses. *Trop Med. Health* **2017**, *45*, 32. [CrossRef] [PubMed]

96. Yang, S.; Xu, M.; Lee, E.M.; Gorshkov, K.; Shiryaev, S.A.; He, S.; Sun, W.; Cheng, Y.S.; Hu, X.; Tharappel, A.M.; et al. Emetine inhibits Zika and Ebola virus infections through two molecular mechanisms: Inhibiting viral replication and decreasing viral entry. *Cell Discov* **2018**, *4*, 31. [CrossRef] [PubMed]

97. Tang, H.; Hammack, C.; Ogden, S.C.; Wen, Z.; Qian, X.; Li, Y.; Yao, B.; Shin, J.; Zhang, F.; Lee, E.M.; et al. Zika virus infects human cortical neural progenitors and attenuates their growth. *Cell Stem Cell* **2016**, *18*, 587–590. [CrossRef] [PubMed]

98. Leonardi, W.; Zilbermintz, L.; Cheng, L.W.; Zozaya, J.; Tran, S.H.; Elliott, J.H.; Polukhina, K.; Manasherob, R.; Li, A.; Chi, X.; et al. Bithionol blocks pathogenicity of bacterial toxins, ricin, and Zika virus. *Sci. Rep.* **2016**, *6*, 34475. [CrossRef] [PubMed]

99. Villareal, V.A.; Rodgers, M.A.; Costello, D.A.; Yang, P.L. Targeting host lipid synthesis and metabolism to inhibit dengue and hepatitis c viruses. *Antivir. Res.* **2015**, *124*, 110–121. [CrossRef] [PubMed]

100. Garavito, R.M.; Mulichak, A.M. The structure of mammalian cyclooxygenases. *Annu. Rev. Biophys. Biomol. Struct.* **2003**, *32*, 183–206. [CrossRef] [PubMed]

101. Opie, L.H. Present status of statin therapy. *Trends Cardiovasc. Med.* **2015**, *25*, 216–225. [CrossRef] [PubMed]

102. Merino-Ramos, T.; Vazquez-Calvo, A.; Casas, J.; Sobrino, F.; Saiz, J.C.; Martin-Acebes, M.A. Modification of the host cell lipid metabolism induced by hypolipidemic drugs targeting the acetyl coenzyme a carboxylase impairs West Nile virus replication. *Antimicrob. Agents Chemother.* **2015**, *60*, 307–315. [CrossRef] [PubMed]

103. Heaton, N.S.; Perera, R.; Berger, K.L.; Khadka, S.; Lacount, D.J.; Kuhn, R.J.; Randall, G. Dengue virus nonstructural protein 3 redistributes fatty acid synthase to sites of viral replication and increases cellular fatty acid synthesis. *Proc. Natl. Acad. Sci. USA* **2010**, *107*, 17345–17350. [CrossRef] [PubMed]

104. Martin-Acebes, M.A.; Blazquez, A.B.; Jimenez de Oya, N.; Escribano-Romero, E.; Saiz, J.C. West nile virus replication requires fatty acid synthesis but is independent on phosphatidylinositol-4-phosphate lipids. *PLoS ONE* **2011**, *6*, e24970. [CrossRef] [PubMed]

105. Perera, R.; Riley, C.; Isaac, G.; Hopf-Jannasch, A.S.; Moore, R.J.; Weitz, K.W.; Pasa-Tolic, L.; Metz, T.O.; Adamec, J.; Kuhn, R.J. Dengue virus infection perturbs lipid homeostasis in infected mosquito cells. *PLoS Pathog.* **2012**, *8*, e1002584. [CrossRef] [PubMed]

106. Merino-Ramos, T.; Jimenez de Oya, N.; Saiz, J.C.; Martin-Acebes, M.A. Antiviral activity of nordihydroguaiaretic acid and its derivative tetra-*O*-methyl nordihydroguaiaretic acid against West Nile virus and Zika virus. *Antimicrob. Agents Chemother.* **2017**, *61*. [CrossRef] [PubMed]

107. Pascoalino, B.S.; Courtemanche, G.; Cordeiro, M.T.; Gil, L.H.; Freitas-Junior, L. Zika antiviral chemotherapy: Identification of drugs and promising starting points for drug discovery from an FDA-approved library. *F1000Research* **2016**, *5*, 2523. [CrossRef] [PubMed]

108. Sarkey, J.P.; Richards, M.P.; Stubbs, E.B., Jr. Lovastatin attenuates nerve injury in an animal model of guillain-barre syndrome. *J. Neurochem.* **2007**, *100*, 1265–1277. [CrossRef] [PubMed]

109. Wichit, S.; Hamel, R.; Bernard, E.; Talignani, L.; Diop, F.; Ferraris, P.; Liegeois, F.; Ekchariyawat, P.; Luplertlop, N.; Surasombatpattana, P.; et al. Imipramine inhibits chikungunya virus replication in human skin fibroblasts through interference with intracellular cholesterol trafficking. *Sci. Rep.* **2017**, *7*, 3145. [CrossRef] [PubMed]

110. Huang, Y.; Li, Y.; Zhang, H.; Zhao, R.; Jing, R.; Xu, Y.; He, M.; Peer, J.; Kim, Y.C.; Luo, J.; et al. Zika virus propagation and release in human fetal astrocytes can be suppressed by neutral sphingomyelinase-2 inhibitor GW4869. *Cell Discov.* **2018**, *4*, 19. [CrossRef] [PubMed]

111. Martin-Acebes, M.A.; Merino-Ramos, T.; Blazquez, A.B.; Casas, J.; Escribano-Romero, E.; Sobrino, F.; Saiz, J.C. The composition of West Nile virus lipid envelope unveils a role of sphingolipid metabolism in flavivirus biogenesis. *J. Virol.* **2014**, *88*, 12041–12054. [CrossRef] [PubMed]

112. Jimenez de Oya, N.; Blazquez, A.B.; Casas, J.; Saiz, J.C.; Martin-Acebes, M.A. Direct activation of adenosine monophosphate-activated protein kinase (AMPK) by PF-06409577 inhibits flavivirus infection through modification of host cell lipid metabolism. *Antimicrob. Agents Chemother.* **2018**, *62*. [CrossRef] [PubMed]

113. Cheng, F.; Ramos da Silva, S.; Huang, I.C.; Jung, J.U.; Gao, S.J. Suppression of Zika virus infection and replication in endothelial cells and astrocytes by PKA inhibitor PKI 14-22. *J. Virol.* **2018**, *92*. [CrossRef] [PubMed]

114. Grant, A.; Ponia, S.S.; Tripathi, S.; Balasubramaniam, V.; Miorin, L.; Sourisseau, M.; Schwarz, M.C.; Sanchez-Seco, M.P.; Evans, M.J.; Best, S.M.; et al. Zika virus targets human STAT2 to inhibit type I interferon signaling. *Cell Host Microbe* **2016**, *19*, 882–890. [CrossRef] [PubMed]

115. Snell, N.J. Ribavirin—Current status of a broad spectrum antiviral agent. *Expert Opin. Pharmacother.* **2001**, *2*, 1317–1324. [CrossRef] [PubMed]

116. Markland, W.; McQuaid, T.J.; Jain, J.; Kwong, A.D. Broad-spectrum antiviral activity of the imp dehydrogenase inhibitor VX-497: A comparison with ribavirin and demonstration of antiviral additivity with alpha interferon. *Antimicrob. Agents Chemother.* **2000**, *44*, 859–866. [CrossRef] [PubMed]

117. Crotty, S.; Cameron, C.E.; Andino, R. Rna virus error catastrophe: Direct molecular test by using ribavirin. *Proc. Natl. Acad. Sci. USA* **2001**, *98*, 6895–6900. [CrossRef] [PubMed]

118. Ortega-Prieto, A.M.; Sheldon, J.; Grande-Perez, A.; Tejero, H.; Gregori, J.; Quer, J.; Esteban, J.I.; Domingo, E.; Perales, C. Extinction of hepatitis c virus by ribavirin in hepatoma cells involves lethal mutagenesis. *PLoS ONE* **2013**, *8*, e71039. [CrossRef] [PubMed]

119. Julander, J.G.; Siddharthan, V.; Evans, J.; Taylor, R.; Tolbert, K.; Apuli, C.; Stewart, J.; Collins, P.; Gebre, M.; Neilson, S.; et al. Efficacy of the broad-spectrum antiviral compound BCX4430 against Zika virus in cell culture and in a mouse model. *Antivir. Res.* **2017**, *137*, 14–22. [CrossRef] [PubMed]

120. Baz, M.; Goyette, N.; Griffin, B.D.; Kobinger, G.P.; Boivin, G. In vitro susceptibility of geographically and temporally distinct Zika viruses to favipiravir and ribavirin. *Antivir. Ther.* **2017**, *22*, 613–618. [CrossRef] [PubMed]

121. Kamiyama, N.; Soma, R.; Hidano, S.; Watanabe, K.; Umekita, H.; Fukuda, C.; Noguchi, K.; Gendo, Y.; Ozaki, T.; Sonoda, A.; et al. Ribavirin inhibits Zika virus (zikv) replication in vitro and suppresses viremia in zikv-infected stat1-deficient mice. *Antivir. Res.* **2017**, *146*, 1–11. [CrossRef] [PubMed]

122. Kim, J.A.; Seong, R.K.; Kumar, M.; Shin, O.S. Favipiravir and ribavirin inhibit replication of Asian and African strains of Zika virus in different cell models. *Viruses* **2018**, *10*, 72. [CrossRef] [PubMed]

123. Tong, X.; Smith, J.; Bukreyeva, N.; Koma, T.; Manning, J.T.; Kalkeri, R.; Kwong, A.D.; Paessler, S. Merimepodib, an impdh inhibitor, suppresses replication of Zika virus and other emerging viral pathogens. *Antivir. Res.* **2018**, *149*, 34–40. [CrossRef] [PubMed]

124. Goebel, S.; Snyder, B.; Sellati, T.; Saeed, M.; Ptak, R.; Murray, M.; Bostwick, R.; Rayner, J.; Koide, F.; Kalkeri, R. A sensitive virus yield assay for evaluation of antivirals against Zika virus. *J. Virol. Methods* **2016**, *238*, 13–20. [CrossRef] [PubMed]

125. Lucas-Hourani, M.; Dauzonne, D.; Jorda, P.; Cousin, G.; Lupan, A.; Helynck, O.; Caignard, G.; Janvier, G.; Andre-Leroux, G.; Khiar, S.; et al. Inhibition of pyrimidine biosynthesis pathway suppresses viral growth through innate immunity. *PLoS Pathog.* **2013**, *9*, e1003678. [CrossRef] [PubMed]

126. Chung, D.H.; Golden, J.E.; Adcock, R.S.; Schroeder, C.E.; Chu, Y.K.; Sotsky, J.B.; Cramer, D.E.; Chilton, P.M.; Song, C.; Anantpadma, M.; et al. Discovery of a broad-spectrum antiviral compound that inhibits pyrimidine biosynthesis and establishes a type 1 interferon-independent antiviral state. *Antimicrob. Agents Chemother.* **2016**, *60*, 4552–4562. [CrossRef] [PubMed]

127. Zhou, T.; Tan, L.; Cederquist, G.Y.; Fan, Y.; Hartley, B.J.; Mukherjee, S.; Tomishima, M.; Brennand, K.J.; Zhang, Q.; Schwartz, R.E.; et al. High-content screening in HPSC-neural progenitors identifies drug candidates that inhibit Zika virus infection in fetal-like organoids and adult brain. *Cell Stem Cell* **2017**, *21*, 274–283.e5. [CrossRef] [PubMed]

128. Cugola, F.R.; Fernandes, I.R.; Russo, F.B.; Freitas, B.C.; Dias, J.L.; Guimaraes, K.P.; Benazzato, C.; Almeida, N.; Pignatari, G.C.; Romero, S.; et al. The Brazilian Zika virus strain causes birth defects in experimental models. *Nature* **2016**, *534*, 267–271. [CrossRef] [PubMed]

129. Garcez, P.P.; Loiola, E.C.; Madeiro da Costa, R.; Higa, L.M.; Trindade, P.; Delvecchio, R.; Nascimento, J.M.; Brindeiro, R.; Tanuri, A.; Rehen, S.K. Zika virus impairs growth in human neurospheres and brain organoids. *Science* **2016**, *352*, 816–818. [CrossRef] [PubMed]

130. Li, C.; Xu, D.; Ye, Q.; Hong, S.; Jiang, Y.; Liu, X.; Zhang, N.; Shi, L.; Qin, C.F.; Xu, Z. Zika virus disrupts neural progenitor development and leads to microcephaly in mice. *Cell Stem Cell* **2016**, *19*, 120–126. [CrossRef] [PubMed]

131. Costa, V.V.; Del Sarto, J.L.; Rocha, R.F.; Silva, F.R.; Doria, J.G.; Olmo, I.G.; Marques, R.E.; Queiroz-Junior, C.M.; Foureaux, G.; Araujo, J.M.S.; et al. *N*-methyl-D-aspartate (NMDA) receptor blockade prevents neuronal death induced by Zika virus infection. *mBio* **2017**, *8*. [CrossRef] [PubMed]

132. Simanjuntak, Y.; Liang, J.J.; Chen, S.Y.; Li, J.K.; Lee, Y.L.; Wu, H.C.; Lin, Y.L. Ebselen alleviates testicular pathology in mice with Zika virus infection and prevents its sexual transmission. *PLoS Pathog.* **2018**, *14*, e1006854. [CrossRef] [PubMed]

133. Contreras, D.; Arumugaswami, V. Zika virus infectious cell culture system and the in vitro prophylactic effect of interferons. *J. Vis. Exp.* **2016**. [CrossRef] [PubMed]

134. Bayer, A.; Lennemann, N.J.; Ouyang, Y.; Bramley, J.C.; Morosky, S.; Marques, E.T., Jr.; Cherry, S.; Sadovsky, Y.; Coyne, C.B. Type iii interferons produced by human placental trophoblasts confer protection against Zika virus infection. *Cell Host Microbe* **2016**, *19*, 705–712. [CrossRef] [PubMed]

135. Jagger, B.W.; Miner, J.J.; Cao, B.; Arora, N.; Smith, A.M.; Kovacs, A.; Mysorekar, I.U.; Coyne, C.B.; Diamond, M.S. Gestational stage and IFN-lambda signaling regulate ZIKV infection in utero. *Cell Host Microbe* **2017**, *22*, 366–376e363. [CrossRef] [PubMed]

136. Savidis, G.; Perreira, J.M.; Portmann, J.M.; Meraner, P.; Guo, Z.; Green, S.; Brass, A.L. The IFITMs inhibit Zika virus replication. *Cell Rep.* **2016**, *15*, 2323–2330. [CrossRef] [PubMed]

137. Pryke, K.M.; Abraham, J.; Sali, T.M.; Gall, B.J.; Archer, I.; Liu, A.; Bambina, S.; Baird, J.; Gough, M.; Chakhtoura, M.; et al. A novel agonist of the TRIF pathway induces a cellular state refractory to replication of zika, chikungunya, and dengue viruses. *mBio* **2017**, *8*. [CrossRef] [PubMed]

138. Kumar, A.; Hou, S.; Airo, A.M.; Limonta, D.; Mancinelli, V.; Branton, W.; Power, C.; Hobman, T.C. Zika virus inhibits type-I interferon production and downstream signaling. *EMBO Rep.* **2016**, *17*, 1766–1775. [CrossRef] [PubMed]

139. Bowen, J.R.; Quicke, K.M.; Maddur, M.S.; O'Neal, J.T.; McDonald, C.E.; Fedorova, N.B.; Puri, V.; Shabman, R.S.; Pulendran, B.; Suthar, M.S. Zika virus antagonizes type I interferon responses during infection of human dendritic cells. *PLoS Pathog.* **2017**, *13*, e1006164. [CrossRef] [PubMed]

140. Chen, J.; Yang, Y.F.; Yang, Y.; Zou, P.; He, Y.; Shui, S.L.; Cui, Y.R.; Bai, R.; Liang, Y.J.; Hu, Y.; et al. AXL promotes Zika virus infection in astrocytes by antagonizing type I interferon signalling. *Nat. Microbiol.* **2018**, *3*, 302–309. [CrossRef] [PubMed]

141. Yockey, L.J.; Jurado, K.A.; Arora, N.; Millet, A.; Rakib, T.; Milano, K.M.; Hastings, A.K.; Fikrig, E.; Kong, Y.; Horvath, T.L.; et al. Type I interferons instigate fetal demise after Zika virus infection. *Sci. Immunol.* **2018**, *3*. [CrossRef] [PubMed]

142. Smith, J.L.; Jeng, S.; McWeeney, S.K.; Hirsch, A.J. A microRNA screen identifies the Wnt signaling pathway as a regulator of the interferon response during flavivirus infection. *J. Virol.* **2017**, *91*. [CrossRef] [PubMed]

143. Arbuckle, J.H.; Gardina, P.J.; Gordon, D.N.; Hickman, H.D.; Yewdell, J.W.; Pierson, T.C.; Myers, T.G.; Kristie, T.M. Inhibitors of the histone methyltransferases EZH2/1 induce a potent antiviral state and suppress infection by diverse viral pathogens. *mBio* **2017**, *8*. [CrossRef] [PubMed]

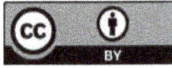

![viruses logo] *viruses*

MDPI

Article

Inhibition of Zika Virus Replication by Silvestrol

Fabian Elgner [1], Catarina Sabino [1], Michael Basic [1], Daniela Ploen [1], Arnold Grünweller [2] and Eberhard Hildt [1,3,*]

[1]   Department of Virology, Paul-Ehrlich-Institut, 63225 Langen, Germany; fabian.elgner@pei.de (F.E.); catarina.sabino@pei.de (C.S.); michel.basic@pei.de (M.B.); daniela.ploen@pei.de (D.P.)
[2]   Pharmazeutische Chemie, Philipps-Universität Marburg, 35037 Marburg, Germany; arnold.gruenweller@staff.uni-marburg.de
[3]   German Center for Infection Research (DZIF), 38124 Braunschweig, Germany
*   Correspondence: eberhard.hildt@pei.de; Tel.: +49-6103-77-2140

Received: 31 January 2018; Accepted: 24 March 2018; Published: 27 March 2018

Abstract: The Zika virus (ZIKV) outbreak in 2016 in South America with specific pathogenic outcomes highlighted the need for new antiviral substances with broad-spectrum activities to react quickly to unexpected outbreaks of emerging viral pathogens. Very recently, the natural compound silvestrol isolated from the plant *Aglaia foveolata* was found to have very potent antiviral effects against the (−)-strand RNA-virus Ebola virus as well as against Corona- and Picornaviruses with a (+)-strand RNA-genome. This antiviral activity is based on the impaired translation of viral RNA by the inhibition of the DEAD-box RNA helicase eukaryotic initiation factor-4A (eIF4A) which is required to unwind structured 5′-untranslated regions (5′-UTRs) of several proto-oncogenes and thereby facilitate their translation. Zika virus is a flavivirus with a positive-stranded RNA-genome harboring a 5′-capped UTR with distinct secondary structure elements. Therefore, we investigated the effects of silvestrol on ZIKV replication in A549 cells and primary human hepatocytes. Two different ZIKV strains were used. In both infected A549 cells and primary human hepatocytes, silvestrol has the potential to exert a significant inhibition of ZIKV replication for both analyzed strains, even though the ancestor strain from Uganda is less sensitive to silvestrol. Our data might contribute to identify host factors involved in the control of ZIKV infection and help to develop antiviral concepts that can be used to treat a variety of viral infections without the risk of resistances because a host protein is targeted.

Keywords: Ziks virus; silvestrol; antiviral; eIF4A; hepatocytes

---

1. Introduction

The Zika virus (ZIKV) is an emerging mosquito-borne virus of the genus *Flavivirus* within the Flaviviridae family. It is closely related to other flaviviruses like dengue virus, West Nile virus, and yellow fewer virus, which are all transmitted by mosquitos and can cause severe pathological effects in infected individuals. The ZIKV genome is a (+)-strand ssRNA of about 11 kb with highly structured untranslated regions (UTRs) on the 5′- and 3′-ends, which are predicted to form hairpin structures and are essential for viral replication and translation [1–3]. The genome acts as a viral mRNA with a single open reading frame that is directly translated into a polyprotein of 3419 or 3410 amino acids for the Africa and French Polynesia strains, respectively [4,5]. This polyprotein is then co- and posttranslational processed by viral and host proteases into three structural proteins (capsid, premembrane, envelope) and seven non-structural proteins (NS1, NS2A, NS2B, NS3, NS4A, NS4B, NS5) [4]. The viral RNA-dependent RNA polymerase NS5 possesses an additional methyltransferase domain which introduces an essential 5′-cap on the viral RNA [6].

The recent outbreak of ZIKV in Brazil, which was associated with severe neurological effects like Guillain-Barré syndrome and microcephaly of newborns if ZIKV infection occurred during pregnancy, prompted the WHO to consider ZIKV infection as a "public health emergency of international concern (PHEIC)". This highlights the need for efficient and well-tolerated antiviral therapies for emerging infectious diseases [7,8]. Such severe pathological effects were not present in patients infected with the original isolate from Uganda but firstly appeared in an outbreak in French Polynesia. The high mutation rate of RNA-viruses like ZIKV offers them the chance to develop escape mutant strains that are resistant to drugs targeting viral proteins. Therefore, a promising strategy is to target host proteins which are essential for the viral life cycle but do not underlie the high viral mutation rate.

Silvestrol is a natural compound of the rocaglate family that can be isolated from the plant *Aglaia foveolata* [9]. It has been identified as a specific inhibitor of the DEAD-box RNA helicase eukaryotic initiation factor-4A (eIF4A), which is part of the heterotrimeric translation initiation complex eIF4F together with the cap binding protein eIF4E and the scaffolding protein eIF4G [10,11]. The complex eIF4F regulates translation by recruiting ribosomes to the 5'-UTR of many mRNAs through binding to m^7GpppN cap structures [12]. The helicase eIF4A unwinds RNA secondary structures to create a binding platform for the 43S preinitiation complex. Silvestrol selectively binds eIF4A, resulting in its depletion from the eIF4F complex due to an increased affinity of eIF4A to its bound mRNA substrate and thus abolishes translation [13]. Silvestrol exhibits anti-tumor activity in many pre-clinical models without showing major toxic side effects [11,14–16]. The proposed mechanism of silvestrol is to inhibit the eIF4A-dependent translation of short-lived key proto-oncogenes such as *c-MYC* and *PIM1*, whose mRNA 5'-UTRs are extended and include regions of stable RNA secondary structures that require unwinding by eIF4A to create a binding platform for the 43S preinitiation complex [17]. Moreover, silvestrol leads to an increased survival rate in several xenograft mouse models and thus was described as a potential novel anticancer drug [14,15,18,19]. In addition, in two recent studies antiviral effects of silvestrol against Ebola, Corona-, and Picornaviruses have been reported. In these systems, silvestrol inhibits the eIF4A-dependent translation of viral mRNAs with extended and structured 5'-UTRs [20–22]. While Ebola virus and Coronavirus are 5'-cap dependently translated, Picornavirus is translated via an eIF4A-dependent internal ribosomal entry site (IRES) [21].

Given the facts that the rocaglate silvestrol inhibits the eIF4A-dependent translation of capped mRNAs with extended 5'-UTRs and the ZIKV genome represents an RNA with these features, this study aims to investigate the effect of silvestrol on the translation and replication of two ZIKV strains.

2. Materials and Methods

2.1. Cell Culture

Human A549 cells were cultured in DMEM supplemented with 4.5 g/L glucose, 10% fectal calf serum (FCS), 2 mM L-Glutamine, 0.1 U/mL Penicillin, and 100 µg/mL Streptomycin. The cells were seeded in a multi-well plate and 6 h later infected with ZIKV strain 976 Uganda (U) (kindly provided by the European Virus Archive) or ZIKV PF13/251013-18 from French Polynesia (FP) (kindly provided by Prof. Didier Musso Institute Louis in Papeete, Malardé, Tahiti) with an multiplicity of infection (MOI) of 0.1. The substances silvestrol (Medchemexpress LLc; purity > 98%) and DMSO (Genaxxon bioscience; purity > 99%) were present in the respective dilutions in the inoculum. The cells were washed once with warm PBS 16 h, 40 h, and 64 h p.i., and covered with fresh DMEM supplemented with the respective substances in the same concentrations to ensure presence of silvestrol during the whole time course. At 24 h, 48 h, or 72 h p.i. the cells were washed with PBS and harvested in peqGOLD TriFast (peqlab Biotechnologie GmbH, Erlangen, Germany) for RNA isolation or RIPA-buffer for protein isolation. The supernatant was harvested for the determination of extracellular viral RNA and particles.

Primary human hepatocytes (PHHs) were isolated and cultivated as described [23,24]. Infection and treatment of the PHHs were performed in accordance with the A549 experiments.

2.2. RNA-Isolation

The intracellular RNA was isolated using peqGOLD Trifast (peqlab Biotechnologie GmbH) according to the manufacturer's instructions.

The extracellular RNA was isolated from the cell culture supernatant after 5 min of centrifugation at $1000 \times g$ with the QIAamp Viral RNA Mini Kit (Qiagen, Hilden, Germany) following the manufacturer's instructions.

2.3. RT-qPCR

Extracellular ZIKV RNA was quantified in a LightCycler480 (Roche) using the Zika Virus detection kit (TIB Molbiol, Berlin, Germany) together with the LightCycler Multiplex RNA Virus Mastermix (Roche, Basel, Switzerland) according to the manufacturer's protocol.

Reverse transcription of the intracellular RNA was performed as described [25]. The cDNA was quantified in a LightCycler480 (Roche) using the SYBR Green Mastermix (Thermo Fisher Scientific, Waltham, MA, USA) and the following primers: ZIKV-fwd (AGATCCCGGCTGAAACACTG), ZIKV_rev (TTGCAAGGTCCATCTGTCCC), hRPL27_fw (AAAGCTGTCATCGTGAAGAAC), hRPL27_rv (GCTGCTACTTTGCGGGGGTAG).

The amount of ZIKV RNA was normalized to the amount of RPL27 transcripts.

2.4. Cell Viability and Cytotoxicity Assays

Cell viability was assessed using the PrestoBlue Cell viability reagent (Thermo Fisher Scientific) as described [26]. In addition, lactate dehydrogenase (LDH)-release was quantified with the LDH Cytotoxicity Detection Kit (Clontech, Mountain View, CA, USA) according to the manufacturer's protocol. LDH-release-assay was performed in DMEM with a reduced amount of FCS (1%) to lower the measurement background. The LDH activity in the supernatant of cells treated with 1% Triton X-100 served as control and reference for normalization. Viability of PHHs was assessed by ALT (alanine aminotransferase) activity measurement of the cell culture supernatant with the Reflotron Plus (Roche) and the respective GPT (ALT) test strips according to the manufacturer's protocol.

2.5. Western Blot

RIPA-Lysates were used to perform SDS-PAGE and Western blot analysis as described [27]. A specific antibody was used to detect the protein NS1 (Biofront technologies, 1225-36, Tallahassee, FL, USA) in the dilution 1:1000. Detection of β-actin with a specific antibody (Sigma Aldrich, A5316, St. Louis, MO, USA) in the dilution 1:10,000 served as loading control. Specific antibodies were used for the detection of PIM1 (Santa Cruz, 12H8), MVP (LRP 1014, Santa Cruz Biotechnology, Heidelberg, Germany), NS3 (8G-2, abcam), and NS5A (described in Reference [28]) Densitometry scans of the membranes with IRDye-coupled secondary antibodies (dilution 1:10,000) were quantified with the software Image Studio (both from Licor, Lincoln, NE, USA).

2.6. Plaque Assay

For titer determination of cell culture supernatants, plaque assays were performed. For this, Vero cells were seeded in a 6-well plate (3×10^5 cells/well) and infected 6 h later with cell culture supernatant in a serial dilution in DMEM. At 2 h p.i. the cells were washed once with PBS and covered with 37 °C pre-warmed DMEM containing 0.4% agarose. After 15 min at room temperature the plates were incubated for 96 h at 37 °C. To visualize the plaques the agarose was removed, cells were fixed with 4% formaldehyde in PBS for 20 min at room temperature, and then stained for 15 min with 0.1% crystal violet in 20% ethanol. Then the cells were washed once with water and the titer (PFU/mL) was determined by counting the plaques in the well with the respective dilution.

2.7. Immunofluorescence Microscopy

The cells were grown on cover slides and fixed with 4% formaldehyde in PBS for 20 min at room temperature. Then the cells were permeabilized with 0.5% Triton X-100 in PBS for 15 min on room temperature. After blocking with 1% BSA in PBS for 15 min at room temperature, the cells were stained with the anti-NS1 antibody (Biofront technologies, 1225-36) in the dilution 1:200 and afterwards with the secondary antibody anti-mouse-AlexaFluor488 (Thermo Fisher Scientific) for 1 h at room temperature in a humid chamber. The secondary antibody dilution was supplemented with DAPI to visualize the nuclei. Finally, the cells were mounted with Mowiol on microscope slides. Immunofluorescence staining was analyzed using a confocal laser scanning microscope (CLSM 510 Meta) with Zen 2009 Software (both from Carl Zeiss, Oberkochen, Germany) and a Cytation5 with the Gen5 Software (both from Biotek, Winooski, VT, USA). For each condition the amount of ZIKV positive cells in at least four fields of view of three experiments were quantified.

2.8. Statistical Analysis

Results are presented as means $\pm$ standard errors of the means (SEMs) from at least three independent experiments. The significance of the results was analyzed by unpaired two-tailed Student's t test, using GraphPad Prism, version 6.07 for Windows (GraphPad Software, San Diego, CA, USA). In all figures the statistical significance is compared to the DMSO control group. Statistical significance is represented in figures as follows:

ns = not significant = $p > 0.05$; * = $p \leq 0.05$; ** = $p \leq 0.01$; *** = $p \leq 0.001$; **** = $p \leq 0.0001$.

3. Results

3.1. Silvestrol Shows a Cytostatic rather than a Cytotoxic Effect in A549 Cells

In a previous study, silvestrol was used for treatment of Ebola virus (EBOV)-infected HuH7-cells in concentrations of 5, 10, and 50 nM [20]. To determine the working concentration of silvestrol in A549 cells, we first analyzed the metabolic activity of these cells treated with different concentrations of silvestrol for 24, 48, and 72 h by PrestoBlue assays. Silvestrol exhibits a concentration-dependent inhibition of the cells metabolism starting with a concentration as low as 5 nM (Figure 1A). To rule out a cytotoxic effect of silvestrol, an LDH release assay was performed to quantify the activity of LDH in the supernatant released from dead cells. For none of the three tested silvestrol concentrations was a cytotoxic effect reflected by an increase in the LDH activity detected after 24 h. After 48 h, no cytotoxic effect was observed for the 5 nM and 10 nM concentrations, while in case of the cells treated with 50 nM silvestrol an increase in the LDH activity was detected. In case of the incubation period for 72 h a weak cytotoxic effect was detectable for the lower concentrations of silvestrol (5 nM and 10 nM), while treatment with 50 nM silvestrol was associated with cytotoxicity (Figure 1B), although there were still a high number of viable intact cells, as reflected by the intact nuclei in the DAPI staining (Figure 2A).

These data demonstrate that silvestrol affects the cellular metabolism in the cancer cell line A549 in a time- and dose-dependent manner and exerts a moderate cytotoxic effect in higher concentrations after 48 h and 72 h.

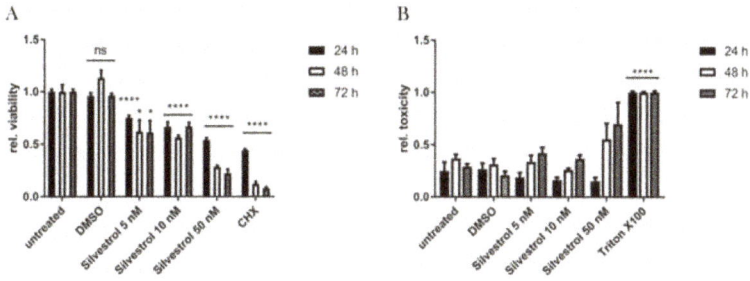

Figure 1. Cytostatic effect of silvestrol in A549 cells. (**A**) Time- and concentration-dependent decrease of cellular metabolic activity after silvestrol treatment in A549 cells determined by the PrestoBlue assay. Cycloheximid (CHX) served as positive control in a concentration of 35 μM to inhibit cell proliferation; (**B**) Lactate dehydrogenase (LDH) release assay with the supernatants of silvestrol treated A549 cells did not show an increased cell death. Treatment with 1% Triton X-100 served as positive control for complete cell death. LDH activity in the samples was normalized to the LDH activity in the supernatant of Triton X-100 treated cells. ns = not significant = $p > 0.05$; * = $p \leq 0.05$; **** = $p \leq 0.0001$.

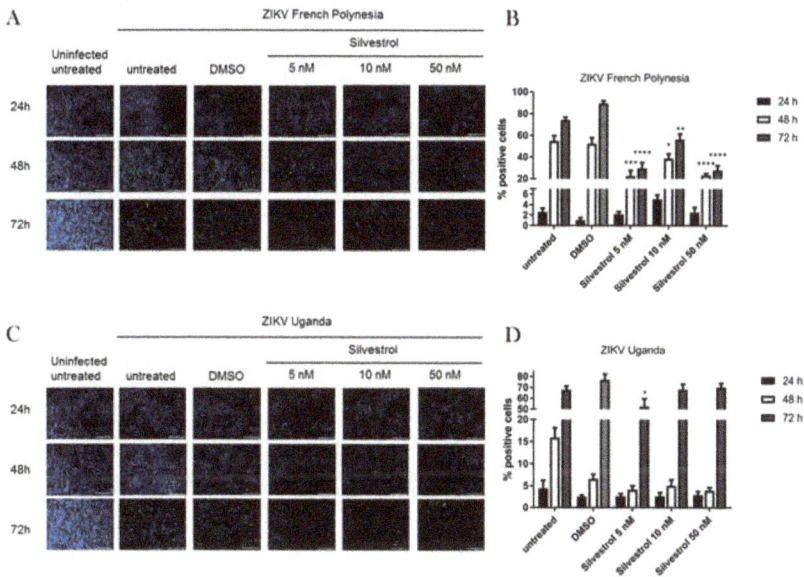

Figure 2. Silvestrol treatment reduces the number of Zika virus (ZIKV) positive cells. (**A**) A549 cells were infected with ZIKV French Polynesia isolate (FP) and treated with the indicated amount of silvestrol. Cells were fixed on the indicated time points and nuclei were stained with DAPI (blue) and NS1 was stained with a specific antibody in green, scale bar = 200 μm; (**B**) Ratio of NS1-positive cells in at least four fields of view of the respective samples exemplary shown in (**A**); (**C**) A549 cells were infected with ZIKV Uganda isolate (U) and treated with the indicated amount of silvestrol. Cells were fixed on the indicated time points and nuclei were stained with DAPI (blue) and NS1 was stained with a specific antibody in green, scale bar = 200 μm; (**D**) Ratio of NS1-positive cells in at least four fields of view of the respective samples exemplary shown in (**C**). * = $p \leq 0.05$; ** = $p \leq 0.01$; *** = $p \leq 0.001$; **** = $p \leq 0.0001$.

3.2. Silvestrol Impairs ZIKV Infection in A549 Cells

To investigate the potential antiviral effect of silvestrol on ZIKV life cycle, A549 cells were infected with two ZIKV strains with an MOI of 0.1 and subsequently treated with silvestrol for 24, 48, and 72 h. The ZIKV strain 976 Uganda (ZIKV U), which did not show neuropathological effects in patients, was compared to the ZIKV strain PF13/251013-18 (ZIKV FP) from French Polynesia, which was the first strain associated with microcephaly. Based on the data from the cytotoxicity and viability assays and in accordance to a previous study, silvestrol was used in concentrations of 5, 10, and 50 nM [20]. The impact on viral life cycle was analyzed by immunofluorescence microscopy using an NS1-specific antiserum (Figure 2A,C). The quantification of the immunofluorescence microscopy reveals for the ZIKV strain French Polynesia a decrease in the number of ZIKV-positive cells and fluorescence intensity as evidenced by the NS1-specific staining after treatment with silvestrol for 48 h and 72 h (Figure 2B). No significant effect could be observed for the ZIKV Uganda strain, except for 5 nM silvestrol at 48 h (Figure 2D).

These data indicate that silvestrol exerts an inhibitory effect on the spread of ZIKV infection in A549 cells.

3.3. Inhibition of ZIKV Replication by Silvestrol

For a more detailed analysis of the effect of silvestrol on the ZIKV life cycle, the amount of intra- and extracellular ZIKV-specific RNA was determined by real-time PCR (RT-qPCR). For both isolates (Uganda isolate (U) and French Polynesia isolate (FP)) a strong decrease of the intra- and extracellular amount of ZIKV-genomes was observed for infected cells that were incubated with 5 nM or 50 nM at all three analyzed points in time (24 h, 48 h, and 72 h). Interestingly, there was no strict dose-effect relation since a weaker (for the intracellular viral RNA, see Figure 3A,B) or almost no effect (for the extracellular viral RNA, see Figure 3C,D) was observed if silvestrol was applied in a 10 nM concentration.

As viral genomes do not directly correspond to infectious viral particles, the impact of silvestrol treatment on the number of released viral particles was determined by plaque assay on Vero cells. Again, for both isolates there was no strict dose-effect relation. In case of cells infected with the French Polynesia isolate for 5 nM and 50 nM silvestrol as compared to the control (DMSO-treated cells), a decrease in the number of released viral particles was observed at 24 and 48 h. Treatment for 72 h with 5 nM silvestrol very efficiently decreased the titer, but no significant effect was observed with 50 nM silvestrol. A similar picture was observed in the case of cells infected with the Uganda strain, but the 72-h treatment did not lead to a reduction in the amount of released viral particles (Figure 3E,F).

The observed lack of a strict dose-effect relation might reflect the equilibrium of silvestrol actions on the one hand directly affecting ZIKV life cycle/replication and on the other hand affecting the antiviral defense mechanisms of the host cell. In this context, it should be considered that silvestrol, as an inhibitor of eIF4A, affects on the one hand the translation of the viral RNA and on the other hand the translation of a variety of host factors. These factors could include RNases, proteasomal, lysosomal, or autophagosomal proteins. If such activities triggering the degradation of viral genomes or viral proteins are impaired, a stabilization of i.e., viral genomes is the consequence that could compensate for the inhibitory effects of silvestrol on other parts of the viral life cycle.

Taken together, these data show that the silvestrol-dependent effects on the ZIKV life cycle do not follow a strict dose-effect relation in A549 cells. While 5 nM and 50 nM silvestrol exerted a strong inhibition of ZIKV replication as reflected by a significantly reduced amount of intra- and extracellular ZIKV genomes, 10 nM silvestrol failed to impair ZIKV replication most likely due to secondary effects in the infected host cell.

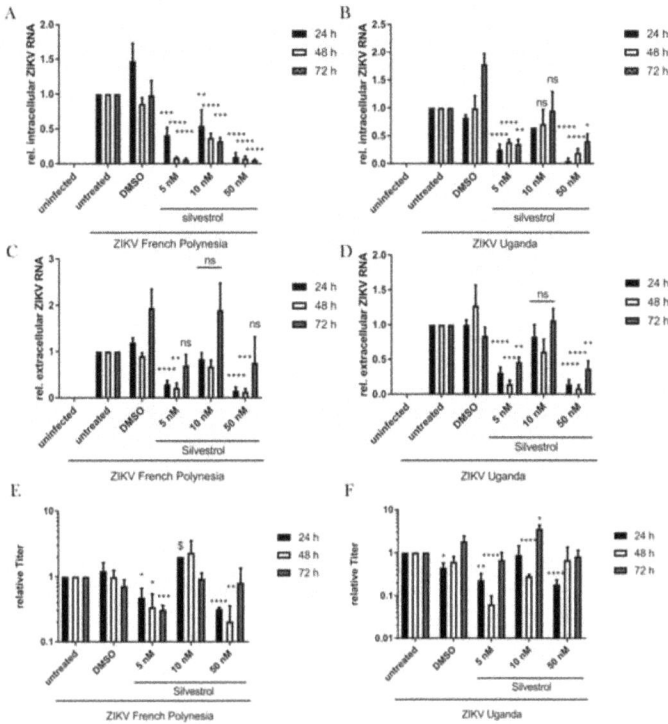

Figure 3. Significant reduction of intra- and extracellular ZIKV RNA levels and released virions. (**A**) Quantification of intracellular ZIKV RNA of A549 cells infected with ZIKV FP and treated with the indicated concentrations of silvestrol. ZIKV RNA was quantified by RT-qPCR and normalized to the amount of RPL27 transcripts; (**B**) Quantification of intracellular ZIKV RNA of A549 cells infected with ZIKV U and treated with the indicated concentrations of silvestrol. ZIKV RNA was quantified by RT-qPCR and normalized to the amount of RPL27 transcripts; (**C**) RT-qPCR quantification of extracellular ZIKV RNA of A549 cells infected with ZIKV FP and treated with the indicated concentrations of silvestrol; (**D**) RT-qPCR quantification of extracellular ZIKV RNA of A549 cells infected with ZIKV U and treated with the indicated concentrations of silvestrol; (**E**) Relative extracellular titers of A549 cells infected with ZIKV FP and treated with the indicated concentrations of silvestrol. Titers were quantified by plaque assay in Vero cells; (**F**) Relative extracellular titers of A549 cells infected with ZIKV U and treated with the indicated concentrations of silvestrol. Titers were quantified by plaque assay in Vero cells. $: only two experiments were performed. ns = not significant = $p > 0.05$; * = $p \leq 0.05$; ** = $p \leq 0.01$; *** = $p \leq 0.001$; **** = $p \leq 0.0001$.

3.4. Silvestrol Inhibits ZIKV Translation by Inhibition of eIF4A

To pinpoint whether silvestrol exerts its direct antiviral effect on the translation of viral proteins due to specific inhibition of the DEAD-box RNA helicase eIF4A, a Western blot analysis of infected and silvestrol-treated A549 cells was performed. The ZIKV protein NS1 was detected with a specific antibody and referred to the β-actin signal. In case of the lowest concentration (5 nM) there was, for both isolates—ZIKV-U and ZIKV-FP—after 24 h, no significant reduction detectable. This may be because only 2% of the cell culture was infected with ZIKV after 24 h (see Figure 2), so the detection of NS1 by Western blot showed only moderate signals, resulting in increased SEM for this time point. However, after 48 h and 72 h a significant reduction in the amount of NS1 was found. This comes along with a dose-dependent reduction of the oncogene PIM1, which is known to be translated in an eIF4A-dependent manner (Figure S1). In case of 50 nM silvestrol, for both isolates a strong reduction in the amount of NS1 was found at all three investigated time points. As described above, again there was no strict dose-effect relation. Thus, for both isolates treated with 10 nM almost no reduction in the amount of NS1 was detectable (Figure 4). This is in accordance to the data described above that show that 10 nM silvestrol leads to a slight increase in the amount of ZIKV-specific RNA. These results indicate that the antiviral effect of silvestrol observed in A549 cells for concentrations of 5 nM and 50 nM is associated with a decreased amount of ZIKV proteins, as shown here by a NS1-specific Western blot.

As a loss in viral protein could also be related to an inhibition of reinfections or the viral replication rather than the translation, according to similar experiments that were performed with a high MOI (MOI = 1). Even higher MOIs would not be beneficial in this system because of the cytopathic effect of ZIKV. Silvestrol is able to decrease the amount of ZIKV RNA and proteins in the same concentration range also at this high MOI, confirming the eIF4A-dependent mechanism of silvestrol (Figure S4).

To test whether this effect is specific to cap-dependent viral translation the effect of silvestrol on hepatitis C virus (HCV), which uses an eIF4A-independent IRES for translation was tested. Indeed, the treatment of HCV-positive Huh7.5 cells did not result in a decrease of the viral proteins (Figure S3). This data confirms the specificity of silvestrol on eIF4A-dependent viral translation.

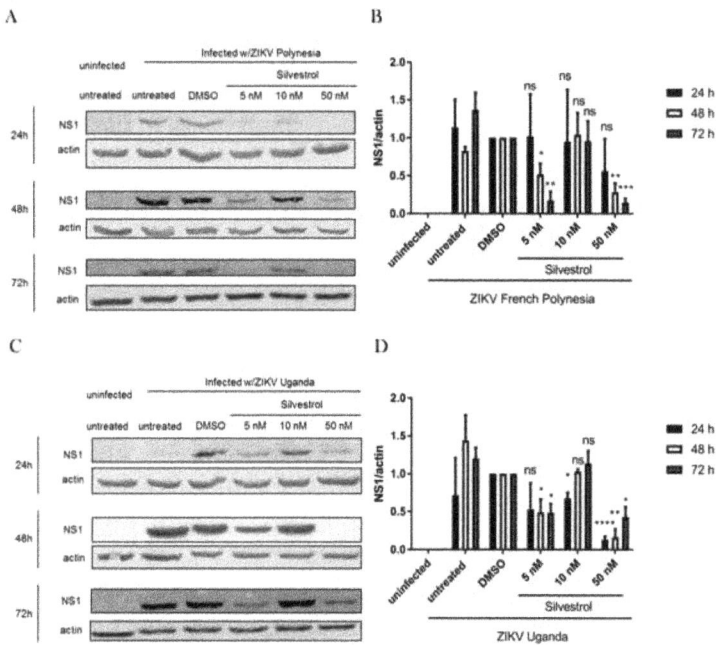

Figure 4. Silvestrol treatment reduces the amount of intracellular NS1 protein. (**A**) A549 cells were infected with ZIKV U and treated with the indicated amount of silvestrol. Cell lysates of the indicated time points were analyzed by Western blot with specific antibodies against NS1 and β-actin; (**B**) Quantification of densitometry scans examples are shown in (**A**); (**C**) A549 cells were infected with ZIKV FP and treated with the indicated amount of silvestrol. Cell lysates of the indicated time points were analyzed by Western blot with specific antibodies against NS1 and β-actin; (**D**) Quantification of densitometry scans examples are shown in (**C**). ns = not significant = $p > 0.05$; * = $p \leq 0.05$; ** = $p \leq 0.01$; *** = $p \leq 0.001$; **** = $p \leq 0.0001$.

3.5. Silvestrol Inhibits ZIKV Replication in Infected Primary Human Hepatocytes

Initially, silvestrol was described as a potential anti-cancer drug due to its inhibitory effect on the proliferation of a variety of cancer cells [11,14,16]. As A549 cells originate from a human lung carcinoma primary, non-transformed cells were used to study the antiviral effect of silvestrol on the ZIKV life cycle to exclude any side effects that are due to the anti-cancer effect of silvestrol. For this purpose, primary human hepatocytes (PHHs) of two different donors were infected with ZIKV FP and subsequently treated with silvestrol. Even though the physiological host cells of ZIKV are thought to be keratinocytes and neurons, in a recent study we found that ZIKV efficiently replicates in hepatocytes [29]. As the isolation and cultivation of primary human hepatocytes (PHHs) is well-established in our lab, we decided to use these cell culture model for human primary cells. Supernatants were harvested after 24 h, 48 h, and 72 h. As primary human hepatocytes are much more resistant to silvestrol [20,30,31], 100 nM silvestrol was tested as the highest concentration. The amount of viral genomes was quantified by RT-qPCR, and the number of infectious viral particles was quantified by plaque assays. The results analyzed after 24 h show that none of the investigated concentrations of silvestrol (5 nM, 10 nM and 100 nM) exhibited a significant reduction in the amount of viral genomes. However, after 48 h and 72 h a strong and significant reduction of the number of released viral genomes was observed (Figure 5A–C).

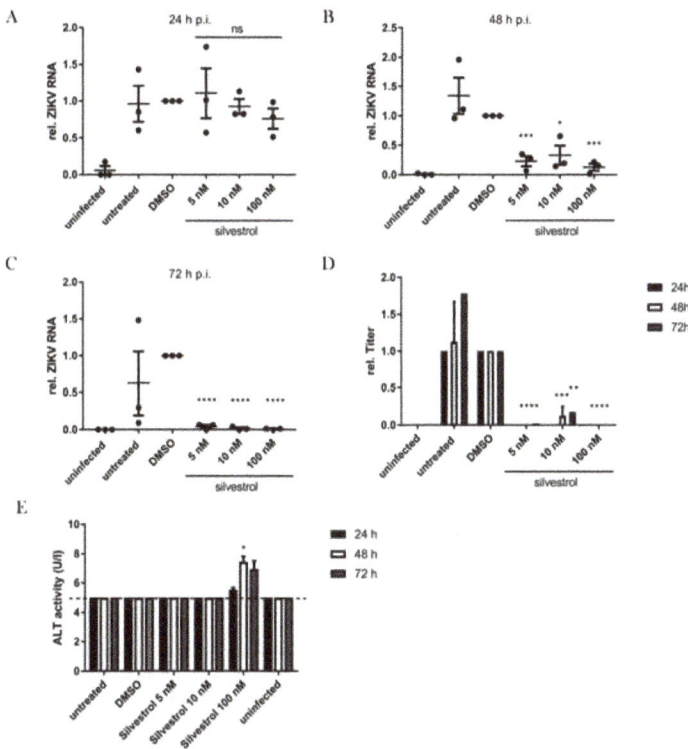

Figure 5. Silvestrol exerts an anti-ZIKV effect also in primary cells. Primary human hepatocytes were infected with ZIKV FP and treated with the indicated concentrations of silvestrol. The extracellular ZIKV RNA was quantified by RT-qPCR after 24 (**A**), 48 (**B**), and 72 h (**C**); (**D**) Extracellular titers of infected and treated primary human hepatocytes (PHHs) after 48 and 72 h. Shown are titers from just one PHH donor quantified by plaque assay in Vero cells; (**E**) ALT activity in PHH supernatants. ns = not significant = $p > 0.05$; * = $p \leq 0.05$; ** = $p \leq 0.01$; *** = $p \leq 0.001$; **** = $p \leq 0.0001$.

Quantification of the number of infectious viral particles in the supernatant confirmed this. For all three investigated time points, the number of infectious ZIKV particles was strongly decreased and in some cases even below the detection limit, reflecting a strong inhibitory potential (Figure 5D). Interestingly, as observed for the A549 cells, there was no strict dose-effect relation as in case of the cells treated with 10 nM silvestrol. ZIKV particles were detectable in the supernatant but in a strongly reduced amount as compared to the control. The ALT activity in the supernatants of the PHHs, as a measure of cytotoxicity, was below the detection limit of 5 U/L in most samples and only slightly increased in case of 100 nM silvestrol (Figure 5E). However, sera of male humans with ALT activities above 41 U/L are considered to represent liver damage, hence the obtained ALT activities of about 7 U/L do not correspond to cytotoxicity. To address the toxicity of silvestrol on primary cells in more detail, brightfield imaging and PrestoBlue assays were performed with treated cells as well. Both readouts confirmed the toxic effect of 100 nM silvestrol on the PHHs at 48 h and 72 h of treatment (Figure S2). However, the lower concentrations are not toxic to the cells but show a remarkably reduction of the viral load.

These data confirm that the specific inhibition of eIF4A-dependent translation affects ZIKV replication in a complex interplay between direct inhibition of the viral life cycle on the one hand and interference with cellular antiviral mechanisms on the other hand.

4. Discussion

The Zika viral genome is a (+)-strand ssRNA and therefore serves directly as a template for protein biosynthesis by the cellular translation machinery. As the ZIKV genome has an exposed and structured 5'-UTR and its translation depends on the 5'-cap introduced by the viral NS5 protein, eIF4A is expected to be required to initiate the translation of the viral polyprotein by unwinding the RNA secondary structures [6,21,32]. For EBOV, a (−)-strand ssRNA virus, a significant antiviral effect of silvestrol was observed. In the EBOV system, silvestrol inhibits the eIF4A-dependent translation of viral mRNAs with extended and structured 5'-UTRs [20].

Indeed, the natural compound silvestrol, if used in 5 nM and 50 nM concentrations, exerts a significant antiviral effect on ZIKV-infected A549 cells. This effect was observed for both analyzed Zika virus strains (ZIKV-U and ZIKV-FP). As silvestrol is well characterized to inhibit eIF4A-dependent protein synthesis, these data suggest that translation of the ZIKV genome is eIF4A-dependent and can be blocked by silvestrol [13]. To prove the inhibitory effect of silvestrol on eIF4A-dependent translation in the used system, the amount of the oncogene PIM1 was determined by Western blot, which decreases in a concentration-dependent manner by silvestrol treatment (Figure S1). Futhermore, the lack of an inhibitory effect of silvestrol on the IRES-dependent translation of HCV underlines the proposed eIF4A-dependent antiviral mechanism of silvestrol in the case of ZIKV (Figure S3).

Both ZIKV strains possess a stable and long stem-loop structure in their 5'-UTR, but the secondary structure of the Uganda strain seems to be much more stable, as predictions with several online tools show [1]. This higher stability would imply a higher dependency of the helicase activity of eIF4A to initiate the translation of the Uganda strain genome. Hence, a stronger antiviral effect of silvestrol would be expected. In general, we did not observe a different effectivity of silvestrol on the ZIKV Uganda strain, except in the quantification of the infectious titer. Concerning the number of positive cells, silvestrol seems even to be less effective as mentioned before. This could be partially explained by the fact that ZIKV-U represents a very early isolate that might have acquired cell culture adaptive mutations and therefore might have better replication efficiency [33]. The ZIKV strain PF13/251013-1 was isolated in 2007 and therefore is not as well adapted to cell cultures as the ancestor virus from Uganda [34]. Furthermore, the unwinding of 5'-UTR with higher stability may require additional helicase activities such as DDX3, so inhibiting eIF4A alone might not be sufficient to inhibit the translation of these RNAs. Uncovering the detailed features of a silvestrol-sensitive 5'-UTR structure will be of future interest. However, the more sensitive readout via RT-qPCR clearly shows a significant antiviral effect of silvestrol on ZIKV U, which suggests that viral translation is also inhibited in this strain.

To investigate the specificity of the observed effects, cell viability and toxicity assays were performed. In the cell viability assay (PrestoBlue assay), which measures metabolic activity of the cells, a time- and concentration-dependent decrease of the metabolic activity was observed by silvestrol (Figure 1A). This is in accordance with former publications as well as the microscopic images in this study (Figure 2), which show a decreased proliferation of tumor cell lines by silvestrol [14]. However, no cytotoxicity was observed by silvestrol treatment in the LDH-release assay for the 24-h and 48-h incubation periods (Figure 1B). This was expected, as the inhibition of eIF4A by different substances did not show a cytotoxic effect in previous studies [35]. Therefore, the antiviral effect of silvestrol on the Zika virus at these time points is not based on cytotoxicity and can also not be explained by a minor cytostatic effect. Moreover, the amount of the NS1 protein and the ZIKV genomes were normalized on the housekeepers β-actin and RPL27, respectively, to rule out possible secondary effects. The specificity of silvestrol on the ZIKV translation is further underlined by using primary human hepatocytes infected with the French Polynesia strain (Figure 5). These cells are not based on tumor cell lines and therefore show no growth inhibition by silvestrol. No increased ALT activity and no morphological effect were observed due to silvestrol treatment (Figure 5E). Remarkably, 100 nM silvestrol showed a toxic effect on PHHs of some donors, which could be explained by a oncogenic predisposition of these cells as donors suffered from hepatocellular carcinomas (Figure S2). The strong effect of silvestrol on ZIKV is even more pronounced in these cells.

Of course, on first glance the lack of a clear dose-effect relation is surprising. However, it should be considered that silvestrol, as an inhibitor of eIF4A, affects on the one hand the translation of the viral RNA and on the other hand the translation of cellular mRNAs, and thus the expression of a variety of host factors. From the mass spectrometry data of cellular lysates of A549 cells, the cellular major vault protein (MVP) was identified to be downregulated by silvestrol treatment (submitted). This was confirmed by Western blot and immunofluorescence analysis, which showed a decreased amount of MVP and a translocation from the cytoplasm to the perinuclear region (Figure S5). As MVP is supposed to exert its antiviral effect by affecting IRF7 and interferon type I cytoplasmic signaling, a decreased amount of the protein and a withdrawal of MVP from the cytoplasm would affect the its capacity to deregulate these cytoplasmic antiviral signaling cascades. As MVP is part of an antiviral interferon-cascade, a decreased amount of this protein in the cytoplasm could explain the partial recovery of ZIKV at 10 nM silvestrol [36]. However further experiments have to be performed to characterize the potential antiviral effect of MVP on ZIKV and to study the impact of MVP on the ZIKV life cycle in detail.

Surprisingly, there was a concentration-dependent effect of silvestrol in A549 cells infected with a comparably high MOI of 1 (Figure S4). This might indicate that in low MOI infections, the antiviral effect (of e.g., MVP) inhibits the spread of the virus which cannot be seen with a high MOI, because reinfections are rare.

Interestingly MVP could not be detected in HCV-positive Huh7.5 cells (Figure S3). This is not surprising, since Huh7.5 cells bear mutations in the antiviral interferon-pathway (e.g., RIG-I) which confers the susceptibility of those cells to HCV. In line with this, no increase of viral proteins was observed with silvestrol treatment because cellular antiviral proteins cannot be affected.

In light of the complex interplay of silvestrol in inhibiting the pathogenic and host translation of some antiviral proteins, a direct application of silvestrol in clinics might be difficult. However, this study identified eIF4A as a cellular factor that can be targeted to inhibit ZIKV spread.

A comparison of the antiviral effects of cells treated with 5 nM or 50 nM to the effects observed for cells treated with 10 nM silvestrol showed the lack of a dose-effect relation. This atypical course reflects a complex interplay between direct effects on ZIKV translation and the translation of anti-viral factors. There is a variety of host factors triggering an antiviral response, such as RNases, and proteasomal, lysosomal, or autophagosomal proteins. If the translation of these antiviral activities involved i.e.,

Viruses **2018**, *10*, 149

in the degradation of viral genomes or viral proteins is impaired, a stabilization of viral genomes is the consequence. This increased stability leads to elevated genome levels and thereby could compensate for the inhibitory effects of silvestrol in other parts of the viral life cycle, such as impaired translation.

5. Conclusions

Taken together, this study gives evidence that silvestrol has the potential to exert a potent antiviral effect on the pathogenic ZIKV. It might contribute to identify host factors involved in the control of ZIKV infection and so might help to develop antiviral concepts that can be used to treat a variety of viral infections without the risk of resistances as a host protein is targeted.

Supplementary Materials: The following are available online at http://www.mdpi.com/1999-4915/10/4/149/s1, Figure S1. Silvestrol inhibits eIF4A-dependent translation. A549 cells were treated with the indicated amount of silvestrol. Cell lysates of the indicated time points were analyzed by Western blot with specific antibodies against PIM1 and β-actin; Figure S2. Toxic effect of 100 nM silvestrol in primary human hepatocytes. PHHs were treated with the indicated concentrations of silvestrol. At 24 h, 48 h, and 72 h post treatment, PrestoBlue assay (A) and brightfield imaging (B) were performed; Figure S3. No inhibiting effect of silvestrol on the IRES-dependent translation of HCV. Huh7.5 cells were transfected with the full-length HCV genome Jc1 and 72 h post-transfection treated with the indicated concentrations of silvestrol. (A) Cells lysates of the indicated time points were analyzed by Western blot with specific antibodies against NS3, NS5A, and β-actin. (B) Quantification of NS3 of densitometry scans exemplary shown in A). (C) Quantification of NS5A of densitometry scans exemplary shown in (A); Figure S4. Silvestrol exerts its antiviral effect also with higher MOI. (A) Quantification of intracellular ZIKV RNA of A549 cells infected with ZIKV FP (MOI = 1) and treated with the indicated concentrations of silvestrol. ZIKV RNA was quantified by RT-qPCR and normalized to the amount of RPL27 transcripts; (B) Quantification of intracellular ZIKV RNA of A549 cells infected with ZIKV U (MOI = 1) and treated with the indicated concentrations of silvestrol. ZIKV RNA was quantified by RT-qPCR and normalized to the amount of RPL27 transcripts; (C) RT-qPCR quantification of extracellular ZIKV RNA of A549 cells infected with ZIKV FP (MOI = 1) and treated with the indicated concentrations of silvestrol; (D) RT-qPCR quantification of extracellular ZIKV RNA of A549 cells infected with ZIKV U (MOI = 1) and treated with the indicated concentrations of silvestrol; (E) Western blot analysis of A549 cells infected with ZIKV FP (MOI = 1) and treated with the indicated concentrations of silvestrol; (F) Quantification of NS1 of densitometry scans exemplary shown in (E); (G) Western blot analysis of A549 cells infected with ZIKV U (MOI = 1) and treated with the indicated concentrations of silvestrol; (H) Quantification of NS1 of densitometry scans exemplary shown in (G); Figure S5. Silvestrol decreases the amount of the antiviral protein MVP. A549 cells were treated with the indicated concentrations of silvestrol. (A) Twenty-four hours after treatment, cells were fixed with ice-cold ethanol. Nuclei were stained with DAPI (blue) and MVP was stained with an antibody (red); (B) cell lysates were analyzed by Western blot analysis with antibodies against MVP and actin.

Acknowledgments: The authors thank Gert Carra for his excellent technical support and Dagmar Fecht-Schwarz for her critical reading of the manuscript. Moreover, the authors thank the PHH Core Facility of Florian Vondran at the Medizinische Hochschule Hannover for isolating and sharing the PHHs. We thank Didier Musso (Director of the Research and Diagnosis Laboratory, Institute Louis Malardé in Papeete, Tahiti) for donating the ZIKV Polynesia strain (PF 13/251013-18). This publication was supported by the European Virus Archive goes Global (EVAg) project that has received funding from the European Union's Horizon 2020 research and innovation program under grant agreement No 653316. Based on this funding, EVAg provided the ZIKV strain Uganda (strain 976). This work was supported by a grant from the Federal Ministry of Health (BMG) to E.H. A.G. and E.H. obtained funding from the LOEWE Center DRUID (Novel Drug Targets against Poverty-Related and Neglected Tropical Infectious Diseases).

Author Contributions: Eberhard Hildt, Arnold Grünweller, and Fabian Elgner conceived and designed the experiments; Fabian Elgner, Michael Basic and Catarina Sabino performed the experiments; Fabian Elgner and Daniela Ploen analyzed the data; Fabian Elgner and Eberhard Hildt wrote the paper.

Conflicts of Interest: The authors declare no conflict of interest.

References

1. Göertz, G.P.; Abbo, S.R.; Fros, J.J.; Pijlman, G.P. Functional RNA during Zika virus infection. *Virus Res.* 2017. [CrossRef] [PubMed]
2. Heinz, F.X.; Stiasny, K. The Antigenic Structure of Zika Virus and Its Relation to Other Flaviviruses: Implications for Infection and Immunoprophylaxis. *Microbiol. Mol. Biol. Rev.* **2017**, *81*. [CrossRef] [PubMed]
3. Zhu, Z.; Chan, J.F.-W.; Tee, K.-M.; Choi, G.K.-Y.; Lau, S.K.-P.; Woo, P.C.-Y.; Tse, H.; Yuen, K.-Y. Comparative genomic analysis of pre-epidemic and epidemic Zika virus strains for virological factors potentially associated with the rapidly expanding epidemic. *Emerg. Microbes Infect.* **2016**, *5*, e22. [CrossRef] [PubMed]

4. Kuno, G.; Chang, G.-J.J. Full-length sequencing and genomic characterization of Bagaza, Kedougou, and Zika viruses. *Arch. Virol.* **2007**, *152*, 687–696. [CrossRef] [PubMed]

5. Baronti, C.; Piorkowski, G.; Charrel, R.N.; Boubis, L.; Leparc-Goffart, I.; de Lamballerie, X. Complete coding sequence of zika virus from a French polynesia outbreak in 2013. *Genome Announc.* **2014**, *2*. [CrossRef] [PubMed]

6. Coutard, B.; Barral, K.; Lichière, J.; Selisko, B.; Martin, B.; Aouadi, W.; Lombardia, M.O.; Debart, F.; Vasseur, J.-J.; Guillemot, J.C.; et al. Zika Virus Methyltransferase: Structure and Functions for Drug Design Perspectives. *J. Virol.* **2017**, *91*. [CrossRef] [PubMed]

7. Cao-Lormeau, V.M.; Blake, A.; Mons, S.; Lastere, S.; Roche, C.; Vanhomwegen, J.; Dub, T.; Baudouin, L.; Teissier, A.; Larre, P.; et al. Guillain-Barré Syndrome outbreak associated with Zika virus infection in French Polynesia: A case-control study. *Lancet* **2016**, *387*, 1531–1539. [CrossRef]

8. Victora, C.G.; Schuler-Faccini, L.; Matijasevich, A.; Ribeiro, E.; Pessoa, A.; Barros, F.C. Microcephaly in Brazil: How to interpret reported numbers? *Lancet* **2016**, *387*, 621–624. [CrossRef]

9. Kim, S.; Hwang, B.Y.; Su, B.-N.; Chai, H.; Mi, Q.; Kinghorn, A.D.; Wild, R.; Swanson, S.M. Silvestrol, a potential anticancer rocaglate derivative from Aglaia foveolata, induces apoptosis in LNCaP cells through the mitochondrial/apoptosome pathway without activation of executioner caspase-3 or -7. *Anticancer Res.* **2007**, *27*, 2175–2183. [PubMed]

10. Chu, J.; Galicia-Vázquez, G.; Cencic, R.; Mills, J.R.; Katigbak, A.; Porco, J.A.; Pelletier, J. CRISPR-Mediated Drug-Target Validation Reveals Selective Pharmacological Inhibition of the RNA Helicase, eIF4A. *Cell Rep.* **2016**, *15*, 2340–2347. [CrossRef] [PubMed]

11. Bordeleau, M.-E.; Robert, F.; Gerard, B.; Lindqvist, L.; Chen, S.M.H.; Wendel, H.-G.; Brem, B.; Greger, H.; Lowe, S.W.; Porco, J.A.; et al. Therapeutic suppression of translation initiation modulates chemosensitivity in a mouse lymphoma model. *J. Clin. Investig.* **2008**, *118*, 2651–2660. [CrossRef] [PubMed]

12. Pelletier, J.; Graff, J.; Ruggero, D.; Sonenberg, N. Targeting the eIF4F translation initiation complex: A critical nexus for cancer development. *Cancer Res.* **2015**, *75*, 250–263. [CrossRef] [PubMed]

13. Sadlish, H.; Galicia-Vazquez, G.; Paris, C.G.; Aust, T.; Bhullar, B.; Chang, L.; Helliwell, S.B.; Hoepfner, D.; Knapp, B.; Riedl, R.; et al. Evidence for a functionally relevant rocaglamide binding site on the eIF4A-RNA complex. *ACS Chem. Biol.* **2013**, *8*, 1519–1527. [CrossRef] [PubMed]

14. Kogure, T.; Kinghorn, A.D.; Yan, I.; Bolon, B.; Lucas, D.M.; Grever, M.R.; Patel, T. Therapeutic potential of the translation inhibitor silvestrol in hepatocellular cancer. *PLoS ONE* **2013**, *8*, e76136. [CrossRef] [PubMed]

15. Wolfe, A.L.; Singh, K.; Zhong, Y.; Drewe, P.; Rajasekhar, V.K.; Sanghvi, V.R.; Mavrakis, K.J.; Jiang, M.; Roderick, J.E.; van der Meulen, J.; et al. RNA G-quadruplexes cause eIF4A-dependent oncogene translation in cancer. *Nature* **2014**, *513*, 65–70. [CrossRef] [PubMed]

16. Cencic, R.; Carrier, M.; Galicia-Vázquez, G.; Bordeleau, M.-E.; Sukarieh, R.; Bourdeau, A.; Brem, B.; Teodoro, J.G.; Greger, H.; Tremblay, M.L.; et al. Antitumor activity and mechanism of action of the cyclopentabbenzofuran, silvestrol. *PLoS ONE* **2009**, *4*, e5223. [CrossRef] [PubMed]

17. Hinnebusch, A.G.; Ivanov, I.P.; Sonenberg, N. Translational control by 5′-untranslated regions of eukaryotic mRNAs. *Science* **2016**, *352*, 1413–1416. [CrossRef] [PubMed]

18. Lucas, D.M.; Edwards, R.B.; Lozanski, G.; West, D.A.; Shin, J.D.; Vargo, M.A.; Davis, M.E.; Rozewski, D.M.; Johnson, A.J.; Su, B.-N.; et al. The novel plant-derived agent silvestrol has B-cell selective activity in chronic lymphocytic leukemia and acute lymphoblastic leukemia in vitro and in vivo. *Blood* **2009**, *113*, 4656–4666. [CrossRef] [PubMed]

19. Schatz, J.H.; Oricchio, E.; Wolfe, A.L.; Jiang, M.; Linkov, I.; Maragulia, J.; Shi, W.; Zhang, Z.; Rajasekhar, V.K.; Pagano, N.C.; et al. Targeting cap-dependent translation blocks converging survival signals by AKT and PIM kinases in lymphoma. *J. Exp. Med.* **2011**, *208*, 1799–1807. [CrossRef] [PubMed]

20. Biedenkopf, N.; Lange-Grünweller, K.; Schulte, F.W.; Weißer, A.; Müller, C.; Becker, D.; Becker, S.; Hartmann, R.K.; Grünweller, A. The natural compound silvestrol is a potent inhibitor of Ebola virus replication. *Antivir. Res.* **2017**, *137*, 76–81. [CrossRef] [PubMed]

21. Müller, C.; Schulte, F.W.; Lange-Grünweller, K.; Obermann, W.; Madhugiri, R.; Pleschka, S.; Ziebuhr, J.; Hartmann, R.K.; Grünweller, A. Broad-spectrum antiviral activity of the eIF4A inhibitor silvestrol against corona- and picornaviruses. *Antivir. Res.* **2017**, *150*, 123–129. [CrossRef] [PubMed]

22. Rubio, C.A.; Weisburd, B.; Holderfield, M.; Arias, C.; Fang, E.; DeRisi, J.L.; Fanidi, A. Transcriptome-wide characterization of the eIF4A signature highlights plasticity in translation regulation. *Genome Biol.* **2014**, *15*, 476. [CrossRef] [PubMed]

23. Himmelsbach, K.; Sauter, D.; Baumert, T.F.; Ludwig, L.; Blum, H.E.; Hildt, E. New aspects of an anti-tumour drug: Sorafenib efficiently inhibits HCV replication. *Gut* **2009**, *58*, 1644–1653. [CrossRef] [PubMed]

24. Weiss, T.S.; Pahernik, S.; Scheruebl, I.; Jauch, K.-W.; Thasler, W.E. Cellular damage to human hepatocytes through repeated application of 5-aminolevulinic acid. *J. Hepatol.* **2003**, *38*, 476–482. [CrossRef]

25. Masoudi, S.; Ploen, D.; Kunz, K.; Hildt, E. The adjuvant component α-tocopherol triggers via modulation of Nrf2 the expression and turnover of hypocretin in vitro and its implication to the development of narcolepsy. *Vaccine* **2014**, *32*, 2980–2988. [CrossRef] [PubMed]

26. Elgner, F.; Ren, H.; Medvedev, R.; Ploen, D.; Himmelsbach, K.; Boller, K.; Hildt, E. The intra-cellular cholesterol transport inhibitor U18666A inhibits the exosome-dependent release of mature hepatitis C virus. *J. Virol.* **2016**, *90*, 11181–11196. [CrossRef] [PubMed]

27. Ploen, D.; Hafirassou, M.L.; Himmelsbach, K.; Sauter, D.; Biniossek, M.L.; Weiss, T.S.; Baumert, T.F.; Schuster, C.; Hildt, E. TIP47 plays a crucial role in the life cycle of hepatitis C virus. *J. Hepatol.* **2013**, *58*, 1081–1088. [CrossRef] [PubMed]

28. Bürckstümmer, T.; Kriegs, M.; Lupberger, J.; Pauli, E.K.; Schmittel, S.; Hildt, E. Raf-1 kinase associates with Hepatitis C virus NS5A and regulates viral replication. *FEBS Lett.* **2006**, *580*, 575–580. [CrossRef] [PubMed]

29. Himmelsbach, K.; Hildt, E. Identification of various cell culture models for the study of Zika virus. *World J. Virol.* **2018**, *7*, 10–20. [CrossRef] [PubMed]

30. Su, B.-N.; Chai, H.; Mi, Q.; Riswan, S.; Kardono, L.B.S.; Afriastini, J.J.; Santarsiero, B.D.; Mesecar, A.D.; Farnsworth, N.R.; Cordell, G.A.; et al. Activity-guided isolation of cytotoxic constituents from the bark of Aglaia crassinervia collected in Indonesia. *Bioorg. Med. Chem.* **2006**, *14*, 960–972. [CrossRef] [PubMed]

31. Zhu, J.Y.; Lavrik, I.N.; Mahlknecht, U.; Giaisi, M.; Proksch, P.; Krammer, P.H.; Li-Weber, M. The traditional Chinese herbal compound rocaglamide preferentially induces apoptosis in leukemia cells by modulation of mitogen-activated protein kinase activities. *Int. J. Cancer* **2007**, *121*, 1839–1846. [CrossRef] [PubMed]

32. Muthukrishnan, S.; Both, G.W.; Furuichi, Y.; Shatkin, A.J. 5′-Terminal 7-methylguanosine in eukaryotic mRNA is required for translation. *Nature* **1975**, *255*, 33–37. [CrossRef] [PubMed]

33. Dick, G.W.A.; Kitchen, S.F.; Haddow, A.J. Zika Virus (I). Isolations and serological specificity. *Trans. R. Soc. Trop. Med. Hyg.* **1952**, *46*, 509–520. [CrossRef]

34. Laughhunn, A.; Santa Maria, F.; Broult, J.; Lanteri, M.C.; Stassinopoulos, A.; Musso, D.; Aubry, M. Amustaline (S-303) treatment inactivates high levels of Zika virus in red blood cell components. *Transfusion* **2017**, *57*, 779–789. [CrossRef] [PubMed]

35. Chu, J.; Pelletier, J. Targeting the eIF4A RNA helicase as an anti-neoplastic approach. *Biochim. Biophys. Acta* **2015**, *1849*, 781–791. [CrossRef] [PubMed]

36. Liu, S.; Hao, Q.; Peng, N.; Yue, X.; Wang, Y.; Chen, Y.; Wu, J.; Zhu, Y. Major vault protein: A virus-induced host factor against viral replication through the induction of type-I interferon. *Hepatology* **2012**, *56*, 57–66. [CrossRef] [PubMed]

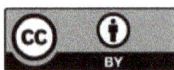

viruses

MDPI

Article

The Oxysterol 7-Ketocholesterol Reduces Zika Virus Titers in Vero Cells and Human Neurons

Katherine A. Willard [1], **Christina L. Elling** [2], **Steven L. Stice** [2] and **Melinda A. Brindley** [3,*]

1   Department of Infectious Diseases, College of Veterinary Medicine, University of Georgia,
    Athens, GA 30602, USA; katherine.willard@duke.edu
2   Department of Animal and Dairy Science, Regenerative Bioscience Center, College of Agriculture and
    Environmental Science, University of Georgia, Athens, GA 30602, USA;
    christina.elling@ucdenver.edu (C.L.E.); sstice@uga.edu (S.L.S.)
3   Department of Infectious Diseases, Department of Population Health, Center for Vaccines and Immunology,
    College of Veterinary Medicine, University of Georgia, Athens, GA 30602, USA
*   Correspondence: mbrindle@uga.edu; Tel.: +1-706-542-5796

Received: 13 November 2018; Accepted: 29 December 2018; Published: 30 December 2018

Abstract: Zika virus (ZIKV) is an emerging flavivirus responsible for a major epidemic in the Americas beginning in 2015. ZIKV associated with maternal infection can lead to neurological disorders in newborns, including microcephaly. Although there is an abundance of research examining the neurotropism of ZIKV, we still do not completely understand the mechanism by which ZIKV targets neural cells or how to limit neural cell infection. Recent research suggests that flaviviruses, including ZIKV, may hijack the cellular autophagy pathway to benefit their replication. Therefore, we hypothesized that ZIKV replication would be impacted when infected cells were treated with compounds that target the autophagy pathway. We screened a library of 94 compounds known to affect autophagy in both mammalian and insect cell lines. A subset of compounds that inhibited ZIKV replication without affecting cellular viability were tested for their ability to limit ZIKV replication in human neurons. From this second screen, we identified one compound, 7-ketocholesterol (7-KC), which inhibited ZIKV replication in neurons without significantly affecting neuron viability. Interestingly, 7-KC induces autophagy, which would be hypothesized to increase ZIKV replication, yet it decreased virus production. Time-of-addition experiments suggest 7-KC inhibits ZIKV replication late in the replication cycle. While 7-KC did not inhibit RNA replication, it decreased the number of particles in the supernatant and the relative infectivity of the released particles, suggesting it interferes with particle budding, release from the host cell, and particle integrity.

Keywords: Zika virus; antiviral compounds; neural cells; viral replication

1. Introduction

Zika virus (ZIKV) is an emerging arbovirus that gained public attention in 2015 when maternal infection in the Americas was causally associated with congenital birth defects, including microcephaly [1]. ZIKV belongs to the *Flaviviridae* family and is related to other important human pathogens, including dengue (DENV), yellow fever (YFV) and West Nile (WNV). ZIKV is an enveloped virus with a positive-sense RNA genome that translates into a single polypeptide, which is later cleaved into three structural and seven nonstructural viral proteins. Upon binding to host cell receptors, the cell engulfs virions through clathrin-mediated endocytosis [2]. Low pH in the endosome triggers viral-cellular membrane fusion, releasing the viral RNA genome into the host cell cytoplasm [2]. Transcription occurs in the cytoplasm and translation of ZIKV proteins occurs on membrane scaffolds near the endoplasmic reticulum (ER) [3].

Autophagy is a normal cellular process used to recycle cytoplasmic components in eukaryotic cells. The autophagy pathway is activated by mTOR [4]. This activation signals the production of lipid membranes that engulf targeted cytoplasmic components, forming autophagosome vesicles. Eventually, the autophagosomes fuse with lysosomes to form autophagolysosomes, which degrade cargo and prepare it to either be recycled or ejected from the cell [4]. Because cells always contain components that need to be recycled, the autophagy pathway is constantly on at a basal level. Different stimuli or stresses, such as pathogen infection, can alter basal levels of autophagy. For example, selectively encasing intercellular bacteria and targeting them for autophagic degradation is part of the innate immune response pathway for dealing with *Salmonella enterica* serovar Typhimurium and *Mycobacterium tuberculosis* [5,6].

While the host can utilize this pathway to rid itself of some pathogens, many flaviviruses, including Dengue, Hepatitis C, and Zika viruses, hijack this process to benefit their own replication [4,7–9]. The autophagy process mobilizes cellular membranes. Flaviviruses replicate on membranes and appear to benefit from initiating early cellular autophagy processes [7,10]. Chemical inducers of autophagy, such as rapamycin, slightly increase levels of viral RNA and infectious particle production [11–13]. In addition, chemical inhibitors of autophagy decrease particle production [12,13]. Some autophagy inhibitors, such as bafilomycin A, prevent the acidification of autophagolysosomes. Such compounds do not selectively block acidification of only autophagolysosomes, but also alter the pH of other endosomal vesicles. Because flavivirus entry requires an acidic endosome environment to trigger membrane fusion, some of the drugs may be inhibiting initial entry. Therefore, their effects on autophagy may be unrelated to the flavivirus inhibition. Flavivirus replication appears to be enhanced when the autophagy pathway is started, but is stalled and autolysosome degradation is blocked [4].

Autophagy also affects other aspects of cell biology that may influence viral pathogenesis, including induction of the interferon response [14]. However, depending on the location and timing of infection, autophagy can also be antiviral. For instance, experiments in *Drosophila* indicate that ZIKV infection in the brain induces an NF-κB/dSTING (*Drosophila* stimulator of interferon genes) signaling pathway, which induces autophagy and protects against ZIKV infection [15]. Therefore, autophagy can be very consequential to viral replication and may play a role in ZIKV pathogenesis [4].

Since autophagy and ZIKV replication are intertwined, small molecules that induce or inhibit stages of the autophagy pathway may alter ZIKV production and spread in host cells. To elucidate these interactions, we screened a library of 94 autophagy inducers or inhibitors in Vero and C6/36 cells infected with ZIKV. Surprisingly, only about 30% of compounds reduced ZIKV titer by at least one log compared to control. We performed subsequent experiments in both Vero cells and human neurons with the compounds that reduce ZIKV replication without inhibiting cell viability. We identified one compound, 7-ketocholesterol (7-KC), which effectively reduced ZIKV titer in human neurons without affecting cellular viability. 7-KC blocked late stages of ZIKV replication, suggesting it reduces particle integrity and budding efficiency from host cells.

2. Materials and Methods

2.1. Cell Lines

Vero cells were maintained in DMEM with 5% fetal bovine serum (FBS) at 37 °C, 5% CO_2. C6/36 *Ae. albopictus* cells (ATCC CRL-1660) were maintained in L-15 Leibovitz Medium with L-glutamine and 10% FBS at 28 °C. Human neurons were made by differentiating hNP1 cells and were obtained from ArunA Biomedical, Inc. [16]. Neurons were maintained in medium containing AB2™ basal medium supplemented with ANS™ neural supplement (both from ArunA Biomedical Inc. Athens, GA, USA), 2 mM L-glutamine (Gibco, ThermoFisher, Waltham, MA, USA), 2 U/mL penicillin (Gibco, ThermoFisher, Waltham, MA, USA), 2 µg/mL streptomycin (Gibco, ThermoFisher, Waltham, MA, USA), and 10 ng/mL leukemia inhibitory factor (LIF) (Millipore, Billerica, MA, USA) and plated on cell culture dishes coated with Matrigel 1:100 (B&D, Franklin Lakes, NJ, USA).

2.2. Virus Isolates

ZIKV SPH is a low-passage (<5), Asian-lineage isolate derived from an infected patient in Brazil in 2015 and obtained from the Oswaldo Cruz Foundation (FIOCRUZ). ZIKV IbH 30656 (ATCC # VR-182) is a highly-passaged, African-lineage isolate derived from a human patient in Nigeria in 1968. Following its initial isolation, IbH was extensively passaged in mouse brains.

2.3. Reagents

We used the Enzo Screen-Well Autophagy Library for these experiments (category number: BML-2837-0100; Lot number: 03181609B; Version 1.5). The compounds came resuspended at 10 mM in dimethyl sulfoxide (DMSO). To prevent DMSO related toxicity, we diluted the stocks 1:1000 and screened the compounds at a final concentration of 10 μM. DMSO was included in all of our untreated controls.

2.4. Autophagy Compound Library Screen

Vero and C6/36 cells were plated at densities of 1.5×10^5 cells/well and 2×10^5 cells/well, respectively in 24-well plates. The cells were incubated for 2–4 h and then treated with the autophagy compounds at a final concentration of 10 μM. Immediately after treatment, the cells were infected with ZIKV (MOI 0.1). Vero cells were incubated for 40 h and the C6/36 cells for 96 h, then supernatants were collected and titrated by determining the 50% tissue culture infective dose (TCID$_{50}$) according to the Spearman-Karber method [17,18]. Results from treated cells were compared to results from DMSO controls.

2.5. Autophagy Detection

Vero cells were plated at densities of 3×10^5 cells/well in 12-well plates. The cells were incubated for 2–4 h and then treated with the autophagy compounds at a final concentration of 10 μM. Twenty-four hours following treatment, the cells were lifted in trypsin, washed in PBS, and stained with the CYTO-ID Autophagy Detection Kit 2.0 (Enzo, Farmington, NY, USA). The autophagy activity factor (AAF) [19] was determined by comparing the green mean fluorescence intensities (MFI) of treated and DMSO control cells using the formula:

$$AAF = 100 \times \left(\frac{MFItreated - MFIcontrol}{MFItreated} \right)$$

2.6. Cell Viability

Vero and C6/36 cells were plated at densities of 1.5×10^4 cells/well and 2×10^4 cells/well, respectively in 96-well plates. The cells were incubated for 2–4 h and then treated with the autophagy compounds at a final concentration of 10 μM. Vero cells were incubated for 40 h and the C6/36 cells incubated for 96 h. Metabolic activity (ATP abundance), which correlates to cell viability, was determined with CellTiter-Glo Luminescent Cell Viability Assay (Promega, Madison, WI, USA) and a Glomax plate reader per the manufacturer's instructions. The experiment was repeated at least three independent times. Results from treated cells were compared to results from DMSO controls.

2.7. Human Neuron Response to Autophagy Compounds

The human PSC line WA09 (WiCell 0062, Madison, WI, USA) was used to derive human neural progenitor cells (hNP1TM 00001) as previously described [16]. ArunA Biomedical, Inc. (Athens, GA, USA) differentiated the hNP1 cells into neurons and we cultured the neurons as previously described [20]. Before plating neurons, each well was coated with Matrigel (1:100 dilution; (B&D, Franklin Lakes, NJ, USA) and incubated for at least 30 min at room temperature. After incubation, the Matrigel was removed and the wells were washed twice with PBS. Neurons were immediately plated at densities of 2×10^5 cells/well in 24-well plates and 3×10^4 cells/well in 96-well plates. The following day cells were treated with 10 μM final concentration of compounds, and the 24-well plate was infected with ZIKV SPH (MOI 1.0). The infected/compound-treated neurons were incubated for 4 days then the supernatants were collected and neuron viability was determined as described above. The compound-treated supernatants were titrated via $TCID_{50}$.

2.8. 7-Ketocholesterol Dose-Response

Vero cells were plated at 1.5×10^5 cells/well in a 24-well plate and 1.5×10^4 cells/well in a 96-well plate and incubated for 16 h. Cells were treated with the indicated concentration of 7-KC or DMSO control. The cells in the 24-well plate were immediately infected with MOI 1 of ZIKV SPH. After 2 h, the infectious media was removed and replaced with the same concentrations of 7-KC treated media as indicated. The cell supernatants were collected 24 h following infection and titers were reported in $TCID_{50}$ units. ZIKV titers from 7-KC treated cells were compared to those from DMSO-treated controls.

2.9. 7-Ketocholesterol Time-of-Addition

Vero cells at a density of 3×10^5 cells/well in 24-well plates were treated with either 10 μM of 7-KC or 30 mM of ammonium chloride under the following conditions: 2 h prior to ZIKV infection, at the same time as ZIKV infection, 2 h following ZIKV infection, or 6 h following ZIKV infection. Regardless of treatment condition, the cells were infected with ZIKV SPH MOI 0.1 for 2 h. After 2 h, the infectious media was removed and replaced with fresh media. For the cells treated at the same time as infection, the fresh media was re-treated with the compounds at the same concentrations as above. The supernatants were collected at 24 hours post infection (hpi) and titers were reported in $TCID_{50}$ units. ZIKV titers from treated cells were compared to those from controls, which were treated with either DMSO or DMEM at the time of infection and retreated after the media change.

2.10. 7-Ketocholesterol and ZIKV Pre-Incubation

Vero cells were plated at 1.5×10^5 cells/well in a 24-well plate and incubated for 18 h. The next day, ZIKV stock was pre-incubated with 200 μM of 7-KC for 1 h at room temperature. After incubation, the ZIKV/7-KC mixture was diluted and added to the Vero cells. The dilution resulted in an infection at MOI 0.1 and final concentration of 7-KC was approximately 0.2 μM (below the active range of 7-KC as determined by our dose-response curve). The cell supernatants were collected at 40 hpi and titers were determined. Pre-incubation results were compared to DMSO controls.

2.11. qRT-PCR

Vero cells were infected with ZIKV SPH and treated with compounds in the same manner as the time-of-addition experiment. Supernatants and cellular lysates were collected at 24 hpi. Viral RNA was isolated using the ZR Viral RNA kit (Zymo, Irvine, CA, USA) and cellular RNA was isolated with the RNAeasy Mini kit (Qiagen, Hilden, Germany). Both total and viral RNA samples were reverse-transcribed (RT) to cDNA (High Capacity RNA-to-cDNA Kit, Applied Biosystems, Foster City, CA, USA). To quantify the copies of ZIKV genomes we used the cDNA in a quantitative PCR (qPCR) reaction assay using TaqMan Gene Expression Master Mix (Applied Biosystems, ThermoFisher, Waltham, MA, USA), primers and probes (F: ZIKV 1086, R: ZIKV 1162c, ZIKV 1107-FAM; TaqMan MGB Probe; Invitrogen Custom Primers) [21]. Each sample was analyzed in duplicate, and each plate contained a DNA plasmid standard curve (ZIKV molecular clone), no template, and no primer controls. ZIKV copy numbers were extrapolated from the generated standard curve using the Applied Biosystems protocol. The limit of detection was experimentally established to be 30 copies (10^{-16} g). Final copy numbers were adjusted by back-calculations to the total RNA and cDNA volume and expressed as copies per sample.

2.12. Chemical Structures

We created chemical structures using PyMOL version 2.1.1. Structure files were downloaded from Pubchem (https://pubchem.ncbi.nlm.nih.gov/).

2.13. Statistics

All experiments were performed in at least three independent trials. We assessed variation across trials using the standard error of the mean. We used the student's unpaired *t*-test to test for significance when comparing data plotted on a linear scale and Welch's *t*-test of unequal variance when data is plotted on a log-scale. Significance values are: * $p < 0.05$; ** $p < 0.01$; *** $p < 0.001$; NS- not significant.

3. Results

3.1. Autophagy Compound Screen in Vero Cells

We tested the ability of the Enzo Screen-Well Autophagy Library (94 compounds listed in Table 1) to reduce ZIKV titer in mid-logarithmic growth phase (40 h post infection) [22], without negatively impacting viability compared to controls in Vero cells. These compounds produced a wide range of effects on ZIKV titer, though only approximately 30% were able to decrease ZIKV titer by at least one log compared to control (Figure 1A). Similar to previously published data, treatment with the prototypical autophagy inducer rapamycin increased ZIKV titers whereas the prototypical autophagy inhibitor hydroxychloroquine decreased titers [11–13]. Of the 94 compounds, three (amiodarone-HCl, 7-ketocholesterol, and licochalcone A) reduced ZIKV titer to below 10% of control while maintaining cell viability above 80% of control (Figure 1B).

Table 1. Summary of autophagy compound screen.

# [a]	Name	Type [b]	ZIKV SPH Relative Titer in Vero Cells [c]	Vero Viability [d]	ZIKV SPH Relative Titer in C6/36 Cells [c]	C6/36 Viability [d]
1	Bafilomycin A1	H	0.0 ± 0	55.7 ± 9.5	0.0 ± 0	36 ± 6.1
2	Rapamycin	D	167.9 ± 44.4	66.0 ± 2.6	75.7 ± 47.7	59 ± 7.3
3	Timosaponin A-III	D	0.0 ± 0	38.7 ± 11.9	13.0 ± 5.2	67 ± 3.6
4	3-Methyladenine	H	73.4 ± 4.9	90.7 ± 1.8	155.3 ± 41	120 ± 15.6
5	PI-103	D	42.3 ± 20.6	43.7 ± 6.4	46.2 ± 13.3	39 ± 8.9
6	LY294002	H	264.3 ± 182.9	56.0 ± 6	548.4 ± 221	97 ± 17.2
7	Lithium Chloride	D	85.4 ± 18.7	87.0 ± 1	167.9 ± 68.4	111 ± 10.7
8	L-690,330	D	40.7 ± 10.6	93.7 ± 3.5	66.8 ± 2.6	87 ± 4.6
9	Wortmannin	H	46.9 ± 9	79.0 ± 3.1	190.1 ± 57.8	105 ± 5.5
10	Sodium Valproate	D	110.8 ± 80.4	92.7 ± 1.2	111.4 ± 20.7	111 ± 6.2
11	Verapamil·HCl	D	92.9 ± 20.8	87.7 ± 0.9	89.0 ± 40.8	71 ± 2.9
12	SP600125	H	26.5 ± 15	66.0 ± 2.1	50.3 ± 19.8	132 ± 9
13	Chloroquine	H	109.0 ± 65	89.7 ± 4.4	126.5 ± 44.8	81 ± 17.1
14	Loperamide HCl	D	11.7 ± 3.3	66.7 ± 17.4	0.1 ± 0.1	12 ± 6.1
15	Amiodarone HCl	D	6.3 ± 3.6	84.0 ± 8.2	2.0 ± 0.5	44 ± 15.3
16	Nimodipine	D	32.5 ± 7.3	92.0 ± 1.5	26.9 ± 13.6	41 ± 8.4
17	Nitrendipine	D	66.0 ± 27.1	88.7 ± 1.9	219.7 ± 44.4	62 ± 10.5
18	Niguldipine	D	0.2 ± 0.1	30.0 ± 14.2	0.0 ± 0	5 ± 2.1
19	Penitrem A	D	34.9 ± 10.4	78.3 ± 6.4	29.8 ± 6.4	43 ± 8.1
20	Ionomycin	D	0.0 ± 0	27.7 ± 10.4	0.0 ± 0	1 ± 0.3
21	Rotenone	D	1.8 ± 0.9	61.3 ± 7.7	0.1 ± 0.1	17 ± 5.8
22	TTFA	D	24.4 ± 7.6	90.0 ± 3.5	72.8 ± 9.6	78 ± 19.9
23	Fluspirilene	D	2.5 ± 0.6	56.7 ± 16	1.0 ± 0.7	26 ± 10.3
24	Hydroxychloroquine	H	14.7 ± 7.3	85.3 ± 8.4	25.1 ± 12.6	35 ± 9.7
25	Norclomipramine HCl	H	3.9 ± 0.5	48.7 ± 22.9	13.4 ± 8.7	19 ± 8.9
26	Trifluoperazine·2HCl	D	2.8 ± 0.7	51.0 ± 22.1	0.3 ± 0.3	10 ± 3.8
27	Sorafenib tosylate	D	5.8 ± 1.8	58.3 ± 9.9	9.4 ± 8.8	23 ± 8.8
28	Niclosamide	D	0.1 ± 0	29.7 ± 3.8	0.1 ± 0	2 ± 0.3
29	Rottlerin	D	10.3 ± 5	80.7 ± 8.5	30.3 ± 16.9	40 ± 8.4
30	Caffeine	D	80.6 ± 20.9	104.7 ± 8.6	138.4 ± 37.7	83 ± 4.6

Table 1. *Cont.*

#[a]	Name	Type[b]	ZIKV SPH Relative Titer in Vero Cells[c]	Vero Viability[d]	ZIKV SPH Relative Titer in C6/36 Cells[c]	C6/36 Viability[d]
31	Metformin·HCl	D	122.3 ± 41.5	92.3 ± 4.2	75.8 ± 19.2	64 ± 10.3
32	Clonidine·HCl	D	65.4 ± 17.3	97.7 ± 2.6	95.9 ± 53.4	69 ± 5.4
33	Rilmenidine	D	191.2 ± 49.5	97.0 ± 2	161.0 ± 58.1	79 ± 8.3
34	2′,5′-Dideoxyadenosine	D	93.3 ± 31.9	95.0 ± 1.5	317.4 ± 161.9	118 ± 15
35	Suramin·6Na	D	107.4 ± 44.8	92.0 ± 1.2	86.6 ± 23.2	86 ± 8.4
36	(±)Bay K8644	H	34.9 ± 15.2	94.0 ± 3	39.4 ± 10.7	53 ± 11.1
37	Forskolin	H	139.0 ± 32.1	74.7 ± 3.7	302.5 ± 18.3	94 ± 12
38	Pimozide	D	77.9 ± 15.5	90.0 ± 5.7	109.0 ± 22	49 ± 3.6
39	STF-62247	D	45.0 ± 21.4	77.3 ± 11.7	169.8 ± 45.9	49 ± 9.3
40	Spermidine	D	115.0 ± 44.9	78.0 ± 17	90.2 ± 57.4	70 ± 3
41	FK-866	D	7.3 ± 6.5	32.7 ± 2.7	92.7 ± 32.4	48 ± 5.5
42	Tamoxifen citrate	D	3.3 ± 2.3	60.7 ± 18.4	8.2 ± 7.3	32 ± 11.9
43	Minoxidil	D	60.4 ± 27.2	96.3 ± 3.2	145.7 ± 16.6	72 ± 2.6
44	Imiquimod	D	228.5 ± 139.8	91.3 ± 1.2	72.5 ± 18.4	37 ± 8.1
45	Imatinib mesylate	D	91.2 ± 60	81.0 ± 10.7	5.3 ± 2.2	19 ± 5.4
46	AG112	D	77.7 ± 38.2	96.7 ± 3.7	85.5 ± 21.3	80 ± 5.8
47	SU11652	D	0.1 ± 0	1.0 ± 0	0.0 ± 0	1 ± 0
48	Dibutyryl cAMP·Na	H	60.6 ± 36.7	98.3 ± 4.4	142.6 ± 63.9	117 ± 10.7
49	Rolipram	H	103.8 ± 26.8	91.0 ± 3.2	215.4 ± 74.8	127 ± 12.1
50	SB202190	D	13.3 ± 4.2	74.3 ± 5.2	25.9 ± 7.4	44 ± 7.9
51	Brefeldin A	D	5.4 ± 4.9	17.0 ± 2.1	123.5 ± 25	91 ± 8.4
52	Tunicamycin	D	0.5 ± 0.5	56.3 ± 8.7	1.8 ± 0.8	47 ± 7.6
53	Thapsigargin	D	0.4 ± 0.4	38.0 ± 10.5	0.0 ± 0	23 ± 3.9
54	A23187	D	0.5 ± 0.5	17.0 ± 6.7	0.0 ± 0	1 ± 0
55	Capsaicin	D	76.9 ± 29.6	91.7 ± 2.4	48.1 ± 12	66 ± 7.2
56	Dihydrocapsaicin	D	28.7 ± 10.5	92.3 ± 3.8	64.1 ± 16	61 ± 2.2
57	Glucosamine HCl	D	51.8 ± 11.8	99.3 ± 1.9	242.1 ± 45.8	88 ± 5.2
58	DTT	D	60.2 ± 20.1	93.0 ± 1.5	145.7 ± 16.6	79 ± 4.4
59	Deoxycholate·Na	D	76.6 ± 16.6	95.3 ± 2.6	90.6 ± 12.5	83 ± 1
60	8-CPT-cAMP·Na	H	107.8 ± 65.3	92.7 ± 0.7	60.1 ± 18.3	75 ± 3.7
61	EHNA·HCl	H	81.0 ± 7.6	92.3 ± 2	36.4 ± 9.1	55 ± 4.2
62	ABC294640·HCl	D	51.7 ± 29.2	87.7 ± 6.8	26.0 ± 10.8	32 ± 3.5
63	Licochalcone A	D	7.2 ± 2.9	100.7 ± 9.4	51.8 ± 28.5	43 ± 2
64	Curcumin	D	24.1 ± 11.3	75.3 ± 11.3	0.3 ± 0.2	3 ± 0.7
65	Plumbagin	D	0.1 ± 0	2.0 ± 0	21.4 ± 17.5	49 ± 1.5
66	6-Gingerol	D	99.9 ± 63.9	100.0 ± 2.5	109.3 ± 9.3	55 ± 11
67	Akt Inhibitor X·HCl	D	3.5 ± 3.3	32.3 ± 14.2	0.0 ± 0	7 ± 1.9
68	PMSF	D	89.0 ± 7	98.3 ± 2	258.0 ± 145.2	81 ± 6.4
69	MG132	D	0.1 ± 0.1	10.7 ± 2.8	9.5 ± 7.1	31 ± 5.7
70	ALLN	D	123.3 ± 27.3	75.0 ± 17.1	41.6 ± 0.6	49 ± 6.6
71	7-Ketocholesterol	D	7.5 ± 1.3	93.0 ± 4	9.8 ± 3.3	36 ± 5.1
72	SB-216763	H	41.6 ± 30.6	80.0 ± 9	54.0 ± 21.7	63 ± 3.6
73	Tolazamide	H	176.8 ± 50.9	99.0 ± 1.5	120.1 ± 33.7	113 ± 7.3
74	17-AAG	D	36.4 ± 20.8	56. 7 ± 11.8	18.2 ± 11.2	79 ± 16.4
75	Geldanamycin	D	108.4 ± 39.4	61.3 ± 5.7	25.8 ± 14.5	45 ± 5.8
76	C1	D	119.3 ± 34.4	97.3 ± 2.4	101.2 ± 29.5	55 ± 1.7
77	Z36	D	0.1 ± 0.1	0.7 ± 0.3	0.0 ± 0	0 ± 0
78	Rockout	D	169.6 ± 69.3	87.7 ± 3.8	96.2 ± 44.2	76 ± 5.2
79	Go6850	D	1.3 ± 0.9	36.0 ± 9	1.4 ± 1.4	21 ± 0
80	2-Deoxyglucose	D	99.7 ± 15.4	98.7 ± 0.9	108.8 ± 61.2	73 ± 1
81	Etoposide	D	134.0 ± 34.3	84.0 ± 3.6	736.8 ± 89.3	119 ± 12.5
82	SMER28	D	65.0 ± 5.6	92.7 ± 3.5	38.7 ± 12.2	36 ± 5.3
83	Trehalose	D	107.1 ± 16.9	97.7 ± 1.5	245.7 ± 101.3	99 ± 2.9
84	Quinine HCl·2H2O	H	180.2 ± 70.4	89.7 ± 2.7	123.0 ± 28	54 ± 4.6
85	AICAR	H	112.3 ± 32.3	90.0 ± 11.1	252.0 ± 115	125 ± 16.4
86	C2-dihydroceramide	D	36.5 ± 3	101.3 ± 3.7	262.1 ± 51.7	97 ± 5.8
87	Temozolomide	D	89.9 ± 17.5	104.7 ± 1.9	218.7 ± 49.8	113 ± 9.2
88	Resveratrol	D	67.5 ± 13.2	87.3 ± 2.3	154.6 ± 62	81 ± 7.5
89	Staurosporine	D	0.1 ± 0	14.0 ± 1.5	0.0 ± 0	16 ± 5.3
90	PD-98059	H	101.0 ± 23.3	90.7 ± 1.3	197.3 ± 40	93 ± 8.4
91	Anisomycin	H	0.0 ± 0	12.7 ± 4.3	0.0 ± 0	7 ± 0.9
92	Cycloheximide	H	0.0 ± 0	37.3 ± 6.2	0.0 ± 0	24 ± 3.5
93	Pifithrin-μ	H	38.5 ± 12.4	49.0 ± 15	75.3 ± 27.5	72 ± 3.2
94	Nocodazole	H	28.4 ± 23.9	56.0 ± 9.6	182.0 ± 39.5	58 ± 2.9

[a] Compounds are numbered based on the Enzo library and correlate to Figures 1A and 3A. [b] Autophagy inducers are labeled D whereas autophagy inhibitors are labeled H; [c] All values are displayed as percent of untreated control ± the standard error of the mean (SEM) from three independent trials. Viral inhibition is color coded as follows: compounds resulting in >90% of control are highlighted in red, between 10–90% are in yellow, and compounds that dropped titers below 10% are in green. [d] All values are displayed as percent of untreated control ± the standard error of the mean (SEM) from three independent trials. Cell viability data is color coded as compounds that retained >80% viability are in blue and compounds with <80% viability are in grey.

Amiodarone-HCl, 7-ketocholesterol, and licochalcone A are all characterized as autophagy inducers. Based on previous work, autophagy inducers would be predicted to increase ZIKV titers. However, amiodarone-HCl, 7-ketocholesterol, and licochalcone A decreased ZIKV titers in our assay. To confirm that these compounds induced autophagy in the Vero cells, we stained treated cells with CYTO-ID, a dye that binds to autophagic vesicles [19]. We detected increased fluorescence when cells were treated with rapamycin as well as with amiodarone-HCl, 7-ketocholesterol, and licochalcone A, confirming the compounds induce autophagy in Vero cells (Table 2). Amiodarone-HCl treatment in particular led to a very large increase in fluorescence intensity. While rapamycin and licochalcone A both induce autophagy through mTOR signaling, amiodarone-HCl induces autophagy through mTOR independent pathways [23].

Table 2. Autophagy activity factor.

Compound	Autophagy Activity Factor (AAF)
DMSO	−0.85
Rapamycin	7.74
Amiodarone HCl	60.40
Licochalcone A	12.33
7-Ketocholesterol	27.01

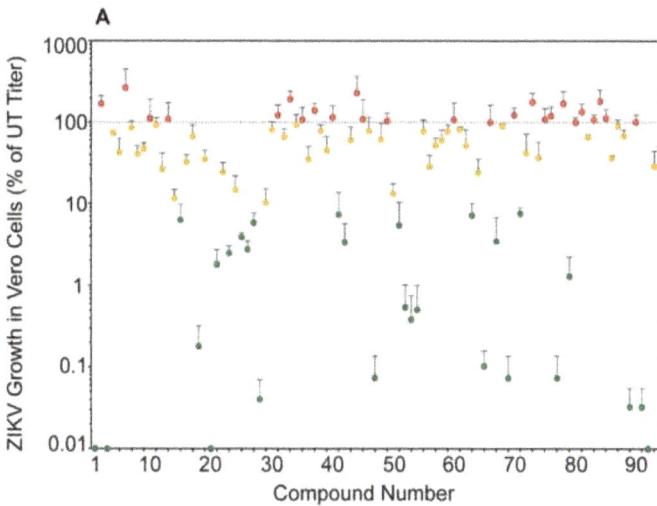

Figure 1. *Cont.*

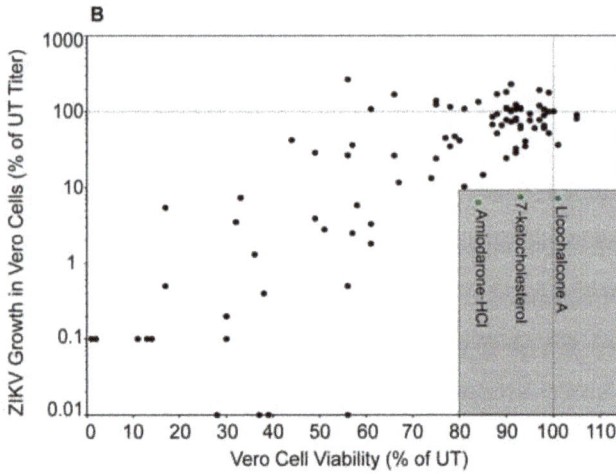

Figure 1. Autophagy compound screen in Vero cells. (**A**) ZIKV SPH growth in compound-treated Vero cells as a percent of ZIKV titer in untreated Vero cells. Red symbols represent compounds that increased ZIKV titer compared to the untreated control, yellow symbols represent compounds that reduced titer between 10 and 99% of control, and green symbols represent compounds that reduced ZIKV titer below 10% of control (at least 1 log of viral growth). Error bars represent the standard error of the mean (SEM) from three independent trials. The compounds are numbered according to Table 1. (**B**) ZIKV growth in Vero cells versus viability of compound-treated Vero cells. The shaded box represents the zone in which ZIKV titer is reduced to 10% or lower than the untreated control and cell viability is at least 80% of control. Compounds that meet these criteria are in green and labeled with their names.

3.2. Autophagy Compound Screen in Vero Cells Infected with ZIKV IbH

There are two genetic lineages of ZIKV [24], and isolates from these different lineages can produce distinct phenotypes in infected cells [20,22,25,26]. Therefore, we tested the ability of a subset of 22 autophagy compounds to inhibit African lineage ZIKV IbH in Vero cells (Figure 2). We chose this subset based on our results with SPH; one third of the compounds decreased SPH titer below 10%, one third decreased SPH titer between 10 and 99%, and the final one third increased SPH titer compared to control. These compounds affected African-lineage IbH replication in a manner similar to the effects on ZIKV-SPH (Figure S1). Thus, the compounds effect on ZIKV replication is not lineage specific. While amiodarone-HCl, 7-ketocholesterol, and licochalcone A all reduced ZIKV IbH titers, only 7-KC dropped titers more than a log compared to control. Because we did not identify major differences in ZIKV titer across lineages, we continued with Asian-lineage ZIKV SPH for the remainder of our experiments.

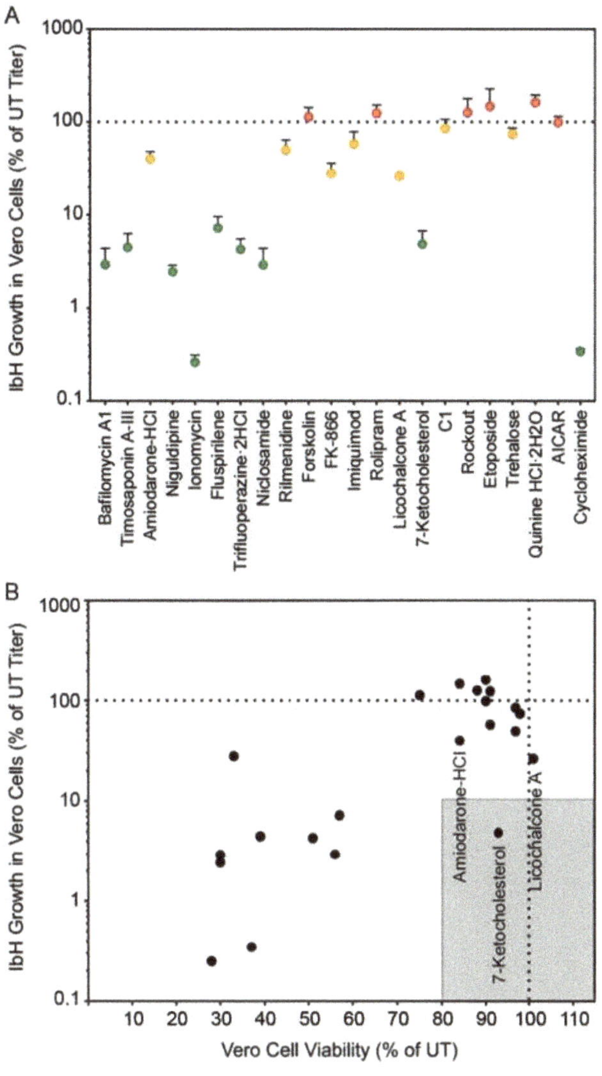

Figure 2. African- lineage ZIKV IbH growth in compound-treated Vero cells as a percent of ZIKV titer in untreated Vero cells (**A**). The color-codes are the same as in Figure 1A. (**B**) ZIKV IbH growth in Vero cells versus viability of compound-treated Vero cells. The shaded box represents the zone in which ZIKV titer is reduced to 10% or lower than the untreated control and cell viability is at least 80% of control.

3.3. Autophagy Compound Screen in C6/36 Cells

ZIKV is transmitted primarily by *Aedes* mosquitoes and the virus must infect and replicate in mosquito cells to be transmitted. To determine if the autophagy compound panel altered ZIKV replication in mosquito cells in a similar manner to mammalian cells, we performed the screen in C6/36 *Aedes albopictus* cells. Because mosquito cells have a slower metabolic rate, cellular viability and viral titers were examined 96 h post-infection/treatment [22]. Once again, the autophagy compounds produced a wide range of effects on SPH titer (Figure 3A). However, unlike in Vero cells, we did not identify any compounds that reduced ZIKV titer to below 10% of control while maintaining viability above 80% of control (Figure 3B). Some compounds did not produce the expected results. For example, rapamycin which increase particle production in Vero cells, slightly decreased titers in C6/36 cells. Interestingly, more compounds increased SPH titer in C6/36 cells compared to Vero cells (Figures 2A and 3A, Figure S2, Table 1). While 27 compounds in Vero cells produced virus >90% of control, 38 compounds behaved similarly in C6/36 cells. The insect and mammalian autophagy pathways are highly conserved [27] and many of the autophagy altering compounds affected ZIKV replication in Vero and C6/36 cells in a similar fashion (Figure S2). However we found opposing effects with some compounds. Cell type specific cytotoxicity may explain many of the differences observed. For example, brefeldin A was toxic in Vero cells, resulting in little virus production, yet brefeldin A did not alter viral titers or cell viability in C6/36 cells. While amiodarone HCl, licochalcone A, and 7-ketocholesterol (7-KC) inhibited ZIKV replication in both Vero and C6/36 cells, they were more toxic to the C6/36 cells. Many compounds resulted in significant cell death in the C6/36 cells and may be related to the increased time period the cells were exposed to the compounds. We did not identify any compounds that inhibited viral replication without significantly affecting cell viability.

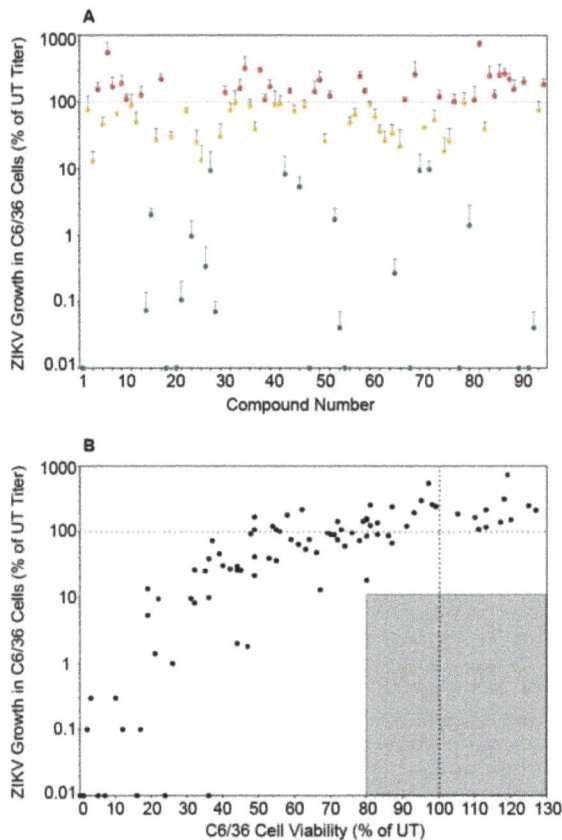

Figure 3. Autophagy compound screen in C6/36 cells. (A) ZIKV growth in compound-treated C6/36 cells as a percent of ZIKV titer in untreated C6/36 cells. The labels and color-codes are the same as in Figure 1A. (B) ZIKV growth in C6/36 cells versus viability of compound-treated C6/36 cells. As in Figure 1, the shaded box represents the zone in which ZIKV titer is reduced to 10% or lower than the untreated control and cell viability is at least 80% of control. No compounds fit these criteria in C6/36 cells.

3.4. Autophagy Compound Screen in Human Neurons

The three compounds that reduced ZIKV titer without impacting Vero cell viability were further characterized to determine these compounds' abilities to inhibit ZIKV replication in human neurons, a cell line more relevant to clinical ZIKV infection. We performed this screen with neurons derived from human neural progenitor cells, which have been characterized in previous ZIKV experiments [20]. Of these three compounds, only 7-ketocholesterol (7-KC) reduced ZIKV titer without significantly decreasing neuron viability (Figure 4A,B). Structurally, 7-KC is very similar to cholesterol, a major component of cellular membranes; the only difference between the two compounds is an extra oxygen molecule on 7-KC compared to cholesterol (Figure 4C). The addition of a cholesterol-like molecule could alter cellular membrane composition, which could block one of the many stages in ZIKV replication that relies on membranes, including entry, genome replication, or budding from the host cell.

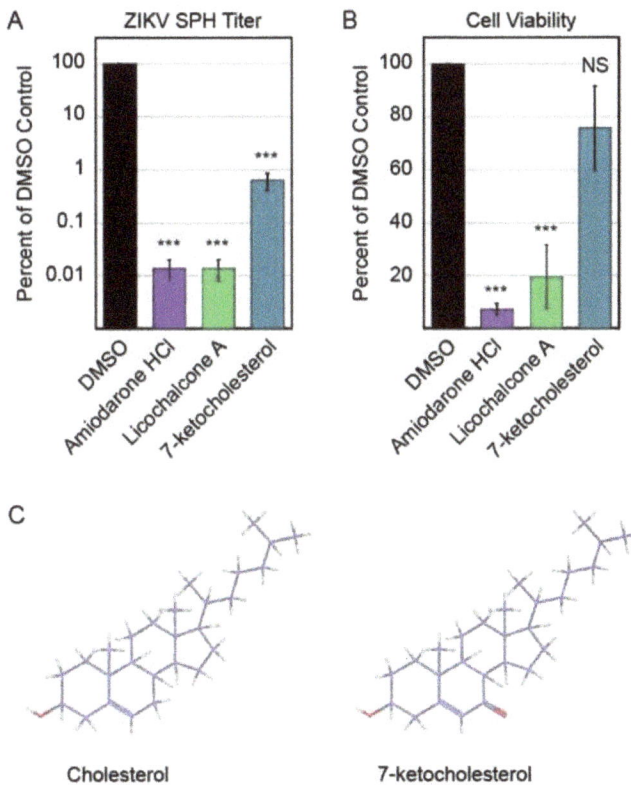

Figure 4. Autophagy compound screen in human neurons. (**A**) Impact of autophagy compounds on ZIKV replication in neurons and (**B**) neuron viability. (**C**) Chemical structure of cholesterol (PubChem CID 5997) versus 7-ketocholesterol (PubChem CID 91474). Carbon atoms are shaded in purple, hydrogen atoms are shaded in grey, and oxygen atoms are shaded in red.

3.5. 7-Ketocholesterol Dose-Response

We generated a dose-response curve to determine the IC50 and range of activity of 7-KC in Vero cells (Figure 5). The IC50 of 7-KC for ZIKV SPH is 4.064 μM, and Vero cells remained more than 80% viable at all 7-KC concentrations tested (0–27 μM). Because of the high cell viability, we were not able to generate a full viability curve over the range of active 7-KC doses, suggesting there is a large range of activity between cell viability and viral inhibition.

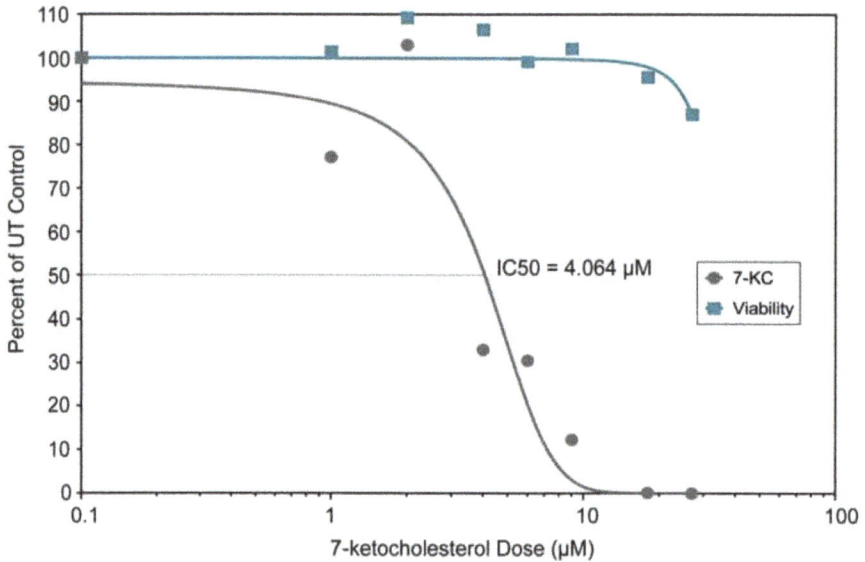

Figure 5. Dose-response curve and viability of Vero cells treated with varying doses (0–27 µM) of 7-ketocholesterol. The curves were generated by GraphPad Prism version 7.04 using the log (inhibitor) vs. normalized response variable slope regression. The regression curve estimates the IC50 at 4.064 µM (R^2 = 0.9078). The cell viability did not drop below 80% preventing us from determining the EC50.

3.6. 7-Ketocholesterol Time-of-Addition

To help elucidate the mechanism by which 7-KC inhibits ZIKV replication, we performed a time-of-addition experiment to determine when 7-KC was most effective at inhibiting ZIKV replication. First, we determined if 7-KC directly impacts ZIKV infectivity through a virucidal effect. ZIKV stock was preincubated with a high concentration (200 µM) of 7-KC for 1 h. This mixture was then diluted onto Vero cells so that the 7-KC concentration was below the active range as determined by the dose-response curve (Figure 5). Therefore, any viral inhibition would be caused by 7-KC virucidal effect and not by 7-KC activity within the host cell. As shown in Figure 6A, 7-KC preincubation with ZIKV SPH did not reduce viral titers compared to controls suggesting 7-KC modifies the infected host cell in a way that limits ZIKV replication.

Cells were treated with 7-KC or ammonium chloride 2 h before infection, at the time of infection, and 2, 6, 12, and 18 h following infection. Ammonium chloride raises lysosomal pH, preventing flavivirus entry [28] and was used as an entry inhibitor control. Ammonium chloride treatment 2 h prior to infection and at the time of infection inhibited ZIKV replication, but it was less inhibitory when added later in infection. Interestingly, pre-treating cells with 7-KC 2 h before infection did not reduce viral titers, yet treatment with 7-KC at the time of infection, at 2 hpi, or at 6 hpi all decreased ZIKV titers by 90% (Figure 6B). ZIKV inhibition continued even 12 h after infection, while 18 h after infection only showed a slight decrease in titer. It may take some time for 7-KC treatment to take effect, and adding the drug at 18 hpi (only 6 h before virus was collected) may allow some virions to be produced before the drug was added. These results suggest that 7-KC does not inhibit ZIKV entry and instead inhibits a downstream step in the replication pathways such as viral replication or budding.

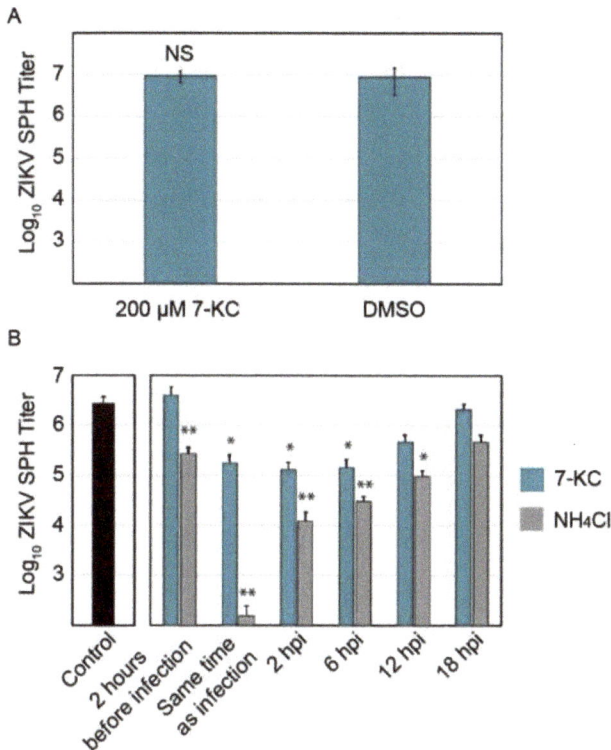

Figure 6. Analysis of 7-ketocholesterol inhibition of ZIKV SPH replication. (**A**) ZIKV SPH preincubation with 200 μM of 7-KC before Vero cell infection. (**B**) 7-KC versus ammonium chloride time-of-addition assay in Vero cells. Error bars represent the SEM. *, $p < 0.05$; **, $p < 0.01$.

3.7. 7-Ketocholesterol qRT-PCR

Time-of-addition experiments demonstrate that 7-KC is able to reduce virus production even when added 6 h following infection, suggesting that the compound most likely affects ZIKV production late in the infection cycle. To examine the levels of viral RNA production, we isolated total RNA from infected cells and quantified the number of viral genome copies present. The levels of ZIKV RNA were not significantly altered in the presence of 7-KC (Figure 7A), suggesting 7-KC does not alter RNA production. Although the levels of RNA found in the cells were not significantly different, the number of viral genome copies in the supernatant was reduced, suggesting a budding or release defect. When we compared the number of genomes in the supernatant to the amount in the cells, 7-KC treatment decreases budding/release efficiency to approximately 30% of untreated cells (Figure 7B). While this defect could account for a slight decrease in virion production, it alone could not cause the greater than 90% decrease in infectious virions. Therefore, we hypothesized that the particles budding from the 7-KC treated cells may be less infectious than ZIKV produced from untreated cells. We determined the specific infectivity of the particles by comparing the infectious titer to the number of genome copies in the supernatant samples (Figure 7C). Particles produced in cells treated with 7-KC were significantly less infectious than the DMSO control. Only 1 in approxiamately 9000 genomes were infectious when 7-KC was present compared to 1 in 1200 of control.

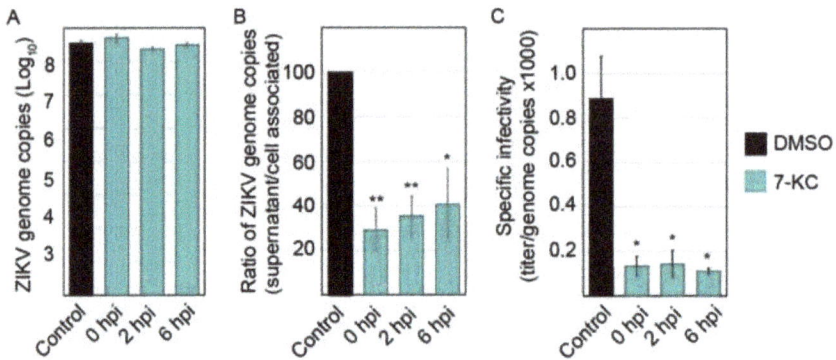

Figure 7. 7-KC reduced ZIKV budding efficiency and infectious virion production. (A) ZIKV infection was inhibited by adding 7-KC at the indicated time points following infection. Twenty-four hours post infection (hpi), total cellular RNA was harvested and ZIKV genomes were quantified using q-RT-PCR. 7-KC did not significantly alter the level of ZIKV genomes in the cells. (B) ZIKV genome copies present in the supernatants were also quantified. To determine the budding/release efficiency we compared the number of genomes present in the supernatant to cell associated genomes and determined the budding efficiency based on DMSO control. (C) ZIKV produced in the presence of 7-KC is less infectious than virus grown in DMSO control cells. The specific infectivity of the virions was determined by comparing the titer to the number of genome copies found in the supernatant ($\times 1000$). Each RNA sample was run in triplicate during each trial for a total of 3 trials. *, $p < 0.05$; **, $p < 0.01$.

4. Discussion

To further our understanding of how ZIKV replication interacts with the autophagy pathway, we examined ZIKV replication in the presence of 94 autophagy inducers and inhibitors. Most compounds did not affect ZIKV replication or substantially reduce cell viability, preventing us from assessing the compounds' effect on replication. When comparing the effects of the compounds in the mammalian and mosquito cell lines, we observed a similar pattern of inhibition for the most part (Figure S2). Some compounds had cell-type specific cytotoxicity which frequently explained any differences in trends. The number of compounds that did not significantly alter ZIKV replication surprised us. While all the compounds in the library have been shown to alter the autophagy pathway, some of the compounds effects may be indirect. Rapamycin, the prototypical autophagy inducer increased ZIKV production in Vero cells, yet slightly decreased production in C6/36 cells. Hydroxychloroquine blocked ZIKV spread in a mouse model [12] and we found it decreased titers in both Vero and C6/36 cells. While trehalose, an autophagy inducer, has been suggested to block ZIKV transmission [29], it was not able to reduce ZIKV titers in Vero or C6/36 cells.

Three compounds, amiodarone-HCl, 7-ketocholesterol, and licochalcone A, inhibited ZIKV replication in Vero cells without reducing cell viability, but neurons only remained viable when treated with 7-KC. 7-KC was also the only compound that reduced ZIKV IbH by more than 90% of control. 7-KC is an oxysterol formed by oxidation of cholesterol [30] and is a major component of oxidized lipoprotein found in atherosclerotic plaque [31]. 7-KC is a biomarker for oxidative stress and elevated levels are observed in blood samples of cancer patients and patients with inflammation [32–34]. Although the mechanism remains unclear, sub-toxic levels of 7-KC activates PI3K/mTOR signaling, inducing autophagy [35]. 7-KC has also been linked to enhancing intracellular hydrogen peroxide levels, triggering autophagy [36]. While low concentrations of 7-KC are associated with autophagy induction, high concentrations are cytotoxic and induce apoptosis [36]. Most of the existing research on this compound focuses on it association with atherosclerosis [37], a condition characterized by hardened, plaque-filled arterial walls caused by oxysterol buildup over time [31]. 7-KC also induces inflammation through TLR4 signaling [38]. Currently there is no literature examining

Viruses **2019**, *11*, 20

7-KC and antiviral activity against enveloped viruses, however one study examining oxysterols and non-enveloped viruses found 7-KC had no activity against human papillomavirus and human rotavirus with minor activity for human rhinovirus [39].

7-KC will incorporate into cellular lipids and disrupt normal lipid order [40,41], which can impair phagocytosis [42]. A similar oxidized cholesterol-based compound, 25-hydroxycholesterol (25-HC), reduced ZIKV titers in vitro and in vivo by inhibiting viral entry [43]. 25-HC may modify host membranes, preventing efficient fusion [43]. Due to the similar make-up of 25-HC and 7-KC one might predict it would also decrease viral entry. However, our time-of-addition studies suggests 7-KC does not block viral entry or RNA production, but a late stage in viral replication such as viral budding or particle release from the cell. In addition to decreasing the efficiency of particle release, the particles that are released into the supernatant are less infectious.

Interestingly, 7-KC induces autophagy [36], and because ZIKV replication is enhanced by autophagy induction, one could suggest that 7-KC should increase ZIKV titers. 7-KC's role in inducing autophagy and the antiviral activity we observed may not be related. While 7-KC may increase autophagy flux through activating PI3K/mTOR, its effects on disrupting lipid order may have more profound consequences on ZIKV spread. ZIKV replication, budding, maturation, and release all rely on host lipids and the cellular secretory pathway [44]. Particle infectivity was altered when the infected cells were treated with 7-KC, but the compound had no virucidal effect on intact particles. This suggests that the 7-KC may significantly alter the lipid environment in the organelles that are critical for budding and trafficking of ZIKV.

In conclusion, we identified 7-ketocholesterol as an inhibitor of ZIKV replication in both Vero cells and human neurons. While antiviral, 7-KC only dropped viral titers by an order of magnitude, suggesting the compound would not be clinically relevant. However, we believe that 7-KC will be a useful tool to examine the lipids involved in ZIKV particle production and further explore ZIKV budding and trafficking mechanisms.

Supplementary Materials: The following are available online at http://www.mdpi.com/1999-4915/11/1/20/s1; Figure S1: Comparison of autophagy compounds' effects on ZIKV SPH and IbH; Figure S2: Comparison of the autophagy compounds' effects on ZIKV SPH in Vero and C6/36 cells.

Author Contributions: M.A.B. and K.A.W. conceived and designed the experiments; K.A.W. performed the experiments; M.A.B. and K.A.W. analyzed the data; C.L.E. and S.L.S. contributed reagents/materials/analysis tools; K.A.W. and M.A.B. wrote the paper.

Funding: Work was supported by laboratory start-up funds provided by the University of Georgia.

Acknowledgments: We would like to thank members of the Brindley lab for scientific consultation.

Conflicts of Interest: The authors declare no conflict of interest.

References

1. Broutet, N.; Krauer, F.; Riesen, M.; Khalakdina, A.; Almiron, M.; Aldighieri, S.; Espinal, M.; Low, N.; Dye, C. Zika Virus as a Cause of Neurologic Disorders. *N. Engl. J. Med.* **2016**, *374*, 1506–1509. [CrossRef] [PubMed]

2. Persaud, M.; Martinez-Lopez, A.; Buffone, C.; Porcelli, S.A.; Diaz-Griffero, F. Infection by Zika viruses requires the transmembrane protein AXL, endocytosis and low pH. *Virology* **2018**, *518*, 301–312. [CrossRef] [PubMed]

3. Rossignol, E.D.; Peters, K.N.; Connor, J.H.; Bullitt, E. Zika virus induced cellular remodelling. *Cell. Microbiol.* **2017**, *19*. [CrossRef] [PubMed]

4. Chiramel, A.I.; Best, S.M. Role of autophagy in Zika virus infection and pathogenesis. *Virus Res.* **2018**, *254*, 34–40. [CrossRef] [PubMed]

5. Knodler, L.A.; Celli, J. Eating the strangers within: Host control of intracellular bacteria via xenophagy. *Cell. Microbiol.* **2011**, *13*, 1319–1327. [CrossRef] [PubMed]

6. Kimmey, J.M.; Stallings, C.L. Bacterial Pathogens versus Autophagy: Implications for Therapeutic Interventions. *Trends Mol. Med.* **2016**, *22*, 1060–1076. [CrossRef] [PubMed]

7. Richards, A.L.; Jackson, W.T. How positive-strand RNA viruses benefit from autophagosome maturation. *J. Virol.* **2013**, *87*, 9966–9972. [CrossRef] [PubMed]

8. Heaton, N.S.; Randall, G. Dengue virus-induced autophagy regulates lipid metabolism. *Cell Host Microbe* **2010**, *8*, 422–432. [CrossRef]

9. Zhang, Z.W.; Li, Z.L.; Yuan, S. The Role of Secretory Autophagy in Zika Virus Transfer through the Placental Barrier. *Front. Cell. Infect. Microbiol.* **2016**, *6*, 206. [CrossRef]

10. Blazquez, A.B.; Escribano-Romero, E.; Merino-Ramos, T.; Saiz, J.C.; Martin-Acebes, M.A. Stress responses in flavivirus-infected cells: Activation of unfolded protein response and autophagy. *Front. Microbiol.* **2014**, *5*, 266. [CrossRef]

11. Hamel, R.; Dejarnac, O.; Wichit, S.; Ekchariyawat, P.; Neyret, A.; Luplertlop, N.; Perera-Lecoin, M.; Surasombatpattana, P.; Talignani, L.; Thomas, F.; et al. Biology of Zika Virus Infection in Human Skin Cells. *J. Virol.* **2015**, *89*, 8880–8896. [CrossRef] [PubMed]

12. Cao, B.; Parnell, L.A.; Diamond, M.S.; Mysorekar, I.U. Inhibition of autophagy limits vertical transmission of Zika virus in pregnant mice. *J. Exp. Med.* **2017**, *214*, 2303–2313. [CrossRef] [PubMed]

13. Liang, Q.; Luo, Z.; Zeng, J.; Chen, W.; Foo, S.S.; Lee, S.A.; Ge, J.; Wang, S.; Goldman, S.A.; Zlokovic, B.V.; et al. Zika Virus NS4A and NS4B Proteins Deregulate Akt-mTOR Signaling in Human Fetal Neural Stem Cells to Inhibit Neurogenesis and Induce Autophagy. *Cell Stem Cell* **2016**, *19*, 663–671. [CrossRef] [PubMed]

14. Chang, Y.P.; Tsai, C.C.; Huang, W.C.; Wang, C.Y.; Chen, C.L.; Lin, Y.S.; Kai, J.I.; Hsieh, C.Y.; Cheng, Y.L.; Choi, P.C.; et al. Autophagy facilitates IFN-gamma-induced Jak2-STAT1 activation and cellular inflammation. *J. Biol. Chem.* **2010**, *285*, 28715–28722. [CrossRef] [PubMed]

15. Liu, Y.; Gordesky-Gold, B.; Leney-Greene, M.; Weinbren, N.L.; Tudor, M.; Cherry, S. Inflammation-Induced, STING-Dependent Autophagy Restricts Zika Virus Infection in the Drosophila Brain. *Cell Host Microbe* **2018**, *24*, 57–68.e3. [CrossRef] [PubMed]

16. Shin, S.; Mitalipova, M.; Noggle, S.; Tibbitts, D.; Venable, A.; Rao, R.; Stice, S.L. Long-term proliferation of human embryonic stem cell-derived neuroepithelial cells using defined adherent culture conditions. *Stem Cells* **2006**, *24*, 125–138. [CrossRef] [PubMed]

17. Hamilton, M.A.; Russo, R.C.; Thurston, R.V. Trimmed Spearman-Karber Method for Estimating Median Lethal Concentrations in Toxicity Bioassays. *Environ. Sci. Technol.* **1977**, *11*, 714–719. [CrossRef]

18. Spearman, C. The Method of 'Right and Wrong Cases' ('Constant Stimuli') without Gauss's Formulae. *Br. J. Psychol.* **1908**, *2*, 227–242. [CrossRef]

19. Chan, L.L.; Shen, D.; Wilkinson, A.R.; Patton, W.; Lai, N.; Chan, E.; Kuksin, D.; Lin, B.; Qiu, J. A novel image-based cytometry method for autophagy detection in living cells. *Autophagy* **2012**, *8*, 1371–1382. [CrossRef]

20. Goodfellow, F.T.; Willard, K.A.; Wu, X.; Scoville, S.; Stice, S.L.; Brindley, M.A. Strain-Dependent Consequences of Zika Virus Infection and Differential Impact on Neural Development. *Viruses* **2018**, *10*, 550. [CrossRef]

21. Lanciotti, R.S.; Kosoy, O.L.; Laven, J.J.; Velez, J.O.; Lambert, A.J.; Johnson, A.J.; Stanfield, S.M.; Duffy, M.R. Genetic and serologic properties of Zika virus associated with an epidemic, Yap State, Micronesia, 2007. *Emerg. Infect. Dis.* **2008**, *14*, 1232–1239. [CrossRef] [PubMed]

22. Willard, K.A.; Demakovsky, L.; Tesla, B.; Goodfellow, F.T.; Stice, S.L.; Murdock, C.C.; Brindley, M.A. Zika Virus Exhibits Lineage-Specific Phenotypes in Cell Culture, in Aedes aegypti Mosquitoes, and in an Embryo Model. *Viruses* **2017**, *9*, 383. [CrossRef] [PubMed]

23. Lin, C.W.; Chen, Y.S.; Lin, C.C.; Chen, Y.J.; Lo, G.H.; Lee, P.H.; Kuo, P.L.; Dai, C.Y.; Huang, J.F.; Chung, W.L.; et al. Amiodarone as an autophagy promoter reduces liver injury and enhances liver regeneration and survival in mice after partial hepatectomy. *Sci. Rep.* **2015**, *5*, 15807. [CrossRef] [PubMed]

24. Haddow, A.D.; Schuh, A.J.; Yasuda, C.Y.; Kasper, M.R.; Heang, V.; Huy, R.; Guzman, H.; Tesh, R.B.; Weaver, S.C. Genetic characterization of Zika virus strains: Geographic expansion of the Asian lineage. *PLoS Negl. Trop. Dis.* **2012**, *6*, e1477. [CrossRef] [PubMed]

25. Shao, Q.; Herrlinger, S.; Zhu, Y.N.; Yang, M.; Goodfellow, F.; Stice, S.L.; Qi, X.P.; Brindley, M.A.; Chen, J.F. The African Zika virus MR-766 is more virulent and causes more severe brain damage than current Asian lineage and dengue virus. *Development* **2017**, *144*, 4114–4124. [CrossRef] [PubMed]

26. Simonin, Y.; Loustalot, F.; Desmetz, C.; Foulongne, V.; Constant, O.; Fournier-Wirth, C.; Leon, F.; Moles, J.P.; Goubaud, A.; Lemaitre, J.M.; et al. Zika Virus Strains Potentially Display Different Infectious Profiles in Human Neural Cells. *EBioMedicine* **2016**, *12*, 161–169. [CrossRef] [PubMed]

27. Moy, R.H.; Cherry, S. Antimicrobial autophagy: A conserved innate immune response in Drosophila. *J. Innate Immun.* **2013**, *5*, 444–455. [CrossRef] [PubMed]
28. Sanchez-San Martin, C.; Liu, C.Y.; Kielian, M. Dealing with low pH: Entry and exit of alphaviruses and flaviviruses. *Trends Microbiol.* **2009**, *17*, 514–521. [CrossRef]
29. Yuan, S.; Zhang, Z.W.; Li, Z.L. Trehalose May Decrease the Transmission of Zika Virus to the Fetus by Activating Degradative Autophagy. *Front. Cell. Infect. Microbiol.* **2017**, *7*, 402. [CrossRef]
30. Shinkyo, R.; Xu, L.; Tallman, K.A.; Cheng, Q.; Porter, N.A.; Guengerich, F.P. Conversion of 7-dehydrocholesterol to 7-ketocholesterol is catalyzed by human cytochrome P450 7A1 and occurs by direct oxidation without an epoxide intermediate. *J. Biol. Chem.* **2011**, *286*, 33021–33028. [CrossRef]
31. Brown, A.J.; Jessup, W. Oxysterols and atherosclerosis. *Atherosclerosis* **1999**, *142*, 1–28. [CrossRef]
32. Arca, M.; Natoli, S.; Micheletta, F.; Riggi, S.; Di Angelantonio, E.; Montali, A.; Antonini, T.M.; Antonini, R.; Diczfalusy, U.; Iuliano, L. Increased plasma levels of oxysterols, in vivo markers of oxidative stress, in patients with familial combined hyperlipidemia: Reduction during atorvastatin and fenofibrate therapy. *Free Radic. Biol. Med.* **2007**, *42*, 698–705. [CrossRef] [PubMed]
33. Rodriguez, I.R.; Larrayoz, I.M. Cholesterol oxidation in the retina: Implications of 7KCh formation in chronic inflammation and age-related macular degeneration. *J. Lipid Res.* **2010**, *51*, 2847–2862. [CrossRef] [PubMed]
34. Thanan, R.; Oikawa, S.; Hiraku, Y.; Ohnishi, S.; Ma, N.; Pinlaor, S.; Yongvanit, P.; Kawanishi, S.; Murata, M. Oxidative stress and its significant roles in neurodegenerative diseases and cancer. *Int. J. Mol. Sci.* **2014**, *16*, 193–217. [CrossRef] [PubMed]
35. Wang, S.F.; Chou, Y.C.; Mazumder, N.; Kao, F.J.; Nagy, L.D.; Guengerich, F.P.; Huang, C.; Lee, H.C.; Lai, P.S.; Ueng, Y.F. 7-Ketocholesterol induces P-glycoprotein through PI3K/mTOR signaling in hepatoma cells. *Biochem. Pharmacol.* **2013**, *86*, 548–560. [CrossRef] [PubMed]
36. He, C.; Zhu, H.; Zhang, W.; Okon, I.; Wang, Q.; Li, H.; Le, Y.Z.; Xie, Z. 7-Ketocholesterol induces autophagy in vascular smooth muscle cells through Nox4 and Atg4B. *Am. J. Pathol.* **2013**, *183*, 626–637. [CrossRef] [PubMed]
37. Lyons, M.A.; Brown, A.J. 7-Ketocholesterol. *Int. J. Biochem. Cell Biol.* **1999**, *31*, 369–375. [CrossRef]
38. Huang, J.D.; Amaral, J.; Lee, J.W.; Rodriguez, I.R. 7-Ketocholesterol-induced inflammation signals mostly through the TLR4 receptor both in vitro and in vivo. *PLoS ONE* **2014**, *9*, e100985. [CrossRef]
39. Civra, A.; Cagno, V.; Donalisio, M.; Biasi, F.; Leonarduzzi, G.; Poli, G.; Lembo, D. Inhibition of pathogenic non-enveloped viruses by 25-hydroxycholesterol and 27-hydroxycholesterol. *Sci. Rep.* **2014**, *4*, 7487. [CrossRef]
40. Massey, J.B.; Pownall, H.J. The polar nature of 7-ketocholesterol determines its location within membrane domains and the kinetics of membrane microsolubilization by apolipoprotein A-I. *Biochemistry* **2005**, *44*, 10423–10433. [CrossRef]
41. Magenau, A.; Benzing, C.; Proschogo, N.; Don, A.S.; Hejazi, L.; Karunakaran, D.; Jessup, W.; Gaus, K. Phagocytosis of IgG-coated polystyrene beads by macrophages induces and requires high membrane order. *Traffic* **2011**, *12*, 1730–1743. [CrossRef] [PubMed]
42. Lu, S.M.; Fairn, G.D. 7-Ketocholesterol impairs phagocytosis and efferocytosis via dysregulation of phosphatidylinositol 4,5-bisphosphate. *Traffic* **2018**, *19*, 591–604. [CrossRef] [PubMed]
43. Li, C.; Deng, Y.Q.; Wang, S.; Ma, F.; Aliyari, R.; Huang, X.Y.; Zhang, N.N.; Watanabe, M.; Dong, H.L.; Liu, P.; et al. 25-Hydroxycholesterol Protects Host against Zika Virus Infection and Its Associated Microcephaly in a Mouse Model. *Immunity* **2017**, *46*, 446–456. [CrossRef] [PubMed]
44. Sager, G.; Gabaglio, S.; Sztul, E.; Belov, G.A. Role of Host Cell Secretory Machinery in Zika Virus Life Cycle. *Viruses* **2018**, *10*, 559. [CrossRef] [PubMed]

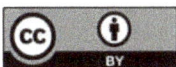

MDPI

Review

External Quality Assessment (EQA) for Molecular Diagnostics of Zika Virus: Experiences from an International EQA Programme, 2016–2018

Oliver Donoso Mantke [1,*], Elaine McCulloch [1], Paul S. Wallace [1], Constanze Yue [2],
Sally A. Baylis [2] and Matthias Niedrig [3]

[1] Quality Control for Molecular Diagnostics (QCMD), Unit 5, Technology Terrace, Todd Campus,
     West of Scotland Science Park, Glasgow G20 0XA, UK; ElaineMcCulloch@qcmd.org (E.M.);
     PaulWallace@qcmd.org (P.S.W.)
[2] Division of Virology, Paul-Ehrlich-Institut (PEI), Federal Institute for Vaccines and Biomedicines,
     63225 Langen, Germany; Constanze.Yue@pei.de (C.Y.); Sally.Baylis@pei.de (S.A.B.)
[3] Robert Koch-Institut (RKI), 13353 Berlin, Germany; niedrigm@rki.de
*   Correspondence: OliverDonoso@qcmd.org

Received: 27 July 2018; Accepted: 12 September 2018; Published: 13 September 2018

Abstract: Quality Control for Molecular Diagnostics (QCMD), an international provider for External Quality Assessment (EQA) programmes, has introduced a programme for molecular diagnostics of Zika virus (ZIKV) in 2016, which has been continuously offered to interested laboratories since that time. The EQA schemes provided from 2016 to 2018 revealed that 86.7% (92/106), 82.4% (89/108), and 88.2% (90/102) of the participating laboratories reported correct results for all samples, respectively in 2016, 2017, and 2018. The review of results indicated a need for improvement concerning analytical sensitivity and specificity of the test methods. Comparison with the outcomes of other EQA initiatives briefly summarized here show that continuous quality assurance is important to improve laboratory performance and to increase preparedness with reliable diagnostic assays for effective patient management, infection and outbreak control.

Keywords: Zika virus; mosquito-borne flavivirus; emerging arbovirus; outbreak control; molecular diagnostics; laboratory preparedness; assay standardization; external quality assessment; EQA; QCMD

---

1. Introduction

Zika virus (ZIKV) is a mosquito-borne flavivirus which had been considered to have low pathogenicity, with only very sporadic human cases and outbreaks reported in the past [1]. In 2015, ZIKV was first detected in patients in Brazil, which was a viral strain of the Asian lineage [2,3]. After introduction into South America, the virus has spread rapidly in over 48 countries and territories in the Americas, with over 220,000 confirmed autochthonous cases and over 3500 confirmed congenital cases associated with ZIKV infection [4]. During this rapid emergence, the World Health Organization (WHO) declared a Public Health Emergency of International Concern (PHEIC) in response to a cluster of microcephaly cases among newborns and other neurological disorders, like Guillain-Barré syndrome, in adults [5]. In accordance with the situation, the WHO assigned the development, assessment and validation of ZIKV diagnostic assays as a priority [6]. The PHEIC declaration ended in November 2016 with a longer-term programmatic approach for control and prevention [7].

Laboratory preparedness with access to reliable diagnostic assays, when facing an outbreak of arboviral infections and increase of international travel, is a key issue for patient management, infection and outbreak control worldwide [8–13]. Since the beginning of the ZIKV outbreak many diagnostic tests, mostly molecular in-house assays, have been developed [6,14–16]. Molecular methods are preferred for laboratory diagnosis of acute cases, especially in the early stage of arboviral infection [17]. Specific assays have been published for Asian and African ZIKV strains targeting several genomic regions including the envelope and NS5 [14,15,17]. Several months after the initial outbreak, there are also some commercial molecular assays available for ZIKV genome detection which have received regulatory approval [6,18,19].

Quality Control for Molecular Diagnostics (QCMD) is an international provider for External Quality Assessment (EQA) programmes covering a comprehensive range of infectious diseases [20]. The aims of QCMD's EQA programmes are to help monitor and improve laboratory quality by assessing a laboratory's use of molecular diagnostic technologies within the routine clinical setting. Participation in EQA programmes is a requirement for achieving accreditation/certification according to the International Organization for Standardization (ISO) 15189 ('Medical laboratories–requirements for quality and competence' [21]) or equivalent regulatory requirements. After the declaration of the PHEIC related to ZIKV in February 2016, QCMD rapidly introduced an EQA programme for molecular diagnostics of ZIKV in August 2016 to support the laboratory's requirements and provide appropriate proficiency testing options from then on. Here we review the results of the EQA schemes performed from 2016 to 2018 showing need for improvement concerning analytical sensitivity and specificity of the test methods.

2. The QCMD Zika Virus EQA Programme, 2016–2018

QCMD distributes the EQA programme for molecular diagnostics of ZIKV to registered laboratories annually. The annual EQA schemes have different panel compositions comprising eight to 12 lyophilized samples with samples containing cell culture-derived, inactivated African- and Asian-lineage ZIKV at different concentrations, specificity controls covering a range of related flaviviruses and other arboviruses, and negative samples with transport medium only. Furthermore, each QCMD panel includes the first WHO international standard (IS) for ZIKV for molecular assays, developed by the Paul-Ehrlich-Institut (PEI code number 11468/16 [22]) which allows traceability of EQA materials and comparability of laboratory performance in order to resolve the lack of assay standardization [23]. This material was officially established as WHO IS by the WHO Expert Committee on Biological Standardization in October 2016, however the candidate material had been made available prior to its establishment as the WHO IS for proficiency testing, assay development and clinical use because of the urgent need for quality-assured diagnostics [6].

All EQA programme and panel design specifications are defined by QCMD in close collaboration with Scientific Experts in the field, based on epidemiological, clinical and/or technical aspects. Participating laboratories are expected to test each panel using their routine molecular assays and workflows, and to report their results together with information of the applied extraction and amplification methods through the online reporting system to QCMD [20].

The panel compositions and performances for 2016–2018 are shown in Table 1. Participation has been relatively high since the introduction of the EQA programme, with 106 (116 datasets), 108 (114 datasets), and 102 (112 datasets) participating laboratories from around 37 countries worldwide, including those in affected geographical regions (with up to 17% of participating laboratories from affected countries like Brazil, Mexico, Panama), respectively, in 2016, 2017 and 2018. The results were predominantly generated by commercial assays with 54.3% (2016), 57.0% (2017), and 52.7% (2018) of the submitted datasets. No remarkable difference in performance between in-house and commercial assays were observed, however for some specific commercial assays analytical challenges could be identified concerning sensitivity with lower sample concentrations as well as specificity issues producing false positive results (data not specified). Please note that these observations do not allow a solid and statistically assured statement as EQA studies per se are not appropriate for assay validation.

Table 1. Quality Control for Molecular Diagnostics (QCMD) Zika Virus External Quality Assessment (EQA) Programme. Panel compositions and performances, 2016–2018.

(A) Data and Results on the Individual EQA Sample Level

Sample Content	Target Concentration [log₁₀ IU/mL]	EQA Scheme 2016			EQA Scheme 2017			EQA Scheme 2018		
		Assigned as Sample	Percentage Correct [%]	Datasets# (n)	Assigned as Sample	Percentage Correct [%]	Datasets# (n)	Assigned as Sample	Percentage Correct [%]	Datasets# (n)
ZIKV MR766	4.7	ZIKA16-08	97.4	116	ZIKA17S-07	97.4	114	ZIKA18S-05	97.3	112
ZIKV MR766	4.7	ZIKA16-09	99.1	116	-	-	-	-	-	-
ZIKV MR766	3.7	ZIKA16-10	95.7	116	ZIKA17S-06	95.6	114	ZIKA18S-04	95.5	112
ZIKV MR766	2.7	ZIKA16-02	93.1	116	ZIKA17S-03	89.5	114	ZIKA18S-06	89.3	112
ZIKV 11474/16	5.7	ZIKA16-04	100	116	-	-	-	-	-	-
ZIKV 11474/16	3.7	-	-	-	ZIKA17S-01	94.7	114	ZIKA18S-01	93.8	112
ZIKV 11468/16	5.7	ZIKA16-06	100	116	ZIKA17S-05	99.1	114	ZIKA18S-03	97.3	112
ZIKV 11468/16	4.7	ZIKA16-03	100	116	ZIKA17S-04	96.5	114	ZIKA18S-02	94.6	112
ZIKV 11468/16	3.7	-	-	-	-	-	-	ZIKA18S-07	98.2	112
Non-Zika flaviviruses	-	ZIKA16-01	94.8	116	ZIKA17S-02	98.2	114	-	-	-
Chikungunya virus	-	ZIKA16-07	96.6	116	-	-	-	-	-	-
Transport medium	-	ZIKA16-05	97.4	116	ZIKA17S-08	96.5	114	ZIKA18S-08	100	112

(B) Overall Qualitative Performance for the Core Sample Panel

	EQA Scheme 2016	EQA Scheme 2017	EQA Scheme 2018
Percentage [%] of datasets with All Core samples correct	86.2 (10/10 core samples) 116 datasets#	82.5 (8/8 core samples) 114 datasets#	85.7 (8/8 core samples) 112 datasets#

Positive samples contained different concentrations of Zika virus strain Uganda MR766 provided by the Robert Koch-Institut (RKI) (representing the African lineage), ZIKV reference material 11474/16 prepared by the Paul-Ehrlich-Institut (PEI) (from French Polynesian ZIKV strain PF13/251013-18, representing the Asian lineage), or WHO IS preparation 11468/16 developed by PEI (from French Polynesian ZIKV strain PF13/251013-18, representing the Asian lineage) [24,25]. Negative samples contained a mixed sample of flaviviruses other than ZIKV (dengue virus serotype 2, DENV-2; West Nile virus strain NY99, WNV-NY99 and yellow fever virus 17D, YFV-17D) and/or a sample with chikungunya virus (CHIKV) for specificity control, and a sample with transport medium only (which was used as sample matrix for the EQA samples). All cell culture–derived arboviral samples were inactivated and lyophilized. # A dataset is defined as one qualitative laboratory result per sample and applied workflow.

In the EQA schemes of 2016–2018, all samples were designated by the QCMD Scientific Experts as Core proficiency samples, which are expected to be correctly reported by the participating laboratories within the EQA challenge in order to show an acceptable level of proficiency/successful participation. The percentage of datasets with All Core samples correctly reported were 86.2% (2016), 82.5% (2017), and 85.7% (2018) (see Table 1). At the laboratory level, these were 86.7% (92/106), 82.4% (89/108), and 88.2% (90/102), respectively. Incorrect results (including false positive or not determined) were reported for the true negative sample containing transport medium only (2.6% in 2016; 3.5% in 2017; 0.0% in 2018), for a specificity negative sample containing a mixture of flaviviruses other than ZIKV (5.2% in 2016; 1.8% in 2017; 1.8% in 2018), and for a specificity negative sample containing chikungunya virus (3.4%, only included in 2016).

Review of the three QCMD EQA schemes performed between 2016 and 2018 demonstrate that the overall qualitative performance of participating laboratories for molecular diagnostics of ZIKV was at an acceptable level. However, analytical sensitivity and specificity remain a challenge. False positive results may lead to misdiagnosis and potentially affect clinical decisions. Processes should be reviewed by laboratories reporting false positive results. The risk of a false negative result was a concern for a small number of laboratories and may result in failure to detect a ZIKV in low concentration in infected patients during the acute phase of the disease. Laboratories who were unable to detect the lower concentrated samples should strive to improve the sensitivity of the ZIKV molecular assay used.

3. Review of Results from Other EQA Initiatives

To date, a further three EQA activities for ZIKV molecular diagnostics performed by different groups have been identified showing similar observations as mentioned above [26–28].

Fischer et al. [26] conducted an EQA study for Brazilian laboratories in 2017. Fifteen laboratories participated in this study applying their routine molecular diagnostics for ZIKV on a panel comprising 12 lyophilized samples with inactivated full virus spiked into arbovirus-negative human plasma. The panel included four ZIKV-positive samples with 10^3–10^6 RNA copies/mL (representing the African and Asian lineage, including the outbreak strain in the Americas) to assess sensitivity, seven different arbovirus-positive samples (chikungunya virus, CHIKV; dengue viruses, DENV-2 & DENV-4; Japanese encephalitis virus, JEV; St. Louis encephalitis virus, SLEV; West Nile virus, WNV; yellow fever virus, YFV) for specificity control, and a negative plasma sample. In addition, the WHO IS [24] as well as a ZIKV armored RNA standard available at the EVAg portal (European Virus Archive goes Global) were provided as references for quantification of the ZIKV-positive samples. Only 27.0% (four of 15 laboratories) reported correct results for all samples, while 73.0% (11/15) had limited sensitivity (correctly testing only the two samples with the highest ZIKV concentration) and/or specificity (including false positive results from ZIKV-negative samples).

Abdad et al. [27] pointed out how important it is to continually offer and expand an EQA initiative for emerging arboviruses which helps to assess the laboratory performance and to increase the preparedness in a certain region. The WHO Regional Office for the Western Pacific Region (WPR) started with an EQA pilot for two participating laboratories in 2011, including only dengue virus, and developed it to a global EQA programme for arbovirus diagnostics (including CHIKV, DENV, YFV, and ZIKV) with participation of 96 laboratories worldwide (of which 25 were coming from 19 countries in the WPR) in 2016. In 2016, the panels contained blinded samples with different concentrations for the four targeted arboviruses and were shipped to the participants between November and December. For ZIKV, 72.0% (18 of 25 laboratories of the WPR) reported correct results in all samples, while 28.0% (seven) had at least one false result which was not further specified.

Charrel et al. [28] published an EQA study that was performed by the Emerging Viral Diseases Expert Laboratory Network (EVD-LabNet, Rotterdam, The Netherlands) in October/November 2016 to assess and to improve the capability of European reference and expert laboratories for ZIKV molecular detection. Fifty laboratories (reporting 85 datasets) from 31 countries took part in this study, using mostly in-house assays (72.0% of the submitted datasets). The panel consisted of 12 lyophilized samples with inactivated virus spiked into plasma or urine, including six ZIKV-positive samples with 10^3-10^9 copies/mL (representing the African and Asian lineage, including the outbreak strain in the Americas; calibrated using in vitro-transcribed ZIKV RNA), three different arbovirus-positive samples (CHIKV, YFV, DENV-1), and three negative plasma or urine samples. Based on the submitted results, all samples were assigned as core samples, having a ZIKV status scored correctly by >50% of the participating laboratories. The study revealed that only 40.0% of the laboratories (20/50), representing 45.0% of the countries, achieved a sufficient analytical performance. 60.0% of the laboratories (30/50) had a need to improve their molecular ZIKV detection in relation with specificity, but more obviously with sensitivity as only half of the laboratories correctly scored the sample with the lowest concentration.

4. Conclusions

Although the comparison of the recent results from the QCMD Zika Virus EQA Programme done for 2016–2018 with the briefly summarized outcomes of the other EQA initiatives for ZIKV molecular diagnostics shows great variations in laboratory performance with 27.0–88.2% of participating laboratories reporting correct results for all samples, all EQAs indicate that there is a clear need to improve sensitivity and specificity of ZIKV molecular assays.

The ZIKV molecular diagnostics would benefit greatly from the use of standards and controls in order to ensure that laboratories would also detect lower viral loads as known from the literature [17,29,30] to avoid false negative results during acute infection. The continued use of the WHO IS as included in the QCMD EQA programme for molecular diagnostics of ZIKV will help to support assay standardization and to improve quality performance of molecular ZIKV diagnostics.

As ZIKV and other arboviruses (e.g., DENV, CHIKV) co-circulate affecting many endemic countries and at-risk countries globally, being a risk for local populations and international travelers, it is important that laboratories can accurately detect and differentiate to avoid false positive results, potentially having serious consequences for patients as exemplified by a dramatic increase in abortion requests in South America during the 2016 ZIKV outbreak [31]. Regular participation in EQA schemes by laboratories is important to monitor the improvement in laboratory performance; also, for laboratories outside endemic regions a regular EQA participation would provide confidence in tests when positive samples are not routinely seen.

Laboratories should be aware of the limitation of their assays and perform their own validation and verification in line with ISO 15189 and other requirements. Continually offered EQA programmes for arbovirus diagnostics are an important tool to improve laboratory performance and to increase preparedness having quality-assured assays disponible for effective patient management, infection and outbreak control.

Author Contributions: EQA Programme Planning & Design, O.D.M. and E.M.; EQA Project Management, O.D.M. and E.M.; Resources & Supervision, P.S.W.; Technical Contributions, C.Y.; Material Acquisition, Testing & Scientific Advice, S.A.B. and M.N.; Writing-Manuscript, O.D.M.; Writing-Review & Editing, all.

Funding: This research received no external funding.

Acknowledgments: We thank former and current QCMD staff members from EQA Administration, EQA Operations, EQA Project Management, IT & Informatics and Technical Support who supported the EQA programme activities. Special thanks to Pranav Patel (TIB MOLBIOL, Berlin, Germany) who contributed to the material assessment.

Conflicts of Interest: The authors declare no conflict of interest.

References

1. Baud, D.; Gubler, D.J.; Schaub, B.; Lanteri, M.C.; Musso, D. An update on Zika virus infection. *Lancet* **2017**, *390*, 2099–2109. [CrossRef]
2. De Oliveira, W.K.; de França, G.V.A.; Carmo, E.H.; Duncan, B.B.; de Souza Kuchenbecker, R.; Schmidt, M.I. Infection-related microcephaly after the 2015 and 2016 Zika virus outbreaks in Brazil: A surveillance-based analysis. *Lancet* **2017**, *390*, 861–870. [CrossRef]

3. Weaver, S.C.; Costa, F.; Garcia-Blanco, M.A.; Ko, A.I.; Ribeiro, G.S.; Saade, G.; Shi, P.Y.; Vasilakis, N. Zika virus: History, emergence, biology, and prospects for control. *Antivir. Res.* **2016**, *130*, 69–80. [CrossRef] [PubMed]
4. Pan American Health Organization (PAHO); World Health Organization (WHO). *Cumulative Cases: Zika Suspected and Confirmed Cases Reported by Countries and Territories in the Americas, 2015–2017*; Updated as of 4 January 2018; PAHO/WHO: Washington, DC, USA, 2017; Available online: www.paho.org/hq/index. php?option=com_content&view=article&id=12390&Itemid=42090&lang=en (accessed on 16 February 2018).
5. World Health Organization (WHO). *WHO Statement on the First Meeting of the International Health Regulations (2005) (IHR 2005) Emergency Committee on Zika Virus and Observed Increase in Neurological Disorders and Neonatal Malformations*; WHO: Geneva, Switzerland, 2016; Available online: www.who.int/news-room/detail/01-02-2016-who-statement-on-the-first-meeting-of-the-international-health-regulations-(2005)-(ihr-2005)-emergency-committee-on-zika-virus-and-observed-increase-in-neurological-disorders-and-neonatal-malformations (accessed on 16 February 2018).
6. Chua, A.; Prat, I.; Nuebling, C.M.; Wood, D.; Moussy, F. Update on Zika Diagnostic Tests and WHO's Related Activities. *PLoS Negl. Trop. Dis.* **2017**, *11*, e0005269. [CrossRef] [PubMed]
7. World Health Organization (WHO). *Fifth Meeting of the Emergency Committee under the International Health Regulations (2005) Regarding Microcephaly, Other Neurological Disorders and Zika Virus*; WHO: Geneva, Switzerland, 2016; Available online: www.who.int/news-room/detail/18-11-2016-fifth-meeting-of-the-emergency-committee-under-the-international-health-regulations-(2005)-regarding-microcephaly-other-neurological-disorders-and-zika-virus (accessed on 16 February 2018).
8. Wilder-Smith, A.; Preet, R.; Renhorn, K.E.; Ximenes, R.A.; Rodrigues, L.C.; Solomon, T.; Neyts, J.; Lambrechts, L.; Willison, H.; Peeling, R.; et al. ZikaPLAN: Zika Preparedness Latin American Network. *Glob. Health Action* **2017**, *10*, 1398485. [CrossRef] [PubMed]
9. Mögling, R.; Zeller, H.; Revez, J.; Koopmans, M.; ZIKV Reference Laboratory Group; Reusken, C. Status, quality and specifc needs of Zika virus (ZIKV) diagnostic capacity and capability in National Reference Laboratories for arboviruses in 30 EU/EEA countries, May 2016. *Eurosurveillance* **2017**, *22*, 30609.
10. Escadafal, C.; Gaayeb, L.; Riccardo, F.; Pérez-Ramírez, E.; Picard, M.; Dente, M.G.; Fernández-Pinero, J.; Manuguerra, J.C.; Jiménez-Clavero, M.Á.; Declich, S.; et al. Risk of Zika virus transmission in the Euro-Mediterranean area and the added value of building preparedness to arboviral threats from a One Health perspective. *BMC Public Health* **2016**, *16*, 1219. [CrossRef] [PubMed]
11. Madad, S.S.; Masci, J.; Cagliuso, N.V., Sr.; Allen, M. Preparedness for Zika Virus Disease—New York City, 2016. *Morb. Mortal. Wkly. Rep. (MMWR)* **2016**, *65*, 1161–1165. [CrossRef] [PubMed]
12. Squires, R.C.; Konings, F.; World Health Organization Regional Office for the Western Pacific Zika Incident Management Team. Preparedness for Zika virus testing in the World Health Organization Western Pacific Region. *West. Pac. Surveill. Response J.* **2016**, *7*, 44–47. [CrossRef] [PubMed]
13. Petersen, E.; Wilson, M.E.; Touch, S.; McCloskey, B.; Mwaba, P.; Bates, M.; Dar, O.; Mattes, F.; Kidd, M.; Ippolito, G.; et al. Rapid Spread of Zika Virus in The Americas—Implications for Public Health Preparedness for Mass Gatherings at the 2016 Brazil Olympic Games. *Int. J. Infect. Dis.* **2016**, *44*, 11–15. [CrossRef] [PubMed]
14. Theel, E.S.; Hata, D.J. Diagnostic Testing for Zika Virus: A Postoutbreak Update. *J. Clin. Microbiol.* **2018**, *56*, e01972-17. [CrossRef] [PubMed]
15. Charrel, R.N.; Leparc-Goffart, I.; Pas, S.; de Lamballerie, X.; Koopmans, M.; Reusken, C. Background review for diagnostic test development for Zika virus infection. *Bull. World Health Organ.* **2016**, *94*, 574–584. [CrossRef] [PubMed]
16. Corman, V.M.; Rasche, A.; Baronti, C.; Aldabbagh, S.; Cadar, D.; Reusken, C.B.E.M.; Pas, S.D.; Goorhuis, A.; Schinkel, J.; Molenkamp, R.; et al. Clinical Comparison, Standardization and Optimization of Zika Virus Molecular Detection. Bulletin World Health Organization. 2016. Available online: www.who.int/bulletin/online_first/16-175950.pdf (accessed on 26 April 2016).
17. Corman, V.M.; Rasche, A.; Baronti, C.; Aldabbagh, S.; Cadar, D.; Reusken, C.B.E.M.; Pas, S.D.; Goorhuis, A.; Schinkel, J.; Molenkamp, R.; et al. Assay optimization for molecular detection of Zika virus. *Bull. World Health Organ.* **2016**, *94*, 880–892. [CrossRef] [PubMed]
18. Zika Diagnostic Tests Currently Authorized under EUA. Available online: www.fda.gov/EmergencyPreparedness/Counterterrorism/MedicalCountermeasures/MCMIssues/ucm485199.htm#eua (accessed on 10 June 2018).

19. Landry, M.L.; St. George, K. Laboratory Diagnosis of Zika Virus Infection. *Arch. Pathol. Lab. Med.* **2017**, *141*, 60–67. [CrossRef] [PubMed]

20. Quality Control for Molecular Diagnostics (QCMD). Available online: www.qcmd.org/index.php?pageId= 45&pageVersion=EN (accessed on 25 May 2018).

21. International Organization for Standardization (ISO). *ISO 15189:2012: Medical Laboratories—Requirements for Quality and Competence*; ISO: Geneva, Switzerland, 2012; Available online: www.iso.org/obp/ui/#iso:std:iso: 15189:ed-3:v2:en (accessed on 16 February 2018).

22. Paul-Ehrlich-Institut. *1st World Health Organization International Standard for Zika Virus RNA for Nucleic Acid Amplification Techniques (NAT)-Based Assays*; PEI Code 11468/16, Version 1.3; Paul-Ehrlich-Institut: Langen, Germany, 2016; Available online: www.pei.de/SharedDocs/Downloads/EN/who/11468-16-ifu.pdf?__ blob=publicationFile&v=5 (accessed on 16 February 2018).

23. Baylis, S.A.; McCulloch, E.; Wallace, P.; Donoso Mantke, O.; Niedrig, M.; Blümel, J.; Yue, C.; Nübling, C.M. External Quality Assessment (EQA) of Molecular Detection of Zika Virus: Value of the 1st World Health Organization International Standard. *J. Clin. Microbiol.* **2018**, *56*, e01997-17. [CrossRef] [PubMed]

24. Baylis, S.A.; Hanschmann, K.O.; Schnierle, B.S.; Trosemeier, J.H.; Blumel, J.; Zika Virus Collaborative Study Group. Harmonization of nucleic acid testing for Zika virus: Development of the 1st World Health Organization International Standard. *Transfusion* **2017**, *57*, 748–761. [CrossRef] [PubMed]

25. Trösemeier, J.H.; Musso, D.; Blümel, J.; Thézé, J.; Pybus, O.G.; Baylis, S.A. Genome sequence of a candidate World Health Organization reference strain of Zika virus for nucleic acid testing. *Genome Announc.* **2016**, *4*, 00917-16. [CrossRef] [PubMed]

26. Fischer, C.; Pedroso, C.; Mendrone, A., Jr.; de Filippis, A.M.B.; Vallinoto, A.C.R.; Ribeiro, B.M.; Marques, E.T.A., Jr.; Campos, G.S.; Viana, I.F.T.; Levi, J.E.; et al. External Quality Assessment for Zika Virus Molecular Diagnostic Testing, Brazil. *Emerg. Infect. Dis.* **2018**, *24*, 888–892. [CrossRef] [PubMed]

27. Abdad, M.Y.; Squires, R.C.; Cognat, S.; Oxenford, C.J.; Konings, F. External quality assessment for arbovirus diagnostics in the World Health Organization Western Pacific Region, 2013–2016: Improving laboratory quality over the years. *West. Pac. Surveill. Response J.* **2017**, *8*, 27–30. [CrossRef] [PubMed]

28. Charrel, R.; Mögling, R.; Pas, S.; Papa, A.; Baronti, C.; Koopmans, M.; Zeller, H.; Leparc-Goffart, I.; Reusken, C.B. Variable Sensitivity in Molecular Detection of Zika Virus in European Expert Laboratories: External Quality Assessment, November 2016. *J. Clin. Microbiol.* **2017**, *55*, 3219–3226. [CrossRef] [PubMed]

29. Froeschl, G.; Huber, K.; von Sonnenburg, F.; Nothdurft, H.D.; Bretzel, G.; Hoelscher, M.; Zoeller, L.; Trottmann, M.; Pan-Montojo, F.; Dobler, G.; et al. Long-term kinetics of Zika virus RNA and antibodies in body fluids of a vasectomized traveller returning from Martinique: A case report. *BMC Infect. Dis.* **2017**, *17*, 55. [CrossRef] [PubMed]

30. Mansuy, J.M.; Mengelle, C.; Pasquier, C.; Chapuy-Regaud, S.; Delobel, P.; Martin-Blondel, G.; Izopet, J. Zika Virus Infection and Prolonged Viremia in Whole-Blood Specimens. *Emerg. Infect. Dis.* **2017**, *23*, 863–865. [CrossRef] [PubMed]

31. Aiken, A.R.; Scott, J.G.; Gomperts, R.; Trussell, J.; Worrell, M.; Aiken, C.E. Requests for Abortion in Latin America Related to Concern about Zika Virus Exposure. *N. Engl. J. Med.* **2016**, *375*, 396–398. [CrossRef] [PubMed]

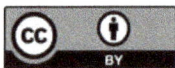

MDPI

Article

Simultaneous Detection of Different Zika Virus Lineages via Molecular Computation in a Point-of-Care Assay

Sanchita Bhadra [1,*], Miguel A. Saldaña [2], Hannah Grace Han [1], Grant L. Hughes [3,†] and Andrew D. Ellington [1]

[1] Department of Molecular Biosciences, College of Natural Sciences, The University of Texas at Austin, Austin, TX 78712, USA; whitehannahhan@gmail.com (H.G.H.); ellingtonlab@gmail.com (A.D.E.)

[2] Department of Microbiology and Immunology, University of Texas Medical Branch, Galveston, TX 77555, USA; misaldan@utmb.edu

[3] Department of Pathology, Institute for Human Infections and Immunity, Center for Tropical Diseases, Center for Biodefense and Emerging Infectious Disease, University of Texas Medical Branch, Galveston, TX 77555, USA; Grant.Hughes@lstmed.ac.uk

* Correspondence: sanchitabhadra@utexas.edu; Tel.: +1-512-471-6445

† Present Address: Department of Vector Biology and Department of Parasitology, Liverpool School of Tropical Medicine, Pembroke Place, Liverpool L3 5QA, UK.

Received: 20 October 2018; Accepted: 11 December 2018; Published: 14 December 2018

Abstract: We have developed a generalizable "smart molecular diagnostic" capable of accurate point-of-care (POC) detection of variable nucleic acid targets. Our isothermal assay relies on multiplex execution of four loop-mediated isothermal amplification reactions, with primers that are degenerate and redundant, thereby increasing the breadth of targets while reducing the probability of amplification failure. An easy-to-read visual answer is computed directly by a multi-input Boolean OR logic gate (gate output is true if either one or more gate inputs is true) signal transducer that uses degenerate strand exchange probes to assess any combination of amplicons. We demonstrate our methodology by using the same assay to detect divergent Asian and African lineages of the evolving Zika virus (ZIKV), while maintaining selectivity against non-target viruses. Direct analysis of biological specimens proved possible, with crudely macerated ZIKV-infected *Aedes aegypti* mosquitoes being identified with 100% specificity and sensitivity. The ease-of-use with minimal instrumentation, broad programmability, and built-in fail-safe reliability make our smart molecular diagnostic attractive for POC use.

Keywords: point-of-care diagnostics; isothermal nucleic acid amplification; nucleic acid computation; nucleic acid strand exchange; zika virus; mosquito; mosquito surveillance; multiplex nucleic acid detection; boolean logic-processing nucleic acid probes

---

1. Introduction

While point-of-care (POC) diagnostic assays can be performed at or near the site of sample acquisition, they have for the most part been considered to be relatively simplistic tests that provide relatively little information to a clinician or public health worker. Familiar examples include electrochemical sensors for glucose [1] or rapid immunoassays for metabolites such as human chorionic gonadotropin (the canonical pregnancy test) [2], and pathogens, either directly (influenza viruses and Zika virus) or via immune responses (antibodies against HIV-1/2) [3–5]. The range of conditions and pathogens that could be tested for could likely be greatly expanded by developing POC diagnostics for nucleic acids [3] that would have greater sensitivity and accuracy. However, the current gold standard for molecular diagnostics, the quantitative polymerase chain reaction (qPCR), requires significant technical expertise and expensive and cumbersome equipment. Even portable instruments, such the Cepheid GeneXpert Omni, cost several thousand dollars and rely on expensive qPCR cartridge consumables for individual tests.

In contrast, isothermal nucleic acid amplification tests (iNAATs) have been developed that rival PCR in sensitivity, cost far less, and do not necessarily rely on complex instrumentation [6]. To further the adoption of these assays, we and others have begun to develop "smart molecular diagnostics" that can integrate information at the molecular level. For example, to increase signal specificity, a variety of sequence-specific probes, including molecular beacons, nuclease-dependent probes, and fluorescence resonance energy transfer (FRET) pairs have been adapted to isothermal amplification assays such as rolling circle amplification (RCA), recombinase polymerase amplification (RPA), or loop-mediated amplification (LAMP) [7–9]. More recently, RNA-guided CRISPR (Clustered Regularly Interspaced Short Palindromic Repeats) enzymes, such as Cas13a and Cas12a, have been used to signal the presence of isothermally generated amplicons [10,11].

In our own previous work, we developed oligonucleotide strand displacement (OSD) probes [12] that were triggered by strand exchange reactions with transiently single-stranded stem-loop sequences [13]. This led to the exquisitely sensitive detection of LAMP amplicons without interference [14]. Loop-mediated amplification-OSD assays that can work with crude samples are especially appealing for POC use [15,16]. These assays have been coupled to highly-sensitive and reliable "yes/no" output signals such as fluorescence, glucose, or hCG (human chorionic gonadotropin) that can be readily read using off-the-shelf cellphones, glucometers, or pregnancy test strips, respectively [14,15,17–21]. Toehold switch RNA sensors have also been used to link iNAATs with in vitro reporter protein translation, leading to colorimetric signals [22].

Even as these iNAAT tests move towards wider adoption, they all still face the same problem as other POC assays, in that the answers they give are relatively simplistic. However, given that the strand exchange reactions that underlie OSD probes were originally derived from far more complex DNA computations [12,23–25], it may be possible to go beyond mere improvements in specificity and to integrate additional desirable features directly into the molecular diagnostic itself, such that the reaction helps to "compute" its own outcome. As examples, we have previously developed strand exchange computation modules that can quantitate inputs to isothermal amplification reactions [26], or that can integrate multiple molecular signals via Boolean logic operations [19].

We now attempt to take on real-world problems with computations that are embedded in the smart molecular diagnostics themselves. It is unfortunately a fundamental fact that diagnostic targets often evolve faster than assays designed to detect them. The resulting target sequence variations can easily prevent recognition of assay primers and probes, leading to test failure and false negative readouts, a problem which to date can only be solved via regular (and impractical) assay updates [27,28]. For instance, primers and probes for all eight published reverse transcription (RT) qPCR assays (qRT-PCR) for Zika virus (ZIKV) were found to have numerous mismatches with multiple ZIKV genomes sequenced from recent outbreaks [29]. Although most mismatched alleles were common among all outbreak samples and had likely appeared prior to entry of ZIKV into the Americas, new mutations were also found. Most of these were detected in fewer than 10% of samples, but one new mutation appeared in as many as 29% of the samples [29]. These data suggest that continuing viral genome evolution could lead to accumulation of mismatches with diagnostic assay oligonucleotides, which might in turn decrease amplification efficiency and assay sensitivity [30–32]. Limited sensitivity of diagnostic tests combined with relatively low viral loads may cause a significant number of ZIKV-infected patients to remain undiagnosed [28].

To overcome this problem and increase the overall accuracy of POC nucleic acid testing we have engineered additional computations into our smart molecular diagnostics that can compute the presence of almost any ZIKV variant. Strategic degenerate bases in 21 multiplex primers allow the amplification of multiple ZIKV viral genes and gene variants in four, simultaneous LAMP reactions. The presence of any positive signal is calculated by multi-input Boolean "OR"-gated logic processors in a single reaction that directly analyzes crude biological samples and provides a visual yes/no readout for any ZIKV variant within 60–90 min. As with previous LAMP-OSD assays, the exquisite sequence-specificity of oligonucleotide strand exchange probes ensures signal specificity, while the built-in assay redundancy of the molecular logic processors guards against false negatives.

To demonstrate the utility of this smart molecular diagnostic we detected both Asian and African lineage ZIKVs, which can differ by as much as 12% [33], and cleanly distinguished them from otherwise related and often co-circulating dengue virus (DENV) and chikungunya virus (CHIKV). Pilot studies with un-infected and ZIKV-infected *Aedes aegypti* mosquitoes suggest that the integrated computations performed by our smart molecular diagnostic yielded results that are on par with qRT-PCR and demonstrate 100% specificity and sensitivity.

2. Materials and Methods

2.1. Chemicals and Reagents

All chemicals were of analytical grade and were purchased from Sigma–Aldrich (St. Louis, MO, USA) unless otherwise indicated. All enzymes and related buffers were purchased from New England Biolabs (NEB, Ipswich, MA, USA) unless otherwise indicated. All oligonucleotides and gene blocks (summarized in Supplementary Tables S1–S4) were obtained from Integrated DNA Technologies (IDT, Coralville, IA, USA). Virus genomic RNA and inactivated virions (Supplementary Table S5) were obtained from BEI Resources (Manassas, VA, USA).

2.2. Cloning of gBlocks and PCR Amplification of Transcription Templates

The gBlock double stranded DNA surrogates of ZIKV sequences were designed to include a T7 RNA polymerase promoter at their 5′-ends. These gBlocks were cloned into the pCR2.1-TOPO vector (Fisher Scientific, Hampton, NH, USA) by Gibson assembly (NEB) according to the manufacturer's instructions [34]. Cloned plasmids were selected and maintained in an *E. coli* Top10 strain. Plasmid minipreps prepared from these strains using Qiagen miniprep kit (Qiagen, Valencia, CA, USA). All gBlock inserts were verified by Sanger sequencing at the Institute of Cellular and Molecular Biology Core DNA Sequencing Facility.

For performing in vitro run-off transcription, ZIKV gene segments cloned in a pCR2.1-TOPO vector were amplified from sequenced plasmids by PCR using Phusion DNA polymerase. The PCR products were verified by agarose gel electrophoresis and then purified using the Wizard SV gel and PCR clean-up system (Promega, Madison, WI, USA), according to the manufacturer's instructions.

2.3. In Vitro Transcription

Some 1000 ng of purified linear, double-stranded DNA transcription templates were transcribed using the HiScribe T7 High Yield RNA synthesis kit (NEB) according to the manufacturer's instructions. Transcription was allowed to occur at 37 °C for 2 h. Subsequently the transcription reactions were incubated with 2 units of DNase I (NEB) at 37 °C for 30 min to degrade the template DNA prior to RNA gel purification.

2.4. Denaturing Polyacrylamide Gel Electrophoresis and RNA Gel Purification

Denaturing 8% polyacrylamide gels containing 7 M urea were prepared using 40% acrylamide and bis-acrylamide solution, 19:1 (Bio-Rad) in 1× TBE buffer (89 mM Tris Base, 89 mM Boric acid, 2 mM EDTA, pH 8.0) containing 0.04% ammonium persulphate and 0.1% TEMED (N,N,N′,N′-Tetramethylethylenediamine). An equal volume of 2× denaturing dye (7 M urea, 1× TBE, 0.1% bromophenol blue) was added to the RNA samples. These were incubated at 65 °C for 3 min followed by cooling to room temperature before electrophoresis. The RNA bands were demarcated using UV shadowing. Desired bands were excised from the gel and the RNA was eluted twice into Tris-EDTA (TE) (10:1, pH 7.5) buffer (10 mM Tris-HCl, pH 7.5, 1 mM EDTA, pH 8.0) by incubation at 70 °C and 1000 rpm for 20 min. Acrylamide traces were removed by filtering eluates through Ultrafree-MC centrifugal filter units (EMD Millipore, Billerica, MA, USA) followed by precipitation with 2× volume of 100% ethanol in the presence of both 15 µg GlycoBlue (Thermo Fisher Scientific, Waltham, MA, USA) and 0.3 M sodium acetate, pH 5.2. RNA pellets were washed once in 70% ethanol. Dried pellets of purified RNA were resuspended in 0.1 mM EDTA and stored at −80 °C.

2.5. LAMP Primer and Strand Exchange Probe Design

Zika virus genomic sequences were analyzed for variation using the National Center for Biotechnology Information (NCBI) Virus Variation Resource [35]. Zika virus sequences were also compared to related and co-circulating viruses, such as DENV and CHIKV, using MUSCLE [36,37]. Four relatively conserved genomic regions in ZIKV *capsid*, *NS1*, *NS3*, and *NS5* genes were chosen for primer design. The Primer Explorer v5 LAMP (loop-mediated isothermal amplification) primer design software (Eiken Chemical Co., Tokyo, Japan) was used for generating LAMP primer sets composed of the outer primers F3 and B3 and the inner primers FIP (forward inner primer) and BIP (backward inner primer). Primer design was constrained to include at least a 40 base pair (bp) gap between the F1 and F2 as well as between the B1 and B2 priming sites. Loop primers and stem primers were manually designed. Primer specificity for ZIKV isolates and a corresponding lack of significant cross-reactivity to other nucleic acids of human or pathogenic origin was further assessed using NCBI BLAST [38,39]. Polymorphic loci in the primers were substituted with degenerate bases, although some polymorphisms near the 5'-end of F3 or B3 or near the middle of FIP or BIP were ignored to reduce the degeneracy burden and to ensure efficient amplification [17]. Our previous work had shown that such mismatches minimally disrupted LAMP primer efficiency [17].

The nucleic acid circuit design software NUPACK [40] was used to design four OSD probes, each specific to one of the four ZIKV amplicons, according to our previously published design rules [14]. Unique, fluorophore-labeled OSD strands were designed to bind between B1 and B2 sequences of *NS5* and *NS3* amplicons and between F1 and F2 sequences of *NS1* and *capsid* amplicons. The quencher-labeled OSD strands were designed to be partially complementary to the fluorophore-labeled strand. Single-stranded toeholds at the 3'-end or 5'-end of fluorophore-labeled strands were designed to be 10 or 13 nucleotides long. All 3'-OH ends were blocked with inverted deoxythymidine (dT) to prevent extension by DNA polymerase. Polymorphic loci in all four OSD probes were substituted with appropriate degenerate bases. These degenerate OSD probe strands were then used as a basis for designing the two-input 2GO and four-input 4GO probes. The web application NUPACK was used to visualize and optimize probe architecture with variables such as buffer composition, temperature, and oligonucleotide concentrations.

2.6. Assembly of Strand Exchange Probes

The OSD probes were prepared by annealing 1 µM of the fluorophore-labeled OSD strand with 5 µM of the quencher-labeled strand in 1× isothermal buffer (NEB: 20 mM Tris-HCl, 10 mM $(NH_4)_2SO_4$, 50 mM KCl, 2 mM $MgSO_4$, 0.1% Tween 20, pH 8.8 at 25 °C). Annealing was performed by denaturing the oligonucleotide mix at 95 °C for 1 min followed by slow cooling at the rate of 0.1 °C/s to 25 °C. Excess annealed probe was stored at −20 °C.

The CAN3.2GO probe was assembled by annealing 4 µM of CAN3.2GO.Gate oligonucleotide with 6 µM of the quencher-labeled CAN3.2GO.Q oligonucleotide and 2 µM of the fluorophore-labeled CAN3.2GO.FAM oligonucleotide. Similarly, the N1N5.2GO probe was assembled by annealing 6 µM of N5N1.2GO.Gate oligonucleotide with 8 µM of the quencher-labeled N5N1.2GO.Q oligonucleotide and 2 µM of the fluorophore-labeled N5N1.2GO.FAM oligonucleotide. The three oligonucleotide components of each 2GO probe were mixed in 1× isothermal buffer supplemented with 8 mM $MgSO_4$ and incubated for 1 min at 95 °C. The mixture was then slowly cooled at the rate of 0.1 °C/s to 25 °C. Excess annealed 2GO probes were stored at −20 °C.

The 4GO probe was assembled by annealing 4 µM of the 4GO.S1 strand, 1 µM of the fluorophore-labeled 4GO.S2 strand, 4 µM of the quencher-labeled 4GO.S3 strand, 4 µM of the 4GO.S4 strand, and

3 µM of the 4GO.S5 strand. All oligonucleotides were mixed in 1× isothermal buffer supplemented with 8 mM MgSO$_4$ and incubated for 1 min at 95 °C. The mixture was then slowly cooled at the rate of 0.1 °C/s to 25 °C. Excess annealed 4GO probes were stored at −20 °C.

2.7. RT-LAMP Assay

All RT-LAMP assays were assembled in 25 µL reactions containing 1× isothermal buffer supplemented with 1.4 mM deoxyribonucleotides (dNTPs), 0.4 M betaine, 6 mM additional MgSO$_4$, 16 units of Bst 2.0 DNA polymerase (NEB), and 7.5 units of warmstart RTx reverse transcriptase (NEB). Reactions containing primers for only one target gene were appended with 2.4 µM each of a single type of FIP and BIP primer (*NS5* assay utilized 4.8 µM BIP), 1.2 µM of the corresponding loop primer, 1.2 µM of the corresponding stem primer (only for the *capsid* assay), and 0.6 µM each of the corresponding F3 and B3 primer. Primer-containing multiplex LAMP reactions received 0.6 µM of each of the four FIP and BIP primers (*NS5* BIP primer was added at 1.2 µM concentration), 0.3 µM of each of the four loop primers, 0.3 µM of the *capsid* stem primer, and 0.15 µM each of the four F3 and B3 primers. The total primer content of these multiplex assays was similar to individual primer concentrations used in LAMP reactions for single target genes. Control assays lacking primers received equivalent volume of TE 10:0.1 buffer (10 mM Tris, pH 7.5, and 0.1 mM EDTA pH 8.0).

Loop-mediated amplification assays read using OSD reporters received 200 nM of the fluorophore-labeled strand annealed with a five-fold excess of the complementary quencher-labeled strand (see Section 2.6.). Multiplex LAMP-OSD assays received 50 nM of each of the four fluorophore-labeled OSD strands pre-annealed individually with five-fold excess of their corresponding quencher-labeled complementary strands.

Assays analyzed using 2GO probes were supplemented with 50 mM trehalose and 100 nM of the fluorophore-labeled probe strand pre-annealed with the complementary gate and quencher-labeled oligonucleotides as described in Section 2.6. Multiplex assays read using the complete bipartite signal transducer contained 100 nM each of both CAN3.2GO and N1N5.2GO probes. Assays read using 4GO probes were also supplemented with 50 mM trehalose along with 80 nM of the fluorophore-labeled strand annealed with the remaining four strands of the 4GO probe as described in Section 2.6.

Real-time measurement of fluorescence accumulation was performed using the LightCycler96 real-time PCR machine (Roche, Basel, Switzerland). Reactions were subjected to isothermal amplification by programming 45 cycles of 150 sec at 65 °C (step 1) followed by 30 sec at 65 °C (step 2). Fluorescence was measured in the FAM (Fluorescein) channel during step 2 of each amplification cycle. Post-amplification reporter fluorescence was also monitored by programming the LightCycler96 to hold the assays at 37 °C for 40 min.

Loop-mediated amplification-based assays intended for visual readout and smartphone imaging were assembled in 0.2 mL optically clear thin-walled tubes with low auto-fluorescence (Axygen, Union City, CA, USA). Following 90–120 min of incubation in a 65 °C heat block, the reactions were imaged at room temperature using an unmodified iPhone 6 and an UltraSlim-LED (light emitting diode) transilluminator (Syngene, Frederick, MD, USA). In some experiments, our previously described in-house 3D-printed imaging device [15] was used for fluorescence visualization and smartphone imaging. Briefly, this device uses Super Bright Blue 5-mm light emitting diodes (LED) (Adafruit, New York, NY, USA) to excite fluorescence. Two cut-to-fit layers of inexpensive >500 nm bandpass orange lighting gel sheets (Lee Filters, Burbank, CA, USA) placed on the observation window filter the fluorescence for observation and imaging.

The following ZIKV templates were analyzed by LAMP-OSD, LAMP-2GO, and LAMP-4GO assays: (i) zero to several thousands of copies of ZIKV synthetic RNA or genomic RNA in TE 10:0.1 buffer. Zika virus genomic RNA preparations, obtained from BEI Resources, were contained in a background of cellular nucleic acid and carrier RNA that were isolated from preparations of cell lysates and supernatants from *Cercopithecus aethiops* kidney epithelial cells (Vero 76, clone E6: ATCC ® CRL-1586™) infected with specific ZIKV (Supplementary Table S5); (ii) ZIKV virions in TE 10:0.1 buffer; (iii) un-infected and

ZIKV-infected *Ae. aegypti* mosquitoes (see Section 2.10.). Negative controls included (i) assays without any templates; (ii) assays with non-specific templates including synthetic RNA, DENV genomic RNA, and CHIKV genomic RNA; and (iii) assays with non-specific amplicons (generated by substituting with a non-specific template and its cognate LAMP primer set).

2.8. TaqMan qRT-PCR Analysis

The previously reported ZIKV NS2b-specific TaqMan qRT-PCR assay (Supplementary Table S4) [41] was performed using either the Evoscript RNA Probes Master (Roche, Basel, Switzerland) or the TaqMan RNA-to-Ct 1-Step Kit (Thermo Scientific, Waltham MA, USA). Standard curves were prepared using a ten-fold dilution series of 10^5 to 10 copies of a synthetic RNA template (Supplementary Table S4). Reactions without any templates served as negative controls. These templates were subjected to one-step qRT-PCR in 10 μL reactions containing 800 nM each of forward (Zika4481_F) and reverse (Zika4552c_R) primers along with 200 nM of the TaqMan probe (Zika4507cTqMFAM). Amplification was performed by adding either (i) 2 μL of the 5× Evoscript RNA probes Master or (ii) 0.25 μL of the 40X TaqMan RT Enzyme Mix (Thermo Scientific) along with 5 μL of the 2× TaqMan RNA-to-Ct 1-Step master mix. Reactions were incubated for 30 min at 60 °C followed by 10 min at 95 °C. Subsequently 45 cycles of 15 sec at 95 °C and 30 sec at 55 °C were performed. TaqMan fluorescence was measured during the second step of each cycle. Reactions containing Evoscript RNA Probes Master were analyzed using the LightCycler96 qPCR machine while TaqMan RNA-to-Ct 1-Step assays were performed on the StepOnePlus real-time PCR machine (Thermo Scientific).

2.9. Analysis of ZIKV Virions

Heat-inactivated virions of Asian ZIKV strain PRVABC59 (BEI Resources, Manassas, VA, USA) were used as templates for LAMP-based assays and for one-step qRT-PCR. Virions were diluted in TE 10:0.1 buffer prior to being directly added to LAMP-based and qRT-PCR reactions.

2.10. Rearing and Analysis of ZIKV-Infected Mosquitoes

Aedes aegypti mosquitoes were reared under conventional conditions in the insectary at the University of Texas medical Branch, Galveston, TX, USA. To obtain ZIKV-infected insects, mosquitoes were starved for a period of 24 hours and then offered a sheep blood meal (Colorado Serum Company, Denver, CO, USA) containing 10^6 virions using a hemotek membrane system (Hemotek). Un-infected mosquitoes received a blood meal that did not contain virus. After 14 days, mosquitoes were collected and immediately frozen at −80 °C. Prior to molecular testing, each mosquito was heated for 10 min at 60 °C in order to inactivate the Zika virus [42] for compliance with biosafety level 2 requirements. Each mosquito was then manually crushed in a 1.7 mL microcentrifuge tube using a disposable micropestle (Fisherbrand™ RNase-Free Disposable Pellet Pestles, Catalog number 12-141-364, Fisher Scientific, Hampton, NH, USA). Each macerated mosquito was re-suspended in 100 μL water. A 2 μL aliquot of this mosquito sample was directly assessed by *Ae. aegypti coi* LAMP-OSD assay in both primer-containing and primer-free reactions. For ZIKV LAMP-based reactions and qRT-PCR assays, 3 μL mosquito samples were directly used as sources of templates. Both primer-containing and primer-less LAMP-based assays were operated.

3. Results

3.1. Degenerate LAMP-OSD Assays for Detection of Asian and African Lineage ZIKV

Zika virus has an ~10 kilobase RNA genome encoding a polyprotein that is cleaved into ten structural and non-structural (NS) proteins: 5′-Capsid (C)-preMembrane (prM)-Envelope (E)-NS1-NS2A-NS2B-NS3-NS4A-NS4B-NS5-3′. Zika virus clusters into two African lineages and one Asian lineage that includes the current epidemic strains [33]. The Asian and African lineages of ZIKV show 0.2% to 10.6% intra-lineage and 4.5% to 12.1% inter-lineage nucleotide variation [33].

The epidemic strains have accumulated additional changes and have potentially undergone multiple natural recombinations [33,43]. The strains are likely continuing to evolve, presenting a challenging target for surveillance and diagnostics. Here, we designed four reverse transcription (RT) LAMP assays to amplify relatively conserved regions in four ZIKV genes—*capsid* (CA), *NS1*, *NS3*, and *NS5*. Each individual assay included two inner primers (FIP and BIP), two outer primers (B3 and F3), and one loop primer (LP). The CA LAMP assay utilized an additional sixth primer, termed stem primer [44] (SP), complementary to the target region between F1 and B1 priming sites (Figure 1A). Specific nucleotide positions within these primers were substituted with degenerate nucleobases to allow pairing with variant ZIKV RNA (Supplementary Table S1). The NS3 LAMP primer set had the lowest degeneracy with only 10 positions varying between two nucleobases and one position varying between three nucleobases. Twelve positions in the NS1 LAMP primer set varied between two nucleobases. The CA LAMP primers had a slightly higher degeneracy with 13 polymorphic positions varying between two bases. The NS5 primer set was the most degenerate with 15, 6, and 1 positions varying between two, three, or four bases, respectively.

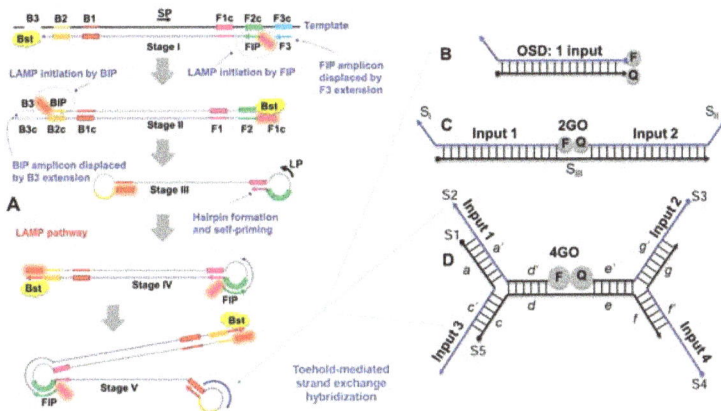

Figure 1. Schematic depicting (**A**) loop-mediated isothermal amplification (LAMP) integrated with (**B**) one-, (**C**) two-, or (**D**) four-input oligonucleotide strand exchange signal transducers. LAMP uses 2 inner (FIP and BIP) and 2 outer (F3 and B3) primers along with the optional stem (SP) and loop (LP) primers to prime strand displacement DNA amplification by Bst DNA polymerase. The resulting continuous amplification (initiated by both new primer-binding and by self-priming) generates double-stranded concatameric amplicons containing single-stranded loops to which non-priming oligonucleotide strand exchange signal transducers can hybridize. The one-input OSD signal transducer composed of one long and one short DNA strand can hybridize to a single LAMP amplicon loop sequence leading to separation of the fluorophore (F) and quencher (Q). The OR Boolean logic processing two-input strand exchange transducer, 2GO, is composed of two labeled strands, S_I and S_{II}, and a third bridging strand S_{III}. Either S_I and/or S_{II} can hybridize to their specific LAMP loop sequences resulting in separation of F and Q. The four-input 4GO probe composed of 5 DNA strands (S1–S5) can hybridize to any combination of up to four different LAMP amplicon loops and perform an OR Boolean operation to produce fluorescence signal. The 4GO probe is denoted in terms of lettered domains (*a–g*), each of which represents a short fragment of DNA sequence in an otherwise continuous oligonucleotide strand. Complementarity is denoted by a single prime symbol.

To ensure readout specificity, individual hemiduplex OSD probes [14] were designed for each of the four ZIKV LAMP amplicons (Figure 1B). To facilitate detection of LAMP amplicons from different viral lineages, probe nucleotide positions corresponding to polymorphic target loci were substituted with degenerate bases (Supplementary Table S2). The NS3 OSD probe was the least degenerate with only two positions in the long and the short probe strands varying between two bases. The *capsid*

OSD probe contained two nucleotide variations at four and two positions in the long and the short strand, respectively. Three positions in both the long and the short strands of the *NS5* OSD probe varied between two bases. The *NS1* OSD probes displayed the greatest degeneracy with four positions in both the long and the short strands varying between two bases.

Performance of these four degenerate reverse transcription LAMP-OSD assays was optimized in individual amplification reactions containing different amounts of synthetic target RNA derived from ZIKV genomic sequences (Supplementary Table S3). All four assays could detect a few hundred copies of synthetic target RNA within 60 min without producing spurious signal (Figure 2). Furthermore, the high signal amplitude and low noise allowed simple yes/no visual readouts and cellphone imaging of these assays—target RNA yielded bright visible fluorescence while assays lacking specific templates remained dark (Figure 2).

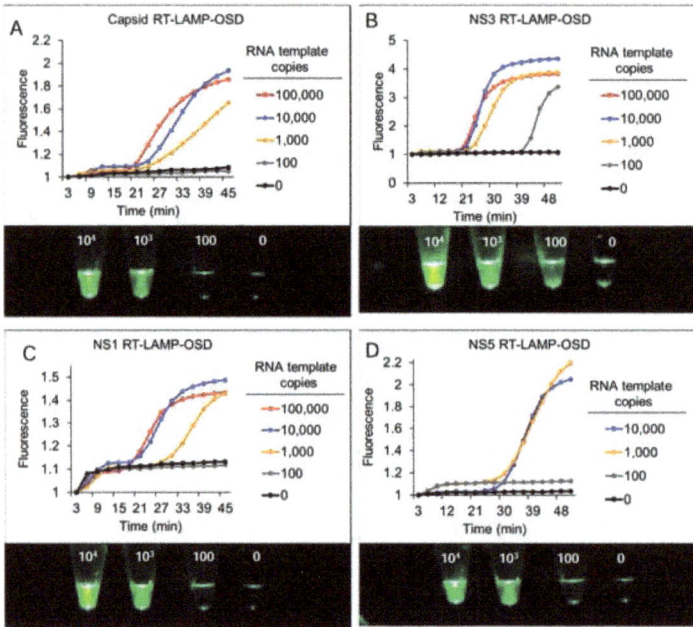

Figure 2. Detection of Zika virus *capsid*, *NS1*, *NS3*, and *NS5* genes using real-time and visually-read reverse transcription LAMP-OSD assays. Indicated copies of *capsid* (**A**), *NS3* (**B**), *NS1* (**C**), and *NS5* (**D**) synthetic RNA templates were amplified by degenerate LAMP-OSD assays specific to each template. OSD fluorescence signals measured in real-time during LAMP amplification are depicted as red (10^5 template copies), blue (10^4 template copies), orange (10^3 template copies), gray (100 template copies), and black (0 template copies; 10^6 non-template RNA) traces. The *x*-axis depicts the duration of LAMP amplification. OSD fluorescence was also imaged at amplification endpoint using a cellphone (images depicted at the bottom of each panel). Numbers on each assay tube in these images indicate the RNA template copies used. Representative results from three replicate experiments are depicted.

To verify that all the four assays could identify both Asian and African lineage ZIKV genomes we individually challenged *NS1*, *NS3*, *NS5*, and *CA* LAMP-OSD assays with genomic RNA from nine Asian ZIKV, and two African ZIKV strains (Supplementary Table S5). Reaction specificity was assessed by seeding duplicate assays with genomic RNA of related dengue virus (DENV) serotypes 1–4 and chikungunya virus (CHIKV) that often co-circulate with ZIKV [45]. Endpoint OSD fluorescence in all LAMP assays seeded with Asian or African ZIKV genomes was significantly elevated above background noise in assays seeded with DENV or CHIKV genomic RNA (Figure 3). These results demonstrate that all four degenerate LAMP-OSD assays were capable of lineage-independent ZIKV detection without cross-reaction with or interference from non-target nucleic acids. In contrast, LAMP-OSD assays containing non-degenerate versions of the same primers demonstrated reduced breadth of detection. The *capsid* and *NS3* assays recognized only Asian lineages. The *NS1* assay recognized all Asian lineage and one of the two African lineage ZIKV genomes. Meanwhile, the *NS5* assay recognized both the African lineage genomes while failing to give a signal with any Asian lineage ZIKV (Supplementary Figure S1).

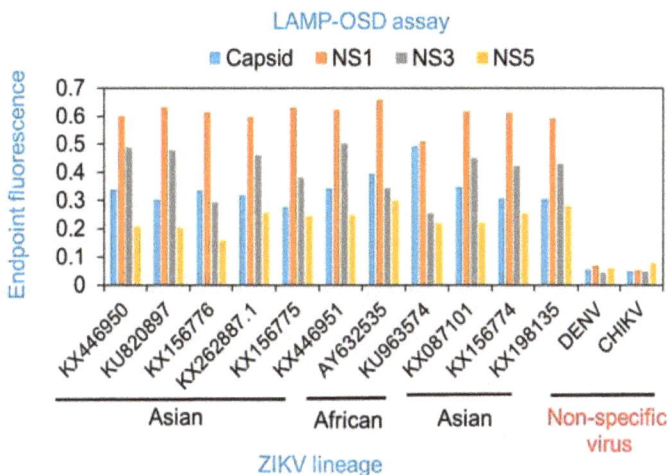

Figure 3. Detection of Asian and African lineage ZIKV using degenerate reverse transcription LAMP-OSD assays. Genomic RNA from DENV, CHIKV, or Asian or African lineage ZIKV (indicated by their GenBank accession numbers) were used as templates for amplification in degenerate RT-LAMP-OSD assays for Zika virus *capsid*, *NS1*, *NS3*, and *NS5* genes. OSD fluorescence signals measured at amplification endpoint using LightCycler 96 real-time PCR machine are depicted as blue (*capsid*), orange (*NS1*), gray (*NS3*), and yellow (*NS5*) bars. Representative results from three replicate experiments are depicted.

3.2. Multiplex LAMP with Degenerate Primers and OSD Probes

To create a multiplex, internally redundant assay that simultaneously amplifies and detects *CA*, *NS1*, *NS3*, and *NS5* sequences, all 21 LAMP primers and 4 hemi-duplex OSD reporters were combined in a single reaction (multiplex LAMP-OSD). To verify that each individual reverse transcription LAMP-OSD reaction was functional in this multiplex environment, replicate multiplex assays were supplemented with all 21 primers but only a single type of OSD reporter at a time. In the presence of all four ZIKV synthetic RNA templates, multiplex LAMP-OSD demonstrated exponential fluorescence accumulation. Despite co-mingling of multiple degenerate primers and OSD probes, no spurious signals were observed in the absence of specific templates (Figure 4A). As a result, brightly fluorescent ZIKV-positive assays containing only a few hundred copies of ZIKV templates could be readily distinguished from dark ZIKV-negative reactions by simple visual examination (Figure 4B). Each individual LAMP assay was functional in the multiplex assay, as indicated by accumulation of fluorescence in multiplex LAMP-OSD reactions probed with individual OSD reporters (Figure 4C–F). The multiplex LAMP-OSD assay could also readily identify the more complex ZIKV genomic RNA from both Asian and African lineages without cross-reaction with DENV and CHIKV genomic nucleic acids (Figure 4G).

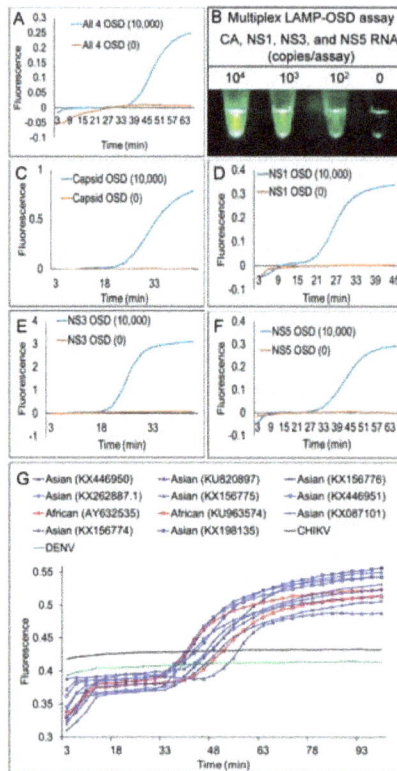

Figure 4. Simultaneous detection of four Zika virus genes using multiplex reverse transcription degenerate LAMP-OSD (multiplex LAMP-OSD) assay. (**A**) Real-time multiplex LAMP-OSD—synthetic RNA mixtures containing indicated copies of each of the four ZIKV synthetic RNA templates (*CA*, *NS1*, *NS3*, and *NS5*) were amplified using multiplex LAMP-OSD assays containing 21 degenerate primers and 4 degenerate OSD probes for simultaneous LAMP amplification and sequence-specific detection of all four ZIKV targets. OSD fluorescence signals measured in real-time during LAMP amplification are depicted as blue (10,000 copies each of *CA*, *NS1*, *NS3*, and *NS5* RNA) and orange (0 ZIKV RNA; 10^6 copies of DENV RNA) traces. The *x*-axis depicts the duration of LAMP amplification. (**B**) Endpoint multiplex LAMP-OSD assay with visual detection—synthetic RNA mixtures containing indicated copies of each of the four ZIKV synthetic RNA templates (*CA*, *NS1*, *NS3*, and *NS5*) were amplified using degenerate multiplex LAMP-OSD assays. OSD fluorescence was imaged after 90 min of amplification using a cellphone. Numbers above each assay tube indicate the RNA template copies used. The reaction with '0' ZIKV RNA received 10^6 copies of DENV RNA. (**C-F**) Performance of individual assays in the multiplex LAMP-OSD system—synthetic RNA mixtures containing indicated copies of each of the four ZIKV synthetic RNA templates (*CA*, *NS1*, *NS3*, and *NS5*) were amplified using multiplex LAMP-OSD assays containing LAMP primers for all four targets but only one type of OSD for either *capsid* (**C**), *NS1* (**D**), *NS3* (**E**), or *NS5* (**F**) amplicons. OSD fluorescence signals measured in real-time during LAMP amplification are depicted as blue (10,000 copies each of *CA*, *NS1*, *NS3*, and *NS5* RNA) and orange (0 ZIKV RNA; 10^6 copies of DENV RNA) traces. The *x*-axis depicts the duration of LAMP amplification. (**G**) Detection of Asian and African lineage ZIKV genomic RNA using degenerate multiplex LAMP-OSD assays. Genomic RNA from DENV, CHIKV, or Asian or African lineage ZIKV (indicated by their GenBank accession numbers) were used as templates for amplification. Real-time OSD fluorescence signals are depicted as blue (Asian), red (African), black (CHIKV), and green (DENV) traces. The *x*-axis depicts the duration of LAMP amplification. For all experiments, representative results from three replicate tests are depicted.

3.3. Multiplex LAMP with Degenerate Primers and Four-Input Logic-Processing Probes

After functionally verifying the feasibility of multiplex reverse transcription LAMP-OSD using degenerate primers and OSD probes, we sought to reduce reaction cost and enhance assay versatility by replacing the four individual OSD probes with a single four-input OR Boolean logic-processing strand exchange probe (4GO) that would "compute" the presence of ZIKV by simultaneously looking across *CA*, *NS1*, *NS3*, and *NS5* amplicons for similarity to the probe. Unlike four individual OSDs that required a combination of 8 fluorophore or quencher-labeled oligonucleotides, the three-way junction 4GO probe would need a single fluorophore-quencher pair (Figure 1). If either *CA*, *NS1*, *NS3*, or *NS5* amplicon was similar enough to initiate strand exchange, the fluorophore would separate from the quencher and the 4GO probe would light up.

The 4GO probe was composed of 5 oligonucleotides (S1–S5) with a total of 19 degenerate loci that varied between two nucleobases (Supplementary Table S2). Oligonucleotides S1–S4, designed based on validated degenerate OSD sequences, served as strand exchange probes for *NS1*, *NS5*, *CA*, and *NS3* amplicons, respectively. The S5 strand acted as a scaffold for 4GO probe assembly (Figure 1D). Domain *c* at the 5'-end of S5 was complementary to domain *c'* in S1, while domain *f* at the 3'-end of S5 was complementary to domain *f'* of the S4 strand. The intervening region of S5 contained two short target-independent sequences—domain *d* complementary to domain *d'* at the fluorophore-labeled 5'-end of S2 and domain *e* complementary to domain *e'* at the quencher-labeled 3'-end of S3. Concomitant hybridization of S2 and S3 to S5 would juxtapose the fluorophore and quencher leading to loss of signal. However, at temperatures ≥20 °C, pairing of S2 and S5 was contingent upon formation of a three-way junction with S1 via interactions between complementary S2 domain *a'* with S1 domain *a* and S5 domain *c* with S1 domain *c'*. Similarly, stable interaction of S3 and S5 was dependent upon a three-way hybridization with S4. As a result, strand exchange between the 4GO probe and any one or more of the ZIKV amplicons would separate the fluorophore-bearing S2 from quencher-labeled S3. For example, the *NS5* LAMP amplicon loop would directly remove S2 from the 4GO probe. Meanwhile, by binding S1, the *NS1* amplicons would destroy the three-way junction between S1, S2, and S5. Consequently, the 4GO probe would transduce the presence of one or any combination of the four ZIKV amplicons into a single-channel endpoint fluorescence that could be easily read at ambient temperature.

To test 4GO probe function, multiplex reverse transcription LAMP reactions containing all 21 degenerate primers and the degenerate 4GO probe (multiplex LAMP-4GO) were spiked with a single type or a combination of all four of the ZIKV synthetic RNA templates *NS1*, *NS3*, *NS5*, and *CA*. As a control to assess signal specificity, duplicate reactions were assembled using a non-specific RNA template and its cognate LAMP primers that would lead to generation of non-specific LAMP amplicons. Following LAMP amplification, 4GO probe fluorescence was found to be elevated in all reactions containing even a few hundred copies of at least one of the ZIKV templates (Figure 5A–E). This ZIKV-specific signal remained consistently above noise generated in the absence of specific amplicons. These results demonstrate that the 4GO probe was able to function specifically in multiplex LAMP to identify and signal the presence of a few hundred copies of one or all four ZIKV amplicons without interference from non-specific templates or amplicons.

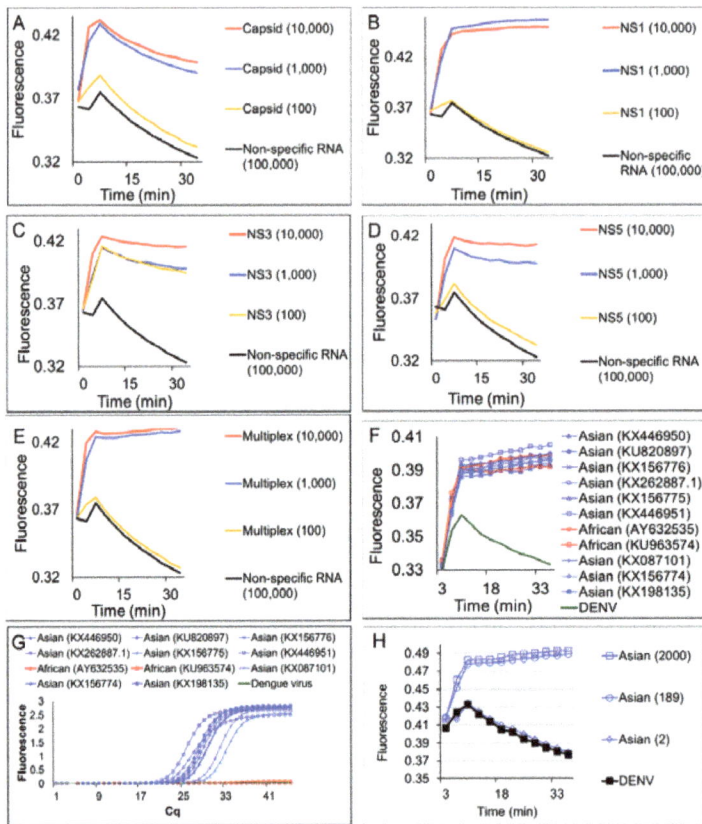

Figure 5. Simultaneous detection of four Zika virus genes using degenerate 4GO probes and multiplex degenerate reverse transcription LAMP (multiplex LAMP-4GO) assays. Indicated copies of *capsid*, *NS1*, *NS3*, and *NS5* synthetic target RNA were amplified either individually (panels **A–D**, respectively) or as a mixture (panel **E**) using multiplex LAMP-4GO assays containing LAMP primers for all four ZIKV targets and the four-input 4GO probe. 4GO probe fluorescence, measured in real-time at 37 °C after 90 min of LAMP amplification, is depicted as red (10,000 template copies), blue (1,000 template copies), yellow (100 template copies), and black (non-specific LAMP primers with 10^5 copies of its target RNA) traces. The *x*-axis depicts the duration of endpoint signal measurement. (**F**) Detection of Asian and African lineage ZIKV genomic RNA using degenerate multiplex LAMP-4GO assays. Genomic RNA from DENV, or Asian or African lineage ZIKV (indicated by their GenBank accession numbers) were used as templates for amplification. 4GO probe fluorescence, measured in real-time at 37 °C after 90 min of LAMP amplification, is depicted as blue (Asian), red (African), and green (DENV) traces. The x-axis depicts the duration of endpoint signal measurement. (**G**) Detection of Asian and African lineage ZIKV genomic RNA using TaqMan qRT-PCR assay specific for Asian lineage ZIKV NS2b gene. Same amount of viral genomic RNA as was used in panel **F** were amplified and real-time measurements of assay fluorescence are depicted as blue (Asian), red (African), and green (DENV) traces. (**H**) Detection limit of degenerate multiplex LAMP-4GO assay for ZIKV genomic RNA. Indicated copies of an Asian lineage ZIKV genome or non-specific DENV genomes were amplified using multiplex LAMP-4GO assays. 4GO probe fluorescence, measured in real-time at 37 °C after 90 min of LAMP amplification, is depicted as blue (Asian) and black (DENV) traces with template copies indicated by open squares (2000 genomes), open circles (189 genomes), and open diamonds (2 genomes). The *x*-axis depicts the duration of endpoint signal measurement. For all experiments, representative results from three replicate tests are depicted.

The 4GO probes were also able to specifically identify all nine Asian and both African ZIKV strains tested without cross reaction with related viruses (Figure 5F). Endpoint fluorescence signals in all degenerate multiplex LAMP-4GO assays seeded with Asian or African lineage ZIKV genomic RNA were consistently elevated above background noise in assays containing non-specific DENV genomes. In contrast, a previously reported Asian ZIKV *NS2b* gene-specific TaqMan qRT-PCR assay [41] was able to detect only Asian lineage viral genomes while failing to amplify African lineage genomic RNA (Figure 5G). Asian genomic RNA copy numbers estimated from this qRT-PCR assay (Supplementary Figure S2) suggested that multiplex LAMP-4GO assays could readily detect a few hundred copies of viral genomes (Figure 5H). These results demonstrate that a single assay comprised of 21 degenerate LAMP primers and a five-stranded degenerate logic processing strand exchange probe could reliably detect viral variants within a genus and distinguish them from related viruses. Furthermore, by integrating signals from four separate inputs into one output via a single fluorophore-quencher pair, the five-stranded 4GO probe could capture the viral diversity at a fraction of the cost of four individually-labeled OSD probes.

3.4. Multiplex LAMP with Degenerate Primers and Two-Input Logic-Processing Probes

Our results demonstrated that the multiplex LAMP-4GO assay could specifically identify both Asian and African ZIKV without non-specific signaling. However, a fluorimeter was necessary for assay readout due to the relatively high background noise of the 4GO probe. Therefore, we sought to further engineer the logic processing probe in order to achieve a signal-to-noise ratio that could be visually discriminated and thereby allowed easy "yes/no" assay readout in austere conditions without complex instruments. We surmised that the fluorophore was insufficiently quenched in the five-stranded 4GO probe due to its high degeneracy level. To reduce probe degeneracy, we engineered a bipartite four-input signal processor composed of two OR gated strand exchange modules (2GO) (Figure 1C). Each 2GO probe was comprised of three degenerate oligonucleotides (S_I–S_{III}) that were partially complementary to each other. The 5'-ends of both S_I strands were labeled with the same type of fluorophore while the 3'-ends of S_{II} strands were labeled with the corresponding quencher molecules. Simultaneous hybridization of S_I and S_{II} to the unlabeled S_{III} strand would juxtapose the fluorophore and quencher resulting in loss of signal. Short single-stranded toeholds at the 3'- and 5'-ends of S_I and S_{II}, respectively, could independently initiate strand exchange with their cognate target sequences resulting in separation of the fluorophore from the quencher and a concomitant rise in signal. For instance, the CAN3.2GO probe fluorescence would increase if it underwent strand exchange with either CA or N3 amplicons. Similarly, the N1N5.2GO probe would signal if either or both *NS1* and *NS5* amplicons were present.

To functionally verify the bipartite signal processor, reverse transcription LAMP assays containing the degenerate CAN3.2GO or the NS1NS5.2GO probes were supplemented with primers specific to either ZIKV *NS1*, *NS3*, *NS5*, or *CA* genes. At amplification endpoint, fluorescence of CAN3.2GO probe increased only in assays containing CA or *N3* amplicons (Figure 6A). Meanwhile the N1N5.2GO probe was activated only in the presence of *NS1* or *NS5* sequences. Both probes remained quenched in the presence of non-specific LAMP amplicons. Moreover, amplicon-specific 2GO probe fluorescence could be readily distinguished from non-specific noise simply by direct visual examination of assay tubes or their cellphone images (Figure 6B).

The complete multiplex assay system (multiplex LAMP-2GO) containing 21 degenerate LAMP primers and the bipartite signal processor (CAN3.2GO + N1N5.2GO) was tested using different amounts of a synthetic RNA mixture containing all four ZIKV templates (*NS1*, *NS3*, *NS5*, and *CA*). Assays containing only a few hundred copies of ZIKV RNA produced bright fluorescence that could be readily captured using unmodified smartphone camera (Figure 6C). In contrast, assays containing non-specific amplicons remained dark thereby allowing easy visual distinction from ZIKV-positive assays.

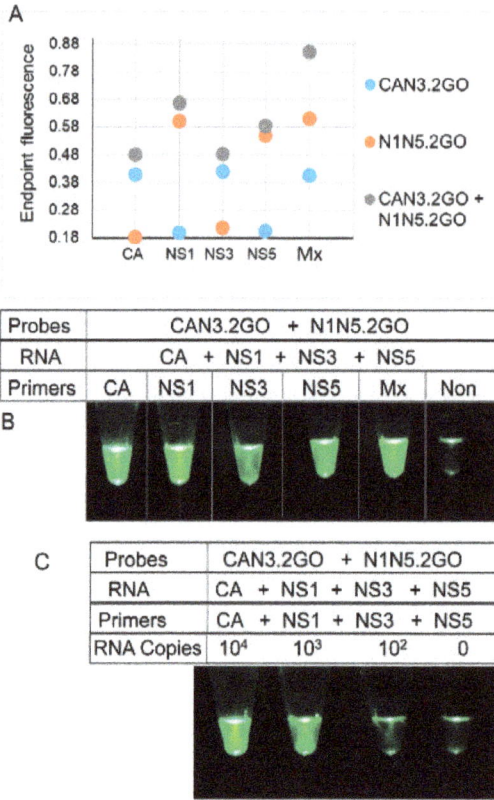

Figure 6. Detection of ZIKV RNA using two-input 2GO probes and degenerate reverse transcription LAMP. (**A**) Sequence-dependent activation of 2GO probes—synthetic RNA mixtures of 10^6 copies of *CA*, *NS1*, *NS3*, and *NS5* RNA were amplified using individual or multiplex (Mx) degenerate LAMP assays containing either one or both CAN3.2GO and N1N5.2GO probes. 2GO probe fluorescence signals measured at amplification endpoint using LightCycler 96 real-time PCR machine are depicted as blue (LAMP with only CAN3.2GO), orange (LAMP with only N1N5.2GO), and gray (LAMP with both CAN3.2GO and N1N5.2GO) dots. LAMP primer specificities are indicated on the *x*-axis. (**B**) Visual readout of degenerate LAMP-2GO assays. Cellphone image depicts 2GO probe fluorescence at amplification endpoint in individual or multiplex ZIKV LAMP assays containing both CAN3.2GO and N1N5.2GO probes and 10^6 copies of all four synthetic ZIKV RNA and a non-specific LAMP assay ("Non") containing its cognate RNA. (**C**) Detection limit of visually-read degenerate multiplex LAMP-2GO assays. Cellphone image depicts endpoint 2GO probe fluorescence of multiplex degenerate RT-LAMP assays containing primers and indicated template RNA copies of all four ZIKV targets. The reaction without any ZIKV RNA contained a non-specific RNA and its cognate LAMP primers. For all experiments, representative results from three replicate tests are depicted.

Similar to LAMP-OSD and multiplex LAMP-4GO assays, multiplex LAMP-2GO assays could also detect all nine Asian and both African ZIKV strains tested while suppressing spurious signal from dengue viruses (serotypes 1–4) (Figure 7A). Examination of endpoint smartphone images of multiplex LAMP-2GO assays revealed that as few as 189 copies of a representative Asian ZIKV genomic RNA (quantified using NS2b-specific TaqMan qRT-PCR) could be reliably identified using simple yes/no visual readout of presence or absence of fluorescence (Figure 7B and Supplementary Figure S2).

Similarly, African ZIKV genomic RNA could also be detected using smartphone imaged multiplex LAMP-2GO assays (Figure 7B).

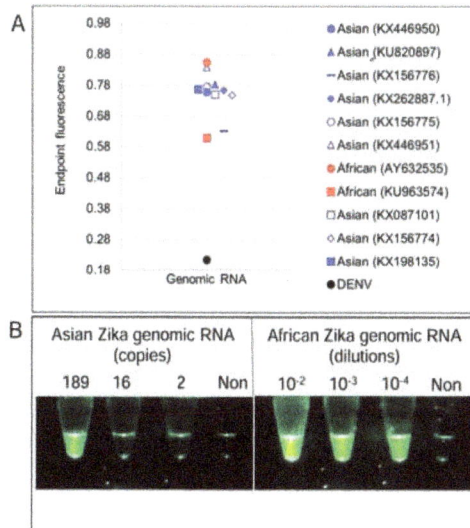

Figure 7. Detection of Asian and African lineage ZIKV genomes using degenerate multiplex LAMP-2GO assays. (**A**) Genomic RNA from DENV, or Asian or African lineage ZIKV (indicated by their GenBank accession numbers) were used as templates for amplification. 2GO probe fluorescence signals measured at amplification endpoint using LightCycler 96 real-time PCR machine are depicted as blue (Asian ZIKV), red (African ZIKV), and black (DENV) markers. (**B**) Detection limit of degenerate multiplex LAMP-2GO assay for ZIKV genomic RNA. Indicated copies of an Asian lineage ZIKV genome (left panel), indicated dilutions of an African ZIKV genome (right panel), and non-specific DENV genomes ("Non") were amplified using multiplex LAMP-2GO assays. 2GO probe fluorescence was imaged at amplification endpoint using a cellphone. For all experiments, representative results from three replicate tests are depicted.

3.5. Identification of ZIKV-Infected Mosquitoes using Cellphones and Smart Molecular Diagnostics

To evaluate assay performance in natural biological matrices, *Ae. aegypti* mosquitoes were fed a blood meal spiked with ZIKV virions and then individually tested for viral nucleic acids after 14 days. Half of these mosquitoes that were exposed to ZIKV generated bright endpoint fluorescence in both *NS1* LAMP-OSD and *capsid* LAMP-OSD assays as well as in multiplex LAMP-2GO assays (Figure 8, Supplementary Figure S3). Parallel tests performed in the absence of primers, and hence, absence of LAMP amplification and concomitant probe activation, revealed negligible signal inflation due to sample auto-fluorescence, indicating the positive LAMP signal was due to these mosquitoes developing a viral infection. These mosquitoes also tested positive by ZIKV NS2b TaqMan qRT-PCR assay and were found to contain ~6 × 10^3 to 4 × 10^5 NS2b RNA copies per mosquito (Figure 8). Since only a 1/33 fraction of each mosquito was used for a LAMP test, these results suggest that the LAMP-based assays were able to generate a readily discernable bright visible fluorescence starting from as few as 190 copies of ZIKV genomic material embedded in crude virus-infected mosquito matrix.

Capsid and *NS1* LAMP-OSD assays and multiplex LAMP-2GO assays of the remaining half of the ZIKV-fed mosquitoes remained as dark as primer-less assays (Supplementary Figure S3). Our LAMP-based assays were in 100% agreement with TaqMan qRT-PCR, which also failed to detect ZIKV nucleic acids in these ZIKV-fed mosquitoes (Figure 8). These results suggest an absence of detectable infection in these mosquitoes, which is consistent with previously reported infection rates [46–50].

Specificity of LAMP-based assays was confirmed by analyzing six additional age-matched *Ae. aegypti* mosquitoes that had not received a ZIKV-spiked blood meal and were negative for ZIKV when tested by qRT-PCR. None of the uninfected mosquitoes triggered a false positive signal; LAMP assays containing these uninfected mosquitoes remained indistinguishable from primer-less assays (Supplementary Figure S3).

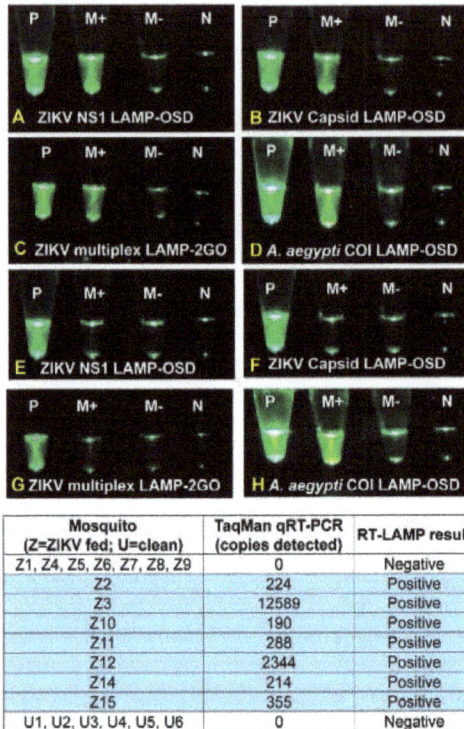

Mosquito (Z=ZIKV fed; U=clean)	TaqMan qRT-PCR (copies detected)	RT-LAMP result
Z1, Z4, Z5, Z6, Z7, Z8, Z9	0	Negative
Z2	224	Positive
Z3	12589	Positive
Z10	190	Positive
Z11	288	Positive
Z12	2344	Positive
Z14	214	Positive
Z15	355	Positive
U1, U2, U3, U4, U5, U6	0	Negative

Figure 8. Detection of Zika virus-infected mosquitoes using individual- and multiplex degenerate reverse transcription LAMP assays. Zika virus-infected (panels **A–D**) and uninfected (panels **E–H**) *Aedes aegypti* mosquitoes were directly analyzed using *NS1* and *capsid* LAMP-OSD assays or with multiplex LAMP-2GO assays. As a positive control, mosquitoes were tested using the *A. aegypti coi* LAMP-OSD assay (panels **D** and **H**). Smartphone images acquired after 2 h of amplification are depicted. P: positive control; M+: mosquito analyte with LAMP primers; M-: mosquito analyte without LAMP primers; N: no template control. Results of NS2b TaqMan qRT-PCR analysis of all mosquitoes are tabulated.

Absence of signal in ZIKV-uninfected mosquitoes was not due to inhibition of amplification. Both ZIKV-infected and uninfected mosquitoes generated bright fluorescence when tested using a LAMP-OSD assay for *Ae. aegypti* mitochondrial cytochrome oxidase I (*coi*) gene [16] (Figure 8, Supplementary Figure S3).

These results indicate that our smart molecular diagnostic assays perform at par with qRT-PCR for direct analysis of ZIKV virions in infected mosquitoes. Similar to *capsid* and *NS1* LAMP-OSD assays, the multiplex LAMP-2GO assays operated without discernible inhibition or spurious actuation in this complex milieu and demonstrated 100% specificity and 100% sensitivity for viral detection.

4. Discussion

While iNAATs have potential as POC diagnostics, they often lack the versatility and intelligence to deal with genetically variable and rapidly evolving targets. To fill this need we have created a smart molecular diagnostic composed of a parallel set of degenerate primers that can readily amplify variant targets. Degenerate LAMP primers have been successfully used by other groups as well [51–55]. Moreover, the resulting multiplex amplicons are integrated into a single readout via a multiplex OR-gated strand exchange logic processor that "computes" and returns the presence of a target relative to even closely related non-target sequences. The fact that multiple, different amplification reactions can be carried out in parallel, and yet the user need only attend to the final, fluorescent signal, highlights the power of the diagnostic, and presages the possibility of even more complex integration of molecular signals. For example, strand exchange nucleic acid computation has allowed (i) analysis of repetitive DNA targets of greater than 500 nucleotides in length with single nucleotide specificity, using "modular probes" composed of multiple short oligonucleotides that undergo competitive hybridization [56]; (ii) sensing and imaging of nucleic acids, enzymes, small molecules, proteins, and tumor cells via hairpin oligonucleotide probes and the hybridization chain reaction (HCR) [57]; and (iii) coupling nucleic acid detection to translational reporters via amplicon-mediated strand displacement reactions that couple to reporter protein production in a cell-free translation system [22].

More importantly, integration of strand exchange nucleic acid logic computation in a single tube with LAMP did not significantly compromise the robustness of LAMP, which has been previously shown to function in the presence of untreated biological fluids [58,59]. Our smart molecular diagnostic performed with little or no error in inclement environments, such as with crude preparations of macerated mosquitoes. The LAMP-based smart molecular assays of ZIKV-infected and un-infected mosquitoes could be performed with results that were on par with those obtained by qPCR analyses. As few as 190 copies of ZIKV RNA could be readily identified using multiplex LAMP-2GO assays without any false positive reactions. These assays were equally adept at identifying both Asian and African lineages of ZIKV without cross-reaction with related or co-circulating viruses. The assay thus enhances the programmability and signal processing capability of LAMP-based tests, which like many other isothermal molecular diagnostics are truly capable of performing in demanding field conditions. For instance, LAMP has been found to be a field-friendly diagnostic test for diseases such as malaria [60] and tuberculosis [61]. Similarly, RPA has demonstrated near 100% sensitivity and specificity in field tests for detection of many viruses, bacteria, and parasites [62–64]. Another iNAAT termed, isothermal nicking enzyme amplification reaction (NEAR), was automated on the Clinical Laboratory Improvement Amendments (CLIA)—waived portable device Alere i (Alere, Scarborough, MA) and is being used for POC diagnosis of infectious agents such as influenza viruses [65].

Overall, though, our envisioned smart molecular diagnostics methodology has much greater versatility for field use going forward. For instance, most field applications of RPA involve purification of nucleic acid analytes from clinical specimens. In contrast, our reactions can directly analyze crude biospecimens without necessitating complicated sample preparation and nucleic acid purification. Field applications of RPA and NEAR typically employ commercial instruments costing a few thousand dollars for assay readout [64] whereas our assay requires a simple 3D printed box for visual "yes/no" score for the presence or absence of visual fluorescence signal at endpoint. We have previously demonstrated execution of our LAMP-based assays using chemical heat from commercial hand warmers [15]. Our single temperature assay should also be amenable for incubation in other chemical heaters for LAMP, such as the NINA (non-instrumented nucleic acid amplification) heater [66], as well as commercial electrical heat blocks.

Most importantly, existing iNAATs lack design considerations to counter target variability, a deficiency that may reduce sensitivity [65], and in extreme cases lead to assay failure. For example, RPA uses a recombinase enzyme to facilitate invasion of double stranded templates by primers, which are then extended by a strand displacing DNA polymerase resulting in signal amplification [8]. Amplicon detection is typically achieved using fluorophore-labeled probes that are measured using fluorimetry or converted to a color readout using lateral flow assays [8,67]. Nicking enzyme amplification reaction relies on DNA nicking and extension reactions using nicking enzymes and strand displacing DNA polymerase to achieve exponential amplification of target DNA or RNA [68]. The resulting amplicons are typically converted to a fluorescence signal using cleavage probes. Neither configuration would be particularly suitable for degenerate priming and/or strand exchange computations, as opposed to our internally redundant Boolean logic processing assay.

In conclusion, our smart molecular diagnostic overcomes the principal challenges faced by most iNAATs—non-specific amplification, false negatives, and false positives—while maintaining an easy-to-use user-interface. This assay methodology should be of greatest utility for the development of disposable point-of-care devices. Despite performing multi-component analytical operations, the molecular computations are hidden from the user in a single assay that can both directly receive the sample and emanate visual results. We have previously demonstrated that strand exchange modules are compatible with preparation of lyophilized LAMP assay mixes [15]—a common mode of extended storage and commercial application of LAMP tests [69–73]. These various features should minimize device intricacies, and in turn reduce cost, especially since only two protein enzymes and a single fluorophore-quencher pair are required. Most importantly, the molecular probes can be configured to capture both current and future fast-evolving targets, such as Zika viruses, with both greater breadth and greater accuracy than existing tests.

Supplementary Materials: The following are available online at http://www.mdpi.com/1999-4915/10/12/714/s1, Supplementary Table S1: Primers used for single and multiplex Zika LAMP assays, Supplementary Table S2: Strand exchange probes used in this study, Supplementary Table S3: LAMP synthetic template RNA sequences, Supplementary Table S4: Zika NS2b qRT-PCR primers, TaqMan probe, and RNA template, Supplementary Table S5: Virions and viral genomic RNA samples used in this study, Supplementary Figure S1: Detection of Zika virus genomic RNA using non-degenerate LAMP primers. Supplementary Figure S2: Estimation of template copies in Asian lineage ZIKV genomic RNA and ZIKV virions, Supplementary Figure S3. Detection of Zika virus infected mosquitoes using single- and multiplex degenerate LAMP assays.

Author Contributions: Conceptualization, S.B., G.L.H., and A.D.E.; Methodology, S.B. and G.L.H.; Validation, S.B. and H.G.H.; Formal Analysis, S.B.; Investigation, S.B., M.A.S., H.G.H.; Resources, S.B., M.A.S., G.L.H., and A.D.E.; Data Curation, S.B. and G.L.H; Writing—Original Draft Preparation, S.B.; Writing—Review & Editing, S.B., G.L.H. and A.D.E.; Visualization, S.B.; Supervision, S.B. and G.L.H; Project Administration, G.L.H. and A.D.E.; Funding Acquisition, A.D.E. and G.L.H.

Funding: This work was supported by a Bill and Melinda Gates Foundation grant (OPP1128792) and the National Science Foundation BEACON (DBI-0939454) grant to ADE and a National Institute of Allergy and Infectious Diseases Small Business Innovation Research grant (R43 AI131948) to ADE and GLH. GLH was also supported by the Wolfson Foundation and Royal Society; National Institutes of Health grants (R21AI138074, R21AI124452 and R21AI129507); a University of Texas Rising Star award; the Western Gulf Center of Excellence for Vector-borne Diseases (Centers for Disease Control and Prevention grant CK17-005); the Robert J. and Helen Kleberg Foundation; and the Gulf Coast Consortia. MS was supported by a National Institutes of Health T32 fellowship (2T32AI007526). The papers contents are solely the responsibility of the authors and do not necessarily represent the official views of the Centers for Disease Control and Prevention or the Department of Health and Human Services.

Conflicts of Interest: The authors declare no conflict of interest.

References

1. Bruen, D.; Delaney, C.; Florea, L.; Diamond, D. Glucose sensing for diabetes monitoring: Recent developments. *Sensors* **2017**, *17*, 1866. [CrossRef] [PubMed]
2. Gnoth, C.; Johnson, S. Strips of hope: Accuracy of home pregnancy tests and new developments. *Geburtshilfe Frauenheilkd.* **2014**, *74*, 661–669. [CrossRef] [PubMed]
3. Kozel, T.R.; Burnham-Marusich, A.R. Point-of-care testing for infectious diseases: Past, present, and future. *J. Clin. Microbiol.* **2017**, *55*, 2313–2320. [CrossRef] [PubMed]
4. Kaushik, A.; Tiwari, S.; Jayant, R.D.; Vashist, A.; Nikkhah-Moshaie, R.; El-Hage, N.; Nair, M. Electrochemical biosensors for early stage zika diagnostics. *Trends Biotechnol.* **2017**, *35*, 308–317. [CrossRef] [PubMed]
5. Kaushik, A.; Yndart, A.; Kumar, S.; Jayant, R.D.; Vashist, A.; Brown, A.N.; Li, C.Z.; Nair, M. A sensitive electrochemical immunosensor for label-free detection of zika-virus protein. *Sci. Rep.* **2018**, *8*, 9700. [CrossRef] [PubMed]

6. Craw, P.; Balachandran, W. Isothermal nucleic acid amplification technologies for point-of-care diagnostics: A critical review. *Lab Chip* **2012**, *12*, 2469–2486. [CrossRef] [PubMed]
7. Nilsson, M.; Gullberg, M.; Dahl, F.; Szuhai, K.; Raap, A.K. Real-time monitoring of rolling-circles amplification using a modified molecular beacon design. *Nucleic Acids Res.* **2002**, *30*, e66. [CrossRef]
8. Piepenburg, O.; Williams, C.H.; Stemple, D.L.; Armes, N.A. DNA detection using recombination proteins. *PLoS Boil.* **2006**, *4*, e204. [CrossRef] [PubMed]
9. Kubota, R.; Jenkins, D.M. Real-time duplex applications of loop-mediated amplification (LAMP) by assimilating probes. *Int. J. Mol. Sci.* **2015**, *16*, 4786–4799. [CrossRef] [PubMed]
10. Chen, J.S.; Ma, E.; Harrington, L.B.; Da Costa, M.; Tian, X.; Palefsky, J.M.; Doudna, J.A. CRISPR-Cas12a target binding unleashes indiscriminate single-stranded DNase activity. *Science* **2018**, *360*, 436–439. [CrossRef]
11. Gootenberg, J.S.; Abudayyeh, O.O.; Kellner, M.J.; Joung, J.; Collins, J.J.; Zhang, F. Multiplexed and portable nucleic acid detection platform with Cas13, Cas12a, and Csm6. *Science* **2018**, *360*, 439–444. [CrossRef] [PubMed]
12. Zhang, D.Y.; Seelig, G. Dynamic DNA nanotechnology using strand-displacement reactions. *Nat. Chem.* **2011**, *3*, 103–113. [CrossRef] [PubMed]
13. Notomi, T.; Okayama, H.; Masubuchi, H.; Yonekawa, T.; Watanabe, K.; Amino, N.; Hase, T. Loop-mediated isothermal amplification of DNA. *Nucleic Acids Res.* **2000**, *28*, e63. [CrossRef] [PubMed]
14. Jiang, Y.S.; Bhadra, S.; Li, B.; Wu, Y.R.; Milligan, J.N.; Ellington, A.D. Robust strand exchange reactions for the sequence-specific, real-time detection of nucleic acid amplicons. *Anal. Chem.* **2015**, *87*, 3314–3320. [CrossRef]
15. Jiang, Y.S.; Riedel, T.E.; Popoola, J.A.; Morrow, B.R.; Cai, S.; Ellington, A.D.; Bhadra, S. Portable platform for rapid in-field identification of human fecal pollution in water. *Water Res.* **2017**, *131*, 186–195. [CrossRef] [PubMed]
16. Bhadra, S.; Riedel, T.E.; Saldaña, M.A.; Hegde, S.; Pederson, N.; Hughes, G.L.; Ellington, A.D. Direct nucleic acid analysis of mosquitoes for high fidelity species identification and detection of Wolbachia using a cellphone. *PLoS Negl. Trop. Dis.* **2018**. [CrossRef] [PubMed]
17. Bhadra, S.; Jiang, Y.S.; Kumar, M.R.; Johnson, R.F.; Hensley, L.E.; Ellington, A.D. Real-time sequence-validated loop-mediated isothermal amplification assays for detection of Middle East respiratory syndrome coronavirus (MERS-CoV). *PLoS ONE* **2015**, *10*, e0123126. [CrossRef]
18. Jung, C.; Ellington, A.D. Diagnostic applications of nucleic acid circuits. *Acc. Chem. Res.* **2014**, *47*, 1825–1835. [CrossRef]
19. Du, Y.; Hughes, R.A.; Bhadra, S.; Jiang, Y.S.; Ellington, A.D.; Li, B. A sweet spot for molecular diagnostics: Coupling isothermal amplification and strand exchange circuits to glucometers. *Sci. Rep.* **2015**, *5*, 11039. [CrossRef]
20. Li, B.; Ellington, A.D.; Chen, X. Rational, modular adaptation of enzyme-free DNA circuits to multiple detection methods. *Nucleic Acids Res.* **2011**, *39*, e110. [CrossRef]
21. Allen, P.B.; Arshad, S.A.; Li, B.; Chen, X.; Ellington, A.D. DNA circuits as amplifiers for the detection of nucleic acids on a paperfluidic platform. *Lab Chip* **2012**, *12*, 2951–2958. [CrossRef] [PubMed]
22. Pardee, K.; Green, A.A.; Takahashi, M.K.; Braff, D.; Lambert, G.; Lee, J.W.; Ferrante, T.; Ma, D.; Donghia, N.; Fan, M.; et al. Rapid, low-cost detection of Zika virus using programmable biomolecular components. *Cell* **2016**, *165*, 1255–1266. [CrossRef]
23. Qian, L.; Winfree, E. Scaling up digital circuit computation with DNA strand displacement cascades. *Science* **2011**, *332*, 1196–1201. [CrossRef] [PubMed]
24. Qian, L.; Winfree, E.; Bruck, J. Neural network computation with DNA strand displacement cascades. *Nature* **2011**, *475*, 368–372. [CrossRef] [PubMed]
25. Zhang, D.Y.; Turberfield, A.J.; Yurke, B.; Winfree, E. Engineering entropy-driven reactions and networks catalyzed by DNA. *Science* **2007**, *318*, 1121–1125. [CrossRef] [PubMed]
26. Jiang, Y.S.; Stacy, A.; Whiteley, M.; Ellington, A.D.; Bhadra, S. Amplicon competition enables end-point quantitation of nucleic acids following isothermal amplification. *ChemBioChem* **2017**. [CrossRef]
27. Faria, N.R.; Quick, J.; Claro, I.M.; Theze, J.; de Jesus, J.G.; Giovanetti, M.; Kraemer, M.U.G.; Hill, S.C.; Black, A.; da Costa, A.C.; et al. Establishment and cryptic transmission of Zika virus in brazil and the Americas. *Nature* **2017**, *546*, 406–410. [CrossRef] [PubMed]
28. Corman, V.M.; Rasche, A.; Baronti, C.; Aldabbagh, S.; Cadar, D.; Reusken, C.B.; Pas, S.D.; Goorhuis, A.; Schinkel, J.; Molenkamp, R.; et al. Assay optimization for molecular detection of Zika virus. *Bull. World Health Organ.* **2016**, *94*, 880–892. [CrossRef]

29. Metsky, H.C.; Matranga, C.B.; Wohl, S.; Schaffner, S.F.; Freije, C.A.; Winnicki, S.M.; West, K.; Qu, J.; Baniecki, M.L.; Gladden-Young, A.; et al. Zika virus evolution and spread in the Americas. *Nature* **2017**, *546*, 411–415. [CrossRef] [PubMed]

30. Kwok, S.; Kellogg, D.E.; McKinney, N.; Spasic, D.; Goda, L.; Levenson, C.; Sninsky, J.J. Effects of primer-template mismatches on the polymerase chain reaction: Human immunodeficiency virus type 1 model studies. *Nucleic Acids Res.* **1990**, *18*, 999–1005. [CrossRef] [PubMed]

31. Petruska, J.; Goodman, M.F.; Boosalis, M.S.; Sowers, L.C.; Cheong, C.; Tinoco, I., Jr. Comparison between DNA melting thermodynamics and DNA polymerase fidelity. *Proc. Natl. Acad. Sci. USA* **1988**, *85*, 6252–6256. [CrossRef] [PubMed]

32. Lemmon, G.H.; Gardner, S.N. Predicting the sensitivity and specificity of published real-time PCR assays. *Ann. Clin. Microbiol. Antimicrob.* **2008**, *7*, 18. [CrossRef] [PubMed]

33. Zhu, Z.; Chan, J.F.; Tee, K.M.; Choi, G.K.; Lau, S.K.; Woo, P.C.; Tse, H.; Yuen, K.Y. Comparative genomic analysis of pre-epidemic and epidemic Zika virus strains for virological factors potentially associated with the rapidly expanding epidemic. *Emerg. Microbes Infect.* **2016**, *5*, e22. [CrossRef] [PubMed]

34. Gibson, D.G.; Young, L.; Chuang, R.Y.; Venter, J.C.; Hutchison, C.A.; Smith, H.O. Enzymatic assembly of DNA molecules up to several hundred kilobases. *Nat. Methods* **2009**, *6*, 343–345. [CrossRef] [PubMed]

35. Hatcher, E.L.; Zhdanov, S.A.; Bao, Y.; Blinkova, O.; Nawrocki, E.P.; Ostapchuck, Y.; Schaffer, A.A.; Brister, J.R. Virus variation resource—Improved response to emergent viral outbreaks. *Nucleic Acids Res.* **2017**, *45*, D482–D490. [CrossRef] [PubMed]

36. Edgar, R.C. Muscle: Multiple sequence alignment with high accuracy and high throughput. *Nucleic Acids Res.* **2004**, *32*, 1792–1797. [CrossRef] [PubMed]

37. Edgar, R.C. Muscle: A multiple sequence alignment method with reduced time and space complexity. *BMC Bioinform.* **2004**, *5*, 113. [CrossRef] [PubMed]

38. Altschul, S.F.; Gish, W.; Miller, W.; Myers, E.W.; Lipman, D.J. Basic local alignment search tool. *J. Mol. Biol.* **1990**, *215*, 403–410. [CrossRef]

39. Altschul, S.F.; Madden, T.L.; Schaffer, A.A.; Zhang, J.; Zhang, Z.; Miller, W.; Lipman, D.J. Gapped blast and psi-blast: A new generation of protein database search programs. *Nucleic Acids Res.* **1997**, *25*, 3389–3402. [CrossRef]

40. Zadeh, J.N.; Steenberg, C.D.; Bois, J.S.; Wolfe, B.R.; Pierce, M.B.; Khan, A.R.; Dirks, R.M.; Pierce, N.A. Nupack: Analysis and design of nucleic acid systems. *J. Comput. Chem.* **2011**, *32*, 170–173. [CrossRef]

41. Waggoner, J.J.; Pinsky, B.A. Zika virus: Diagnostics for an emerging pandemic threat. *J. Clin. Microbiol.* **2016**, *54*, 860–867. [CrossRef]

42. Muller, J.A.; Harms, M.; Schubert, A.; Jansen, S.; Michel, D.; Mertens, T.; Schmidt-Chanasit, J.; Munch, J. Inactivation and environmental stability of Zika virus. *Emerg. Infect. Dis.* **2016**, *22*, 1685–1687. [CrossRef] [PubMed]

43. Faye, O.; Freire, C.C.; Iamarino, A.; de Oliveira, J.V.; Diallo, M.; Zanotto, P.M.; Sall, A.A. Molecular evolution of Zika virus during its emergence in the 20(th) century. *PLoS Negl. Trop. Dis.* **2014**, *8*, e2636. [CrossRef]

44. Gandelman, O.; Jackson, R.; Kiddle, G.; Tisi, L. Loop-mediated amplification accelerated by stem primers. *Int. J. Mol. Sci.* **2011**, *12*, 9108–9124. [CrossRef]

45. Faria, N.R.; Azevedo, R.; Kraemer, M.U.G.; Souza, R.; Cunha, M.S.; Hill, S.C.; Theze, J.; Bonsall, M.B.; Bowden, T.A.; Rissanen, I.; et al. Zika virus in the Americas: Early epidemiological and genetic findings. *Science* **2016**, *352*, 345–349. [CrossRef] [PubMed]

46. Ciota, A.T.; Bialosuknia, S.M.; Zink, S.D.; Brecher, M.; Ehrbar, D.J.; Morrissette, M.N.; Kramer, L.D. Effects of Zika virus strain and Aedes mosquito species on vector competence. *Emerg. Infect. Dis.* **2017**, *23*, 1110–1117. [CrossRef] [PubMed]

47. Chouin-Carneiro, T.; Vega-Rua, A.; Vazeille, M.; Yebakima, A.; Girod, R.; Goindin, D.; Dupont-Rouzeyrol, M.; Lourenco-de-Oliveira, R.; Failloux, A.B. Differential susceptibilities of *Aedes aegypti* and *Aedes albopictus* from the Americas to Zika virus. *PLoS Negl. Trop. Dis.* **2016**, *10*, e0004543. [CrossRef]

48. Weger-Lucarelli, J.; Ruckert, C.; Chotiwan, N.; Nguyen, C.; Garcia Luna, S.M.; Fauver, J.R.; Foy, B.D.; Perera, R.; Black, W.C.; Kading, R.C.; et al. Vector competence of American mosquitoes for three strains of Zika virus. *PLoS Negl. Trop. Dis.* **2016**, *10*, e0005101. [CrossRef]

49. Diagne, C.T.; Diallo, D.; Faye, O.; Ba, Y.; Faye, O.; Gaye, A.; Dia, I.; Faye, O.; Weaver, S.C.; Sall, A.A.; et al. Potential of selected Senegalese *Aedes* spp. Mosquitoes (diptera: Culicidae) to transmit Zika virus. *BMC Infect. Dis.* **2015**, *15*, 492. [CrossRef]

50. Roundy, C.M.; Azar, S.R.; Rossi, S.L.; Huang, J.H.; Leal, G.; Yun, R.; Fernandez-Salas, I.; Vitek, C.J.; Paploski, I.A.; Kitron, U.; et al. Variation in *Aedes aegypti* mosquito competence for Zika virus transmission. *Emerg. Infect. Dis.* **2017**, *23*, 625–632. [CrossRef]

51. Nunes, M.R.; Vianez, J.L., Jr.; Nunes, K.N.; da Silva, S.P.; Lima, C.P.; Guzman, H.; Martins, L.C.; Carvalho, V.L.; Tesh, R.B.; Vasconcelos, P.F. Analysis of a reverse transcription loop-mediated isothermal amplification (RT-LAMP) for yellow fever diagnostic. *J. Virol. Methods* **2015**, *226*, 40–51. [CrossRef] [PubMed]

52. Poon, L.L.; Leung, C.S.; Chan, K.H.; Lee, J.H.; Yuen, K.Y.; Guan, Y.; Peiris, J.S. Detection of human influenza a viruses by loop-mediated isothermal amplification. *J. Clin. Microbiol.* **2005**, *43*, 427–430. [CrossRef] [PubMed]

53. Mamba, T.S.; Mbae, C.K.; Kinyua, J.; Mulinge, E.; Mburugu, G.N.; Njiru, Z.K. Lateral flow Loop-Mediated isothermal amplification test with stem primers: Detection of cryptosporidium species in Kenyan children presenting with diarrhea. *J. Trop. Med.* **2018**, *2018*, 7659730. [CrossRef] [PubMed]

54. Blaser, S.; Diem, H.; von Felten, A.; Gueuning, M.; Andreou, M.; Boonham, N.; Tomlinson, J.; Muller, P.; Utzinger, J.; Frey, J.E.; et al. From laboratory to point of entry: Development and implementation of a loop-mediated isothermal amplification (LAMP)-based genetic identification system to prevent introduction of quarantine insect species. *Pest Manag. Sci.* **2018**, *74*, 1504–1512. [CrossRef] [PubMed]

55. Ge, Y.; Zhou, Q.; Zhao, K.; Chi, Y.; Liu, B.; Min, X.; Shi, Z.; Zou, B.; Cui, L. Detection of influenza viruses by coupling multiplex reverse-transcription loop-mediated isothermal amplification with cascade invasive reaction using nanoparticles as a sensor. *Int. J. Nanomed.* **2017**, *12*, 2645–2656. [CrossRef] [PubMed]

56. Wang, J.S.; Yan, Y.H.; Zhang, D.Y. Modular probes for enriching and detecting complex nucleic acid sequences. *Nat. Chem.* **2017**, *9*, 1222–1228. [CrossRef] [PubMed]

57. Bi, S.; Yue, S.; Zhang, S. Hybridization chain reaction: A versatile molecular tool for biosensing, bioimaging, and biomedicine. *Chem. Soc. Rev.* **2017**, *46*, 4281–4298. [CrossRef]

58. Francois, P.; Tangomo, M.; Hibbs, J.; Bonetti, E.J.; Boehme, C.C.; Notomi, T.; Perkins, M.D.; Schrenzel, J. Robustness of a loop-mediated isothermal amplification reaction for diagnostic applications. *FEMS Immunol. Med. Microbiol.* **2011**, *62*, 41–48. [CrossRef]

59. Ebbinghaus, P.; von Samson-Himmelstjerna, G.; Krucken, J. Direct loop-mediated isothermal amplification from *Plasmodium chabaudi* infected blood samples: Inability to discriminate genomic and cDNA sequences. *Exp. Parasitol.* **2012**, *131*, 40–44. [CrossRef]

60. Cook, J.; Aydin-Schmidt, B.; Gonzalez, I.J.; Bell, D.; Edlund, E.; Nassor, M.H.; Msellem, M.; Ali, A.; Abass, A.K.; Martensson, A.; et al. Loop-mediated isothermal amplification (LAMP) for point-of-care detection of asymptomatic low-density malaria parasite carriers in Zanzibar. *Malar. J.* **2015**, *14*, 43. [CrossRef]

61. Nakiyingi, L.; Nakanwagi, P.; Briggs, J.; Agaba, T.; Mubiru, F.; Mugenyi, M.; Ssengooba, W.; Joloba, M.L.; Manabe, Y.C. Performance of loop-mediated isothermal amplification assay in the diagnosis of pulmonary tuberculosis in a high prevalence TB/HIV rural setting in Uganda. *BMC Infect. Dis.* **2018**, *18*, 87. [CrossRef]

62. Xing, W.; Yu, X.; Feng, J.; Sun, K.; Fu, W.; Wang, Y.; Zou, M.; Xia, W.; Luo, Z.; He, H.; et al. Field evaluation of a recombinase polymerase amplification assay for the diagnosis of *Schistosoma japonicum* infection in Hunan province of China. *BMC Infect. Dis.* **2017**, *17*, 164. [CrossRef] [PubMed]

63. Escadafal, C.; Faye, O.; Sall, A.A.; Faye, O.; Weidmann, M.; Strohmeier, O.; von Stetten, F.; Drexler, J.; Eberhard, M.; Niedrig, M.; et al. Rapid molecular assays for the detection of yellow fever virus in low-resource settings. *PLoS Negl. Trop. Dis.* **2014**, *8*, e2730. [CrossRef] [PubMed]

64. Daher, R.K.; Stewart, G.; Boissinot, M.; Bergeron, M.G. Recombinase polymerase amplification for diagnostic applications. *Clin. Chem.* **2016**, *62*, 947–958. [CrossRef] [PubMed]

65. Nolte, F.S.; Gauld, L.; Barrett, S.B. Direct comparison of Alere i and cobas Liat Influenza A and B tests for rapid detection of influenza virus infection. *J. Clin. Microbiol.* **2016**, *54*, 2763–2766. [CrossRef] [PubMed]

66. LaBarre, P.; Hawkins, K.R.; Gerlach, J.; Wilmoth, J.; Beddoe, A.; Singleton, J.; Boyle, D.; Weigl, B. A simple, inexpensive device for nucleic acid amplification without electricity-toward instrument-free molecular diagnostics in low-resource settings. *PLoS ONE* **2011**, *6*, e19738. [CrossRef]

67. Powell, M.L.; Bowler, F.R.; Martinez, A.J.; Greenwood, C.J.; Armes, N.; Piepenburg, O. New Fpg probe chemistry for direct detection of recombinase polymerase amplification on lateral flow strips. *Anal. Biochem.* **2018**, *543*, 108–115. [CrossRef]

68. Maples, B.K.; Holmberg, R.C.; Miller, A.P.; Provins, J.W.; Roth, R.B.; Mandell, J.G. Nicking and Extension Amplification Reaction for the Exponential Amplification of Nucleic Acids. U.S. Patent 20090017453A1, 15 January 2009.

69. Carter, C.; Akrami, K.; Hall, D.; Smith, D.; Aronoff-Spencer, E. Lyophilized visually readable loop-mediated isothermal reverse transcriptase nucleic acid amplification test for detection Ebola Zaire RNA. *J. Virol. Methods* **2017**, *244*, 32–38. [CrossRef]

70. Chen, H.W.; Ching, W.M. Evaluation of the stability of lyophilized loop-mediated isothermal amplification reagents for the detection of *Coxiella burnetii*. *Heliyon* **2017**, *3*, e00415. [CrossRef]

71. Wong, Y.P.; Othman, S.; Lau, Y.L.; Radu, S.; Chee, H.Y. Loop-mediated isothermal amplification (LAMP): A versatile technique for detection of micro-organisms. *J. Appl. Microbiol.* **2018**, *124*, 626–643. [CrossRef]

72. Howson, E.L.A.; Armson, B.; Madi, M.; Kasanga, C.J.; Kandusi, S.; Sallu, R.; Chepkwony, E.; Siddle, A.; Martin, P.; Wood, J.; et al. Evaluation of two lyophilized molecular assays to rapidly detect foot-and-mouth disease virus directly from clinical samples in field settings. *Transbound. Emerg. Dis.* **2017**, *64*, 861–871. [CrossRef] [PubMed]

73. Lucchi, N.W.; Gaye, M.; Diallo, M.A.; Goldman, I.F.; Ljolje, D.; Deme, A.B.; Badiane, A.; Ndiaye, Y.D.; Barnwell, J.W.; Udhayakumar, V.; et al. Evaluation of the *Illumigene malaria* LAMP: A robust molecular diagnostic tool for malaria parasites. *Sci. Rep.* **2016**, *6*, 36808. [CrossRef] [PubMed]

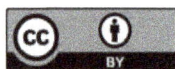

viruses

MDPI

Article

Comparative Evaluation of Indirect Immunofluorescence and NS-1-Based ELISA to Determine Zika Virus-Specific IgM

Fernando De Ory [1,2,*], María Paz Sánchez-Seco [1], Ana Vázquez [1,2], María Dolores Montero [3], Elena Sulleiro [4], Miguel J. Martínez [5], Lurdes Matas [2,6], Francisco J. Merino [7] and Working Group for the Study of Zika Virus Infections [†]

[1] Laboratorio de Serología y Arbovirus, Centro Nacional de Microbiología, Instituto de Salud Carlos III, Majadahonda 28220, Spain; paz.sanchez@isciii.es (M.P.S.-S.); a.vazquez@isciii.es (A.V.)

[2] Centro de Investigación Biomédica en Red en Epidemiología y Salud Pública, Instituto de Salud Carlos III, Madrid 28029, Spain; lmatas.germanstrias@gencat.cat

[3] Hospital Universitario La Paz, Madrid 28046, Spain; mdolores.montero@salud.madrid.org

[4] Hospital Vall d'Hebron, Barcelona 08035, Spain; esulleir@vhebron.net

[5] Hospital Clínic, Barcelona 08036, Spain; myoldi@clinic.cat

[6] Hospital Universitari Germans Trias i Pujol, Badalona 08916, Spain

[7] Hospital Severo Ochoa, Leganés 28911, Spain; franciscojesus.merino@salud.madrid.org

* Correspondence: fory@isciii.es; Tel.: +34-91-8223630

† Working Group for the Study of Zika Virus Infections (WGSZVI): Elena Sáez, BR Salud, Hospital Infanta Sofía, San Sebastián de los Reyes; Mercedes Rodríguez Pérez, Hospital Universitario Central de Asturias; Carlos Gustavo Cilla, Hospital de Donostia; José Cobos Dorado, Megalab, Madrid; Jorge Cabrera, Hospital do Meixoeiro, Vigo; Marta Domínguez Gil-González, Hospital Universitario Del Río Hortega, Valladolid; Juan Carlos Galán, Hospital Ramón y Cajal, Madrid; María Nieves Gutiérrez Zufiaurre, Hospital Clínico, Salamanca; María José Goyanes, Hospital General Universitario Gregorio Marañón, Madrid; Carolina Campelo, Fundación Hospital Alcorcón; Mirian Blasco Alberdi, Hospital San Pedro, Logroño; Bartolomé Carrilero Fernández, Hospital Universitario Virgen de la Arrixaca, Murcia; Rodolfo Copado Carretero, Hospital General de Lanzarote; María Teresa Durán Valle, Hospital de Móstoles; Ricardo Fernández Roblas, Fundación Jiménez Díaz, Madrid; Isabel García Bermejo, Hospital de Getafe; José Ignacio García Cía, Unilabs, Madrid; Araceli Hernández Betancor, Hospital Universitario Insular de Gran Canaria, Las Palmas; Isabel Cristina López Mestanza, Hospital Santa Bárbara, Soria; Lourdes Roc Alfaro, Hospital Universitario Miguel Servet, Zaragoza; Giovani Fedele, Centro Nacional de Microbiología; Luis Antonio Arroyo Pedrero, Hospital Rafael Méndez, Lorca; Rafael Benito Ruesca, Hospital Clínico Universitario Lozano Blesa, Zaragoza; Buenaventura Buendía, Hospital de la Princesa, Madrid; Alejandro González Praetorius, Hospital Universitario de Guadalajara; Miriam Hernández Porto, Hospital Universitario de Canarias, La Laguna; Adoración Hurtado Hernández, Hospital Can Misses, Ibiza; Marta Lalana Garcés, Hospital de Barbastro; Ana Isabel López López, Labco General Lab, Pozuelo de Alarcón; Paloma Martín Cordero, Hospital Infanta Cristina, Badajoz; Rosario Millán Pérez, Hospital Puerta de Hierro, Majadahonda; Laura Molina Esteban, Hospital de Fuenlabrada; Francisco Javier Ramos Germán, Hospital Obispo Polanco, Teruel; Montserrat Ruiz García, Hospital General Universitario de Elche; Pino del Carmen Suárez, Hospital General de Fuerteventura; César Gómez Hernando, Hospital Virgen de la Salud, Toledo; Mariano Andreu López, Hospital General Universitario, Alicante; Noelia Arenal Andrés, Hospital Santos Reyes, Aranda de Duero; Francisco José Arjona Zaragozi, Hospital de la Marina Baixa, Villajoyosa; Elvira Baos Muñoz, Hospital Clínico San Carlos, Madrid; Xavier Casal Martínez, Hospital Nostra Senyora de Meritxell, Andorra; Amparo Coira Nieto, Complejo Hospitalario Xeral-Calde, Lugo; David Navalpotro, Consorcio Hospital General Universitario, Valencia; Alfredo Esteban Martín, Hospital de León; Mónica Gozalo Margüello, Hospital Universitario Marqués de Valdecilla, Santander; Susana Hernando Real, Hospital General de Segovia; María Jesús Lezaun Bugui, Hospital Galdakao-Usansolo; Elisa Martínez Alfaro y Juan Carlos Segura Luque, Complejo Hospitalario Universitario de Albacete; María Mateo Maestre, Hospital Central de la Defensa, Madrid; Ana MíguezSantiyán, Centro de Salud Pública de Valencia; Alfredo Pérez Rivilla, Hospital 12 de Octubre, Madrid; Mercedes Pérez Ruiz, Hospital Universitario Virgen de las Nieves; Isabel Polo Vigas, Complejo Hospitalario de Navarra; Carmen Raya Fernández, Hospital El Bierzo, Ponferrada; Rafael Sánchez Arroyo, Hospital Nuestra Señora de Sonsoles; María Reyes Sánchez

Flórez, Complejo Hospitalario Universitario Nuestra Señora de Candelaria, Santa Cruz de Tenerife; Matilde Trigo Daporta, Complejo Hospitalario de Pontevedra; Emilio David Valverde Romero, Hospital de León; Silvia Rojo Rello, Hospital Clínico Universitario, Valladolid; María José Rodríguez Escudero, Hospital General Virgen de la Luz, Cuenca; Francisco Salva, Hospital Universitario Son Espases, Palma de Mallorca; Juan Carlos Sanz, Laboratorio de Salud Pública, Comunidad de Madrid, and Teodora Minguito, Francisca Molero, Jesús María de la Fuente, Laura Herrera, Pilar Balfagón, María Lourdes Hernández, María Ángeles Murillo and María Concepción Perea, Centro Nacional de Microbiología.

Received: 23 May 2018; Accepted: 30 June 2018; Published: 19 July 2018

Abstract: Differential diagnosis of the Zika virus (ZIKV) is hampered by cross-reactivity with other flaviviruses, mainly dengue viruses. The aim of this study was to compare two commercial methods for detecting ZIKV immunoglobulin M (IgM), an indirect immunofluorescence (IIF) and an enzyme immunoassay (ELISA), using the non-structural (NS) 1 protein as an antigen, both from EuroImmun, Germany. In total, 255 serum samples were analyzed, 203 of which showed laboratory markers of ZIKV infections (PCR-positive in serum and/or in urine and/or positive or indeterminate specific IgM). When tested with IIF, 163 samples were IgM-positive, while 13 samples were indeterminate and 78 were negative. When IIF-positive samples were tested using ELISA, we found 61 positive results, 14 indeterminate results, and 88 negative results. Among the indeterminate cases tested with IIF, ELISA analysis found two positive, two indeterminate, and nine negative results. Finally, 74 of the 78 IIF-negative samples proved also to be negative using ELISA. For the calculations, all indeterminate results were considered to be positive. The agreement, sensitivity, and specificity between ELISA and IIF were 60.2%, 44.9%, and 94.9%, respectively. Overall, 101 samples showed discrepant results; these samples were finally classified on the basis of other ZIKV diagnostic approaches (PCR-positive in serum and/or in urine, IgG determinations using IIF or ELISA, and ZIKV Plaque Reduction Neutralization test—positive), when available. A final classification of 228 samples was possible; 126 of them were positive and 102 were negative. The corresponding values of agreement, sensitivity, and specificity of IIF were 86.0%, 96.8%, and 72.5%, respectively. The corresponding figures for ELISA were 81.1%, 65.9%, and 100%, respectively. The ELISA and IIF methods are both adequate approaches for detecting ZIKV-specific IgM. However, considering their respective weaknesses (low sensitivity in ELISA and low specificity in IIF), serological results must be considered jointly with other laboratory results.

Keywords: Zika virus; dengue viruses; flavivirus; ELISA; indirect immunofluorescence; plaque reduction neutralization test; polymerase chain reaction; cross-reactions

---

1. Introduction

The Zika virus (ZIKV) is a mosquito-transmitted virus belonging to the flavivirus genus. This genus includes other human pathogens, such as the dengue virus (DENV), the West Nile virus, and the yellow fever virus. ZIKV shares some clinical and microbiological characteristics with DENV, making its diagnosis difficult.

Firstly, both viruses cause an exanthematic febrile disease, characterized by the presence of arthralgia and retroocular pain, although there are differential signs or symptoms, such as rash with pruritus, conjunctivitis, and limb edema (characteristic of ZIKV disease), or leucopenia/thrombocytopenia (characteristic of dengue) [1,2]. Secondly, they share a vector (mosquitoes of the genus, *Aedes*) and, consequently, a distribution area [3]. Thirdly, both viruses, as well as other flaviviruses, share antigenic reactivity, resolved in serological cross-reactivity when measuring specific antibodies [4]. For these reasons, it is important to have specific serological assays that can facilitate an adequate differential diagnosis.

Indirect immunofluorescence (IIF) is widely used to detect ZIKV antibodies, using ZIKV-infected cells to identify class-specific antibodies. However, using this approach, the high degree of cross-reactivity between ZIKV and other flaviviruses makes correct serological diagnosis difficult. The ZIKV non-structural (NS) 1 protein was identified as being largely specific to the virus [5], and, as a consequence, new ELISA assays were developed. Although some studies evaluated the use of ELISA reagents for determining immunoglobulin M (IgM) against ZIKV [6–12], no comparisons with IIF are available.

The aim of this study was to evaluate the comparative performance characteristics of an NS1 antigen-based ELISA and an IIF assay for identifying ZIKV-specific IgM. For this purpose we used a large panel of samples that were well characterized by molecular and serological approaches, including a real-time molecular assay, IgM and IgG ELISA, and the plaque reduction neutralization test (PRNT).

2. Materials and Methods

2.1. Samples

A total of 255 serum samples received in our laboratory were included in the study. Of these, 239 samples showed markers of ZIKV infection, including 203 cases from 201 adults (66 men, 135 women (30 pregnant)) and two newborns. The samples were received over a period of 18 months (1 January 2016–31 July 2017). The study was approved by the Ethical Committee of the Institute of Health Carlos III (code: CEI PI 64_2018). All patients had recently traveled to one or more Latin American countries. The samples were grouped as described below.

1. Seventy-one paired samples from 35 cases (three samples were available from one case):

    (a) Four cases (eight samples) were PCR-positive (using real-time PCR) in serum and urine, and ZIKV IgM-positive using IIF (five samples).
    (b) Five cases (10 samples) had a positive result with PCR in serum (one of them was negative in urine), and two samples from two cases were ZIKV IgM-positive using IIF.
    (c) Nine cases (19 samples) were PCR-positive only in urine (six were negative in serum), and ZIKV IgM-positive in eight (eight positive and four indeterminate samples).
    (d) The remaining 17 cases (34 samples; three with a PCR-negative result in serum and one in urine) were IgM-positive or indeterminate in at least one sample. Seven of them were ZIKV IgM-positive in acute and convalescent samples. Three cases showed seroconversion of ZIKV IgM. Of these, both samples of one case were indeterminate, and in the other case, the acute sample was indeterminate and the convalescent sample was positive. Finally, five cases (indeterminate to positive (two cases), positive to indeterminate (one case), positive to negative (one case), and indeterminate to negative (one case)), showed the presence of DENV IgM (four cases) or DENV IgG seroconversion (one case).

2. One hundred and sixty-eight samples:

    (a) Twenty-three samples were ZIKV IgM-positive, of which PCR was positive in serum and urine (one case), in serum only (eight cases), or in urine only (14 cases).
    (b) One hundred and one samples gave a positive result for ZIKV IgM; PCR was carried out in serum and urine in 28 of them, all of which gave a negative result.
    (c) Forty-four samples were negative for ZIKV IgM using IIF, with a positive PCR result in serum and urine (six cases), in serum only (15 cases), or in urine only (23 cases).

The remaining 16 samples came from recent dengue infections (nine samples from eight patients), as diagnosed by IgM detection, or past dengue infections (seven samples), as confirmed by IgG detection in the absence of IgM. These samples were taken during 2012, before the ZIKV epidemic in the Americas. The patients reported recent travel to Latin American countries. When tested for ZIKV IgM using IIF, two samples were positive, another two were indeterminate, and one other gave an uninterpretable result, with a strong background and no specific fluorescence.

2.2. Methods

ZIKV-specific IgM and IgG were tested using IIF with commercial reagents (Arbovirus Fever Mosaic 2, catalog #FR2668-1010-1G and #FR2668-1010-1M for IgG and IgM, respectively, obtained from EuroImmun, Lübeck, Germany). For testing IgM, samples were pretreated with an anti-human IgG (RF Absorbent, reference OUCG, Siemens, Marburg, Germany), to remove the interference due to the presence of rheumatoid factor and specific IgG to avoid false-positive results. Briefly, samples pretreated with a ten-fold dilution were incubated for 30 min at 37 °C in wells of slides containing ZIKV-infected cells. After washing with phosphate-buffered saline (PBS), pH 7.2, supplemented with Tween 20 (PBS-Tween), an anti-human IgM (goat)-fluorescein isothiocyanate conjugate was added to the wells and incubated as before. After the final washing, the slides were mounted in glycerol buffered with PBS, pH 8.4, and read in an inverted fluorescence microscope (Zeiss Axiovert 25, Jena, Germany) equipped with a mercury vapor lamp HBO50 (Osram, Munich, Germany), at a magnification of 200×. Samples showing fine-to-coarse granular cytoplasmic structures and/or net-like fluorescence with a dense perinuclear reactivity were considered to be positive. The kit included positive and negative controls. The results obtained using IIF were read by two different people. Samples where interpretations differed between the two assessors were considered to be indeterminate.

Dengue virus serology was done using commercial ELISA tests. Immunoglobulin M was determined with the Panbio Dengue IgM Capture ELISA, catalog #01PE20, while DENV IgG was determined with the Panbio Dengue IgG Indirect ELISA, catalog #01PE30, both obtained from Standard Diagnostics Inc., Geonggi-do, South Korea. Dengue virus assays use DENV 1–4 antigens, recombinant in the case of the IgM assay. Dengue virus IgM was confirmed using a background assay, as described elsewhere [13]. The ZIKV PRNT was assessed with an in-house test using Vero E6 cells and 100 tissue infective infectious dose 50% of ZIKV (African strain MR-766, isolated from a rhesus monkey in the Zika Forest, Uganda, in 1947, and maintained in our laboratory in Vero E6 cells). For neutralizing antibodies, samples were tested following titration in two-fold dilutions from 1/8. Samples were considered positive if neutralization of viral growth at a dilution greater than 128-fold was observed; samples with titers between eight-fold and 128-fold were considered indeterminate, while samples with a titer less than eight-fold were considered negative. Zika virus RNA was determined using a commercial assay of real-time PCR (RealStar®Zika Virus, altona Diagnostics, Hamburg, Germany, catalog number: 774AD-591013) [14].

The assay under evaluation was an ELISA using the NS1 protein (recombinant) from the virus (ELISA Zika virus IgM, catalog number EI 2668-9601 M, EuroImmun) as the antigen. Briefly, samples diluted 100-fold in a buffer containing anti-human IgG (goat) were incubated with the immobilized antigen NS1 for 1 h at 37 °C. The plate was washed three times, and an anti-human IgM (goat) peroxidase conjugate was added. After incubating for 30 min at room temperature and washing as before, a solution of 3, 3′, 5, 5′ tetramethylbenzidine/H_2O_2 was added as the enzyme substrate. The reaction was stopped with 0.5 M H_2SO_4, and the plate was read at 450 nm. A calibrator containing ZIKV-specific IgM included in the kit was tested in each run to define the cut-off of the test. Samples with absorbance/cut-off values greater than 1.1 were considered positive, and values less than 0.8 were considered negative. All other values were regarded as indeterminate.

All tests using commercial reagents were done strictly following the manufacturer's instructions.

To establish the comparison, all indeterminate results using either IIF or ELISA were considered as positive.

3. Results

Overall, in the IIF assay, 163 samples were ZIKV IgM-positive, 13 were indeterminate, and 78 were negative. The result from the remaining sample could not be interpreted, and was excluded from the analysis.

The general comparison between IIF and ELISA for detecting ZIKV-specific IgM is illustrated in Table 1. Excluding the sample with an uninterpretable result, the ELISA test showed 67 samples to be positive, 16 to be indeterminate, and 171 to be negative.

Out of 163 positive IIF samples, 61 were positive, 14 were indeterminate, and 88 were negative with ELISA. Of the 13 indeterminate IIF samples, two were positive, two were indeterminate, and nine were negative with ELISA. Finally, 74 of the 78 IIF-negative samples were also negative with ELISA, while four were positive (Table 1).

Table 1. Results of ELISA compared with indirect immunofluorescence (IIF).

		Indirect Immunofluorescence			
		Positive	Indeterminate	Negative	Uninterpretable
	Positive	61	2	4	0
ELISA	Indeterminate	14	2	0	0
	Negative	88	9	74	1

Considering all indeterminate results to be positive, the comparison of ELISA and IIF provided values of agreement of 60.2% (95% confidence intervals (CIs): 53.9–66.2%; 153/254), a sensitivity of 44.9% (95% CIs: 37.5–52.5%; 79/176), and a specificity of 94.9% (95% CIs: 86.7–98.3%; 74/78).

All positive and indeterminate results with both IIF and ELISA were considered as true positives, and the samples showing a negative result with both assays were considered as negative. One hundred and one samples showed discrepant results with the two assays (listed in Tables 2–4). The samples were finally classified considering other specific ZIKV diagnostic approaches (PCR-positive in serum and/or in urine, IgG determinations using IIF or ELISA, and ZIKV PRNT-positive), when available.

Table 2. Discrepant results finally classified as negative.

Number	ZIKV IgM		Other Results *	Final Classification
	IIF	ELISA		
#1	POS	NEG	Acute sample. DENV (NS1 Ag & IgM)	Negative (dengue)
#2	IND	NEG	Acute sample. DENV (NS1 Ag & IgM). PRNT ind (9 dao)	Negative (dengue)
#3	POS	NEG	Follow-up sample. DENV (IgM). PRNT neg (45 dao)	Negative
#4	POS	NEG	Single sample. DENV (NS1 Ag & IgM). PRNT neg	Negative (dengue)
#5	POS	NEG	Single sample. PCR neg (serum & urine), PRNT neg, DENV (IgM)	Negative (dengue)
#6	POS	NEG	Single sample. PCR neg (serum), PRNT neg, DENV (IgM)	Negative (dengue)
#7–#9	IND	NEG	Single sample. DENV (IgM). Sample from 2012	Negative (dengue)
#10	POS	NEG	Acute sample. DENV (IgM). Sample from 2012	Negative (dengue)
#11, #12	POS	NEG	Single sample. PCR neg (serum & urine), PRNT neg	Negative
#13, #14	POS	NEG	Single sample. PCR neg (serum)	Negative
#15	POS	NEG	Single sample. PCR neg (urine)	Negative
#16–#28	POS	NEG	Single sample. PRNT neg	Negative

* dao: days after onset; PRNT: plaque reduction neutralization test; ind: indeterminate result; pos: positive; neg: negative; ZIKV: Zika virus; DENV: dengue virus; NS1 Ag: non-structural protein 1 antigen; IgM: immunoglobulin M.

Table 3. Discrepant results finally classified as positive.

Number	ZIKV IgM		Other Results *	Final Classification
	IIF	ELISA		
#29	POS	NEG	Acute sample. PCR pos (serum) (1 dao)	Positive
#30	POS	NEG	Follow-up sample (180 dao)	Positive
#31	IND	NEG	Acute sample. PCR pos (urine) (n dao)	Positive
#32	POS	NEG	Follow-up sample. PRNT pos (n+18 dao)	Positive
#33	POS	NEG	Acute sample. PCR pos (urine) (n dao)	Positive
#34	IND	NEG	Follow-up sample. PRNT pos (n+25 dao)	Positive
#35	IND	NEG	Acute sample. PCR pos (urine) (7 dao)	Positive
#36	POS	NEG	Follow-up sample. PRNT ind (33 dao)	Positive

Table 3. *Cont.*

Number	ZIKV IgM		Other Results *	Final Classification
	IIF	ELISA		
#37	POS	NEG	Acute sample. PRNT pos (n dao)	Positive
#38	POS	NEG	Follow-up sample. PRNT pos (n+12 dao)	Positive
#39	POS	NEG	Acute sample. PRNT pos (50 dao)	Positive
#40	IND	NEG	Follow-up sample. PRNT pos (78 dao)	Positive
#41	POS	NEG	Acute sample. IgG SC (IIF & ELISA)	Positive
#42	POS	NEG	Convalescent sample. PRNT pos. PCR pos (urine)	Positive
#43	POS	NEG	Convalescent sample. PCR neg (serum). Acute sample: IgM pos (IIF & ELISA)	Positive
#44	IND	NEG	Convalescent sample. Acute sample: IgM ind (ELISA)	Positive
#45	POS	NEG	Convalescent sample. Acute sample: IgM ind (IIF); pos (ELISA)	Positive
#46	POS	NEG	Convalescent sample. IgM SC (IIF). PRNT pos. Acute sample: PCR pos (serum & urine)	Positive
#47, #48	POS	NEG	Convalescent sample. IgG SC (ELISA)	Positive
#49	IND	NEG	Acute sample. PCR pos (urine)	Positive
#50	POS	NEG	Single sample. PCR pos (urine & serum)	Positive
#51	POS	NEG	Single sample. PCR pos (serum). PRNT pos	Positive
#52–#54	POS	NEG	Single sample. PCR pos (serum)	Positive
#55	POS	NEG	Single sample. PCR pos (urine). PRNT pos	Positive
#56–#59	POS	NEG	Single sample. PCR pos (urine)	Positive
#60–#71	POS	NEG	Single sample. PRNT pos	Positive
#72	NEG	POS	Convalescent sample. IgG SC (IIF & ELISA). PCR pos (urine)	Positive
#73	NEG	POS	Convalescent sample. Acute sample: IgM ind (IIF); pos (ELISA)	Positive
#74, #75	NEG	POS	Single sample. PCR pos (urine)	Positive

* SC: seroconversion.

Table 4. Unclassifiable discrepant results.

Number	ZIKV IgM		Other Results	Final Classification
	IIF	ELISA		
#76	POS	NEG	Acute sample. PRNT ind	Unclassifiable
#77	POS	NEG	Follow-up sample. PRNT ind	Unclassifiable
#78	POS	NEG	Single sample. PCR neg (serum& urine), PRNT ind	Unclassifiable
#79	POS	NEG	Single sample. PRNT ind. PCR neg (serum)	Unclassifiable
#80–#91	POS	NEG	Single sample. PRNT ind	Unclassifiable
#92–#99	POS	NEG	Single sample. No more results	Unclassifiable
#100	POS	NEG	Single sample. PCR neg (serum), PRNT pos. DENV (IgM pos, NS1 Ag neg)	Unclassifiable
#101	POS	NEG	Single sample. PRNT ind. DENV (IgM pos)	Unclassifiable

Firstly, 28 discrepant samples, all with a positive (25 samples) or indeterminate (3 samples) result using IIF were finally classified as negative (Table 2). Ten of them (#1 to #10, Table 2) came from dengue cases, since they showed either DENV IgM and NS1 antigens (samples #1, #2, and #4), or DENV IgM in a follow-up sample (#3), or DENV IgM with ZIKV PRNT-negative and ZIKV PCR-negative in serum and urine (#5) or in serum only (#6), or DENV IgM in samples taken in 2012, before the outbreak of ZIKV in the Americas in 2015 (four samples, #7 to #10). Two additional cases tested negative for ZIKV PCR in urine and serum, and for ZIKV PRNT (#11, #12), while three more were negative for ZIKV PCR in serum (#13 and #14) or in urine (#15), and the remaining 13 samples (#16 to #28) were negative for PRNT.

Secondly, 47 samples with discrepant results were finally classified as positive (Table 3). Of these, 43 were positive (37 samples) or indeterminate (6 samples) using IIF and negative using ELISA, and four were positive using ELISA and negative using IIF. Of the samples giving a positive or indeterminate result using IIF, 12 were paired samples (#29 to #40, Table 3) from six cases that were positive (eight samples, #29, #30, #32, #33, #36, #37, #38, and #39) or indeterminate (four samples, #31, #34, #35, and #40) using IIF. Of these, four cases gave a positive result for ZIKV PCR three cases in urine (with a positive PRNT assay result in two of them) and one in serum. Two other paired samples were ZIKV PRNT-positive in acute and convalescent samples. Sample #41 was an acute sample whose corresponding convalescent sample showed IgG seroconversion with both ELISA and IIF. Samples #42 to #48 were convalescent ones, showing either a ZIKV PCR-positive result in urine and an PRNT-positive result (#42), or a positive or indeterminate result using IIF and/or ELISA in the corresponding acute samples (#43, #44, and #45), or seroconversion of IgM (#46) or IgG (#47 and #48). Sample #49 was an acute sample with a ZIKV PCR-positive result in urine. Samples #50 to #71 were single samples that were ZIKV PCR-positive in urine and serum (#50), ZIKV PCR-positive in serum and ZIKV PRNT-positive (#51), ZIKV PCR-positive in serum (#52, #53, and #54), ZIKV PCR-positive in urine and PRNT-positive (#55), and ZIKV PCR-positive in urine (#56, #57, #58, and #59). Samples #60 to #71 were single samples for which a single positive result in the ZIKV PRNT assay was demonstrated.

Of the four samples showing a positive result using ELISA but a negative one using IIF, two were convalescent samples showing a ZIKV PCR-positive result in urine and IgG seroconversion (#72), or an IgM-positive result using ELISA and an indeterminate result using IIF in the acute sample (#73). The latter samples were two single samples from cases that were ZIKV PCR-positive in urine (#74 and #75).

Finally, the other 26 samples showing discrepant results were considered unclassifiable, because not enough results were available (Table 4).

Thus, a final classification was possible for 228 samples (126 positive and 102 negative; Table 5). Indirect immunofluorescence showed 86% agreement (95% CIs: 80.6–90.1%; 196/228), 96.8% sensitivity (95% CIs: 91.6–99.0%; 122/126), and 72.5% specificity (95% CIs: 62.7–80.7%; 74/102). ELISA, on the other hand, showed 81.1% agreement (95% CIs: 75.3–85.9%; 185/228), 65.9% sensitivity (95% CIs: 56.8–73.9%; 83/126), and 100% specificity (95% CIs: 95.5–100%; 102/102).

Table 5. Performance characteristics of IIF and ELISA after the final classification of samples.

		Final Classification	
		Positive (126)	Negative (102)
Indirect	Positive	122	28
Immunofluorescence	Negative	4	74
ELISA	Positive	83	0
	Negative	43	102

4. Discussion

The best definition of a clinical case of ZIKV in areas with concurrent circulation of other flaviviruses is the presence of a rash with pruritus or conjunctival hyperemia, in the absence of any other general clinical manifestations [2]. However, there are difficulties in the differential diagnosis of individual cases with other arboviruses, especially DENV, due to the cross-reactions between the members of the flavivirus genus, and the chikungunya virus. Thus, the main problem in comparatively evaluating serological assays for ZIKV assays is the correct classification of cases. In the presented study, samples giving the same result with the compared methods were considered as true, as was the case in 153 samples (60.2%) of those analyzed, having obtained 101 discrepant results using IIF and ELISA. For the final classification of the discrepant results, the results of other infection markers (PCR-positive in urine and serum and/or IgG seroconversion and/or PRNT-positive for ZIKV, and IgM and/or IgG seroconversion and/or NS1 antigen detection for DENV) were taken into consideration when they were available. In this way, discrepant samples were finally classified as negative (28 samples; Table 3) or positive (47 samples; Table 4), while a definitive classification of the remaining 26 samples was not possible (Table 5). After the final classification of the discrepancies, the NS1-based ELISA showed excellent specificity when applied to samples that were received by the laboratory for the diagnosis of ZIKV infection. The high specificity obtained was consistent with that previously reported for the ELISA assay evaluated here [6–9], as well as for other tests based on the NS1 protein [9,10]. It is of particular note that the specificity of ELISA is markedly higher than that of IIF (Table 5).

The sensitivity, on the other hand, was lower using ELISA than with the IIF test. The figure obtained here for ELISA (65.9%) was better than those previously reported in the literature: 20.7% [10]; 32% [9]; 54% [8], and 58.8% [7]. The differences in sensitivity could be related to the different approaches used to establish the comparisons in the various reports. The lower sensitivity of ELISA in relation to IIF could be explained by the fact that only one protein (NS1) acted as an antigen in ELISA in contrast to the whole virus in IIF, or by the kinetics of the antibodies against NS1, which could be delayed in relation to the antibodies detected against the complete virus, as detected in the IIF assay. In order to assess this aspect, the dates of bleeding of the paired samples showing discrepant results, and those which were finally classified as positive (samples #29 to #40, Table 3) were reviewed. Follow-up samples were taken between 12 days and 180 days after the first sample was taken, and in none of the six cases was the follow-up sample positive using ELISA. Therefore, it does not seem likely that the lower sensitivity of ELISA compared with that of IIF is related to a deferred response of the ZIKV IgG to the NS1 antigen.

The cross-reactivity between ZIKV and DENV, as well as that with other flaviviruses, as consistently reported [6,12], is of particular note. This issue is of particular interest, since patients with prior dengue infections were reported to not develop an IgM response against ZIKV NS1 [15]. Of the cases analyzed with a unique IIF-positive result for ZIKV IgM, 12 showed markers of recent DENV infection, either in samples that were classified as ZIKV-negative (#1 to #10, Table 2) or that were unclassifiable (#100 and #101, Table 4). All cases produced by DENV, included in Table 2, were confirmed as false-positive in IIF, since they showed markers of DENV infection, by IgM (all cases) and, more importantly, by detection of the NS1 antigen of DENV (samples #1, #2, and #4), in the absence of other markers of ZIKV infection. Also of interest are the IIF-positive results in the samples showing DENV IgM taken before the epidemic of the virus in the Americas (samples #7 to #10, Table 2). Nevertheless, ZIKV and DENV double infections cannot be completely ruled out; this seems to be the case for samples #100 and #101 (Table 4), which were considered as unclassifiable. Thus, the ELISA technique was confirmed as being more specific than IIF, and appeared not to be affected by the cross-reaction when analyzing cases of DENV infection, even in the presence of the DENV NS1 antigen. The specificity of the IIF and ELISA assays should be the subject of a broader study, including not only cases of DENV and ZIKV, but also, at least, cases of yellow fever.

In conclusion, the ELISA and IIF methods could both be adequate approaches for detecting ZIKV-specific IgM. However, considering their respective weaknesses (sensitivity in ELISA and specificity in IIF), serological results must be considered in the context of clinical and epidemiological data, and of other laboratory results.

Author Contributions: Conceptualization, F.d.O. Investigation, F.d.O., M.P.S.-S., and A.V. Methodology, M.D.M., E.S., M.J.M., L.M., and F.J.M. Writing—original draft, F.d.O. Writing—review and editing, F.d.O., M.P.S.-S., and A.V.

Acknowledgments: The study was partially financed by a contract between the ISCIII and Euroimmun Diagnostics España SLU (MVP216/17), and by ISCIII, project RD16CIII/0003/0003, "Red de Enfermedades Tropicales", Subprogram RETICS Plan Estatal de I+D+I 2013-2016, and co-funded by FEDER "Una manera de hacer Europa" and project PI16CIII/00037.

Conflicts of Interest: The founding sponsors had no role in the design of the study, in the collection, analyses, or interpretation of data, in the writing of the manuscript, or in the decision to publish the results.

References

1. Bachiller-Luque, P.; Dominguez-Gil-González, M.; Alvarez-Manzanares, J.; Vázquez, A.; de Ory, F.; Sánchez-Seco Fariñas, M.P. First case of Zika virus infection imported to Spain. *Enferm. Infecc. Microbiol. Clin.* **2016**, *34*, 243–246. [CrossRef] [PubMed]
2. Braga, J.U.; Bressan, C.; Dalvi, A.P.R.; Calvet, G.A.; Daumas, R.P.; Rodrigues, N.; Wakimoto, M.; Nogueira, R.M.R.; Nielsen-Saines, K.; Brito, C.; et al. Accuracy of Zika virus disease case definition during simultaneous Dengue and Chikungunya epidemics. *PLoS ONE* **2017**, *12*, e0179725. [CrossRef] [PubMed]
3. Epelboin, Y.; Talaga, S.; Epelboin, L.; Dusfour, I. Zika virus: An updated review of competent or naturally infected mosquitoes. *PLoS Negl. Trop. Dis.* **2017**, *11*, e0005933. [CrossRef] [PubMed]
4. Priyamvada, L.; Hudson, W.; Ahmed, R.; Wrammert, J. Humoral cross-reactivity between Zika and dengue viruses: Implications for protection and pathology. *Emerg. Microbes Infect.* **2017**, *6*, e33. [CrossRef] [PubMed]

5. Stettler, K.; Beltramello, M.; Espinosa, D.A.; Graham, V.; Cassotta, A.; Bianchi, S.; Vanzetta, F.; Minola, A.; Jaconi, S.; Mele, F.; et al. Specificity, cross-reactivity, and function of antibodies elicited by Zika virus infection. *Science* **2016**, *353*, 823–826. [CrossRef] [PubMed]

6. Huzly, D.; Hanselmann, I.; Schmidt-Chanasit, J.; Panning, M. High specificity of a novel Zika virus ELISA in European patients after exposure to different flaviviruses. *Euro. Surveill.* **2016**, *21*. [CrossRef] [PubMed]

7. Steinhagen, K.; Probst, C.; Radzimski, C.; Schmidt-Chanasit, J.; Emmerich, P.; van Esbroeck, M.; Schinkel, J.; Grobusch, M.P.; Goorhuis, A.; Warnecke, J.M.; et al. Serodiagnosis of Zika virus (ZIKV) infections by a novel NS1-based ELISA devoid of cross-reactivity with dengue virus antibodies: A multicohort study of assay performance, 2015 to 2016. *Euro. Surveill.* **2016**, *21*, 30426. [CrossRef] [PubMed]

8. Kadkhoda, K.; Gretchen, A.; Racano, A. Evaluation of a commercially available Zika virus IgM ELISA: Specificity in focus. *Diagn. Microbiol. Infect. Dis.* **2017**, *88*, 233–235. [CrossRef] [PubMed]

9. Safronetz, D.; Sloan, A.; Stein, D.R.; Mendoza, E.; Barairo, N.; Ranadheera, C.; Scharikow, L.; Holloway, K.; Robinson, A.; Traykova-Andonova, M.; et al. Evaluation of 5 commercially available Zika virus immunoassays. *Emerg. Infect. Dis.* **2017**, *23*, 1577–1580. [CrossRef] [PubMed]

10. Wong, S.J.; Furuya, A.; Zou, J.; Xie, X.; Dupuis, A.P., II; Kramer, L.D.; Shi, P.Y. A Multiplex Microsphere Immunoassay for Zika Virus Diagnosis. *EBioMedicine* **2017**, *16*, 136–140. [CrossRef] [PubMed]

11. Granger, D.; Hilgart, H.; Misner, L.; Christensen, J.; Bistodeau, S.; Palm, J.; Strain, A.K.; Konstantinovski, M.; Liu, D.; Tran, A.; et al. Serologic testing for Zika virus: Comparison of three Zika virus IgM-screening enzyme-linked immunosorbent assays and initial laboratory experiences. *J. Clin. Microbiol.* **2017**, *55*, 2127–2136. [CrossRef] [PubMed]

12. Pasquier, C.; Joguet, G.; Mengelle, C.; Chapuy-Regaud, S.; Pavili, L.; Prisant, N.; Izopet, J.; Bujan, L.; Mansuy, J.M. Kinetics of anti-ZIKV antibodies after Zika infection using two commercial enzyme-linked immunoassays. *Diagn. Microbiol. Infect. Dis.* **2018**, *90*, 26–30. [CrossRef] [PubMed]

13. Domingo, C.; de Ory, F.; Sanz, J.C.; Reyes, N.; Gascón, J.; Wichmann, O.; Puente, S.; Schunk, M.; López-Vélez, R.; Ruíz, J.; et al. Molecular and serological markers of acute dengue infection in naïve and flavivirus vaccinated travellers. *Diagn. Microbiol. Infect. Dis.* **2009**, *65*, 42–48. [CrossRef] [PubMed]

14. L'Huillier, A.G.; Lombos, E.; Tang, E.; Perusini, S.; Eshaghi, A.; Nagra, S.; Frantz, C.; Olsha, R.; Kristjanson, E.; Dimitrova, K.; et al. Evaluation of Altona Diagnostics RealStar Zika virus reverse transcription-PCR test kit for Zika virus PCR testing. *J. Clin. Microbiol.* **2017**, *55*, 1576–1584. [CrossRef] [PubMed]

15. Barzon, L.; Percivalle, E.; Pacenti, M.; Rovida, F.; Zavattoni, M.; Del Bravo, P.; Cattelan, A.M.; Palù, G.; Baldanti, F. Virus and antibody dynamics in travelers with acute Zika virus infection. *Clin. Infect. Dis.* **2018**, *66*, 1173–1180. [CrossRef] [PubMed]

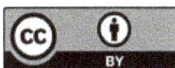

![viruses logo] *viruses*

MDPI

Article

Development and Characterization of Double-Antibody Sandwich ELISA for Detection of Zika Virus Infection

Liding Zhang [†], Xuewei Du [†], Congjie Chen, Zhixin Chen, Li Zhang, Qinqin Han, Xueshan Xia *, Yuzhu Song * and Jinyang Zhang *[iD]

Faculty of Life Science and Technology, Kunming University of Science and Technology,
727 Jingming South Road, Kunming 650500, China; lidingzhang@aliyun.com (L.Z.); xueweidu@126.com (X.D);
kmustccj@163.com (C.C.); arnoldchen1997@gmail.com (Z.C.); lilizhang7102@foxmail.com (L.Z.);
qqhan10@kmust.edu.cn (Q.H.)
* Correspondence: oliverxia2000@aliyun.com (X.X.); syzzam@126.com (Y.S.); jyzhang@kmust.edu.cn (J.Z.);
Tel./Fax: +86-871-6593-9528 (J.Z.)
† These authors contributed equally to this work.

Received: 26 October 2018; Accepted: 13 November 2018; Published: 15 November 2018

check for updates

Abstract: Zika virus (ZIKV) is an emerging mosquito-transmitted flavivirus that can cause severe disease, including congenital birth defect and Guillain−Barré syndrome during pregnancy. Although, several molecular diagnostic methods have been developed to detect the ZIKV, these methods pose challenges as they cannot detect early viral infection. Furthermore, these methods require the extraction of RNA, which is easy to contaminate. Nonstructural protein 1 (NS1) is an important biomarker for early diagnosis of the virus, and the detection methods associated with the NS1 protein have recently been reported. The aim of this study was to develop a rapid and sensitive detection method for the detection of the ZIKV based on the NS1 protein. The sensitivity of this method is 120 ng mL^{-1} and it detected the ZIKV in the supernatant and lysates of Vero and BHK cells, as well as the sera of tree shrews infected with the ZIKV. Without the isolation of the virus and the extraction of the RNA, our method can be used as a primary screening test as opposed to other diagnosis methods that detect the ZIKV.

Keywords: NS1 protein; Zika virus; diagnosis; monoclonal antibodies; ELISA

1. Introduction

The Zika virus (ZIKV), a new arbovirus, is a member of the *Flavivirus* genus of the Flaviviridae family. It was initially isolated from a macaque in 1947 in the Zika Forest of Uganda [1]. With fewer than 20 humans documented infected with the ZIKV, it received almost no attention before 2007. During this time, the ZIKV silently circulated in many parts of Africa and Asia without causing severe diseases or large outbreaks [2]. In 2015, an outbreak in Northeast Brazil led to an alarming number of babies born with microcephalus [3]. During this recent outbreak, many devastating severe diseases, including the Guillain−Barré syndrome in adults and congenital malformations in the fetuses of infected pregnant women such as microcephaly and fetal demise, were caused by the ZIKV [2,4,5]. Recently, the ZIKV has been recognized as a significant threat to global public health [6]. The disease was present in large parts of the Americas, the Caribbean, and also the Western Pacific region of Southern Asia during 2015 and 2016 [7,8]. Thereafter, the ZIKV spread rapidly and large-scale outbreaks were documented in other regions of the world [9]. As of April 2016, there were approximately 1.5 million people confirmed to be infected with the ZIKV. More than 46 countries have reported cases of ZIKV infections. In China, 13 ZIKV cases have been documented, and the possibility of new outbreaks still exists [10].

Mosquitoes of the *Aedes* species represent the main vector of transmission; however, it is possible to become infected with the ZIKV by exposure to blood, as well as perinatal and sexual contact [11,12]. Currently, there is no cure for ZIKV infection and no vaccine is available. Furthermore, rapid, efficient and easy-to-use kits are scarce [13]. Therefore, the early diagnosis of the ZIKV infection is the most effective way to treat patients and to control future outbreaks.

Presently, several studies have reported the methods used to detect the ZIKV. Using specific primers of viral RNAs for a highly-sensitive and simple experiment, the RT-qPCR assay was considered as a preferred diagnostic method. However, the false-negative results arising from new strains and the false-positive results arising from sample contamination still exist [14]. Therefore, other methods are needed to verify the accuracy of the RT-qPCR assay. Furthermore, there are other serological methods for detecting either ZIKV antigens (e.g., NS1) or immunoglobulins (e.g., IgG and IgM antibodies (Abs)). Due to the fact that IgM/IgG Abs, which are produced approximately seven days after the onset of symptoms, vary from patient to patient [15,16]. Thus, these methods are not suitable for the early diagnosis of ZIKV infection.

Nonstructural protein 1 (NS1) is an important protein secreted by cells infected with the virus, and it interacts with the host. It forms the homologous dimers within cells and binds to the type of adipocyte membrane system that participates in viral replication [17]. Furthermore, NS1 is a soluble protein that is secreted, suggesting that the virus can escape the immune system to strengthen interactions with the host [18,19]. More importantly, as the main antigen, NS1 can induce the production of Abs, which is important in early diagnosis of viral markers [20].

Currently, the early detection of the ZIKV largely depends on the NS1 protein, as several studies have reported that its level remains elevated up to nine days for Dengue, which is more sensitive than the other ZIKV proteins [21–24]. The detection of the ZIKV antigen for the development of a diagnostic method has not yet been reported, so the development of a ZIKV detection kit based on a specific monoclonal antibody (mAb) is absolutely critical [16].

In this study, we developed a rapid and sensitive method to detect the ZIKV in the supernatants and lysates of Vero and BHK cells, as well as the sera of tree shrew. Due to the short window for the detection of the ZIKV, it is presently difficult to diagnose patients with traditional methods [25,26]. Thus, we developed a double-antibody sandwich ELISA (DAS-ELISA) to detect the ZIKV-NS1 protein in individuals newly infected with the ZIKV and to assist the other screening methods used for detection. This method can effectively improve the diagnosis accuracy.

2. Materials and Methods

2.1. Expression and Purification of the NS1 Protein

The nucleotide sequence of the ZIKV-NS1 protein (Accession number: MG674719.1) was used to design the primers for the amplification of NS1. Total RNA was extracted from the supernatant of ZIKV infected Vero cells using the TIANamp Virus DNA/RNA Kit (TIANGEN, Beijing, China) and PCR was carried out to amplify the *NS1* gene with the specific primers 5′-GGAATTCGGGATGTTGGGTGTTCAGT-3′ (forward; underlined, *EcoR* I site) and 5′-CCGCTCGAGTTACGCTGTCACCACAGACCT-3′ (reverse; underlined, *Xho* I site). The amplified *NS1* gene product was digested with *EcoR* I and *Xho* I, and ligated into the pET-32a (+) to generate the recombinant cloning plasmid pET-32a (+)-NS1. The recombinant NS1 protein was expressed in BL21 (DE3) cells. Nickel-nitrilotriacetic acid (Ni2+-NTA) agarose resin was used to purify the NS1 proteins from the insoluble fraction of induced *E. coli* cells.

2.2. Ethics Statement

The animal study was approved by the Kunming University of Science and Technology with permit number: KMUST2018-0053. All experimental procedures involving mice and rabbits were performed in accordance with the regulations prescribed by the Administration of Laboratory Animals.

2.3. Production of Monoclonal and Polyclonal Antibodies Against the ZIKV-NS1 Protein

The production of mAb and polyclonal antibody (pAb) against ZIKV-NS1 protein was performed as previously described by our laboratory [27,28]. After repeated immunizations in rabbits, the polyclonal antiserum against the ZIKV-NS1 protein was successfully prepared. After the last immunization, the spleen cells of mice were collected and fused with SP2/0 cells. The fused cells were cultured in RPMI 1640 containing 20% FBS (Gbico, Gaithersburg, MD, USA) and hypoxanthine-aminopterin-thymidine (Sigma, Ronkonkoma, NY, USA) for one to two weeks. The ELISA and the indirect immunofluorescent assay were used to determine the presence of ZK-NS1-specific Abs in the hybridoma supernatants. Immunoglobulin G (IgG) from nine mAbs and the pAb were purified using protein A sepharose (GE Healthcare, Chicago, IL, USA).

2.4. Detection of Recombinant ZIKV-NS1 Protein by the DAS-ELISA

To screen a pair of Abs for the development of the DAS-ELISA, nine mAbs were conjugated with HRP, respectively. Horse radish peroxidase (HRP) labeled Abs and the pAb R1 were prepared pairwise combinatorial testing for pre-experiment. The pAb R1 was diluted to a final concentration of 10 μg mL^{-1} with CBS buffer (CBS; NaHCO$_3$ 17.84 mM, Na$_2$CO$_3$ 27.64 mM, pH 9.6) and the wells of 96 plate were coated with 100 μL coated for 2 h at 37 °C. The wells were blocked with 200 μL blocking buffer (5% skim milk in PBS-T) for 2 h at 37 °C. Thereafter, 2 μg recombinant ZIKV-NS1 protein was added to each well and incubated for 2 h at 37 °C. The wells were washed three times with PBS-T (PBS-T; KCl 2.7 mM, KH$_2$PO$_4$ 2 mM, NaCl 137 mM, Na$_2$HPO$_4$ 10 mM, 0.05% Tween$-$20, pH 7.4), and then 2A7, 4G6, 3F1, 1F4, 3G12, 2C4, 1G2, 2C9, and 1F12 (all conjugated with HRP) were diluted to a final concentration of 1.4 μg mL^{-1} with blocking buffer. Thereafter, 100 μL of each mAb was added into each well, and the plate was incubated for 1 h at 37 °C. The wells were washed three times with PBS-T, 100 μL of the soluble TMB substrate solution (TIANGEN, Beijing, China) was added into each well and incubated for 20 min at 37 °C. Lastly, 50 μL of stopping buffer (2 M H$_2$SO$_4$) was added to terminate the reaction, and the optical density of each well was then measured at 450 nm using a microplate reader (Bio-Rad, Hercules, CA, USA).

2.5. Titer and Binding Affinity of mAb 1F12 and pAb R1 Based on the ELISA

An indirect enzyme-linked immunosorbent assay (ELISA) was used to determine the titer of mAb 1F12 and pAb R1. The wells of a 96-well plate were coated with 1 μg of the recombinant NS1 protein, and incubated for 2 h at 37 °C. The wells were washed three times with PBS-T, and then blocked with 200 μL of blocking buffer for 2 h at 37 °C. Thereafter, 100 μL of mAb 1F12 or pAb R1 at different dilutions (from 1:100 to 1:409,600) were added into each well, and the plate was incubated for 2 h at 37 °C. The wells were washed as described above, and then goat anti-mouse IgG (H + L) HRP or goat anti-rabbit IgG (H + L) HRP (GenScript, Piscataway, NJ, USA) was diluted to a final concentration of 2 μg mL^{-1} with blocking buffer. Thereafter, 100 μL of the secondary Ab was added into each well. The blank control well was incubated with 5% skimmed milk. The optical density of each well was measured at 450 nm using a microplate reader. The binding affinity of mAb 1F12 and pAb R1 were determined by the ELISA as described above.

2.6. Western Blot Assay

To characterize the reactivity and specificity of mAb 1F12 and pAb R1, Vero cells infected and mock-infected with ZIKV were harvested, and the proteins were separated by SDS-PAGE and transferred to nitrocellulose (NC) membranes. The membranes were blocked with blocking buffer for 2 h at 37 °C. Subsequently, the membranes were probed with mAb 1F12 or pAb R1 diluted to a final concentration of 1.4 μg mL^{-1} with blocking buffer and incubated for 2 h at 37 °C. Thereafter, the membranes were incubated with HRP-conjugated secondary Abs (diluted as above) for 1 h at 37 °C.

After each incubation step, the membranes were washed five times with PBS-T. Finally, the EasySee Western Blot Kit (TransGen, Beijing, China) was used to detect the immunoreactive proteins.

2.7. Indirect Immunofluorescent Assay

For the immunofluorescent assay, ZIKV infected and mock-infected Vero cells were cultured for 48 h and fixed with pre-chilled acetone-methanol (1/1) for 20 min at −20 °C. After fixation, the cells were blocked with blocking buffer for 1 h at 37 °C. Subsequently, the cells were incubated with mAbs 2A7, 4G6, 3F1, 1F4, 3G12, 2C4, 1G2, 2C9, 1F12, or pAb R1 diluted to a final concentration of 1.4 µg mL^{-1} with blocking buffer, and 100 µL of each primary Ab was added into each well. The plate was incubated for 2 h at 37 °C. Finally, fluorescein isothiocyanate (FITC)-conjugated goat anti-mouse immunoglobulin G (Abcam, Cambridge, UK) was diluted to a final concentration of 1 µg mL^{-1} with blocking buffer, and 100 µL of the secondary Ab was added into each well. The plate was incubated for 1 h at 37 °C. After each incubation step, the cells were washed five times with PBS-T. Lastly, 200 µL of PBS was added into each well for fluorescent detection at 488 nm using the Leica DMI3000B microscope (Buffalo Grove, IL, USA).

2.8. Establishment of the DAS-ELISA Based on pAb R1 and mAb 1F12 Probe

To establish the DAS-ELISA, 1 µg of pAb R1 was diluted in CBS buffer and incubated for 2 h at 37 °C. The wells of a 96-well plate were blocked with blocking buffer for 1 h at 37 °C. Thereafter, the ZIKV-NS1 protein was added into each well, and the plate was incubated for 2 h at 37 °C. The wells were washed three times with PBS-T. Thereafter, mAb 1F12-HRP was diluted as described above and 100 µL of the secondary Ab was added into each well, followed by incubation for 1 h at 37 °C. After washing, 100 µL of TMB was added into each well, and the plate was incubated for 15 min at 37 °C. Lastly, 50 µL of stopping buffer (2M H$_2$SO$_4$) was added to terminate the reaction. The optical density of each well was measured at 450 nm using a microplate reader. A yellow-colored reaction and a high absorbance reading were indicative of a positive reaction, whereas a clear-colored reaction and a low absorbance reading were indicative of a negative reaction.

2.9. Specificity and Sensitivity of the DAS-ELISA

The specificity and sensitivity for the ZIKV-NS1 protein were determined based on the calibration curve of the DAS-ELISA. Vero cells were infected with four similar flavivirus (DEN-1, DEN-2, DEN-3, and JEV). The natural NS1 protein in cell culture supernatant was used to determine the specificity of the DAS-ELISA. Four similar flavivirus and the ZIKV were added into each well precoated with pAb R1, and the plate was incubated for 2 h at 37 °C. Thereafter, mAb-HRP probes were added and recognized with the antigen. After washing the plate three times with PBS-T, 100 µL of TMB was added, and the plate was incubated at 37 °C. Negative and positive samples could be easily distinguished by the naked eye after 15 min. The optical density of each well was measured using a microplate reader. The sensitivity of the DAS-ELISA was established using the recombinant ZIKV-NS1 protein serially diluted in water, for the final concentrations of NS1 protein from 500 µg mL^{-1} to 0.122 µg mL^{-1}. The following steps were the same as those previously described.

2.10. Application of the DAS-ELISA for the Detection of ZIKV Infection in Cells and Tree Shrews

The test for the application of the DAS-ELISA, supernatants, and cell lysates from Vero and BHK cells, as well as sera from three tree shrew infected with ZIKV were used. In brief, Vero and BHK cells were infected with one multiplicity of infection (MOI) and cultured in the presence of 1% FBS. The supernatants and cell lysates of infected Vero and BHK cells were collected at different times (12, 24, 36, 48, 60, and 72 h) and used for the DAS-ELISA assay. On the other hand, tree shrews were subcutaneous inoculated with 1×10^6 PFU of the ZIKV. Tree shrews' sera were collected at different infection times (from 1 to 15 days) and used for the DAS-ELISA assay described above.

3. Results

3.1. Expression and Purification of the ZIKV-NS1 Protein

The *ZIKV-NS1* gene was amplified from the cDNA of infected cells and cloned into the pET-32a (+) expression vector. The pET-32a-NS1 plasmid was transformed into *E. coli* Rosetta (DE3) cells, and the transformation was confirmed by PCR (Figure 1A, lane 1). Thereafter, the recombinant NS1 protein was expressed after induction with 1.0 mM IPTG for 10 h at 20 °C (Figure 1B, lane 1). The expressed NS1 protein was purified using a Ni2+-NTA resin column (Figure 1B, lane 3).

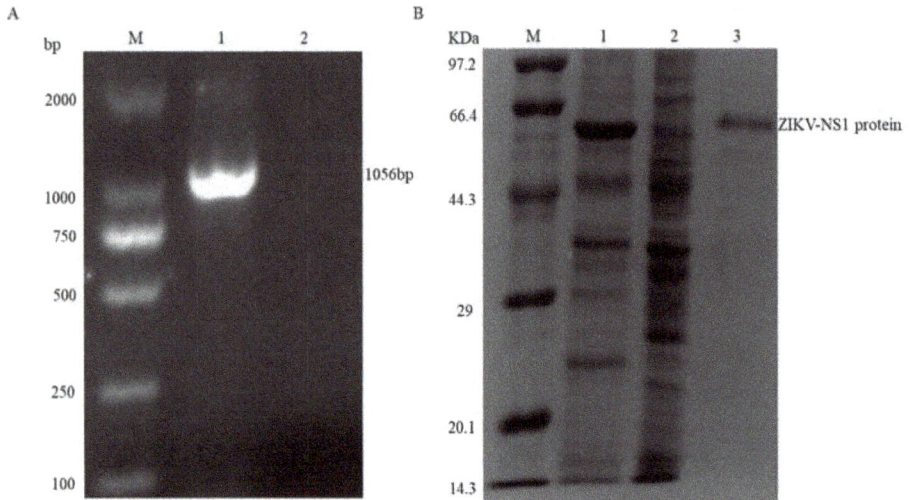

Figure 1. Analysis of the recombinant vector construction and expression of recombinant ZIKV-NS1 protein. (**A**) Identification of the positive clone of pET-32a-NS1 by bacteria polymerase chain reaction, lane 1: positive clone; lane 2: blank control. (**B**) Lane 1: *E. coli* was induced with IPTG; lane 2: *E. coli* before induced; lane 3: the purified ZIKV-NS1 after dialysis.

3.2. Evaluation of the Rabbit Antiserum

The recombinant NS1 protein was used as an immunogen for immunization. After repeated immunizations in rabbits, the antiserum was produced. The reactivity and specificity of the rabbit antiserum were evaluated by immunofluorescent and Western blot assays. As shown in Figure 2A, the anti-ZIKV-NS1 serum (R1) reacted with the native NS1 protein in ZIKV infected cells, and the negative control was not. The Western blot results showed that the rabbit pAb R1 specifically recognized the recombinant NS1 protein, as well as the native NS1 protein in cells infected with the ZIKV (Figure 2C,D).

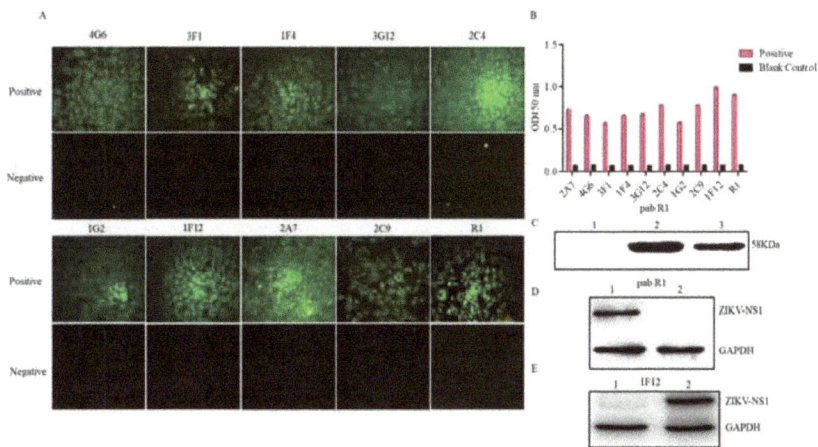

Figure 2. Evaluation of the pAb R1 and mAbs against ZIKV-NS1 protein. (**A**) Indirect immunofluorescent assay of the mAbs and pAb R1, Scale bar = 100 μm. (**B**) ELISA test of the mAbs and pAb R1. (**C**) Western blot analysis of the pAb R1; lane 1: *E. coli* Rosetta (DE3) without IPTG; lane 2: *E. coli* Rosetta (DE3) induced with IPTG; lane 3: the purified ZIKV-NS1. (**D**) ZIKV infected (lane 1) and mock-infected Vero cells (lane 2) were used for Western blot analysis using pAb R1. (**E**) Mock-infected (lane 1) and ZIKV infected Vero cells (lane 2) were used for Western blot analysis using mAb 1F12.

3.3. Characterization of the Ascites Against NS1 Protein

Ascites of the nine hybridomas were prepared and purified using protein A Sepharose. The reactivity and specificity of the nine ascites were determined using an immunofluorescent assay and an ELISA. All mAbs were further verified by the immunofluorescent assay. The results showed that all Abs recognized the native NS1 protein in cells infected with the ZIKV, and the negative control had no fluorescence (Figure 2A). Furthermore, the results of the ELISA assay showed that the nine mAbs reacted with the recombinant NS1 protein (Figure 2B).

3.4. Establishment of the DAS-ELISA

Several Ab pairs were screened to develop the DAS-ELISA. In brief, the mAbs were labeled with HRP probe and used for ELISA (Figure 3A). Thereinto, HRP-labeled mAbs (2A7, 4G6, 3F1, 1F4, 3G12, 2C4, 1G2, 2C9, and 1F12) and unlabeled pAb R1 were prepared in different combinations for the pre-experiment. The absorbance values indicated that R1 and 1F12 were more effective than the other combinations (Figure 3B). Besides, R1 and 1F12 were titrated by the ELISA (Figure 3C,D). Horse radish peroxidase (HRP) labeled mAb 1F12 and pAb R1 were used for subsequent specificity and affinity experiments. The K_D values of HRP-labeled mAb 1F12 and pAb R1 were measured using an affinity test, and the results were analyzed by non-linear regression using software GraphPad Prism 6. Their K_D values were calculated as $K_D = 1.77 \pm 0.206$ nM for the HRP-labeled mAb 1F12 and $K_D = 0.868 \pm 0.0816$ nM for pAb R1 (Figure 3E). Lastly, pAb R1 and mAb 1F12 were purified, and their purity was confirmed by SDS-PAGE (Figure 3F). According to Figures 3 and 3, pAb R1 functioned as the capture Ab and mAb 1F12 functioned as the signal Ab, and they were the best combination for detecting the ZIKV.

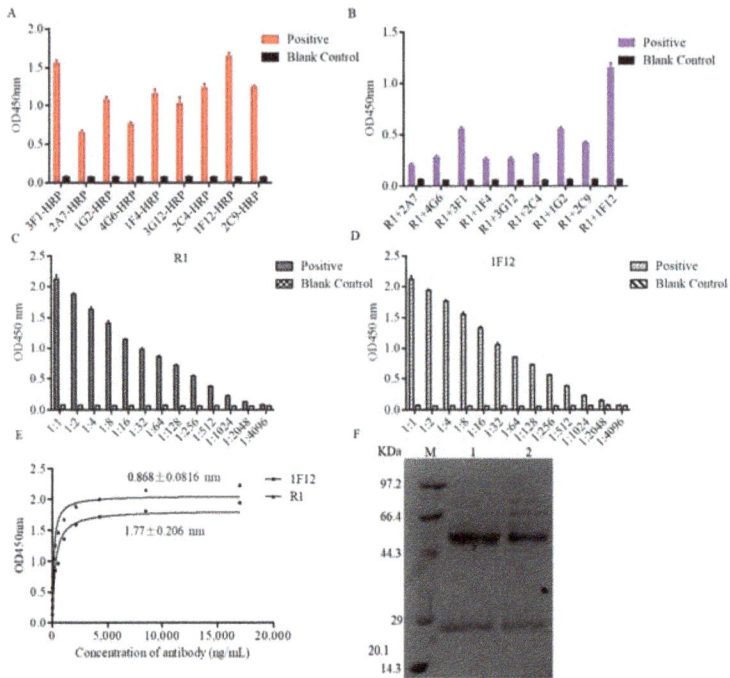

Figure 3. Characteristics of the key components of the DAS-ELISA. (**A**) The reactivity of nine mAbs conjugated with HRP, 5% skimmed milk as the blank control. (**B**) Nine different groups for DAS-ELISA, the blank control was 5% skimmed milk. The titer of pAb R1 (**C**) and mAb 1F12 (**D**) at different dilution ratios were determined by ELISA, 5% skimmed milk as the blank control. (**E**) The saturation curves for determination of the dissociation constants of mAb 1F12 and pAb R1. (**F**) SDS-PAGE analysis of purified mAb 1F12 (lane 1) and pAb R1 (lane 2).

3.5. *Optimization Operations*

To achieve a high sensitivity, a short detection time, and a low cost, the individual steps of the DAS-ELISA were optimized. Firstly, a suitable buffer for pAb R1 was identified using three commonly employed coating buffers (PBS buffer, TBS buffer, and CBS buffer). As shown in Figure 4A, CBS buffer had the highest coating efficiency. Secondly, the time and temperature for the immobilization of pAb R1 onto the plate were optimized. Figure 4B showed that the absorbance was higher at 37 °C than at 4 °C with increasing incubation time from 60 to 120 min. However, there was no significant difference when the incubation time or temperature was raised. Thirdly, the optimal concentration of pAb R1 and mAb 1F12 was determined when R1 and HRP-1F12 Ab s were serially diluted and incubated with a fixed amount of the recombinant NS1 protein, respectively. The results showed that the capturing efficiency of the R1 and HRP-1F12 Ab s increased between 10 µg mL^{-1} and 15 µg mL^{-1}. There was no obvious change in the curve at concentrations greater than 10 µg mL^{-1} and 15 µg mL^{-1}, respectively (Figure 4C,D). Moreover, we also established the temperature and time of antigen binding for pAb R1. The results of the ELISA indicated that the antigen was able to be completely bound by R1 at 37 °C (Figure 4E). Lastly, the binding of the HRP-1F12 probe to the recombinant NS1 protein was investigated when pAb R1 was combined with the NS1 protein and the HRP-1F12 antibody were added into the wells, and incubated at 37 °C or 4 °C, for different time periods. The results showed that the suitable time and temperature were 1 h at 37 °C (Figure 4F).

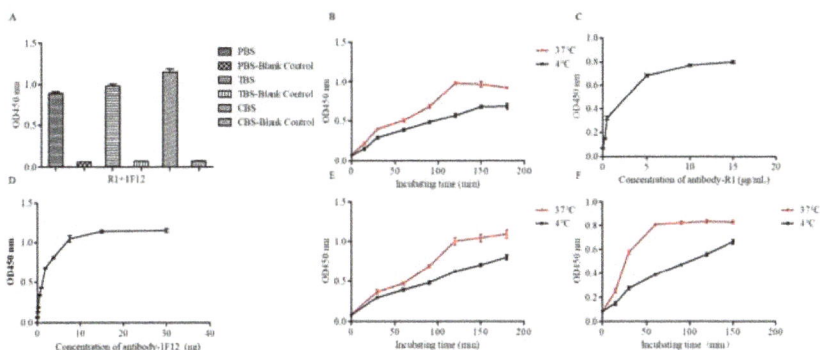

Figure 4. Optimization operations of DAS-ELISA. Optimum coating solution (**A**), coating temperatures and times (**B**) of pAb R1. Optimum working concentration of pAb R1 (**C**) and HRP-labeled mAb 1F12 (**D**). (**E**) Optimum incubating temperatures and times of antigen. (**F**) Optimum incubating times and temperatures of mAb 1F12-HRP probe.

3.6. The Specificity and Sensitivity of ZIKV Detection by DAS-ELISA

The specificity of the DAS-ELISA was evaluated with others similar flaviviruses. As shown in Figure 5A,B, the presence of the ZIKV and the recombinant ZIKV-NS1 protein were defined by the yellow color and the optical density of the solution, respectively. At the same time, the sensitivity of the DAS-ELISA was established using the recombinant NS1 protein serially diluted from 500 µg mL^{-1} to 0.122 µg mL^{-1}. Figure 5C,D clearly show that the color of the solution and the optical density gradually reduced with decreasing concentrations of the recombinant NS1 protein. Figure 5E shows a good linear relationship when the concentration of the NS1 protein ranged from 500 µg mL^{-1} to 0.122 µg mL^{-1}, with a correlation coefficient of 0.9984. Within this range, the DAS-ELISA is useful for quantitative analysis, with a sensitivity of 0.122 µg mL^{-1}.

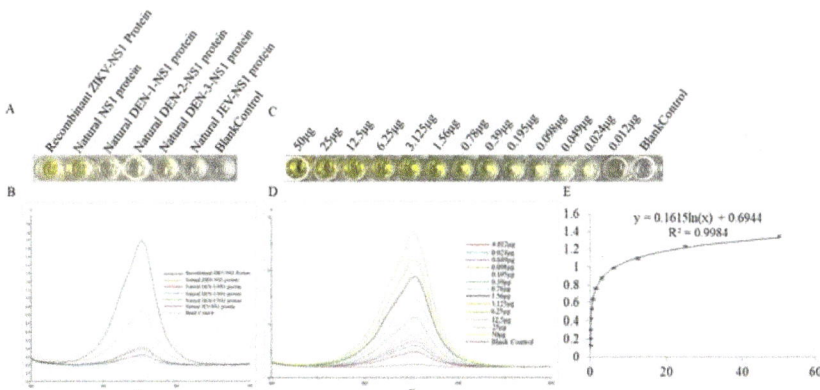

Figure 5. Specificity and sensitivity of the DAS-ELISA. (**A**) Specificity of the DAS-ELISA: well 1 represents the recombinant ZIKV-NS1 protein; well 2 represents the natural NS1 protein in the cell culture supernatant that infected with ZIKV; well 3−6 represent the natural NS1 protein in the cell culture supernatant infected with DEN-1, DEN-2, DEN-3, and JEV, respectively; and well 7 represents the blank control. (**B**) Optical density for the detection of different viruses. (**C**) Sensitivity of the DAS-ELISA: well 1−13 represent the different concentrations of recombinant ZIKV-NS1 proteins (500 µg mL^{-1}–0.122 µg mL^{-1}), well 14 represents the blank control. (**D**) Optical density for the detection of different concentrations of recombinant ZIKV-NS1 protein (500 µg mL^{-1}–0.122 µg mL^{-1}). (**E**) The plotted linear curve based on the different concentrations of recombinant ZIKV-NS1 protein.

3.7. Application of the DAS-ELISA for ZIKV Detection in the Supernatants, Cell Lysates of Cells, and the Sera of Tree Shrews

To test the application of the DAS-ELISA, supernatants, and lysates from Vero and BHK cells, as well as sera of tree shrews infected with ZIKV were used. In brief, Vero and BHK cells were infected with viruses at one multiplicity of infection (MOI). The supernatants of the infected cells were collected at different infection times and concentrated. Thereafter, 100 µL of the supernatant or cell lysates was used for DAS-ELISA assay, respectively. The results of the DAS-ELISA showed that the supernatants and lysates of Vero and BHK cells collected at 12 h, 24 h, 36 h, 48 h, 60 h, and 72 h were detectable (Figure 6A–D). Furthermore, the ZIKV was used to infect tree shrews. Thereafter, tree shrews' sera were collected at different infection times for DAS-ELISA. Figure 6E,F shows that the DAS-ELISA detected the ZIKV, even at eight days after infection. Moreover, the ZIKV-infected supernatants and sera were used for RT-qPCR using specific primers and probes (Table 1) to confirm the existence of ZIKV (Figure 6G,H), whereas the Western blot assay was carried out to detect the NS1 protein in the supernatants and lysates of cells (Figure 6I).

Table 1. Primers used for RT-qPCR.

Name	Sequence	Length (bp)
ZIKV-ASF	GGTCAGCGTCCTCTCTAATAAACG	24
ZIKV-ASR	GCACCCTAGTGTCCACTTTTTCC	23
ZIKV-Probe	FAM-AGCCATGACCGACACCACACCGT-BQ1	23

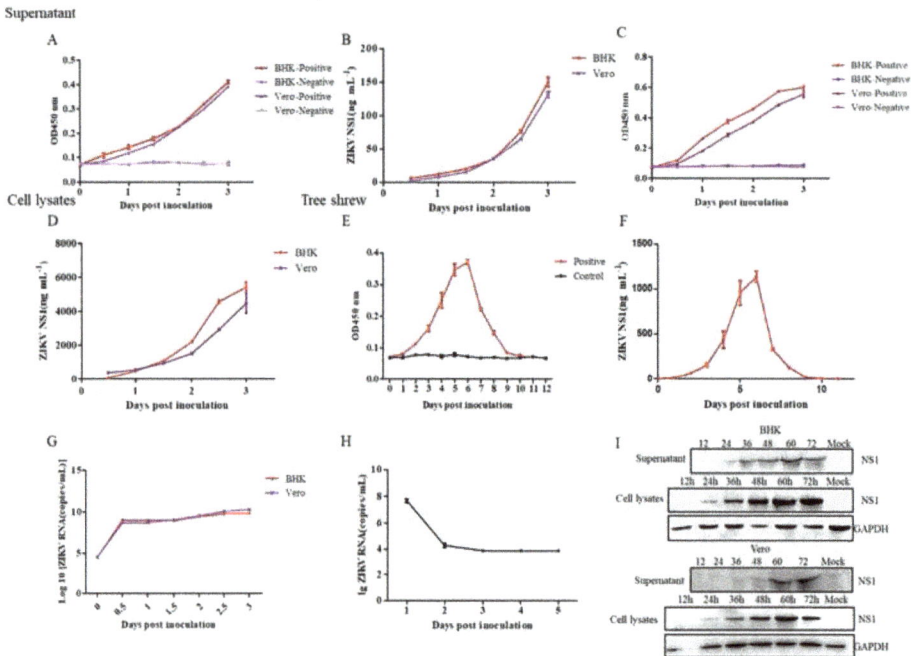

Figure 6. Detection of the ZIKV-NS1 protein in cell culture supernatants and lyates, as well as sera of animal infection model by the DAS-ELISA. Supernatants (**A,B**) and cell lysates (**C,D**) of Vero and BHK cells infected with ZIKV from 12, 24, 36, 48, 60, and 72 h were detected by DAS-ELISA. (**E,F**) Sera of tree shrews infected with ZIKV from 1 to 12 days were detected by DAS-ELISA. A Real-time quantitative reverse transcription polymerase chain reaction analysis of the supernatant of Vero, BHK (**G**) and the sera of tree shrews (**H**) after infected with ZIKV. (**I**) Western blot assay of supernatants and cell lysates of BHK and Vero cells infected with ZIKV.

4. Discussion

The ZIKV is an emerging mosquito-transmitted flavivirus that causes severe disease, including congenital birth defects during pregnancy [3]. Recently, an outbreak of the ZIKV in Northeast Brazil led to an alarming number of babies born with microcephaly in this region [29]. Based on the current clinical manifestations, it is very difficult to detect the ZIKV, especially in the early stages of infection. Regardless, the early diagnosis of ZIKV infection is important because it is a major factor in the treatment of patients and in the control of future outbreaks [30].

Traditional diagnostic methods that involve serological techniques and virus isolation are considered as the golden methods. However, these methods are time consuming, with low specificity. Fluorescence quantitative polymerase chain reaction (PCR) has been widely used in the detection of the ZIKV, due to its high sensitivity and specificity [31]. Although this method is reliable, most regions of the world do not have access to the expensive equipment, as well as the stable power required to operate the system. Due to the limited window period of virus detection, it is difficult to diagnose patients one to two weeks after the onset of symptoms [25,32].

Thus, it is very important that this issue of virus detection be addressed. A rapid, accurate, and sensitive diagnostic technique is urgently needed for early detection of ZIKV-infected patients, which can effectively control ZIKV transmission.

In this study, the NS1 protein was purified and used as antigen to immunize rabbit and mice. Nine mAbs and one pAb were prepared and screened using ELISA, Western blot, and indirect immunofluorescent assay. Based on the two Abs, the DAS-ELISA was developed for the detection of the ZIKV-NS1 protein. The specificity and sensitivity of the DAS-ELISA were successfully demonstrated. Moreover, the practical application of the DAS-ELISA was also determined using the supernatants and lysates from Vero and BHK cells, as well as the serum of tree shrews that were infected with ZIKV. Moreover, all samples used for the DAS-ELISA assay were screened by RT-qPCR and Western blot to confirm the existence of the ZIKV. The results showed that ZIKV existed in the supernatants of infected Vero, BHK cells, and the sera of infected tree shrews. In addition, we observed the natural ZIKV-NS1 protein secreted into the cell culture supernatant. Furthermore, the ZIKV tree shrew model confirmed the accuracy of the DAS-ELISA we established. Figure 6E,F revealed that the native ZIKV-NS1 protein was present in the serum from two to eight days after infection. However, we found that the RNA of the ZIKV was detectable by RT-qPCR at three days after infection in tree shrews, and it was undetectable after three days. Compared to RT-qPCR, the DAS-ELISA can monitor the presence of the NS1 protein from two to eight days. Therefore, the DAS-ELISA developed here can accurately and quickly detect the ZIKV.

Due to the lack of human clinical samples, we could not use the DAS-ELISA to screen the sera from patients infected with the ZIKV. In cases requiring the screening of clinical samples, the sera of ZIKV-infected patients were collected and added for DAS-ELISA according to the above procedures. Positive results were defined as the ratio of the value to the background value that was greater than 2.1, which was biologically significant. Furthermore, the positive results could be judged by the naked eye, as the solution was yellow after adding 50 μL of 2 M H_2SO_4. The DAS-ELISA developed here, like many other rapid detection methods, is not guaranteed to generate accurate diagnoses 100% of the time. Regardless of the positive results obtained from nucleic acid tests, the DAS-ELISA or another assays, still requires a second or even a third method to confirm the results.

In conclusion, a rapid, sensitive, and reliable method for the detection of ZIKV antigens was developed based on the sandwich ELISA. By targeting the NS1 protein, two Abs were prepared and screened by the DAS-ELISA. The specificity, sensitivity, and practical application of the DAS-ELISA were successfully established for monitoring ZIKV infection. Therefore, the DAS-ELISA developed in this work can serve as a potential tool for monitoring the virus in a variety of clinical samples and guiding the timely treatment of patients.

Author Contributions: L.Z., X.D. designed and drafted the work. L.Z., X.D., C.C., Z.C., L.Z., and Q.H. performed the experiments, analyzed the data, and interpreted the results. J.Z., Y.S., and X.X. designed the work and revised it critically.

Funding: This research was funded by National Natural Science Foundation of China grant number [81860625, U1702282], Applied Basic Research Projects of Yunnan Province grant number [2018FB128].

Conflicts of Interest: The authors declare no conflict of interest.

References

1.   Dick, G.W.A.; Kitchen, S.F.; Haddow, A.J. Zika Virus (I). Isolations and serological specificity. *Trans. R. Soc. Trop. Med. Hyg.* **1952**, *46*, 509–520. [CrossRef]

2.   Rasmussen, S.A.; Jamieson, D.J.; Honein, M.A.; Petersen, L.R. Zika Virus and Birth Defects—Reviewing the Evidence for Causality. *N. Engl. J. Med.* **2016**, *374*, 1981–1987. [CrossRef] [PubMed]

3.   Coyne, C.B.; Lazear, H.M. Zika virus- reigniting the TORCH. *Nat. Rev. Microbiol.* **2016**, *14*, 707–715. [CrossRef] [PubMed]

4.   Brasil, P.; Pereira, J.P., Jr.; Moreira, M.E.; Nogueira, R.M.R.; Damasceno, L.; Wakimoto, M.; Rabello, R.S.; Valderramos, S.G.; Halai, U.A.; Salles, T.S. Zika Virus Infection in Pregnant Women in Rio de Janeiro. *N. Engl. J. Med.* **2016**, *375*, 2321–2334. [CrossRef] [PubMed]

5.   Caolormeau, V.M.; Blake, A.; Mons, S.; Lastère, S.; Roche, C.; Vanhomwegen, J.; Dub, T.; Baudouin, L.; Teissier, A.; Larre, P. Guillain-Barre Syndrome outbreak associated with Zika virus infection in French Polynesia: A case-control study. *Lancet* **2016**, *387*, 1531–1539. [CrossRef]

6.   Heymann, D.L.; Hodgson, A.; Sall, A.A.; Freedman, D.O.; Staples, J.E.; Althabe, F.; Baruah, K.; Mahmud, G.; Kandun, N.; Vasconcelos, P.F.C. Zika virus and microcephaly: Why is this situation a PHEIC. *Lancet* **2016**, *387*, 719–721. [CrossRef]

7.   Fauci, A.S.; Morens, D.M. Zika Virus in the Americas—Yet Another Arbovirus Threat. *N. Engl. J. Med.* **2016**, *374*, 601–604. [CrossRef] [PubMed]

8.   Maurer-Stroh, S.; Mak, T.M.; Ng, Y.K.; Phuah, S.P.; Huber, R.G.; Marzinek, J.K.; Holdbrook, D.A.; Lee, R.T.; Cui, L.; Lin, R.T. South-east Asian Zika virus strain linked to cluster of cases in Singapore, August 2016. *Eurosurveillance* **2016**, *21*, 3407. [CrossRef] [PubMed]

9.   Johansson, M.A.; Mier-Y-Teran-Romero, L.; Reefhuis, J.; Gilboa, S.M.; Hills, S.L. Zika and the Risk of Microcephaly. *N. Engl. J. Med.* **2016**, *375*, 1–4. [CrossRef] [PubMed]

10.   Zhang, Y.; Chen, W.; Wong, G.; Bi, Y.; Yan, J.; Yi, S.; Chen, E.; Hao, Y.; Lou, X.; Mao, H. Highly diversified Zika viruses imported to China, 2016. *Protein Cell* **2016**, *7*, 461–464. [CrossRef] [PubMed]

11.   Haddow, A.D.; Schuh, A.J.; Yasuda, C.Y.; Kasper, M.R.; Heang, V.; Huy, R.; Guzman, H.; Tesh, R.B.; Weaver, S.C. Genetic characterization of Zika virus strains: Geographic expansion of the Asian lineage. *PLoS Negl. Trop. Dis.* **2012**, *6*, e1477. [CrossRef] [PubMed]

12.   Ibrahim, N.K. Zika virus: Epidemiology, current phobia and preparedness for upcoming mass gatherings, with examples from World Olympics and Pilgrimage. *Pak. J. Med. Sci.* **2016**, *32*, 1038–1043. [CrossRef] [PubMed]

13.   Bhavani, K.G.; Krishna, K.B.M.; Srinivasu, N.; Ramachandran, D.; Raman, N.V.V.S.S.; Babu, B.H. Determination of genotoxic impurity in atazanavir sulphate drug substance by LC-MS. *J. Pharm. Biomed. Anal.* **2017**, *132*, 156–158.

14.   Nicolini, A.M.; Mccracken, K.E.; Yoon, J.Y. Future developments in biosensors for field-ready Zika virus diagnostics. *J. Biol. Eng.* **2017**, *11*, 7. [CrossRef] [PubMed]

15.   Musso, D.; Gubler, D.J. Zika Virus. *Clin. Microbiol. Rev.* **2016**, *29*, 487–524. [CrossRef] [PubMed]

16.   Brooks, J.T. Update: Interim Guidance for Prevention of Sexual Transmission of Zika Virus—United States, July 2016. *Morb. Mortal. Wkly. Rep.* **2016**, *65*, 323–325. [CrossRef] [PubMed]

17.   Suthar, M.S.; Diamond, M.S.; Gale, M., Jr. West Nile virus infection and immunity. *Nat. Rev. Microbiol.* **2013**, *11*, 115–128. [CrossRef] [PubMed]

18.   Klema, V.; Padmanabhan, R.; Choi, K. Flaviviral Replication Complex: Coordination between RNA Synthesis and 5'-RNA Capping. *Viruses* **2015**, *7*, 4640–4656. [CrossRef] [PubMed]

19. Brown, W.C.; Akey, D.L.; Konwerski, J.R.; Tarrasch, J.T.; Skiniotis, G.; Kuhn, R.J.; Smith, J.L. Extended surface for membrane association in Zika virus NS1 structure. *Nat. Struct. Mol. Biol.* **2016**, *23*, 865–867. [CrossRef] [PubMed]

20. Young, P.R.; Hilditch, P.A.; Bletchly, C.; Halloran, W. An Antigen Capture Enzyme-Linked Immunosorbent Assay Reveals High Levels of the Dengue Virus Protein NS1 in the Sera of Infected Patients. *J. Clin. Microbiol.* **2000**, *38*, 1053–1057. [PubMed]

21. Cecchetto, J.; Fernandes, F.C.B.; Lopes, R.; Bueno, P.R. The capacitive sensing of NS1 Flavivirus biomarker. *Biosens. Bioelectron.* **2017**, *87*, 949–956. [CrossRef] [PubMed]

22. Parkash, O.; Shueb, R.H. Diagnosis of Dengue Infection Using Conventional and Biosensor Based Techniques. *Viruses* **2015**, *7*, 5410–5427. [CrossRef] [PubMed]

23. Wong, S.J.; Furuya, A.; Zou, J.; Xie, X.; Ii, A.P.D.; Kramer, L.D.; Shi, P.Y. A Multiplex Microsphere Immunoassay for Zika Virus Diagnosis. *Ebiomedicine* **2017**, *16*, 136–140. [CrossRef] [PubMed]

24. Stettler, K.; Beltramello, M.; Espinosa, D.A.; Graham, V.; Cassotta, A.; Bianchi, S.; Vanzetta, F.; Minola, A.; Jaconi, S.; Mele, F. Specificity, cross-reactivity and function of antibodies elicited by Zika virus infection. *Science* **2016**, *353*, 823–826. [CrossRef] [PubMed]

25. Musso, D.; Roche, C.; Nhan, T.X.; Robin, E.; Teissier, A.; Caolormeau, V.M. Detection of Zika virus in saliva. *J. Clin. Virol.* **2015**, *68*, 53–55. [CrossRef] [PubMed]

26. Bingham, A.M. Comparison of Test Results for Zika Virus RNA in Urine, Serum, and Saliva Specimens from Persons with Travel-Associated Zika Virus Disease—Florida, 2016. *Morb. Mortal. Wkly. Rep.* **2016**, *65*, 475–478. [CrossRef] [PubMed]

27. Jin, Z.; Sun, T.; Xia, X.; Wei, Q.; Song, Y.; Han, Q.; Chen, Q.; Hu, J.; Zhang, J. Optimized Expression, Purification of Herpes B Virus gD Protein in Escherichia coli, and Production of Its Monoclonal Antibodies. *Jundishapur J. Microbiol.* **2016**, *9*, e32183. [CrossRef] [PubMed]

28. Zhang, L.; Chen, C.; Dai, L.; Zhang, L.; Xu, K.; Song, Y.; Xia, X.; Han, Q.; Chen, Q.; Zhang, J. Efficient Capture and Detection of Zika Virion by Polyclonal Antibody Against Prokaryotic Recombinant Envelope Protein. *Jundishapur J. Microbiol.* **2018**, *11*, e68858. [CrossRef]

29. Musso, D.; Nilles, E.J.; Cao-Lormeau, V.M. Rapid spread of emerging Zika virus in the Pacific area. *Clin. Microbiol. Infect.* **2014**, *20*, O595–O596. [CrossRef] [PubMed]

30. Lee, K.H.; Zeng, H. Aptamer-Based ELISA Assay for Highly Specific and Sensitive Detection of Zika NS1 Protein. *Anal. Chem.* **2017**, *89*, 12743–12748. [CrossRef] [PubMed]

31. Langerak, T.; Yang, H.; Baptista, M.; Doornekamp, L.; Kerkman, T.; Codrington, J.; Roosblad, J.; Vreden, S.G.; De Bruin, E.; Mogling, R.; et al. Zika Virus Infection and Guillain-Barre Syndrome in Three Patients from Suriname. *Front. Neurol.* **2016**, *7*, 233. [CrossRef] [PubMed]

32. Gourinat, A.C.; O'Connor, O.; Calvez, E.; Goarant, C.; Dupontrouzeyrol, M. Detection of Zika Virus in Urine. *Emerg. Infect. Dis.* **2015**, *21*, 84–86. [CrossRef] [PubMed]

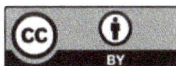

![viruses logo] *viruses*

MDPI

Article

Detection of Specific ZIKV IgM in Travelers Using a Multiplexed Flavivirus Microsphere Immunoassay

Carmel T. Taylor * , Ian M. Mackay , Jamie L. McMahon, Sarah L. Wheatley, Peter R. Moore, Mitchell J. Finger, Glen R. Hewitson and Frederick A. Moore

Public Health Virology, Forensic and Scientific Services, Queensland Health, Coopers Plains, Queensland, 4108, Australia; ian.mackay@health.qld.gov.au (I.M.M.); Jamie.McMahon@health.qld.gov.au (J.L.M.); Sarah.Wheatley@health.qld.gov.au (S.L.W.); Peter.Moore2@health.qld.gov.au (P.R.M.); Mitchell.Finger@health.qld.gov.au (M.J.F.); Glen.Hewitson@health.qld.gov.au (G.R.H.); Frederick.Moore@health.qld.gov.au (F.A.M.)
* Correspondence: carmel.taylor@health.qld.gov.au

Received: 28 March 2018; Accepted: 10 May 2018; Published: 12 May 2018

Abstract: Zika virus (ZIKV) has spread widely in the Pacific and recently throughout the Americas. Unless detected by RT-PCR, confirming an acute ZIKV infection can be challenging. We developed and validated a multiplexed flavivirus immunoglobulin M (IgM) microsphere immunoassay (flaviMIA) which can differentiate ZIKV-specific IgM from that due to other flavivirus infections in humans. The flaviMIA bound 12 inactivated flavivirus antigens, including those from ZIKV and yellow fever virus (YFV), to distinct anti-flavivirus antibody coupled beads. These beads were used to interrogate sera from patients with suspected ZIKV infection following travel to relevant countries. FlaviMIA results were validated by comparison to the ZIKV plaque reduction neutralization test (PRNT). The results highlight the complexity of serological ZIKV diagnosis, particularly in patients previously exposed to, or vaccinated against, other flaviviruses. We confirmed 99 patients with ZIKV infection by a combination of RT-PCR and serology. Importantly, ZIKV antibodies could be discriminated from those ascribed to other flavivirus infections. Serological results were sometimes confounded by the presence of pre-existing antibodies attributed to previous flavivirus infection or vaccination. Where RT-PCR results were negative, testing of appropriately timed paired sera was necessary to demonstrate seroconversion or differentiation of recent from past infection with or exposure to ZIKV.

Keywords: Zika virus; serology; flavivirus; microsphere immunoassay; validated; optimised; dengue virus

1. Introduction

Zika virus (ZIKV) is an arthropod-borne virus (arbovirus) assigned to the genus *Flavivirus* of the family *Flaviviridae*. The virus was identified in 1947 in Uganda [1]. Following outbreaks in western Pacific and southern Pacific regions, ZIKV has been grouped into three genetically distinct lineages, East African, West African and Asian. Most infections have been reported to be asymptomatic [2]. When present, signs and symptoms are nonspecific and overlap with those due to other often co-circulating arboviruses including dengue virus (DENV) [3]. A suspected human case of ZIKV disease may include rash, fever, conjunctivitis, arthralgia, arthritis, myalgia, headache, malaise and fatigue [4]. After an outbreak in French Polynesia in 2013–2014, neurological complications and congenital cerebral malformations were identified [3,5]. From 2015, a relationship between ZIKV, congenital infection and central nervous system malformation and disease became known as congenital Zika virus syndrome [6–8]. Where resources permit, PCR-based molecular diagnostics are used to support clinical decision-making by detecting acute infection. Molecular methods to detect arboviruses are less effective when samples have low viral loads such as occurs during the short-lived viremia caused by ZIKV. Serology extends the infection identification window but is often cross-reactive; that is, antibodies triggered by one flavivirus infection may react with various other flaviviruses. In some instances, an extended panel of serological virus testing may assist in getting a specific diagnosis.

We previously described an IgM capture ELISA (MAC-ELISA) which could sensitively and specifically differentiate between infections due to any of the four DENV serotypes, Japanese encephalitis virus (JEV), Murray Valley encephalitis virus (MVEV), Kunjin virus (KUNV), Alfuy virus (ALFV), Kokobera (KOKV) and Stratford virus (STRV) [9]. We subsequently developed a novel multiplexed flavivirus IgM typing microsphere immunoassay (flaviMIA) to replace the MAC-ELISA, with the inclusion of YFV and eventually, in response to the sudden outbreak across the South Pacific region, ZIKV. We use the flaviMIA diagnostic assay to differentiate IgM antibodies to locally acquired and commonly imported flaviviruses [10].

We describe the development, validation, challenges and application of the flaviMIA consisting of a panel of 12 flaviviruses which are either endemic or relevant to travelers visiting or returning to Australia. The flaviMIA allows identification of plaque reduction neutralization test (PRNT)-confirmed ZIKV-specific IgM among sera sent to a public health virology laboratory for characterization.

2. Materials and Methods

2.1. Bead Coupling to Monoclonal Antibody for FlaviMIA

Bio-Plex Pro Magnetic carboxylated beads (Bio-Rad, Hercules, CA, USA) were coupled to the 6B6C-1 flavivirus monoclonal antibody [11] using a Bio-Plex Amine Coupling Kit (Bio-Rad, USA). Generally, 1.25×10^6 beads were coupled to approximately 10–12 µg of antibody. The antibody was either purified in-house from stocks of murine ascitic fluid, or obtained commercially (Millipore, Burlington, MA, USA). Coupled microspheres were stored at 4 °C at approximately 10^7 beads per mL.

2.2. Production of Purified Whole Virus Antigen Preparations for FlaviMIA

ZIKV strain MR766 was sourced from the American Type Culture Collection (Manassas, VA, USA). This was the only strain available at short notice permitting us to rapidly develop tests in response to a public health need. The literature suggests there is only a single serotype of ZIKV and there is no evidence that different phylogenetic lineages react differently to IgG and IgM [12]. The vaccine strain of YFV (17D) was used to prepare YFV antigen. Other flaviviruses (DENV serotypes 1–4, JEV, MVEV, KUNV, ALFV, KOKV and STRV) were as described previously [9,13]. ZIKV was cultured in the C6/36 mosquito cell line for seven days in Gibco Opti-MEM Reduced Serum Medium (Thermo Fisher Scientific, Waltham, MA) + 0.2% Bovine Serum Albumin Fraction V (Thermo Fisher Scientific, Waltham, MA, USA) followed by virus inactivation for 24 h using binary ethyleneimine (BEI) prepared from 2-Bromoethylamine hydrobromide (Sigma-Aldrich, St. Louis, MO, USA [14]). ZIKV was concentrated from the supernatant using Amicon Ultra 3 kDa centrifugal filters (Millipore, USA), following which the viral inactivation was confirmed by three serial passages in C6/36 cells followed by immunofluorescence testing using a panel of monoclonal antibodies. The other flaviviruses were prepared by cross-flow filtration and inactivated as previously described [14]. Where required, the preparations were further concentrated using Amicon filters as described above. Mock (control) preparations were created from uninfected cells.

2.3. Binding of Flavivirus Preparations to Monoclonal Antibody-Coupled Microspheres for FlaviMIA

Each inactivated virus preparation was pre-titrated to determine optimal working dilution by flaviMIA testing of serial two-fold dilutions against known positive human sera and selecting the dilution giving maximum reactivity. Each virus preparation was diluted to 4 mL in MIA buffer (PBS + BSA (Sigma-Aldrich, USA) + ProClin300 (Sigma-Aldrich, USA) as a preservative) then mixed with its corresponding 6B6C-1-coupled beadset at 1:20. The virus–bead mixes were stored in light-resistant 4 mL bottles (Amber bottles, Nalgene, Rochester, NY, USA) which were incubated at room temperature on a shaker for several hours after which they were stored at 4 °C.

2.4. Reference Sera

Because infections by various viruses included in the flaviMIA occur infrequently (e.g., MVEV, ALFV, and STRV), characterized clinical reference sera are rare and often unavailable commercially.

Where possible, reference sera were sourced from IgM positive patients with RT-PCR-confirmed recent flavivirus infections who were willing to donate a large volume of sera for laboratory quality assurance purposes. When this was not possible, control sera were constructed by pooling reactive patient samples.

2.5. Flavivirus Screening Assays

Patient serum samples referred to our laboratory from public hospitals or private diagnostic laboratories specifically for flavivirus serology were first screened for flavivirus IgG and IgM by in-house ELISAs (Figure 1). These ELISAs employ a pool of flaviviruses, as listed above, prepared using pre-titrated antigens at equivalent dilutions, combined into a 100 mL volume in 1× Milk Diluent (prepared from Milk Diluent/Blocking Solution Concentrate (Kirkegaard & Perry Laboratories, Gaithersburg, MD, USA)). A control pool was prepared from a mock antigen preparation from uninfected cells at the same combined dilution as the viral antigens. Specimens which exhibited flavivirus IgG reactivity in the absence of IgM by ELISA were reported as resulting from probable past flavivirus infections and a follow-up specimen was requested. Specimens giving positive results in the flavivirus IgM MAC-ELISA were then tested by flaviMIA to determine the specificity of the IgM, if possible (Figure 1).

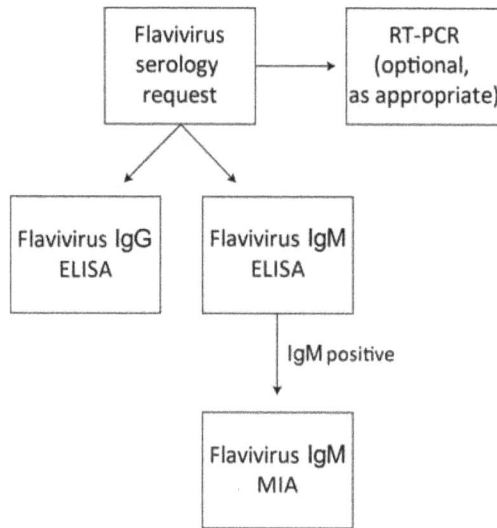

Figure 1. Test algorithm for flavivirus serology requests. When requested, sera are screened for flavivirus IgG and IgM by in-house ELISAs employing a pool of purified flaviviruses. Specimens determined to be reactive or equivocal in the flavivirus MAC-ELISA are then tested by the multiplexed flavivirus IgM typing microsphere immunoassay (flaviMIA). Specific RT-PCR tests may also be conducted on the sample as appropriate.

Upon request, sera were also tested using two real-time RT-PCRs targeting the Asian lineage ZIKV non-structural protein 1 or envelope gene (Figure S1) [10]. A validated, previously described African lineage ZIKV real-time RT-PCR assay was available if travel history indicated a need. Both RT-PCRs were challenged using samples known to be positive for Chikungunya virus, each of the four DENV serotypes as well as a range of related sample types submitted for viral investigations of patients with related clinical presentations. Both tests were 100% specific. Briefly, 5 μL of RNA extracted from patient samples using the BioRobot® Universal System and QIAamp One-For-All Nucleic Acid Kit, (Qiagen, Hilden, Germany) or EZ1 and Virus Mini Kit v2.0, (Qiagen, Hilden, Germany) were added to 15 μL RT-PCR reactions (SSIII Platinum One-Step qRT-PCR System, Invitrogen, Carlsbad, CA, USA; oligonucleotide sequences described previously [10]) and amplified using a RotorGene thermal cycler (Qiagen, Hilden, Germany). Samples were reverse transcribed for 5 min at 50 °C, incubated at 95 °C for 2 min, and then subjected to 40 cycles of 95 °C for 3 s and 60 °C for 30 s.

2.6. Flavivirus-Specific IgM Serology—FlaviMIA

Flavivirus IgM ELISA-positive serum specimens were treated with rheumatoid factor (RF) removal reagent (RF absorbent, Dade Behring, Deerfield, IL, USA) to remove potentially interfering IgG and rheumatoid factor. This was performed in a microtiter plate with 5 μL serum diluted 1:20 in 95 μL MIA buffer. RF removal reagent was added (100 μL) to each well, followed by incubation at room temperature for 15 min and a final dilution of 1:800 in MIA buffer.

The flaviMIA antibody binding reaction was then performed in 96-well filter plates (Millipore, USA), in wells pre-wetted with PBS-Tween. Each flavivirus and control beadset were further diluted 1:20 in MIA buffer in sufficient volume for the number of samples being tested. The bead mixture was added to the wells of the plate at 100 μL per well followed by washing in PBS-Tween using a Bio-Plex Pro II washer. Diluted sera were added to the plate, along with a specific positive control serum for each virus, and a negative serum in duplicate. The plate was incubated at room temperature with shaking for 45 min after which the washing was repeated. Phycoerythrin-labelled donkey anti-human IgM antibody (Jackson Immuno Research, West Grove, PA, USA) was diluted to previously-determined optimal concentration in MIA buffer and added to each well of the plate. Incubation and wash steps were repeated and the beads were resuspended in each well by addition of 150 μL MIA buffer.

The plate was read on a Bio-Plex 200 instrument (Bio-Rad, USA), with 100 beads per well read in 100 μL of buffer using Bio-Plex Manager® software (Version 6.0, Bio-Rad, Hercules, CA, USA). Results were exported to Microsoft Excel® and presented graphically for easier determination of specificity and analysis. A mean fluorescent intensity (MFI) cut-off of 2000 units was assigned based on comparison to RT-PCR-confirmed dengue sera; values above 2000 were considered a positive result. Specificity determinations were based on the MFI result of one viral beadset preparation being 1.5 times higher than the MFI of any other beadset in the panel. Where a single virus-specific IgM could not be determined, i.e., if there was reactivity to two or more flaviviruses in the panel (excluding between dengue serotypes) the result was reported as "cross-reactive" (Figure 2). This cross-reactivity is known to occur in human sera following infection with a single virus, but the possibility of co-infection with at least two viruses is also known to occur and should be considered a possibility.

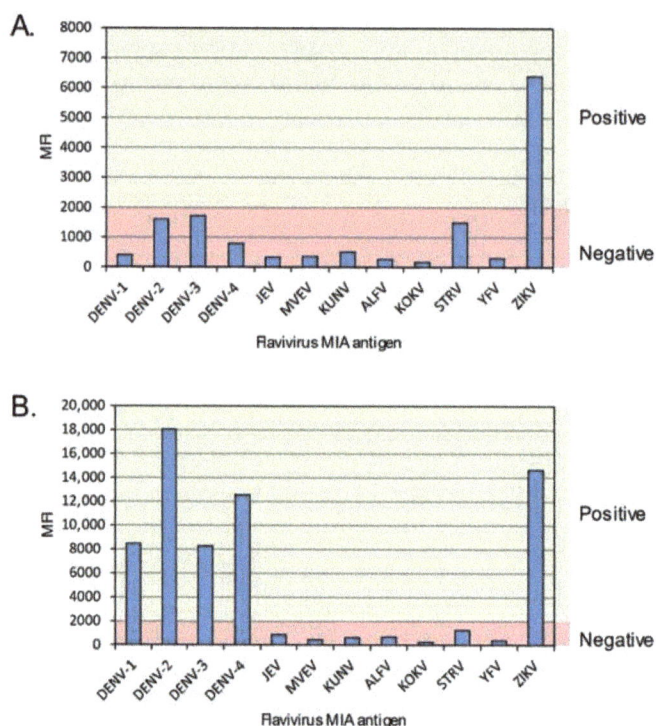

Figure 2. Multiplexed flavivirus IgM microsphere immunoassay (flaviMIA) result examples highlighting specific and cross-reactive IgM reactivity. (**A**) The intensity of the anti-ZIKV IgM signal, reported as mean fluorescence intensity (MFI, *y*-axis) compared to 11 other viruses (*x*-axis) used in the flaviMIA defined this sample from Patient Reference No. 7 as clearly containing ZIKV-specific IgM. (**B**) This ZIKV RNA positive representative sample from Patient Reference No. 11 was classified as having cross-reactive IgM towards both ZIKV and DENV. Red shading indicates the MFI signal range from a seronegative result; green shading indicates the region into which seropositive results fall. DENV, Dengue virus; JEV, Japanese encephalitis virus; MVEV, Murray Valley encephalitis virus; KUNV, Kunjin virus; ALFV, Alfuy virus; KOKV, Kokobera virus; STRV, Stratford virus; YFV, Yellow fever virus; ZIKV, Zika virus.

2.7. ZIKV PRNT

Because PRNT is considered a gold standard assay for confirmation of flavivirus antibodies, a ZIKV PRNT was conducted to interrogate ZIKV results from the ZIKV component of the flaviMIA. Sera were screened at a dilution of 1:10 after incubation at 37 °C for 90 min with an equivalent volume of diluted ZIKV MR766 whole virus antigen preparation. Serum from a confirmed ZIKV Asian lineage infected patient was used as a positive control and a pool of flavivirus negative sera was used as the negative control. ZIKV was pre-titrated to give approximately 75 plaques per well of a 6-well plate. After incubation, 100 μL of each serum/virus mix was inoculated in duplicate into 6-well plates seeded one day previously with Vero cells (ATCC® CCL-81™). Following virus absorption for 60 min, the cells were overlaid with a medium containing Gibco Opti-MEM (Thermo Fisher Scientific, Waltham, MA, USA), 3% foetal bovine serum (In Vitro Technologies, Noble Park North, Australia) and 1.5% carboxymethylcellulose (Sigma Aldrich, USA). The Vero cell plates were then incubated for seven days, after which the supernatant was removed and the cells washed with PBS and stained with naphthalene black stain (0.1% (*w/v*) naphthol Blue Black, 6% (*v/v*) glacial acetic acid, 1.36% sodium acetate). Plaques were counted and sera (at 1:10) demonstrating >90% plaque neutralization by comparison of plaque counts in duplicate "no antibody" control wells were reported as positive.

3. Results

3.1. FlaviMIA Validation

For the purpose of validation of the assay for ZIKV diagnosis, 38 acute phase sera and 25 convalescent phase (collected > 7 days after the first) sera from patients positive for ZIKV (RT-PCR or PRNT confirmed cases) but who have no serological evidence of previous flavivirus infection (primary ZIKV cases), 834 acute and convalescent-phase sera known to be positive for one of nine other flaviviruses and 70 flavivirus IgG and IgM screening ELISA negative sera were analyzed by flaviMIA (Table S1). The sensitivity was found to be 47.4% for acute sera and 100% for convalescent sera. Specificity of the assay was found to be 100%. The flaviMIA processing time varies depending on number of samples per run, but can be completed in as little as 2.5 h.

A strain from the ZIKV Asian lineage [15] was isolated from an infected traveler and used to create a purified whole virus antigen preparation to test representative sera to investigate whether both lineages performed similarly. Parallel testing of serum from six ZIKV-infected patients showed no significant titer differences between the African lineage and Asian lineage antigens (less than a two-fold difference in PRNT$_{90}$ titer).

3.2. Analysis of Patient Samples

In responding to clinical and public health need, our laboratory has identified a total of 101 patients with flaviMIA results indicating specific IgM to ZIKV (Table 1). Of these, 43 were determined to be recent primary ZIKV infections (no serological evidence of previous flavivirus infection, Group 1) and 21 were recent secondary infections (flavivirus IgG or IgM in the acute sample suggestive of previous infection by, or vaccination with, another flavivirus, Group 2). A further 14 were determined as past ZIKV infections with persistent IgM as no change in antibody level was detected between acute and convalescent paired sera (Group 3). Two patients had serological results consistent with a recent dengue infection with a history of ZIKV infection, however concurrent infection with both viruses could not be excluded (Group 4). For 19 patients, ZIKV specific IgM was detected by flaviMIA and confirmed by PRNT, however, in the absence of a convalescent specimen collected ≥7 days post-onset, ZIKV infection could not be determined as having occurred recently (Group 5). A further two patients were found to be flaviMIA positive with ZIKV specific IgM but were neither RT-PCR nor PRNT positive and therefore could not be confirmed as ZIKV positive. One of these (Reference No. 56) was identified as a false ZIKV IgM positive as seroconversion was not demonstrated. The other (Reference No. 77) may have been collected too early in infection for neutralizing antibodies to be detected, but could not be excluded as a false positive.

3.3. Patients with Recent Primary ZIKV Infections

Of the 43 patients determined as having recent primary ZIKV infection, 23 (53.5%) had acute samples which were negative by flaviMIA while 20 (46.5%) were positive. All but one of the positive sera had specific ZIKV IgM. Twenty-eight (65.1%) of the 43 patients had a follow-up sample collected. In 27 patients, the flaviMIA was specific for ZIKV, while the other patient exhibited cross-reactivity to other flaviviruses (ZIKV positive, but reactivity also detected to DENV, JEV, ALFV and STRV).

Table 1. Laboratory data for 101 patients with flaviMIA results indicating specific IgM to ZIKV.

Group Reference Number	Laboratory Reference No.	Sex	Age	Flavivirus IgG ELISA Result 1st Sample	Flavivirus IgG ELISA Results 2nd Sample	FlaviMIA Result 1st Sample	FlaviMIA Result 2nd Sample	SI	RT-PCR Result	PRNT Result	Year/Travel Region
Group 1: recent ZIKV infection—primary											
#1	1	M	40	Negative	Positive	Negative	Positive (ZIKV specific)	19	Not detected	Positive	2013 Thailand
#2	2	M	34	Negative	Positive	Negative	Positive (ZIKV specific)	14	Not detected	Positive	2013 Vietnam
#3	3	M	30	Negative	nss	Negative	nss	n/a	ZIKV RNA detected	Insufficient	2014 Cook Islands
#4	7	M	58	Negative	Positive	Negative	Positive (ZIKV specific)	6	ZIKV RNA detected	Positive	2014 Cook Islands
#5	9	M	32	Negative	nss	Negative	nss	n/a	ZIKV RNA detected	Negative	2014 Cook Islands
#6	12	M	38	Negative	nss	Negative	nss	n/a	ZIKV RNA detected	Insufficient	2014 Cook Islands
#7	13	M	79	Negative	nss	Negative	nss	n/a	ZIKV RNA detected	Insufficient	2014 Cook Islands
#8	14	M	24	Negative	Negative	Negative	Positive (ZIKV specific)	4	ZIKV RNA detected	Negative	2014 Cook Islands
#9	15	F	7	Negative	Positive	Negative	Positive (ZIKV specific)	35	Not detected	Positive	2014 Country of travel not identified
#10	16	F	37	Negative	Positive	Positive (ZIKV specific)	Positive (ZIKV specific)	15	Not detected	Positive	2014 Country of travel not identified
#11	19	F	42	Negative	Positive	Negative	Positive (cross-reactive)	19	ZIKV RNA detected	Positive	2014 Vanuatu
#12	20	F	43	Negative	Positive	Negative	Positive (ZIKV specific)	16	Not detected	Positive	2015 Bali
#13	26	M	48	Negative	nss	Negative	nss	n/a	ZIKV RNA detected	Negative	2015 Solomon Islands
#14	27	M	45	Negative	nss	Negative	nss	n/a	ZIKV RNA detected	Negative	2015 Solomon Islands
#15	29	M	33	Negative	Positive	Positive (ZIKV specific)	Positive (ZIKV specific)	15	ZIKV RNA detected	Positive	2015 Solomon Islands
#16	30	M	52	Negative	nss	Positive (ZIKV specific)	nss	n/a	Not detected	Positive	2015 Solomon Islands
#17	32	M	29	Negative	Positive	Negative	Positive (ZIKV specific)	91	Not detected	Positive	2015 Solomon Islands
#18	33	F	22	Negative	Positive	Negative	Positive (ZIKV specific)	10	ZIKV RNA detected	Positive	2015 Vanuatu
#19	34	F	33	Negative	nss	Positive (ZIKV specific)	nss	n/a	ZIKV RNA detected	Positive	2015 Vanuatu
#20	47	F	30	Negative	Positive	Positive (ZIKV specific)	Positive (ZIKV specific)	14	Not detected	Positive	2016 Fiji
#21	52	F	22	Negative	Positive	Positive (ZIKV specific)	Positive (ZIKV specific)	17	Not detected	Positive	2016 Fiji
#22	53	F	62	Negative	Positive	Positive (ZIKV specific)	Positive (ZIKV specific)	16	Not detected	Positive	2016 Fiji
#23	57	F	17	Negative	Positive	Positive (ZIKV specific)	Positive (ZIKV specific)	24	Not detected	Positive	2016 Fiji/Samoa
#24	60	M	50	Negative	nss	Negative	nss	n/a	ZIKV RNA detected	Insufficient	2016 Guyana
#25	61	M	30	Negative	Positive	Positive (ZIKV specific)	Positive (ZIKV specific)	26	ZIKV RNA detected	Positive	2016 Jamaica
#26	64	F	33	Negative	nss	Positive (ZIKV specific)	nss	n/a	ZIKV RNA detected	Negative	2016 Mexico
#27	65	F	33	Negative	Positive	Negative	Positive (ZIKV specific)	14	Not detected	Positive	2016 Mexico
#28	68	M	37	Negative	Positive	Positive (ZIKV specific)	Positive (ZIKV specific)	8	Not detected	Positive	2016 Mexico
#29	69	F	42	Negative	Positive	Positive (ZIKV specific)	Positive (ZIKV specific)	21	Not detected	Positive	2016 Mexico
#30	71	F	21	Negative	nss	Positive (ZIKV specific)	nss	n/a	Not detected	Positive	2016 Nicaragua
#31	74	F	28	Negative	Positive	Negative	Positive (ZIKV specific)	16	ZIKV RNA detected	Positive	2016 Samoa
#32	76	F	2	Negative	nss	Positive (ZIKV specific)	nss	n/a	ZIKV RNA detected	Positive	2016 Samoa
#33	81	F	28	Negative	Positive	Positive (ZIKV specific)	Positive (ZIKV specific)	15	Not detected	Positive	2016 Solomon Is
#34	84	F	43	Negative	Positive	Positive (ZIKV specific)	Positive (ZIKV specific)	14	Not detected	Positive	2016 Thailand
#35	86	F	37	Negative	nss	Negative	Positive (ZIKV specific)	46	ZIKV RNA detected	Positive	2016 Tonga

Table 1. *Cont.*

Group Reference Number	Laboratory Reference No.	Sex	Age	Flavivirus IgG ELISA Result (1st Sample)	Flavivirus IgG ELISA Results (2nd Sample)	FlaviMIA Result (1st Sample)	FlaviMIA Result (2nd Sample)	SI	RT-PCR Result	PRNT Result	Year/Travel Region
Group 1: recent ZIKV infection—primary											
#36	88	F	52	Negative	nss	Negative	nss	n/a	ZIKV RNA detected	Negative	2016 Tonga
#37	89	F	23	Negative	Positive	Positive (cross-reactive)	Positive (ZIKV specific)	14	Not detected	Positive	2016 Tonga
#38	92	M	41	Negative	Negative	Positive (ZIKV specific)	Positive (ZIKV specific)	11	Not detected	Positive	2016 Tonga
#39	94	M	43	Negative	Positive	Positive (ZIKV specific)	Positive (ZIKV specific)	94	ZIKV RNA detected	Positive	2016 Vanuatu/Fiji
#40	95	F	56	Negative	nss	Negative	nss	n/a	ZIKV RNA detected	Negative	2016 Vietnam
#41	97	F	71	Negative	Positive	Positive (ZIKV specific)	Positive (ZIKV specific)	12	Not detected	Positive	2017 Country of travel not identified
#42	99	F	49	Negative	nss	Negative	nss	n/a	Not detected	Positive	2017 Cuba
#43	100	M	33	Negative	Positive	Negative	Positive (ZIKV specific)	20	ZIKV RNA detected	Positive	2017 Cuba
Group 2: recent ZIKV infection—secondary											
#1	4	F	42	Positive	nss	Positive (cross-reactive)	nss	n/a	ZIKV RNA detected	Positive	2014 Cook Islands
#2	5	M	30	Positive	nss	Positive (ZIKV specific)	nss	n/a	ZIKV RNA detected	Negative	2014 Cook Islands
#3	6	F	43	Positive	nss	Positive (cross-reactive)	nss	n/a	ZIKV RNA detected	Insufficient	2014 Cook Islands
#4	8	F	65	Positive	Positive	Positive (DENV-4 specific)	Positive (ZIKV specific)	23	ZIKV RNA detected	Positive	2014 Cook Islands
#5	10	F	38	Positive	Positive	Negative	Positive (DENV-2 specific)	20	ZIKV RNA detected	Positive	2014 Cook Islands
#6	11	M	31	Positive	Positive	Positive (DENV-2 specific)	Positive (cross-reactive)	23	ZIKV RNA detected	Positive	2014 Cook Islands
#7	23	F	51	Positive	Positive	Negative	Positive (cross-reactive)	30	ZIKV RNA detected	Positive	2015 El Salvador
#8	24	M	55	Positive	Positive	Negative	Positive (ZIKV specific)	25	Not detected	Positive	2015 Samoa
#9	25	M	46	Positive	nss	Negative	nss	n/a	ZIKV RNA detected	Insufficient	2015 Solomon Islands
#10	28	F	26	Positive	nss	Negative	nss	n/a	ZIKV RNA detected	Positive	2015 Solomon Islands
#11	36	M	54	Positive	Positive	Negative	Positive (cross-reactive)	13	ZIKV RNA detected	Positive	2016 Bali
#12	38	M	25	Negative	nss	Positive (YFV specific)	nss	n/a	ZIKV RNA detected	Negative	2016 Colombia
#13	45	M	42	Positive	Positive	Positive (ZIKV specific)	Positive (ZIKV specific)	15	ZIKV RNA detected	Positive	2016 El Salvador
#14	46	F	45	Positive	Positive	Negative	Positive (ZIKV specific)	13	ZIKV RNA detected	Positive	2016 Fiji
#15	62	F	25	Positive	Positive	Positive (ZIKV specific)	Positive (ZIKV specific)	14	ZIKV RNA detected	Positive	2016 Mexico
#16	63	M	34	Positive	nss	Positive (ZIKV specific)	nss	n/a	ZIKV RNA detected	Negative	2016 Mexico
#17	75	M	52	Positive	nss	Positive (ZIKV specific)	nss	n/a	ZIKV RNA detected	Positive	2016 Samoa
#18	82	F	60	Positive	Positive	Negative	Positive (ZIKV specific)	22	ZIKV RNA detected	Positive	2016 Solomon Islands
#19	83	F	30	Negative	Positive	Positive (YFV specific)	Positive (ZIKV specific)	18	ZIKV RNA detected	Positive	2016 Thailand
#20	85	F	71	Positive	Positive	Positive (ZIKV specific)	Positive (ZIKV specific)	13	ZIKV RNA detected	Positive	2016 Tonga
#21	87	M	34	Positive	nss	Negative	nss	n/a	ZIKV RNA detected	Insufficient	2016 Tonga

Table 1. *Cont.*

Group Reference Number	Laboratory Reference No.	Sex	Age	Flavivirus IgG ELISA Result	Flavivirus IgG ELISA Results	FlaviMIA Result	FlaviMIA Result	SI	RT-PCR Result	PRNT Result	Year/Travel Region
Group 3: patients with past ZIKV infection											
#1	18	M	77	Positive	Positive	Positive (ZIKV specific)	Positive (ZIKV specific)	11	Not detected	Positive	2014 Papua New Guinea
#2	21	M	43	Positive	Positive	Positive (ZIKV specific)	Positive (ZIKV specific)	30	Not tested	Positive	2015 Brazil
#3	37	F	68	Positive	Positive	Positive (ZIKV specific)	Positive (ZIKV specific)	9	Not tested	Positive	2016 Caribbean
#4	39	F	23	Positive	Positive	Positive (ZIKV specific)	Positive (ZIKV specific)	26	Not detected	Positive	2016 Colombia
#5	40	M	35	Positive	Positive	Positive (ZIKV specific)	Positive (ZIKV specific)	22	Not detected	Positive	2016 Country of travel not identified
#6	41	F	39	Positive	Positive	Positive (ZIKV specific)	Positive (ZIKV specific)	14	Not detected	Positive	2016 Country of travel not identified
#7	43	F	61	Positive	Positive	Positive (ZIKV specific)	Positive (ZIKV specific)	17	Not detected	Positive	2016 Curacao
#8	51	F	23	Positive	Positive	Positive (ZIKV specific)	Positive (ZIKV specific)	17	Not detected	Positive	2016 Fiji
#9	67	M	48	Positive	Positive	Positive (ZIKV specific)	Positive (ZIKV specific)	28	Not detected	Positive	2016 Mexico
#10	72	M	88	Positive	Positive	Positive (ZIKV specific)	Positive (ZIKV specific)	9	Not detected	Positive	2016 No recent travel
#11	73	M	82	Positive	Positive	Positive (ZIKV specific)	Positive (ZIKV specific)	20	Not detected	Positive	2016 No recent travel
#12	80	M	73	Positive	Positive	Positive (ZIKV specific)	Positive (ZIKV specific)	36	Not detected	Positive	2016 Solomon Is
#13	90	M	27	Positive	Positive	Positive (cross-reactive)	Positive (ZIKV specific)	14	Not detected	Positive	2016 Tonga
#14	91	F	27	Positive	Positive	Positive (ZIKV specific)	Positive (ZIKV specific)	10	Not detected	Positive	2016 Tonga
Group 4: patients with ZIKV/DENV IgM											
#1	17	F	43	Positive	nss	Positive (ZIKV specific)	nss	n/a	Not detected	Positive	2014 Maldives
#2	22	M	78	Positive	Positive	Positive (ZIKV specific)	Positive (ZIKV/DENV)	16	Not tested	Positive	2015 Burma
Group 5: patients with recent or past ZIKV infection											
#1	31	M	37	Positive	nss	Positive (ZIKV specific)	nss	n/a	Not detected	Positive	2015 Solomon Islands
#2	35	F	34	Positive	nss	Positive (ZIKV specific)	nss	n/a	Not tested	Positive	2015 Vanuatu
#3	42	M	31	Positive	nss	Positive (ZIKV specific)	nss	n/a	Not detected	Positive	2016 Country of travel not identified
#4	44	F	57	Positive	Positive	Positive (ZIKV specific)	Positive (ZIKV specific)	6	Not detected	Positive	2016 Dominican Republic
#5	48	F	25	Positive	nss	Positive (ZIKV specific)	nss	n/a	Not detected	Positive	2016 Fiji
#6	49	M	56	Positive	nss	Positive (ZIKV specific)	nss	n/a	Not detected	Positive	2016 Fiji
#7	50	F	41	Positive	nss	Positive (ZIKV specific)	nss	n/a	Not detected	Positive	2016 Fiji
#8	54	M	12	Positive	nss	Positive (ZIKV specific)	nss	n/a	Not tested	Positive	2016 Fiji
#9	55	F	31	Positive	nss	Positive (ZIKV specific)	nss	n/a	Not tested	Positive	2016 Fiji
#10	58	M	54	Positive	nss	Positive (ZIKV specific)	nss	n/a	Not detected	Positive	2016 Fiji/Tonga 2016
#11	59	F	30	Positive	nss	Positive (ZIKV specific)	nss	n/a	Not tested	Positive	Guatemala/Belize
#12	66	F	25	Positive	nss	Positive (ZIKV specific)	nss	n/a	Not detected	Positive	2016 Mexico

Table 1. Cont.

Group Reference Number	Laboratory Reference No.	Sex	Age	Flavivirus IgG ELISA Result	Flavivirus IgG ELISA Results	FlaviMIA Result	FlaviMIA Result	SI	RT-PCR Result	PRNT Result	Year/Travel Region
Group 5: patients with recent or past ZIKV infection											
#13	70	F	36	Positive	nss	Positive (ZIKV specific)	nss	n/a	Not detected	Positive	2016 Mexico
#14	78	M	73	Positive	nss	Positive (ZIKV specific)	nss	n/a	Not detected	Positive	2016 Samoa
#15	79	F	27	Positive	nss	Positive (ZIKV specific)	nss	n/a	Not detected	Positive	2016 Solomon Is
#16	93	F	31	Positive	nss	Positive (ZIKV specific)	nss	n/a	Not detected	Positive	2016 Tonga
#17	96	M	32	Positive	nss	Positive (ZIKV specific)	nss	n/a	Not detected	Positive	2016 Vietnam/Myanmar
#18	98	F	20	Positive	nss	Positive (ZIKV specific)	nss	n/a	Not detected	Positive	2017 Country of travel not identified
#19	101	F	36	Positive	nss	Positive (ZIKV specific)	nss	n/a	Not tested	Positive	2017 Fiji
Group 6: patients with unconfirmed ZIKV infection/false positives											
#1	56	M	16	Negative	Negative	Positive (ZIKV specific)	Positive (ZIKV specific)	12	Not detected	Negative	2016 Fiji
#2	77	F	52	Negative	nss	Positive (ZIKV specific)	nss	n/a	Not detected	Negative	2016 Samoa

SI, sampling interval; nss, no specimen submitted; n/a, not applicable.

3.4. Patients with Recent Secondary ZIKV Infections

Our laboratory also tested samples from 21 patients whose results indicated that infection with ZIKV was secondary to a previous flavivirus infection. Previous infection was determined by the presence of flavivirus IgG (detected by ELISA) concurrent with the detection of ZIKV RNA or in one case (Reference No. 24) Flavivirus IgG in the absence of IgM within five days of return from overseas travel. Of the 21 acute sera, nine (42.9%) were negative and the remainder were positive by flaviMIA. Six of the flaviMIA positive sera were ZIKV IgM specific, two were cross-reactive between ZIKV and at least one other virus, while the remainder had IgM that specifically reacted to either DENV-2 or DENV-4 (both suggesting previous infection with these dengue serotypes) and two to YFV (consistent with previous vaccination with YFV associated with travel to South America). Unfortunately, these prior infections could not be confirmed (by PRNT) owing to routinely insufficient sample volume, however pre-existing specific antibodies were confirmed by indirect fluorescent antibody test.

A convalescent serum sample was collected from 12 of the patients and each was tested in parallel with its paired acute serum to demonstrate change in antibody levels. Eight of the follow-up sera were positive and specific for ZIKV IgM including the acute sample with initial DENV-4 IgM (Reference No. 8), three from initially negative patients, three from the initially ZIKV-specific patients, and from one patient whose acute sample was YFV IgM reactive (Reference No. 83). Three further patients had cross-reactive IgM in the convalescent sample, two from initially negative patients (Reference No. 23 and 36) and one from the DENV-2 specific patient (Reference No. 11). One convalescent specimen (Reference No. 10) was DENV-2 specific by flaviMIA with ZIKV infection clearly demonstrated by both RNA detection and PRNT. Co-infection of ZIKV and DENV in this patient cannot be excluded, although DENV RNA was not detected.

3.5. Patients with Past ZIKV Infection

Past ZIKV infection was demonstrated in 14 patients by parallel testing demonstrating stable antibody levels between the samples. One of the 14 acute samples had cross-reactive IgM (Reference No. 90) while the remainder were ZIKV IgM specific. All convalescent sera were ZIKV-IgM specific and all were confirmed by PRNT.

3.6. Patients with ZIKV/DENV IgM

Patient Reference No. 17 had a single sample which was DENV-1 RNA positive, but the flaviMIA result was ZIKV IgM specific. The sample was also positive by ZIKV PRNT, suggesting previous infection or exposure to ZIKV. Balmaseda et al. reported DENV-1 to be the most common DENV to cross-react with ZIKV [16].

Patient Reference No. 22 was found to have ZIKV-specific IgM and ZIKV neutralizing antibodies in the acute sample, while the flaviMIA result on the convalescent sample showed cross-reactive IgM between ZIKV and DENV. This result is suggestive of dengue infection secondary to an earlier infection or exposure to ZIKV.

4. Discussion

Huge numbers of suspected ZIKV infections were recorded across the Americas in 2015 and 2016 but most were not confirmed by laboratory methods. This and other regions have co-circulating viruses which can produce a clinically indistinguishable initial picture to that from ZIKV infection. Laboratory methods are the only way to ensure accurate diagnoses. With the discovery of congenital Zika virus syndrome, robust diagnosis to support patient prognosis has become more urgent however, definitive results require a complex and resource intensive process. Molecular methods used on serum samples rapidly, sensitively and accurately identify ZIKV RNA but suffer from the short window of detection using sera. Whole blood and urine may extend this window over testing of sera alone [17,18].

Other researchers have described new serological tests incorporating panels of flaviviruses but these usually include fewer virus targets than we have, are region-specific, or use recombinant rather than whole-virus antigens [16,19–22]. One MIA method included an avidity determination step to reduce weaker, presumably less specific, false positive reactions, to good effect in known ZIKV or DENV infected returning travelers or among Swedish blood donors [23]. However, this method yielded low MFI values compared to the flaviMIA. Avidity testing also aided a new microarray platform which performed better on convalescent than acute samples [22]. New and traditional culture-based methods have also been described, but results can take days rather than hours, may remain unclear without additional testing and generally only account for a subset of flaviviruses [24]. Each of these approaches has advantages and disadvantages but it is important to include a well characterized specimen panel assembled from travelers with a potentially complex history of past flavivirus exposures.

Paired sera, collected two weeks apart, are essential for antibody-based identification of virus infection and serology is important to support the diagnosis of ZIKV infection. Despite only 60.6% of our sera being paired, the addition of a convalescent sample frequently permitted clarification of an initially unclear result as when IgM persisted from a past flavivirus infection or vaccination. This has been reported by others [25]. Hence, an acute and a convalescent serum pair are desirable to measure a seroconversion, a significant rise in specific antibody titer or a drop in titer against an unexpected virus. Reactive flavivirus serology results on single samples cannot be reliably interpreted [24]. For some patients with a clinical picture of ZIKV but a negative or equivocal or cross-reactive result from an acute serum, collecting a convalescent serum can mean prolonging the final result. This is especially unsatisfactory for pregnant women. Alternative rapid methods are needed, or testing of whole blood or urine samples using RT-PCR, which are known to contain signs of virus for longer than serum.

In our study, a combination of RT-PCR and flavivirus serology identified and confirmed the presence of ZIKV infection in 99 suspected cases. By combining molecular and serological techniques, we could differentiate primary from secondary infections and recent from past infections in most cases as described by others [26]. The difficulties of flavivirus laboratory investigations were exemplified by results from two patients with evidence of past exposure to DENV (they were defined as secondary flavivirus infections because of the presence of DENV IgG who were producing IgM which was specific to DENV but not to the RT-PCR-positive current ZIKV infection. This may represent a new DENV co-infection but is more likely to be evidence of "original antigenic sin" [27,28]; the anamnestic production of antibody to a past (DENV) infection, resulting from a new yet different (ZIKV) infection prior to the development of specific antibodies to the more recently encountered virus. Either outcome would be unsurprising in travelers from geographic regions where a range of arboviruses may co-circulate. Possible ZIKV co-infections are being reported more often as investigations broaden and more inclusive testing protocols are employed [29–31]. A multifaceted approach to testing, rather than reliance solely on RT-PCR or serology, would ideally improve results [32].

Patients originating from some areas of the world may have been exposed to multiple flaviviruses over a lifetime. Among primary ZIKV infections, we found antibody reactivity by flaviMIA was usually specific when follow-up samples were available and collected within a relevant time-frame from onset of disease. In the case of secondary infections however, results were often less clear, with the earliest detected antibody often directed towards a presumed earlier virus, or to prior YFV vaccination.

The flaviMIA is a specialized technique requiring an experienced laboratory. The use of a multi-target antibody testing protocol such as this for screening samples from patients with suspected flavivirus infections benefits from including viral targets most appropriate to a patient's exposure history [13].

The results of our study suggest that all patients with suspected ZIKV infection should have a submitted specimen tested initially by RT-PCR (see Supplementary Materials). Where RNA is detected, ZIKV infection is confirmed without further testing. However, where specimens are negative by RT-PCR (due to late collection, poor sample quality or low viral load), then the flaviMIA is useful to determine presence and specificity of flavivirus IgM. In some cases, PRNT may be required to confirm ZIKV infection. We suggest that a minimum of 1 mL of serum be supplied for testing to ensure sufficient is available for all tests that may be required.

Our in-house flaviMIA protocol affords broad concurrent flavivirus serodiagnostic capacity. In our professional laboratory setting, it proved easy to use, was amenable to high throughput testing, had a short turnaround time and generated reproducible results. The flaviMIA was rapid in both analysis time and in interpretation of results. However, our results highlight the complexities of flavivirus diagnostic serology, which can be confounded by several factors including the presence of cross-reactive antibodies and high titers of specific antibody to antigenically different viruses that have resulted from recent or concurrent infection, vaccination or because of an anamnestic response triggered by a new ZIKV infection.

Supplementary Materials: The following are available online at http://www.mdpi.com/1999-4915/10/5/253/s1, Figure S1: Comprehensive testing algorithm for ZIKV requests, Table S1: Validation of flaviMIA.

Author Contributions: C.T.T. and I.M.M. analyzed the data and wrote the paper. C.T.T. conceived, designed, and performed MIA and PRNT experiments. J.L.M., S.L.W., P.R.M., M.J.F., G.R.H and F.A.M. performed the experiments and contributed to the manuscript.

Acknowledgments: We thank our client laboratories and the staff of Public Health Virology for support with specimen handling, serological and molecular testing, and tissue culture, and David Warrilow for proof-reading the manuscript.

Conflicts of Interest: The authors declare no conflict of interest.

References

1. Dick, G.W.; Kitchen, S.F.; Haddow, A.J. Zika Virus (I). Isolations and serological specificity. *Trans. R. Soc. Trop. Med. Hyg.* **1952**, *46*, 509–520. [CrossRef]

2. Duffy, M.R.; Chen, T.H.; Hancock, W.T.; Powers, A.M.; Kool, J.L.; Lanciotti, R.S.; Pretrick, M.; Marfel, M.; Holzbauer, S.; Dubray, C.; et al. Zika virus outbreak on Yap Island, federated states of Micronesia. *N. Engl. J. Med.* **2009**, *360*, 2536–2543. [CrossRef] [PubMed]

3. Besnard, M.; Eyrolle-Guignot, D.; Guillemette-Artur, P.; Lastere, S.; Bost-Bezeaud, F.; Marcelis, L.; Abadie, V.; Garel, C.; Moutard, M.L.; Jouannic, J.M.; et al. Congenital cerebral malformations and dysfunction in fetuses and newborns following the 2013 to 2014 Zika virus epidemic in French Polynesia. *Eur. Commun. Dis. Bull.* **2016**, *21*. [CrossRef] [PubMed]

4. World Health Organization. Zika Virus Disease Interim Case Definition. 12 February 2016. Available online: http://who.int/csr/disease/zika/case-definition/en/ (accessed on 5 July 2016).

5. Musso, D.; Nilles, E.J.; Cao-Lormeau, V.M. Rapid spread of emerging Zika virus in the Pacific area. *Clin. Microbiol. Infect.* **2014**, *20*, 595–596. [CrossRef] [PubMed]

6. Oliveira Melo, A.S.; Malinger, G.; Ximenes, R.; Szejnfeld, P.O.; Alves Sampaio, S.; Bispo de Filippis, A.M. Zika virus intrauterine infection causes fetal brain abnormality and microcephaly: Tip of the iceberg? *Ultrasound Obstet. Gynecol.* **2016**, *47*, 6–7. [CrossRef] [PubMed]

7. Hubner, R. Zika virus—Brazil (16): (Pernambuco) Microcephaly Cause Determined. Available online: http://promedmail.org/post/20151118.3799192 (accessed on 18 November 2015).

8. Pan American Health Organization. Epidemiological Update Neurological Syndrome, Congenital Anomalies, and Zika Virus Infection. 17 January 2016. Available online: http://www.paho.org/hq/index.php?option=com_docman&task=doc_view&Itemid=270&gid=32879&lang=en (accessed on 5 July 2016).

9. Taylor, C.; Simmons, R.; Smith, I. Development of immunoglobulin M capture enzyme-linked immunosorbent assay to differentiate human flavivirus infections occurring in Australia. *Clin. Diagn. Lab. Immunol.* **2005**, *12*, 371–374. [CrossRef] [PubMed]

10. Pyke, A.T.; Daly, M.T.; Cameron, J.N.; Moore, P.R.; Taylor, C.T.; Hewitson, G.R.; Humphreys, J.L.; Gair, R. Imported Zika virus infection from the Cook Islands into Australia, 2014. *PLoS Curr.* **2014**, *6*. [CrossRef] [PubMed]

11. Roehrig, J.T.; Mathews, J.H.; Trent, D.W. Identification of epitopes on the E glycoprotein of Saint Louis encephalitis virus using monoclonal antibodies. *Virology* **1983**, *128*, 118–126. [CrossRef]

12. Dowd, K.A.; DeMaso, C.R.; Pelc, R.S.; Speer, S.D.; Smith, A.R.; Goo, L.; Platt, D.J.; Mascola, J.R.; Graham, B.S.; Mulligan, M.J.; et al. Broadly neutralizing activity of Zika virus-immune sera identifies a single viral serotype. *Cell Rep.* **2016**, *16*, 1485–1491. [CrossRef] [PubMed]

13. Basile, A.J.; Horiuchi, K.; Panella, A.J.; Laven, J.; Kosoy, O.; Lanciotti, R.S.; Venkateswaran, N.; Biggerstaff, B.J. Multiplex microsphere immunoassays for the detection of IgM and IgG to arboviral diseases. *PLoS ONE* **2013**, *8*, e75670. [CrossRef] [PubMed]

14. Pyke, A.T.; Phillips, D.A.; Chuan, T.F.; Smith, G.A. Sucrose density gradient centrifugation and cross-flow filtration methods for the production of arbovirus antigens inactivated by binary ethylenimine. *BMC Microbiol.* **2004**, *4*, 3. [CrossRef] [PubMed]

15. Pyke, A.T.; Moore, P.R.; Hall-Mendelin, S.; McMahon, J.L.; Harrower, B.J.; Constantino, T.R.; van den Hurk, A.F. Isolation of Zika virus imported from Tonga into Australia. *PLoS Curr.* **2016**, *8*. [CrossRef]

16. Balmaseda, A.; Zambrana, J.V.; Collado, D.; Garcia, N.; Saborio, S.; Elizondo, D.; Mercado, J.C.; Gonzalez, K.; Cerpas, C.; Nunez, A.; et al. Comparison of four serological methods and two RT-PCR assays for diagnosis and surveillance of Zika. *J. Clin. Microbiol.* **2018**. [CrossRef] [PubMed]

17. Mansuy, J.M.; Mengelle, C.; Pasquier, C.; Chapuy-Regaud, S.; Delobel, P.; Martin-Blondel, G.; Izopet, J. Zika virus infection and prolonged viremia in whole-blood specimens. *Emerg. Infect. Dis.* **2017**, *23*, 863–865. [CrossRef] [PubMed]

18. Lum, F.M.; Lin, C.; Susova, O.Y.; Teo, T.H.; Fong, S.W.; Mak, T.M.; Lee, L.K.; Chong, C.Y.; Lye, D.C.B.; Lin, R.T.P.; et al. A sensitive method for detecting Zika virus antigen in patients' whole-blood specimens as an alternative diagnostic approach. *J. Infect. Dis.* **2017**, *216*, 182–190. [CrossRef] [PubMed]

19. Wong, S.J.; Furuya, A.; Zou, J.; Xie, X.; Dupuis, A.P., 2nd.; Kramer, L.D.; Shi, P.Y. A multiplex microsphere immunoassay for Zika virus diagnosis. *EBioMedicine* **2017**, *16*, 136–140. [CrossRef] [PubMed]

20. Balmaseda, A.; Stettler, K.; Medialdea-Carrera, R.; Collado, D.; Jin, X.; Zambrana, J.V.; Jaconi, S.; Cameroni, E.; Saborio, S.; Rovida, F.; et al. Antibody-based assay discriminates Zika virus infection from other flaviviruses. *Proc. Natl. Acad. Sci. USA* **2017**, *114*, 8384–8389. [CrossRef] [PubMed]

21. Steinhagen, K.; Probst, C.; Radzimski, C.; Schmidt-Chanasit, J.; Emmerich, P.; van Esbroeck, M.; Schinkel, J.; Grobusch, M.P.; Goorhuis, A.; Warnecke, J.M.; et al. Serodiagnosis of Zika virus (ZIKV) infections by a novel NS1-based ELISA devoid of cross-reactivity with dengue virus antibodies: A multicohort study of assay performance, 2015 to 2016. *Eur. Commun. Dis. Bull.* **2016**, *21*. [CrossRef] [PubMed]

22. Zhang, B.; Pinsky, B.A.; Ananta, J.S.; Zhao, S.; Arulkumar, S.; Wan, H.; Sahoo, M.K.; Abeynayake, J.; Waggoner, J.J.; Hopes, C.; et al. Diagnosis of Zika virus infection on a nanotechnology platform. *Nat. Med.* **2017**, *23*, 548–550. [CrossRef] [PubMed]

23. Ronnberg, B.; Gustafsson, A.; Vapalahti, O.; Emmerich, P.; Lundkvist, A.; Schmidt-Chanasit, J.; Blomberg, J. Compensating for cross-reactions using avidity and computation in a suspension multiplex immunoassay for serotyping of Zika versus other flavivirus infections. *Med. Microbiol. Immunol.* **2017**. [CrossRef] [PubMed]

24. Shan, C.; Ortiz, D.A.; Yang, Y.; Wong, S.J.; Kramer, L.D.; Shi, P.Y.; Loeffelholz, M.J.; Ren, P. Evaluation of a novel reporter virus neutralization test for serological diagnosis of Zika and dengue virus infection. *J. Clin. Microbiol.* **2017**, *55*, 3028–3036. [CrossRef] [PubMed]

25. Hennessey, M.J.; Fischer, M.; Panella, A.J.; Kosoy, O.I.; Laven, J.J.; Lanciotti, R.S.; Staples, J.E. Zika virus disease in travelers returning to the United States, 2010–2014. *Am. J. Trop. Med. Hyg.* **2016**, *95*, 212–215. [CrossRef] [PubMed]

26. Schilling, S.; Ludolfs, D.; van An, L.; Schmitz, H. Laboratory diagnosis of primary and secondary dengue infection. *J. Clin. Virol.* **2004**, *31*, 179–184. [CrossRef] [PubMed]

27. Halstead, S.B.; Rojanasuphot, S.; Sangkawibha, N. Original antigenic sin in dengue. *Am. J. Trop. Med. Hyg.* **1983**, *32*, 154–156. [CrossRef] [PubMed]

28. Lanciotti, R.S.; Kosoy, O.L.; Laven, J.J.; Velez, J.O.; Lambert, A.J.; Johnson, A.J.; Stanfield, S.M.; Duffy, M.R. Genetic and serologic properties of Zika virus associated with an epidemic, Yap State, Micronesia, 2007. *Emerg. Infect. Dis.* **2008**, *14*, 1232–1239. [CrossRef] [PubMed]

29. Furuya-Kanamori, L.; Liang, S.; Milinovich, G.; Soares Magalhaes, R.J.; Clements, A.C.; Hu, W.; Brasil, P.; Frentiu, F.D.; Dunning, R.; Yakob, L. Co-distribution and co-infection of chikungunya and dengue viruses. *BMC Infect. Dis.* **2016**, *16*, 84. [CrossRef] [PubMed]

30. Villamil-Gomez, W.E.; Rodriguez-Morales, A.J.; Uribe-Garcia, A.M.; Gonzalez-Arismendy, E.; Castellanos, J.E.; Calvo, E.P.; Alvarez-Mon, M.; Musso, D. Zika, dengue, and chikungunya co-infection in a pregnant woman from Colombia. *Int. J. Infect. Dis.* **2016**, *51*, 135–138. [CrossRef] [PubMed]

31. Waggoner, J.J.; Gresh, L.; Vargas, M.J.; Ballesteros, G.; Tellez, Y.; Soda, K.J.; Sahoo, M.K.; Nunez, A.; Balmaseda, A.; Harris, E.; et al. Viremia and clinical presentation in nicaraguan patients infected with Zika virus, chikungunya virus, and dengue virus. *Clin. Infect. Dis.* **2016**, *63*, 1584–1590. [CrossRef] [PubMed]

32. Faccini-Martinez, A.A.; Botero-Garcia, C.A.; Benitez-Baracaldo, F.C.; Perez-Diaz, C.E. With regard about the case of dengue, chikungunya and Zika co-infection in a patient from Colombia. *J. Infect. Public Health* **2016**, *9*, 687–688. [CrossRef] [PubMed]

![viruses logo] *viruses*

MDPI

Article

The Application and Interpretation of IgG Avidity and IgA ELISA Tests to Characterize Zika Virus Infections

Fátima Amaro [1,2], María P. Sánchez-Seco [2,3], Ana Vázquez [2,3,4], Maria J. Alves [3,5], Líbia Zé-Zé [5], Maria T. Luz [5], Teodora Minguito [2], Jesús De La Fuente [2] and Fernando De Ory [2,3,4,*]

[1]   European Programme for Public Health Microbiology Training (EUPHEM), European Centre for Disease Prevention and Control (ECDC), 17165 Solna, Sweden; fatima.f.amaro@gmail.com
[2]   National Centre for Microbiology, Institute of Health Carlos III, 28220 Majadahonda, Spain; paz.sanchez@isciii.es (M.P.S.-S.); a.vazquez@isciii.es (A.V.); teoml@isciii.es (T.M.); jfuentel@isciii.es (J.D.L.F.)
[3]   Virored-Network for Emerging Viruses; m.joao.alves@insa.min-saude.pt
[4]   Centro de Investigación Biomédica en Red de Epidemiología y Salud Pública (CIBERESP), 28029 Madrid, Spain
[5]   National Institute of Health Doutor Ricardo Jorge, Centre for Vectors and Infectious Diseases Research 2965-575 Águas de Moura, Portugal; libia.zeze@insa.min-saude.pt (L.Z.-Z.); teresa.luz@insa.min-saude.pt (M.T.L.)
*   Correspondence: fory@isciii.es; Tel.: +34-918223630

Received: 16 October 2018; Accepted: 27 December 2018; Published: 20 February 2019

Abstract: In the absence of viremia, the diagnostics of Zika virus (ZIKV) infections must rely on serological techniques. In order to improve the serological diagnosis of ZIKV, ZIKV-IgA and ZIKV-IgG avidity assays were evaluated. Forty patients returning from ZIKV endemic areas, with confirmed or suspected ZIKV infections were studied. Samples were classified as early acute, acute and late acute according to the number of days post illness onset. Low avidity IgG was only detected at acute and late acute stages and IgA mostly at the early acute and acute stages. The date of sampling provides useful information and can help to choose the best technique to use at a determined moment in time and to interpret low avidity IgG and IgA results, improving the serological diagnosis of ZIKV.

Keywords: Zika virus; dengue virus; secondary infections; cross-reactions; IgA; IgG avidity tests

---

1. Introduction

Zika virus (ZIKV), an emerging flavivirus transmitted mainly by mosquitos from the genus *Aedes*, is a cause of public health concern. Prior to 2015, ZIKV outbreaks occurred in Africa, Southeast Asia, and the Pacific Islands. In May 2015, the Pan American Health Organization issued an alert regarding the first confirmed ZIKV infections in Brazil [1]. Between 2015 and 2016, large outbreaks occurred in many countries in South and Central America as well as in the Caribbean [2]. Travelling for work or tourism between Portugal and Spain and Latin America is very common. Portugal reported ZIKV infections imported from Brazil for the first time in June 2015 [3]. In Spain, the first case of imported ZIKV infection was confirmed in January 2016 [4]. Shortly after, in March 2016, vertical transmission in an imported case was detected, in a 17-week pregnant woman [5].

ZIKV disease can be diagnosed within two weeks after onset of symptoms in serum or plasma, and up to three weeks in urine by real-time PCR (RT-PCR) [6]. However, in the absence of detectable ZIKV RNA or available molecular techniques, the only diagnostic methodology available is serology.

The current knowledge on ZIKV antibody kinetics is still limited. In addition, the cross-reactivity between ZIKV and other flaviviruses complicates serology. Thus, a positive result should always be confirmed by neutralization tests (NT), and even this assay is not always able to provide a definitive determination of the specific flavivirus causing the infection, particularly in individuals with a history of flavivirus infection or vaccination [6,7].

The co-circulation of DENV and ZIKV in some regions and the possibility of reinfections by the four DENV serotypes and/or ZIKV highlight the need for reliable serological tests when no molecular tools are available, or when viremia drops to undetectable levels in the patients. One way of discriminating infections between related viruses is to characterize IgG avidity [8]. Immunoglobulin G avidity is low after primary antigenic challenge but increases throughout progressively during subsequent weeks and months due to affinity maturation and antigen-driven B-cell selection. Avidity assays have been used to differentiate between acute or primary infection and persistent infection, recurrent infection, or reactivated disease in a number of infections and have been successfully used for flaviviruses such as West Nile and dengue viruses [8–12]. On the other hand, the IgA response has also been used as an indicator of recent and active infections in dengue and West Nile cases [13,14]. The objective of this study was to evaluate ZIKV IgG avidity and ZIKV IgA in their application of diagnosis of ZIKV infections.

2. Materials and Methods

2.1. Studied Samples

A total of 79 serum samples, collected from 56 individuals were analyzed. These included 62 samples from 40 patients returning from ZIKV endemic areas in 2015–2016 and received for ZIKV diagnostics at the National Health institutes in Portugal and Spain. As controls, 16 patients (17 samples) with known recent or past DENV infection (15 collected in 2012, before the outbreak in the Americas, and one in 2016), were studied. The study was approved by the Ethical Committee of the Institute of Health Carlos III (code: CEI PI 70_2018).

These patients were organized in three groups: (I) 29 patients (43 samples) with ZIKV infection (cases confirmed by positive RT-PCR in at least one of the available samples for each patient) (Table 1); (II) 11 patients (19 samples) with serological suspicion of ZIKV infection (seroconversion and/or positive IgG and IgM and negative RT PCR) (Table 2); (III and IV) the control group, including patients with known recent (nine patients, 10 samples) or past (seven patients, seven samples) DENV infection (Table 3).

Time elapsed after illness onset (days post symptom onset, dpso) was available for 60 samples (39 patients) in groups I and II, allowing us to classify the samples according to their infectious stage as early acute ($\leq$5 dpso, $n = 18$), acute (6–20 dpso, $n = 25$) and late acute (>20 dpso, $n = 17$) [7,15].

2.2. Serological Diagnostic

IgM and IgG for DENV were determined using commercial ELISA (Panbio, Standard Diagnostics Inc., Geonggi-do, South Korea) (Spanish samples) or by in-house immunofluorescence as previously described [3] (Portuguese samples); IgM and IgG for ZIKV were determined using commercial ELISA kits (Euroimmun, Lübeck, Germany). DENV IgM in ELISA was confirmed by a background assay as described [10].

ZIKV-IgG avidity and ZIKV-IgA were tested by ELISA (Euroimmun, Lübeck, Germany) according to the manufacturer's instructions. Samples with ratio avidity index (RAI) lower than 40% were regarded as having low avidity and those with RAI higher than 60% as having high avidity. Values between 40% and 60% were considered equivocal. Serum dilutions started at 1:101. As advised, when the OD was >1.2 without urea treatment and the RAI was >60%, we did fourfold dilutions, until the OD was <1.2, to avoid false high avidity results, according to manufacturer´s instructions. Whenever the OD reached a value of less than 0.140 without urea treatment after tentative dilutions, we considered as the final result the RAI's of the last dilution with a valuable result. Results were deemed as inconclusive when IgG dropped to a negative value after the next dilution. For the ZIKV

IgA assay samples were classified according to the ratio referred to a calibrator as positive (ratio was >1.1), equivocal (0.8–1.1) or negative (<0.8). All ZIKV ELISA tests were based on the NS1 protein.

Neutralizing antibodies were detected by an in house neutralization test, using Vero E6 cells and 100 TCID50% of ZIKV (strain MR-766). Samples were titrated in two-fold dilutions from 1/32. neutralization titers <1/32 were considered indicative of the absence of ZIKV neutralizing antibodies.

Specificity and sensitivity were calculated for ZIKV-IgG avidity and ZIKV-IgA. These parameters were also calculated for both techniques together, considering as positive the patients positive for both approaches.

2.3. Molecular Diagnostics

RT PCR for ZIKV was performed with RealStar®Zika Virus (altona Diagnostics, Hamburg, Germany) at Institute of Health Carlos III (Spain) or with the RT-PCR as previously described [16] at the National Institute of Health Dr. Ricardo Jorge (Portugal). Positive results were confirmed in a second amplification using the method described by Balm and co-workers with slight modifications [17]. The performance in both countries has been evaluated through external quality assays [18] showing equivalent results.

3. Results

All patients in whom ZIKV infection was confirmed or suspected were infected in countries from the Caribbean, South and Central America except for patient P4 who had sexually acquired the infection (Tables 1 and 2).

In group I (Table 1), regarding dpso, from 29 RT PCR positive samples, 15 were classified as early acute infections, 13 as acute and only one patient, a pregnant woman, presented a positive RT PCR result in a late acute infection (32 dpso). IgM was present in 14 samples (from 13 patients), ranging from 3–58 dpso (median 20), one at the early acute stage, six at acute stage and seven at the late acute stage. IgG was detected in 23 samples from 21 patients, ranging from 3–261 dpso (median 11), four at the early acute stage, 10 at the acute stage and nine at the late acute stage. Nine samples (from nine patients) presented low avidity (7–58 dpso, median = 21), three at acute and six at the late acute stage. Two patients presented high avidity results, at a late acute stage (36 and 261 dpso). IgA was present in 19 samples from 17 patients, ranging from 3–27 dpso (median 10), three at the early acute stage, 13 at acute stage and three at late acute stage. In this group, five samples from five patients presented DENV IgM positive results and 28 samples from 21 patients were positive for DENV IgG.

In group II (Table 2), there were 10 samples (from eight patients) with IgM positive results (9–45 dpso; median = 15). Eight of those samples were collected at acute stage, one at a late acute stage and one was unknown. Regarding IgG, 14 samples (10 patients) were positive (10–76 dpso; median = 24.5), six at acute stage, six at late acute stage and two unknown. Low avidity was observed in nine samples (8 patients; 10–49 dpso; median = 17.5) five at the acute stage and three at the late acute stage. A high avidity result was presented by a patient at 19 dpso (late acute stage). IgA was present in 11 samples from nine patients (7–19 dpso; median = 13), one at the early acute stage and eight at the acute stage. In Group II, three patients also showed DENV IgM and 15 samples (9 patients) presented DENV IgG.

Table 1. Group I-PCR and serological results for patients with ZIKV infection.

Group	ID/Sample Number	Country of Infection	DPSO	PRNT (ZIKV)	ZIKV RT-PCR	ZIKV IgM Ratio (ELISA)	ZIKV IgG Ratio (ELISA)	ZIKV RAI (Last Dilution)	IgA Ratio (ELISA)	DENV IgM *	DENV IgG *
I	P1/S1	Venezuela	32	ND	Pos (u)	Neg	Neg	L (35.9)	Neg	ND	Neg
I	P1/S2		58	ND	ND	Pos (2.0)	Pos (3.9)		Equiv (1.0)	ND	Pos
I	P2/S1	Honduras	7	ND	Pos (s)	Neg	Neg	L (33.4)	Neg	Neg	Neg
I	P2/S2		21	Pos	ND	Pos (2.5)	Pos (3.9)		Neg	ND	Pos
I	P3/S1	Dominican Republic	3	Pos	Pos (u)	Neg	Neg	L (18.2)	Neg	Neg	Neg
I	P3/S2		12	Pos	Neg (s)	Pos (3.5)	Pos (1.3)		Pos (2.6)	ND	Neg
I	P4/S1	Sexual transmission	0	ND	Pos (u)	Neg	Neg		Neg	ND	Pos
I	P4/S2		12	ND	Neg (s)	Pos (1.4)	Pos (2.9)	L (15.6)	Pos (5.3)	ND	Pos
I	P5/S1		0	ND	Pos (u)	Neg	Neg		Neg	ND	Pos
I	P5/S2	Brazil	32	ND	ND	Pos (1.7)	Pos (2.8)	L (38.6)	Neg	ND	Pos
I	P6/S1		4	ND	Pos (b,u)	Neg	Neg		Neg	Neg *	Pos *
I	P6/S2	Unk	26	ND	ND	Pos (1.2)	Pos (3.2)	L (38.8)	Neg	Neg *	Pos *
I	P7/S1	Brazil	4	ND	Pos (b)	Neg	Neg		Neg	Neg *	Pos *
I	P7/S2		7	ND	ND	Neg	Neg	Equiv (53.6)	Pos (4.2)	Neg *	Pos *
I	P8/S1	Honduras	4	ND	Pos (u)	Neg	Pos (6.9)	Equiv (40.6)	Neg	Neg *	Pos
I	P9/S1	Honduras	3	Pos	Pos (u)	Neg	Pos (3.3)	Inc (72.6)	Pos (2.7)	Neg *	Pos
I	P10/S1	Venezuela	11	Pos	Pos (u)	Neg	Pos (6.4)	Equiv (41.3)	Pos (2)	ND	Pos
I	P11/S1	Mexico	1	ND	Pos (u)	Neg	Pos (4.6)	Neg	Neg	ND	Neg
I	P12/S1	Colombia	7	Pos	Pos (u)	Pos (6.4)	Pos (2.7)	L (24.3)	Pos (2.9)	Neg	Neg
I	P13/S1	Colombia	3	ND	Pos (u)	Pos (2.4)	Pos (2.2)	Equiv (54.6)	Pos (1.2)	ND	Pos
I	P14/S1	Martinica	7	ND	Pos (u)	Neg	Neg		Neg	Neg *	Pos *
I	P14/S2		21	ND	ND	Pos	Equiv (1.0)	Inc (71.3)	Neg	Neg *	Pos *
I	P15/S1	Brazil	12	ND	Pos (u)	Neg	Pos (6.2)	Inc (73.7)	Pos (4.6)	Neg *	Pos *
I	P16/S1	Brazil	20	ND	Pos (u)	Neg	Pos (5.9)	Inc (64.6)	Pos (1.7)	Neg *	Pos *
I	P17/S1	Brazil	3	ND	Pos (u)	Neg	Neg		Neg	Neg *	Neg *
I	P18/S1	Brazil	5	ND	Pos (b,u)	Neg	Neg		Neg	Neg *	Neg *
I	P19/S1	Unk	19	ND	Pos (u)	Pos (1.4)	Neg		Pos (1.2)	Neg *	Pos *
I	P20/S1	Brazil	3	ND	Pos (u)	Neg	Neg		Neg	Neg *	Neg *
I	P21/S1	Bolivia	6	Pos	Pos (u)	Neg	Pos (5.1)	Equiv (51.0)	Pos (4.7)	Neg	Pos
I	P21/S2		27	Pos	ND	Neg	Pos (5.7)	Equiv (57.8)	Pos (1.2)	Neg	Pos
I	P22/S1	Dominican Republic	7	ND	Pos (u)	Neg	Pos (7.1)	Equiv (53.9)	Pos (2.6)	Neg	Pos
I	P22/S2		36	ND	ND	Neg	Pos (6.2)	H (80.4)	Neg	ND	Pos
I	P23/S1	unk	9	ND	Pos (u)	Neg	Neg		Neg	Neg *	Neg *
I	P24/S1	unk	10	ND	Pos (u)	Neg	Neg		Neg	Neg *	Pos *
I	P25/S1	Colombia	<20	ND	Pos (s)	Neg	Pos (2.8)	Equiv (59)	Pos (1.2)	Neg *	Pos *
I	P26/S1	Venezuela	4	ND	Pos (u)	Neg	Pos (5.0)	Equiv (43.5)	Pos (3.4)	Pos	Pos
I	P27/S1	Brazil	3	ND	Pos (u)	Neg	Neg		Neg	Neg *	Neg *
I	P27/S2		9	ND	ND	Neg	Neg		Pos (2.6)	Pos *	Neg *
I	P27/S3	Brazil	261	ND	ND	Pos (4.6)	Pos (1.4)	H (72.8)	Neg	Neg *	Pos *
I	P28/S1		5	ND	Pos (u)	Neg	Neg		Neg	Neg *	Neg *
I	P28/S2	Brazil	21	ND	ND	Pos (3.5)	Pos (1.7)	L (29.4)	Pos (4.4)	Pos *	Pos *
I	P29/S1		6	ND	Pos (u)	Pos (2.6)	Equiv (1.0)	Equiv (54.8)	Pos (4.8)	Neg *	Pos *
I	P29/S2	Colombia	24	ND	ND	Pos (2.0)	Pos (1.5)	L (33.4)	Pos (4.3)	Pos *	Pos *

DPSO—Days post illness onset; Equiv—Equivocal; Inc—inconclusive; L—low avidity; ND—not determined; Neg—negative result; Pos—positive result; PRNT—plaque reduction neutralization test; RAI—Relative avidity index; unk—unknown; (b)—blood sample; (s)—serum sample; (u)—urine sample. DENV IgM and IgG: the samples marked * were tested by IIF, the remaining by ELISA.

Table 2. Group II. Patients with serological suspicion of ZIKV infection.

Group	ID/Sample Number	Country of Infection	DPSO	PRNT (ZIKV)	ZIKV RT-PCR	ZIKV IgM Ratio (ELISA)	ZIKV IgG Ratio (ELISA)	ZIKV RAI (Last Dilution)	IgA Ratio (ELISA)	DENV IgM *	DENV IgG *
II	P30/S1	Dominican Republic	4	ND	ND	Neg	Neg		Neg	Neg	Neg
II	P30/S2		32	ND	ND	Neg	Pos (2.9)	L (30.4)	Neg	Neg	Neg
II	P31/S1	Brazil	≤7	ND	ND	Equiv (1.1)	Neg		Pos (1.2)	Neg	Pos
II	P31/S2		≤18	Pos	ND	Pos (4.6)	Pos (3.1)	L (16.1)	Pos (5.1)	ND	Pos
II	P32/S1	Venezuela	2	ND	ND	Neg	Neg		Neg	Neg	Pos
II	P32/S2		19	Pos	ND	Pos (1.3)	Pos (6.1)	H (65.8)	Pos (5.0)	Neg	Pos
II	P33/S1	Unk	9	ND	Neg (b)	Pos (2.57)	Neg	L (32.4)	Pos (4.1)	Neg *	Neg *
II	P33/S2		30	ND	ND	Equiv (1.0)	Pos (2.9)	L (30.2)	Neg	Neg *	Neg *
II	P34/S1	Venezuela	49	Pos	ND	Neg	Pos (2.9)	Equiv (44.9)	Neg	Pos	Pos
II	P34/S2		76	Pos	ND	Neg	Pos (3.6)		Neg	Neg	Pos
II	P35/S1	Colombia	unk	Pos	Neg (s)	Pos (7.4)	Pos (3.7)	L (23.4)	Pos (4.1)	Pos	Pos
II	P36/S1	Brazil	10	ND	Neg (b,u)	Pos (2.5)	Pos (1.4)	L (31.6)	Pos (5.2)	Pos	Pos
II	P37/S1	Brazil	13	ND	Neg (b)	Pos (4.2)	Neg		Pos (1.3)	Neg *	Pos *
II	P38/S1	Brazil	13	ND	Neg (b)	Pos (2.8)	Pos (1.9)	L (18.2)	Pos (5.1)	Neg *	Pos *
II	P38/S2		15	ND	ND	Pos (1.6)	Pos (3.0)	L (29.4)	Pos (2.47)	Neg *	Pos *
II	P39/S1	Dominican Republic	17	ND	Neg (s)	Pos (2.4)	Pos (3.8)	L (38.1)	Pos (4.55)	ND	Pos *
II	P39/S2		45	Pos	Neg	Pos (2.5)	Pos (2.8)	Equiv (45.5)	Equiv (0.97)	ND	Pos
II	P40/S1	Dominican Republic	unk	ND	ND	Equiv (1.0)	Pos (6.4)	Inc (72.5)	Pos (1.96)	ND	Pos
II	P40/S2		67*	ND	Neg (s)	Neg	Pos (6.1)	H (68.6)	Neg	ND	Pos

DPSO—Days post illness onset; Equiv—Equivocal; Inc—inconclusive; L—low avidity; ND—not determined; Neg—negative result; Pos—positive result; PRNT—plaque reduction neutralization test; RAI—Relative avidity index; unk—unknown. (b)—blood sample; (s)—serum sample; (u)—urine sample. DENV IgM and IgG: the samples marked * were tested by IIF, the remaining by ELISA.

In group III (Table 3), three patients showed ZIKV low avidity IgG (P44/S1, P45/S1 and P52/S1, and three were equivocal (P42/S1, P53/S1 and P56/S1). In relation to ZIKV IgA, only one sample (P56/S1) showed an equivocal result. All the other samples were negative for IgA.

Figure 1A,B summarize the serological results for samples from groups I and II for low avidity IgG and IgA, respectively, related to the ZIKV infectious stages.

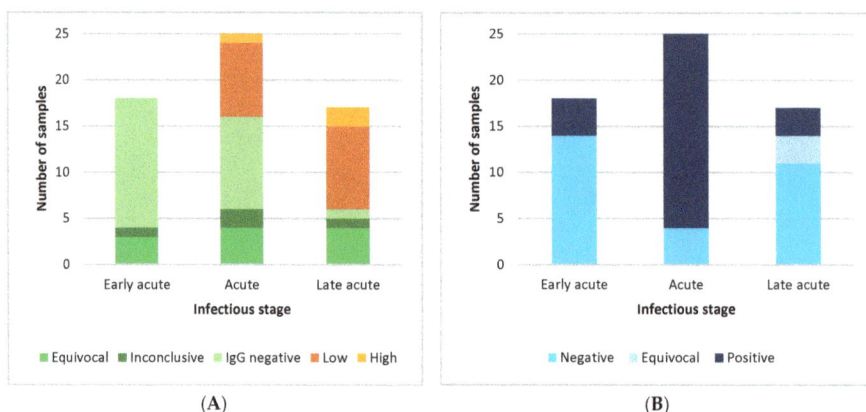

(A) (B)

Figure 1. Serological testing in patients from groups I and II. (**A**) ZIKV IgG avidity results; (**B**) ZIKV IgA Results.

In their application to identify ZIKV recent infection cases, the avidity IgG testing showed a sensitivity value of 42.5% (17/40), (95% confidence interval [CI]: 28.5–57.8), being the specificity 62.5 (10/16) (95%CI: 38.6–81.5). Regarding ZIKV-IgA, sensitivity was 65% (26/40) (95%CI: 49.5–77.9) and specificity was 93.8% (15/16) (95%CI: 71.7–98.9). For both approaches simultaneously, the corresponding figures were 25% (10/40) (95% CI 14.2–40.2) and 100% (16/16) (CI95%: 80.6–100).

4. Discussion

All patients with suspected or confirmed ZIKV infection had traveled to countries with co-circulation of ZIKV and DENV. In our study five ZIKV PCR positive patients also presented with DENV-IgM positive results and/or low avidity and/or IgA positive results for ZIKV. Similar results were also obtained in Group II, with three patients presenting serological positive samples for both viruses. Steinhagen et al. [7], using the same assay we used here (NS1-based ELISA's), found no cross-reactivity between ZIKV and DENV IgM. As such, our results can lead us to the suspicion of co-infection or, at least, shortly followed sequential infections with both viruses. Two cases of co-infection have already been reported in Pernambuco, Brazil, during a DENV outbreak in 2016 [19]. Other two in New Caledonia, 2014, one of those being autochthonous and the other a patient returning from the French Polynesia [20]. However, cross reactivity between ZIKV and DENV is well known [21,22]. In one study, sera from both DENV-naive and DENV pre-immune ZIKV patients strongly bound to ZIKV as well as DENV, with cross-reactive antibodies targeting both E and NS1 proteins. The four patient samples in that study were from primary ZIKV cases, where infection occurred during travel to ZIKV-afflicted areas [21]. Moreover, Lanciotti and colleagues [23] suggested that if ZIKV is causing secondary infections in a population with DENV (or other flaviviruses) background immunity, extensive cross-reactivity in the dengue IgM assay can occur. In this way, ultimate confirmation of co-infection would only rely on PCR positive results for both viruses. Unfortunately, by the time of this study, there was no sample available to perform DENV PCR. All these facts reinforce the need for serological tools to understand the time of infection in the absence of active viremia. This discrimination is very important due to the clinical role of ZIKV infections in pregnancy, which can result in fetal malformations, or in men that can transmit the virus sexually [24,25].

Overall, we had positive ZIKV-IgM results from day three to day 45. A recent similar study reported positive ZIKV-IgM results as early as day two and until 42 dpso [26]. Then again, Kadkhoda et al., using the same assay were able to detect positive IgM only at five dpso, testing a limited number of samples (*n* = 13) [27]. In the present study, ZIKV IgM was not detected in 13 out of 29 PCR positive patients. For seven of those 14 patients, the antibodies probably had not yet reached detectable levels, since samples were collected at the early acute stage (≤5 dpso), as previously reported [7] but we also cannot also exclude that the sensitivity of the technique may play its role in the results. Also, intrinsic immune factors cannot be discarded and might account for differences between individuals or populations, as reported by Lustig and colleagues who observed that ZIKV-IgM kinetics differed in Israeli, European and Chilean travelers [26]. Alternatively, the absence of IgM anti-ZIKV at acute stages concomitantly with high IgG ratio in some patients, may indicate a secondary infection. According to our cases, an IgG ratio > 2.0 was often associated with equivocal or inconclusive avidity IgG results and accompanied by a negative ZIKV-IgM result. Similar results were reported for DENV, where in secondary infections, the IgM response was variable or absent, accompanied by a dramatic increase in IgG antibodies [7,28]. Analogous kinetics has also been observed for ZIKV primary and secondary infections during the ZIKV epidemic in Micronesia in 2007 [23]. All these results strongly suggest than previous flavivirus infection could have an important impact on the interpretation of ZIKV avidity assay. According to the manufacturer of the kit, false high avidity values may be recorded due to high levels of antibodies, which may have been the case of patient P32, Table 2, whose follow up sample was taken 19 dpso. In contrast, the high avidity result for sample P27/S3, (Table 1), was expected since it represented a follow up sample taken nine months after onset of symptoms.

In relation to IgA testing, positive results were obtained in nine samples (eight patients) from ZIKV infections, negative for IgM, two of them at the early acute stage, suggesting that IgA is detectable before IgM. Interestingly, Balmaseda and colleagues suggested that detection of IgA is more sensitive than IgM [29]. The majority of our ZIKV IgA positive results were obtained in samples collected at the early acute and acute stages and only three at the late acute stage (S21/S2, 27 dpso, P28/S2, 21 dpso and P29/S2, 24 dpso, Table 1). Individual kinetics may be observed but, in general, IgA seems to be of rapid appearance and short duration. As an example, in patient P33 with available paired samples (Table 2), there was a positive IgA result on day nine which turned negative on day 30. These results are in accordance with previous studies for other flaviviruses [13,14,27]. These facts can indicate that ZIKV IgA might support recent ZIKV infection, thereby adding a tool for acute ZIKV infection diagnostics with acceptable specificity and high sensitivity, as suggested by Zhang and colleagues [30].

Nearly all the patients in Group II showed some indicators of recent ZIKV infection even though samples had not been tested or were PCR-negative (Table 2). Thus, all the patients in this group could be considered infected by ZIKV.

In groups III and IV (recent and past DENV infections) three patients showed ZIKV low avidity IgG (samples P44/S1, P45/S1 and P52/S1, Table 3). One of them, P44, worked on a cruise ship and was exposed to DENV, acquiring the infection during the outbreak occurred in Madeira Island [31]; this patient could have travelled to various countries and been exposed to other flaviviruses, namely by vaccination for Yellow Fever, Japanese Encephalitis or Tick-Borne Encephalitis viruses. For the other two patients there was no available information and thus we cannot totally exclude the possibility of a ZIKV infection in none of them, in despite of the year in which the samples were taken (before the Zika outbreak in the Americas). The three low and three equivocal ZIKA avidity results from Table 3, that are from patients assumed to have solely a dengue or other flavivirus infection, illustrates the on-going cross-reactivity within the flavivirus group. No positive results were obtained using the IgA assay (only a sample showed an equivocal one), thus ensuring the specificity of this approach.

Table 3. PCR and serological results for patients with recent DENV infections (Group III) and with past DENV infections (Group IV).

Group	ID/Sample Number	DPSO	Country of Infection	PRNT (ZIKV)	ZIKV RT-PCR	ZIKV IgM Ratio (ELISA)	ZIKV IgG Ratio (ELISA)	ZIKV RAI (Last Dilution) (ELISA)	IgA Ratio (ELISA)	DENV IgM (ELISA)	DENV IgG (ELISA)
III	P41/S1	Unk	Unk	ND	ND	Neg	Neg		Neg	Pos	Neg
III	P42/S1	Unk	Unk	ND	ND	Neg	Pos (1.5)	Equiv (45.2)	Neg	Pos	Pos
III	P43/S1	Unk	Cambodia	ND	ND	Neg	Neg		Neg	Pos	Pos
III	P44/S1	Unk	Cruise with a stop at Madeira Island	ND	ND	Neg	Pos (2.9)	L (27.4)	Neg	Pos	Pos
III	P45/S1	Unk	Americas	ND	ND	Neg	Pos (1.3)	L (10.4)	Neg	Pos	Pos
III	P46/S1	Unk	Unk	ND	ND	Neg	Neg		Neg	Pos	Pos
III	P47/S1	Unk	Dominican Republic	ND	ND	Neg	Neg		Neg	Pos	Pos
III	P48/S1	Unk	Unk	ND	ND	Neg	Neg		Neg	Neg	Pos
III	P49/S1	8	Unk	ND	ND	Neg	Neg		Neg	ND	Pos
III	P49/S2	13	Unk	ND	ND	Neg	Equiv (0.9)		Neg	Pos	Pos
IV	P50/S1	Unk	Cambodia	ND	ND	Neg	Neg		Neg	Neg	Pos
IV	P51/S1	Unk	Unk	ND	ND	Neg	Neg		Neg	Neg	Pos
IV	P52/S1	Unk	Unk	ND	ND	Neg	Pos (1.5)	L (39.4)	Neg	Neg	Pos
IV	P53/S1	Unk	Unk	ND	ND	Neg	Pos (1.2)	Equiv (41.8)	Neg	Neg	Pos
IV	P54/S1	Unk	Venezuela	ND	ND	Neg	Neg		Neg	Neg	Pos
IV	P55/S1	Unk	Unk	ND	ND	Neg	Neg		Neg	Neg	Pos
IV	P56/S1	Unk	Unk	ND	ND	Neg	Pos (1.4)	Equiv (41.2)	Equiv (0.96)	Neg	Pos

DPSO—Days post illness onset; Equiv—Equivocal; Inc—inconclusive; L—low avidity; ND—not determined; Neg—negative result; Pos—positive result; PRNT—plaque reduction neutralization test; RAI—Relative avidity index; unk—unknown.

536

The main limitation of this paper was the selection of samples, especially the controls. Control cases were retrospectively selected as having a recent or past DENV infection, prior to the ZIKV epidemics in the Americas. This selection was based on the fact that both viruses share epidemiological and clinical issues, and a high degree of cross reactivity. Furthermore, the selection of the controls did not consider the time elapsed after the onset, making difficult the comparison of cases and controls. The selection of samples has, as well, impact on the sensitivity and specificity of the assays in evaluation, being especially important for the calculation of specificity.

5. Conclusions

Simultaneous ZIKV IgM, low avidity IgG and IgA positive results seem to corroborate a recent ZIKV infection. However, the serological diagnosis of ZIKV in symptomatic patients should be supported by careful inquiry at the time of admission. The date of symptom onset together with the date of sample collection thus provides useful information and may help interpret ZIKV low avidity IgG and IgA. In the early acute and acute stages of the infection, IgA tests seem to be more valuable, while low avidity IgG appears to be more useful at the acute and late acute stages. Lastly, the combined use of both techniques seems preferable in order to avoid false positive results. Further studies, with a larger number of patients, with follow up samples, would be necessary to clarify the kinetics of ZIKV antibodies, and the maturation of IgG avidity.

Author Contributions: F.A. and F.D.O. designed the study, analyzed the data, and drafted the manuscript. M.T.L., J.D.L.F. and T.M. performed the serology of ZIKV and DENV. M.P.S.-S., A.V. performed and analyzed results of virus neutralization experiments and RT-PCR in samples from Spain. M.J.A., M.T.L. and L.Z.-Z. performed and analyzed results of ZIKV RT-PCR in samples from Portugal. All authors revised and approved the final version of the manuscript.

Funding: This work has been partially funded by the ISCIII Project "PI16CIII/00037".

Acknowledgments: We would like to thank Aftab Jasir, Natacha Milhano, and Sonia Vázquez for the review of the manuscript.

Conflicts of Interest: The authors declare no conflict of interest

References

1. Pan American Health Organization, Regional Office of the WHO (PAHO/WHO). Alerta Epidemiológica. Infección por virus Zika, 7 de Mayo de 2015. Available online: http://www.paho.org/hq/index.php?option=com_docman&task=doc_view&Itemid=270&gid=30076&lang=es (accessed on 10 May 2017).
2. Centers for Disease Prevention and Control. All Countries & Territories with Active Zika Virus Transmission. 2016. Available online: http://www.cdc.gov/zika/geo/active-countries.html (accessed on 14 February 2017).
3. Zé-Zé, L.; Prata, M.B.; Teixeira, T.; Marques, N.; Mondragão, A.; Fernandes, R.; Saraiva da Cunha, J.; Alves, M.J. Zika virus infections imported from Brazil to Portugal, 2015. *IDCases* **2016**, *4*, 46–49. [CrossRef] [PubMed]
4. Bachiller-Luque, P.; Domínguez-Gil González, M.; Álvarez-Manzanares, J.; Vázquez, A.; De Ory, F.; Sánchez-Seco Fariñas, M.P. First case of imported Zika virus infection in Spain. *Enferm. Infecc. Microbiol. Clin.* **2016**, *34*, 243–246. [CrossRef] [PubMed]
5. Perez, S.; Tato, R.; Cabrera, J.J.; Lopez, A.; Robles, O.; Paz, E.; Coira, A.; Sanchez-Seco, M.P.; Vazquez, A.; Carballo, R.; et al. Confirmed case of Zika virus congenital infection, Spain, March 2016. *Eurosurveillance* **2016**, *21*. [CrossRef] [PubMed]
6. Centers for Disease Prevention and Control. Guidance for U.S. Laboratories Testing for Zika Virus Infection. 2016; 16p. Available online: https://www.cdc.gov/zika/pdfs/laboratory-guidance-zika.pdf (accessed on 18 April 2017).
7. Steinhagen, K.; Probst, C.; Radzimski, C.; Schmidt-Chanasit, J.; Emmerich, P.; van Esbroeck, M.; Schinkel, J.; Grobusch, M.P.; Goorhuis, A.; Warnecke, J.M.; et al. Serodiagnosis of Zika virus (ZIKV) infections by a novel NS1-based ELISA devoid of cross-reactivity with dengue virus antibodies: A multicohort study of assay performance, 2015 to 2016. *Eurosurveillance* **2016**, *21*. [CrossRef] [PubMed]

8. de Souza, V.A.; Fernandes, S.; Araújo, E.S.; Tateno, A.F.; Oliveira, O.M.; Oliveira, R.R.; Pannuti, C.S. Use of an immunoglobulin G avidity test to discriminate between primary and secondary dengue virus infections. *J. Clin. Microbiol.* **2004**, *42*, 1782–1784. [CrossRef] [PubMed]

9. Fox, J.L.; Hazell, S.L.; Tobler, L.H.; Busch, M.P. Immunoglobulin G avidity in differentiation between early and late antibody responses to West Nile virus. *Clin. Vaccine Immunol.* **2006**, *13*, 33–36. [CrossRef] [PubMed]

10. Domingo, C.; de Ory, F.; Sanz, J.C.; Reyes, N.; Gascón, J.; Wichmann, O.; Puente, S.; Schunk, M.; López-Vélez, R.; Ruiz, J.; et al. Molecular and serologic markers of acute dengue infection in naive and flavivirus-vaccinated travelers. *Diagn. Microbiol. Infect. Dis.* **2009**, *65*, 42–48. [CrossRef] [PubMed]

11. Levett, P.N.; Sonnenberg, K.; Sidaway, F.; Shead, S.; Niedrig, M.; Steinhagen, K.; Horsman, G.B.; Drebot, M.A. Use of immunoglobulin G avidity assays for differentiation of primary from previous infections with West Nile virus. *J. Clin. Microbiol.* **2005**, *43*, 5873–5875. [CrossRef] [PubMed]

12. Matheus, S.; Deparis, X.; Labeau, B.; Lelarge, J.; Morvan, J.; Dussart, P. Discrimination between primary and secondary dengue virus infection by an immunoglobulin G avidity test using a single acute-phase serum sample. *J. Clin. Microbiol.* **2005**, *43*, 2793–2797. [CrossRef] [PubMed]

13. Talarmin, A.; Labeau, B.; Lelarge, J.; Sarthou, J.L. Immunoglobulin A-specific capture enzyme-linked immunosorbent assay for diagnosis of dengue fever. *J. Clin. Microbiol.* **1998**, *36*, 1189–1192. [PubMed]

14. Prince, H.E.; Lapé-Nixon, M. Evaluation of a West Nile virus immunoglobulin A capture enzyme-linked immunosorbent assay. *Clin. Diagn. Lab. Immunol.* **2005**, *12*, 231–233. [CrossRef] [PubMed]

15. Pan American Health Organization, Regional Office of the WHO (PAHO/WHO). Zika Virus (ZIKV) Surveillance in the Americas: Interim Guidance for Laboratory Detection and Diagnosis. 2015. Available online: http://www.paho.org/hq/index.php?option=com_docman&task=doc_view&gid=30176&Itemid=270~{}%208 (accessed on 13 June 2017).

16. Faye, O.; Diallo, D.; Diallo, M.; Weidmann, M.; Sall, A.A. Quantitative real-time PCR detection of Zika virus and evaluation with field-caught mosquitoes. *Virol. J.* **2013**, *10*, 311. [CrossRef] [PubMed]

17. Balm, M.N.; Lee, C.K.; Lee, H.K.; Chiu, L.; Koay, E.S.; Tang, J.W. A diagnostic polymerase chain reaction assay for Zika virus. *J. Med. Virol.* **2012**, *84*, 1501–1505. [CrossRef] [PubMed]

18. Charrel, R.; Mögling, R.; Pas, S.; Papa, A.; Baronti, C.; Koopmans, M.; Zeller, H.; Leparc-Goffart, I.; Reusken, C.B. Variable Sensitivity in Molecular Detection of Zika Virus in European Expert Laboratories: External Quality Assessment, November 2016. *J. Clin. Microbiol.* **2017**, *55*, 3219–3226. [CrossRef] [PubMed]

19. Pessôa, R.; Patriota, J.V.; de Souza, M.D.L.; Felix, A.C.; Mamede, M.; Sanabani, S.S. Investigation into an outbreak of Dengue-like Illness in Pernambuco, Brazil, revealed a cocirculation of Zika, Chikungunya, and Dengue Virus Type 1. *Medicine* **2016**, *95*. [CrossRef] [PubMed]

20. Dupont-Rouzeyrol, M.; O'Connor, O.; Calvez, E.; Daurès, M.; John, M.; Grangeon, J.P.; Gourinat, A.C. Co-infection with Zika and dengue viruses in 2 patients, New Caledonia, 2014. *Emerg. Infect. Dis.* **2015**, *21*, 381–382. [CrossRef] [PubMed]

21. Stettler, K.; Beltramello, M.; Espinosa, D.A.; Graham, V.; Cassotta, A.; Bianchi, S.; Vanzetta, F.; Minola, A.; Jaconi, S.; Mele, F.; et al. Specificity, cross-reactivity and function of antibodies elicited by Zika virus infection. *Science* **2016**. [CrossRef] [PubMed]

22. Priyamvada, L.; Hudson, W.; Ahmed, R.; Wrammert, J. Humoral cross-reactivity between Zika and dengue viruses: Implications for protection and pathology. *Emerg. Microbes Infect.* **2017**, *6*, e33. [CrossRef] [PubMed]

23. Lanciotti, R.S.; Kosoy, O.L.; Laven, J.J.; Velez, J.O.; Lambert, A.J.; Johnson, A.J.; Stanfield, S.M.; Duffy, M.R. Genetic and serologic properties of Zika virus associated with an epidemic, Yap State, Micronesia, 2007. *Emerg. Infect. Dis.* **2008**, *14*, 1232–1239. [CrossRef] [PubMed]

24. Krauer, F.; Riesen, M.; Reveiz, L.; Oladapo, O.T.; Martínez-Vega, R.; Porgo, T.V.; Haefliger, A.; Broutet, N.J.; Low, N. WHO Zika Causality Working Group. Zika Virus Infection as a Cause of Congenital Brain Abnormalities and Guillain-Barré Syndrome: Systematic Review. *PLoS Med.* **2017**, *14*, e1002203. [CrossRef] [PubMed]

25. Mead, P.S.; Hills, S.L.; Brooks, J.T. Zika virus as a sexually transmitted pathogen. *Curr. Opin. Infect. Dis.* **2018**, *31*, 39–44. [CrossRef] [PubMed]

26. Lustig, Y.; Zelena, H.; Venturi, G.; Van Esbroeck, M.; Rothe, C.; Perret, C.; Koren, R.; Katz-Likvornik, S.; Mendelson, E.; Schwartz, E. Sensitivity and Kinetics of an NS1-Based Zika Virus Enzyme-Linked Immunosorbent Assay in Zika Virus-Infected Travelers from Israel, the Czech Republic, Italy, Belgium, Germany, and Chile. *J. Clin. Microbiol.* **2017**, *55*, 1894–1901. [CrossRef] [PubMed]

27. Kadkhoda, K.; Gretchen, A.; Racano, A. Evaluation of a commercially available Zika virus IgM ELISA: Specificity in focus. *Diagn. Microbiol. Infect. Dis.* **2017**, *88*, 233–235. [CrossRef] [PubMed]

28. Teles, F.R.; Prazeres, D.M.; Lima-Filho, J.L. Trends in dengue diagnosis. *Rev. Med. Virol.* **2005**, *15*, 287–302. [CrossRef] [PubMed]

29. Balmaseda, A.; Guzmán, M.G.; Hammond, S.; Robleto, G.; Flores, C.; Téllez, Y.; Videa, E.; Saborio, S.; Pérez, L.; Sandoval, E.; et al. Diagnosis of dengue virus infection by detection of specific immunoglobulin M (IgM) and IgA antibodies in serum and saliva. *Clin. Diagn. Lab. Immunol.* **2003**, *10*, 317–322. [CrossRef] [PubMed]

30. Zhang, B.; Pinsky, B.A.; Ananta, J.S.; Zhao, S.; Arulkumar, S.; Wan, H.; Sahoo, M.K.; Abeynayake, J.; Waggoner, J.J.; Hopes, C.; et al. Diagnosis of Zika virus infection on a nanotechnology platform. *Nat. Med.* **2017**, *23*, 548–550. [CrossRef] [PubMed]

31. Alves, M.J.; Fernandes, P.L.; Amaro, F.; Osorio, H.; Luz, T.; Parreira, P.; Andrade, G.; Zé-Zé, L.; Zeller, H. Clinical presentation and laboratory findings for the first autochthonous cases of dengue fever in Madeira island, Portugal, October 2012. *Eurosurveillance* **2013**, *18*, 20398. [PubMed]

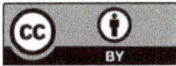

MDPI

St. Alban-Anlage 66

4052 Basel

Switzerland

Tel. +41 61 683 77 34

Fax +41 61 302 89 18

www.mdpi.com

Viruses Editorial Office

E-mail: viruses@mdpi.com

www.mdpi.com/journal/viruses

www.ingramcontent.com/pod-product-compliance
Lightning Source LLC
Chambersburg PA
CBHW051701210326
41597CB00032B/5325